MOSBY'S
PARAMEDIC
TEXTBOOK

About the Author and Contributors

Mick J. Sanders received his paramedic training in 1978 from St. Louis University Hospitals. He earned a Bachelor of Science degree in 1982 and a Master of Science degree in 1983 from Lindenwood College in St. Charles, Missouri. For the past 15 years, he has worked in various health care systems as a field paramedic, emergency department paramedic, and EMS instructor. Since 1981, Mr. Sanders has served as a Training Specialist with the Bureau of Emergency Medical Services, Missouri Department of Health.

Physician Advisers

Lawrence M. Lewis, MD, FACEP, had his medical school training at the University of Miami School of Medicine and completed a residency in Internal Medicine at Washington University. He has been an active staff emergency physician at St. Louis University for 14 years and currently is the Director of the Emergency Medicine Division at that institution.

Gary Quick, MD, FACEP, is an Associate Professor of Surgery and Chief of the Section of Emergency Medicine and Trauma at the University of Oklahoma Health Sciences Center in Oklahoma City. Dr. Quick is a career emergency physician with over 20 years in clinical practice as well as extensive education and research experience.

Contributing Editor

Kim McKenna, RN, CEN, EMT-P, has practiced in intensive care, emergency nursing, and prehospital education since her graduation in 1977 from nursing school in Ottawa, Canada. For the past 7 years, she has been involved in prehospital education, including 4 years as the primary instructor of a paramedic training program. Ms. McKenna is currently an Education Coordinator in the Office of Paramedic Education and a staff nurse in the Emergency Department at St. John's Mercy Medical Center in St. Louis, Missouri.

MOSBY'S PARAMEDIC TEXTBOOK

MICK J. SANDERS, EMT-P, MSA
Training Specialist
Bureau of Emergency Medical Services
Missouri Department of Health
Jefferson City, Missouri

PHYSICIAN ADVISERS

LAWRENCE M. LEWIS, MD, FACEP
Director
Emergency Medicine Division
St. Louis University
St. Louis, Missouri

GARY QUICK, MD, FACEP
Associate Professor of Surgery
Chief, Section of Emergency
Medicine and Trauma
University of Oklahoma
Health Sciences Center
Oklahoma City, Oklahoma

CONTRIBUTING EDITOR

KIM McKENNA, RN, CEN, EMT-P
Education Coordinator
Office of Paramedic Education
Staff Nurse, Emergency Department
St. John's Mercy Medical Center
St. Louis, Missouri

*with 717 illustrations,
including 576 in color*

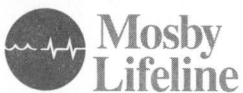
Mosby
Lifeline

St. Louis Baltimore Berlin Boston Carlsbad Chicago London Madrid
Naples New York Philadelphia Sydney Tokyo Toronto

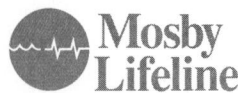

Dedicated to Publishing Excellence

Executive Editor: Claire Merrick
Senior Developmental Editor: Cecilia F. Reilly
Developmental Editor: Nancy J. Peterson
Editorial Assistant: Carla Goldberg
Project Manager: Carol Sullivan Wiseman
Senior Production Editor: Pat Joiner
Cover Design: GW Graphics & Publishing
Designer: Betty Schulz
Manufacturing Supervisor: Theresa Fuchs

Credits and permissions for all tables, illustrations, and other materials appear on pp. 1013 through 1015.

Printed in the United States of America

Composition by The Clarinda Company

Printing/binding by Von Hoffmann Press

Mosby–Year Book, Inc.
11830 Westline Industrial Drive
St. Louis, Missouri 63146

Library of Congress Cataloging in Publication Data
Sanders, Mick J.
    Mosby's paramedic textbook / Mick J. Sanders ; physician advisors, Gary Quick,
Lawrence M. Lewis ; contributing editor, Kim McKenna.
        p.   cm.
    Includes bibliographical references and index.
    ISBM 0-8016-4315-5
    1. Medical emergencies.   2. Emergency medical services.   3. Emergency medical
technicians.   I. Quick, Gary.   II. Lewis, Lawrence M.   III. McKenna, Kim.
IV. Title.   V. Title: Paramedic textbook.
    [DNLM: 1. Emergency Medical Services—methods.   2. Emergency Medical Technicians.
3. Emergencies.   WX 215 S215m 1994]
    RC86.7.S26   1994
    616.02'5—dc20
    DNLM/DLC   94-5630
    for Library of Congress   CIP

94 95 96 97 98 / 9 8 7 6 5 4 3 2 1

*Dedicated to my family,
and in loving memory
of my father.*

FOREWORD

Lawrence M. Lewis, MD, FACEP
Gary Quick, MD, FACEP

The field of medicine is rapidly changing. In few places is this more evident than in the prehospital evaluation and management of critically injured patients. Not since the advent of sophisticated EMS systems in the late '60s and early '70s has so much attention and recognition been given to prehospital care providers. What has led to this resurgence in the importance of emergency medical services?

Technological improvements in the ability to diagnose and treat previously fatal or crippling diseases have focused prehospital and emergency department care providers on salvaging tissue, whether it be myocardium or cerebral cortex. The mantra of the cardiologist that "time is muscle" is echoed by neurologists and remains the first commandment in the care of trauma and cardiac arrest victims.

Several studies show that the prehospital recognition of acute myocardial infarction significantly shortens the time to thrombolysis for eligible patients. Research in the area of drugs that slow or halt cerebral damage from ischemia is also proceeding rapidly. These drugs may need to be given within a window of minutes rather than hours.

As time constraints increasingly become the critical factor in our ability to provide effective treatment, more and more physicians are recognizing the fact that prehospital care providers are the primary link in the chain of medical care.

Every paramedic, emergency nurse, and emergency physician must recognize that a broad knowledge base and an expanding array of procedural skills are critical to the clinical armamentarium of the practicing paramedic. Hazardous materials, once considered an esoteric subject, are now a part of everyday life. Mass-casualty incidents are another challenging reality of our times. Few physicians will acquire the field expertise in securing scene safety, extricating victims, managing hazardous materials, and mastering disaster preparedness that most paramedics develop over their careers.

Thus the time has come to incorporate the extensive knowledge and procedural expertise required of a paramedic into a comprehensive textbook. Through our extensive review and feedback, we assisted Mick Sanders in the task of producing such a work, one that addresses the growing needs of the professionals who practice the specialty of prehospital care. Using the U.S. Department of Transportation curriculum as a guide, we have extensively covered the objectives of paramedic training with examples, illustrations, diagrams, charts, and tables that greatly enhance understanding and retention of the material. In addition, a detailed discussion of anatomical and physiological principles provides the foundation for a continuously growing knowledge base. This offers the paramedic student and the seasoned professional a deeper level of understanding of disease processes manifesting as clinical symptoms in their patients.

For the paramedic student striving for initial mastery of the paramedic knowledge base or the seasoned paramedic who seeks understanding of the complex presentations of disease and injury in the prehospital arena, *Mosby's Paramedic Textbook* sets a new standard of excellence and merits a prominent location in your professional library.

FOREWORD

Chip Boehm, RN, EMT-P
Training Coordinator
Maine Emergency Medical Services
Vice-Chair
National Council of State EMS Training Coordinators

Although EMS is nearing its third decade, it is still a young profession. As members of this field, we have witnessed numerous changes, some of which are now coming full circle.

In the early days, the concept of patient care known as *load and go* meant simply placing a victim on a stretcher and racing to the hospital as fast as the hearse or ambulance would allow. Then came the provision of on-scene emergency medical care and safe transportation by an emergency medical technician. As the field has evolved, the scope of EMS care has expanded to include an increasing number of advanced life-support skills. We have refined our system to care for trauma and medical patients with rapid assessment and transport skills, with the goal of providing care within a 10-minute window.

Other concepts in EMS have evolved as well. The initial focus on retrospective quality assurance has grown to incorporate quality improvement and the current concept of total quality management.

Initially, our goal was simply to decrease the number of people who were dying on the highways and from sudden cardiac arrest. Now, the majority of patients we care for, while experiencing legitimate crises, are not truly at death's door.

As medical technology has improved, life expectancy has increased. Thus we see the graying of America, which has changed the types of calls we receive and the care we provide. As medical diseases and conditions are being treated with advanced technology, the need for long-term care has significantly grown. This has in turn increased the need for EMS and the incidence of patients requiring care on a repeated basis.

Clearly, the changes in the nation are reflected in the patient population we treat. How will these changes impact our roles as EMS providers? What specific changes will we see in the next 20 years?

Medical care as a whole is going through a paradigm shift. For EMS, this means asking some tough questions about the services we provide. What will be the focus of emergency care? How will health care reform impact EMS? Will EMS fit into a managed health care system? Will community paramedicine become a viable option in the overall health care system changes? Can EMS be cost effective? In the past, we have aimed 90% of our resources at approximately 10% of our patients. What about the other 90%? With health care costs out of control, we find ourselves asking difficult questions such as, "We can save this life, but at what cost?"

Statistically, advanced life support does not change mortality; yet it remains the standard of care. There is currently a tremendous push to increase the amount of research in EMS. These scientific studies will certainly shape the future of EMS, in both operations and administration. As a paramedic, your part in gathering the data necessary to improve our profession is crucial.

Because the last revision of the U.S. Department of Transportation guidelines for paramedic education was 8 years ago, EMS educators have had to ensure that their own curriculum remains up to date. As an EMS provider, educator, and administrator, Mick Sanders brings more than 15 years of experience to this textbook. *Mosby's Paramedic Textbook* goes a step farther than the standard DOT objectives and keeps us on the cutting edge of the profession.

The content of the text follows a logical order in presenting material for the student. This is one of the major strengths of the book. Chapters are consistent, easy to follow, and designed with the student in mind, with chapter objectives assisting the reader in identifying and anticipating the required knowledge.

All of the chapters have been developed with most current EMS issues at the forefront. The stress management, overview of human systems and cardiovascular sections in particular are the most comprehensive and up-to-date available. The content in the overview of human systems chapter enables the student to apply knowledge of normal body systems to pathophysiology under abnormal conditions.

Mosby's Paramedic Textbook not only imparts what is required to be a paramedic, but also builds the foundation of knowledge required to be an *excellent* paramedic. For the new student, this text will provide the initial infrastructure of education. For the experienced provider, it will be a valuable resource to keep abreast of our evolving field.

Remember, EMS education does not stop with course completion or certification or licensure. For EMS providers, it is a lifelong process.

PREFACE

Prehospital emergency medical services has come to be recognized as a specialized health care field that is composed of highly trained individuals dedicated to saving lives. Unique to this profession are the men and women who perform technical patient care procedures outside of a hospital environment and away from on-site physician supervision. Therefore the training, expertise, and assessment skills required of the paramedic set EMS apart from other health care professions. This textbook was written by a paramedic, for the paramedic, with this perspective in mind.

Mosby's Paramedic Textbook offers the paramedic student a single and complete text that encompasses the many aspects of prehospital care. The material is presented in a manner that reflects the growth of the EMS profession and the paramedic's level of involvement in today's emergency care systems. *Mosby's Paramedic Textbook* follows the EMT-Paramedic National Standard Curriculum as developed by the U.S. Department of Transportation and prepares the paramedic student for licensure, certification, or both. The material has been extensively reviewed by my physician advisers, a contributing editor, other emergency physicians, national EMS organizations, and a multitude of EMS experts throughout the country.

● ORGANIZATION

The textbook is divided into six divisions. Division One explains the paramedic's role and the unique aspects of the prehospital environment, such as medical-legal considerations, EMS communications, rescue management, and major incident response. Division Two provides an introduction to patient assessment and emergency care, including airway management, shock, and emergency pharmacology. Division Three is a thorough presentation of trauma, soft tissue injuries, and burns. Division Four addresses the many types of medical emergencies encountered in pre-

hospital care, including respiratory and cardiovascular emergencies, diabetes, toxicology, infectious diseases, and emergencies unique to pediatric and geriatric patients. Division Five is dedicated to obstetrical and gynecological emergencies and neonatal resuscitation. Division Six describes patients with behavioral emergencies and the crisis intervention that may be required while providing emergency care. The textbook is also accompanied by a student workbook designed to provide the student with a means to measure his or her understanding of the core material.

Each chapter of *Mosby's Paramedic Textbook* begins with an introduction and a list of guidelines that provide an overview of the material to be presented. This allows the student to view the content and progression of each chapter in an easy-to-follow format. Key terms are included to highlight terminology and concepts critical to providing emergency care. Each chapter concludes with a summary that reviews the focus of the chapter and a reference list that can be used as a resource for supplemental reading. *Mosby's Paramedic Textbook* also includes the following features that promise to make this textbook a leader in EMS education:

- *Hazardous materials chapter.* A separate chapter on hazardous materials has been included to better prepare the paramedic for emergency response to hazardous materials incidents. The chapter presents training requirements as published by the Occupational Safety and Health Administration and the Environmental Protection Agency, methods of product identification, health hazards, and the importance of personal safety during a hazardous materials response.
- *Overview of human systems chapter.* An overview of human anatomy and physiology is presented early in the textbook. This chapter is an easily located reference to anatomical structures and their functions that can be reviewed throughout the course of study.
- *Emergency Drug Index.* The Emergency Drug In-

dex details specific information on more than 70 emergency drugs. It provides a quick source of reference for a drug's onset and duration, indications, contraindications, adverse reactions, drug interactions, dosage and administration, and special considerations for use. The Emergency Drug Index will be a useful reference for paramedic students and practicing paramedics.

- *Advanced ECG interpretation.* All cardiac rhythms and dysrhythmias are presented in Leads I, II, III, and MCL_1, to enhance assessment of the cardiac patient. In addition, the paramedic student will be introduced to advanced electrophysiology, 12-lead ECG monitoring, thrombolytic therapy, and current treatment modalities as recommended by the American Heart Association.
- *Full-color illustrations.* More than 700 tables, charts, line drawings, and photographs have been included in the text to illustrate anatomy, physiology, and patient-management guidelines. Specialized equipment and step-by-step demonstrations of practical skills are also presented in full color to demonstrate state-of-the-art emergency care procedures.
- *Sidebars.* These expand on interesting, relevant information.
- *Notes.* Boxed notes highlight vital information and words of warning.
- *Bibliography and expanded glossary.* An extensive bibliography is included to reflect up-to-date references used to develop this textbook. The expanded glossary contains more than 1900 medical terms presented within the text.

Finally, you may have noticed something unique about the design of this book, particularly the division opener pages. We decided to use portraits and quotations from paramedics from around the country to illustrate a concept that lies at the very heart of this book: Behind all of the high-tech equipment, the standards and protocols that guide our profession, and the quick, efficient skills that mark our patient care are *real people*. Too often, paramedic education focuses on memorizing technical content and practicing skills while the human element of providing patient care under often adverse circumstances is lost.

Clearly, it takes a special person with an outstanding level of dedication to be a paramedic. This book is for you.

Paramedic students, practicing paramedics, prehospital nurses, and educators will find this to be an excellent resource. *Mosby's Paramedic Textbook* addresses trends in prehospital management of trauma and nontraumatic illnesses, emergency cardiac care, and the many operations of an advanced EMS system. Most important, this textbook will serve as a valuable tool in preparing emergency care providers for their future in emergency medical services.

Mick J. Sanders

AUTHOR ACKNOWLEDGMENTS

Mosby's Paramedic Textbook has resulted from the combined efforts of many talented individuals. In addition to my physician advisers, **Larry Lewis** and **Gary Quick,** and the national experts who reviewed the manuscript, I wish to make special note of the following people who helped to make this textbook possible:

Kim McKenna, RN, CEN, EMT-P, for her knowledge, expertise, and unfailing desire to make this textbook a reality. I owe Kim a great deal and will always be in debt to her for her contributions and the emotional support she provided during this project.

Nancy Peterson, for her tireless work as developmental editor, her personal interest in the manuscript, and her wonderful sense of humor in dealing with the complexities of this text.

Claire Merrick, executive editor, and the production staff at **Mosby,** especially **Pat Joiner** and **Betty Schulz,** for their desire to bring this project to completion.

I also want to thank the following people, who supplied the "finishing touches" to the manuscript:

Don McKenna, for his excellent photography

Mark Wieber, for the beautiful illustrations

Dwight Polk, for his careful review of the art

Julie Long, who supplied the simulated ECGs

Bill Raynovich, who carefully reviewed the final draft

Acadian Ambulance Service, Inc.; Larry Ashby; Thomas Cooper; William Greenblatt; Ken Hines; O'Fallon Fire Protection District; Ronald Olschwanger; St. Louis City EMS; James Silvernail; and **Colin Williams,** for supplying emergency scene photographs.

Chris Arter, Larry Ashby, Rosalyn Golden, Jason Herin, Julie Hull, Sue Lakebrink, Frank Lipski, Mindy McCoy, Ginny and **Becky McKenna, Steve Sanneman, Lance Varga, Joel Vanderploeg,** and **Monroe Yancie,** for posing as models for the textbook photographs.

Kevin Agard, Bob Booth, Patricia Dukes, Sherri Gastler, Rick Gower, Neil Holtz, Ray McDowell, Linda McIntosh, Grace Richeson, Ben Sarro, Mike Sturgill, and **Lori Thompson,** for providing portraits and quotes of "real life" paramedics.

The many physicians, hospitals, and equipment manufacturers for supplying illustrations to accompany the text.

And special thanks to **David S. Becker, Willard G. Denney,** and **Jason T. White,** whose contributions are too numerous to mention.

PUBLISHER ACKNOWLEDGMENTS

The editors wish to acknowledge and thank the many reviewers of this book, who devoted countless hours to intensive review. Their comments were invaluable in helping develop and fine tune this manuscript.
Organizations and individuals who took part in this extensive project were:

National Association of EMTs
Society of Paramedics
Instructor/Coordinators Society

National Council of State EMS
Training Coordinators

National Association of EMS
Physicians

Thomas F. Anderson, PhD, RRT
(Chapter 12)
Program Director, Respiratory Therapy
St. Louis Community College
St. Louis, Missouri

Doug Austin, Jr.
EMS Training Services Coordinator
Health/EMS Division
King County EMS Division
Seattle, Washington

Vatche H. Ayvazian, MD (Chapter 16)
Chief, Division of Burn Surgery
St. John's Mercy Medical Center
St. Louis, Missouri

John Barrett, MD (Chapter 13)
Cook County Hospital
Chicago, Illinois

John E. Blue, II, EMT-P, BS
Director, Emergency Medical Services
Education
Gadsden State Community College
Anniston, Alabama

Chip Boehm, RN, EMT-P
Training Coordinator
Maine Emergency Medical Services
Vice-Chair
National Council of State EMS Training
Coordinators
Augusta, Maine

Kevin Brown, MD, MPH
Attending Physician, Emergency
Department
Mount Sinai Medical Center
New York, New York

Jeffrey A. Crill, RN, EMT-P (Chapters 11, 12, 13, 15)
Staff Development Specialist, Medical
Transportation Services
North Memorial Medical Center
Robbinsdale, Minnesota

David DaBell, MD
Emergency Medicine
St. John's Mercy Medical Center
St Louis, Missouri

Alice "Twink" Dalton
Paramedic Nurse Coordinator
Omaha Fire Division
Prehospital Education Department
Creighton University
Omaha, Nebraska

Theodore R. Delbridge, MD
Division of Emergency Medicine
University of Pittsburgh
Pittsburgh, Pennsylvania

Linda D. Dodge
Executive Director
Colorado Trauma Institute
Denver, Colorado

Robert Elling, MPA, NREMT-P
Senior EMS Representative
NYS EMS Program
Albany, New York

Franklin E. Foster, JD
EMS Legal Specialist
State of Missouri Department of Health
Bureau of Emergency Medical Services
Jefferson City, Missouri

Bill Garcia, MICP
Paramedic Field Training Officer
Hartson Medical Services
San Marcos, California

Mike Gray (Chapter 4)
Communications Coordinator
Bureau of Emergency Medical Services
Missouri Department of Health
Jefferson City, Missouri

Janet A. Head, RN, MS
Chair, Community Health, Education &
Preventive Medicine
Kirksville College of Osteopathic
Medicine
Kirksville, Missouri

Kenneth Hines
Assistant Chief
Boone County Fire Protection District
Columbia, Missouri

Steven Kidd
Lieutenant
Orange County Fire/Rescue
Orlando, Florida

Mark A. Kirk, MD
Assistant Director of Clinical Toxicology
Department of Emergency Medicine
Charlotte, North Carolina

Kevin Kraus, BS, EMT-P
New York State Disaster Preparedness
Commission
Clifton Park, New York

Richard A. Lazar
Attorney at Law
Law Offices of Richard A. Lazar
Portland, Oregon

Mark Lockhart, NREMT-P
Director, Department of Paramedic
Education
St. John's Mercy Medical Center
St. Louis, Missouri

Julie Long
Paramedic Instructor
Paramedic Education Department
St. John's Mercy Medical Center
St. Louis, Missouri

Glenn H. Luedtke, NREMT-P
Director, Cape & Islands EMS System
Hyannis, Massachusetts

Mary Beth Michos, RN
Chief EMS Division and Specialty
Teams Coordinator
Department of Fire and Rescue Services
Montgomery County Government
Rockville, Maryland

Gary P. Morris
Deputy Fire Chief
Phoenix, Arizona Fire Department
Phoenix, Arizona

Keith Neely, EMT-P, MPA
Assistant Professor, Emergency
    Medicine
Director, Emergency Medical
    Communication
Oregon Health Sciences University
Portland, Oregon

Gregory Noll
Hildebrand and Noll Associates, Inc.
Laurel, Maryland

Michael P. Peppers, PharmD
Clinical Coordinator, Department of
    Pharmacy
Mineral Area Regional Medical Center
Farmington, Missouri

Dwight Polk, BA, NREMT-P
Paramedic Program Coordinator
University of Maryland, Baltimore
    County
Department of Emergency Health
    Services
Baltimore, Maryland

William Raynovich
Director of Prehospital Services
The Reading Hospital and Medical
    Center
West Reading, Pennsylvania

Lou E. Romig, MD, FAAP
Pediatric Emergency Specialist and
    EMS Liaison
Emergency Medicine Division
Miami Children's Hospital
Miami, Florida

José V. Salazar, BA, NREMT
President
Emergency Med-Care Specialties
Queens Village, New York

Randy L. Sanders
Captain, O'Fallon Fire Protection
    District
O'Fallon, Missouri

Carol J. Shanaberger
Attorney at Law, EMT-P
Lakewood, Colorado

JoAnn Shew, RN, CS, MSN
Psychiatric Clinical Nurse Specialist
Nursing Service Department
St. John's Mercy Medical Center
St. Louis, Missouri

John Sinclair
Battalion Chief
EMS Division
Pierce County Fire District #9
Puyallup, Washington

Todd M. Stanford, BS, PA-C, MICP
Physician's Assistant
Emergency Department
United Hospital Center
Clarksburg, West Virginia

Andrew W. Stern, NREMT-P, MPA
Senior Paramedic
Town of Colonie Emergency
Medical Services
Town of Colonie
Albany, New York

Mike Taigman
Corporate Director of Quality
    Improvement
MedTrans and Subsidiaries
San Francisco, California

Vickie H. Taylor
Licensed Clinical Social Worker
Woodbridge, Virginia

Michael W. Turner
General Manager
Communications/Administration
    Department
Central County Emergency 911
Ballwin, Missouri

Patricia L. Westbrook, MS, CCC
Audiologist
San Antonio, Texas

Jason T. White
Paramedic, Gold Cross Ambulance
EMS Instructor, Medical Center of
    Independence, Missouri
Independence, Missouri

Sherrie C. Wilson, EMT-P, I/C
Executive Director
Emergency Management Resources
Dallas, Texas

Monroe Yancie, NREMT-P
EMS Training Officer
City of St. Louis—Emergency Medical
    Service
St. Louis, Missouri

Rodney C. Zerr (Chapter 4)
Communications Coordinator
St. Charles County Ambulance District
St. Peters, Missouri

CONTENTS

DIVISION THREE   TRAUMA

THE PREHOSPITAL ENVIRONMENT

DIVISION ONE

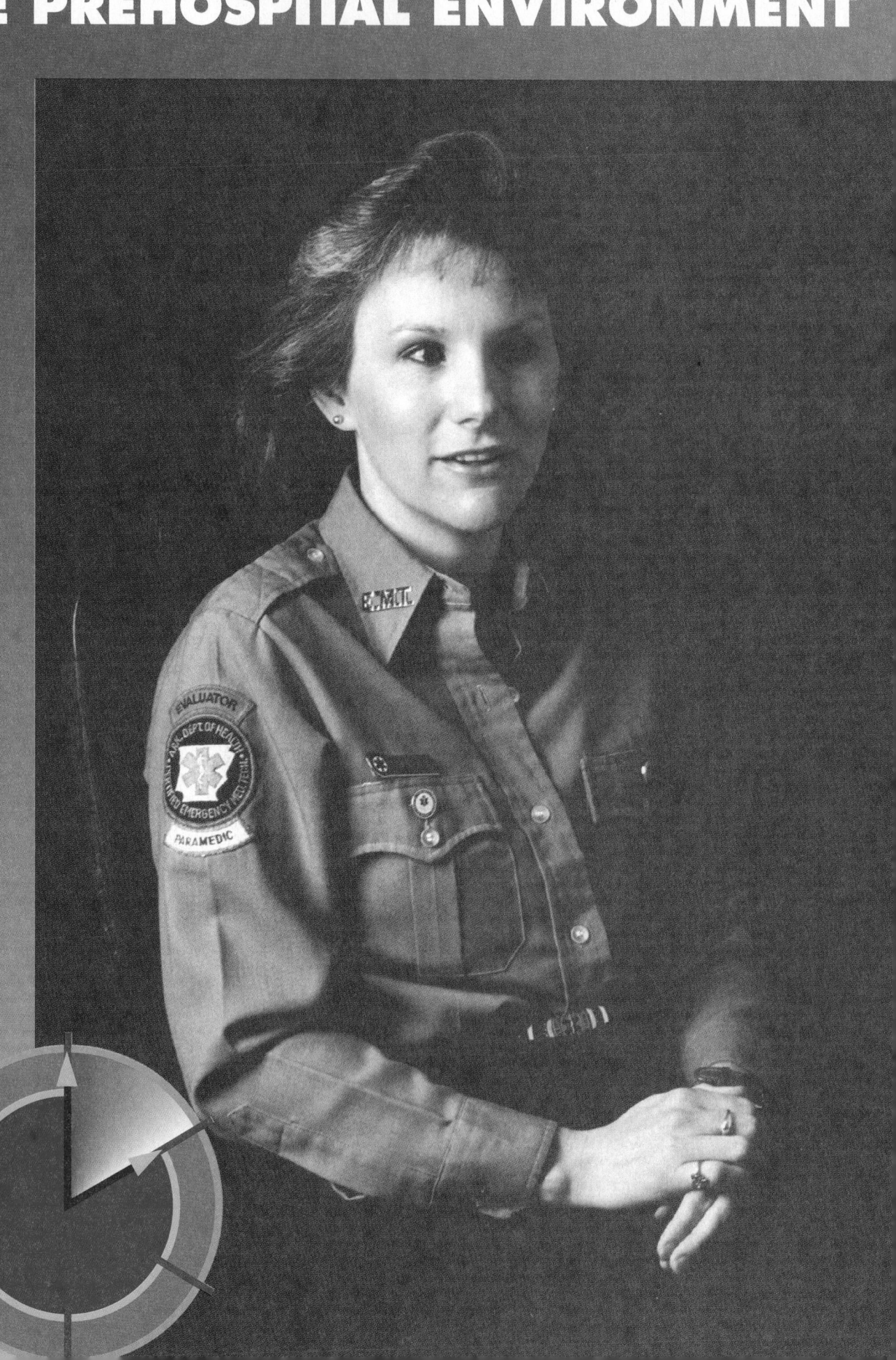

What you are required to do as a para-medic may surprise you. Your role will go far beyond the medical knowledge you gain in paramedic training. It will call on your concern, compassion and under-standing of others.

Grace Richeson, NREMT-P
Assistant Coordinator Cherokee Village Ambulance Service
Cherokee Village, Arkansas

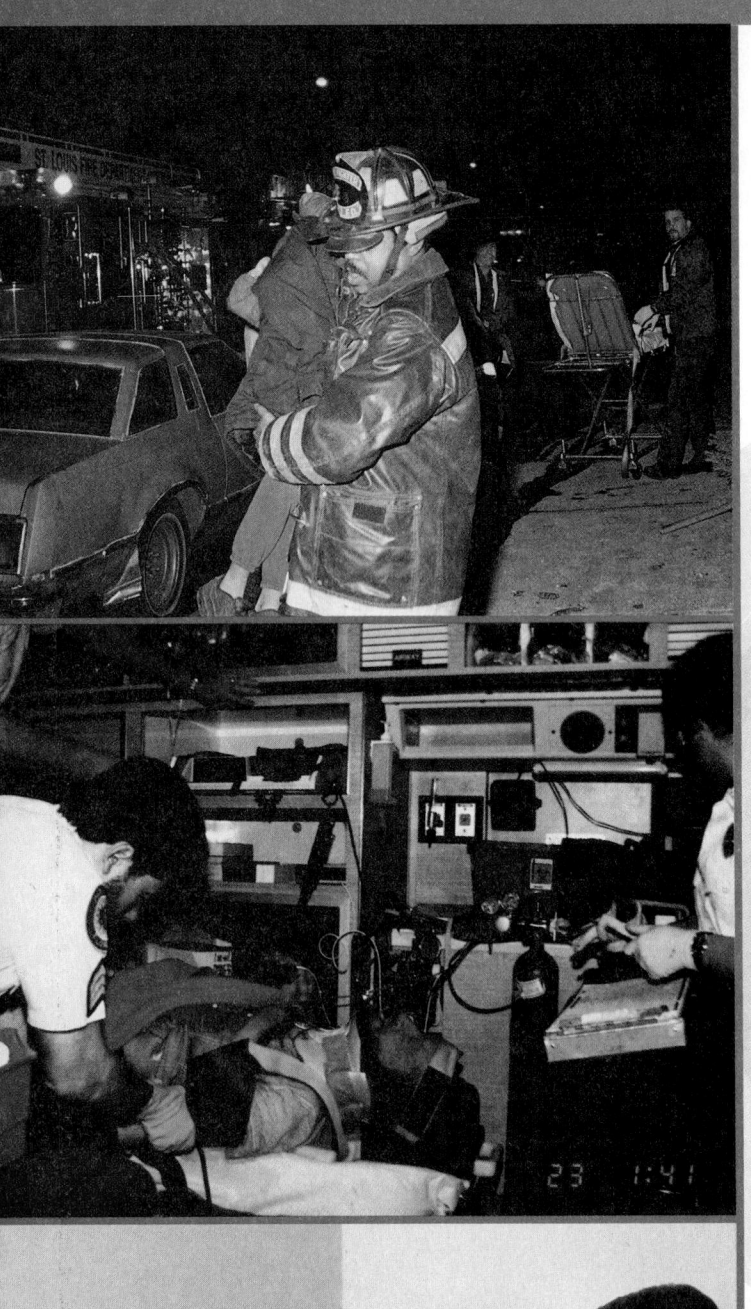

Advanced **emergency medical services (EMS)** plays a key role in the health care delivery system of the United States and much of the world. In just over two decades, emergency medical technicians (EMTs), paramedics, physicians, nurses, dispatchers, and many other dedicated specialists have extended the art and science of emergency medicine into the prehospital setting.

● THE HISTORY OF EMS

It is difficult to assign a specific time and place to the birth of organized prehospital emergency care. However, EMS seems to have its roots in military history. Ancient paintings of Roman battlegrounds suggest that certain warriors were charged with caring for the injured. The first "ambulance" is believed to have been a covered cart used by Napoleon's surgeons to transport wounded soldiers to treatment areas during the Crimean War between 1854 and 1856.[1]

Medical care progressed rapidly during World War I, when it was necessary to care for soldiers wounded by machine guns and massive bombardment. World War II saw the development of air medical transport systems; during the Korean conflict, helicopters were used to evacuate wounded soldiers. In the Vietnam conflict, the concepts of immediate care and rapid evacuation by well-trained corpsmen were further expanded. These military efforts to care for wounded soldiers led to the development of prehospital emergency care as it is known today.

Physicians and nurses have long staffed ambulances in the United States and other countries. France, Russia, and the United States employed nurses and physicians on horse-drawn ambulances in the late 1800s and early 1900s.[2] Through

BOX 1-1

Landmarks in the Development of EMS

1966: *Accidental Death and Disability: The Neglected Disease of Modern Society* was published by the National Academy of Sciences–National Research Council's (NAS/NRC) Committee on Trauma and Shock. This document stressed the difference that quality initial emergency care and transportation could make in the survival of critically injured patients.

1966: The Highway Safety Act of 1966 directed states to develop an effective EMS program or be subject to loss of up to 10% of their federal highway construction funds. This program was administered by the secretary of transportation and charged the U.S. Department of Transportation–National Highway Traffic Safety Administration (DOT-NHTSA) with responsibility for helping states develop their EMS programs.

1968: "9-1-1" was designated as the universal emergency telephone number by the American Telephone and Telegraph Company.

1969: DOT-NHTSA developed the Basic Training Course for EMTs.

1969: *Ambulance Design Criteria,* a report to DOT-NHTSA, was developed by the Committee on Ambulance Design Criteria to complement the NAS/NRC's *Medical Requirements for Ambulance Design and Equipment* (1968). This document recommended ambulance design standards and emergency equipment. The NHTSA agreed to issue matching federal funds to states that purchased vehicles meeting these standards.

1970: The National Registry of Emergency Medical Technicians was organized. The Registry was formed to standardize education, examinations, and certification of EMTs on a national level.

1972: President Nixon directed the Department of Health, Education, and Welfare to develop new ways to organize EMS. This resulted in $8.5 million in contracts being awarded to develop a model EMS system.

1973: The "Star of Life" was adopted as the official symbol for EMS.

1973: The Emergency Medical Services Systems Act identified the key components of the EMS system. It also mandated that emergency medical care programs funded by the Department of Health and Human Services plan and implement a systems approach for emergency response and immediate care.

1974: The first National EMS Week was proclaimed by President Gerald Ford.

1975: The National Association of Emergency Medical Technicians was founded.

1975: The American Medical Association accepted and approved the EMT–P role as an emergency health occupation.

1977: National training standards for the EMT–P were developed and tested for 2 years by more than 40 EMT training agencies throughout the United States.

1980: The federal Department of Health and Human Services released *Position Paper on Trauma Center Designation,* which included trauma centers within EMS systems. Facilities were also categorized.

1986: The 1976 Public Safety Officer's Act (SB 1479) was amended to expand the $50,000 compensation to include survivors of rescue squad and ambulance crew members and public safety department volunteers killed in the line of duty. (It was amended in 1990.)

1990: President George Bush signed the Trauma Care Systems Planning and Development Act of 1990 (HR 1602). The bill provides for annual grants to states based on geographic and population size to help establish and improve trauma systems.

1991: Occupational Exposure to Blood-borne Pathogens; Final Rule (CFR 29 1910.1030) established standards for workplace protection from blood-borne diseases.

most of the early twentieth century and up to the mid-1960s, however, prehospital care in the United States was typically provided by funeral directors and volunteers untrained in emergency care. Most patients received only minimal stabilization at the scene and were hurriedly transported to the nearest hospital.

Modern EMS Systems

In 1965, more than 50,000 people died in traffic accidents in the United States, which prompted the U.S. Congress to pass the Highway Safety Act of 1966. This act provided a major impetus for EMS to emerge as a nationwide system and formulated the blueprint for improving prehospital emergency medical care. As a result, standards were established that recommended all ambulances be equipped with specific lifesaving equipment and be staffed with two people trained in emergency care (Box 1-1).

In 1969, the federal Department of Transportation developed a basic training course for EMTs, and plans were made to upgrade EMS to provide advanced life support (ALS) by emergency medical technician–paramedics (EMT–Ps). Although the EMT–P's role would be years in the making, by the early 1980s there were three categories of EMTs in EMS systems throughout the country: the EMT–basic (EMT–B, formerly known as *EMT–A*), the EMT–intermediate (EMT–I), and the EMT–P.

There are more than 500,000 basic level and intermediate EMTs and paramedics in the United States. More than 12,000 ground and air ambulance services operate some 35,000 emergency vehicles.[3,4] It has also been estimated that over half of all American families now live within 10 minutes of a paramedic unit.[5] Through the efforts of organizations such as the American National Red Cross, the American Heart Association, the Ambulance Association of America, the American College of Emergency Physicians, the Committee on Trauma of the American College of Surgeons, the Committee on Injuries of the American Academy of Orthopaedic Surgeons, and the work of many other groups and dedicated individuals, EMS in the United States has developed into a sophisticated system for providing prehospital emergency care.

● LEVELS OF LICENSURE AND CERTIFICATION

Since the initial training programs were developed, many changes have taken place in the classroom and clinical requirements for EMTs and paramedics. This is to be expected because EMTs must receive training that covers both advances in medical technology and the growing responsibility for care and transportation of the sick and injured. Currently, more than 30 levels of EMTs practice in the United States, with **licensure** and **certification/registration** permitting varied types and degrees of practice and **reciprocity** between states. However, only four levels are generally recognized nationally: EMT–B, EMT–I, EMT–Defibrillation (EMT–D), and EMT–P.

EMT–Basic

The EMT–B has completed the basic National Standard Training Course or its equivalent and is trained in all phases of basic life support, including use of the pneumatic antishock garment. In addition to patient care education, EMT–Bs receive training in ambulance vehicle operations (emergency driving responses, tactics, techniques, and maintenance).

EMT–Intermediate

The EMT–I is a state or nationally certified EMT–B who has completed the National Standard Training Course for EMT–I or its equivalent. This course includes additional training in ALS procedures, including the use of the esophageal obturator airway, the esophageal gastric tube airway, and intravenous therapy.

EMT–Defibrillation

The EMT–D is a state or a nationally certified EMT–B who has completed the additional training in the use of cardiac defibrillators. The national standard training curriculum for EMT–Ds was developed by the American Heart Association in 1990. This level of training has become a recognized classification in nearly all 50 states.

The EMT Oath

Be it pledged as an Emergency Medical Technician, I will honor the physical and judicial laws of God and man. I will follow that regimen which, according to my ability and judgment, I consider for the benefit of my patients and abstain from whatever is deleterious and mischievous, nor shall I suggest any such counsel. Into whatever homes I enter, I will go into them for the benefit of only the sick and injured, never revealing what I see or hear in the lives of men.

I shall also share my medical knowledge with those who may benefit from what I have learned. I will serve unselfishly and continuously in order to help make a better world for all mankind.

While I continue to keep this oath unviolated, may it be granted to me to enjoy life and the practice of the art, respected by all men, in all times. Should I trespass or violate this oath, may the reverse be my lot. So help me God.

Charles Gillespie, M.D.

EMT–Paramedic

The EMT–P is a state or nationally certified EMT–B who has completed the National Standard Training Course for EMT–P or its equivalent. Paramedics are trained in all aspects of BLS and ALS procedures relevant to prehospital emergency care. Per the Department of Transportation, the role of the paramedic includes the ability to[6]:

- Recognize a medical emergency; assess the situation; manage emergency care, and if needed, extricate the patient; coordinate efforts with those of other agencies involved in care and transportation of the patient; and establish rapport with the patient and others to lessen the crisis.
- Assign priorities of emergency treatment and record and communicate data to the designated medical direction authority.
- Initiate and continue emergency medical care under medical direction, which includes recognizing presenting conditions and initiating

appropriate invasive and noninvasive management (for example, surgical and medical emergencies, airway and respiratory problems, cardiac dysrhythmias, cardiac standstill, psychological crisis), and assess patient response to that medical therapy, modifying it as required under the direction of a physician or other authorized personnel.
- Exercise personal judgment if medical direction is interrupted by communication failure or in cases of immediate life-threatening conditions; under these circumstances, emergency care can be rendered as specifically authorized in advance.
- Direct and coordinate patient transport by selecting the best available methods in conjunction with medical direction.
- Document details related to the patient's emergency care and the incident.
- Direct the maintenance and preparation of emergency care equipment and supplies.

● RELICENSURE AND RECERTIFICATION

The mechanisms for maintaining licensure, certification, or both, vary by state and may include the requirements of the National Registry of EMTs. Most licensures and certifications are considered in effect for a 2- to 3-year period, and many states require continuing education or refresher training and skill proficiency (for example, a required number of intravenous lines and intubations) for EMS relicensure or recertification. This process may also include reexamination.

Continuing Education

Continuing education is essential for all health care professionals and is needed to meet the goal of delivering high-quality patient care. Some skills learned during the primary course of study may be infrequently used, and new information, procedures, and resources that enhance patient care are continuously being developed. Continuing education provides a way for the EMS professional to maintain state-of-the-art knowledge and skills. Continuing education may take many forms, including the following:

- Conferences and seminars
- Lectures and workshops
- Quality-improvement reviews
- Skill laboratories
- Certification and recertification programs
- Journal studies
- Videotape presentations
- Independent study

● EMS PROVIDERS AS HEALTH CARE PROFESSIONALS

Rigorous training and performance standards have helped to establish EMTs and paramedics as health care professionals. However, issues such as medical direction, liability, quality improvement, licensing and recertification, reliability, and response times continue to be important areas of concern.

Membership and participation in professional EMS organizations, involvement in community education, and medical research and publication in EMS journals help promote the professional status of the paramedic (Box 1-2). These activities expose the paramedic to current trends in emergency care, to continuing education, and to resource experts, and they provide for national representation in other health care organizations.

Professional Ethics

Ethics, the study of standards, conduct, and moral judgment, is difficult to teach and cannot be mastered within a paramedic training program. Nevertheless, the paramedic is expected to perform duties that may involve conflicts in moral judgment. Examples include issues involving patient confidentiality, patient rights, field testing of experimental drugs or procedures, and honoring a "do not resuscitate" order. The difficulties these issues can present are compounded by the prehospital environment; emergencies often occur remote from medical direction and ancillary resources.

BOX 1-2

Sampling of National EMS Organizations and Associations

- American Ambulance Association (AAA)
- American College of Emergency Physicians (ACEP)
- Association of Air Medical Services (AAMS)
- National Association of EMS Physicians (NAEMSP)
- National Association of Emergency Medical Technicians (NAEMT)
- National Association of Search and Rescue (NASAR)
- National Association of State EMS Directors (NASEMSD)
- National Council of State EMS Training Coordinators (NCSEMSTC)
- National Flight Paramedic Association (NFPA)
- National Registry of Emergency Medical Technicians (NREMT)

During the past 20 years, a branch of ethics dealing with medical issues, **bioethics,** has evolved. Studying bioethics helps the health care provider deal with dilemmas associated with performing duties regarding conflicting professional, legal, and moral accountability.

Professional Accountability

As a professional, the paramedic must conform to a standard established by his or her level of training and regional practice. Responsibilities include commitment to high-quality patient care, continuing education, skill proficiency, and licensure, certification, or both. By seeking licensure, certification, or both, the paramedic demonstrates to the medical community and the lay public that he or she has completed specific training programs and therefore has the knowledge required to perform specific duties. The paramedic is accountable by law to that level of training and that standard of care.

The EMT Code of Ethics

Professional status as an Emergency Medical Technician and Emergency Medical Technician–Paramedic is maintained and enriched by the willingness of the individual practitioner to accept and fulfill obligations to society, other medical professionals, and the profession of Emergency Medical Technician. As an Emergency Medical Technician at the basic level or an Emergency Medical Technician–Paramedic, I solemnly pledge myself to the following code of professional ethics:

A fundamental responsibility of the Emergency Medical Technician is to conserve life, to alleviate suffering, to promote health, to do no harm, and to encourage the quality and equal availability of emergency medical care.

The Emergency Medical Technician provides services based on human need, with respect for human dignity, unrestricted by consideration of nationality, race, creed, color, or status.

The Emergency Medical Technician does not use professional knowledge and skills in any enterprise detrimental to the public well-being.

The Emergency Medical Technician respects and holds in confidence all information of a confidential nature obtained in the course of professional work unless required by law to divulge such information.

The Emergency Medical Technician, as a citizen, understands and upholds the law and performs the duties of citizenship; as a professional, the Emergency Medical Technician has the never-ending responsibility to work with concerned citizens and other health care professionals in promoting a high standard of emergency medical care to all people.

The Emergency Medical Technician shall maintain professional competence and demonstrate concern for the competence of other members of the Emergency Medical Services health care team.

An Emergency Medical Technician assumes responsibility in defining and upholding standards of professional practice and education.

The Emergency Medical Technician assumes responsibility for individual professional actions and judgment, both in dependent and independent emergency functions, and knows and upholds the laws which affect the practice of the Emergency Medical Technician.

An Emergency Medical Technician has the responsibility to be aware of and participate in matters of legislation affecting the Emergency Medical Technician and the Emergency Medical Services System.

The Emergency Medical Technician adheres to standards of personal ethics which reflect credit upon the profession.

Emergency Medical Technicians, or groups of Emergency Medical Technicians, who advertise professional services, do so in conformity with the dignity of the profession.

The Emergency Medical Technician has an obligation to protect the public by not delegating to a person less qualified any service which requires the professional competence of an Emergency Medical Technician.

The Medical Technician will work harmoniously with, and sustain confidence in, Emergency Medical Technician associates, the nurse, the physician, and other members of the emergency medical services health care team.

The Emergency Medical Technician refuses to participate in unethical procedures and assumes the responsibility to expose incompetence or unethical conduct of others to the appropriate authority in a proper and professional manner.

Legal Accountability

Through patient-care activities, the paramedic assumes a distinct role in the health care legal system. Although lawsuits involving prehospital providers have been relatively few, the number is increasing. In addition to providing good patient care, the paramedic must consider the importance of this legal accountability as it relates to professional ethics.

Moral Accountability

A paramedic's actions must also be morally acceptable. Combining moral, legal, and professional accountability may be difficult in an emergency setting, and at times the paramedic must draw on personal beliefs to resolve conflicts among these roles and responsibilities and to decide on a course of action.

These conflicts cannot be satisfactorily addressed in a textbook. However, awareness of these issues will perhaps provide the impetus for thought and meaningful discussion during the course of paramedic training. As bioethics continues to develop, it is hoped that the special needs of the prehospital provider will receive their due consideration.

REFERENCES

1. Roush W, editor: *Principles of EMS systems, a comprehensive text for physicians,* Dallas, 1989, American College of Emergency Physicians.
2. Haller J: The beginnings of urban ambulance service in the United States and England, *J Emerg Med* 8:743, 1990.
3. *Emergency medical services transportation systems and available facilities,* Lexington, Mass, 1988, National EMS Clearinghouse.
4. *Training and certification of EMS personnel,* Lexington, Mass, 1989, National EMS Clearinghouse.
5. Brief history of EMS, *JEMS* S-11, Aug 1989.
6. *Emergency medical technician-paramedic national standard curriculum,* Washington, DC, 1985, US Government Printing Office.-

Summary

In recent years, the paramedic has become a recognized professional member of the emergency health care team. With that recognition comes a number of responsibilities. These include a dedication to patient care; professional, legal, and moral accountability; and a commitment to maintain the knowledge and skills required of the emergency care provider.

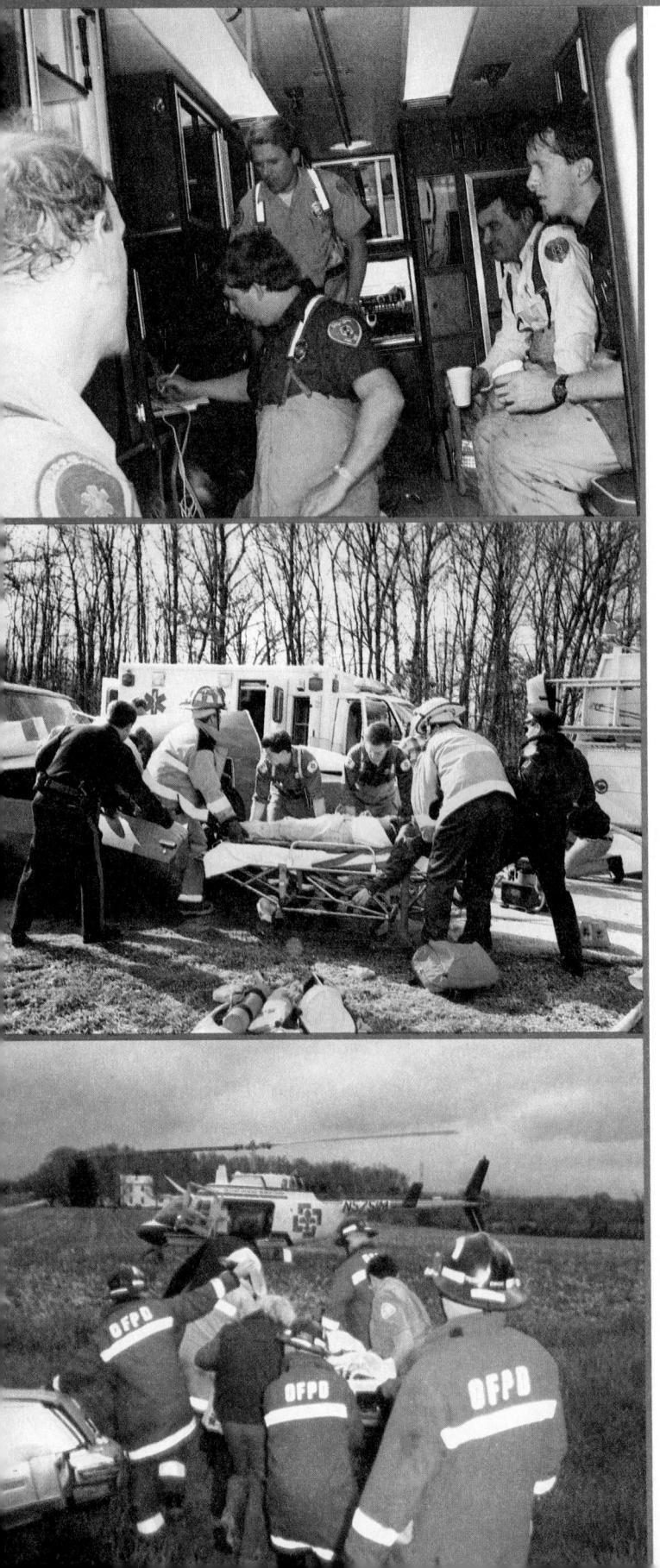

Emergency medical services (EMS) is more than rapid transport to a medical facility. It is a complex system that involves 15 nationally recognized components[1] (Box 2-1). The EMS response begins with the recognition that an emergency exists and continues until all prehospital and in-hospital patient care activities have been delivered. The paramedic crew is but one part of the human and technological resources required for total emergency patient care (Fig. 2-1).

As a paramedic, you should be able to:

1. Describe citizen involvement in the EMS system.
2. Identify how the public can gain access to the EMS system.
3. Distinguish between patient groups who need brief scene care and those who need extended scene care.
4. Describe the benefits of each aspect of off-line and on-line medical direction.
5. Discuss the appropriate transfer of responsibility for patient care in the receiving emergency department.
6. Discuss the benefits of prehospital call reviews.
7. List standards that influence ambulance design and equipment requirements.
8. Outline the factors that must be considered when determining effective ambulance placement in the community.
9. Describe the advantages and disadvantages of air medical transport.
10. Identify the components of an EMS system that may interact in a patient care situation.

● CITIZEN INVOLVEMENT

Although emergency public safety services are highly visible in the community, the public is generally not aware of the complexities involved in providing these services. Citizens expect police and fire protection and a quick response with qualified personnel when emergency medical care is needed. These expectations result from the reputation built on years of service, public relations activities, press coverage, and national media attention. The public expectations also result from public financial support in the form of taxes, donations, subscriptions for service, and user fees.

The Public's Role in EMS

The public's involvement in EMS goes beyond funding. Citizens are often at the scene of an accident or illness and play an important role in recognizing the need for emergency services. In addition, citizens sometimes administer first aid, help secure the scene and gain access to the patient, and can be instrumental in managing a crisis.

Educating the public is fundamental to developing an effective EMS system. More than 40 million Americans have been trained in cardiopulmonary resuscitation (CPR) through the American Red Cross and the American Heart Association.[2] These successful training programs are now being

KEY TERMS

off-line medical direction: The establishment and monitoring of all medical components of an EMS system, including protocols, standing orders, educational programs, and the quality and delivery of on-line medical direction.

on-line medical direction: The direct supervision of prehospital patient care activities by a physician or physician designee.

standing orders: Specific treatment protocols that may be used by prehospital emergency care providers in the absence of on-line medical direction when delay in treatment would harm the patient.

treatment protocols: Guidelines that define the scope of prehospital intervention practiced by emergency care providers.

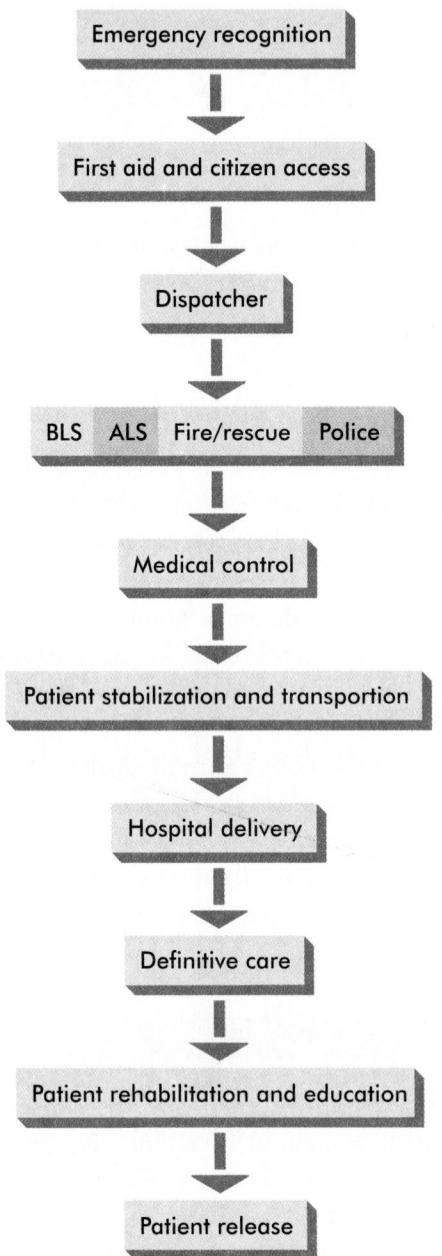

Fig. 2-1 Process of patient care through the EMS system.

BOX 2-1

15 Components of an EMS System

1. Man power
2. Training
3. Communications
4. Transportation
5. Facilities
6. Critical care units
7. Public safety agencies
8. Consumers
9. Access to care
10. Transfer of patients
11. Medical record-keeping
12. Consumer information and education
13. Review and evaluation
14. Disaster linkage
15. Mutual aid

sponsored by many organizations, including the YMCA and YWCA; local EMS, law enforcement, and fire service agencies; local hospitals; public service organizations; and industry. By participating in these training programs, paramedics help prepare the public to respond appropriately to any medical emergency. In addition, paramedic involvement in public education builds support for EMS.

9-1-1: Activating the EMS System

In 1967, the President's Commission on Law Enforcement and Administration of Justice recommended that a single telephone number be established for reporting emergencies. In 1968, the American Telephone and Telegraph Company (AT&T) designated 9-1-1 as the universal emergency number. Through community education, public service announcements, and television programming, 9-1-1 has gained national recognition.

The 9-1-1 emergency telephone number provides easy access to public safety services, such as fire service, law enforcement, and EMS, throughout much of the country. The availability of emergency access via 9-1-1 continues to expand across the country as areas adopt the system. In areas that do not have 9-1-1, access to emergency phone numbers should be made as simple as possible. This can be accomplished through public awareness programs, telephone stickers, telephone book covers, and similar means. Other methods of activating an emergency response include firebox pull stations, citizens band radios, and mobile cellular telephones. Chapter 4 further addresses the 9-1-1 system.

● PREHOSPITAL CARE

The importance of an informed public trained in CPR and emergency first aid and in activating the EMS system has been well established. Several other aspects of prehospital care and crisis intervention, however, must occur before the paramedic crew arrives.

Emergency Dispatch Communications

An effective communications system coordinates an emergency response. After the emergency is recognized, communication centers are contacted through emergency telephone numbers or radio communications. The communications specialist (dispatcher) serves as the primary contact with the public and directs the appropriate agencies (ground and air ambulances, fire departments, law enforcement, utility services) to the scene. Some communications system specialists are also trained to provide emergency medical instructions by phone at the time of the call for help (see Chapter 4).

First Responder Emergency Care

In 1973, the Department of Transportation–National Highway Traffic Safety Administration (DOT-NHTSA) published a training program designed to reduce injuries and deaths on the nation's highways. This program, now known as *First Responder: Emergency Medical Care Training*, has been implemented by many law enforcement, fire service, industry, and other interested groups.

First responders are trained in emergency care with an emphasis on their role in the EMS system. Because they are often the first to arrive at the scene of an accident or an illness, first responders have become an integral part of an effective EMS response team.

Treatment and Transportation

Seriously ill or injured patients may require prehospital intervention and stabilization involving both basic life support (BLS) and advanced life support (ALS) skills. Depending on the circumstances (for example, entrapment, distance to the hospital, availability of ALS), initial prehospital care may be limited to providing comfort and reassurance. It could also require spinal immobilization, airway protection, or a wide range of other procedures, including endotracheal intubation, intravenous cannulation, medication administration, defibrillation, and external cardiac pacing.

The American Heart Association (AHA) recommends that BLS capabilities and early defibrillation be available to out-of-hospital cardiac arrest victims within 4 minutes, followed by ALS capabilities within 8 minutes.[2] The AHA has estimated that implementing these lifesaving resources could save up to 200,000 lives per year.[2] This emphasizes once again the importance of early recognition and initiation of BLS by the general public and/or ancillary public services as part of the EMS system (Fig. 2-2).

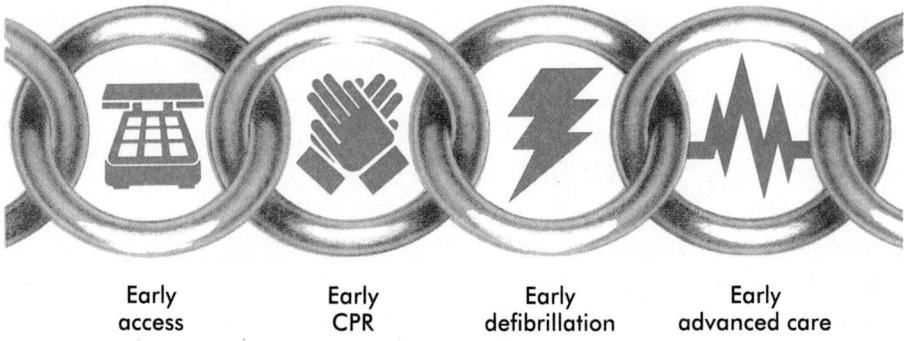

Early access   Early CPR   Early defibrillation   Early advanced care

Fig. 2-2 Chain of survival metaphor. (Reproduced with permission. *Guidelines for Cardiopulmonary Resuscitation and Emergency Cardiac Care*, 1992. © Copyright American Medical Association.)

Great technological advances have been made in emergency cardiac care. Through a medical control authority, paramedics are performing emergency procedures that truly extend the resources of the emergency department into the community. Some patients, however, require definitive treatment, such as surgery, and cannot be stabilized in the field. For these patients (estimated to be 5% of all trauma cases[3]), rapid assessment and stabilization of the airway and cervical spine and rapid and safe transport to an appropriate medical facility are the goals of prehospital care. It is the EMS responder's duty to recognize these patients and to prevent delays in transportation.

● MEDICAL DIRECTION FOR EMS

Medical direction (medical control) means "the direction and quality assurance of health care delivery in an EMS system."[4] Medical direction is a critical component in EMS. It is this relationship between the physician and EMS provider that permits delivery of advanced prehospital care.

There are two types of medical direction—on-line and off-line. When the paramedic crew contacts the hospital by radio or telephone, patient information is transmitted and orders are received through direct, on-line communication with a physician or physician designee, such as a registered nurse or paramedic trained to provide ALS orders in the medical direction system. **On-line medical direction** permits monitoring of prehospital patient care and emergency department preparation for the patient's arrival. On-line medical direction is the most common format for receiving medical orders.

Administrative **off-line medical direction** is often provided by an advisory group or medical director responsible for the quality of medical care delivered by an EMS system. It may include the authority to establish **treatment protocols** and **standing orders** for treatment and triage of prehospital patients (see Chapter 6).

Treatment protocols are guidelines that define the scope of prehospital intervention for EMS providers. They are developed by the medical direc-

Physicians at the Scene

If a non–medical direction physician or the patient's private physician is present at the scene of an emergency, medical direction should be contacted. Written policies developed by many EMS agencies require that the scene physician establish communication with the on-line medical direction physician so that decisions can be made regarding legal responsibility for the patient's care. With the approval of medical direction, an on-scene physician may assume responsibility for patient management. However, if a scene physician attempts to direct patient care in opposition to medical direction, law enforcement should be requested to ensure scene safety and uninterrupted emergency care.

tor of the ALS service or by representatives of a regional EMS advisory group. Standing orders are more specific than treatment protocols and are normally included in a protocol when a delay in treatment would harm the patient. Most protocols and standing orders comply with national standards (for example, the AHA standards for advanced cardiac life support or the American College of Surgeons standards for advanced trauma life support), state EMS Medical Practice Acts, and regional guidelines.

Written protocols define the standard of care for paramedic crews and on-line physicians. Situations in which the paramedic crew functions strictly by protocol are usually limited (for example, intubation of a nonbreathing patient, first-line medication administration in cardiac arrest, situations in which radio contact has failed and a delay in treatment could compromise patient outcome).

● HOSPITAL CARE

When the patient is delivered to the emergency department, patient care resources expand to include physicians, nurses, technicians, ancillary support staff (counselors, social workers, and others), secretaries, medical record staff, and diagnostic services, such as those provided by laboratory, radiology, and cardiopulmonary departments. Resources available beyond the emergency department include surgery, intensive care, physical therapy, pharmacy, patient education, nutrition services, and many others. Prehospital care is important in reducing morbidity and mortality, but field personnel are only part of a comprehensive EMS system.

Categorization of Hospital Resource Capabilities

Categorization of hospital emergency services was recommended by the American Medical Association in the early 1970s.[5] In 1990, *Resources for Optimal Care of the Injured Patient* was published by the Task Force of the American College of Surgeons (ACS) Committee on Trauma. It described three levels of trauma centers based on resources, admissions, staff, research, and education involvement.

A level I institution can provide total care for every aspect of injury and is uniquely qualified to care for the most severely injured patient, especially in the surgical critical care setting, followed by level II and level III facilities. Categorization of hospital resources identifies hospitals capable of handling trauma patients and enables EMS providers to rapidly transport patients to appropriate medical facilities. Based on ACS guidelines, some government agencies have designated certain institutions as trauma centers. Other specialized care facilities, such as pediatric trauma centers, burn centers, hyperbaric centers, and poison treatment centers, provide care for critically ill or injured patients with special needs.

The ACS Committee on Trauma also established guidelines for field triage, interhospital triage to specialized care facilities, and mass casualty triage. These criteria are based on the patient's condition, mechanism of injury, injury severity indices, and available patient care resources.

Emergency Department Delivery

When the ambulance arrives at the receiving hospital, the patient must be "transferred" to the emergency department staff. This involves the physical transfer of the patient, patient care equipment, and personal belongings. EMS providers must also give a verbal report outlining patient information, including the patient's chief complaint, vital signs, present and past medical histories, medications, allergies, clinical data, treatment rendered, and any changes in status during the course of treatment. Responsibility for patient responsibility care is also transferred at this time; in this manner, patient care responsibility is shared with other members of the health care team.

Other EMS-Related Duties

After the paramedic crew has finished the patient care activities, they must complete their paperwork. This may involve gathering patient information for record-keeping and billing purposes and completing all of the prehospital documents needed for the patient's hospital medical record.

The emergency vehicle must be cleaned, disinfected, and made ready for another response. Equipment, fluids, and medications must also be replaced before the next call. These duties should be completed promptly so that the paramedic crew can be available for service.

Prehospital Call Reviews

Reviewing the emergency call is invaluable in identifying difficulties in a particular patient care situation and planning for future EMS responses.

Patient Follow-Up

Information on a patient's progress after hospitalization can be of educational benefit to the EMS crew. It provides valuable feedback on initial emergency care efforts and a more complete view of long-term patient care. Patients should be followed up through a special hospital liaison, EMS training coordinator, supervisor, or service medical director; patient confidentiality, however, should be maintained.

● GROUND AMBULANCE VEHICLE STANDARDS

In 1968, the National Academy of Sciences–National Research Council (NAS–NRC) prepared a document for the U.S. Department of Health, Education, and Welfare entitled *Medical Requirements for Ambulance Design and Equipment* (supplemented in 1969 by a report entitled *Ambulance Design Criteria*). These documents recommended ambulance design standards, including size, shape, color, electrical systems, and emergency equipment, and led to the development of the current federal specifications used by many states for their ambulance licensure requirements.

KKK Standards

The national standards developed by NAS-NRC and NHTSA are known as the *KKK Standards* (specifications KKK-A-1822C, 1990). They are the foundation of uniformity among ambulance vehicles and provide for the adoption of future advances in EMS equipment. The KKK specifications pertain to the following three basic ambulance designs (Fig. 2-3):

Type I   Conventional truck cab–chassis with modular ambulance body

Type II   Standard van, forward control integral cab-body ambulance

Type III   Specialty van, forward control integral cab-body ambulance

In 1970, the ACS Committee on Trauma also issued a list of "essential equipment" to be carried on ambulance vehicles. The recommendations included ALS equipment, emergency drugs, and fluids to be used in ALS procedures.

Emergency Vehicle Placement

In the 1970s, when standards were being set by the Department of Transportation, guidelines were provided for establishing ambulance services. The two measures recommended to help determine service needs were the availability of an ambulance to answer an emergency response and the average response time to the emergency scene.

In recent years, methods for estimating needs have shifted toward determining the percentage of compliance in providing EMS services within time frames that meet national standards (for example, the AHA recommendation that ALS be available at the scene within 8 minutes of a cardiac arrest). These estimates are affected by geographical area, topographical area, population, traffic conditions, time of day, and appropriate

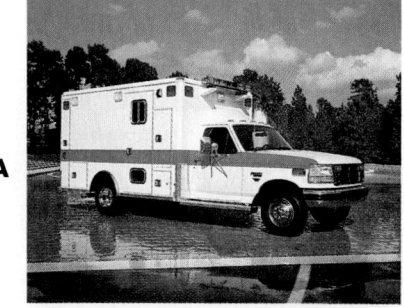

A

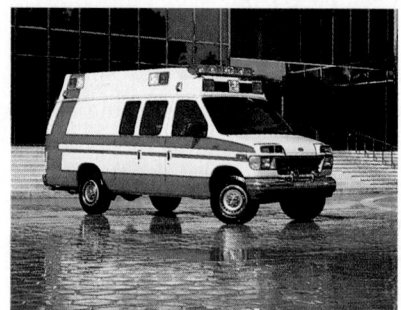

B

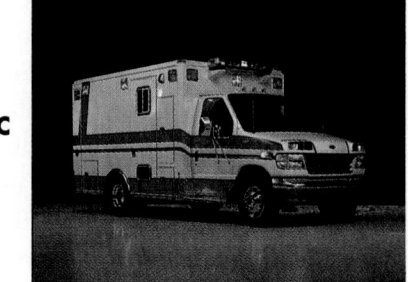

C

Fig. 2-3 Basic ambulance designs. **A,** Type I. **B,** Type II. **C,** Type III.

placement of emergency vehicles within a community. These strategies are based on call volumes and locations and may use computers and other sophisticated technologies to formalize strategic unit deployment and decrease response times.

● AIR MEDICAL SERVICES

Air evacuation, like many other aspects of prehospital emergency care, is rooted in military history. During the Prussian siege of Paris in 1870, soldiers and civilians were evacuated by a hot-air balloon, and in 1928, a Marine pilot used an engine-powered aircraft to evacuate wounded in Nicaragua.[6] The first full-scale use of motorized aircraft for medical evacuation, however, did not occur until 1950 during the Korean conflict.

The experience gained in Korea was the basis for developing helicopter rescue in Vietnam. The Bell UH-1H Huey, a helicopter with specially designed rescue equipment and a sophisticated communications system, ensured that no soldier in Vietnam was more than 35 minutes away from surgical treatment.[7] The Huey could transport up to four patients and crew and could fly 137 mph for up to 3 hours without refueling. For the first time in history, helicopter power and payload capabilities allowed resuscitative measures during flight. During the Vietnam conflict, helicopters transported nearly 1 million casualties. Since the 1960s, the field of air medical services has continued to grow, and there are now approximately 200 civilian EMS flight programs throughout the United States.[8]

Utilization of Air Medical Services

Criteria for requesting air medical services to the scene of an emergency must be developed by the appropriate authority of the local EMS system. As a rule, air transportation should be considered when emergency personnel have found that (1) the time needed to transport a patient by ground to an appropriate facility poses a threat to the patient's survival and recovery; (2) weather, road, or traffic conditions would seriously delay the patient's access to ALS; or (3) critical care personnel and equipment are needed to adequately care

---

BOX 2-2

Advantages and Disadvantages of Air Medical Services

Advantages

- Transports are rapid and usually smooth.
- Access to accident sites is quick.
- Traffic, trains, mountains, ship canals, and other barriers can be avoided.
- Travel is still possible when road conditions are unfavorable.
- Sophisticated communication equipment is available.
- Ground ambulances are not detained for long periods.
- Quality of care is improved in rural areas where only BLS is available.
- There are fewer air ambulance crashes than ground ambulance crashes.

Disadvantages

- In urban settings, ground ambulances are usually faster within a 30-mile range.
- If the helicopter is on another flight, no other aircraft may be available.
- Inclement weather may prevent the aircraft from traveling.
- High noise level may limit or prevent communication with the patient or crew.
- Space and weight restrictions may limit access to the patient and restrict the crew, patients, and equipment that can be carried.
- Helicopter transports are more expensive than transports by ground ambulance.
- Helicopter crashes have fewer survivors.

---

for the patient during transport (Box 2-2). Other factors relating to the consideration of air medical transport are addressed in Chapter 6.

Fixed Wing

Fixed-wing aircraft services are not usually as high-profile as helicopters. However, they may be

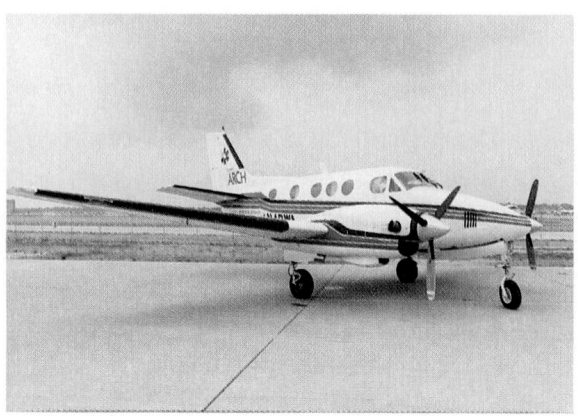

Fig. 2-4 Fixed-wing aircraft.

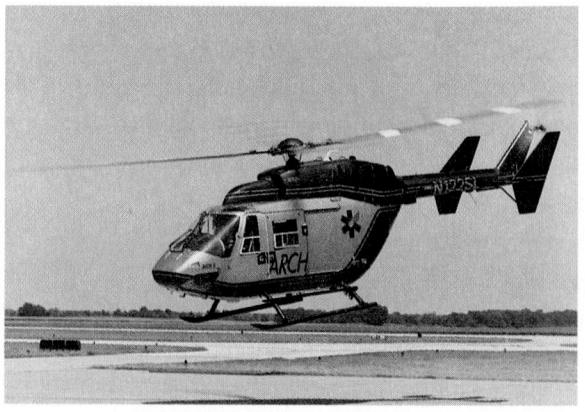

Fig. 2-5 Rotary-wing aircraft.

the primary means of emergency transport in remote regions, such as parts of Alaska. In addition, these aircraft are frequently used for interhospital transfer of patients and vital organ delivery when the distance is greater than 100 miles (Fig. 2-4).

Rotary Wing

Helicopters used in EMS have either one or two engines. In general, single-engine helicopters require less time to start, use less fuel, and cost less to operate. Twin-engine helicopters offer an increased safety margin and usually allow for increased payload, but they require more maintenance and more time to start than single-engine aircraft (Fig. 2-5).

Air Medical Crew Members and Training

The staffing of air ambulances includes a pilot and various health care professionals (such as EMTs, EMT–Ps, respiratory therapists, nurses, and physicians) with specialized training in flight physiology. Guidelines for personnel qualifications have been established by the ACS Committee on Trauma and the Association of Air Medical Services.

The DOT-NHTSA funded the development of the *Air Medical Crew National Standard Curriculum* in 1988. These documents were designed to be used as an adjunct to the existing DOT curricula for the EMT, EMT–I, and EMT–P. The air medical curriculum was printed in 1988 and has been used by many flight programs to teach flight physiology, aircraft components and construction, safety regulations, aviation and navigation terminology, and operational safety.

REFERENCES

1. Federal Emergency Management Agency: *Introduction to emergency medical services*, Emmitsburg, Md, 1984, The Agency.
2. American Heart Association: *Textbook of advanced cardiac life support*, ed 2, Dallas, 1990, The Association.
3. Committee on Trauma, American College of Surgeons: *Resources for optimal care of the injured patient*, Chicago, 1990, The College.
4. Roush W, editor: *Principles of EMS systems*, Dallas, 1989, American College of Emergency Physicians.
5. Kuehl A, editor: *EMS medical directors' handbook*, National Association of EMS Physicians, St Louis, 1989, Mosby.
6. US Department of Transportation, National Highway Traffic Safety Administration: *Air medical crew national standard curriculum*, Washington, DC, 1988, The Department.
7. Lenworth M, Bennett B, editors: Helicopter EMS, *Emerg Care Q* 2(2):11, 1986.
8. Hospital aviation survey: annual transport statistics, *Hosp Aviat* March, 1989.

Summary

An effective EMS system involves many facets of health care delivery and reflects a combined effort of many organizations, agencies, and specially trained individuals. Citizen involvement, communications, medical direction, and the talents of prehospital and in-hospital medical personnel enable the EMS system to have a positive impact on health care delivery in this country.

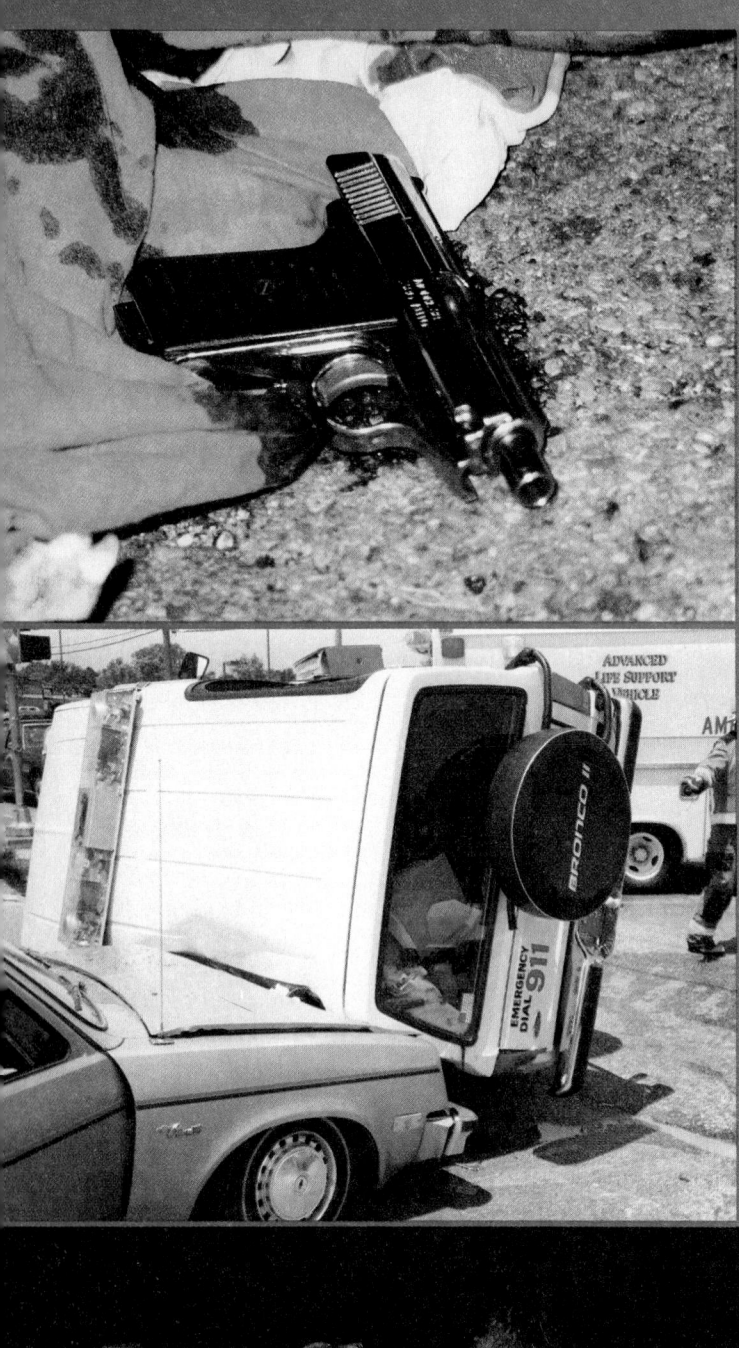

In recent years, the U.S. legal system has been active on issues pertaining to medical malpractice. Historically, only hospitals and physicians were involved in litigation because volunteers were relatively well protected from lawsuits and EMS personnel were not expected to meet professional standards of patient care. With today's state and national certifications, licensure, and the EMS workers' affiliation with traditional health care professionals, however, prehospital providers have legitimate concerns about medical liability.

OBJECTIVES

As a paramedic, you should be able to:

1. Describe the four elements involved in a claim of negligence.
2. Define common medical-legal terms that apply to prehospital situations involving patient care.
3. Describe measures paramedics may take to protect themselves from claims of negligence.
4. List situations that the paramedic is legally required to report in most states.
5. Describe the paramedic's responsibilities with regard to patient confidentiality.
6. Describe the process for obtaining expressed, informed, and implied consent.
7. Describe actions to be taken in a refusal-of-care situation.
8. List uses of the prehospital care report.
9. Detail the components of the narrative report.
10. Discuss the implications of Good Samaritan legislation.

● THE LEGAL SYSTEM

The structure of the legal system in the United States is composed of legislative law, administrative regulations, common law, and criminal law. Legislative law is made by legislative branches of government, such as city councils, district boards, general assemblies, and Congress. The power of these bodies to make law is defined by statutes, state constitutions, and in the case of Congress, the U.S. Constitution.

Administrative regulations are developed as part of a governmental agency (which is created by the legislature) to provide details about the function and process of the law. For example, a state may pass legislation that sets general requirements for EMT and paramedic licensure. The specific requirements are often defined through administrative regulations authorized by the statute. These regulations are enacted by state and federal administrative agencies through a process called *rulemaking* and may address areas such as examinations, licenses, and maintenance of records. These agencies may also hold disciplinary hearings regarding revocation or suspension of licenses. An example of a regulatory agency is a state EMS bureau.

Common law (case law) is based on the decisions of the state and federal judicial systems. With reference to patient care activities, these court decisions may offer guidance in defining acceptable conduct and **negligence** and in interpreting statutes and regulations applicable to EMS.

KEY TERMS

abandonment: Terminating medical care without legal excuse or turning care over to less-qualified personnel, thereby injuring the patient.

implied consent: Presuming that an unconscious or incompetent person would consent to lifesaving care.

informed consent: Consent obtained from a patient after explaining all facts necessary for the patient to make a reasonable decision.

negligence: Failure to use such care as a reasonably prudent EMS provider would use in similar circumstances or a deviation from a standard of care.

prehospital care report: A document used in the prehospital setting to record all patient care activities and circumstances related to an emergency response.

Criminal law is the portion of the legal system in which government officials prosecute individuals for violating the laws enacted to protect society.

> **NOTE:**
> Laws pertaining to patient care delivery vary by state. Every paramedic should be aware of his state's Medical Practice Act and other regulatory statutes. Paramedics should consult with a private attorney or the state Attorney General's office (or its equivalent) to clarify state laws and their application to EMS activities. The information contained in this chapter is general information and is not intended to be a complete guide to any state's legislative system, EMS laws, or regulations.

Civil Lawsuits

Most prehospital patient care activities that result in litigation are civil suits. A civil lawsuit is a "private" complaint brought by a person, known as a *plaintiff*, against another individual, the "defendant," for an alleged illegal act or wrongdoing, termed a *tort*, for which the plaintiff requests the court to award damages. Civil lawsuits may be resolved by a trial in which evidence is presented to a judge or jury. Compensatory damages may be awarded.

Criminal Lawsuits

In a criminal lawsuit, government representatives, such as county prosecutors, district attorneys, or the state Attorney General's office, file criminal charges against a defendant. These criminal actions seek to enforce standards established by statute that define certain conduct as public wrongs. In criminal cases, it is not a private complaint but rather a public complaint because the wrong is considered to have been committed against the public. Criminal cases may result in fines, imprisonment, or both.

Criminal statutes do not always require proof of intent or intentional conduct (criminal intent) for an activity to be considered criminal in nature. EMS personnel who, for example, have a motor vehicle crash as a result of reckless driving while responding to an emergency may face civil and criminal actions. Therefore excessive speed, failure to consider road and weather conditions, and inappropriate use or nonuse of sirens and lights are important issues to all emergency drivers. The paramedic should be well aware of state motor vehicle codes and laws pertaining to emergency vehicle operations.

● NEGLIGENCE

Lawsuits involving patient care usually result from civil claims of negligence: the failure to act as a reasonable, prudent EMT or paramedic would act in similar circumstances. In most states, four elements must be proved for negligence to exist:

1. There was a duty to act.
2. There was a breach of duty by not acting or failing to act in a reasonable, prudent manner, whereby the required standard of care was not observed.
3. There was damage to the patient.
4. The breach was the proximate cause of the damage.

Duty To Act

EMTs and paramedics, whether paid or volunteer, assume a "duty" to provide emergency care while working for an EMS service, provided that emergency assistance was requested. In most states, off-duty EMTs and paramedics have no such duty to act. However, if emergency care is initiated by an off-duty EMT or paramedic, that EMS provider becomes obligated by law to care for that patient just as if he or she were on duty. Once an EMS provider undertakes the duty to act, the provider must *continue to act* until patient care responsibilities have been transferred to another health care worker with equal or greater competence, or it is abundantly clear that the patient no longer needs assistance.

It should be noted that the delegation of scope of practice between a physician and a paramedic is usually only effective when the paramedic is on-duty. Therefore an off-duty paramedic who provides emergency care must usually act in a BLS capacity unless there is written authorization from medical control for ALS procedures to be performed while off duty.

Breach of Duty

If the plaintiff can prove that the paramedic had a duty to act, he or she must also prove that the duty was breached or violated for negligence to exist. As previously stated, the EMT or paramedic assumes the duty of providing the reasonable and acceptable standard of care that any other similarly trained EMT or paramedic would provide under similar circumstances. Many states consider national standards when defining acceptable care. If written national or state standards have been violated, it may be easier for the plaintiff to prove breach of duty.

Damage to the Patient

The third element of negligence is proof that the plaintiff suffered compensable damages. Examples include medical expenses, lost earnings, pain and suffering, and wrongful death. Punitive damages may also be awarded in excess of compensable damages to punish the wrongdoer and to deter others from causing similar harm in the future. Punitive damages are not generally covered by malpractice insurance (see unit on malpractice insurance, p. 27).

Proximate Cause

Finally, the plaintiff must prove that the negligent act caused the injury or worsened an already present injury and that the injury or additional harm was foreseeable to the paramedic. The element of proximate cause is sometimes difficult to establish and often involves expert witnesses who address issues of duty, standard of care, and conflicting views of causation. For example, was a cervical spine injury caused by the motor vehicle crash, or was it the result of rescue efforts by the EMS crew? Most authorities stress that a paramedic's best protection against such claims is training, competent patient care skills, and thorough documentation of all patient care activities.

Additional Examples of Negligence

Areas for potential negligent conduct other than direct patient care activities include (1) patient transportation to a medical facility contrary to medical control advice, trauma center designation criteria, or other known special patient care needs and facility capabilities; (2) failure to maintain equipment, supplies, or vehicles; and (3) driving negligently or recklessly.

● ADDITIONAL AREAS OF LIABILITY

Nearly anyone can be sued, regardless of the legitimacy of the complaint. A lawsuit itself is not an indication of guilt or wrongdoing unless the allegations are proven. Other areas in which EMS providers may incur liability include:

- **Abandonment:** Inappropriate termination of medical care or turning care over to less-qualified personnel, thereby injuring the patient.
- Assault: Creating apprehension, or unauthorized handling and treatment of a patient.
- Battery: Physical contact with a person without his or her consent and without legal justification.
- False imprisonment: Intentional and unjustifiable detention of a person.
- Invasion of privacy: Without legal justification making public details of a person's private life that might reasonably expose that person to ridicule, notoriety, or embarrassment.
- Libel: Writing false statements about someone, knowing them to be false, with malicious

intent or with reckless disregard of the falsity.
- Slander: Verbally making false statements about a person, knowing them to be false, with malicious intent or with reckless disregard of the falsity.

● OTHER SIGNIFICANT LAWS

Paramedics and other health care professionals may be required by law to report cases of abuse or neglect of children and older adults and cases involving rape, gunshot wounds, stab wounds, animal bites, and certain communicable diseases. The paramedic should be familiar with these laws and follow local protocol established by medical control and the EMS agency (Box 3-1).

● PATIENT CONFIDENTIALITY

Some states prohibit physicians from revealing patient information without the patient's consent. In most states, EMS providers do not have this legal obligation but rather have an ethical obligation to protect a patient's privacy. Information obtained from a patient (for example, a patient history of communicable disease) can usually be conveyed without the patient's permission to other health care providers involved in the patient's care. Similarly, information obtained from a pa-

---

BOX 3-1

Cases Reportable Under Law in Most States

- Neglect or abuse of children
- Neglect or abuse of older adults
- Rape
- Gunshot wounds
- Stab wounds
- Animal bites
- Certain communicable diseases

---

tient regarding an accident or crime may be reported to law enforcement personnel and testified to in court. The paramedic should recall, however, that there is potential liability for invasion of privacy, libel, or slander if personal information is released with malicious intent or reckless disregard or to people not legally entitled to the information.

● PATIENT RIGHTS

Patient rights have been defined and clarified by legislation and the judicial system through malpractice litigation. A competent patient's right to decide what medical care he or she will receive is a fundamental concept of law and medical practice.[1]

Informed Consent

Informed consent is patient consent signifying that the patient knows, understands, and agrees to the patient care rendered. Verbal or written consent to the treatment is called *expressed consent*. For consent to be considered informed, the patient must be aware of the following:
- The nature of the illness or injury
- The recommended treatment and associated risks
- The alternative treatment and risks involved
- The danger of refusing treatment

Although EMS providers must generally obtain a patient's consent before initiating treatment, EMTs and paramedics are not obligated to obtain the same degree of informed consent as other health care providers, particularly in an emergency. In these situations, the patient must only agree or at least not object to the general nature of the treatment.

Implied Consent

The concept of **implied consent** presumes that unconscious or mentally impaired people needing immediate emergency care would consent to lifesaving treatment if they were able to do so. Unconscious patients and victims of shock, head injury, and alcohol or drug intoxication are examples of patients to whom emergency care should be delivered in the absence of informed consent.

Special Consent Situations

Situations may occur in which obtaining consent for treatment is difficult (for example, emergencies involving minors, mentally incompetent adults, institutionalized patients, prisoners). In these cases, consent for medical care may need to be obtained from a parent, legal guardian, representative of a state agency, or another legal authority. If a delay in obtaining consent would be life threatening, however, the patient should be treated. EMS personnel should be familiar with state laws governing these unique circumstances, and EMS systems should have protocols covering such situations.

Refusal of Care

A mentally competent adult has the right to refuse medical care, even if the decision could result in death or permanent disability. Refusal of care may be based on religious beliefs, fear, or lack of understanding of medical procedures. The paramedic should be sensitive to these concerns and carefully explain a procedure and answer any questions the patient has. Involving medical control, law enforcement, family members, and friends at the scene may help persuade the patient to accept care and transportation. Despite these efforts, however, some patients still refuse treatment. If this occurs, the paramedic crew should leave the patient with the understanding that he or she can call again for help, despite the initial refusal. Cases involving refusal of care are a significant cause of lawsuits against EMS agencies.

When dealing with any patient who refuses care, the paramedic should document thoroughly. The paramedic crew should obtain names and addresses of others who witnessed the event and all attempts made to obtain consent. In addition, the paramedic should advise the patient of the medical risks associated with refusal of care and record that the advice was provided. Law enforcement officers and other allied professionals should be requested to make similar documentation of the event. Many EMS systems require the paramedic to obtain a signature from the patient refusing care, transportation, or both.

Some EMS systems require EMS crews to contact medical control and review the case with the physician or nurse. Medical control personnel may also discuss the situation with the patient while the call is recorded. This policy may be useful in suppressing legal action, but the most critical legal document of refusal is the written **prehospital care report** prepared by the paramedic.

Law enforcement assistance may be required when dealing with unruly or potentially violent patients who are not able to make rational, informed decisions regarding their care. Examples include patients with behavioral emergencies and those with altered levels of consciousness caused by injury, substance abuse, or illness. Most law enforcement agencies have the authority to place the patient in "protective custody," thereby permitting treatment. EMS personnel should only become involved in restraining a patient when it can be done safely and only if there is reason to suspect that the patient is a threat to himself or herself or others (see Chapter 30).

Patient Self-Determination

In December 1991, a federal law known as the *Patient Self-Determination Act of 1990* required all institutions that accept Medicare or Medicaid to recognize any kind of "advance directive," such as durable power of attorney for health care, or a "do not resuscitate" order.[2] These legal documents are executed to inform health care practitioners of an individual's wishes for treatment or withholding of treatment in case that person becomes incapacitated and unable to communicate those wishes directly. Many states have also enacted legislation regarding "living wills" and the "right to die with dignity" for patients suffering from terminal illness. The EMS service must work closely with medical control to develop procedures and protocols that help EMS providers handle these laws and policies.

If the paramedic crew if dispatched to a dying patient who has requested that he or she not be resuscitated, medical control should be contacted immediately. Decisions can then be made regarding any patient care activities. If it is determined that the patient is not to receive medical intervention to prolong life, the paramedic crew should provide reasonable measures of comfort to the patient and emotional support to family members and loved ones.

● MEDICAL LIABILITY PROTECTION

The paramedic must always remember that he or she is practicing under the extended licensure of the medical control physician. Respect for that relationship is important. The support of medical control and the physician's willingness to extend his or her license in the prehospital setting allow EMS personnel to have an impact on field emergency care.

As previously stated, a paramedic's best protection against potential liability are training, competent patient care skills, and thorough documentation. Training is acquired and patient care skills are developed during the paramedic training program and should be continually monitored by medical control during the paramedic's licensure or certification period. Next to providing good patient care, conscientious written documentation is the paramedic's best protection from liability action.

The Prehospital Care Report

The reasons for thorough, written documentation are many. The prehospital care report is often used by physicians and nurses to better understand the patient's initial condition and the type of care given before hospital treatment. The EMS agency and medical control may also use the report to monitor care in the field and to review emergency calls.

BOX 3-2

Prehospital Care Report Data
- Dates
- Response times
- Difficulties en route
- Communication difficulties
- Scene observations
- Reasons for extended on-scene time
- Prior care provided
- Time of extrication
- Time of patient transport
- Reason for hospital selection (trauma center designation, patient choice, or other concerns)

The prehospital care report gives the writer a means of documenting unique scene situations that may have affected patient care and of tracking particular patient care skills (such as intravenous lines, intubations, defibrillations) that may be required for relicensure or recertification. Some EMS systems also use the report to collect data on matters such as supply inventory, logistic research (response times, number of calls in a given geographical area, similar concerns), and billing information. The report is considered part of the patient's medical record and should be treated accordingly; inappropriate terms and expressions and inaccurate data should be avoided.

The prehospital care report (Box 3-2) should be carefully detailed and legible. Because it is viewed as a legal document, it is best to avoid the use of slang terminology or medical abbreviations that are not universally accepted. The report should include all dates and response times and describe any difficulties encountered while en route and during patient treatment, extrication, and transport. The report should also include observations at the scene, any prior medical care provided (and by whom), and time of patient extrication, if appropriate. The times of all significant occurrences and interventions are useful to the receiving physician and should be recorded.

BOX 3-3

Components of the Narrative Portion of a Prehospital Care Report

- Initial contact
- All patient care activities
- Initial assessment and vital signs
- Chief complaint
- Significant medical history
  - Medications
  - Allergies
- Clock time of hospital contact
  - Requested orders
  - Intravenous therapy
  - Drug therapy
- Medical direction physician name
- Changes in patient status
  - En route to hospital
  - Response to fluids, medications, and other interventions
- Vital sign reassessment
- Electrocardiogram (ECG) interpretation
- Time and condition of patient on delivery
- Name of receiving health care worker
- Signature of paramedic

The narrative portion of the prehospital care report allows for a chronological description of the call (Box 3-3). It should be documented briefly and clearly, using simple words and avoiding abbreviations, unnecessary terms, and duplication of information. A standard format should be established by medical control and followed by the paramedic. This helps ensure completeness and facilitates quality-improvement reviews.

Finally, the prehospital care report should be signed by the writer, listing everyone who participated in caring for the patient before emergency department delivery. In many EMS agencies, a copy of the report is placed in the patient's hospital medical record. Therefore it may be necessary to leave a finished copy with the patient at the receiving hospital. This necessitates developing a systematic approach to completing the report in a timely fashion so that the EMS crew can be available for service.

Government Immunity

Protecting state and other governmental entities from litigation originated from an ancient English common law based on the concept that "the King can do no wrong." In modern law, this means that governmental agencies cannot be held liable for the negligent acts of their employees. Since the 1950s, the trend in many states has been to discard this doctrine or limit the extent of its application. In some states, for example, immunity, if exercised, may only apply to the governmental agency and not to the individual employee or operator of an emergency vehicle. Because governmental immunity statutes vary throughout the country, individual EMS providers may or may not be protected by this statute.

Good Samaritan Legislation

Good Samaritan legislation exists in some form in all 50 states.[3] The intent of these laws is to encourage people to help others without fear of litigation when an emergency arises. As a rule, a person who provides emergency first aid in good faith and in a manner that another person with similar training would provide is covered by these laws. However, these laws do not generally protect health care professionals from acts of gross negligence, reckless disregard, or willful or wanton conduct. They also do not generally apply to paid on-duty EMS employees because they are required to act.

Malpractice Insurance

Adequate professional liability malpractice insurance should be seriously considered by all practicing health care professionals. Policies provide coverage for legal defense as well as potential judgments against the policyholder. Malpractice insurance policies fall into two categories: primary policies and umbrella policies. Primary policies are personal policies that offer certain limits of coverage for the types of risks insured against. For example, a policy with $100,000 policy limits pays up to that amount for covered damages caused by the insured.

Umbrella policies are professional liability insurance carried by a paramedic employer such as an ambulance service or hospital. These policies usually offer additional limits of coverage for on-duty employees who perform activities within the scope of practice that the employer authorizes in policy or protocol. A $1,000,000 umbrella policy, for example, covers damages caused by the insured in excess of those limits contained in the underlying primary policy of insurance. The amount of coverage of these umbrella policies varies by hospital and EMS agency.

If the policy does not cover the individual employee's liability, then separate individual insurance coverage may be desirable. Individual insurance coverage can be obtained from a variety of companies. Group insurance plans are usually less expensive and may provide better coverage than the more expensive individual policies.

● INTERDEPARTMENTAL RELATIONS

Emergency services involve other agencies whose representatives also have a duty and legal responsibility to provide assistance. Fire suppression, extrication, traffic and crowd control, and other fire and law enforcement activities are often needed. EMS personnel must work closely with these agencies for optimal patient care and scene safety. Many fire, police, and EMS agencies work well together. This can only be accomplished through a team approach using communications, coordination of activities, and mutual respect for each other's roles in the chain of emergency services.

REFERENCES

1. Frew S: *Street law: rights and responsibilities of the EMT*, Reston, Va, 1983, Reston Publishing.
2. Hall S: New act compels EMS to define new roles, *JEMS* 17(1):19, 1992.
3. Goldstein A: *EMS and the law*, Bowie, Md, 1983, Robert J Brady.

Summary

Providing emergency services entails numerous responsibilities and legal obligations. The paramedic must be aware of the specific laws and regulations that govern health care activities in his or her state and render emergency treatment in a manner that reflects a commitment to competent patient care delivery.

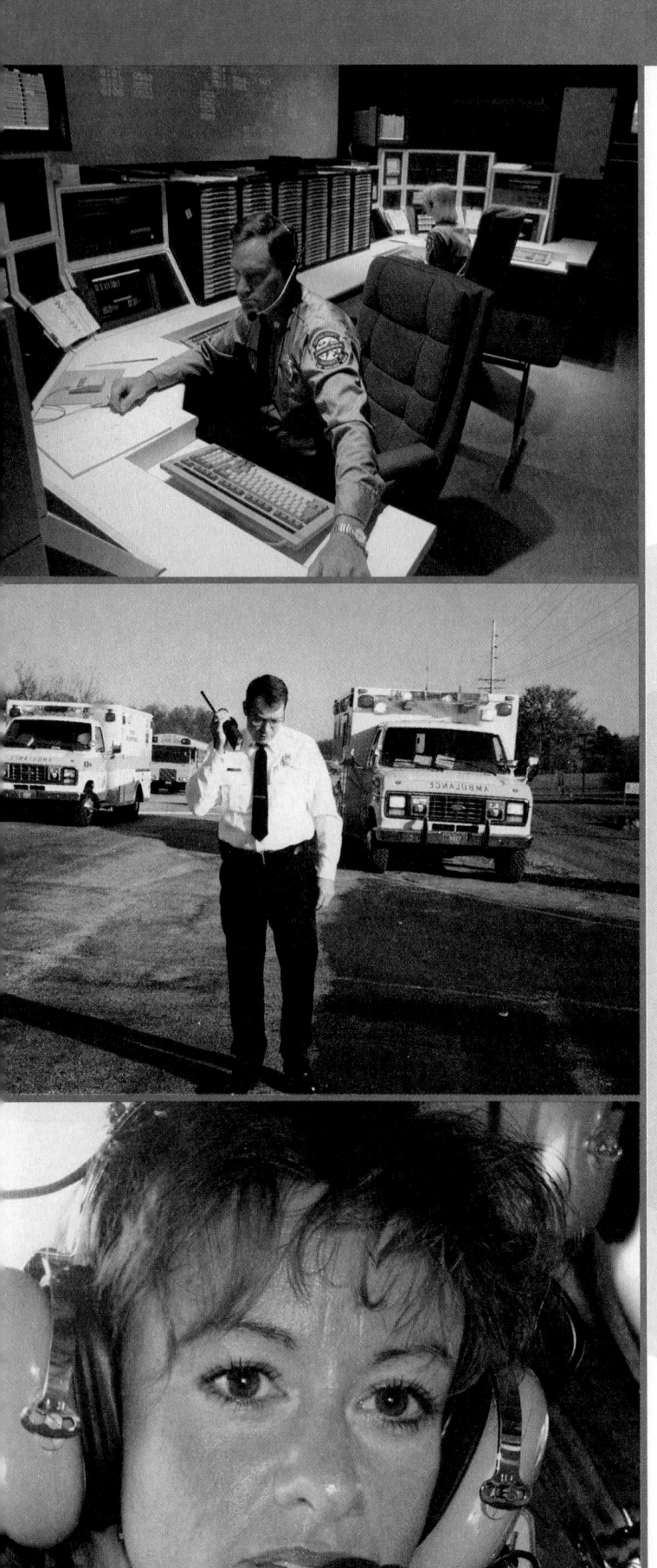

Communications is a vital component of the EMS system. In most urban areas, the public requests assistance via telephone to a communications center. Call takers receive the information, and in the most modern systems, digitalized information about the origin of the call and history of responses to that location is automatically displayed on the console. The call taker then passes the information via digital technology to the dispatcher, who sends a response unit to the scene. The paramedic crew advises the communications center of response and arrival status via radio and contacts medical control for orders and to give status reports. The paramedic must understand the complexities of this communications system.

As a paramedic, you should be able to:

1. Outline the chain of EMS communications.
2. Define common EMS communication terms.
3. Differentiate simple and complex communication systems.
4. Define the functions of key structural and equipment components in an EMS communications system.
5. Discuss how frequency selection influences radio coverage.
6. Describe the role of the Federal Communications Commission (FCC) in EMS communications.
7. Indicate measures for maintaining optimal function of communications equipment.
8. Describe the role of dispatching as it applies to prehospital emergency medical care.
9. Outline techniques for relaying EMS communications clearly and effectively.
10. List various types of documentation and record-keeping that may be required by an EMS agency.

● COMMUNICATION SYSTEMS: EQUIPMENT COMPONENTS

Simple Systems

The minimum radio communication equipment requirements for an ambulance service include a self-contained desktop transceiver with a speaker, microphone, antenna, and a mobile unit and a two-way radio with multiple-frequency capability in the vehicle. Most EMS services also use hand-held portable radios (often termed *portables*) capable of communications contact with the base station and data-recording apparatus for all communications. The portable radio protects the crew and facilitates optimal patient care by permitting continued contact with the communications center and medical direction. The recording apparatus provides medical and legal protection for the service and can verify the communication transmissions when contact is disrupted.

KEY TERMS

duplex: A system with the ability to transmit and receive traffic simultaneously through two different frequencies and that is similar in function to telephone communications in that the two parties can talk simultaneously without blocking either message.

half-duplex: A system that uses two different frequencies, one to transmit, one to receive, that cannot be used simultaneously.

multiplex: A system with the ability to transmit simultaneously two or more different types of information (for example, telemetry and voice) in either or both directions over the same frequency.

simplex: A system with the ability to transmit or receive in one direction at a time; one party transmits, the other receives. Simultaneous transmission cannot occur without blocking a message.

telemetry: The transmission and reception of physiological data such as electrocardiograms by radio or telephone.

Communications Terminology

Amplitude modulation (AM): A transmitted radio frequency carrier fixed in frequency but increasing or decreasing in amplitude in accordance with the strength of the applied audio.

Automatic vehicle location: A radio communications subsystem that uses one or more electronic methods to periodically determine a land, marine, or air vehicle's position and relay that information via radio to a communications center.

Base station: A grouping of radio equipment consisting of at least a transmitter, a receiver, a transmission line, and an antenna located at a specific fixed location.

Carrier: A radio signal of specific frequency generated by a transmitter without audio information imposed on it.

Cellular telephone: An 800- to 900-megahertz (MHz) radio communications system used to access dial-up telephone circuits and vice versa. The system is divided into usually small coverage areas called *cells,* which are interconnected via microwave or dedicated telephone circuits.

Channel: An assigned frequency or pair of frequencies used to carry voice or data communications or both. In EMS, an ALS "MED" channel is a pair of radio frequencies, one used for transmitting, the other for receiving.

Communication: The transmission and reception of information, resulting in common understanding.

Control console: Typically, a desk-mounted, enclosed piece of equipment that contains the mechanical and electronic controls used to operate a radio base station.

Coverage: The area covered by radio communication. The generally accepted national emergency system standard is the "90/90" standard. This means that 90% of the coverage area will have communication 90% of the time. Coverage is usually expressed as dead (no coverage), marginal (spotty), good (few problems), and excellent (no problems).

Dedicated line: A special telephone circuit designated for specific point-to-point communication purposes, such as alerting EMS quarters.

Duplex: A system with the ability to transmit and receive traffic simultaneously through two different frequencies, one to transmit and one to receive. It is similar in function to telephone communications in that two parties on the communications link can talk simultaneously without blocking either message.

Duplex/multiplex: A system with the ability to transmit and receive simultaneously with concurrent transmission of voice and telemetry.

Frequency: The number of repetitive cycles per second completed by a radio wave.

Frequency modulation (FM): A deviation of carrier frequency in accordance with the strength of applied audio. FM is less susceptible to some types of interferences than AM and is typically used in EMS communications.

Half-duplex: A system that uses two different frequencies, one to transmit and one to receive, that cannot be used simultaneously.

Hertz (Hz): A unit of frequency equal to 1 cycle per second.

Interference: Any undesired radio signal on a radio frequency. It may arise from other radio transmitters or other sources of electromagnetic radiation. "Nuisance interference" is interference that can be heard but does not override system signals. "Destructive interference" overrides system signals.

KiloHertz (KHz): A unit of frequency equal to 1000 cycles per second.

MegaHertz (MHz): A unit of frequency equal to 1 million cycles per second. EMS radios transmit and receive on frequencies measured in megaHertz.

Microwave: Radio waves with frequencies of 890 MHz and upward. The signals are generated by special equipment that depends on line-of-sight placement to operate properly. Microwave channels may have a wide band to carry a large number of simultaneous transmissions.

Communications Terminology—cont'd

Mobile data terminal (MDT): A computer, connected through a modem ("black box") with a radio, that sends and receives pretyped messages to printers, computer screens, or both. Some MDTs have graphics (floor plans) and data-base (hazardous materials) capabilities. MDTs rely on a host computer interfaced to a base station.

Mobile relay station: A fixed-base station that automatically retransmits mobile or portable radio communications back to the receiving frequency of other portables, mobiles, and base stations operating in the same system. It is also known as a *repeater*.

Mobile or vehicular repeater: A mobile radio unit capable of automatically retransmitting any radio traffic originated by a hand-held portable, by other mobiles, or by base stations. This repeater may be one way or two way and may be known as a *PAC-RAT* (Motorola) or an *extender*.

Multiplex: A system with the ability to simultaneously transmit two or more different types of information in either or both directions over the same frequency (for example, telemetry and voice).

NiCad batteries: Nickel cadmium rechargeable batteries used in portable radios.

Paging equipment: Equipment typically using tone activation with one-way transmission to receive-only units.

Range: The general perimeter of coverage, beyond which coverage is nonexistent or severely degraded to an unusable level. It is measured in miles.

Special emergency radio service (SERS): A specific group of radio frequencies designated by the FCC.

Simplex: A system with the ability to transmit or receive in one direction at a time; one party transmits, the other receives. Simultaneous transmission cannot occur without blocking a message.

Squelch: A radio receiver circuit used to suppress the audio portion of unwanted radio signals or radio noises below a predetermined carrier strength level.

Telemetry: The transmission and reception of physiological data by radio or telephone (for example, electrocardiograms [ECGs]).

Tone: The audio signal or carrier wave of controlled amplitude and frequency that is used for equipment control purposes or to selectively signal a receiver, such as activating a pager. Tones are measured in Hertz.

Transceiver: A combination transmitter and receiver with a switching circuit or duplexer to use a single antenna.

Trunking system: A radio system consisting of base stations on different channels connected to each other with small computers that work with special mobile and portable signaling to allow multiple simultaneous conversations. Systems are available for VHF, UHF, and 800 MHz.

Ultra high frequency (UHF): This is a radio frequency between 300 and 3000 MHz. The 460 MHz range is most commonly used for EMS communications.

Very high frequency (VHF): This is a radio frequency between 30 and 300 MHz (usually 150-MHz range). The VHF spectrum is further divided into "high" and "low" bands.

Watt: The unit of measurement of a transmitter's power output.

Complex Systems

More sophisticated communication systems can include remote consoles, high-power transmitters, repeaters, satellite receivers, and high-power multifrequency vehicle radios. Some services also use mobile transmitter steering, vehicular repeaters, mobile encode-decode capabilities, mobile data terminals, and microwave links.

Base Stations

Base stations are usually located on a high spot such as a hill, mountain, or tall building for optimal transmission and reception. Base stations are generally connected via telephone lines to dispatch centers, where all elements of the EMS response are coordinated. Depending on locale, one dispatch center may be responsible for all fire, police, and EMS communication activities. Base station transmitters usually have a power output of 45 to 110 watts and must be equipped with a suitable antenna. The maximum allowable base station power is determined by the FCC and is printed on the radio station license.

Mobile Transceivers

Vehicle-mounted transmitters usually operate at lower outputs (typically 40 to 100 watts) than base stations. This output provides a range of 10 to 15 miles over average terrain. Transmission over flat land or water increases this range, and transmission over mountainous terrain, dense foliage, or urban areas with tall buildings decreases the range. Transmitters with higher outputs are available and may provide greater ranges for transmission. Multichannel units are preferred over single-channel radios because of the many channels used in an EMS system.

Portable Transceivers

Portable radios are hand-held or hand-carried devices used when working away from the emergency vehicle. Hand-held units typically have a power output of 1 to 5 watts (with limited range) and hand-carried devices of 10 watts. Many systems boost the signal of these portable radios through a mobile or vehicular repeater. These radios may be single-channel or multichannel units.

Repeaters

Repeaters act as a special type of long-range transceiver. They receive transmissions from a low-power portable or mobile radio on one frequency and simultaneously retransmit it at a higher power on another frequency. Repeaters may be fixed or vehicle mounted; EMS systems commonly use both. Repeaters are necessary for effective radio communications over large geographical areas and are used to increase coverage from portable/mobile-to-portable/mobile. They allow low-power units to hear other radio messages and allow two or more low-power units to communicate with one another when distances or obstructions would normally hinder communication.

Remote Console

Many EMS systems use dispatch services located away from base stations. These remote centers control all base-station functions and are connected via dedicated telephone lines, microwave, or other radio means. Hospitals are also often equipped with a terminal that receives and displays telemetry transmissions as well as providing communications with field paramedic crews. Consoles for these systems include an amplifier, a speaker, a telemetry oscilloscope, a microphone, receiving capabilities, and remote control circuits.

Satellite Receivers

Depending on the geographic area and terrain, satellite receivers are sometimes used to ensure that low-power units are always within communications coverage. The satellite receivers are strategically located and are connected to the base station or repeater by dedicated phone lines, radio, or microwave relay. "Voting systems" automatically select the strongest or best audio signal among multiple satellite receivers and the main base station receiver.

Encoders and Decoders

Selective call encoders are devices that resemble a telephone dial or the buttons of a push-button telephone. When activated, the encoder transmits tone pulses or pairs of tones over the air. Receivers with decoders are programmed to recognize specific codes that open the audio circuits of the receivers. Two-tone sequential paging signals by means of two pairs of specific frequency tones to selectively address pagers and alert monitors. A selective-address system normally incorporates a code for calling all units within radio range (all-call).

Hospitals in certain regions throughout the United States are tied together by radio systems known as *Hospital Emergency Administrative Radio/HEAR* (Motorola) or *Emergency Administrative Communications/EACOM* (General Electric). These radios use 1500-Hz rotary pulse dialing, which transmits specific groups of rotary tone pulses to selectively address hospital-based receivers. Most ambulance services have access to this system.

Cellular Telephones

Some EMS services use cellular telephones as an alternative to dedicated EMS communication systems. In addition to having more channels, cellular telephones provide a secure communications link between EMS personnel and area hospitals. In areas where cellular telephones are available, geographic cells ranging from 2 to 40 square miles are divided into an overlapping network that uses many receiving and transmitting units. Each cell has a mobile telephone switching office (MTSO) that can handle many simultaneous calls and perform automatic "handoffs" to and from other MTSOs as the cellular telephone moves into and out of the individual cells. The overlapping network results in fewer problems with the outside radio transmissions and with physical interference.

Disadvantages of cellular telephone use for emergency services include network usage that might limit channel access or produce problems in maintaining continuous communications in some areas, lack of priority access, and the inability of calls to be monitored by other members of an emergency response team (for example, during a mass casualty incident). Therefore many EMS agencies using cellular telephones have backup radio communication capabilities.

Biotelemetry

Biotelemetry has been used in the prehospital setting since 1967. ECG monitors measure the electrical activity of the patient's heart. These voltage changes modulate an FM subcarrier centered around 1400 Hz, causing a corresponding frequency shift or deviation of the subcarrier. (Most telemetry systems are calibrated so that an ECG output of 1 volt produces a 50-Hz swing in the subcarrier frequency.) Through telemetry equipment, these voltage changes are converted to a variety of audio tones and transmitted to the hospital. The receiver at the hospital converts the audio signal back into measurable voltage changes, producing the ECG tracing on the oscilloscope.

Satellite Terminals

The application of satellite technology is new in emergency response. Portable satellite terminals are being marketed as a means of transmitting important data when other communication systems are not available (for example, during major disasters). Commonly available satellite terminals incorporate ground stations and transportable stations and provide voice, data, and video communications.

● RADIO COMMUNICATIONS

The Federal Communications Commission

Radio communications in the United States is regulated by the FCC. This commission develops rules and regulations for the use of all radio equipment and frequencies. In addition to the FCC, state and local governments may have rules and regulations for radio operation. The paramedic must be knowledgeable about these agencies and

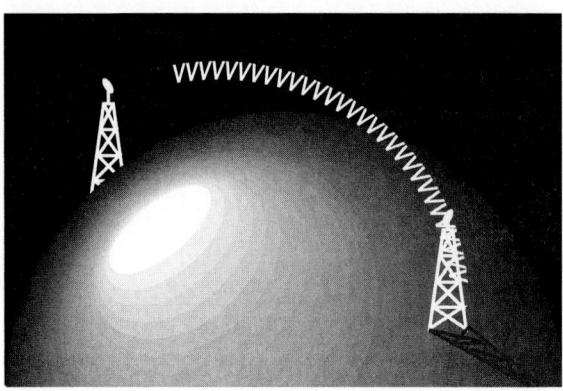

Fig. 4-1 VHF low-band signals follow the curvature of the earth's surface and are subject to noise interference and physical or structural interference.

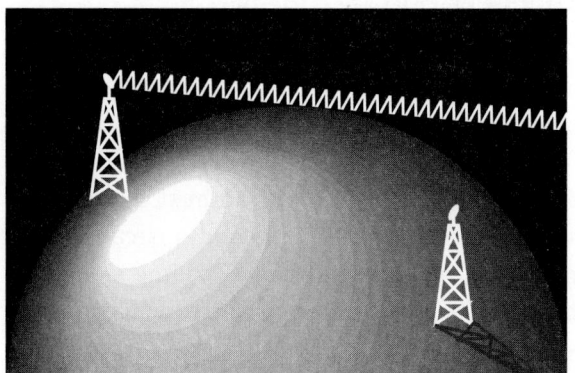

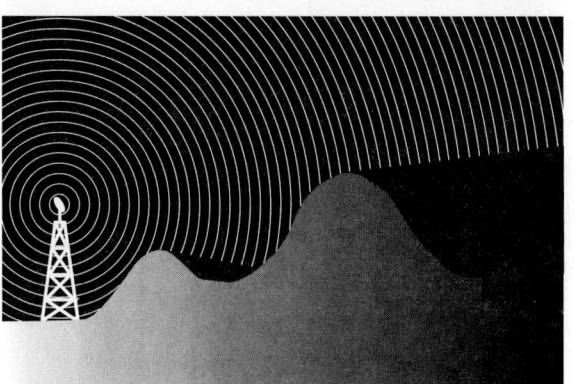

follow their guidelines. The primary functions of the FCC include the following:

- Licensing and frequency allocation
- Establishing technical standards for radio equipment
- Establishing and enforcing rules and regulations for equipment operation, including monitoring frequencies for appropriate usage and spot-checking for appropriate licenses and records

Fig. 4-2 A, VHF high band. High-band signals travel in a straight line and generally allow less range. **B,** Because of their straight-line nature (also referred to as *line-of-sight*), high-band signals are subject to obstruction due to terrain.

EMS Frequency Ranges

For public safety radio, VHF may be defined as VHF low band, 30 to 50 MHz, and VHF high band, 150 to 170 MHz. A number of VHF low-band and VHF high-band frequencies are assigned strictly for two-way use or one-way paging. These frequencies normally operate in a simplex mode. UHF frequencies are used in either half-duplex, duplex, or multiplex modes.

VHF low-band (Fig. 4-1) signals generally have the greatest range and usually cover a greater distance than VHF high band or UHF band. However, these low-band signals follow the curvature of the earth's surface and are therefore subject to noise interference and physical or structural interference. Therefore although this signal has the best range, it may not provide the best coverage.

VHF high-band (Fig. 4-2) signals generally have a medium range and travel in straight lines rather

than following the earth's curvature. This virtual "straight line" characteristic means that high-band signals more easily reflect around buildings and other physical structures and may provide better radio coverage in some areas.

In 1974, the FCC established a structure of radio frequencies called *Special Emergency Radio Services (SERS)*. These frequencies were to be used by EMS, hospitals, school buses, and rescue operations. Of the approximately 75 radio channels in this group, 10 UHF channel pairs were designated for medical communications: 2 for dispatching and 8 for paramedic-to-hospital communications.[1] EMS-only communications were confined to the 450- to 470-MHz UHF frequency band and five VHF frequencies. Table 4-1 lists UHF channels designated for medical communications.

UHF-band signals (Fig. 4-3) generally have a limited range because they are more "straight-line

TABLE 4-1 UHF Channels Designated For Medical Communications

	Base Transmit	Base Receive	Recommended Use
Med 1	463.000	468.000	EMS to medical direction
Med 2	463.025	468.025	EMS to medical direction
Med 3	463.050	468.050	EMS to medical direction
Med 4	463.075	468.075	EMS to medical direction
Med 5	463.100	468.100	EMS to medical direction
Med 6	463.125	468.125	EMS to medical direction
Med 7	463.150	468.150	EMS to medical direction
Med 8	463.175	468.175	EMS to medical direction
Med 9	462.950	467.950	Dispatch
Med 10	462.975	467.975	Dispatch

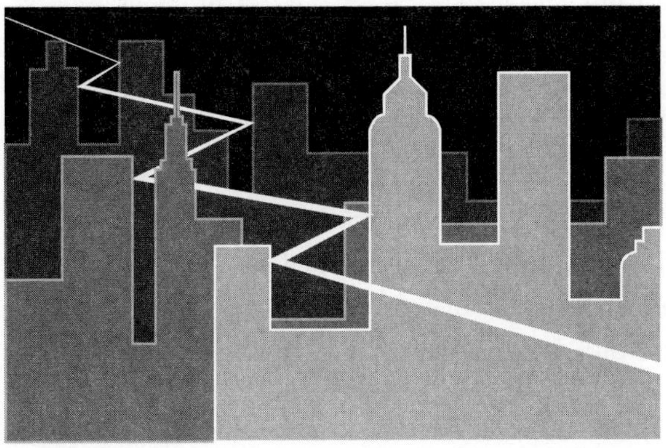

Fig. 4-3 UHF band. These frequencies are more line-of-sight sensitive than high-band frequencies. UHF band frequencies are often the frequencies of choice in metropolitan areas because they reflect readily off objects.

sensitive" than VHF high-band signals. However, the UHF band's ability to reflect or bounce around buildings exceeds that of the VHF high band. In metropolitan areas, UHF may be the most effective frequency. Of the three bands, UHF is the least susceptible to noise interference. In addition, UHF can reach into and out of structures more easily because of its reflective ability and the relationship of wavelength to the radio-frequency–permeable openings in a structure.

Public Safety 800 MHz Frequencies

In recent years, the growth of EMS has resulted in overcrowded frequencies and radio congestion. In 1987, the FCC allocated an additional band, 821

to 824 and 866 to 869 MHz, to SERS assignments to help resolve the communication problems. The 800-MHz signals generally have a limited range because they are more straight line than VHF high-band signals. With the use of repeaters, however, the ability of the 800-MHz band to reflect or bounce around buildings exceeds that of the VHF high band and the UHF 400-MHz band, so the 800-MHz spectrum is best suited for use in urban areas.

In an effort to ensure the efficiency of the 800-MHz band, the FCC has established "trunking" requirements. In the systems required, five or more repeaters, each on a different channel, work together as a group. The trunking system may belong to a single user (such as a specific EMS agency or police department) or may be shared by a number of different public service agencies. When a radio transmission is originated, computerized scanning automatically finds an available repeater in the system and then switches all radios in the fleet to the selected repeater. As one fleet captures an open channel, it locks out all other users who share the system, preventing interference from other agencies.

Several groups have helped the FCC to reorganize frequency management for public service operations and to improve public service agencies' ability to communicate with each other by establishing mutual aid channels and regional plans. The FCC has agreed to establish a new Emergency Medical Radio Service (EMRS) with use limited to those involved in the delivery of emergency medical treatment.[2] In addition, the FCC has reallocated for use by EMRS licensees various channels currently allocated to the SERS and five pairs of 220-MHz narrow-band frequencies. Use of these frequencies will be limited to persons or entities providing basic or advanced life support.

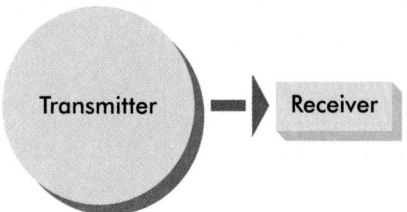

Fig. 4-4 One-way communications is typically used for paging. Required equipment includes a transmitter, a receiver, and a paging receiver, all of which operate on the same frequency.

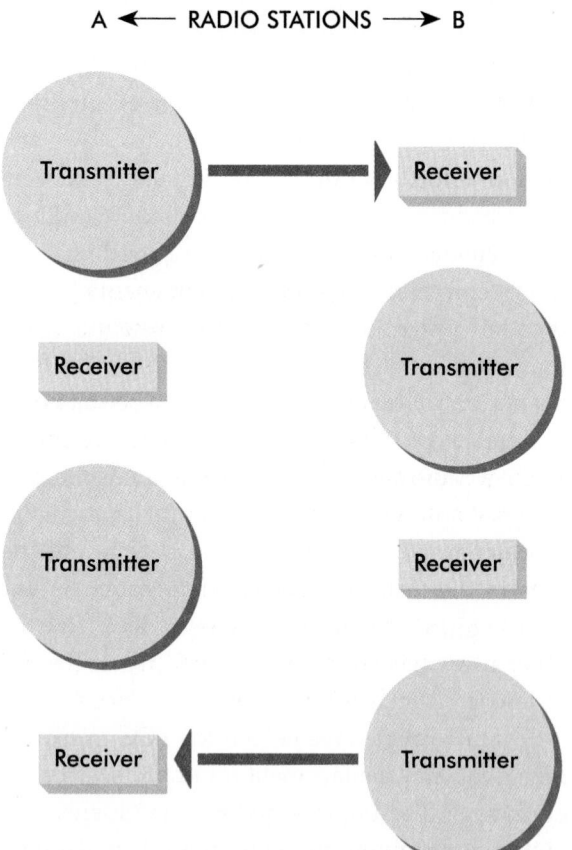

Fig. 4-5 Required equipment for simplex mode includes a transmitter and a receiver at each end of the communications path, both operating on the same frequency. In the simplex mode, only one end may operate at a time.

● OPERATION MODES

One-Way Mode

Generally used for paging, the one-way mode (Fig. 4-4) requires a transmitter, a receiver to monitor the frequency before transmitting, and a paging receiver. All of these elements operate on the same frequency.

Simplex Mode

The **simplex** mode (Fig. 4-5) requires both a transmitter and a receiver at each end of the communications path. Both elements operate on the same frequency, but only one end may operate at a time.

Duplex Mode

Use of two frequencies with a **duplex** device allows both ends to communicate simultaneously. The advantage of this mode (Fig. 4-6) is that either end can interrupt the other or break in (for example, during a two- or three-way conversation).

Half-Duplex Mode

Half-duplex is similar to the duplex mode, but it does not allow the simultaneous or interrupt capability because only one end can transmit and receive at a time.

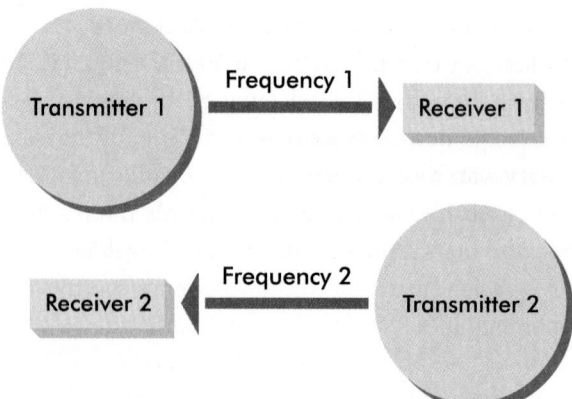

Fig. 4-6 Duplex mode requires two frequencies so that both ends can communicate simultaneously. A half-duplex mode uses the same frequency but does not allow simultaneous or interruption capabilities.

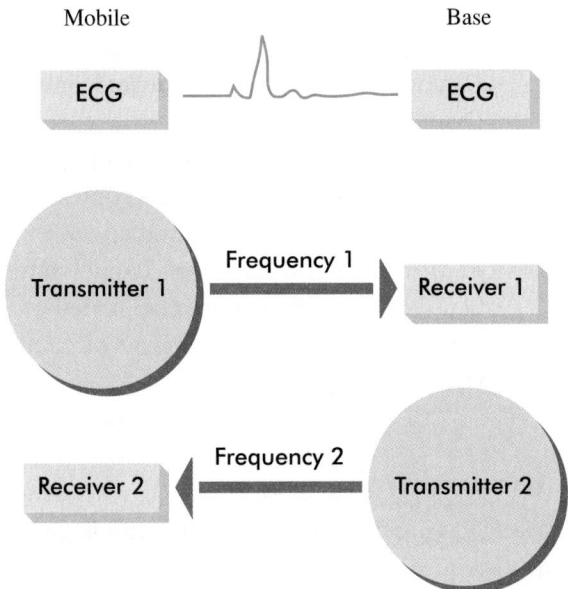

Fig. 4-7 Multiplex mode operates similar to duplex mode with added capabilities, such as simultaneous ECG and voice transmission.

Multiplex Mode

The **multiplex** mode (Fig. 4-7) has the advantage of transmitting telemetry and voice simultaneously from a field unit. This is the most common mode in use today with most paramedic services.

● EQUIPMENT MAINTENANCE

Communications equipment is an important adjunct in providing emergency medical care to patients. Although the manufacturer attempts to provide a durable product, the paramedic should be careful not to subject the equipment to unnecessary harsh conditions such as electrical surges, dust, and dampness. Rough handling and dust are the most frequent causes of equipment failure.

The operator should always follow the recommendations of the manufacturer when cleaning communications equipment. Frequent cleaning improves the equipment's appearance and working life. A slightly damp cloth with very mild detergent is usually adequate to clean the exterior surfaces of radio equipment.

Malfunctioning radio equipment should be reported immediately to an EMS supervisor or licensed radio technician. Daily checking of the equipment at shift change and regular preventative maintenance intervals help ensure operational efficiency.

Portable radios and monitor-defibrillators rely on battery power. These rechargeable batteries must be used properly to maximize battery life and power output. The NiCad rechargeable batteries must be regularly "exercised" for best results. This recharging involves periodic full cycling and discharge of the battery to approximately 1 volt per cell. The paramedic should always follow the manufacturer's recommendations for the use, care, and maintenance of all of the equipment and document and report any irregularities.

● RULES AND OPERATING PROCEDURES

Federal rules and regulations pertaining to EMS communications are contained in *FCC Part 90*. Of particular interest to EMS dispatchers and EMS providers are the following rules and regulations[3]:

- Stations granted frequencies for EMS purposes do not have exclusive right to those frequencies and must coordinate use with other users in the area.
- All transmissions are limited to the minimal practical transmission time, and all of the agencies must employ an efficient operating policy to maximize the use of these frequencies.
- Stations should transmit assigned calls once every 30 minutes during periods of continuous transmission or at the end of each transmission or exchange of transmissions. Call signs should be given in plain English or international Morse code.
- Mobile units need not identify themselves with a call sign if they are listed on the base station license.
- No license or permit is required by individuals operating an EMS station (dispatcher, paramedic, physician).

● DISPATCHING PROCEDURES

Dispatching Responsibilities

The functions of an effective EMS dispatch communications system as defined by the NHTSA include[4]:

- Receive and process calls for EMS assistance. The dispatcher receives and records calls for EMS assistance and selects an appropriate course of action for each call. This function involves obtaining as much information as possible about the emergency event, including name, call back number, and address, and may include dealing with distraught callers.
- Dispatch and coordinate EMS resources. The dispatcher directs the appropriate emergency vehicle(s) to the correct address. In addition, the dispatcher coordinates the movements of emergency vehicles while en route to the scene, to the medical facility, and back to operations base.
- Relay medical information. The dispatcher may provide a telecommunications channel among appropriate medical facilities and EMS personnel, fire, police, rescue workers, and private citizens. The channel may consist of telephone, radio, or biomedical telemetry.
- Coordinate with public safety agencies. The dispatcher provides for communications between public safety units (fire, law enforcement, rescue) and elements of the EMS system to facilitate coordination of services such as traffic control, escort, fire suppression, and extrication. For all of these events to take place in an integrated, well-coordinated system, the dispatcher must know the location and status of all EMS vehicles and the availability of support services. In larger systems, computer-aided dispatching may be used. This advanced technology provides for one or more of the following capabilities or functions:
  - Automatic entry of 9-1-1
  - Automatic interface to automatic vehicle location with or without map display
  - Automatic interface to mobile data terminal
  - Computer messaging among multiple radio operators, call takers, or both
  - Dispatch note taking, reminder aid, or both
  - Display of call information
  - Emergency medical dispatch review
  - Manual or automatic updates of unit status
  - Manual entry of call information
  - Radio control and display of channel status
  - Standard operating procedure review
  - Telephone control and display of circuit status

Dispatcher Training

Many EMS and public service agencies have begun to require specialized training for their dispatch personnel. This training may include the Department of Transportation's training program for emergency medical dispatcher. A base of EMS training helps the dispatcher understand functions of the EMS system, personnel capabilities, and equipment limitations. In addition, it gives the dispatcher the medical background necessary to ask relevant questions regarding the emergency event or the patient's condition. Some systems employ dispatchers trained to provide emergency instructions to the caller while waiting for EMS arrival.

A variety of dispatching systems and procedures are in place throughout the United States. These systems range from very simple "call received—ambulance dispatched" types of programs to the more sophisticated call screening and Medical Dispatch Priority Reference System.

Call Screening

In the call-screening system, a dispatcher, paramedic, or nurse determines what type of assistance is required for a particular emergency call. This may include referring the caller to other services, choosing BLS or ALS response, selecting private or public EMS service, and determining use of lights and sirens. Call screening is considered by some legal authorities to increase the risk of medical liability. Most agencies using this system have built additional safeguards into their program.

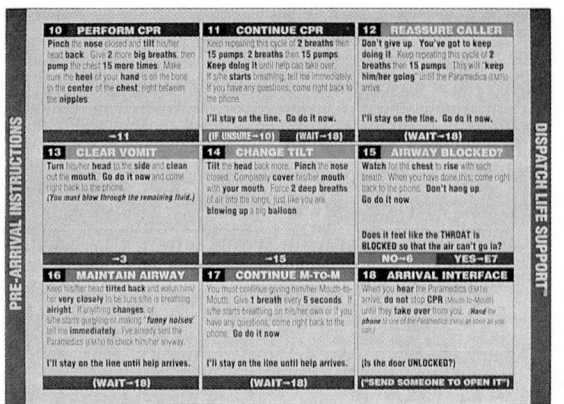

Fig. 4-8 Advanced medical priority dispatch system. **A,** Case entry protocol. **B,** Prearrival instructions.

Medical Dispatch Priority Reference System

The Medical Dispatch Priority Reference System uses trained emergency medical dispatchers and "medical dispatch priority cards" (Fig. 4-8). The priority cards list protocols of four components: key questions, prearrival instructions, dispatch priorities, and response modes. The cards instruct the dispatcher in interviewing the caller, initiating appropriate EMS response, and providing first aid instruction while waiting for EMS arrival. This system has gained wide acceptance and has been adopted in many areas of the United States.

● RECOMMENDED COMMUNICATIONS

Codes

Many EMS agencies use some type of code in radio communications. The FCC has stipulated that EMS frequencies be used only to transmit information pertaining to emergency rescue service. Using communication codes can shorten radio air time, maintain security of transmission, and lessen the possibility of misunderstanding. In addition, communication codes permit transmission of information in a format that is not easily understood by the patient, family, or bystander.

The "10 code" uses the number 10 plus another number to relay a particular message. For ex-

ample, 10-8 may mean a paramedic is in service, and 10-23 may mean he or she has arrived at the scene. Local service protocols dictate whether 10 codes are used. The Associated Public Safety Communications Officers has published a widely used 10 code designed for dispatch use. The disadvantage of such a code is that everyone in the system must be able to understand it. In addition, medical information is usually too complex to convey in coded message. Many EMS services are beginning to use communication codes less frequently, preferring clear English language.

Radio Communication Techniques

Most EMS systems use a standard radio communications protocol that includes the desired format for message transmission and key words and phrases. Following this format aids in professional and efficient radio communications within the system. General guidelines for radio communications include the following:

- Adjust squelch if needed.
- Listen for an open channel before transmitting.
- Press the transmit button for 1 second before speaking.
- Speak at close range, 2 to 3 inches, while talking via microphone.
- Speak slowly and clearly. Enunciate each word distinctly and avoid words that are difficult to hear.

- Speak in a normal pitch without emotion.
- Be brief. Prepare the message before transmitting. Break up long messages into shorter ones.
- Avoid codes unless they are systems approved. Avoid dialect or slang.
- Advise the receiving party when the transmission has been completed.

Relaying Patient Information

A standard format of transmission may be developed as a protocol for some EMS services. This allows efficient use of medical communication systems by limiting radio air time. In addition, physicians can quickly receive information regarding the patient's condition, and the potential for omitting any significant information is lessened.

Patient information can be reported to the hospital or dispatcher by radio or telephone. Although the order of information delivery may vary by EMS system and scenario, the radio report should be brief and concise and contain the following:

- Ambulance service name, unit, and paramedic number or name
- Description of scene or incident
- Patient's age, gender, and approximate weight
- Patient's chief complaint
- Associated symptoms
- Brief history of present illness
- Significant past medical history
- Physical examination findings:
  - Level of consciousness
  - Vital signs
  - Neurological examination
  - General appearance and degree of distress
  - ECG results (if applicable)
  - Trauma Index or Glasgow Coma Scale (if applicable)
  - Other pertinent observations and significant findings
- Any treatment given
- Estimated time of arrival
- Name of private medical physician
- Request for orders or further questions from base hospital physician

When communicating with medical control, the paramedic should repeat all orders received from the physician and question any orders that are unclear or seem inappropriate. The receiving hospital should be kept informed of any changes in patient status before and during transport.

ECG Telemetry

The development of lightweight, portable monitor-defibrillators has improved the quality of care available in the prehospital setting. Through use of this equipment, the paramedic can examine a patient's cardiac activity, interpret the rhythm, and transmit that rhythm through **telemetry** communications to the base hospital.

The use of telemetry varies by EMS system. Most services use cardiac monitors with all trauma and medical patients, but telemetry is usually reserved for the patient who requires management of a rhythm disturbance or 12-lead diagnosis before the administration of some cardiac drugs. Telemetry transmission is limited by excessive use of air time and battery depletion. If telemetry is warranted, 15 to 30 seconds of transmission is usually adequate.

Written Documentation

Documentation of patient care is a vital component of EMS. It provides a record of events and a defense for any future potential litigation. Many legal authorities believe in effect that if it was not written down, it was not done. Written documentation is accordingly a valuable communication tool for the paramedic and EMS service. In addition to the prehospital care report, other types of documentation that may be required by an EMS agency include the following:

- Personnel records documenting training and work assignments
- Call records that list or log dates, times, and other specifics of a call
- Vehicle maintenance records documenting vehicle service at regular intervals
- Vehicle and equipment cleaning records documenting procedures used to disinfect vehicle and emergency equipment

- Drug and equipment inventory records verifying daily checks of drug and fluid expiration, security measures of controlled substances as required by state and federal drug enforcement agencies, and monitor-defibrillator, radio, and telemetry checks
- Incident reports that document problem calls or unusual circumstances
- Records of significant exposures to communicable disease

REFERENCES

1. *E.M.T. paramedic national standard curriculum,* Washington, DC, 1985, US Government Printing Office.
2. Johnson M, Van Cot C: The FCC may be listening, *JEMS* 17(5):19, 1992.
3. *Rules and regulations,* part 90, Washington, DC, 1979, US Government Printing Office.
4. *Course guide dispatcher training program for emergency medical technician,* Washington, DC, 1976, US Government Printing Office.

Summary

Communication is essential for coordinated emergency response and optimal patient care delivery. As a professional, the paramedic is expected to be knowledgeable about the technical aspects of communications equipment and the various rules and regulations governing radio transmission.

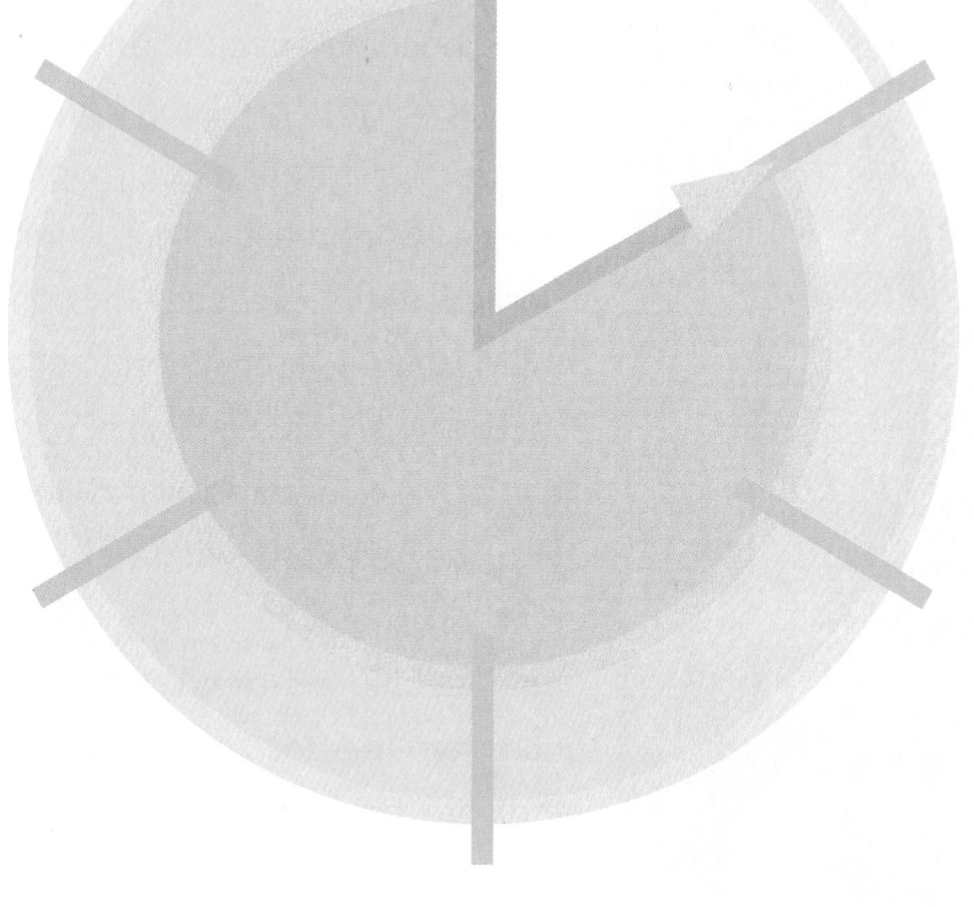

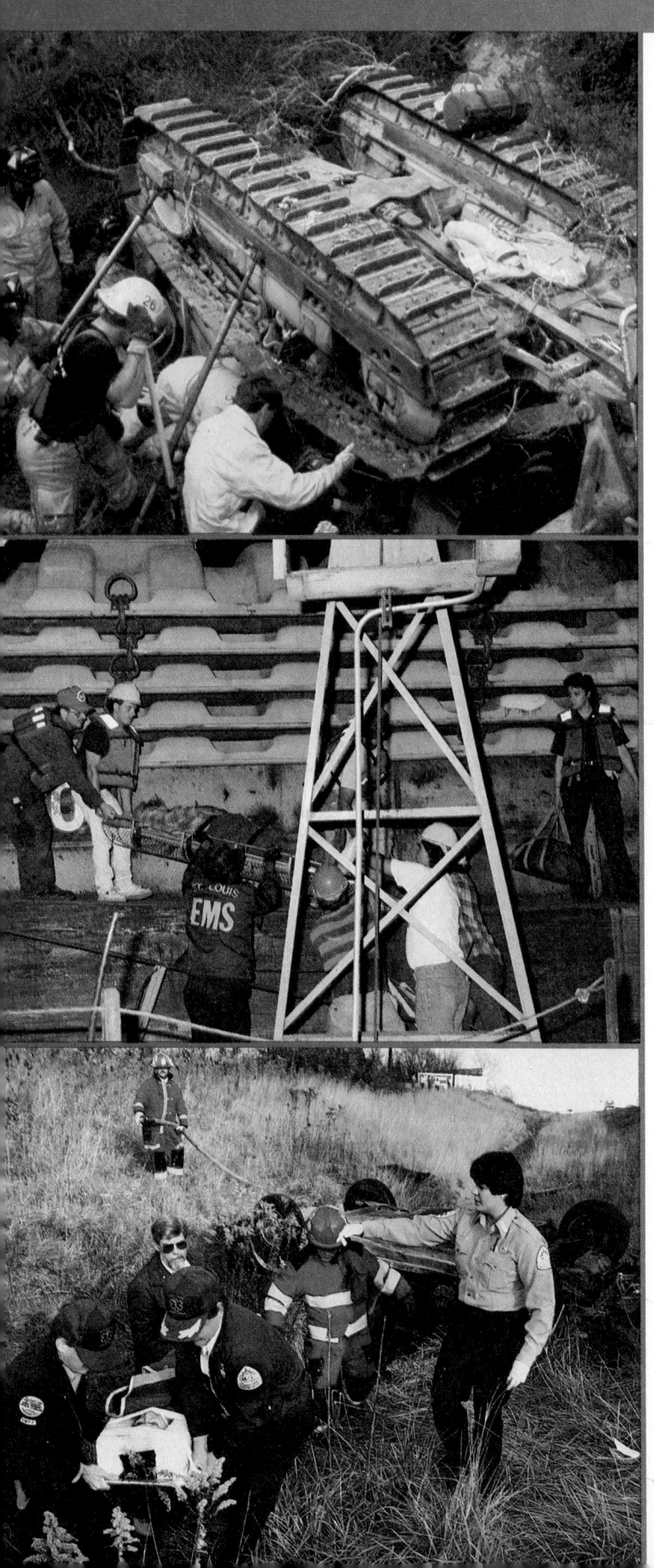

Rescue is defined as "to free from confinement, danger, or evil."[1] Many of the day-to-day activities of EMS providers and other public service agencies are embraced by this definition. In recent years, rescue activities have become specialized. Special techniques are used (for example, for farm rescue, water rescue, wilderness rescue, high-angle rescue, rescue in confined spaces, and search and recovery). Because of the variety of rescue capabilities that may be required within a specific area and the many different techniques involved, this chapter focuses on concepts that are basic to all rescue operations. Class discussion should emphasize the application of these concepts as they pertain to local rescue services.

OBJECTIVES

As a paramedic, you should be able to:

1. Compare the various types of EMS rescue systems found throughout the United States.
2. Describe hazards that may be encountered during rescue situations.
3. List protective clothing and equipment that should be used by EMS personnel during rescue operations.
4. Describe adjuncts that may be used to ensure patient safety during rescue operations.
5. Identify fuel supply hazards.
6. Identify heat source hazards.
7. Discuss safe EMS approach and rescue techniques to be used when an electrical hazard exists.
8. List helpful equipment for vehicle stabilization during rescue operations.
9. Discuss the three elements of the assessment phase.
10. Given a patient care situation, describe the role of EMS in each phase of a rescue operation.

● RESCUE SYSTEMS

Most rescue operations in the United States are provided by systems operations. In this form of rescue management, extrication activities are performed by fire service personnel, specialized units, or both, and patient care activities are the responsibility of EMS providers. In another system, rescue services are provided by fire, EMS, or law enforcement agencies that have "cross-trained" personnel. In this system, roles and responsibilities for rescue and patient care are shared. As in all systems, effectiveness and level of sophistication of a rescue system depend on the dedication of the personnel to the quality of service, as well as training, leadership, interagency cooperation with a clearly defined delineation of each agency's responsibilities, and the organization's financial support.

● SAFETY

Safety during any rescue operation is paramount. Paramedics must be knowledgeable about the rescue system to ensure optimal patient care and scene safety. Many risks are associated with rescue operations. For example, rescues may involve hazardous materials, inclement weather, temperature extremes, fire, toxic gases, unstable structures, heavy equipment, road hazards, and sharp edges and fragments. Initial scene assessment for hazards, personal protective measures, and constant monitoring throughout the operation are essential for every rescue response.

The priorities for safety in any rescue operation begin with personal safety, followed by the safety of the crew, the safety of bystanders, and finally, rescue of the trapped and injured (Box 5-1). The reasons for this order of priority are:

- When the well-trained rescuer acts safely, remaining vigilant of hazards, he or she

KEY TERMS

packaging: The completion of emergency care procedures needed to transfer a patient from the scene to the ambulance.

rescue: To free from confinement or danger.

self-contained breathing apparatus (SCBA): A respiratory protection device that provides an enclosed system of air.

size-up: To quickly assess an emergency scene and determine what resources are needed.

> ### BOX 5-1
>
> ## Priorities for Safety
>
> To respond safely, the rescuer must:
> - Perform an initial scene survey or assessment.
>   - Determine the maximum potential number of people already injured and requiring care and assess the hazards at the scene.
>   - Notify the dispatcher to assign needed resources and alert area hospitals.
>   - Determine the best access routes and staging areas for responders.
> - Secure the area as rapidly as possible, clearing unnecessary people from the scene.
> - Wear protective clothing and use appropriate protective apparatus: coats, headgear, gloves, **self-contained breathing apparatus (SCBA),** eye protection, boots, and similar items.

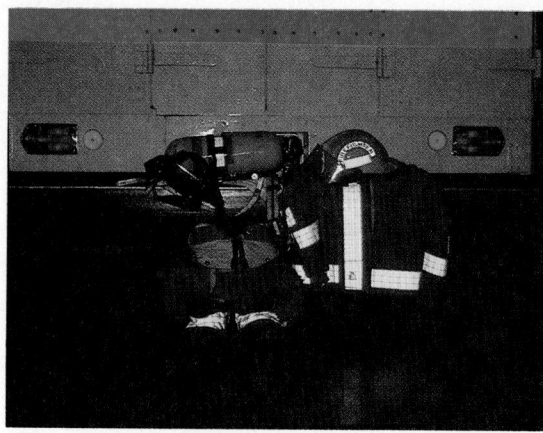

Fig. 5-1 Personal protective equipment.

minimizes the risk of personal injury and of complicating the scene by becoming another patient who requires care and possibly extrication.

- The crew is the support team for the rescuer. Therefore crew safety is essential to ensure an effective operation and provide mutual support for each member of the team. Operating with disregard for the safety of fellow team members increases risk of injuries and complications of the operation.
- Uninvolved people must be evacuated and kept clear of hazards. Bystanders or untrained "helpers" only increase the risk of additional injuries and complications of the rescue operation.
- Rescue of the trapped or injured is the last priority. These people are already trapped or injured. Carrying out the first three priorities safely maximizes the chance for a successful rescue.

Protective Clothing

The standards for protective clothing and personal protection equipment established by the National Fire Protection Association[2] and the Occupational Safety and Health Administration (OSHA)[3,4] have been adopted by many fire and EMS agencies, including a number of municipal and industrial fire services throughout the United States. At a minimum, EMS personnel involved in rescue operations should have access to the following personal protective equipment (Fig. 5-1):

- Impact-resistant protective helmet with ear protection and chin-strap
- Safety goggles with elastic strap and vents to prevent fogging
- Lightweight "turn-out coat" that is puncture resistant
- Slip-resistant, waterproof gloves
- Rubber boots with steel insoles and steel toe protection
- SCBA

Personal Protection from Blood-Borne Pathogens

In addition to the personal protective equipment described above, OSHA's blood-borne pathogens standard established criteria for workplace protection from blood-borne diseases (see universal precautions listed on the inside cover of this text and in Chapter 24).[5] These measures for personal protection should be observed whenever there is a potential for contact with human blood or human body fluids.

● HAZARDS THAT MAY BE ASSOCIATED WITH RESCUE

Hazardous Materials

Emergencies involving any hazardous materials may lead to additional risks and complications. Large geographical areas may be involved, requiring assistance from a number of political subdivisions and public service agencies. If evacuation is necessary, large numbers of people may have to be moved from the hazardous zone. Some of the evacuees may require medical treatment and decontamination (see Chapter 7).

Fire Hazards

A "fire hazard" is a condition that encourages a fire to start or increases the extent or severity of a fire. Fire hazards include fuel supplies, heat sources, oxygen supplies, and chemical reactions. Common fuel supplies and heat source hazards are fuel supply hazards, heat source hazards, and gasoline spills.[6]

Fuel Supply Hazards
- Ordinary combustible solids
- Flammable and combustible liquids
- Combustible gases
- Chemicals
- Dusts
- Metals
- Plastics

Heat Source Hazards
- Chemical heat energy
- Electrical heat energy
- Heat from arcing
- Heat generated by lightning
- Mechanical heat energy
- Nuclear heat energy

Gasoline Spills

Gasoline spills from automobile crashes are a common fire hazard encountered by EMS providers. The chances that flammable liquids will ignite can be reduced by turning off the vehicle ignition switch, forbidding smoking, and avoiding use of flares near the spill. EMS personnel should approach the scene with fire extinguishers and have the extinguishers ready throughout extrication.

It is generally no longer recommended that the car battery of a crashed vehicle be disconnected. An intact electrical system may power electric door locks, windows, seat mechanisms, and trunks. However, if the battery is to be disconnected, the "ground" cable (usually the negative) should be disconnected first. This helps reduce the chance of "sparking," which may ignite spilled fuel or leaking battery gases. Some vehicles have negative electrical ground systems, and others have positive systems. The rescuer should identify the type of system by reading battery markings or locating the ground wires attached to the frame, engine, or body of the vehicle. The battery cable can then be cut or disconnected with bolt or wire cutters. The disconnected cable should be folded back onto itself and securely taped to insulate it from any bare metal contact that might reestablish the electrical ground to the system.

Vehicle fires associated with crashes are usually caused by ruptured fuel tanks and fuel lines ignited during the crash. Paramedics should not attempt to fight fully involved vehicle fires unless they have been trained to do so. If the fire service has not arrived and there are victims in a burning vehicle, the EMS crew should quickly determine whether the victims can be removed. If the victims are trapped and the vehicle is not completely engulfed by flame, paramedics should attempt to stop the fire from spreading by using fire extinguishers.

Burning vehicles present very serious potential hazards and may explode with deadly force at any time. All actions must be directed toward rescuer safety and protection. When it is necessary to approach a burning vehicle, the paramedic should crouch low and approach from the side, staying clear of bumpers that may be compressed or "loaded" from an impact. Personal protective equipment should also be worn to guard against dangerous and caustic smoke.

Fire Extinguishers

Portable fire extinguishers are classified by their anticipated effectiveness in suppressing four classes of fires: class A, ordinary combustibles, class B, flammable liquids; class C, energized electrical equipment; and class D, combustible; metals. ABC-all purpose extinguishers are suitable for more than one class of fire and should be carried by EMS services. These dry chemical extinguishers can be used to suppress fires of ordinary combustible materials, flammable liquids, and electrical equipment. In addition to the letter classifications, class A and B fire extinguishers also receive a numerical rating that designates the size of fire the extinguisher can be expected to suppress. A 20-B extinguisher will generally extinguish 20 times as much fuel as a 1-B extinguisher.

Another type of fire extinguisher, Halon (1211 and 1301), uses liquified compressed gas to suppress fires. This gas leaves little or no residue, does not harm equipment, and is a preferred means of fire suppression in areas that contain computers and other electronic equipment. Halon extinguishers are effective on class B and C fires, but they have a limited range and may be affected by drafts and wind.

Fire-suppression agents work by reducing heat and eliminating the oxygen necessary to maintain combustion. Eliminating oxygen may present danger to the rescuer and the patient, so caution should be taken when working in confined spaces. In addition, crew members and patients should avoid undue exposure to the fumes of any fire-suppression agent, and all rescuers should use appropriate breathing apparatus.

Electrical Hazards

Downed electrical wires are dangerous. Modern transformers are programmed to retest broken circuits at certain time intervals, and "dead" lines may suddenly surge with lethal current. Rescuers must be familiar with the power system in their area and should check with the local power company for information and the availability of training sessions for the response team. Only utility workers and trained rescuers using proper equipment should secure downed electrical wires.

Victims inside a vehicle that is in contact with downed wires should be advised to remain inside unless they are at additional risk of injury (for example, explosion, fire). Leaving the vehicle is dangerous and poses a significant risk of electrical injury.

Rescuers should never approach the patient until the scene is safe. A rescuer who experiences tingling sensations in the soles of the feet, legs, or thorax as he or she enters an area should not proceed. Rather, the rescuer should retreat from the area. When it is absolutely necessary to touch a patient in contact with an electric source, nonconductive equipment such as heavy rubber gloves, leather gauntlets, wooden poles, polypropylene rope, and other specially designed equipment should be used. None of these measures, however, provide absolute safety from electrical injury.

Unstable Vehicles

Unstable vehicles are a common hazard in rescue operations, and all unstable vehicles must be stabilized before access is gained. The mechanism of the accident, position and number of vehicles, and the environment of the scene must all be considered in assessing vehicular stability. Standard methods of stabilizing vehicles include supporting the vehicle with wooden cribbing, wheel chocks, and air bags and securing the vehicle with ropes, cables, and chains to poles, trees, and other vehicles and structures. Fig. 5-2 shows equipment used to stabilize vehicles. Specialized training is required for paramedics involved in this aspect of rescue management.

Air Bag Systems

The concept of air bags as a supplemental restraint system (SRS) was developed by engineers

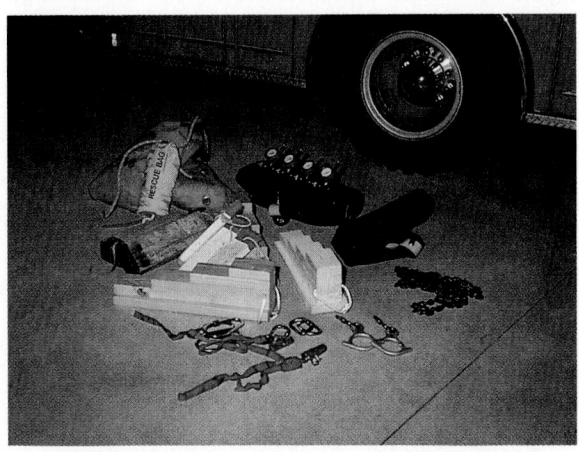

Fig. 5-2 Equipment used to stabilize vehicles.

in 1941. Today, SRS equipment is available from almost all major automobile manufacturers; an estimated 3.3 million air bag systems were installed on 1990 vehicles.

Deployed air bags are not dangerous, but they do produce a residue that can cause minor skin or eye irritation. This residue, which is used to lubricate the bag as it expands, contains cornstarch or talcum powder and a small amount of sodium hydroxide. Nonhazardous irritation from this residue is temporary and can be avoided by wearing gloves and eye protection, by keeping the residue away from the patient's and the rescuer's eyes and wounds, and by thoroughly washing after exposure.

Although it is recommended that emergency personnel be trained in detection and scene management of SRS equipment, rescue guidelines for air bag–equipped cars have been provided by the National Highway Traffic Safety Administration and automobile and air bag manufacturers, coordinated with the U.S. Fire Administration.[7]

Incident With Fire

- Use the normal fire-extinguishing procedures.
- Although heat may trigger an undeployed air bag, it will not cause the activating canister to explode.

Incident With a Deployed Air Bag

- Use normal rescue procedures and equipment.
- Do not delay medical attention.
- Deployed air bags are not dangerous.
- Wear gloves and eye protection.
- Keep residue away from patients' eyes and wounds.
- Remove gloves and wash hands after exposure to residue.

Incident With an Undeployed Air Bag

- An undeployed air bag is unlikely to deploy after a crash.
- When a patient is pinned directly behind an undeployed air bag, special procedures should be followed:
  - Disconnect or cut both battery cables.
  - Avoid placing your body or objects in front of the air bag module (the deployment path of the air bag).
  - Do not mechanically displace or cut through the steering column until after the system has been fully deactivated.
  - Do not cut or drill into the air bag module.
  - Do not apply heat in the area of the steering wheel hub.

Environmental Hazards

Environmental hazards such as earthquakes, tornadoes, hurricanes, floods, and blizzards present clear dangers in rescue operations and often cause mass casualties. Ice, rain, snow, hot and cold temperatures, and other natural weather conditions also complicate emergency scenes and may require sophisticated rescue management. Certain environmental hazards may require highly specialized rescue training (for example, wilderness rescue) and, in some cases, certification (for example, mine rescue).

Safety Operations Management

Managing rescue operations safely requires interagency cooperation and extensive preplanning. Major incident plans involving standard operating procedures and incident command structure should be developed to handle disasters and other emergency scenes. Responding EMS crews and other public service agencies must know the requirements of a safe working environment and the way to acquire resources.

One method of practicing these plans is to activate them on a routine basis (for example, when three or more units are dispatched to a scene). In doing so, the various public service agencies become familiar with what resources should be at the event, what their responsibilities are, and how the resources should be managed.

● SCENE ASSESSMENT (SIZE-UP)

The assessment phase of a rescue requires the paramedic to determine what is needed at a particular emergency event. This activity, commonly referred to as **size-up,** involves quickly gathering facts about the situation, analyzing the problems, and determining the appropriate response. Size-up is a continuous evaluation of the emergency scene that begins the minute the call is received. In addition, the paramedic must be constantly alert to situations that may change the needs of a particular incident. If power lines were downed during extraction, for example, electrical utility services may be needed that were not initially required.

The three elements of the assessment phase are response, other factors, and resources.[8]

Response

During the initial response to an emergency scene, information is often limited. En route, the EMS crew and the dispatcher should gather as much detail about the situation as possible. Essential information includes exact location, type of occupancy (manufacturing, mercantile, residence), number of victims, type of situation, and hazards involved. Weather conditions such as extreme heat or cold, rising water, rain, and high winds can also affect rescue attempts, patient status, and the need to expedite the operation.

Standardized dispatch protocols dictate the initial activation of emergency resources by a prede-

termined system based on the level of the reported event. If the event is a single-vehicle accident, for example, a first-responder fire company and EMS unit are dispatched. If the event is a bus accident with multiple patients, several fire companies and EMS units will respond. As the dispatch center receives information indicating that the event is more or less serious, the dispatch protocol upgrades or downgrades the assignment as needed and advises the responding units of the updated reports.

Other Factors

Another factor to be considered when determining resources for the response is the description of the scene. An emergency in a highly populated area such as a school or shopping mall may require special vehicles and equipment for extrication and fire suppression. An emergency in a rural or wilderness setting may require helicopter rescue or other support resources. If hazardous materials are present, specialized response and decontamination equipment may be needed for bystanders, patients, and rescue personnel.

Time of day may also be a factor when assessing scene requirements. There may, for example, be concern about rush-hour traffic and crowd control; additional lighting may be needed for early morning, evening, or night rescue activities. These and other factors determine the man power requirements and the scene management operations.

Resources

An important component of any emergency response is the available resources. The responding crew may not have the man power, training, or expertise to handle the event. Resources that may be required include the following:

- Additional emergency vehicles for large numbers of patients
- Area hospital availability and personnel
- Air medical services
- Law enforcement
- Fire service for auto extrication, fire suppression, or lighting

- Water rescue, teams with self-contained underwater breathing apparatus (SCUBA), and other specialized rescue units
- Hazardous materials specialists

As previously stated, the ability to quickly and accurately assess an emergency event requires preplanning and the development of a systems approach to the response. For further discussion on incident command systems and major incident management, see Chapter 6.

● GAINING ACCESS

Rapid access to ill or injured patients requiring extrication or rescue is critical to the patient's eventual outcome. With multisystem trauma patients, assessment, stabilization, and extrication should be rapid. However, these procedures must be accomplished with the safety of both the patients and the rescue team as a top priority.

Extrication tools and equipment (Fig. 5-3) can actually cause injuries. To reduce the risk, the paramedic should use the minimum amount of force needed, clear the area of unnecessary people, and keep extraneous noise to a minimum. In addition, a safety officer should remain alert to the stresses of the operation on the rescuers and rotate personnel to avoid heat exposure disorders and injuries from fatigue. Rescuers should wear protective clothing, and protective covering for the patient should be supplied.

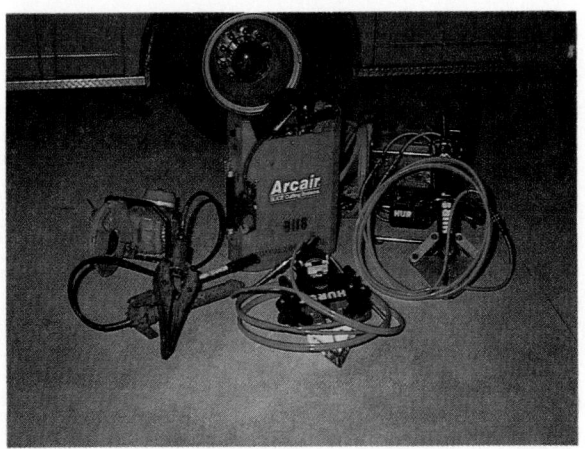

Fig. 5-3 Extrication tools and equipment.

Paramedics may not participate directly in freeing the patient, but they have primary responsibility for patient care and serve an important role as observers for potentially hazardous procedures. The "team concept" is the most important element in any rescue system or operation. Teamwork maximizes safety, efficiency, and effectiveness.

● EMERGENCY CARE

After the team has access to the patient, emergency care procedures can begin. Even when patient care activities are limited by circumstances and working area, it may be possible to begin some stabilization procedures, including spinal immobilization, airway management, oxygen administration, and intravenous fluid therapy.

After the paramedic has access to the patient, the paramedic must perform a rapid primary survey to identify and manage any life-threatening situations. This may entail opening and maintaining the airway with spinal precautions; stabilizing the cervical spine; assessing ventilation and, if necessary, ventilating with positive-pressure breathing; and assessing circulation and, if necessary, controlling external hemorrhage. When the paramedic recognizes rapidly fatal or potentially fatal conditions, a "load and go" approach must be taken. In these situations, expedient extrication and transportation are indicated.

The secondary survey is performed after the primary survey is complete and life-threatening conditions have been stabilized. Another crew member may perform the secondary survey simultaneously if it does not interrupt the primary survey and emergency interventions. The secondary survey includes vital signs and a complete head-to-toe examination (see Chapter 11).

● DISENTANGLEMENT

Disentanglement involves making a pathway through the wreckage of an accident and removing wreckage from patients. It requires extensive training, and EMS personnel should be well aware of the technical expertise available in their area and how to mobilize it. The training and equipment requirements of specialized rescue are beyond the scope of this text.

● PATIENT PACKAGING AND REMOVAL

Physical stabilization and preparation for transport (commonly known as **packaging**) may require special rescue capabilities, such as moving patients over hazardous terrain or lifting patients by hoist to a helicopter. As with all other aspects of rescue operations, coordination of activities and patient care responsibilities among the various agencies offers the greatest chance of a successful outcome.

It is the paramedic's responsibility to ensure that the patient is ready to be removed from the accident scene and is protected from additional injury during disentanglement and egress. The patient should be covered with blankets or tarpaulins and provided with ear and eye protection. In addition, a face mask with supplemental oxygen or air should be applied to protect the patient from toxic fumes, if present.

The patient's airway and cervical spine must be stabilized, intravenous lines and oxygen tubing secured, pneumatic antishock garments applied (per protocol), and the patient immobilized on a long spine board as minimum packaging for transport. When time permits, extremity fractures should be immobilized and open wounds covered with sterile dressings and secured with bandages. A scene delay for patients who require rapid stabilization and transport lessens the patient's chances of survival.

Use of other patient care equipment should be considered as the patient is removed from the area of entrapment. It is important that communication and coordination with other rescuers continue during this process. The exit pathway must be clear and secure, and there should be no additional danger for the patient or the rescuers during the removal phase.

If the patient is to be immediately transported to the ambulance, a wheeled stretcher, basket stretcher, or long spine board should be available. While the patient is transported to the emergency vehicle, the terrain as well as equipment and personnel requirements for moving the patient should be considered. The transport vehicle should be appropriately warmed or cooled based on the needs of the patient and the rescue setting. The rescue is considered complete once the patient is en route to the hospital. As in any other patient transport situation, emergency care is continued by the EMS crew, and medical control is advised of the patient's status.

REFERENCES

1. Neufeldt V, editor: *Webster's new world dictionary,* ed 3, New York, 1988, Simon & Schuster.
2. National Fire Protection Association: *Standard on protective clothing for structural fire fighting* (1971, 1976 rev, 1981), Quincy, Mass, 1975, The Association.
3. Occupational Safety and Health Administration: *Fire brigade regulation,* 29 CFR 1910.156, Washington, DC, 1980, The Administration.
4. Occupational Safety and Health Administration: *Hazardous waste operations and emergency response* (HAZWOPER), standard 1910.120, Washington, DC, 1990, The Administration.
5. Occupational Safety and Health Administration: *Occupational exposure to bloodborne pathogens,* final rule 29 CFR 1910.1030, Washington, DC, 1992, The Administration.
6. *Essentials of fire fighting,* ed 2, Stillwater, Okla, 1983, Fire Protection Publications.
7. *Emergency rescue guidelines for air bag-equipped cars,* Washington, DC, 1990, US Government Printing Office.
8. *E.M.T. paramedic national standard curriculum,* Washington, DC, 1985, US Government Printing Office.

Summary

The need for rescue operations may significantly complicate an EMS response. The paramedic is part of a coordinated team effort that must focus on the elements of a successful rescue operation: personal safety and protection, rapid patient assessment, stabilization, extrication, and transportation.

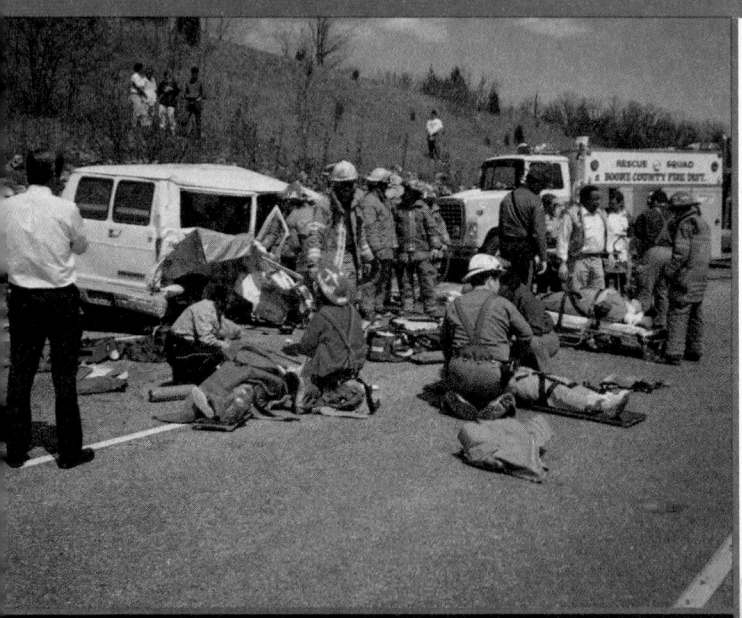

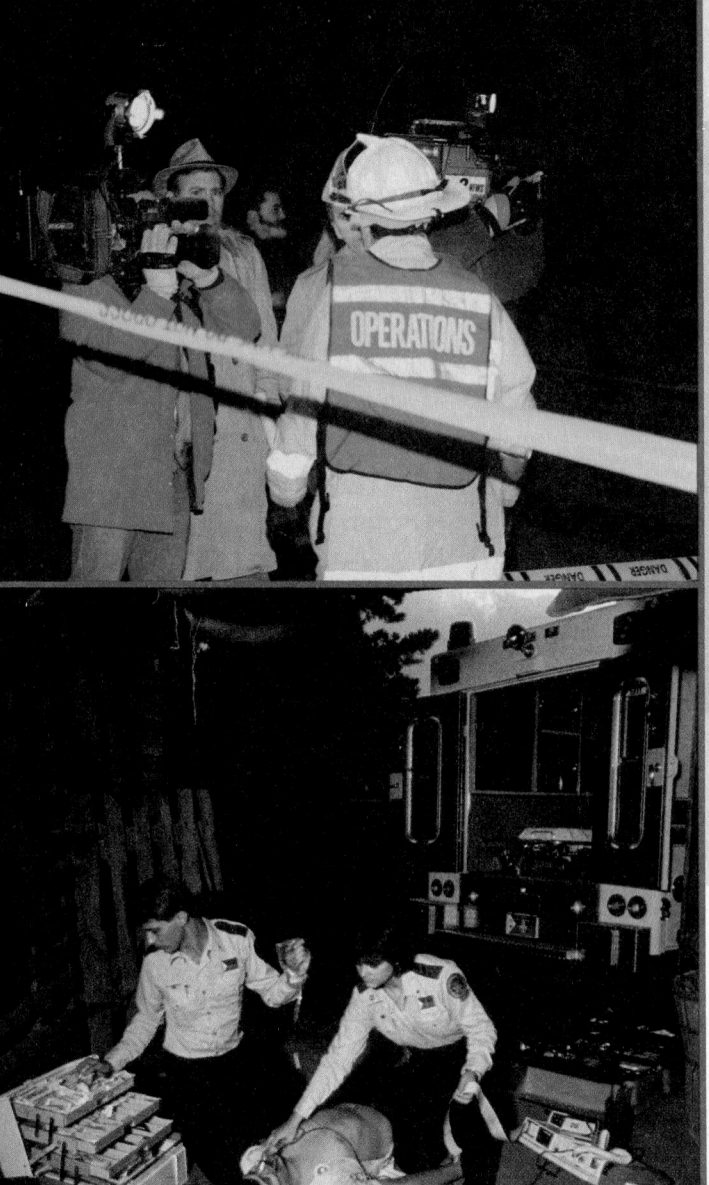

A major incident is an event for which the available resources are insufficient to manage the number of casualties or the nature of the emergency. Major incidents such as highway accidents, air crashes, major fires, train derailments, building collapses, hazardous material releases, earthquakes, tornadoes, and hurricanes stress and may overwhelm local, regional, state, and even national and international resources.

As a paramedic, you should be able to:

1. Describe situations that may be classified as major incidents.
2. Describe how federal agencies and legislation have played a role in the development of the incident command system.
3. Define common terms of the incident command system.
4. Describe critical elements of the incident command system that must be incorporated in the preplanning process.
5. List command responsibilities during a major incident response.
6. Given a major incident, describe sectors that would need to be established and the responsibilities of each.
7. Describe how effective communications can be maintained during a major incident.
8. List common errors of incident command systems.
9. Outline two methods of patient categorization.
10. Describe the process for safely deploying air medical rescue.

● PREPARING FOR A MAJOR INCIDENT

Preparing for a major incident involves three phases: preplanning, scene management, and postdisaster follow-up.

Phase 1: The Preplan

Cooperation and preplanning are crucial in managing a major incident. The preplan must be agreed to by all participating emergency response agencies and address common goals and the specific duties of each group. Multiagency endeavors succeed as a result of frequent meetings and organized practice sessions or exercises. The preplan should include a system of sorting or prioritizing care, treatment, and transportation.

Other considerations in the preplan include identifying hazards within a community, such as manufacturing, storage, and transportation of hazardous materials; fire threats; population base at various times of day; and violence and other potential social problems. An inventory of resources that may be needed during a major incident, including the following, should be made:

- Shelter and mass feeding
- Air evacuation
- Medical equipment and supplies
- Heavy equipment, power generators, and lighting
- Communications
- Law enforcement
- Specialized rescue services

KEY TERMS

incident command system (ICS): A management program designed to control, direct, and coordinate emergency response operations and resources.

major incident: An event for which the resources available are insufficient to manage the number of casualties or the nature of the emergency.

mutual aid: An agreement with neighboring emergency agencies that equipment and manpower can be mutually exchanged when necessary.

sectors: Subdivisions of the incident command system encompassing specific areas of responsibility as deemed necessary by the incident commander.

Phase 2: Scene Management

Phase 2 requires the development of a strategy to manage the emergency scene. A popular management strategy is the **incident command system (ICS).**

Phase 3: Postdisaster Follow-Up

Phase 3 includes a postdisaster review of "lessons learned" from the incident and methods of improvement, such as emergency response, planning, and community protection. This phase should also evaluate stress-related anxiety and illness that may have resulted from the incident among emergency workers.

● THE INCIDENT COMMAND SYSTEM

Historically, emergency management of major incidents often resulted in the response of several different agencies (EMS, fire service, rescue, law enforcement, and others), each performing activities independently, with little or no interagency organization. This made it difficult to determine who was in charge of the scene and to what extent emergency services were needed or were being provided. The ICS was developed to address these concerns and organize interagency functions and responsibilities.

The need for an ICS became apparent in the early 1970s during wildland fires in Southern California. The size of the incident and the multiple agency responses resulted in ineffective communications, lack of accountability, and lack of a well-defined command structure. As a result, the Firefighting Resources of California for Potential Emergencies (FIRESCOPE) was founded, and the original ICS was developed. The ICS evolved into a management plan appropriate for all fire and nonfire emergencies and was later adopted by the National Fire Academy as its model system. Several laws, regulations, standards, and organizations have also helped develop ICS and promote its implementation in disaster planning and operations in emergency services.

● COMPONENTS OF AN ICS

ICS Structure

An effective ICS provides for single jurisdiction and single agency involvement, single jurisdiction and multiagency involvement, and multijurisdiction and multiagency involvement. This organizational structure allows the ICS to adapt to any agency or incident for which emergency management would be needed. The ICS must also be able to expand from dealing with a nonmajor incident to a major incident in a logical manner. The practice of using an ICS as standard operating procedure for small incidents permits a smooth transition when a major incident occurs.

Other components of an effective ICS include common elements in organization, terminology, (Box 6-1) and procedures. The system should be implemented with the least possible disruption to existing systems (EMS, fire, and law enforcement agencies) and should be simple enough to keep operational and maintenance costs to a minimum.

Declaring a Major Incident

Declaring an emergency a major incident is an important phase of the response. If an EMS unit is dispatched to a scene that has this potential, the crew should declare that they are responding to a possible major incident and will confirm on arrival. This information allows other agencies to be contacted and placed on standby and provides time for the availability of other special resources to be determined.

The responding crew should also alert medical control and area hospitals. Receiving hospitals need information on numbers of patients and severity of injuries as soon as possible to prepare for the patients' arrival. A possible major incident should be declared in the following situations[1]:

- Any situation that requires more than two ambulance units for adequate treatment, particularly in rural areas where communities may only have one ambulance
- Any situation involving hazardous or radioactive materials or chemicals

BOX 6-1

ICS Definitions

Apparatus: a vehicle used for fire suppression or rescue that does not include staff vehicles

Command: the individual in charge of the incident scene (also known as the *incident commander*)

Command post: the area from which command directs operations for an incident

Communications center: a facility used to dispatch emergency equipment and coordinate communications between field units and personnel

Medical direction: a process of ensuring that actions taken on behalf of ill or injured people are medically appropriate, including prospective, concurrent, and retrospective aspects of EMS; quality improvement; hiring; and education

Mutual aid: an agreement with neighboring emergency agencies that equipment and manpower can be mutually exchanged when necessary

Sector: a subdivision of the ICS encompassing a specific area of responsibility as deemed necessary by the incident commander

Staging area: a designated area where incident-assigned vehicles are directed and held until needed

• Any situation that requires special EMS resources, such as helicopters, rescue teams, or multiple rescue or extrication units
• Any situation in which when in doubt, a major incident should be declared

● COMMAND RESPONSIBILITIES

Most experts agree that the responsibility of command should belong to *one* individual who has the ability to coordinate a variety of emergency activities. This is the cornerstone of the ICS structure.

Initial command should be determined by a preplanned system of arriving emergency units and personnel (for example, the first or second arriving EMS, fire, or law enforcement unit). The person assuming command must be familiar with the ICS structure and the operating procedures of other responding agencies. It is not necessary that the commander be the individual with the highest rank or most medical training but rather one who is able to effectively manage the emergency scene.

Command organization is an integral component of ICS and must be implemented immediately. The commander must be clearly identified, and all others at the scene must be aware that only one individual is in command. As more qualified individuals arrive, command may be transferred. Once established, command should do the following:

• Assume an effective command mode and position.
• Transmit brief initial radio reports to the communications center.
• Evaluate the situation rapidly.
• Develop a management strategy.
• Request additional resources and provide assignments as necessary.
• Control and assign sectors as required, consistent with the needs of the incident, standard operating procedures, or disaster plans, and provide operating objectives for these sectors.
• Provide continuing effective command and progress reports until relieved by a higher-ranking individual.
• Develop the command organization by delegating authority to subordinates to accomplish incident needs and objectives (by use of sectors).
• Review and evaluate the effectiveness of site operations and revise operations as needed.
• Return units to service and terminate command when appropriate.

● SECTOR RESPONSIBILITIES

In major incidents, a large number of **sectors** may be involved. Examples of sectors include supplies and resources (support sector); helicopter landing zones and vehicle and apparatus arrivals (staging sector); and patient care delivery (treatment sector). It may become necessary to divide the command structure into EMS, fire, and law enforcement operations to oversee the various sectors. However, all sector and operation managers report to *one* individual serving as commander. (Fig. 6-1).

Sector officers must be strong supervisors and managers. Their primary role in ICS is to "make things happen" and ensure that all rescuers in their sector are working toward a common goal.

Sector officers should not become involved in physical tasks (such as carrying litters or operating rescue equipment), because in doing so, they may lose the ability to control and supervise the sector.

General sector responsibilities include the following:

- Accomplishing objectives provided by command
- Monitoring work progress
- Redirecting activities as necessary
- Coordinating related activities with other sectors
- Requesting additional resources as needed for the sector
- Monitoring the welfare of personnel from each sector

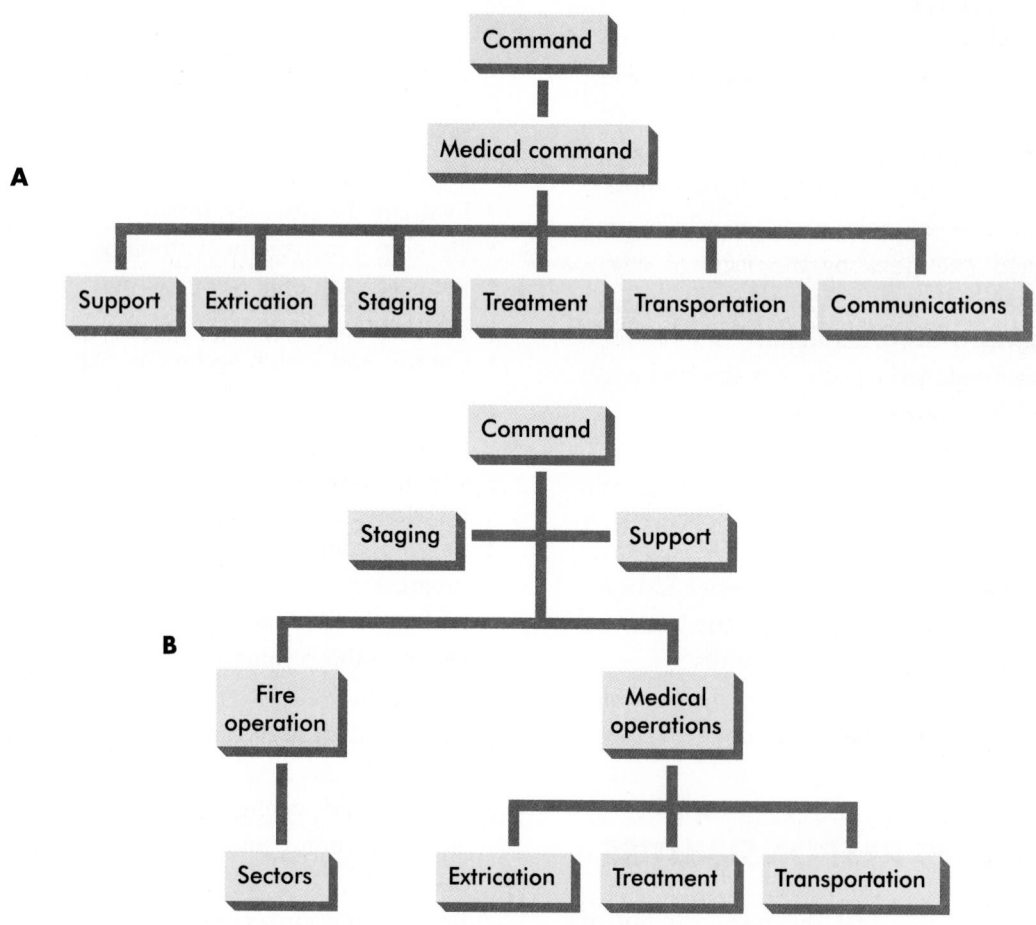

Fig. 6-1 Examples of medical ICS **(A)** and ICS with fire operations **(B).**

- Providing command with frequent reports
- Reallocating resources within the sector

The number of sectors necessary varies based on the scope of the incident. Common sectors and their responsibilities include extrication, treatment, transportation, staging, and support.

Extrication Sector

The extrication sector is responsible for managing entrapped patients at the scene. This involves rescue, initial triage, primary treatment, patient categorization, and initial tagging assignments (for example, the METTAG tagging system) before transferring the patients to the treatment sector. Patient care activities in this sector should include only assessment and treatment of life-threatening situations, such as securing airways, controlling severe bleeding, and covering open chest wounds. In addition, the extrication sector is responsible for site safety and evaluating and directing resources needed for extrication.

Extrication sector responsibilities include the following:

- Determining whether triage and the primary treatment will be conducted onsite or at the treatment sector
- Attaching tagging assignments to injured patients
- Evaluating resources needed for extrication of trapped patients and for their delivery to the treatment sector
- Providing site safety
- Evaluating resources needed for triage and the primary treatment of patients
- Communicating resource requirements to command
- Allocating assigned resources
- Supervising assigned personnel and resources
- Collecting, assembling, and assessing the "walking wounded"
- Reporting progress to command
- Reporting "all clear" to command when all patients have been extricated and delivered to the treatment sector
- Coordinating with other sectors

Treatment Sector

The treatment sector works closely with the extrication sector in patient care delivery. As patients are delivered, they are categorized according to their medical needs. This sector provides advanced care and stabilization until the patients are transported to a medical facility. Most paramedics and hospital personnel are assigned to this area. With large numbers of patients, the area is usually further divided into immediate and delayed treatment zones to help determine priorities in patient transportation. Immediate patients include those with life-threatening injuries; delayed patients include the "walking wounded" and those whose care and transport can be delayed if necessary. It should be noted that triage monitoring is a function of all sectors involving ill or injured patients and is a continuing component of the ICS.

Treatment sector responsibilities include the following:

- Locating a suitable treatment sector area and reporting that location to the extrication sector and command
- Evaluating resources required for patient treatment and reporting these needs to command
- Providing continued triage of patients arriving in the treatment sector
- Providing suitable immediate and delayed treatment areas
- Allocating resources
- Assigning, supervising, and coordinating personnel within the sector
- Reporting progress to command
- Coordinating with other sectors

Transportation Sector

The transportation sector communicates with the receiving hospitals, ambulances, and air medical services for patient transport. This sector must work closely with the treatment sector to determine appropriate destinations for injured patients. The arrival and departure of transfer vehicles must be coordinated with the staging sector.

Transportation sector responsibilities include the following:

- Determining patient transportation needs and obtaining appropriate transportation
- Evaluating resources required to manage patient transportation
- Establishing an ambulance staging area (if command has not already done so) and patient loading areas
- Establishing and operating a helicopter landing zone
- Communicating with hospitals to determine capabilities
- Coordinating patient transportation allocation with the treatment sector and the hospitals
- Reporting resource requirements to command
- Coordinating with other sectors
- Advising command when the last patient has been transported

Staging Sector

Staging sectors are required for large incidents to prevent vehicle congestion and response delays. All emergency vehicles (fire, police, EMS) should report to this sector for direction. Other agencies, such as disaster-relief services and news media, should also be supervised by the staging sector.

Staging sector responsibilities include the following:

- Coordinating with the police department to block streets, intersections, and other areas to facilitate a staging area
- Ensuring that all apparatus is parked in an appropriate manner
- Maintaining a log of all apparatus in the staging area and inventoring all specialized equipment and medical equipment that may be needed
- Reviewing with command what resources must be maintained in staging and coordinating this request with dispatch
- Assuming a visible position for incoming apparatus (for example, leaving emergency lights operating on one apparatus and wearing a sector vest)
- Coordinating with other sectors

Support Sector

The support sector coordinates the gathering and distribution of equipment and supplies for all other sectors. This sector may be responsible for procuring medical supplies from area hospitals, rescue supplies, and other equipment needed at the incident.

Support sector responsibilities include the following:

- Determining the medical supply needs of other sectors
- Establishing a suitable location for supply operations
- Coordinating procurement of medical supplies from hospitals with the transportation sector
- Coordinating procurement of medical supplies that are not available from hospitals
- Reporting additional resource requirements to command
- Allocating supplies and equipment as needed
- Reporting progress to command
- Coordinating with other sectors

● SECTOR IDENTIFICATION

When an ICS is in place, it is imperative that all emergency responders know its organizational structure and the lines of radio communications. Although clothing and identification vary by system, the following guidelines usually apply:

- Color-coded vests identify personnel. For example, the commander may wear a white vest; EMS sector managers, blue vests; fire sector managers, red; law enforcement sector managers, green; and so on.
- With the exceptions of command and sector communications, most communication is face to face. Radio use is intended for command operations.

- Radio communications use operation titles instead of personal or unit names: "EMS sector to command" or "fire sector to law-enforcement sector." This system ensures that all participants can reach the appropriate individual by one radio designation.

Radio Communications

Another key function during a major incident is communications. Preplanning includes identifying the radio frequencies to be used in major incident responses and ways they are to be used. All responding units, for example, should have multichannel radios using a common frequency and separate frequencies for EMS, fire, and other support operations. Sector officers should have portable radios on a channel that permits direct communications with command. These frequencies may be assigned in advance or by the dispatching agency at the time of the incident. In addition, state, regional, and local communication systems should undergo a periodic review that includes the controls for activating communications, sys-

---

Common Failures of Incident Command Systems

Incident Command Failures
- To establish a single, unified command
- To establish staging
- To request additional resources early
- To delegate authority
- To wear identification vests

Dispatch Failures
- To coordinate the response of on-duty and off-duty emergency personnel to the scene

Communications Failures
- To designate a single radio channel for disaster operations
- To adopt standard operating procedures that limit radio traffic during incident operations

Staging Operation Failures
- To establish a central staging area (command)
- To select a large or easily accessible staging area (staging manager)
- To frequently inventory specialized equipment and man power (staging manager)

General Sector Operation Failures
- To provide adequate progress reports to command
- To become involved in physical tasks (sector manager)
- To control the perimeter (law enforcemant)
- To advise command of available man power

Extrication or Rescue Sector Failures
- To triage and tag patients
- To treat patients where they are found rather than stabilizing them and moving them to a treatment area (rescuers)
- To provide adequate safety precautions

Treatment Sector Failures
- To collect patients into an organized treatment area
- To establish a sufficiently large treatment area
- To organize the treatment area and monitor patients
- To effectively coordinate transportation arrangements with the transportation sector

Transportation Sector Failures
- To establish adequate access and egress routes for vehicles
- To have adequate personnel to assist in transportation
- To alert or update hospitals
- To advise hospitals when the last patient is transported

Support Sector Failures
- To plan for the medical supply needs of mass-casualty events
- To provide rapid transport of supplies to the scene

tem frequencies, and portable and mobile radio equipment.

When dealing with various agencies, radio communications must share common terminology. Therefore preplanning may determine that 10-codes are not to be used during a major incident. Other communication considerations are:

- Radio traffic must be clear and concise.
- Messages should be considered and prepared before transmitting.
- The speaker should clearly identify self and unit number or sector.

● TRIAGE AND PATIENT CATEGORIZATION

Triage is a method used to categorize patients for priorities of treatment. The assessment of patient injury severity is based on abnormal physiologic signs, obvious anatomic injury (including mechanism of injury), and concurrent disease factors that might affect the patient's prognosis. It should be stressed that triage is a continuous process during a major incident, and constant monitoring of patient status may indicate a need to change the initial categorization and priority of treatment.

The criteria for triage classifications is determined by the size of the incident, the number of injured patients, and available man power. At present, no national standard guidelines exist for field triage, so the paramedic must be familiar with local methods of patient triage categorization. Two common methods of triage in use throughout the United States are the METTAG system (triage tagging system) and the START (simple triage and rapid transportation) Field Guide.[2]

The METTAG system uses four color tags to alert emergency care personnel and receiving hospital staffs of patient categorization. Red identifies the most critically injured; yellow, less critically injured; green, non–life or limb threatening; and black, patients who have died or have injuries that preclude survival (Fig. 6-2).

The START Field Guide uses a 60-second assessment that evaluates ventilation, perfusion, and mental status. This assessment is used to classify victims as immediate, delayed, or nonsalvageable or dead. The START Field Guide allows rescuers to quickly identify victims at greatest risk of early death and advise other rescuers of the patient's need for stabilization by tagging the patient with color-coded disaster tags (for example, the METTAG tagging system). As in all methods of triage and patient categorization, patients are continuously reevaluated throughout the incident and are retagged as needed (Fig. 6-3).

● AIR MEDICAL TRANSPORT

The availability and use of air medical services varies throughout the United States. Air medical services can provide rapid response time, high-quality medical care, and rapid transport to appropriate care facilities. Helicopters can also provide aerial surveillance and transport of additional personnel and equipment to the emergency scene. Paramedic crews should consult with medical control and follow local protocol regarding use of air medical services.

Notification of Air Medical Services

Requests for air medical services are accepted by most air services from physicians, EMS person-

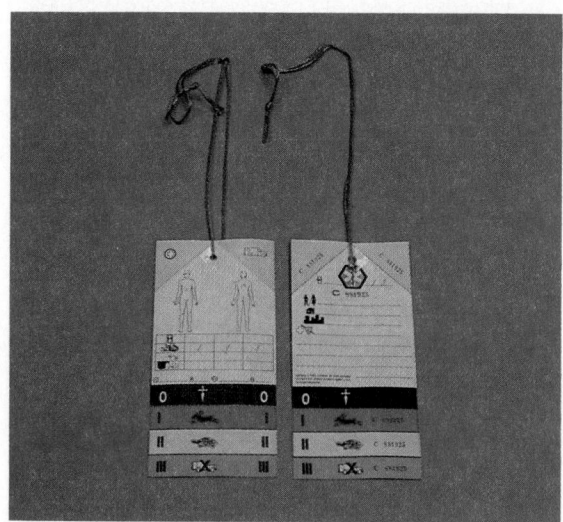

Fig. 6-2 METTAG card.

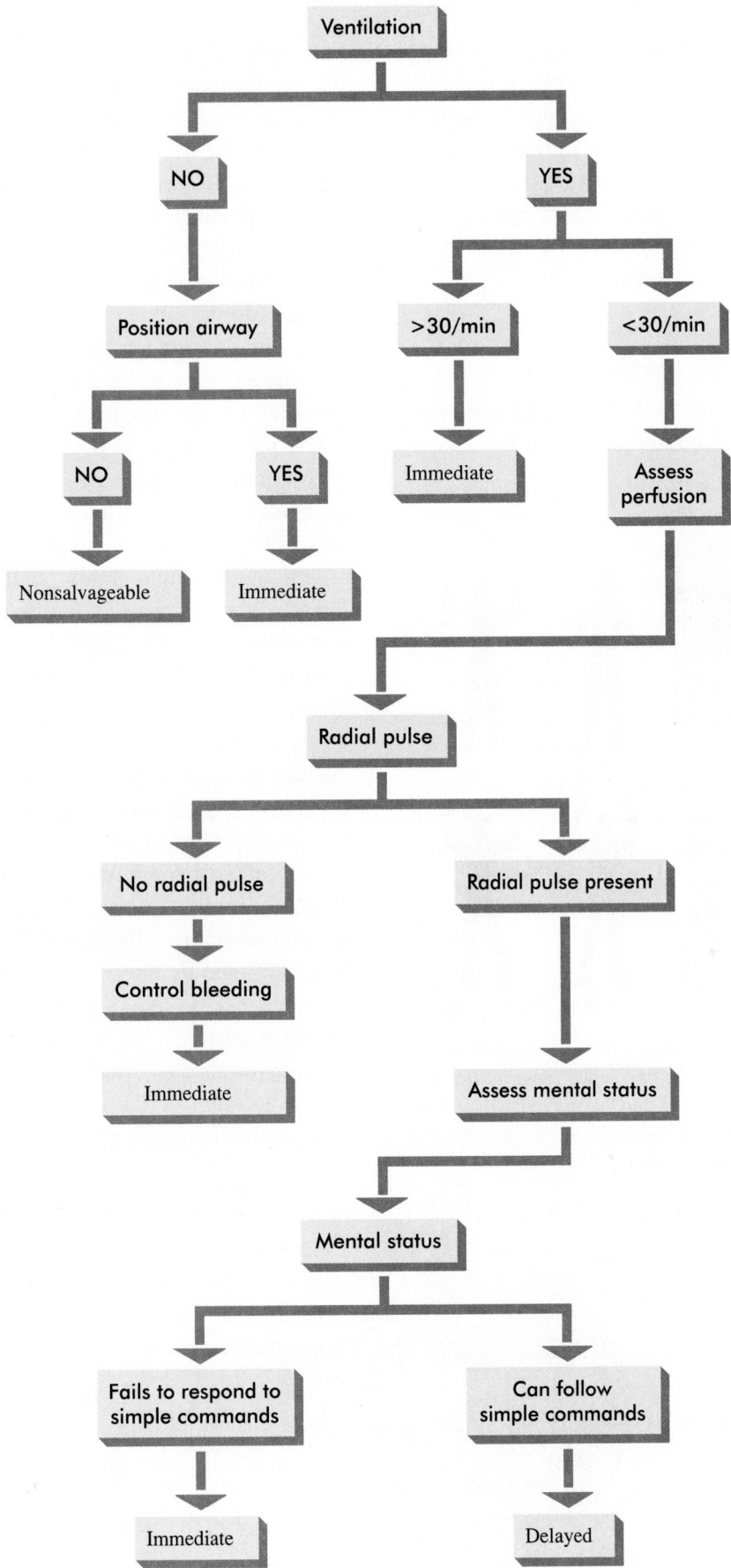

Fig. 6-3 START field guide.

nel, or other public service agency personnel. If the air service is requested, the flight crew should be advised of the type of emergency response, number of patients, location of landing zone (LZ), and any prominent landmarks and hazards (vertical structures, power lines). Direct ground-to-air communications should be available between the LZ officer and the air medical staff.

Landing Site Preparation

Space requirements for helicopter LZ are determined by the size of the aircraft and the time of day. Generally, a daytime LZ must be 60 by 60 feet for single-engine aircraft and 75 by 75 feet for larger (generally twin-engine) aircraft; a nighttime LZ should be 100 by 100 feet.

The ideal LZ should have as few vertical structures as possible. It should be relatively flat and free of high grass, crops, or other factors that may conceal uneven terrain or hinder access. The LZ should also be free of debris that may injure people or damage structures or the helicopter. If patients are close to the LZ, protection should be provided by covering wounds and eyes.

If a nighttime LZ is used, emergency vehicles with lighted bar lights should be situated at the perimeters of the LZ. If white lights are used, they should be directed *down* to the center of the zone as spotlights; white lights (spotlights or headlights) directed toward the aircraft may temporarily blind the pilot. Flares should not be used to identify the LZ, because the downwash may blow the flares from the site and create a fire hazard. Dusty LZs should be wet down by a fire crew, especially if vehicle traffic is moving in the area. This prevents the pilot and vehicle drivers from being temporarily blinded by the dust.

Helpful radio communications with the pilot include notification of wind direction and any possible obstructions or hazards. (Wind direction may be determined by throwing grass or dirt, wetting a finger, or by smoke patterns from flares or smoke canisters.) If hazardous materials are present, the air crew should be advised of the substance, location of the hazardous materials site, and possibility of any patient contamination. The

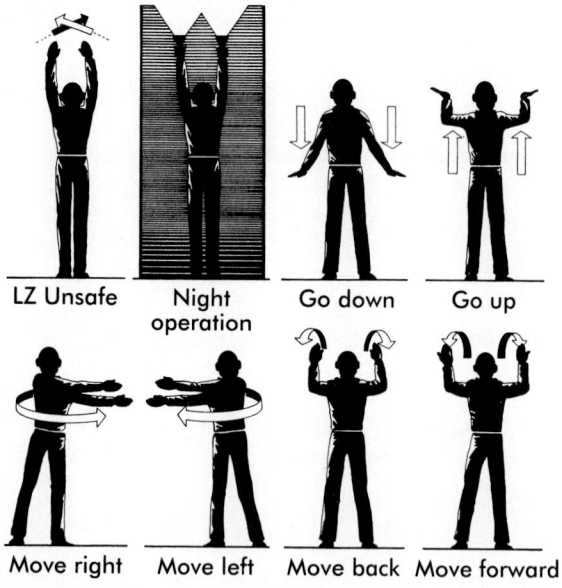

Fig. 6-4 Landing zone hand signals. There are similar positionings for *move back* and *move forward*, but with *move back* the thumbs are in and the signaler waves back to front, and with *move forward* the thumbs are out and the signaler waves front to back.

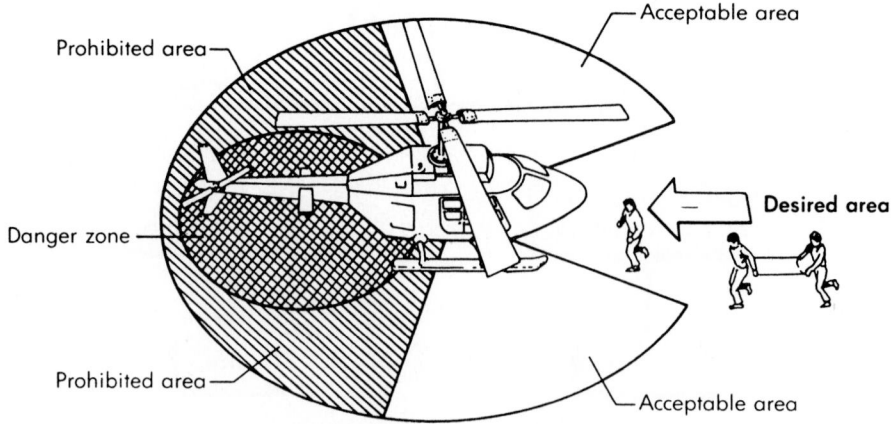

Fig. 6-5 Safe-approach zones.

BOX 6-2

Safety Precautions During Helicopter Landing

- Never allow ground personnel to approach the helicopter unless requested to do so by the pilot or flight crew.
- Allow only necessary personnel to help load or unload patients.
- Secure any loose objects or clothing that could be blown by rotor downwash (stretcher sheets, blankets).
- Allow no smoking.
- After the aircraft is parked, move to the front beyond the perimeter of the rotor blades, and *wait for a signal from the pilot* to approach.
- Approach the helicopter in a crouched position, staying within view of the pilot or other crew members.
- *Never approach the rear of aircraft from any direction.* The tail rotors on most aircraft are near the ground and spin at high RPMs, which makes them virtually invisible. Tail rotor injuries are often fatal.
- Carry long objects horizontally and no more than waist high.
- Depart the helicopter from the front and within view of the pilot.

aircraft should not be permitted to land until all dangers of fire or explosion are eliminated. After the aircraft is coming in to land, one emergency responder should stand facing the LZ so the pilot can see the landing area. LZ hand signals that may be useful to the pilot are illustrated in Fig. 6-4.

Safety Precautions

Everyone should be clear of the touchdown area during takeoffs and landings. A distance of 100 to 200 feet is best (Fig. 6-5). In addition, the precautions in Box 6-2 should be followed.

Patient Preparation

Preparing a patient for air transport requires the following special considerations:
- Airways must be established and secured before loading.
- Pneumatic antishock garments must be applied before loading (per local protocol).
- External cardiopulmonary resuscitation devices should be positioned according to aircraft configuration.
- Restraints or pharmacological control are required for combative patients.

REFERENCES

1. *E.M.T. paramedic national standard curriculum*, Washington, DC, 1985, US Government Printing Office.
2. Hewett C, Schmehl A: *START instructor's manual*, ed 2, Newport Beach, RI, 1984, Hoag Memorial Hospital.

Summary

An emergency response that results in multiagency involvement requires a well-defined command structure to provide organization, effective communications, and accountability. Preplanning, cooperation, and frequent exercises help save lives and make a major incident response workable for all participating agencies.

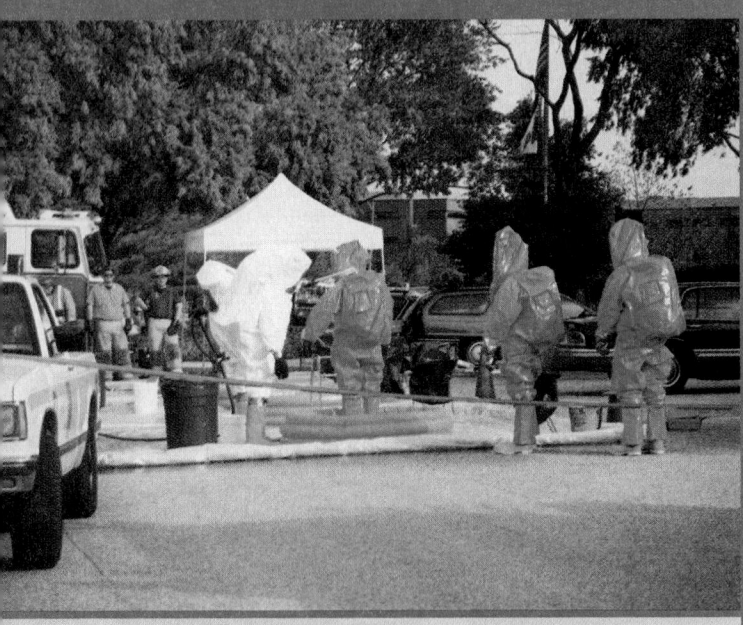

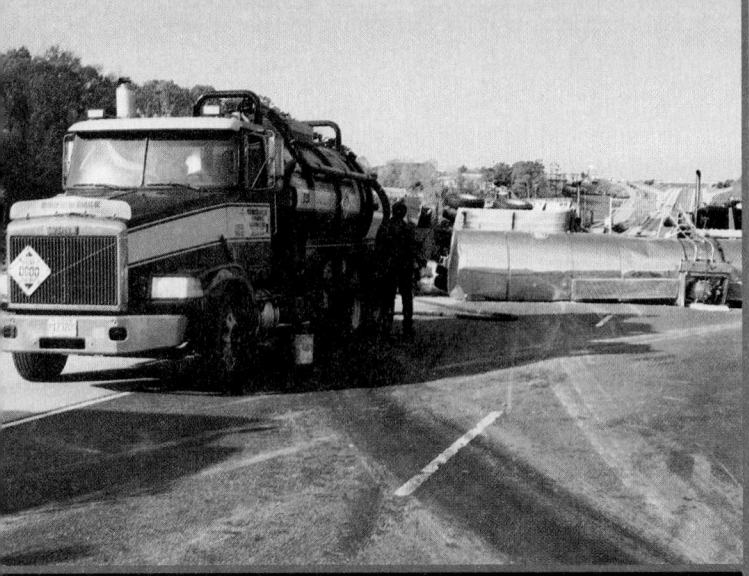

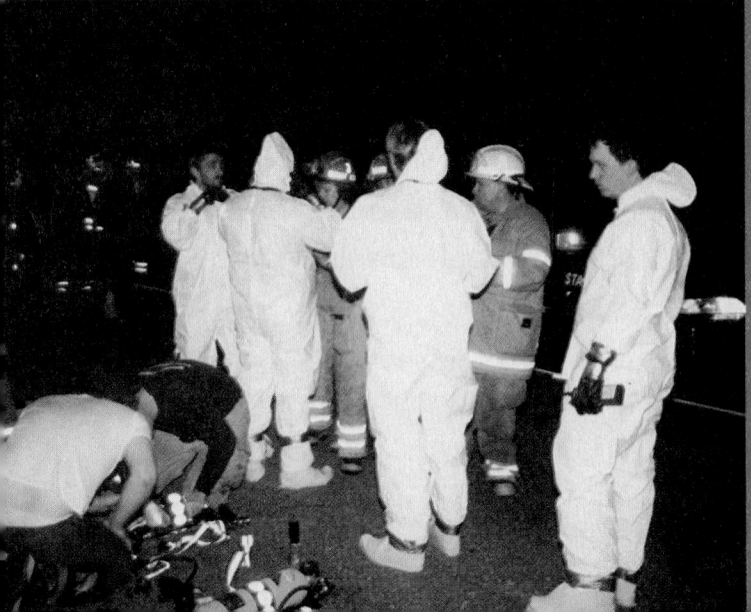

Hazardous materials incidents create additional responsibilities for emergency service providers. Large geographical areas covering several political jurisdictions may be involved, and cooperation in mass evacuations and decontamination may be required. Specialized roles and responsibilities in hazardous material responses include, among others, the recognition and identification of the hazardous material, containment and cleanup of the material, extrication and decontamination of exposed persons, provision of emergency care, and continual medical assessment of team members involved in the incident.

As a paramedic, you should be able to:

1. Define *hazardous materials*.
2. Identify major legislation regarding hazardous materials that influences emergency health care workers.
3. Describe informal and formal means of identifying hazardous materials.
4. List resources for identifying and managing hazardous materials situations.
5. Identify protective clothing and equipment necessary for rescuers responding to various hazardous materials incidents.
6. Describe potential internal damage caused by exposure to hazardous materials.
7. Describe symptoms of exposure to hazardous materials that require intervention.
8. Recognize external symptoms that may present after exposure to corrosive hazardous materials.
9. Outline management techniques for external exposure to corrosive hazardous materials.
10. Describe how radiation causes its harmful effects.
11. Describe emergency care for victims of radiation exposure.
12. Outline the response to a hazardous materials emergency.
13. Describe the three safety zones for a hazardous materials response.
14. Discuss the paramedic's role in medical monitoring at a hazardous materials incident.
15. Describe the emergency management of patients who have been contaminated with hazardous materials.

● THE SCOPE OF HAZARDOUS MATERIALS

A *hazardous material* is defined as "any substance or material capable of posing an unreasonable risk to health, safety, and property."[1] It is estimated that between 5% and 15% of all trucks on the road, at any time, carry hazardous materials. Also, there are approximately 100,000 shippers of hazardous materials and 80,000 carriers, of which most are trucks, transporting hazardous materials of all types. Because emergency responses to vehicular accidents are so common, the potential for exposure to situations involving hazardous materials is great.

In addition to transportation accidents, injury or illness may result from mishaps involving house-

KEY TERMS

CHEMTREC: (Chemical Transportation Emergency Center) A public service of the Chemical Manufacturers Association that provides immediate advice to on-scene personnel regarding hazardous materials management.

placards: Four-sided, diamond-shaped signs displayed on hazardous materials containers that are usually yellow, red, orange, white, or green and contain a four-digit United Nations identification number (UN number) and a legend to indicate container content.

shipping papers: Descriptions of the hazardous materials that include the substance name, classification, and UN identification number. Generally, the papers are required to be carried in the transporting vehicle (motor vehicle, train, vessel, or aircraft).

hold chemicals, pesticides, and industrial toxins. The following statistics emphasize the importance of EMS personnel knowing how to manage hazardous materials exposure:

- The American Association of Poison Control Centers reported over 2 million poisonings during 1990.
- An estimated 100,000 industrial workers are exposed to respiratory irritants each year.
- Some 5000 to 8000 accidental caustic ingestions occur annually in children under the age of 5.
- More than 1 billion pounds of pesticides are produced annually, resulting in 77,000 exposures and 3000 hospitalizations each year.
- The majority of fire-related deaths result from inhalation of toxic products of combustion.

● LAWS AND REGULATIONS

Much attention has been focused on hazardous materials during the past 10 years. Major incidents, such as the Union Carbide disaster in India, the Chernobyl nuclear accident, the Three Mile Island accident, and the need for proper disposal of hazardous wastes have attracted the attention of employee and citizen awareness groups and local, state, and federal officials. This attention has resulted in more laws and regulations to strictly control of hazardous materials.

The Superfund Amendments and Reauthorization Act (SARA) of 1986 established requirements for federal, state, and local governments and industry regarding emergency planning and the reporting of hazardous materials–related incidents. This legislation was designed to help communities better meet their responsibilities in the event of chemical emergencies. SARA helped increase the public's knowledge and access to information on hazardous materials in their community. The act required owners and operators of facilities using or storing any of the 366 extremely hazardous substances on the Environmental Protection Agency (EPA) list[2] to notify the local fire department, the local emergency planning committee, and the state emergency response commission.

In 1989, the *Occupational Safety and Health Administration* and the EPA published rules titled Worker Protection Standards for Hazardous Waste Operations and Emergency Response to govern training requirements, emergency plans, medical checkups, and other safety precautions for workers at uncontrolled hazardous waste sites and those responding to hazardous chemical releases or spills. SARA mandates that states adopt these rules. The training requirements include the following five categories of individuals who may respond to an emergency involving hazardous materials:

1. First-responder awareness. This category pertains to individuals who are likely to witness or discover a hazardous substance release but who do not have emergency-response duties pertaining to hazardous materials as part of their job functions. This applies to most law enforcement officers. Persons in this category must have sufficient training to demonstrate the following:
   a. An understanding of what hazardous materials are and the risks associated with them in an accident
   b. An understanding of the potential outcomes of an emergency in which hazardous materials are present
   c. The ability to recognize the presence of hazardous materials in an emergency
   d. The ability to identify the hazardous materials (if possible)
   e. An understanding of the role of the first responder in the emergency response plan
   f. The ability to recognize the need for additional resources
2. First-responder operations. Individuals are included in this category if they respond to hazardous materials incidents to protect nearby persons, property, or the environment, without trying to stop the hazardous release. Firefighters and EMS personnel are in this category. In addition to the knowledge base of first-responder awareness, these individuals must have training in:
   a. Basic hazard- and risk-assessment techniques
   b. Personal protective clothing and equipment
   c. Basic control, containment, and confinement operations
   d. Basic decontamination procedures

3. Hazardous material technicians. Individuals in this category respond to hazardous materials emergencies for the purpose of stopping the release. Hazardous materials technicians are usually considered to be members of a hazardous materials response team. These individuals have additional training in the following:

a. Emergency response plans

b. The use of survey instruments and equipment to identify hazardous materials

c. Incident command systems

d. Specialized protective clothing and equipment

e. Specialized containment and confinement operations

4. Hazardous materials specialists. The duties of these individuals require specific knowledge of the various hazardous substances. Hazardous materials specialists respond with and provide support to hazardous materials technicians and act as site liaisons with federal, state, and local government authorities. In addition to the knowledge base of the hazardous materials technician, hazardous materials specialists have training in:

a. The use of advanced survey instruments and equipment

b. In-depth hazard and risk assessment

c. The implementation of decontamination procedures

d. Site safety and control

e. Chemical, radiological, and toxicological terminology relevant to hazardous substance behaviors

5. On-scene incident commander. On-scene incident commanders are trained to assume control of a hazardous materials event. In addition to the first-responder awareness level of training, on-scene incident commander's responsibilities include the following:

a. Implementation of an incident command system

b. Implementation of emergency response plans

c. Knowledge of both state and federal regional response teams

d. Knowledge of medical hazards and risks for individuals working in protective clothing and equipment

● IDENTIFYING HAZARDOUS MATERIALS

The two methods used to identify hazardous materials are informal product identification and formal product identification (placards, shipping papers, and other hazardous materials information resources).

Informal Product Identification

Arriving emergency personnel may be able to make some determinations regarding the presence and type of hazardous materials at the scene. Informal methods of identification include the following:

- Visual inspection of the scene with binoculars before entering the site
- Verbal reports by bystanders or other responsible persons
- Occupancy type (intended use of a particular structure [for example, fuel storage, pesticide plant])
- Incident location (probable location for presence of hazardous materials)
- Visual indicators (vapor clouds, smoke, leakage)
- Container characteristics (size, shape, color, deformed containers)
- Senses (peculiar smell)
- Symptoms of victims of exposure

Informal methods of product identification should be used only as a temporary means to determine the presence of any hazardous materials. A product should always be identified formally before any activity that may pose a threat to the safety of all of the emergency responders is undertaken.

Formal Product Identification

Traditionally, hazardous materials have been labeled by one or more of the following six systems:

1. The American National Standards Institute uses a label to identify a specific hazard (such as explosives, flammable liquids, radioactive materials, and so on) as opposed to a specific chemical.

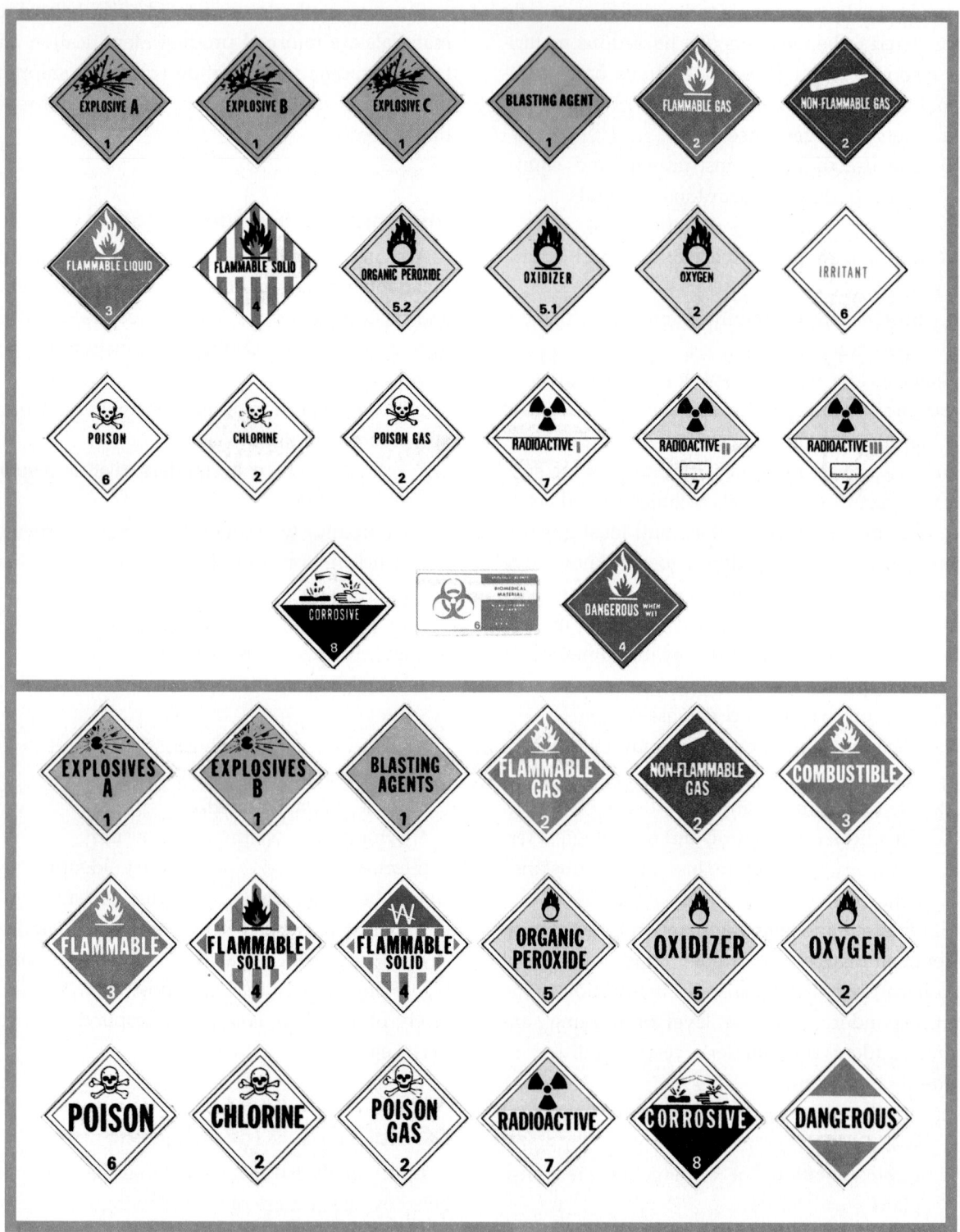

Fig. 7-1 Hazardous materials warning placards and labels.

2. The U.S. Department of Transportation (DOT) uses labels and placards with pictographs and printed hazard categories. In addition, the DOT requires specific information on shipping manifests.
3. The United Nations Labeling System uses pictographs, symbols, or both, similar to those used by the DOT to identify a specific hazard rather than a specific chemical.
4. The International Air Transport Association uses the United Nations pictographs and indicates written emergency precaution measures in case of an incident.
5. The National Fire Protection Association uses color and a numerical rating scale (NFPA 704 System) to identify degree of hazard for health, fire, and reactivity. The diamond-shaped identification symbols are required on fixed facilities by many state and local fire codes.
6. The U.S. Department of Labor requires material safety data sheets (MSDS) for hazardous chemicals that are stored, handled, or used in the workplace.

Placards and Shipping Papers

Although a variety of identification systems may be used, hazardous materials are usually identified through **placards** (Fig. 7-1) and **shipping papers.**

The United Nations class (or division) identification number or North American number (UN/NA number) may be displayed on the bottom of a placard or on the shipping paper after the listed shipping name or names. In certain cases, this class or division number may replace the written name of the hazard class in the shipping paper description.

> **NOTE:**
> Because multiple chemical agents may have the same UN/NA number, it is important to refer to specific guidelines for hazardous material by chemical name in addition to this number.

Meanings of the class and division numbers are shown in Table 7-1.

Material Safety Data Sheets

MSDS are required by OSHA for each chemical produced, stored, used, or transported in the United States. The MSDS are supplied by the manufacturer and contain information for safe and proper handling and storage of the material, as well as information on emergency actions. MSDS also classify the potential of significant health hazards from a particular substance exposure.

The potential health hazard of a material may be defined in several different ways, depending on the degree of inherent toxicity and type of exposure. Although MSDS provide useful information, they should not be used as the sole source of information on health risks or treatment recommendations. Paramedics should consult with medical direction, a poison control center, or another authority.

Other Hazardous Materials Information Resources

A number of resources are available for hazardous materials reference. One such reference is the *Emergency Response Guidebook* published by the DOT. This guidebook lists more than 1000 hazardous materials and appropriate emergency procedures. It includes substance names and identification numbers and is cross-referenced in alphabetical and numerical order. The *Emergency Response Guidebook* is carried in emergency vehicles by many EMS, fire, and other public-service agencies. *It is recommended that product information be referenced through more than one source if time and availability permit.*

Regional poison-control centers have been established throughout most of the United States and are a valuable asset in any EMS system. Many of these centers are available 24 hours a day. They are staffed with specialists who provide information, consultation, treatment recommendations, patient follow-up, and data collection. Poison-control centers are linked to many agencies dealing with toxic substances and are closely tied to all area hospitals. These centers maintain a computerized listing of over 450,000 drugs, toxic substances, and other products.

CHEMTREC (Chemical Transportation Emergency Center), a public service of the Chemical

TABLE 7-1 International Classification System for Hazardous Materials

Class or division numbers may be displayed in the bottom of placards or in the hazardous materials description on shipping papers. In certain cases, a class or division number may replace the written name of the hazard class description on the shipping paper. The class and division numbers have the following meanings:

Class 1   Explosives
Division 1.1   Explosives with a mass explosion hazard
Division 1.2   Explosives with a projection hazard
Division 1.3   Explosives with predominantly a fire hazard
Division 1.4   Explosives with no significant blast hazard
Division 1.5   Very insensitive explosives
Division 1.6   Extremely insensitive explosive articles

Class 2   Gases
Division 2.1   Flammable gases
Division 2.2   Nonflammable gases
Division 2.3   Poison gases
Division 2.4   Corrosive gases (Canadian)

Class 3   Flammable Liquids
Division 3.1   Flashpoint below −18° C (0° F)
Division 3.2   Flashpoint −18° C and above but less than 23° C (73° F)
Division 3.3   Flashpoint of 23° C and up to 61° C (141° F)

Class 4   Flammable Solids, Spontaneously Combustible Materials, Materials That Are Dangerous When Wet
Division 4.1   Flammable solids
Division 4.2   Spontaneously combustible materials
Division 4.3   Materials that are dangerous when wet

Class 5   Oxidizers and Organic Peroxides
Division 5.1   Oxidizers
Division 5.2   Organic peroxides

Class 6   Poisonous and Etiological (Infectious) Materials
Division 6.1   Poisonous materials
Division 6.2   Etiological (infectious) materials

Class 7   Radioactive Materials

Class 8   Corrosives

Class 9   Miscellaneous Hazardous Materials

Manufacturers Association, provides immediate advice to on-scene personnel regarding hazardous materials management. The agency also contacts the shipper of the material for additional assistance and provides follow-up response when appropriate. CHEMTREC operates 24 hours a day, 7 days a week, and can be reached in the United States and Canada through the emergency toll-free number: 1-800-424-9300 (in Alaska 0-202-483-7616.)

CHEMTREC should be contacted as soon as possible during the hazardous materials incident with the name of the substance, its identification number, and the nature of the problem. Involving

CHEMTREC in managing a hazardous materials incident is usually a part of the standard operating procedure of any emergency response team. Other government and private-sector agencies that may offer assistance in a hazardous materials incident are listed on p. 73.

● PERSONAL PROTECTIVE CLOTHING AND EQUIPMENT

The potential for injury from exposure to hazardous materials is related to the toxicity, flammability, and reactivity of a particular substance. It is important that anyone dealing with hazardous materials take precautionary measures, including using the appropriate respiratory devices and wearing protective clothing.

Protective Respiratory Devices

The potential for respiratory system exposure to hazardous materials is of paramount importance to the emergency responder. The respiratory system may be protected by air-purification devices and atmosphere-supplying respiratory equipment.

Air purification relies on respirators or filtration devices to remove particulate matter, gases, or vapors from the atmosphere. These devices do not use a separate source of air and require constant monitoring for contaminants and oxygen levels. As a rule, they are not recommended for use in hazardous materials release.

Atmosphere-supplying devices rely on a separate source of air and provide the highest level of respiratory protection. There are two basic types: self-contained breathing apparatus (SCBA) and air-line respirators. The use of either requires training and recertification as governed by regulations from the Occupational Safety and Health Administration (OSHA).

SCBA provides respiratory protection in oxygen-deficient and toxic atmospheres. Only SCBAs that maintain positive pressure in the face piece during inhalation and exhalation should be used when working with hazardous materials. The SCBA is usually considered an excellent barrier to hazardous environments, but the rescuer should be aware of potential face-piece penetration and contamination by certain toxic substances. Examples include methyl bromide, Telone, and ethyleneimine.

Air-line respirators supply air to the rescuer away from the scene by an air-line hose. These devices are often used at hazardous material sites when extended working times are required. Air-line respirators must have an escape capability for operations in atmospheres classified as immediately dangerous to life and health. Respiratory protection devices that combine SCBAs and air-line hose units are available.

Agencies that Assist in Hazardous Materials Incidents

Federal Agencies
- EPA
- DOT
- National Response Center (NRC)
- United States Coast Guard (USCG)
- Centers for Disease Control (CDC)
- Federal Aviation Administration (FAA)
- United States Armed Forces (Army, Navy, Air Force, Marines)
- U.S. Department of Energy (DOE)

Regional and State Agencies
- State EPA
- State health departments
- National Guard
- State police
- State emergency management agencies

Local Agencies
- Emergency management
- Fire service (HAZMAT units)
- Poison-control center
- Law enforcement agencies
- Public utilities
- Sewage and treatment facilities

Commercial Agencies
- American Petroleum Institute
- Association of American Railroads (AAR) and Hazardous Materials Systems
- Chemical Manufacturers Association
- HELP (Union Carbide's Emergency Response System for company shipments)
- Chevron (provides assistance with Chevron products)
- Railway industry
- Local industry
- Local contractors
- Local carriers and transporters

Classifications of Protective Clothing

Protective clothing is categorized as limited use (disposable) or multiuse (reusable) and is constructed of a variety of materials designed specifically for certain chemical exposures. Examples of this material include Tyvek/Saranex, nitrile rubber, Teflon, and Viton. It should be noted that no single material is compatible with all chemicals, so the manufacturer's guidelines and recommendations must be followed (Box 7-1).

Protective clothing can be classified in generic categories. For the purpose of this text, three general levels of protection are addressed.[3]

> **NOTE:**
> Training in the use of personal protective clothing and equipment should take place in a safe environment before it is used at emergency scenes.

1. Structural firefighting clothing is designed to protect against extremes of temperature, steam, hot water, hot particles, and the ordinary hazards of firefighting. This type of clothing may be used when contact with splashes of extremely hazardous materials is unlikely or when the total atmospheric concentrations do not contain high levels of chemicals that are toxic to the skin.

This classification of clothing usually includes a helmet, positive-pressure SCBA, turnout coat and pants, gloves and boots, and a protective hood made of fire-resistant material (Fig. 7-2). Duct tape or bands of rubber may be wrapped around the clothing where pants and boots, coat and pants, and coat and gloves overlap. This helps prevent dusts, vapors, or splashes of chemicals from entering the protected environment. It should be emphasized that general firefighting clothing is not designed to provide chemical protection.

2. High-temperature protective clothing is designed for use in short-term exposures to high levels of radiant heat. Examples include aircraft firefighting and hazardous incidents involving some petrochemicals. This classification may be further divided into proximity and fire entry suits.

Proximity suits are designed for exposures of short duration and close proximity to flames and radiant heat. These suits are not effective for rescue and are not designed to offer substantial chemical protection. An example of a proximity suit in the protective clothing used for aircraft firefighting.

Fire-entry suits offer complete protection for short-duration entry into a total flame environment. They are effective in rescue operations, but they lack flexibility and reduce rescuer mobility.

BOX 7-1

Forms of Chemical Intrusion

Degradation: the physical destruction or decomposition of a clothing material caused by exposure to chemicals, use, or ambient conditions

Penetration: the flow of a hazardous liquid chemical through zippers, stitched seams, pinholes, or other imperfections in a material

Permeation: the process by which a hazardous liquid chemical moves through a material on a molecular level

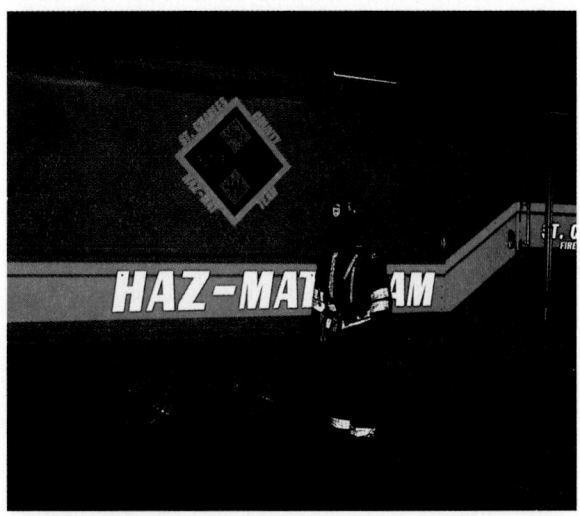

Fig. 7-2 Structural firefighting clothing.

3. Chemical-protective clothing is designed to protect skin and eyes from direct chemical contact. This classification is further divided into chemical splash protection and vapor protective clothing (Fig. 7-3).

Chemical-splash-protective clothing consists of several pieces of special clothing and equipment designed to protect skin and eyes from chemical splashes. This clothing does not provide total body protection from gases or airborne dusts.

Vapor-protective clothing provides total body protection from hostile environments when used with air-supplied respiratory devices. Respiratory protection can be provided by an SCBA that is worn either inside or outside the suit or by an airline hose with emergency escape capabilities (Fig. 7-4).

All avenues through which hazardous materials can enter the body must be protected. The following points should be of particular concern to any rescuer involved in HAZMAT response:

- Protective clothing should not be adversely affected by the hazardous materials involved.
- Protective clothing should seal all exposed skin.
- Contact with the hazardous materials should be of the absolute minimal duration required.
- Protective clothing and equipment should be properly decontaminated or properly discarded.
- Safety standards and methods for cleaning and disposing of clothing and equipment should be strictly followed.

● HEALTH HAZARDS

Hazardous materials may enter the human body through inhalation, ingestion, injection, and absorption. Any of these routes may produce internal and external damage to the rescuer. Exposure to dangerous substances may affect the body in several different ways, producing numerous injuries or illnesses. The following is a brief description of various health hazards. Internal and external injuries associated with hazardous materials exposure are discussed more thoroughly in Chapters 16 and 23.

Internal Damage

Internal damage to the human body from hazardous materials exposure may involve the respiratory tract, central nervous system, or other internal organs. Some substances injure all cells with which they have contact. Others have more direct effect on specific organs (target organs), such as the kidney and liver.

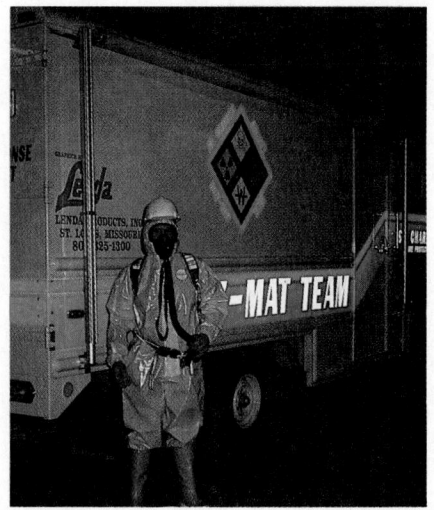

Fig. 7-3 Nonencapsulating protective clothing.

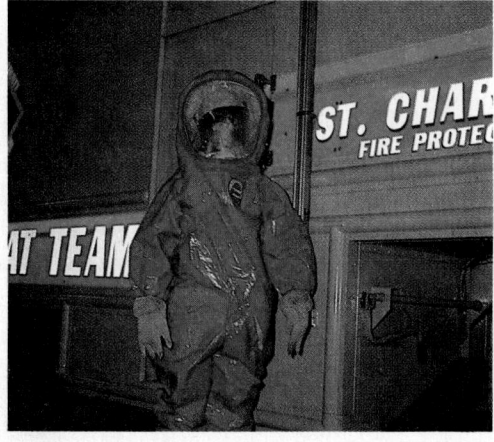

Fig. 7-4 Encapsulating protective clothing.

Depending on the hazardous materials, physical injury may range from minor irritation to more serious complications, including cardiorespiratory compromise and death. Chronic illness (for example, chronic obstructive pulmonary disease) and various forms of cancer may also result. Some substances may have teratogenic or mutagenic consequences, causing abnormal fetal development and changes in gene structure.

Irritants

Respiratory problems are a frequent complaint of rescuers and patients exposed to hazardous materials. Chemical irritants emit vapors that affect the mucous membranes of the body, such as the surfaces of the eyes, nose, mouth, and throat. As these irritants combine with moisture, acidic or alkaline reactions may occur. Exposure to these irritants may result in damage to the upper, lower, and deep respiratory tract. Examples of chemical irritants are hydrochloric acid, halogens, and ozone.

Asphyxiants

Asphyxiants are gases that displace the available oxygen required for respiration by diluting the oxygen concentration in the air. Besides simple asphyxiants such as carbon dioxide, methane, and propane, there are also gases that not only displace oxygen in the air, but also interfere with tissue oxygenation. These are referred to as *blood poisons* or *chemical asphyxiants* because they tend to interrupt the transport or use of oxygen by tissue cells. Through various mechanisms, these toxic gases deprive body tissue of needed oxygen. Examples include hydrogen cyanide, carbon monoxide, and hydrogen sulfide.

Nerve Poisons, Anesthetics, and Narcotics

Nerve poisons, anesthetics, and narcotics act on the nervous system by affecting either the cardiorespiratory regulating mechanisms of the brain or the ability to transmit impulses required for adequate respiratory and circulatory functions.

Nerve poisons were developed by the military and are commonly referred to as *war gases* or *nerve gases*. Similar substances are used in solid pesticides, and exposure to these chemicals may produce fatal complications. Examples of these poisons include parathion and malathion. Although anesthetics and narcotics are less hazardous than nerve poisons, continuous exposure or exposure to large concentrations may produce unconsciousness or death. Examples include ethylene, nitrous oxide, and ethyl alcohol.

Hepatotoxins

Hepatotoxins are substances that cause damage to the liver. The poisons accumulate in the body and destroy the liver's ability to function. Examples include chlorinated and halogenated hydrocarbons.

Cardiotoxins

Cardiotoxins are hazardous materials that may induce myocardial ischemia and cardiac rhythm disturbances. Examples of these substances are aliphatic nitrates, and ethylene glycol dinitrate. Acute myocardial infarction and sudden death have been reported in healthy young persons exposed to these substances. Short-term exposure to fluorocarbons and other halogenated hydrocarbons has also been known to produce cardiac abnormalities.

Nephrotoxins

Nephrotoxins are hazardous materials that are especially destructive to the kidneys. Examples include carbon disulfide, lead, high concentrations of organic solvents, and inorganic mercury. Exposure to carbon tetrachloride used as a solvent or dry-cleaning or fire-extinguishing agent may also produce nephrotoxic effects.

Neurotoxins

Neurological and behavioral toxicity may result from exposure to hazardous substances such as arsenic, lead, mercury, and organic solvents. In some cases, cerebral hypoxia may occur as a result of cellular respiration impaired by decreased oxygenation of blood.

Hemotoxins

Hemotoxins are hazardous substances that may cause the destruction of red blood cells, resulting in hemolytic anemia. Substances that can produce hemolytic anemia include aniline, naphthol, quinones, lead, mercury, arsenic, and copper. Pulmonary edema and cardiac and liver injury may also be caused by hemotoxin exposure.

Carcinogens

Carcinogens are cancer-causing agents, and many hazardous materials are carcinogenic. Although the precise amount of hazardous materials exposure required for cancer to develop is unknown, it is known that short-term exposure to specific agents can produce long-term effects. Disease and complications have been reported 20 years after hazardous materials exposure.

Of particular interest to rescuers involved in firefighting is that all burning fossil and organic fuels produce dioxins, many of which are carcinogens. (For example, burning wood produces carcinogenic formaldehyde.) A positive-pressure SCBA is the most important protective equipment against these carcinogenic vapors and any other respiratory poisons.

General Symptoms of Exposure

Health effects from exposure to hazardous materials vary by individual and depend on the chemical involved, the concentration of the chemical, the duration of exposure, the number of exposures, and the route of entry (inhalation, ingestion, injection, absorption). In addition, personal factors such as an individual's age, gender, general health, allergies, smoking habits, alcohol consumption, and medication influence how an individual is affected.

Various symptoms may result from exposure to hazardous materials. Some symptoms may be delayed or masked by common illnesses such as influenza or by smoke inhalation. If any of the following symptoms is present after exposure to hazardous materials, the rescuer or patient should seek immediate medical attention[4]:

- Confusion, lightheadedness, anxiety, dizziness
- Blurred or double vision
- Changes in skin color or blushing
- Shortness of breath, burning of the upper airway

- Coughing or painful respiration
- Tingling or numbness of extremities
- Loss of coordination
- Seizure
- Nausea, vomiting, abdominal cramping, diarrhea
- Unconsciousness

Any time two or more members of the response team report that they "feel" similar symptoms, a toxic gas should be suspected. EMS responders should always report the onset of symptoms to their crew members, because multiple simultaneous onset is a critical exposure sign.

External Damage

Body surface tissue may be injured by hazardous materials. Many substances have corrosive properties or become corrosive when mixed with water. Exposure to these substances may produce chemical burns and severe tissue damage. Examples include hydrochloric acid, hydrofluoric acid, and caustic soda.

Soft Tissue Damage

Corrosives are acids or bases (alkaline). Exposure to either may cause pain on contact, but alkalis generally burn more extensively than acids. Exposing human tissue to a base corrosive such as lye may result in a breakdown of fatty tissue (liquefaction) that produces a greasy or slick feeling to the skin. These signs should alert the rescuer to seek medical attention. Unless the substance is identified, decontamination should begin by brushing off the powder and flushing the skin with copious amounts of water. Paramedics should never attempt to neutralize an acid or base; doing so could produce great heat and cause further burns. The area should be copiously flushed, and the patient should be transported for care.

Cryogenics are refrigerant liquid gases that can freeze human tissue on contact. These liquids vaporize as soon as they are released from their containers and may cause tissue damage. Extreme caution should be used when near any refrigerated liquids, since they produce freeze burns, frostbite, and other cold-related injuries. Examples include freon, liquid oxygen, and liquid nitrogen.

Chemical Exposure to the Eyes

Chemical exposure to the eyes may cause damage ranging from superficial inflammation, termed *chemical conjunctivitis,* to severe burns. Patients with these conditions have local pain, visual disturbance, lacrimation (tearing), edema, and redness of surrounding tissues. Basic management guidelines include flushing the eyes with water by using a mild flow from a hose, intravenous tubing, or water from a container. The affected eye should be irrigated from the medial to the lateral aspect to avoid flushing the chemical into the unaffected eye. Irrigation should be continued during transport for physician evaluation. If contact lenses are present, they should be removed.

Some EMS services use nasal cannulas to irrigate both eyes simultaneously. The cannula is placed over the bridge of the nose, with the nasal prongs pointing down toward the eyes. The cannula is attached to an intravenous administration set using either normal saline or lactated Ringer's solution, and run continually into both eyes (Fig. 7-5).

Irrigation lenses (Morgan Therapeutic Lens) may be useful for prolonged eye irrigation in adults, provided that edema is absent and there are no lacerations or penetrating wounds of the globe or eyelids. The use of these devices in the

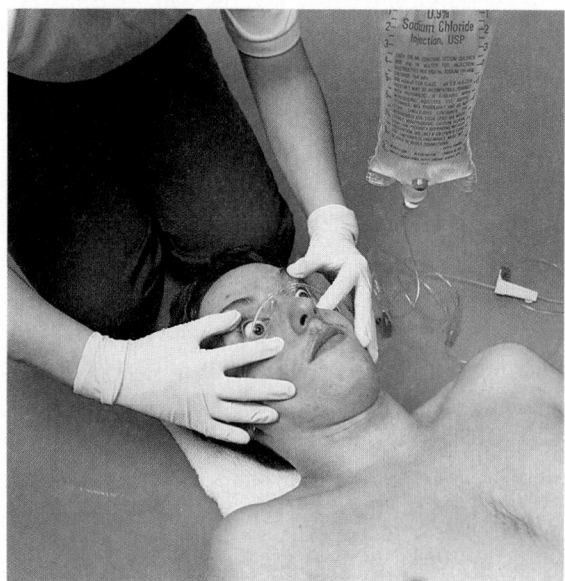

Fig. 7-5 Use of nasal cannula for eye irrigation.

prehospital setting is controversial and requires special training and authorization from medical direction.

● RESPONSE TO HAZARDOUS MATERIALS EMERGENCIES

When EMS is dispatched to a scene involving hazardous materials, decisions must be made regarding rescuer safety, type and degree of the potential hazard, and the involvement of other agencies. As discussed in Chapter 6, preplanning and early coordination of these major incident activities is imperative. In addition, medical control should be advised of the incident as soon as possible so that they can prepare personnel and faculty.

Although the first rescue personnel to arrive at the scene of a hazardous materials incident may not be the most qualified, most communities look to these public-service agencies to provide immediate safety and direction. Therefore the EMS crew must be knowledgeable and proficient in the initial management of hazardous materials incidents.

Responding to the Scene

While en route to the emergency scene, EMS personnel should begin to research hazardous materials references. Most emergency response guides only offer general management objectives. If the product can be identified, the EMS crew should familiarize themselves with potential health hazards, recommended personal protective equipment, initial first aid, and the "safe distance" factor as outlined in the reference guides. After the product is precisely identified, more exact information should be gathered through appropriate HAZMAT agencies (CHEMTREC, poison control).

The scene should be approached cautiously from uphill and upwind. The EMS crew should be alert to environmental clues such as wind direction, unusual odors, leakage, and vapor clouds. Binoculars can be used to initially observe the scene from a safe distance. Emergency vehicles should never be driven through leakage or vapor clouds, and personnel should not enter the incident area until it has been determined that it is safe. In addition to these guidelines, rescuers should[5]:

- Approach cautiously. Resist the urge to rush in; you cannot help others until you know what you are facing.
- Identify the hazards. Placards, container labels, shipping papers, and knowledgeable persons on the scene are valuable information sources. Evaluate all of them, and then consult the recommended guide page before you place yourself or others at risk. Do not be alarmed if new information from a CHEMTREC expert changes some of the emphasis or details of the guide page warnings. You must remember that the guide page provides only the most important information for your initial response with a family or class of hazardous materials. As more accurate, material-specific information becomes available, your response becomes more appropriate for the situation.
- Secure the scene. Without entering the immediate hazard zone, do what you can to isolate the area and ensure the safety of people and the environment. Move and keep people away from the scene and the perimeter. Allow enough room to move and remove your own equipment.
- Obtain help. Advise your headquarters to notify responsible agencies and call for assistance from trained experts through CHEMTREC and the National Response Center, which can be reached through CHEMTREC or dialed directly.
- Decide on site entry. Any efforts you make to rescue persons or protect property or the environment must be weighed against the possibility that you could become part of the problem. Enter the area with the appropriate protective gear (if trained to do so). Above all, *do not walk into or touch spilled material.* Avoid inhalation of fumes, smoke, and vapors, even if no hazardous materials are known to be involved. Do not assume that gases or vapors are harmless because of lack of smell.

Control of the Scene

The first agency to arrive at the scene has several responsibilities. They must detect and identify the materials involved; assess the risk of exposure to rescue personnel and others; consider potential risk of fire or explosion; gather information from on-site personnel or other sources; and confine and control the incident. In addition, a command post should be established per the preplanned ICS structure, and safety distances must be defined.

Safety Zones

After the presence of hazardous materials has been confirmed, the scene should be separated into hot, warm, and cold zones. These safety zones should be established and enforced early in the incident (Fig. 7-6).

The hot zone is the area of the incident that includes the hazardous material and any surrounding area that may be exposed to gases, vapors, mist, dust, or runoff. All rescue personnel and vehicles should be stationed outside of this zone. Anyone entering this zone must wear appropriate protective clothing, and only specially trained EMS personnel should attempt patient care activities in this area. Some EMS agencies and ICS structures refer to the hot zone as a *restricted area* or *red zone.*

The warm zone is a larger area that surrounds the hot zone. Although protective clothing is required, it is usually considered a safer environ-

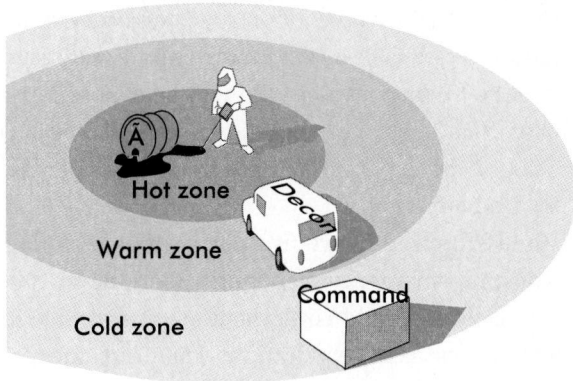

Fig. 7-6 Safety zones for hazardous materials incident.

ment for workers. However, if the hot zone becomes unstable, the warm zone may be exposed to the hazardous materials. It is in this zone that most EMS activities, such as decontamination and patient care procedures, will be performed. Some agencies refer to this zone as a *limited-access* or *yellow zone*.

The cold zone is the area that encompasses the warm zone. It is also restricted to emergency personnel. This area is usually considered safe, requiring only minimal protective clothing. This area contains the command post and other support agencies necessary to control the incident. The cold zone is referred to by some agencies as a *support* or *green zone*.

● MEDICAL SURVEILLANCE

The safety of rescue personnel is of prime importance in any emergency event. Situations involving hazardous materials are among the most dangerous. Therefore a medical surveillance program should be part of any EMS/HAZMAT system and all hazardous materials incidents.

OSHA established the requirement of medical examinations for members of HAZMAT response teams and employees who may have been exposed to hazardous substances during an emergency event. Other components of a HAZMAT medical surveillance program may include any needed medical care, medical monitoring during a hazardous material incident, record-keeping, and periodic evaluation of the surveillance program.

Medical monitoring should include assessment protocols that involve a "presuit" medical examination to establish health history and a vital sign baseline for any rescuer who will be exposed to a hazardous substance. Individuals should be advised of the expected symptoms of illness or exposure before entry.

In addition to injury from hazardous materials exposure, emergency responders working in protective clothing and equipment are susceptible to heat illness and dehydration. Therefore the parameters of the presuit evaluation should include the following:

- Temperature, pulse, respiration, and blood pressure measurements
- Cardiac rhythm
- Weight
- Cognitive and motor skills
- Hydration

After entry into the hazardous environment, medical monitoring should include an assessment of the amount of time a rescuer has been in protective clothing. Rescuers should be observed for any signs of heat-related illness or exposure. If illness or injury is detected at any time during the operation, the rescuer should be removed from the hostile environment for appropriate medical treatment.

After the incident, rescue personnel should be reevaluated using the same parameters as in the presuit examination. This postentry examination determines the rescuer's capability to reenter the operation if needed.

● EMERGENCY MANAGEMENT OF CONTAMINATED PATIENTS

Patient care activities, triage, and evacuation should be a part of a preplanned incident command system structure. Because of the time involved in identifying specific hazardous substances, rescue efforts, decontamination, and possible evacuation, timely treatment of toxic exposures is very important. Some EMS and HAZMAT systems carry antidotes designed for field use in treating chemical exposures. These seven guidelines are general and should not supersede any organizational approach in scene management of hazardous materials incidents or treatment recommendations for chemical exposures:

1. The paramedic should not enter a contaminated area or initiate patient care without adequate personal protective equipment and training specific to the incident.
2. Nonambulatory patients should be removed from the hot zone by trained personnel. Removal is usually performed by fire department personnel, specialized HAZMAT teams, or both. Patient care activities in the hot zone should be limited to gross airway

management, spinal immobilization, and hemorrhage control. Decontamination and additional patient care should be initiated in the warm zone.

3. All patients exposed to the hot zone should be considered contaminated. They should be treated as such until properly assessed and decontaminated.

4. Patient care provisions of airway, breathing, and circulatory support should begin as soon as the patient is contacted amd conditions allow. The product-specific information received from HAZMAT agencies regarding rescuer safety when initiating basic life support procedures should be remembered.

5. Intravenous therapy should be administered only with physician direction. This and other invasive procedures may create a direct route for introducing the hazardous materials into the patient.

6. Decontamination procedures should be initiated without undue exposure to the rescuer. EMS providers assisting in decontamination should be well protected with two to three layers of gloves, head coverings, positive-pressure SCBA, gowns, and shoe coverings.

7. When the hazardous material is a dry agent, the agent should be removed by lightly brushing the material from patient surfaces, making sure not to introduce the contaminant into the patient's airway. Cutting or removing clothing often removes the majority of the contaminating material. After the dry agent has been removed, the decontamination should continue as follows:

   a. Wash the patient with copious amounts of water and mild detergent soap, making sure that all water and runoff is contained in the warm zone. Depending on the exposure, additional patient decontamination procedures may be warranted. Special attention should be paid to irrigation of the eyes, hair, ears, underarms, and pubic areas and thorough cleaning of the body creases of the neck, groin, elbows, and knees. Be careful not to abrade the skin, which may promote absorption of the material involved.

   b. Leave all patient clothing, rescuer clothing, and decontamination equipment in the decontamination area. Safely move the patient to the support zone for further triage, treatment, and transport.

It should be noted that the field decontamination procedures described represent only a gross decontamination. The resources required for complete decontamination are usually unavailable at the emergency scene. Therefore the patient should be isolated from the environment to contain any contamination that has been missed during these procedures. This is accomplished by placing the patient in a body bag to the neck and covering the patient's hair. In the absence of body bags, the victim may be packaged for transport by folding one side of a sheet or blanket over the patient and using the other side to overlap and package the patient. If necessary, the patient's arm may be exposed through an opening in the sheet for vital sign assessment and fluid and drug administration.

Preparing the Ambulance For Patient Transfer

Contamination of ambulances and equipment can be minimized by preparing the vehicle before transporting a contaminated patient. These protective measures include removing all items from cabinets that will be required for patient use and taping all cabinets and doors shut to prevent contaminants from entering. The inner surface of the ambulance should be draped with plastic sheeting.

On arrival at the hospital, the EMS crew should follow the hospital's decontamination protocols. The EMS crew should not return to regular service until rescue personnel, vehicle, and equipment have been monitored for the presence of contamination. Equipment decontamination should follow the recommendations of local, state, and federal authorities, or medical control standard operating procedures. Although specific solutions may be required for a particular hazardous materials exposure, most equipment can be adequately cleaned and made ready for use with soap and water.

● DECONTAMINATION OF RESCUE PERSONNEL AND EQUIPMENT

Ten steps are recommended for proper decontamination at a hazardous materials incident[6]:

1. An entry point where "dirty" personnel and equipment are set up to start the process. Outer gloves and boots are removed and placed in a receptacle.
2. Gross surface contamination are removed generally by washing with copious amounts of water.
3. Contaminated breathing apparatus is removed for personnel who must reenter the dirty area; at this step, they will receive clean breathing apparatus.
4. Protective clothing is removed and handled (store, decontaminated) as required.
5. Other clothing is removed. This step depends on the seriousness of the hazardous materials involved.
6. Personnel wash their bodies using overhead showers. Usually two washings are required.
7. Personnel dry and receive new or clean, noncontaminated clothing.
8. Personnel going through the decontamination system receive medical evaluation.
9. Medical evaluation continues at a medical facility.
10. The decontamination site is cleaned up and materials are properly disposed of.

In addition, the following safety precautions should be followed by any rescuer exposed to hazardous materials:

- Do not touch your face, mouth, nose, or genital area before full body decontamination.
- Shower thoroughly with warm water, surgical soap, sponge, and brush; pay particular attention to hair, body orifices, and any body parts that come in contact with each other (arms and chest, thighs, fingers, toes, and buttocks). Repeat shower and rinse.
- Shampoo hair several times, and rinse thoroughly.
- Avoid shaving, which might introduce contaminated material through the skin.
- Use clean drying towels after each shower.

Care and Maintenance of Clothing and Equipment

After the hazardous materials incident, the rescuer should take the following precautions:

- Properly dispose of any protective clothing that has been torn or worn through.
- Properly and thoroughly clean all clothing and equipment to avoid the possibility of chemical reactions at future incidents and to lessen the potential for chronic exposure to absorbed chemicals. Some hazardous materials produce chemical degradation or permeation of protective clothing and equipment. Therefore product compatibility tables should be evaluated during the decontamination procedure. Decontamination provides no assurance that protective clothing is clean or that the process of chemical permeation has stopped.
- Do not wash or dispose of clothing or equipment at home to avoid exposing family members and contaminating home articles.
- Follow all local codes and laws regarding disposal or decontamination of equipment and clothing.
- Carefully maintain personal SCBA.

● RADIATION HAZARDS

The most common radiation accidents involve sealed radioactive sources used in industrial radiography and nondestructive testing. Victims of these types of accidents rarely require emergency care. However, EMS personnel may frequently be summoned to building fires and transportation accidents involving radioactive materials, so an understanding of the potential hazards of radiation exposure is important.

Characteristics of Radioactive Particles

Radioactive particles are generally classified into three types: alpha, beta, and gamma. Alpha particles are large, travel only a few millimeters, and have minimal penetrating ability. They may be stopped by paper, clothing, or skin and are considered the least dangerous external radiation source. If alpha particles enter the body through inhalation, ingestion, or absorption, however, they can damage internal organs and interfere with the body's chemical functions. Internal exposure to alpha radiation is considered to be the most dangerous form of internal radiation exposure.

Beta particles are 1/7000 the size of alpha particles but have considerably more energy and penetrating power. Beta particles can penetrate subcutaneous tissue and usually enter the body through damaged skin, ingestion, or inhalation. Protection from alpha and beta radiation requires full protective clothing, including a positive-pressure SCBA.

Gamma rays and x-rays are the most dangerous forms of penetrating radiation, requiring lead shields for protection. Gamma rays have 10,000 times the penetrating power of alpha particles and 100 times the penetrating power of beta particles. Protective clothing does not stop gamma rays. Gamma rays constitute both internal and external hazards and may produce localized skin burns and extensive internal damage.

Harmful Effects from Radiation Exposure

Radiation may be classified as nonionizing and ionizing. Nonionizing radiation includes radio waves and microwaves and is not usually considered dangerous. Ionizing radiation is produced by nuclear weapons, reactors, radioactive material, and x-ray machines. Although it is rare, the exposure to ionizing radiation poses a threat to rescue personnel.

The amount of emitted radiation is expressed in roentgens and indicates the ionization produced in the air by gamma or x-radiation. Other units used to measure radiation are the rad (radiation absorbed dose), and the rem (roentgen equivalent man). A rad is a measure of both the amount of ionized radiation being emitted and the amount that has been absorbed and is active within the body tissues. A rem is used to assess the biological effects of the different types of radiation. For emergency purposes, rescue personnel should assume that 1 roentgen = 1 rad = 1 rem.

Doses of less than 100 rem usually do not cause significant acute problems. Doses from 100 to 200 rem may cause symptoms, but are not life threatening. When an exposure of 200 rem is approached, nausea, vomiting, and diarrhea begin within 2 to 4 hours. After an exposure of 450 rems, 50% mortality can be expected within 30 days if no medical care is given. Guidelines for emergency personnel recommend accumulation of not more than 25 rem in general emergency situations and not more than 100 rem to save a life.[7]

Types of Radiation Injury

Victims of radiation accidents rarely show immediate signs or symptoms of exposure. Therefore all victims of possible exposure should be presumed to have a radiation injury until proved otherwise. The harmful effects from radiation may be classified as external irradiation, contamination by radioactive materials, incorporation of radioactive materials, and combined radiation injury.

> **NOTE:**
> An object or a person who has been exposed to radiation is not "radioactive." It is only the *presence* of radioactive residue that poses a threat to rescuers.

External irradiation occurs when all or part of the body is exposed to penetrating radiation from an external source. An example of external irradiation is a medical x-ray. The degree of radiation injury depends on the intensity of radiation, which in turn depends on the duration of exposure and the distance from the source. A patient who has been exposed to large amounts of radiation may have nausea, vomiting, and diarrhea. In severe cases, additional symptoms may include weight loss, hair loss, fever, bleeding, mouth and throat sores, skin burns, lowered body resistance, vesiculation, and ulceration. The effects from this type of radiation are not contagious, and providing emergency care poses no risks to the rescuer.

Contamination occurs when radioactive materials in the form of gases, liquids, or solids are released into the environment, contaminating people internally, externally, or both. When radioactive material remains on the patient's clothing or skin or in open wounds, a potential hazard is present for both the rescuer and the patient. Patients who have been contaminated should be considered medical emergencies and may pose significant risk to emergency providers.

Incorporation refers to the uptake of radioactive materials by body cells, tissues, and target organs such as bone, liver, thyroid, or kidney. Incorporation is impossible unless contamination has occurred.

A combination radiation injury involves external irradiation, contamination, incorporation, or some combination of these. This type of exposure is usually the result of a major incident and may be complicated by a patient's physical injury.

After exposure to radiation, individuals may be at risk for delayed complications, which include cell and chromosomal changes, subsequent reproductive genetic aberrations, cell death, and sterility. In addition, diseases such as anemia and various forms of cancer may develop.

Emergency Response to Radiation Accidents

If the EMS crew has been advised that radioactive materials are present at an emergency scene, they should approach the site with caution. Rescue personnel, emergency vehicles, and the command post should be positioned 200 to 300 feet upwind of the site. Emergency workers should not eat, drink, or smoke at the accident site or in any rescue vehicle. The appropriate local authorities should be contacted (state radiological health office, local specialists), and medical direction should be notified. Protective clothing suitable for other hazardous material releases should be worn by all emergency workers. SCBAs should be used if fire, smoke, or gas is present.

Personal Protection From Radiation

The Federal Emergency Management Agency recommends that basic radiation protection for both the rescuer and the patient include four factors[7]:

1. Time: The less time spent in a radiation field, the less radiation exposure. If adequate personnel are available, a rotating team approach can be used to keep individual radiation exposure to a minimum.

2. Distance: The farther a person from the source of radiation, the lower the radiation dose. Even moving several feet away from a radioactive source greatly reduces the level of exposure.

3. Shielding: The general principle of shielding is that the denser the material, the greater its ability to stop the passage of radiation. Lead shields provide the best protection from exposure. However, vehicles, mounds of dirt, and pieces of heavy equipment placed between the radiation source and the rescuer and victim and the radiation source can also diminish exposure levels. Protective clothing and SCBAs may provide adequate protection from all alpha and some beta radiation, but protective clothing does not prevent penetration of gamma rays. If adequate shielding is not readily available, rescuers should use the time and distance factors to reduce radiation exposure.

4. Quantity: Limiting the amount of radioactive material in a specific area lessens the radiation exposure. Examples include removing contaminated clothing, bagging all contaminated items, and moving containers of radioactive material from the area.

Emergency Care for Victims of Radiation Accidents

As previously stated, patients who have been irradiated are not radioactive. However, when external contamination occurs and radioactive material remains on the patient's clothing and skin or in open wounds, the rescuer should consult with medical direction and follow agency protocol.

With the exception of dealing with contaminants and containing their spread, there are no emergency care procedures specific to radiation injury. All external bleeding should be controlled, the spine immobilized, open wounds covered, and fractures stabilized in normal fashion. The EMS crew should move the patient away from the radiation source as soon as possible. Lifesaving care should not be delayed for patient transfer or decontamination procedures.

Intravenous fluid replacement should be initiated if indicated, using every possible aseptic technique. If an intravenous line is not needed for specific therapy, its use should be avoided because of the possibility of introducing contaminants into the body.

The presence of radiation does not interfere with rescue or extrication equipment and does not influence the extinguishing properties of firefighting products. If nuclear fuels, waste fuels, or nuclear weapons are involved, it is best to let them burn. The contamination at the site may be too high to justify entry. The area should be isolated to 3000 feet or more, especially downwind. State and federal radiological response authorities should be notified.

Radiation Decontamination Procedures

Radiation emergencies involving patients may be defined as either clean, meaning that the patient was exposed but not contaminated, or dirty, meaning that the patient was contaminated. Only properly trained personnel (for example,

HAZMAT teams and qualified county, state, or federal health department personnel) should attempt to decontaminate radiation victims at the scene. If the patient is to be transported to a hospital for decontamination, he or she should be isolated from the environment as previously described, and all patient effects should be transported with the patient.

REFERENCES

1. *Code of federal regulations*, 49 CFR, 173.500, parts 100-177, Washington, DC, 1981, Office of the Federal Register, National Archives and Records Service, General Services Administration.
2. Environmental Protection Agency: *Title III list of lists*, EPA 560/4-90-011, Washington, DC, 1990, US Government Printing Office.
3. Noll G, Hildebrand M, Yvorra J: *Hazardous materials: managing the incident*, Stillwater, Okla, 1988, Fire Protection Publications.
4. *Hazardous materials for first responders*, ed 1, Stillwater, Okla, 1988, Fire Protection Publications.
5. US Department of Transportation: *Emergency response guidebook*, Washington, DC, 1990, The Department.
6. Stutz D, Janusz S: *Hazardous materials injuries: a handbook for pre-hospital care*, ed 2, Beltsville, Md, 1988, Bradford Communications.
7. Ricks R: *Prehospital management of radiation accidents*, Oak Ridge, Ill, 1984, Oak Ridge Associated Universities.

Summary

Hazardous materials are a serious concern to all emergency responders. Successful management of a hazardous materials incident requires training, preplanning, interagency cooperation, and consideration of personal safety.

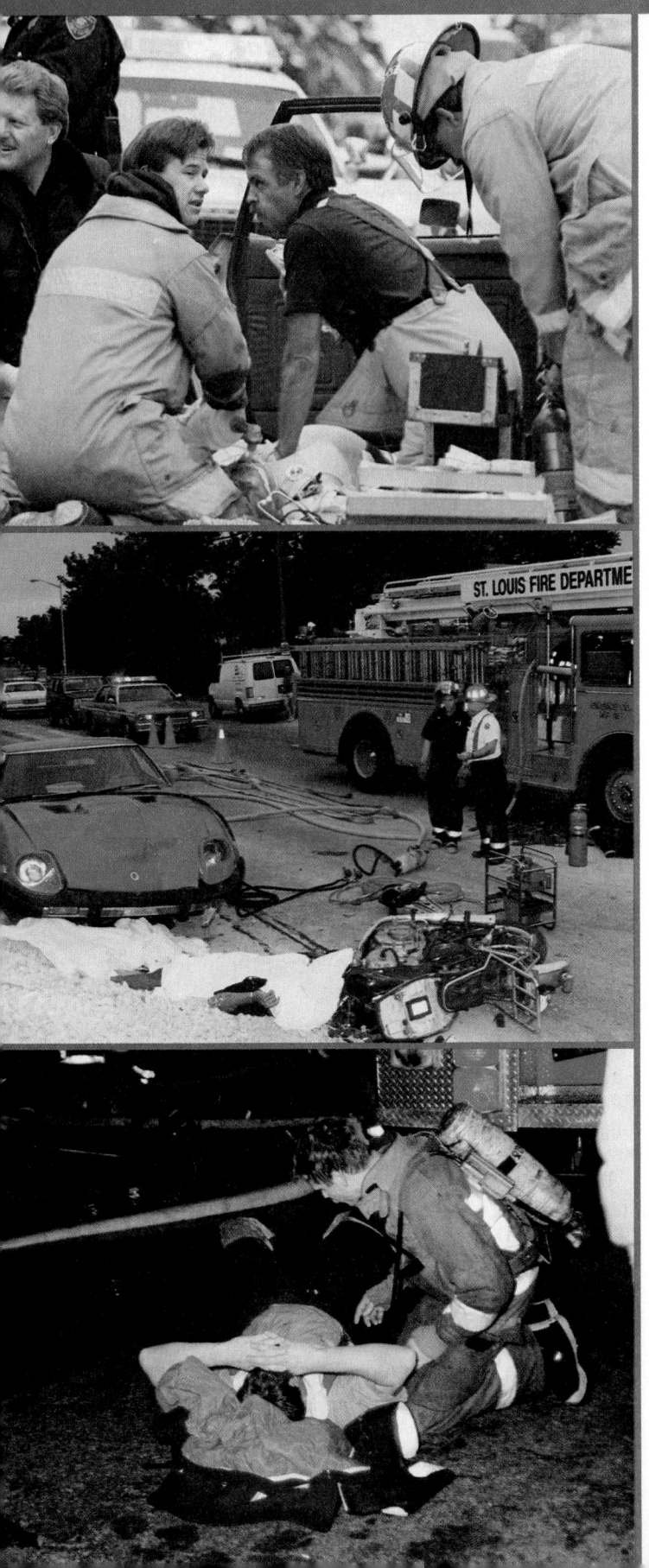

Emergency personnel are frequently exposed to stressful situations and are therefore vulnerable to acute and chronic stress-related disorders. These may involve mental or physical dysfunction or illness. Knowing the causes, signs and symptoms, and management strategies for stress disorders is essential for early recognition and healthy intervention.

As a paramedic, you should be able to:

1. Define *stress* and outline the three phases of the stress response.
2. Define *anxiety*.
3. Differentiate between normal and detrimental reactions to anxiety and stress.
4. Describe the paramedic's management of patients, family members, and bystanders who are encountering a stressful situation.
5. List situations that may provoke job stress for the paramedic.
6. List stress-management techniques.
7. Identify various defense mechanisms.
8. Recognize the five stages of grief that a patient or significant other may experience during death or dying, as described by Dr. Elizabeth Kübler-Ross.
9. Describe appropriate ways to help the patient, family, or significant other deal with a situation in which death is imminent or has occurred.
10. Describe the special needs of children related to their understanding of death and dying.

● STRESS

The term **stress** was coined in its medical usage by Austrian-born Hans Selye, a professor at the University of Montreal, who published a book by that title in 1950.[1] Dr. Selye's studies described body reactions to all types of severe injury, disease, and excessive stimulation or unusual work demands. He noted that in addition to "specific" physical changes in the body, such as a bruise from an injury or the rash from measles, there were also "nonspecific" reactions that increased the body's ability to adapt and reestablish normalcy. Dr. Selye termed these nonspecific reactions *stress*.

A variety of sources can produce stress in EMS. Environmental stress includes such factors as siren noise, inclement weather conditions, confined work spaces, poor scene lighting, spectators, rapid response to the scene, and life-and-death decision making. Psychosocial stress arises from family relationships, conflicts with coworkers, abusive patients, and similar sources. Personality stress is the human element that relates to the way individuals think and feel (for example, the need to be liked, personal expectations, and feelings of guilt and anxiety).

Each person has unique capabilities to deal with stressful situations. Individual reactions to stress

KEY TERMS

anxiety: A state or feeling of apprehension, uneasiness, agitation, uncertainty, and fear resulting from the anticipation of some threat or danger.

autonomic nervous system (ANS): The part of the nervous system that regulates involuntary vital function, including the activity of cardiac muscle, smooth muscle, and glands, and that is subdivided into sympathetic and parasympathetic divisions.

defense mechanism: An unconscious, intrapsychic reaction that offers protection to the self from a stressful situation.

stress: A nonspecific mental or physical strain caused by any emotional, physical, social, economic, or other factor that initiates a physiological response.

stressor: Any factor that causes wear and tear on the body's physical or mental resources.

are "customized" based on previous exposure to a specific type of stress, perception of the stressful event, experience, and personal coping skills. The response to these stresses may be physical, emotional, or both.

Alarm Reaction, the Body's Response to Stress

The human body can quickly prepare itself to do battle or run from danger. This "fight or flight" phenomenon occurs when any emergency situa-

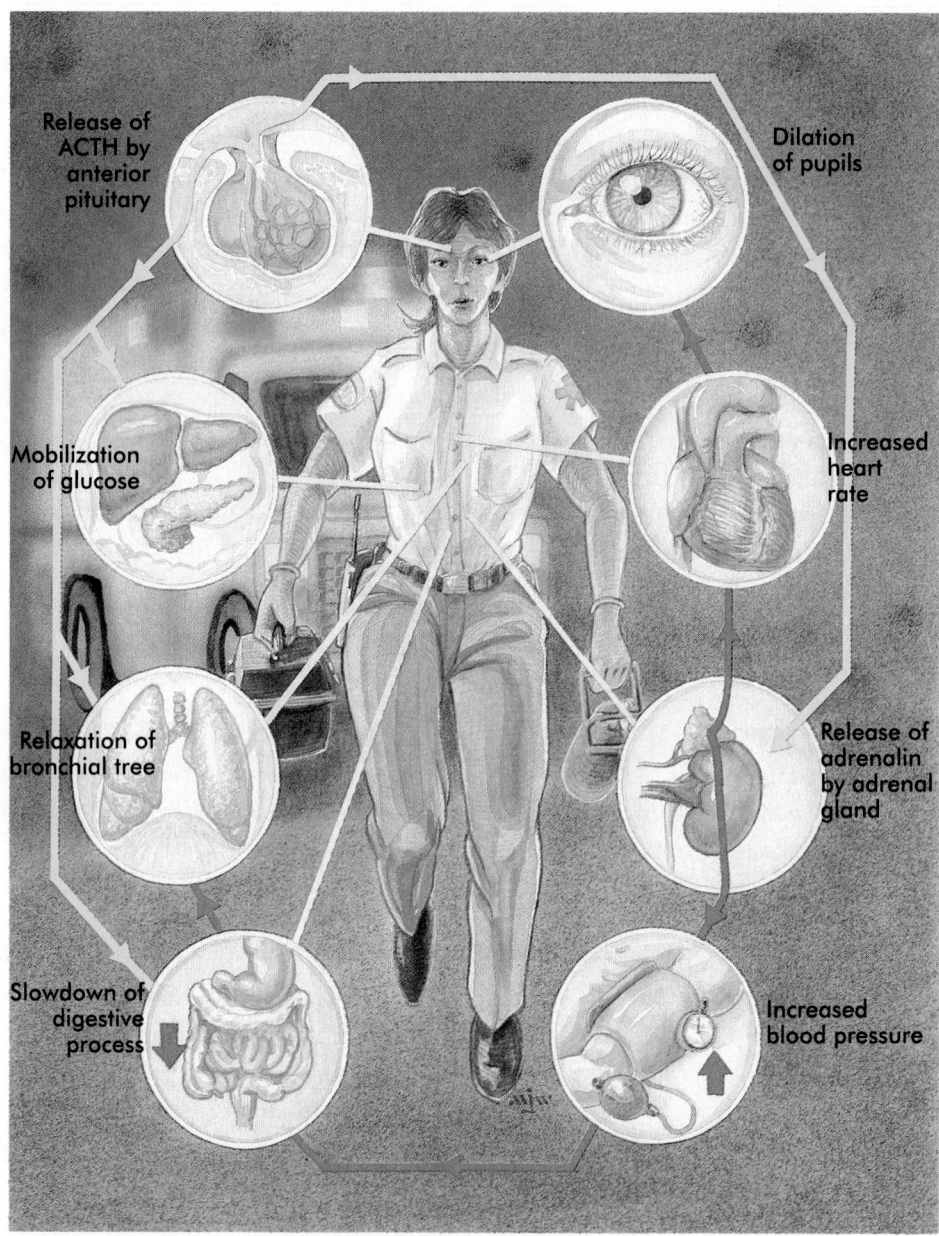

Fig. 8-1 Physiological response to stress. During the alarm reaction, the release of adrenocorticotropic hormone *(yellow)* results in a sympathetic discharge of adrenalin *(red)*. These "stress hormones" stimulate glucose production and cause the heart rate to increase, blood pressure to rise, and pupils to dilate. The bronchial tree relaxes for deep breathing, the digestive process slows, and there is a shift of the blood supply to accommodate clotting mechanisms in case the body is wounded.

tion threatens the individual's safety or comfort. This reaction is considered positive in that it prepares one to be alert and to defend oneself.

Initially, the body's response to stress is unaffected by the type of situation being faced. It reacts equally to events that are pleasant or unpleasant, dangerous or exciting, happy or sad. The purpose of the response is to achieve top physical condition to cope with the event. Examples would be an argument with a co-worker, performing an unfamiliar patient care procedure, and participating in the delivery of a healthy infant.

The alarm reaction is mediated by the **autonomic nervous system (ANS)** and coordinated by the hypothalamus. The hypothalamus triggers the pituitary gland to release adrenocorticotropic hormone (ACTH) into the blood stream. These "stress hormones" stimulate glucose production and increase the blood's concentration of energy-providing nutrients necessary for the response to stress. ACTH also activates the adrenal glands for an intense sympathetic discharge of adrenalin and noradrenalin, which cause heart rate to increase, blood pressure to rise, and the pupils of the eyes to dilate, thereby improving vision. This combination of hormones relaxes the bronchial tree for deeper breathing, increases blood sugar for maximal energy, slows the digestive process, and shifts blood supply to accommodate the clotting mechanism in case the body is wounded. After these physiological events, the body becomes ready for an emergency (fight or flight) and can perform feats of strength and endurance far beyond its normal capacity (Fig. 8-1).

The alarm reaction takes only seconds and occurs to some extent at the body's first exposure to a **stressor.** When the body realizes that a particular event is not dangerous or does not require the alarm reaction, the response stops. The individual begins to adapt to the situation, and bodily functions return to normal.

Stages of Resistance

One of Selye's findings was that the stress response raises the level of resistance to the agent that provoked it and others like it. That is, if a particular stress persists long enough, an individual's reactions change. As the paramedic becomes accustomed to responding to emergency scenes in an ambulance using lights and sirens, for example, the alarm reaction that once occurred is no longer elicited.

Stages of Exhaustion

Initially, the resistance to the stress appears to be above normal, but over time, this coping mechanism becomes exhausted. The EMS provider may appear to be unaffected by the stress of life-threatening emergencies, for example, when in fact all adaptive resources have been used to reach this stage of resistance. Resistance to other types of stress tends to decline as well, and the body may become susceptible to physical and psychological ills. Dr. Selye called this response the *general adaption syndrome* to describe the attempt of body and mind to deal with stressful events (Fig. 8-2).[1]

When individuals are no longer capable of resisting stress, they enter the exhaustion stage in which resistance diminishes and physical and

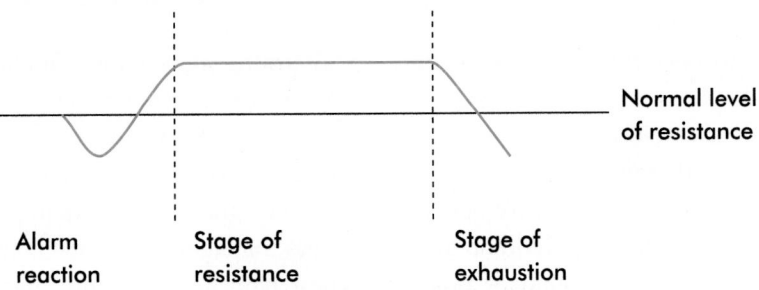

Normal level
of resistance

Alarm reaction | Stage of resistance | Stage of exhaustion

Fig. 8-2 General adaption curve.

psychological activity return to the nonemergency state that existed before the crisis. Rest and recovery follow the exhaustion stage, after which the individual is ready for another "emergency." Some believe that recurrent alarm reactions to chronic stress may lead to "diseases of adaption" such as heart disease, ulcers, hypertension, and renal disease. Sweating, vomiting, hives, and asthma have all been attributed to illness originating from stress.

● ANXIETY

Anxiety is a common symptom of stress and may be defined as "generalized feelings of apprehension."[2] The consequences of anxiety are influenced by the individual's personal perception of the event and each person's internal process of coping with stressful situations.

Sources of anxiety may be internal or external. Internal sources of anxiety may result from conflicts in personal expectations and motivations (for example, an individual who is unhappy with his or her career choice). External sources of anxiety usually involve people and events surrounding the individual. Conflicts with spouses, supervisors, and co-workers are examples of external sources of anxiety.

Feeling anxious in certain situations or unusual circumstances is considered normal. This response provides a warning system that protects an individual from being overwhelmed by a sudden stimulation and from being helpless in critical situations. Some anxiety is adaptive and helps people react appropriately to and cope with many stressful events. It is this adaptive response to anxiety that prepares the paramedic to make quick, appropriate decisions regarding the emergency and to perform at maximal efficiency.

Anxiety that is not effectively reduced by a solution to the conflict or frustration may lead to decreased mental efficiency. Chronic anxiety fails to stimulate coping behavior, and the individual may respond to the conflict by anxious behavior alone. This interferes with thought processes, personal relationships, and work performance. For ex-

ample, a person may develop problems in concentration, lose the ability to trust other people, or become isolated or withdrawn.

Individuals who are frequently exposed to stressful situations or who are unable to cope effectively with stressful events may respond with a chronic state of anxiety. Some of the physical effects of which the individual may be aware follow:

- Heart palpitations
- Difficult or rapid breathing
- Dry mouth
- Chest tightness or pain
- Anorexia (lack or loss of appetite), nausea, vomiting, abdominal cramps, flatulence (excessive air or gas in the stomach or intestinal tract), "butterflies"
- Flushing, diaphoresis, body temperature fluctuation
- Urgency and frequency in urination
- Dysmenorrhea (painful menstruation), decreased sexual drive or performance
- Aching muscles, joints
- Backache, headache

Physical effects that may not be noticeable include the following:

- Increased blood pressure and heart rate
- Blood shunting (diversion of the flow) to muscles
- Increased blood glucose level
- Increased adrenalin production by adrenal glands
- Reduced gastrointestinal peristalsis
- Pupillary dilation

● WARNING SIGNS AND SYMPTOMS OF STRESS

Warning signs of the cumulative nature of stress may be categorized as physical, emotional, cognitive, and behavioral responses.[3] These signals should alert the individual, family members, co-workers, and supervisors to potential problems in stress management. Some warning signs, such as chest pain and difficulty breathing, may require immediate corrective action and medical care; others require less immediate action. Although the presence of one or more warning signs is an indicator of distress, their absence does not preclude the possibility of a stress reaction. Examples of warning signs and symptoms are listed in Box 8-1.

● REACTIONS TO ANXIETY AND STRESS

How those involved in emergency events deal with anxiety depends on past experiences and individual psychological composition. The EMS provider should be aware not only of his or her personal reactions but also of a variety of responses from patients, family members, bystanders, and co-workers. A professional and nonjudgmental attitude in response to these anxiety reactions, combined with a caring and understanding approach, helps make a workable environment.

Patients and family members deserve special consideration as they try to deal with emergency situations. Often, they feel that their lives are out of control, and they may be angry with themselves or others as they try to deal with this loss of control. They may blame themselves for an accident or illness, express feelings of guilt, and be unable to make rational decisions without assistance.

The paramedic should remember that many of these individuals need someone to provide direction. They may require clear instructions regarding what needs to be done and how to do it. Choices and alternatives regarding treatment and medical facilities should be limited and provided at the discretion of the paramedic and medical direction. This form of crisis intervention is an important component of emergency care and is further addressed in Chapter 30.

Bystanders are often involved with an emergency event. They may be passersby who stopped to help or friends and neighbors who have emotional ties to the patient. These people may experience anxiety reactions similar to those of family members. If the bystanders or family members interfere with care or are unable to cope with the event, it will help to have them moved to an area away from patient-care activities. If necessary, law-enforcement assistance should be requested.

No one is immune from the anxiety and stress of emergency situations. Because the paramedic crew has great responsibilities in scene management, it is reasonable to expect that reactions to this anxiety will become evident. The crew may be impatient or short-tempered with one another, and signs of anger or fear may be visible. At times, a crew member may need to leave the environment or collect his or her thoughts before proceeding with emergency care activities. After the call, the paramedic may want to discuss the event with co-workers, a supervisor, or a mental health professional. This communication is positive, and sensitive co-workers can be very helpful in these difficult circumstances.

● PARAMEDIC JOB STRESS

There are many stressors in EMS. Aside from the rigors of providing emergency care and its related stress, other job-related issues must be considered. Examples of these stressors include critically ill and dying patients; pediatric trauma and child abuse; lack of recognition; angry or confused citizens; excessive demands on time, energy, ability, or emotional control; unpredictable changes in work pace; extended periods of time away from family; abusive patients; and dangerous situations. Before choosing a career in EMS, the paramedic must begin to develop an understanding of job-related stress and effective stress management.

Dealing With Job-Related Stress

It has been suggested that certain personalities are attracted to certain types of careers. Many believe that EMS providers, firefighters, police officers, and others in public-safety professions are predisposed to stressful and demanding jobs. However, no personality is immune from potential conflicts in managing stress.

As previously stated, each individual has particular ways to deal with stressful situations. Some coping mechanisms prove beneficial to the individual. For example, many deal with stress by increasing work activity, which results in financial rewards and increased productivity. Other positive coping mechanisms include the ability to find humorous aspects in personal crises and "talking through" stressful situations with family members, friends, and co-workers.

People may also use harmful or negative coping mechanisms. An individual may become withdrawn or use drugs or alcohol. Some have angry outbursts toward family members and co-workers, whereas others may become silent. These negative coping mechanisms threaten interpersonal relationships with co-workers and loved ones and should be considered as signs that an individual is having trouble dealing with stress.

Stress Management

To manage stress effectively, a person must recognize the early warning signs of anxiety that were previously described. Many warning signs appear during the emergency response or within 24 hours after the event. Some responses, however, may be delayed for quite some time and may not appear for months or years after the event. If signs and symptoms of stress-related illness appear, the person should seek appropriate medical or psychological help.

Intervening to alleviate stress is as important as recognizing its warning signals. Stress interventions include awareness of personal limitations; peer counseling and group discussions; proper diet, sleep, and rest; and pursuit of positive activities outside of EMS to balance work and recreation. Although the responsibility for personal health and well-being belongs to the individual, intervention programs may be available through EMS agencies, hospitals, and other groups.

Critical Incident Stress Debriefing

In the early 1970s, the concept of critical incident stress debriefing (CISD) was developed to assist emergency personnel exposed to a major incident. Pioneered by Jeff Mitchell, CISD is based on a partnership of mental health professionals and peer group support. The program is designed to allow emergency workers an opportunity to vent their feelings relating to a particular call or situation that had a powerful emotional impact. Examples include but are not limited to major incidents, death of a coworker on duty, death of a patient as a result of emergency care intervention, the suicide of a co-worker, and the death of children under very tragic circumstances.

CISD helps emergency personnel understand their reactions and reassures them that what they are experiencing is normal and common to most others involved in the incident. The debriefing process may be initiated for a particular individual or may include various members of the emergency team (for example, police, EMS crew members, firefighters, and emergency department staff). CISD also allows for group support and an opportunity to find those who may need short- or long-term therapy. Ideally, CISD teams provide at least 10 basic types of services[3]:

1. Preincident stress training to all personnel
2. On-scene support for obviously distressed personnel
3. Individual consults when only one or two personnel are affected by an incident
4. Defusing services immediately after a large-scale incident
5. Demobilization services after a large-scale incident
6. Formal CISD 24 to 72 hours after an event for any emergency personnel involved in a stressful incident
7. Follow-up services to ensure that personnel are recovering
8. Specialty debriefings to nonemergency groups when no other timely resources are available within the community
9. Support during routine discussions of an incident by emergency personnel
10. Advice to command staff during large-scale events

In addition to CISD, other approaches can help manage stress. These include employee assistance programs, counseling, spouse support programs, family life programs, pastoral services, and periodic stress evaluations. These and other approaches can be valuable resources to the paramedic in understanding and dealing with job-related stress.

● DEFENSE MECHANISMS

Sigmund Freud introduced his theories of psychoanalysis in the 1920s. He believed that conscious thought and behavior accounted for only a small portion of the way individuals react to stressful situations and that most reactions were based on subconscious attempts to lessen stress. These attempts described by Freud and others are known as **defense mechanisms.**

Many authorities believe that subconscious defense mechanisms are constantly used to resolve anxiety and other uncomfortable aspects of daily activity. They are used as a form of self-protection to help the person better adjust to a particular situation. Defense mechanisms common to EMS personnel and other emergency workers include depersonalization (forced emotional estrangement), desensitization (emotional insensitivity), and gallows humor (morbid or cynical humor). Defensive behavior is considered healthy when used to relieve tension or avoid unpleasant emotions but may be overused to a degree that distorts reality.

The *E.M.T. Paramedic National Standard Curriculum* lists the following ten defense mechanisms:

1. Repression. Repression is believed to be the mechanism underlying all other defense mechanisms. Repression is the involuntary attempt to keep certain feelings or memories from reaching conscious awareness. Traumatic events, intolerable and dangerous impulses, and other unacceptable ideas are forced out of consciousness. This defense mechanism may be viewed as a result of an approach-avoidance conflict, which is a conflict between trying to remember or think about something and trying to avoid the topic because it produces fear. Once repressions form, they are usually difficult to abolish. The individual must be reassured that no danger exists in remembering the event. Example: An EMS coworker is killed while working. The partner has no recall of the event from the time they arrived at the scene until after the accident.

2. Regression. Regression is characterized by a return to earlier levels of emotional adjustment. Of all the reactions to anxiety and danger, extreme regression may be the most dramatic and debilitating. The individual returns to an earlier developmental phase of life when tension and conflict could be avoided. Example: A hospitalized patient reduces his self-care responsibilities to those of a child even though still capable of performing care activities.

3. Projection. Projection involves attributing one's own undesirable characteristics, feelings, motives, or desires to someone else. It

may appear as aggression toward others when the problem is actually self-anger. Often, the individual is incorrect in labeling his or her own motives, as well as the motives of others. Example: A paramedic accidentally crashes an emergency vehicle en route to a call. Because of guilt, he feels that others blame him for the accident when in fact he is blaming himself.

4. Rationalization. Rationalizations occur when, as a result of social training, the person feels the need to logically explain his or her behavior because acceptance of the true explanation would provoke anxiety or guilt. The individual is trying to prove that the behavior is "rational" and therefore worthy of the approval of self and others. Rationalization is a commonly used defense mechanism. Example: A paramedic performs a poor secondary assessment on a trauma patient and fails to discover a femur fracture. When questioned by medical direction, she justifies her actions by stating that the police were hurrying her to clear the accident scene.

5. Compensation. Compensation is an attempt to substitute or cover up for a real or imagined weakness by emphasizing a more positive trait, skill, or attribute. Compensatory mechanisms disguise and conceal frustration and consequent anxiety by focusing attention on other behavior. Example: An EMS crew member has weak clinical skills and feels inadequate at emergency scenes. He compensates by becoming an instructor in water rescue.

6. Reaction formation. Reaction formation is a defensive behavior that prevents unacceptable desires from being expressed by exaggerating opposing attitudes and behavior and thereby expressing the opposite of the true motive. The original impulse is still subconsciously present but is masked by actions or attitudes that do not cause anxiety or stress. Example: A paramedic is outwardly friendly to a co-worker whom she dislikes.

7. Sublimation. Sublimation is the modification of unacceptable urges so that they become socially acceptable. It is a form of substitution. Sublimation is considered a defense mechanism, but its functions are believed to extend beyond that of protection. It requires an energy transformation in which instinctual drives are substituted in activities that may produce a higher cultural achievement. Example: An individual with hostile feelings expresses aggression as a literary, music, or art critic.

8. Denial. Denial is a defense mechanism in which elements of reality that would be consciously intolerable are rejected. One is protected from unpleasant reality by refusing to perceive it. There may be denial of the experience itself or the memory of it. Example: An individual who has just lost a loved one may be unable to accept the reality of death. (Denial differs from repression in that an individual who uses repression as a defense mechanism seems to "deliberately" keep his or her feelings or memories at a distance from the conscious mind.)

9. Substitution. This defense mechanism substitutes an alternative activity or goal for an originally desired but unobtainable one. It is similar to another defense mechanism, displacement, and may involve the redirection of an emotion from the original object to a more acceptable substitute object. Substitution often results from frustration. Example: A co-worker is experiencing marital problems and feels that it is unacceptable to argue with his spouse. He substitutes and displaces his anger at work by being irritable and hostile toward other crew members.

10. Isolation. Isolation involves the separation of unacceptable impulses, acts, or ideas from their origin in memory. This defense mechanism removes the emotional charge from the event and prevents feelings from accompanying the memory. Isolation is probably helpful to the EMS providers who must "turn off" feelings until after the emergency call has been completed. Example: An EMS provider who is also a parent renders emergency care to a dying child.

● DEALING WITH DEATH AND DYING

Death and dying will always be part of health care delivery. Even though medical science has given society the ability to postpone death in some instances and perhaps lessen its physical pain, the fight for self-preservation is inevitably lost. This lack of power creates anxiety.

Throughout history, the mystery of death has been at the core of religious systems and philosophical thought. Individual attitudes toward death have been shaped by belief systems, which may include religions that affirm the continuation of a soul or personality. Some believe in the finality of death, others in reincarnation, and still others in a variety of perspectives between these extremes. All belief systems must be respected by health care providers, for this is perhaps the most important factor in the process of dying—the attitudes of the people involved.

Sudden or Anticipated Death

Sudden death is common in prehospital care. It occurs as a result of some cardiac rhythm disturbances, trauma, suicide, and other unexpected causes. EMS providers are prepared for exposure to sudden death. Loved ones and other survivors, however, are not. There is no opportunity to prepare for the event, and the emotional impact can be devastating.

When death has been anticipated for an extended period, the patient and loved ones have had time to prepare themselves. An expected death, however, is sometimes as difficult or more difficult for the survivors as a sudden death. There may have been months and years of serious debilitating illness, physical wasting, psychological changes, and mental deterioration. As family members adjust to their loved one's debilitated state, they may use denial and other defense mechanisms and respond to an anticipated death as they would to a sudden one.

Hospice programs began in England in 1967 and have since become a standard service of many health care institutions in the United States. The purpose of these programs is to help the terminally ill patient, family, and loved ones cope with anticipated death. The hospice philosophy encourages home care for the patient to provide for a more natural environment. In addition, volunteers and health care professionals provide counseling and other psychological support to the patient and family throughout the death process. Hospice programs are well respected in the medical community and play an important role in helping many patients and their families accept death as a natural event in life.

Stages of Grief

In 1968, Elizabeth Kübler-Ross began her work on the psychological aspects of death and dying. Her studies identified five predictable stages of dying, which include denial, anger, bargaining, depression, and acceptance. Kübler-Ross found that patients and loved ones dealing with the death process generally experience the following five stages[4]:

1. Denial, characterized by the feeling "No, not me," is a predictable response to news of a life-threatening illness or situation. The news is so overwhelming that it must be absorbed slowly. The patient seeks other opinions, verifies the accuracy of medical reports, or simply seems to ignore what he or she has been told. Denial is a valuable defense mechanism and is troubling only when there is no indication that the patient understands the seriousness of the situation. Most patients, families, and friends deny death to some degree to continue with the daily business of living.

2. Anger, the "Why me?" phase, is probably the most difficult for persons who care about or are trying to help the dying person. In this phase, all efforts to help or console the person are rejected. This anger is really the anger of the dying person toward all the people who continue to live.

3. Bargaining is reflected in a "Yes, me, but . . ." stance. The reality of being very sick and of probably dying is admitted, but the person tries to bargain for extension or quality of life. These bargains are usually secret, frequently made with God, and rarely kept. For example, a person promises to be a

"perfect patient" if only he or she can live for a son's wedding.

4. Depression is the "Yes, me" reaction to anticipated death. It involves preparing to say and saying goodbye to everything and everyone a person has known and loved. The inherent sadness of this phase is appropriate and should be respected.

5. Acceptance, the simple and quiet "Yes," grows out of a person's conviction that he or she has done what is possible to be ready to die. Personal energy and interpersonal interests decrease significantly. During this phase, relatives and friends usually need more help than the dying person, whose most important wish is not to die alone.

Although paramedics are seldom involved in a particular patient's process of accepting death, they are frequently exposed to the various reactions of patients and families experiencing the death process. For example, denial may be apparent in some family members who do not appear to recognize the seriousness of a situation or acknowledge a situation in which decisions about resuscitation must be made; anger may be directed at the paramedic crew or other health care workers; and bargaining may occur in the form of a mother who says, "Please save my child, and I promise that I'll always make her wear her seat belt!" The paramedic must understand the psychological aspects of the stages of grief.

Patient and Family Needs

Responding crews sometimes find themselves faced with a dying person surrounded by loved ones. In these situations, the emotional needs of the dying patient, family, and loved ones should be of utmost importance to the health care provider. These people often need to be comforted, given privacy, and treated with respect and dignity. Loved ones may need to express feelings of rage, anger, despair, and guilt, and they may need someone to provide control and direction for this solemn event. The role of the paramedic crew in this scenario is important and may be a determining factor in the way survivors adjust to their loss.

It is uncomfortable to be in a situation involving death and dying, and communication with the patient and loved ones is difficult. The following recommendations for communications and activities may help the EMS provider when dealing with dying patients and their families:

- Answer questions for the patient and family, and explain all activities.
- Do not approach the subject of dying; let it come from the patient or family.
- If the patient or family asks you if the patient is going to die, advise that you are doing everything you possibly can but that the situation is critical. This allows a brief time for the patient and family to prepare themselves.
- Do not falsely reassure the patient or family.
- Use compassionate, nonverbal communication (facial expression, touching).
- Offer to contact someone if the patient is alone.
- If family is not present, assure the patient that emergency department personnel will notify them. If they are nearby, encourage them to come to the patient immediately or to meet the patient at the emergency department.
- Allow the family to stay with the patient.

When it is necessary to convey news of a sudden death to family members, the paramedic's initial contact with the family can significantly influence the grief response. The family should be gathered in a private area and advised of the patient's death, with a brief description of the circumstances causing the death. Use the words "death" or "dead," and avoid euphemisms such as "he's passed on," or "she's no longer with us." Be compassionate, and allow time for the news to be absorbed and for questions to be asked. Permit the family to see their relative, and advise them in advance if resuscitation equipment is still connected to the patient. These efforts, combined with empathic communication with the family, help relatives deal with the loss of a loved one.

Special Needs of Children

The way children cope with their own death or the death of a loved one depends on their age, maturity, and understanding of death. The paramedic crew should be particularly sensitive to the emotional needs of children during this crisis. Box 8-2 offers some guidelines for understanding children.[4]

BOX 8-2

Children's and Adolescents' Understanding of Death

Preschoolers (up to age 6)
- View death as temporary and reversible (for example, dead people have "gone to sleep" or "gone away")
- Often are confused about the relationship between illness and death
- May view death as punishment for their own bad thoughts or fulfillment of angry wishes

School-age children (7 to 12 years)
- Begin to realize that death is final and that all living things die
- Feel death happens only to others, never to themselves
- May have nightmares about death

Adolescents (over age 12)
- Understand that death is permanent and irreversible
- Begin to develop and explore personal philosophies of life and death
- Find coping with death especially difficult because they are just beginning to shape their own lives

EMS Provider Needs

It is difficult for anyone to deal with death, and the feelings and emotions of EMS providers must also be considered. The paramedic may experience some of the same stages of grief previously described. These reactions are normal, and a great deal of effort may have to be expended to disguise or suppress these emotions at the scene or while rendering care. However, it is important to discuss these feelings as soon as possible in a constructive way that will lessen the emotional burden.

Other issues related to death and dying may produce additional stress and anxiety for the paramedic crew. Examples include the resuscitation of a terminally ill patient at the request of the family or physician and personal feelings regarding the value and ethics of resuscitation efforts for a patient in a vegetative state. These are sensitive topics and should be addressed through open communication with medical direction.

REFERENCES

1. Selye H: *The stress of life,* New York, 1956, McGraw-Hill.
2. Ruch F, Zimbardo P: *Psychology of life,* ed 8, Glenview, Ill, 1971, Scott, Foresman.
3. Mitchell J, Bray G: *Emergency services stress,* Englewood Cliffs, NJ, 1990, Brady Publishing.
4. Bassuk E, Fox S, Pendergast K: *Behavioral emergencies,* Boston, 1983, Little, Brown.

Summary

Medical and public safety emergencies are stressful events because they often involve fear of the unknown, lack of control, serious illness, and loss of life and property. Important strategies for dealing with EMS-related stress are to recognize the signs and symptoms in the earliest stages and to intervene at the onset of stress-related disorders.

PREPARATORY

DIVISION TWO

IN THIS DIVISION

9 MEDICAL TERMINOLOGY AND THE
   METRIC SYSTEM
10 OVERVIEW OF HUMAN SYSTEMS
11 GENERAL PATIENT ASSESSMENT
12 AIRWAY AND VENTILATION
13 SHOCK
14 EMERGENCY PHARMACOLOGY

People ask, "How do you keep from panicking and do your job?" People fear the unknown or the unfamiliar. I've been provided with knowledge and skills, so I have the confidence to react appropriately during an emergency.

Sherri Gastler, EMT-P
American Medical Transport
Big Springs, Texas

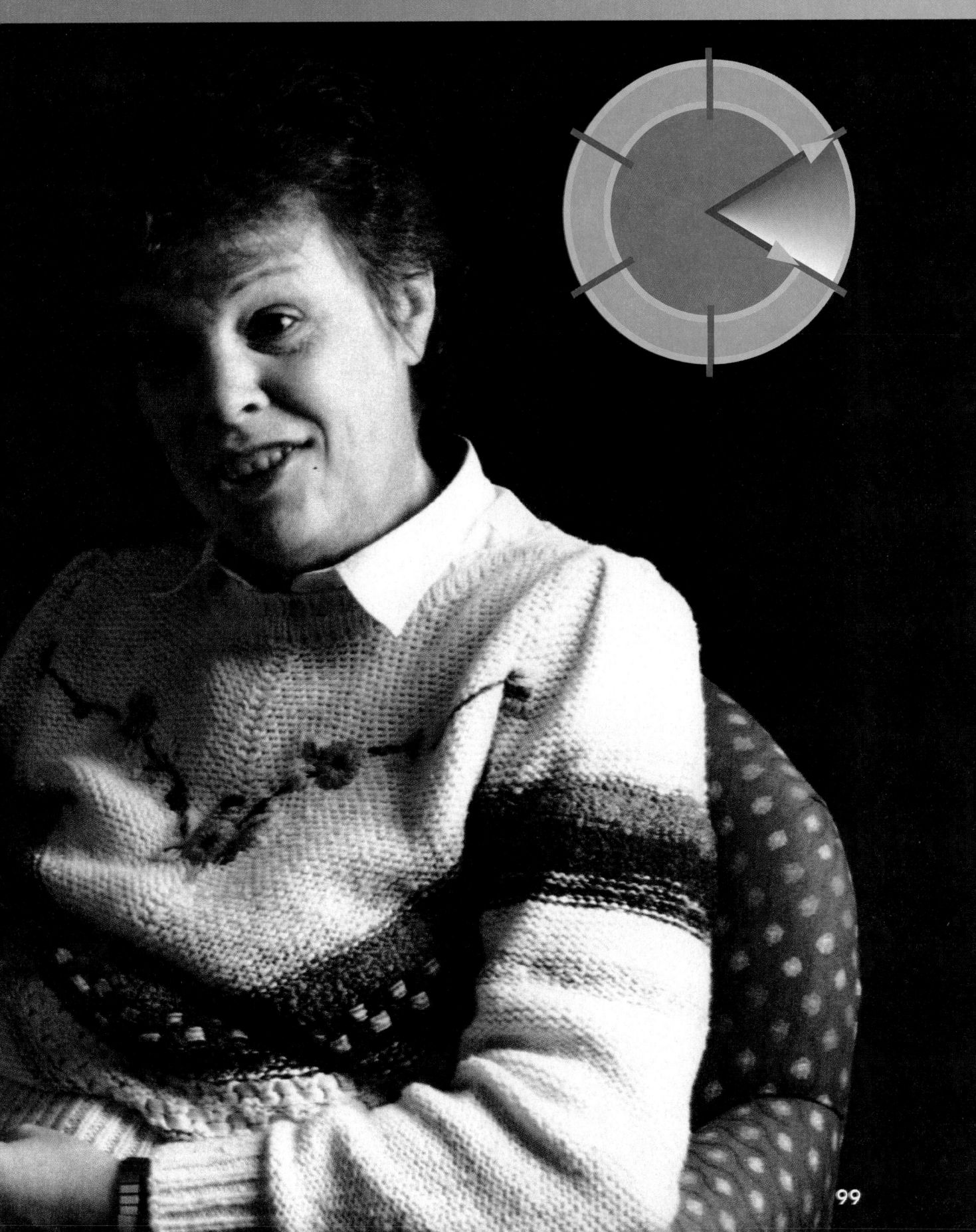

9 MEDICAL TERMINOLOGY AND THE METRIC SYSTEM

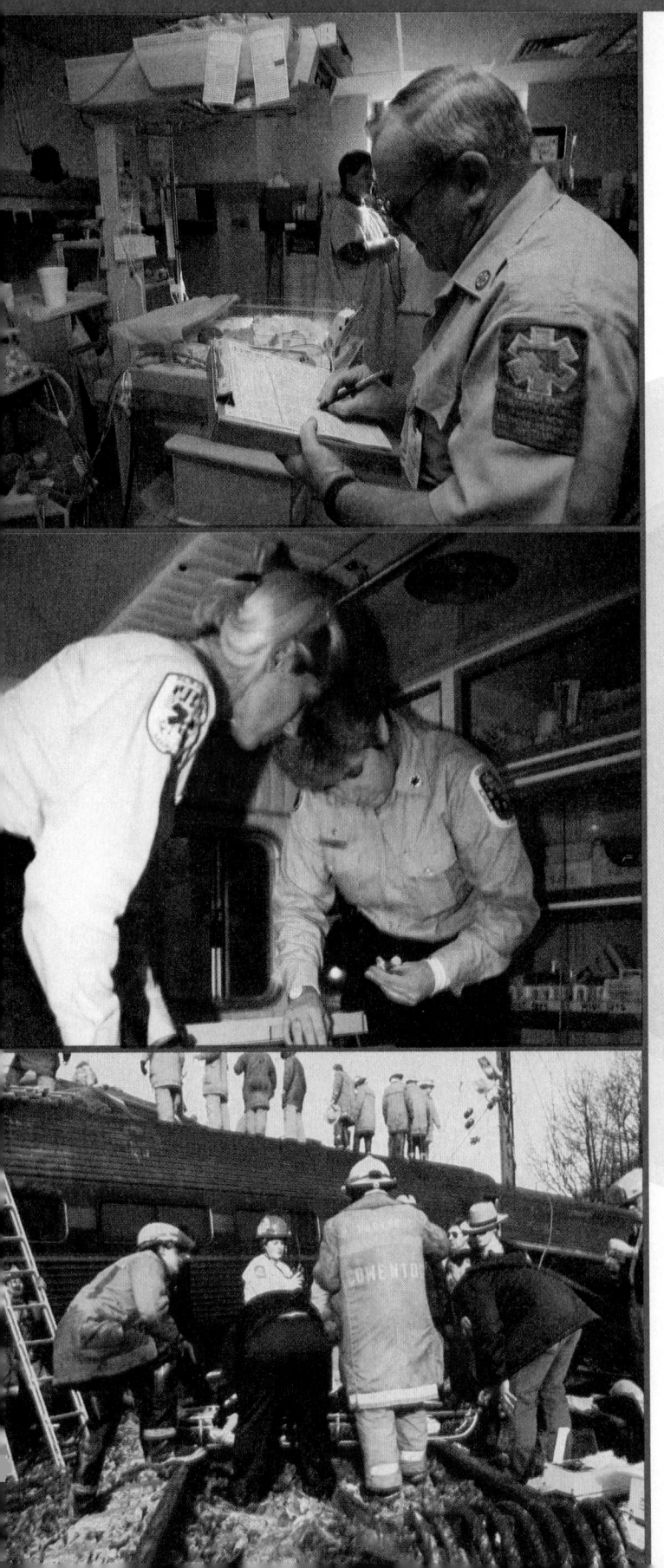

A necessary aspect of providing emergency care is efficient communication with medical control, co-workers, and other health care professionals. This communication may involve conveying patient information, requesting medication orders, and advising medical control of scene activities. Using accepted medical terminology helps bridge the distance between the emergency scene and the emergency department physician or nurse. In addition, medical terminology is universally understood and provides a clear and concise way to document patient care activities. As a member of the health care team, the paramedic must be well versed in the language of medicine.

OBJECTIVES

As a paramedic, you should be able to:
1. Describe the purpose of medical terminology.
2. Identify the function of prefixes, suffixes, and root words as they pertain to medical terminology.
3. Apply and interpret medical terminology based on an understanding of a given list of prefixes, suffixes, and root words.
4. Appropriately document information using accepted medical abbreviations.
5. Document with the metric system, using the current notation and units for a given measurement.

● THE LANGUAGE OF MEDICINE

Most medical terms are derived from Greek, and many have Latin roots. Medical terms are usually composed of a word preceded by a *prefix* (one or more root syllables at the beginning of a word), followed by a *suffix* (one or more root syllables at the end of a word), or both. An understanding of the basic prefixes and suffixes promotes ease of communication with medical terminology.

Prefixes

Prefixes appear at the beginning of a medical word and often describe location and intensity. For example, *abnormal* begins with the prefix *ab,* which means "away from," and is followed by *normal,* which means "within a balance." Therefore *abnormal* describes something that is not within balance. Other common prefixes are listed in Table 9-1.

Suffixes

Suffixes appear at the end of a medical word and often describe the patient's condition or diagnosis. For example, *bronchitis* begins with the root word *bronchi,* which refers to a respiratory structure, and is followed by the suffix *itis,* which means "inflammation." Therefore *bronchitis* would describe inflammation of the patient's bronchi. Other common suffixes are listed in Table 9-2.

Root Words

Root words are medical words that may be combined to describe a particular structure or condition. For example, *cardiopulmonary* begins with a root word *cardio,* which means "heart," and is followed by the root word *pulmonary,* which means "lungs." Therefore *cardiopulmonary* refers to the patient's cardiac and respiratory systems. Other common root words are listed in Table 9-3.

KEY TERMS

gram (g): A metric unit of mass equal to one thousandth of a kilogram.

kilogram (kg): A metric unit of mass equal to 1000 grams or 2.2046 pounds.

liter (l): A metric unit of capacity equal to one cubic decimeter, 61.025 cubic inches, or 1.0567 liquid quarts.

meter (m): A metric unit of length equal to 39.37 inches.

microgram (mcg, μ): A metric unit of mass equal to one millionth of a gram.

milligram (mg): A metric unit of mass equal to one thousandth of a gram.

milliliter (ml): A metric unit of capacity equal to one thousandth of a liter.

TABLE 9-1 Common Prefixes

Prefixes	Meaning	Example
a-, an-	without, lack of	Apnea—without breath Anemia—lack of blood
ad-	to, toward	Adhesion—something stuck to or remaining in close proximity to
angio-	vessel	Angiogram—study of vessels
ante-	before, forward	Antenatal—occurring or formed before birth
anti-	against, opposed to	Antipyretic—against fever
arter-	artery	Arteriogram—study of arteries
arthro-	pertaining to a joint	Arthroscopy—inspection of joint
bi-	two	Bilateral—both sides
bio-	life	Biology—study of life
brady-	slow	Bradycardia—slow heart rate
cardi-	pertaining to the heart	Cardiography—recording the movements of the heart
cerebr-	brain	Cerebral—pertaining to the brain
cerv-	neck	Cervical—pertaining to the neck
chole-	pertaining to bile	Cholelithiasis—stones in the gallbladder
contra-	against, opposite	Contrastimulant—against stimulating
cost-	pertaining to a rib	Costal margin—margin of lower limit of ribs
cyst-	pertaining to the bladder or any fluid-containing sac	Cystitis—inflammation of the urinary bladder
cyt-	cell	Cytology—study of cells
di-	twice, double	Diplopia—double vision
dys-	with difficulty	Dyspnea—difficulty breathing
ecto-	out from	Ectopic—out of place

TABLE 9-2 Common Suffixes

Suffixes	Meaning	Example
-algia	pertains to pain	Neuralgia—pain along a nerve
-centesis	puncturing	Thoracentesis—puncturing of a pleural space
-cyte	cell	Leukocyte—white cell
-ectomy	a cutting out	Tonsillectomy—surgical removal of the tonsils
-emia	blood	Anemia—decrease in blood hemoglobin
-esthesia	sensation	Anesthesia—without sensation
-genic	causing	Carcinogenic—cancer causing
-ology	science of	Psychology—science or study of behavior
-ostomy	creation of an opening	Gastrostomy—artificial opening into the stomach
-osis	condition	Psychosis—condition of the mind
-paresis	weakness	Hemiparesis—one-sided weakness
-phagia	eating	Polyphagia—excessive eating
-pnea	breathing	Dyspnea—difficult breathing
-pathy	disease	Neuropathy—disease of peripheral nerves
-phasia	speech	Aphasia—loss of speech power
-plasty	repair of, tying of	Angioplasty—repair of damaged vessels
-rhythmia	rhythm	Dysrhythmia—variation from a normal rhythm
-rrhagia	bursting forth	Hemorrhage—flowing of blood
-rrhea	flowing	Pyorrhea—discharge of pus
-scopy	examination by inspection	Laparoscopy—examination of the abdominal cavity with a laparoscope
-uria	pertaining to urine	Polyuria—excessive secretion of urine

TABLE 9-3 Common Root Words

Root Words	Meaning	Root Words	Meaning
adeno-	gland	mal-	bad
arter-	artery	menigo-	meninges
arthro-	joint	myo-	muscle
asthenia	weakness	nephro-	kidney
bio-	life	neuro-	nerve
bucc-	cheek	noct-	night
burs-	pouch or sac	oculo-	eye
carc-	cancer	orchi-	testicle
cardio-	heart	osteo-	bone
caut-	to burn	oto-	ear
cephalo-	head	ov-	egg
cerv-	neck	pariet-	wall
chole-	bile	phago-	to eat
chondro-	cartilage	pharyngo-	throat
cysto-	bladder	phlebo-	vein
cyto-	cell	photo-	light
dermo-	skin	pmeumo-	air
edem-	swelling	procto-	rectum
entero-	intestine	pseud-	false
eryth-	red	psych-	mind
eti-	cause	pyo-	pus
febr-	fever	rhino-	nose
flex-	to bend	sclero-	hardness
gastro-	stomach	sept-	wall
glyco-	sugar	somat-	body
gyn-	female	stern-	chest
hemo-	blood	tact-	to touch
hepato-	liver	thoraco-	chest
hydra-	water	uro-	urinary
iod-	distinct	varic-	dilated vein
leuko-	white	vaso-	vessel

● MEDICAL ABBREVIATIONS AND ACRONYMS

Medical abbreviations and acronyms are useful tools for efficient communication and documentation. Communicating and documenting medical information requires thoroughness, precision, and accuracy. Medical abbreviations and acronyms are a form of medical "shorthand" universally understood by other members of the health care team.

Some of the more common medical abbreviations and acronyms are listed in Table 9-4.

NOTE:

Many medical abbreviations and acronyms have common, multiple meanings. For example, the acronym *PE* may be used to describe physical examination, pulmonary edema, or pulmonary embolus. Therefore it is important for every EMS agency or medical control system to approve an abbreviation and acronyms list. This ensures precision in documentation, facilitates patient assessments and patient histories, and may provide for medical-legal protection if cases are reviewed for litigation.

TABLE 9-4 Common Medical Abbreviations and Acronyms

Abbreviation/ Acronym	Meaning	Abbreviation/ Acronym	Meaning
ā	before	L	liter
ALS	advanced life support	Ⓛ	left
AMA	against medical advice	LLQ	left lower quadrant
AMI	acute myocardial infarction	LMP	last menstrual period
AP	anterior-posterior	LOC	level of consciousness, loss of consciousness
ASA	aspirin		
ASHD	atherosclerotic heart disease	LUQ	left upper quadrant
bid	twice a day	mcg, μg	microgram
BLS	basic life support	MCL	modified chest lead
BM	bowel movement	mEq	milliequivalent
BP	blood pressure	mg	milligram
c̄	with	MI	myocardial infarction
Ca	cancer	ml	milliliter
CAD	coronary artery disease	NA	not applicable (available)
cc	cubic centimeter	NG	nasogastric
CC	chief complaint	NKA	no known allergies
CCU	coronary care unit	NPO	nothing by mouth
CHF	congestive heart failure	NTG	nitroglycerin
CNS	central nervous system	N/V	nausea and vomiting
c/o	complains of	O₂	oxygen
CO	carbon monoxide	OB	obstetrics
CO₂	carbon dioxide	OB/GYN	obstetrics/gynecology
COPD	chronic obstructive pulmonary disease	OD	overdose; right eye
		OS	left eye
CPR	cardiopulmonary resuscitation	OU	both eyes
CSF	cerebrospinal fluid	p̄	after
CVA	cerebral vascular accident	PAC	premature atrial contraction
D/C	discontinue	PASG	pneumatic antishock garment
DOA	dead on arrival	PAT	paroxysmal atrial tachycardia
DOE	dyspnea on exertion	PCN	penicillin
DTs	delirium tremens	PE	physical examination, pulmonary edema, pulmonary embolus
Dx	diagnosis		
ECG, EKG	electrocardiogram	PEA	pulseless electrical activity
ED	emergency department	PEARL	pupils equal and reactive to light
ETA	estimated time of arrival	PEEP	positive end expiratory pressure
ETOH	ethyl alcohol	PID	pelvic inflammatory disease
FB	foreign body	PJC	premature junctional contraction
Fx	fracture	PMH	past medical history
GI	gastrointestinal	po	by mouth
g	gram	prn	whenever necessary, as needed
gr	grain	PERL	pupils equal and react to light
GSW	gunshot wound	PROM	premature rupture of membranes
GU	genitourinary	PSVT	paroxysmal supraventricular tachycardia
h, hr	hour		
Hg	mercury	PUD	peptic ulcer disease
HIV	human immunodeficiency virus	PVC	premature ventricular contraction
h/o	history of	q̄	every
Hx	history	qh	every hour
IM	intramuscular	qid	four times each day
IUD	intrauterine device	qtt	drop
IV	intravenous	Ⓡ	right
IVP	IV push	RLQ	right lower quadrant
IVPB	intravenous piggyback	R/O	rule out
JVD	jugular vein destention	ROM	range of motion
kg	kilogram	RUQ	right upper quadrant
KVO	keep vein open	Rx	treatment

TABLE 9-4 Common Medical Abbreviations and Acronyms—cont'd

Abbreviation/ Acronym	Meaning
s̄	without
SIDS	sudden infant death syndrome
SQ	subcutaneous
SL	sublingual
stat	immediately
STD	sexually transmitted disease
SVT	supraventricular tachycadia
TB	tuberculosis
TIA	transient ischemic attack
tid	three times each day
TKO	to keep open
URTI	upper respiratory tract infection
UTI	urinary tract infection
μ	micro
VD	venereal disease
VF	ventricular fibrillation
VT	ventricular tachycardia
WNL	within normal limits
yo	year old
♂	male
♀	female
↑	increasing
↓	decreasing
Δ	change
+	plus-positive
−	minus-negative
±	plus or minus; indefinite, either positive or negative
#	number; pounds
=	equals
≠	not equal to
@	at
%	percentage
°	degree
>	greater than
<	less than

TABLE 9-5 Common Metric Prefixes

Prefix	Meaning
kilo-	1000 times greater
deci-	10 times less
centi-	100 times less
milli-	1000 times less
micro-	1,000,000 times less

● THE METRIC SYSTEM

The metric system of weights and measures was developed by the French in the latter part of the eighteenth century and was declared by Congress to be the official measurement system in the United States in 1866.[1] Although the use of the metric system in the United States is not mandatory, it has been adopted by the medical sciences and pharmacies, in weighing currency at the federal mints, and in the armed forces.

The metric system was originally proposed as a uniform decimal system, with its basic unit derived through a survey of the earth's dimensions. The word *metric* was taken from the basic measure of length of a meter (one ten-millionth of the distance along any meridian from the North Pole to the equator). The updated metric system (1961) is based on the wavelength of light of krypton-86 and on the mass of a cylinder of platinum-iridium alloy. This system became known as the *International System of Units*, abbreviated *SI* for the French name, *Système International d'Unites*. To date, approximately 92% of the countries of the world use the SI system.

Definitions of Units

The basic metric units of measurement are the meter, the liter, and the gram. The meter is the unit for linear measurement, the liter for capacity or volume, and the gram for weight. A meter is slightly longer than a yard; a liter, slightly more than a quart; and a gram, slightly more than the weight of a steel paper clip.

The basic units of the metric system can be divided or multiplied by 10, 100, or 1000 parts to form secondary units that differ from each other by 10 or some multiple of 10. Subdivisions of these basic units are made by moving the decimal point to the left, and multiples of the basic unit are indicated by moving the decimal point to the right. The names of the secondary units are formed by joining Greek or Latin prefixes to the primary unit (Table 9-5).

The **meter (m)** is the unit from which the other metric units are derived (Fig. 9-1). Centimeters

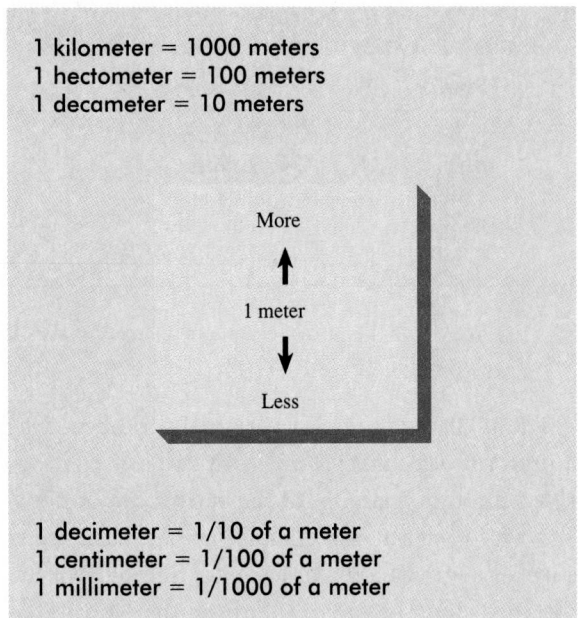

1 kilometer = 1000 meters
1 hectometer = 100 meters
1 decameter = 10 meters

More

↑

1 meter

↓

Less

1 decimeter = 1/10 of a meter
1 centimeter = 1/100 of a meter
1 millimeter = 1/1000 of a meter

Fig. 9-1 The meter for measuring length.

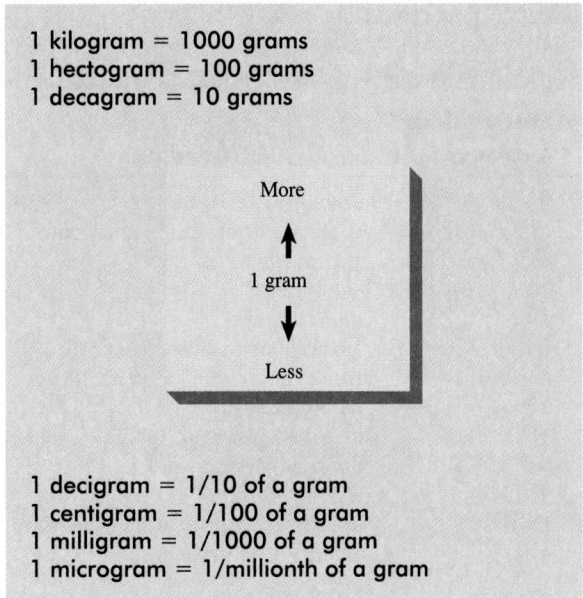

1 kilogram = 1000 grams
1 hectogram = 100 grams
1 decagram = 10 grams

More

↑

1 gram

↓

Less

1 decigram = 1/10 of a gram
1 centigram = 1/100 of a gram
1 milligram = 1/1000 of a gram
1 microgram = 1/millionth of a gram

Fig. 9-3 The gram for measuring weight.

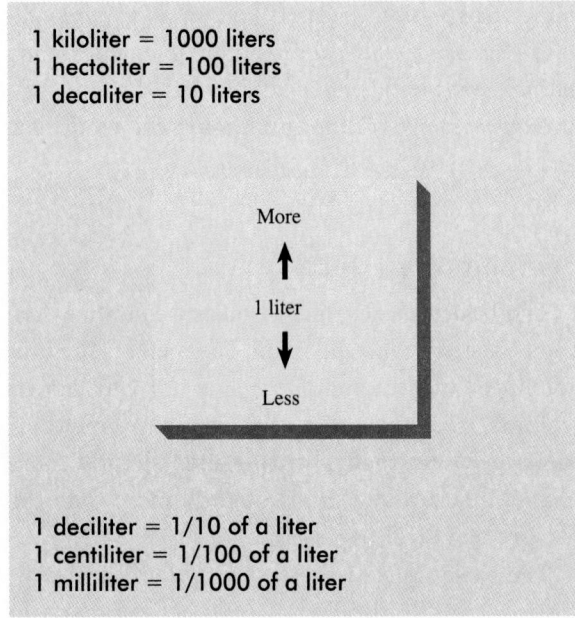

1 kiloliter = 1000 liters
1 hectoliter = 100 liters
1 decaliter = 10 liters

More

↑

1 liter

↓

Less

1 deciliter = 1/10 of a liter
1 centiliter = 1/100 of a liter
1 milliliter = 1/1000 of a liter

Fig. 9-2 The liter for measuring capacity.

(cm) and millimeters (mm) are the primary linear measurements used in medicine. They are used, for example, to measure the size of body organs and to measure blood pressure.

The **liter (L)** is the unit of capacity or volume (Fig. 9-2). Fractional parts of a liter are expressed in **milliliters (ml)** or cubic centimeters (cc). The liter is equal to approximately 1000 ml or 1000 cc. The National Bureau of Standards recommends that the abbreviation *ml* or *mL* be used to express fractional parts of a liter.

The **gram (g)** is the metric unit of weight used in weighing drugs and various pharmaceutical preparations (Fig. 9-3). The gram equals the weight of 1 ml of distilled water at 4° C. A **kilogram** is equal to 2.2 pounds. A **milligram** is equal to one thousandth of a gram. A **microgram** is equal to one millionth of a gram.

Metric Style of Notation

The National Bureau of Standards has recommended the following style of metric notation, except when it conflicts with use of proper English language[2]:

- Units are not to be capitalized (gram, not Gram).
- Periods should not be used with unit abbreviations (ml, not m.l. or ml.).
- A single space should be left between the quantity and the symbol (24 kg, not 24kg).
- Large numbers may be separated into groups of three numbers without commas (25 000, not 25,000).

- As a rule, fractions should not be used, only decimal notation (0.25 kg, not 1/4 kg).
- Numerical quantities less than 1 should have a 0 placed to the left of the decimal point (0.75 mg, not .75 mg).

REFERENCES

1. *Everything you always wanted to know about metrics,* Valdese, 1978, R&R Enterprises.
2. McKenry L, Salerno E: *Mosby's pharmacology in nursing,* ed 18, St Louis, 1992, Mosby.

Summary

A thorough understanding of medical terminology, medical abbreviations, and the metric system is an important tool for the delivery of patient care. Use of these tools permits efficient communication and documentation, physiological measurement, and the administration of medications. Mastery of these skills is necessary for all professional members of the health care team.

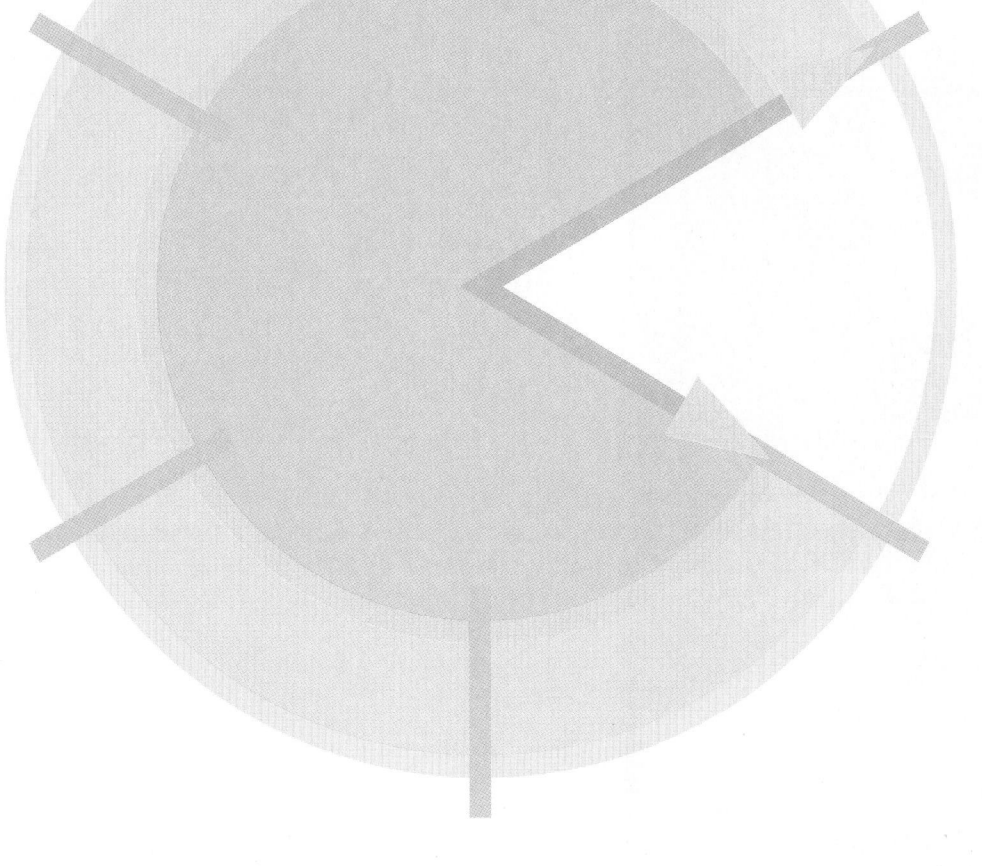

10 OVERVIEW OF HUMAN SYSTEMS

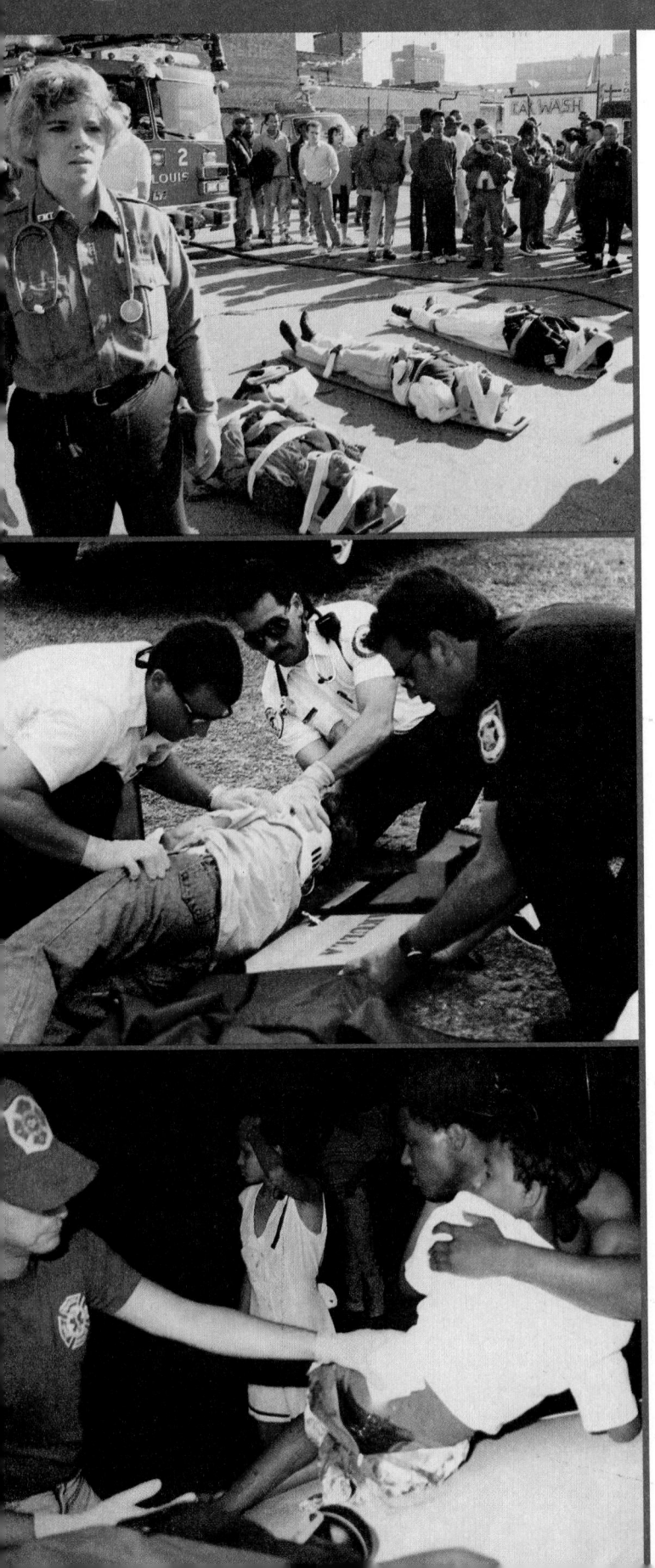

This chapter provides an overview of the structure and function of the human body. A discussion of each major organ system introduces the paramedic to key terms and concepts that will be presented throughout this text as indicated by subject headings of the various chapters.

OBJECTIVES

As a paramedic, you should be able to:

1. Discuss the importance of human anatomy as it relates to the paramedic profession.
2. Describe the anatomical position.
3. Properly interpret anatomical directional terms and body planes.
4. List the structures that compose the axial and appendicular regions of the body.
5. Define the divisions of the abdominal region.
6. List the three major body cavities.
7. Describe the contents of the three major body cavities.
8. Discuss the functions of the following cellular structures: the cytoplasmic membrane, the cytoplasm (and its organelles), and the nucleus.
9. Describe the process by which human cells reproduce.
10. Differentiate and describe the following tissue types: epithelial tissue, connective tissue, muscle tissue, and nervous tissue.
11. For each of the eleven major organ systems in the human body, label a diagram of anatomical structures, list the functions of the major anatomical structures, and explain how the organs of the system interrelate to perform the specified functions of the system.
12. For the special senses, label a diagram of the anatomical structures of the special sense, list the functions of the anatomical structures of each sense, and explain how the structures of the sense interrelate to perform its specified functions.

● OVERVIEW OF THE HUMAN BODY

Human anatomy is the study of how the human body is structurally organized. The paramedic must thoroughly understand human anatomy to organize a patient assessment by body region and to communicate effectively with medical control and other members of the health care team.

Terminology

Directional terms used by the medical profession refer to the human body in the **anatomical position:** a person standing erect with the feet and palms facing the examiner. A patient in the supine position is lying on his or her back (face up). A patient in the prone position is lying on his or her

KEY TERMS

anatomical position: A person standing erect with the feet and palms facing the examiner.

appendicular region: The limbs or extremities.

axial region: The head, neck, thorax, abdomen, and pelvis.

central nervous system (CNS): The brain and spinal cord, which are encased in and protected by bone.

organ: A structure made up of two or more kinds of tissues organized to perform a more complex function than any one tissue can alone.

peripheral nervous system (PNS): A major subdivision of the nervous system consisting of nerves and ganglia.

system: A group of organs arranged to perform a more complex function than any one organ can alone.

stomach (face down). A patient in the lateral recumbent position is lying on his or her right or left side. Regardless of the patient's actual position, information about the patient should always be communicated by referring to the anatomical position (Fig. 10-1).

Directional terms, such as *up* or *down, front* or *back,* and *right* or *left,* are also communicated in anatomical terminology and always refer to the patient, not the examiner (for example, the patient's left arm). Important anatomical terms are listed in Table 10-1.

Anatomical Planes

Internal body structure relationships are classified into anatomical planes or imaginary straight-line divisions of the human body (Fig. 10-2). The sagittal plane runs vertically through the middle

of the body, producing right and left sections. A plane that is to one side of the midline is said to be *parasagittal.* The transverse or horizontal plane divides the body into top and bottom, or superior and inferior sections. The frontal or coronal plane divides the body into front and back, or anterior and posterior positions.

Body Regions

The human body is divided into several regions for the purpose of organizing anatomical structures. The **appendicular region** includes the limbs, or extremities. The **axial region** consists of the head, neck, thorax, abdomen, and pelvis.

The abdomenal is usually divided into four quadrants: the upper right, lower right, upper left, and lower left. The dividing lines consist of two imaginary divisions that run horizontally through the umbilicus and vertically from the xiphoid process through the symphysis pubis (Fig. 10-3).

Body Cavities

The three major cavities of the human body are the thoracic cavity, the abdominal cavity, and the

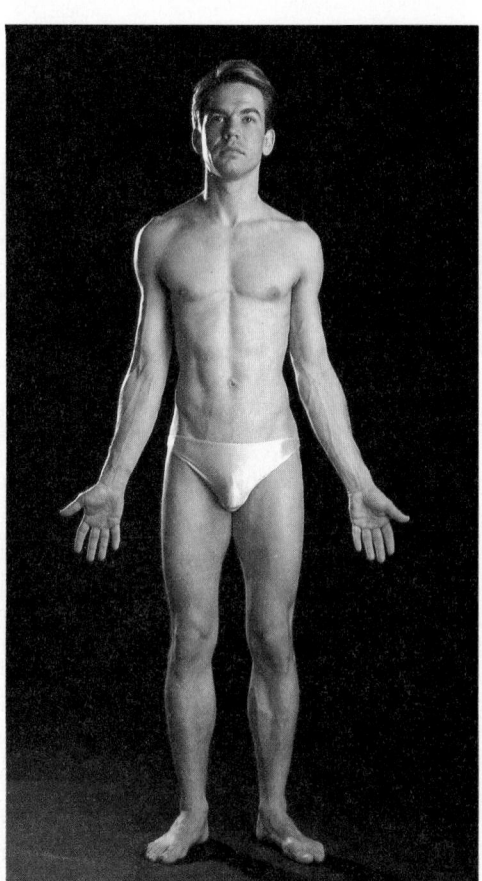

Fig. 10-1 Anatomical position. A human in the anatomical position is standing with the feet and palms of the hands facing forward with the thumbs to the outside.

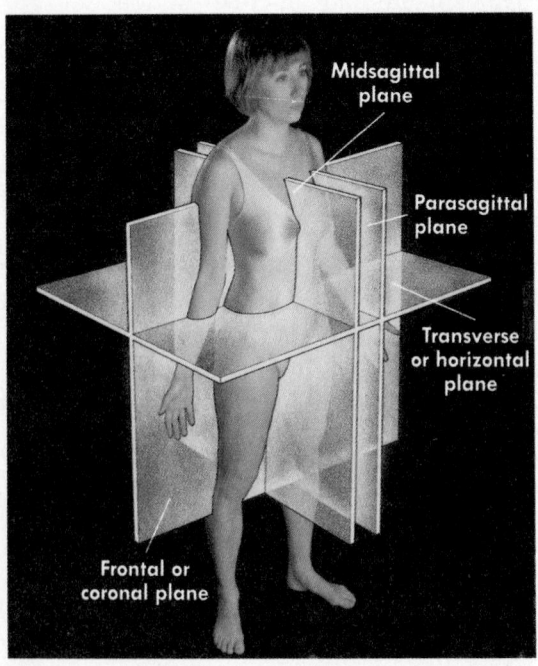

Fig. 10-2 Body planes.

pelvic cavity. The thoracic cavity is divided into two portions by a midline structure known as the *mediastinum*. The mediastinum includes the trachea, esophagus, thymus, heart, and great vessels. The lungs are located on either side of this midline structure. The thoracic cavity is surrounded by the rib cage and is separated from the abdominal cavity by the diaphragm.

The thorax contains two pleural cavities (which contain the lungs) and a pericardial cavity (which contains the heart). These cavities are lined with a serous membrane. The serous membrane that comes in contact with the organ is visceral, and the serous membrane that comes in contact with the cavity wall is parietal. A thin, lubricating film of fluid is produced by these membranes and re-

TABLE 10-1 Directional Terms

Term	Definition	Term	Definition
Left	Toward the left side	Distal	Farther than another structure from the point of attachment to the trunk
Right	Toward the right side	Medial	Toward the midline of the body
Superior	Situated above another structure (usually synonymous with "cephalic")	Lateral	Away from the midline of the body
Inferior	Situated below another structure (usually synonymous with "caudal")	Anterior	The front of the body (synonymous with "ventral")
Cephalic	Toward the head of the body	Posterior	The back of the body (synonymous with "dorsal")
Caudal	Toward the distal end of the spine	Ventral	Pertaining to the front
Proximal	Closer than another structure to the point of attachment to the trunk	Dorsal	Pertaining to the back

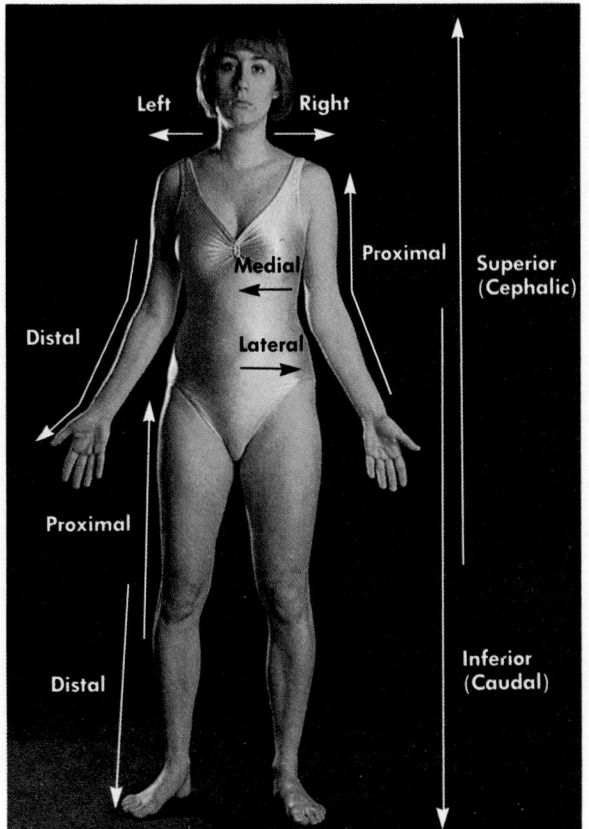

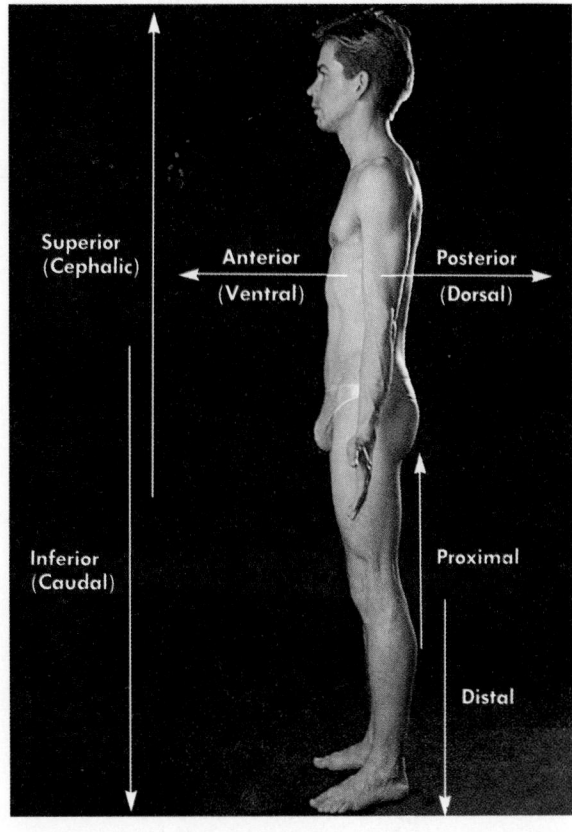

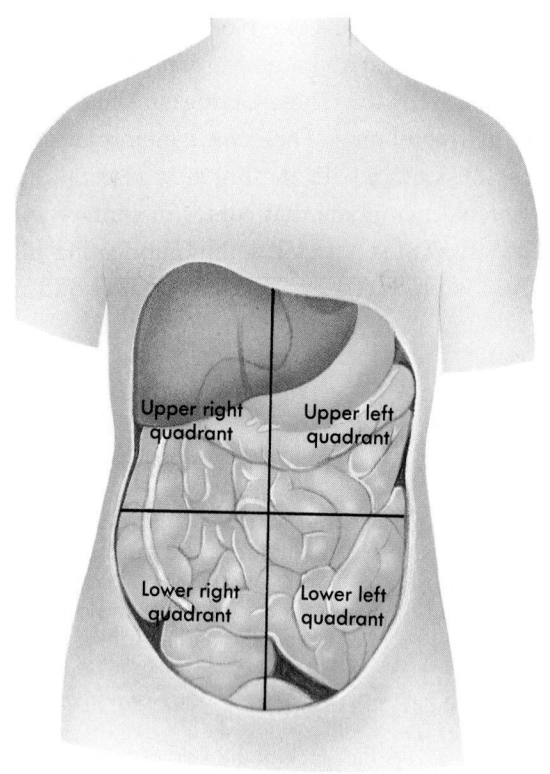

Fig. 10-3 Abdominal quadrants.

duces the friction that occurs during movement of organs against other organs or body cavities.

An imaginary plane separates the abdominal cavity from the pelvic cavity. The division is drawn between the symphysis pubis and the sacral promontory (the projecting portion of the pelvis at the base of the sacrum). The abdominal and pelvic cavities are lined with a thin sheet of membranous tissue that secretes serous fluid. The serous membrane that covers the abdominal organs is known as *visceral peritoneum*. The serous membrane that covers the body cavity wall is known as the *parietal peritoneum*. Peritoneal organs are held in place by connective tissue called *mesentery*. The mesentery anchors some of the abdominal organs to the body wall and provides a pathway for nerves and vessels to reach the organs. Abdominopelvic organs that do not have mesentery or peritoneum are said to be *retroperitoneal* (behind the peritoneum); they include the kidneys, adrenal glands, pancreas, portions of the colon, and the urinary bladder. The pelvic cavity is enclosed by the bones of the pelvis. The abdomi-

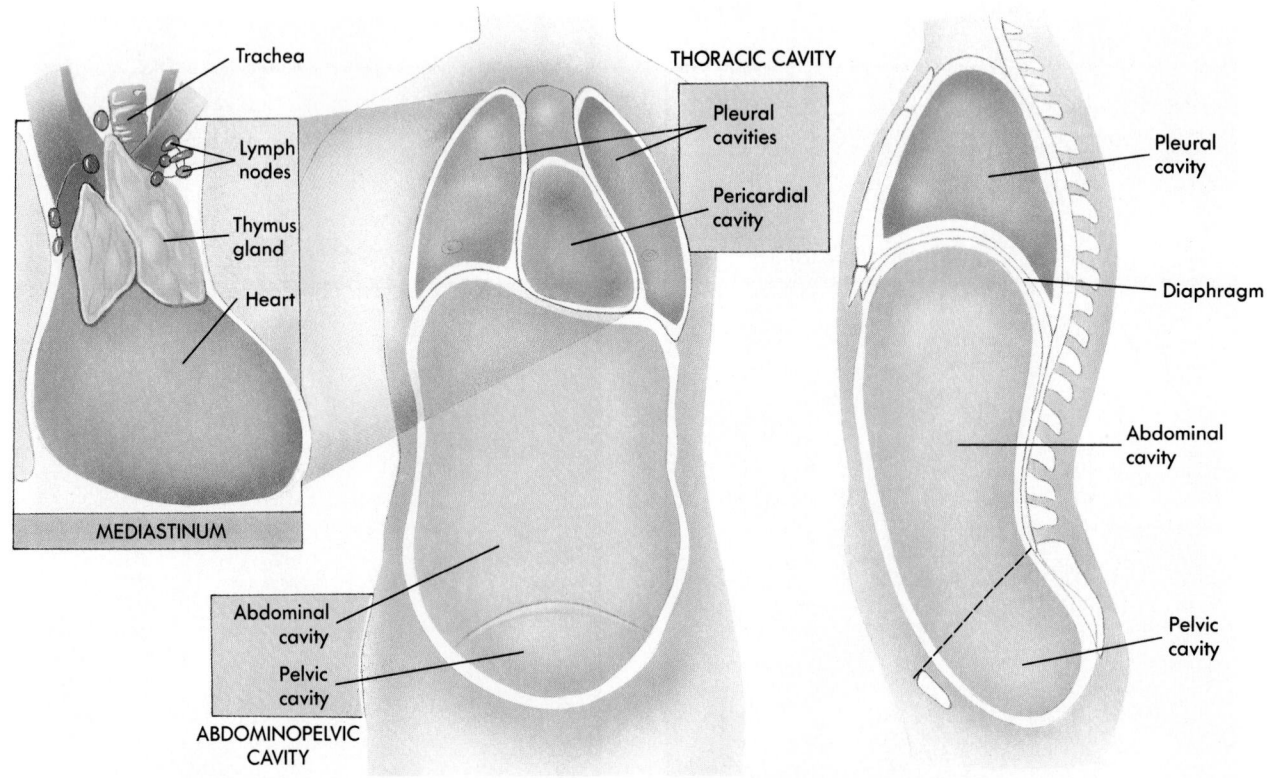

Fig. 10-4 Body cavities. The thoracic cavity includes the two pleural cavities and the pericardial cavity. Some of the contents of the mediastinum are shown on the left. The abdominopelvic cavity contains the abdominal cavity and the pelvic cavity.

nal and pelvic cavities are often referred to collectively as the *peritoneal* or *abdominopelvic cavity* (Fig. 10-4).

● CELL STRUCTURE

Cells are the most basic unit of life. They are highly organized units that are composed of protoplasm, or living matter. The three main parts of all human cells are the cytoplasmic membrane (plasma membrane), the cytoplasm, and the nucleus.

Cytoplasmic Membrane

The cytoplasmic membrane encloses the cytoplasm, forming the outer boundary of the cell. It is believed to have two layers of phosphate-containing fat molecules known as *phospholipids* that form a fluid framework for the cytoplasmic membrane (Fig. 10-5). Substances outside this membrane are considered extracellular (outside of cells) or intercellular (between cells), and substances inside this membrane are intracellular. The functions of the cytoplasmic membrane are to enclose and support the cell contents and to regulate what moves into and out of the cell.

The central layer of the cytoplasmic membrane is a lipid bilayer composed of a double layer of lipid molecules. The lipid bilayer has a liquid quality, and protein molecules "float" on both the inner and the outer surfaces. Some of these proteins have carbohydrate molecules bound to them and are thought to function as membrane channels, carrier molecules, receptor molecules, enzymes, or structural supports in the membrane.

Cytoplasm

Cytoplasm lies between the cytoplasmic membrane and the nucleus. The nucleus can be viewed as a round or spherical structure in the center of the cell. Specialized structures in the cell known as *organelles* are located in the cytoplasm and perform functions important to the cell's survival (Table 10-2 and Fig. 10-6).

The endoplasmic reticulum is a network of connecting sacs or canals that wind through a cell's cytoplasm, serving as a miniature circulatory system for the cell. The tubular passageways or canals in the endoplasmic reticulum carry proteins and other substances through the cytoplasm of the cell from one area to another.

There are two types of endoplasmic reticulum: smooth and rough. Smooth endoplasmic reticulum is found in cells that handle or manufacture fatty substances; it also participates in detoxification processes through the chemical action of enzymes. Rough endoplasmic reticulum is found in

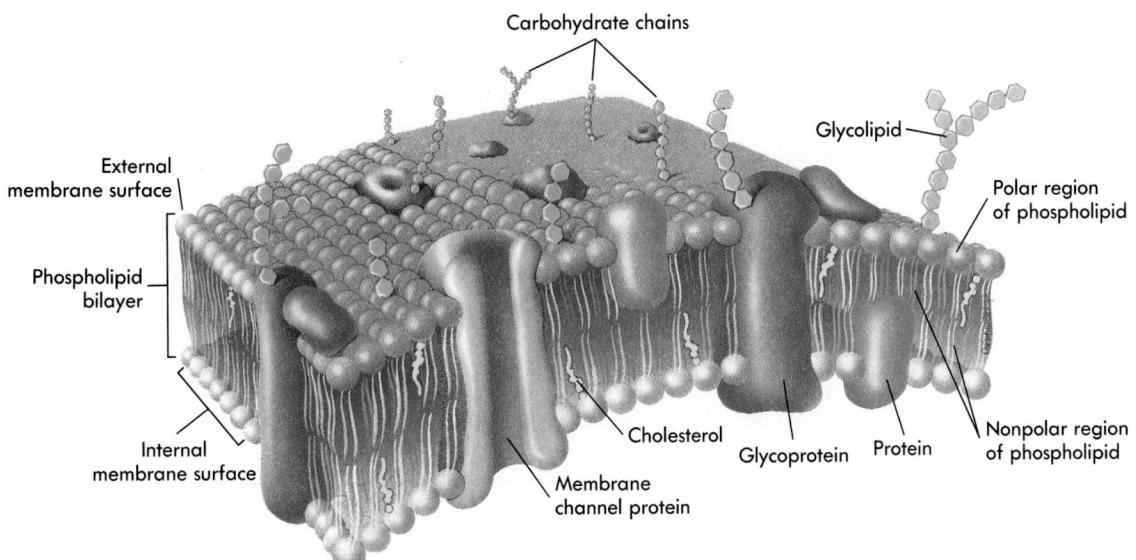

Fig. 10-5 Fluid mosaic model of the plasma membrane.

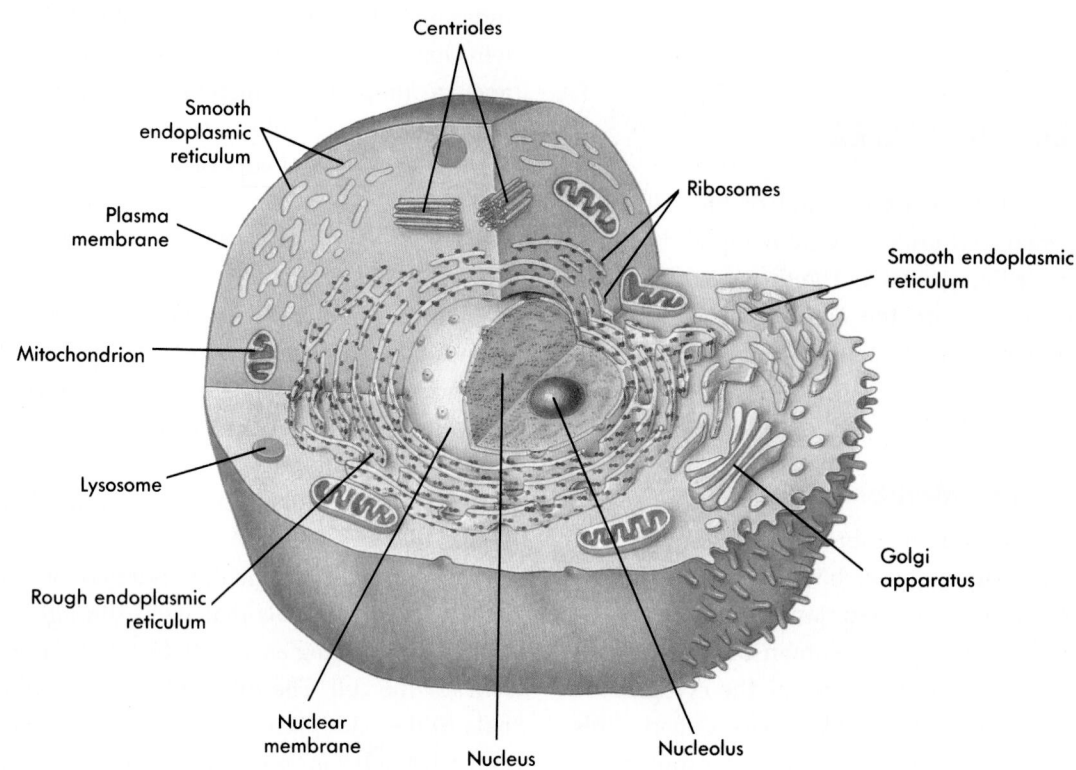

Fig. 10-6 Artist's interpretation of cell structure.

Cell Structure	Function
TABLE 10-2 Some Major Cell Structures and Their Functions	
Plasma membrane	Serves as the boundary of the cell; protein and carbohydrate molecules on the outer surface of plasma membrane perform various functions; for example, they serve as markers that identify cells of each individual or as receptor molecules for certain hormones
Endoplasmic reticulum	Ribosomes attached to rough endoplasmic reticulum synthesize proteins; smooth endoplasmic reticulum synthesizes lipids and certain carbohydrates
Ribosomes	Synthesize proteins; a cell's "protein factories"
Mitochondria	Synthesize adenosine triphosphate; a cell's "powerhouses"
Lysosomes	A cell's "digestive system"
Golgi apparatus	Synthesizes carbohydrate, combines it with protein, and packages the product as globules of glycoprotein
Centrioles	Function in cell reproduction
Cilia	Short, hairlike extensions on the free surfaces of some cells capable of movement
Flagella	Single and much larger projections of cell surfaces than cilia; the only example in humans is the "tail" of a sperm cell
Nucleus	Dictates protein synthesis, thereby playing an essential role in other cell activities, namely, active transport, metabolism, growth, and heredity
Nucleoli	Play an essential role in the formation of ribosomes

cells that manufacture proteins to be secreted for use outside the cell.

Ribosomes are the "factories" in the cells where protein is synthesized. Ribosomes are macromolecules of protein composed of thousands of atoms. They are usually bound to the endoplasmic reticulum but are also found free in cytoplasm. Ribosomes form complexes with strands of ribonucleic acid (RNA), which through the genetic code, provide the blueprint for the new protein. Individual amino acids are attached in long chains with peptide bonds to form the new proteins.

The Golgi apparatus concentrates and packages materials for secretion from the cell. It consists of tiny sacs composed of smooth endoplasmic reticulum that are stacked one on the other near the nucleus. The Golgi apparatus concentrates and in some cases chemically modifies the proteins by synthesizing and attaching carbohydrate molecules to the proteins to form glycoproteins or attaches lipids to proteins to form lipoproteins. These concentrated globules move slowly outward to and through the cell membrane, at which point they break open and spill all of their contents. An example of a Golgi apparatus product is mucus.

Lysosomes are membranous-walled organelles that contain enzymes enabling them to function as intracellular digestive systems. These enzymes include those that digest nucleic acids, proteins, polysaccharides, and lipids. Certain white blood cells have large numbers of lysosomes that contain enzymes to digest phagocytosic bacteria. If tissues are damaged, these powerful enzymes may escape from ruptured lysosome sacs into the cytoplasm, digesting both damaged and healthy cells. Lysosomes also digest organelles of the cell that are no longer functional (autophagia).

The mitochondria ("power plants of the cell") are found throughout the cell and are the site of aerobic oxidation. It is here that energy, derived from the efficient metabolism of nutrients and oxygen via the Krebs' cycle, is used to synthesize high-energy triphosphate bonds (for example, adenosine triphosphate, or ATP). These triphosphate bonds are the energy source for the body's muscles, nerves, and overall function.

Centrioles are paired, rod-shaped organelles that lie at right angles to each other in a specialized zone of cytoplasm known as the centrosome. Each centriole is composed of microtubules that play an important role in the process of cell division.

At some point in their existence, all human cells contain a nucleus in which the genetic material of the cell is located. The nucleus is a large, membrane-bound organelle that ultimately controls all other organelles in the cytoplasm. It may be spherical, elongated, or lobed, depending on the type of cell in which it is found. The nucleus is usually located near the center of the cell, but some cells, such as red blood cells, lose their nucleus as they develop. Other cells, such as certain bone cells, have more than one nucleus.

The cell nucleus is surrounded by a nuclear membrane, which encloses a special type of protoplasm known as *nucleoplasm*. The nucleoplasm contains a number of specialized structures, two of which are the nucleolus and the chromatin granules. The nucleolus consists of deoxyribonucleic acid (DNA), which "programs" the formation of the RNA, and protein, which makes ribosomes. These ribosomes then migrate through the nuclear membrane into the cytoplasm of the cell and produce proteins.

Chromatin granules are threadlike structures made up of proteins and DNA. During cell division, the chromatin condenses to form the 23 pairs of chromosomes characteristic of human cells. The information contained within nuclear DNA determines most of the chemical events that occur within the cell.

Cell Reproduction

All human cells, with the exception of reproductive (sex) cells, reproduce by a process known as *mitosis*. In this process, cells divide to multiply: One cell divides to form two cells. Many cell types in the body (for example, epithelial, liver, and bone marrow cells) undergo cell division throughout the life of the individual. Other cell types (for example, nerve and skeletal muscle cells) divide until near the time of birth.

● TISSUES

Characteristics of cell structure and composition are used to classify tissue types. The four main types of tissue that compose the body's many organs are epithelial, connective, muscle, and nervous tissue.

Epithelial Tissue

Epithelial tissue covers surfaces or forms structures (for example, glands) derived from body surfaces. This tissue consists almost entirely of cells that have little or no intercellular material between them, and they form continuous sheets that contain no blood vessels. Epithelium covers the outside of the body and lines the digestive tract, the vessels, and many body cavities.

Epithelial tissues can be subdivided according to the shape and arrangement of the cells found in each type. If classified according to shape, epithelial cells are squamous (flat and scalelike), cuboidal (cube-shaped), or columnar (more tall than wide). If classified according to arrangement, epithelial cells are simple (a single layer of cells of the same shape), stratified (multiple layers of cells of the same shape), or transitional (several layers of cells of differing shapes).

Connective Tissue

Connective tissue is the most abundant and widely distributed type of tissue in the body. It consists of cells separated from each other by intercellular material known as the *extracellular matrix*. This nonliving matrix gives most connective tissue its fundamental characteristics and is the basis for separating connective tissue into the following seven subgroups:

1. Areolar connective tissue is a loose tissue that consists of delicate webs of fibers and a variety of cells embedded in a matrix of soft, sticky gel. It is the "loose packing" material of most organs and other tissues and attaches the skin to underlying tissues. The areolar connective tissue contains three major types of protein fibers: collagen, reticulum, and elastin.

2. Adipose or fat tissue is a specialized connective tissue that stores lipids. Lipids take up less space per calorie than either carbohydrates or proteins. Therefore adipose tissue not only functions as an insulator and protector but is also a site of energy storage.

3. Fibrous connective tissue consists mainly of bundles of strong, white collagenous fibers arranged in parallel rows. Tendons are composed of this type of connective tissue, which is characterized by strength and inelasticity.

4. Cartilage is composed of cartilage cells (chondrocytes) that are located in tiny spaces and distributed throughout a relatively rigid matrix. The composition of cartilage varies somewhat by its anatomical location and ultimate function. For example, hyaline cartilage, which is present at articulating surfaces, is firm and smooth, whereas fibrocartilage is more flexible and supple. Cartilage constitutes part of the human skeleton and covers the articulating surfaces of bones. In addition, cartilage forms the major skeletal tissue of the embryo before its replacement by bony tissue.

   The type of cartilage depends on the relative amounts of collagen, elastin, and ground substance, which is composed of nonfibrous protein and other organic molecules and fluid. Increased amounts of collagen or elastin function to allow cartilage to spring back after being compressed. Blood vessels do not penetrate the substance of cartilage, so cartilage heals slowly after injury.

5. Bone is a highly specialized form of hard, connective tissue that consists of living cells and mineralized matrix. The strength and rigidity of this matrix allow bone to support and protect other tissues and organs.

   Bones are classified according to their shape. Long bones are longer than they are wide. Examples of long bones are the humerus, ulna, radius, femur, tibia, fibula, and phalanges. Short bones are approximately as broad as they are long. Examples of short bones are the carpal bones of the wrist and the tarsal bones of the ankle. Flat bones have a thin, flattened shape. Examples of flat bones are certain skull bones, ribs, sternum, and scapulae. Irregular bones are those that do not fit the other three categories. Examples of irregular bones include vertebrae and facial bones.

Each growing long bone consists of a diaphysis (shaft), an epiphysis at the end of each bone, and an epiphyseal or growth plate. The epiphyseal plate is the site of bone elongation. When bone growth stops, the epiphyseal plate becomes ossified and is called the *epiphyseal line.* Injury to this area can impair bone growth if not recognized and treated properly.

Bones contain large cavities, such as the medullary cavity in the diaphysis, and smaller cavities, such as in the epiphyses of long bones and throughout the interior of other bones. These spaces are filled with yellow marrow (mainly adipose tissue) or red marrow (the site of blood formation). Blood supply to most bones is excellent, so some bones, such as the tibia, are a suitable choice for venous access via intraosseous infusion.

Bones may be further classified as cancellous or spongy bone and compact bone. Cancellous bone has spaces between the plates of the bone and resembles a sponge. Compact bone is essentially solid. Unlike cartilage, bone has a rich blood supply and can repair itself much more readily than cartilage.

6. Blood is a unique connective tissue because the matrix between the cells is liquid. The liquid matrix of blood allows it to flow rapidly through the body, carrying nutrients, oxygen, waste products, and other materials.

7. Hemopoietic tissue is the connective tissue found in the marrow cavities of bones and in such organs as the spleen, tonsils, and lymph nodes. This connective tissue is responsible for the formation of blood cells and lymphatic system cells that are important in the body's defense against disease.

Muscle Tissue

Muscle tissue is a contractile tissue that is responsible for movement. It is highly specialized to contract or shorten forcefully. Muscle tissue is responsible for all of the mechanical processes providing motion for the body. Muscle tissue is classified as skeletal, cardiac, and smooth or visceral muscle, according to both anatomical location and function. When classified according to its appearance, muscle is either striated or nonstriated. When classified according to its function, muscle is either voluntary (consciously controlled) or involuntary (not normally consciously controlled). The three types of muscles are striated voluntary (skeletal) muscle, striated involuntary (cardiac) muscle, and nonstriated involuntary (smooth) muscle.

Skeletal muscle attaches to bones and represents a large portion of the human body's total weight. Contraction of these muscles is responsible for body movement. Cardiac muscle is the muscle of the heart. Contraction of the cardiac muscle pumps blood throughout the body. Smooth muscle is widespread throughout the body and is responsible for a wide variety of functions. Examples include movement in the digestive, urinary, and reproductive systems.

Nervous Tissue

The nervous tissue is characterized by the ability to conduct electrical signals, which are known as *action potentials.* The nervous tissue consists of two basic kinds of cells: neurons and neuroglia.

Neurons, or nerve cells, are the actual conducting cells of nervous tissue. They are composed of three major parts: cell body, dendrite, and axon. The cell body contains the nucleus and is the site of general cell functions. Dendrites and axons are nerve cell processes (projections of cytoplasm surrounded by membrane). Dendrites receive electrical impulses and conduct them toward the cell body. Axons usually conduct impulses away from the cell body. There are many different sizes and shapes of neurons, especially in the brain and spinal cord.

Neuroglia are the support cells of the brain, spinal cord, and peripheral nerves. These cells are divided into several subgroups that nourish, protect, and insulate neurons.

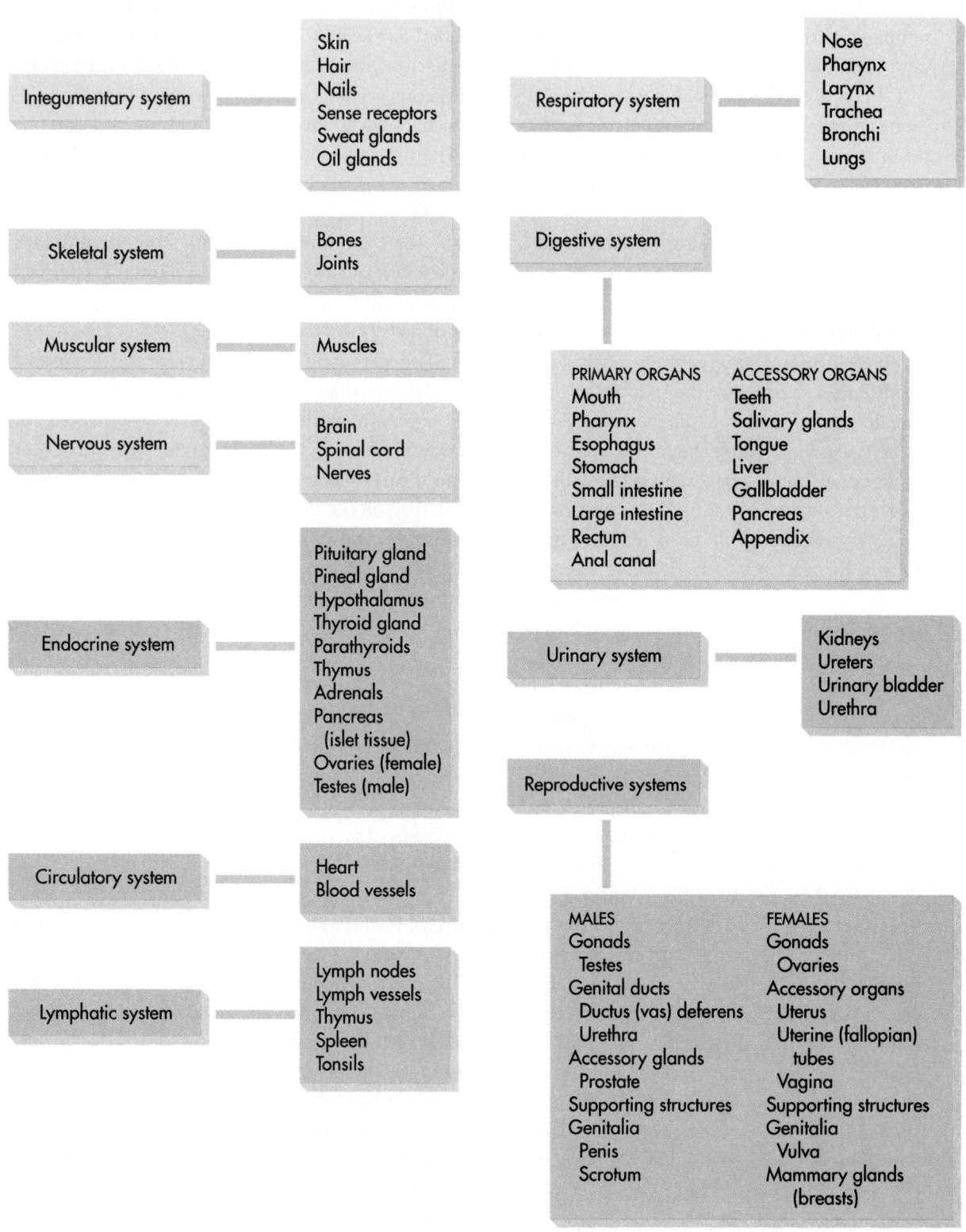

Fig. 10-7 Body systems and their organs.

● ORGAN SYSTEMS OF THE BODY

An **organ** is a structure made up of two or more kinds of tissues organized to perform a more complex function than can any one tissue alone. A **system** is a group of organs arranged to perform a more complex function than can any one organ alone (Fig. 10-7). Eleven major organ systems compose the human body:

1. Integumentary
2. Skeletal
3. Muscular
4. Nervous
5. Endocrine
6. Circulatory
7. Lymphatic
8. Respiratory
9. Digestive
10. Urinary
11. Reproductive

The Integumentary System

The integumentary system is the largest organ system of the body. It consists of the skin and accessory structures such as hair, nails, and a variety of glands. The functions of the integumentary system include protecting the body against injury and dehydration, defense against invading microorganisms, and temperature regulation.

Skin

The skin is a sheetlike organ composed of two distinct layers of tissue: the epidermis and the dermis (Fig. 10-8). The epidermis is the outermost layer of skin, consisting of tightly packed epithelial cells. Cells of the innermost layer of the epidermis have the ability to undergo mitosis and to repair themselves if injured. This characteristic makes it possible for the body to maintain an effective barrier against infection, even when subjected to injury and normal wear and tear.

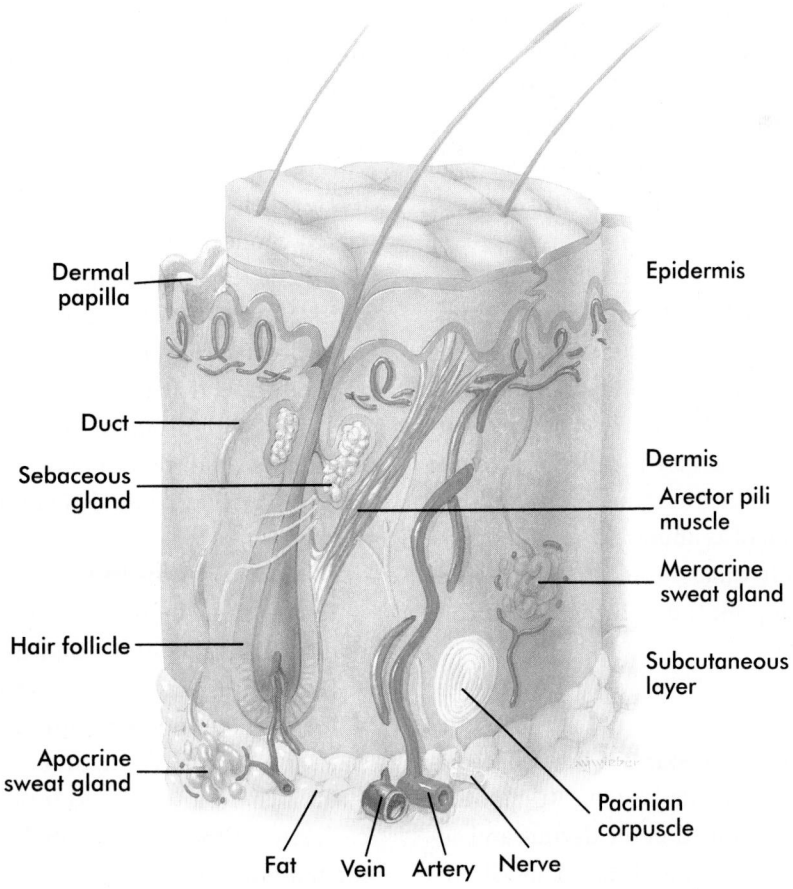

Dermal papilla

Duct

Sebaceous gland

Hair follicle

Apocrine sweat gland

Epidermis

Dermis

Arector pili muscle

Merocrine sweat gland

Subcutaneous layer

Pacinian corpuscle

Fat   Vein   Artery   Nerve

Fig. 10-8 Microscopic view of the skin.

The dermis is the deeper of the two layers of skin, made up largely of connective tissue. It is much thicker than the epidermis and contains collagenous and elastic fibers. The dermis also contains a specialized network of nerves and nerve endings that provide sensory information about pain, pressure, touch, and temperature. At various levels of the dermis are muscle fibers, hair follicles, sweat and sebaceous glands, and many blood vessels.

The layers of skin are supported by a thick layer of loose connective tissue and fat known as *subcutaneous tissue*. Subcutaneous tissue insulates the body from temperature extremes, serves as a source of stored energy, and acts as a shock absorber to protect underlying tissue from injury.

Hair

Hair growth begins when cells of the epidermal layer of the skin grow down into the dermis, forming a small tube called the *hair follicle*. The growth of the hair begins from a small, cap-shaped cluster of cells called the *hair papilla*. The part of the hair that lies hidden in the follicle is known as the *root*, and the visible part is called the *shaft*. Smooth muscles known as *arrector pili* are associated with each hair follicle. Movement of the hair follicle by the arrector pili produces a pressure on the skin ("goose bumps") and pulls the hairs upward.

Nails

Nails are produced by cells in the epidermis. The visible part of the nail is the nail body. The root of the nail lies in a groove and is hidden by a fold of skin known as the *cuticle*. The crescent-shaped white area of the nail is called the *lunula* and is most visible on the thumbnail. The nail bed that lies under the nail is abundant in blood vessels. In healthy individuals, this layer of epithelium appears to be pink through the translucent nail body.

Glands

The major glands of the skin are the sebaceous glands and the sweat glands (see Fig. 10-8). Most sebaceous glands are located in the dermis and secrete oil (sebum) for the hair and skin. This oil prevents drying and protects against some bacteria.

Sebum secretion increases during adolescence, stimulated by increased blood levels of the sex hormones. Other skin glands include the ceruminous glands of the external auditory meatus, which produce cerumen (earwax), and the mammary glands.

Sweat (sudoriferous) glands are the most numerous skin glands. They are usually classified as merocrine and apocrine according to their mode of secretion. Merocrine sweat glands are the most common and open directly onto the surface of the skin through sweat pores. The coiled portion of the gland produces a fluid that is mostly water but also contains some salts (mainly sodium chloride) and small amounts of ammonia, urea, uric acid, and lactic acid. As the body temperature rises, the sweat glands produce sweat, which evaporates and cools the body.

Apocrine glands usually open into hair follicles. These glands are found in the axillae and genitalia and around the anus. They become active at puberty from the influence of sex hormones. Apocrine glands secrete an organic substance that is odorless when released but is quickly metabolized by bacteria to cause body odor.

The Skeletal System

The skeletal system consists of bones and associated connective tissues, including cartilage, tendons, and ligaments. The skeletal system provides a rigid framework for support and protection and provides a system of levers on which muscles act to produce body movements. The skeletal system contains 206 individual bones. The named bones are divided into two categories: the axial skeleton and the appendicular skeleton (Fig. 10-9).

The Axial Skeleton

The axial skeleton consists of the skull, hyoid bone, vertebral column, and thoracic cage.

The skull is composed of 28 separate bones divided into the following groups: the auditory ossicles, the cranial vault, and the facial bones (Fig. 10-10). There are six auditory ossicles (three on each side of the head) located inside the cavity of the temporal bone. The auditory ossicles function in hearing.

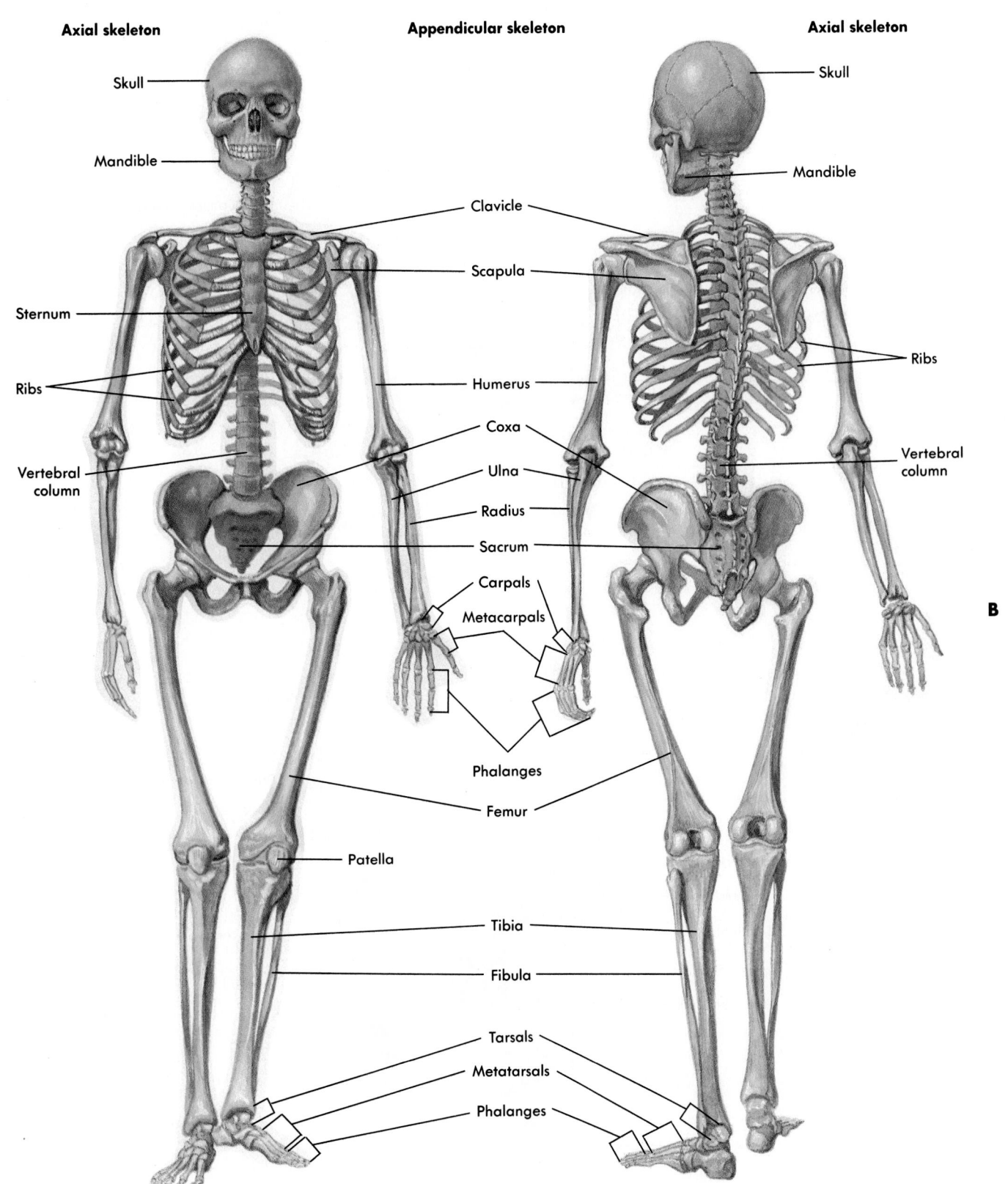

Fig. 10-9 Anterior **(A)** and posterior **(B)** view of the skeleton.

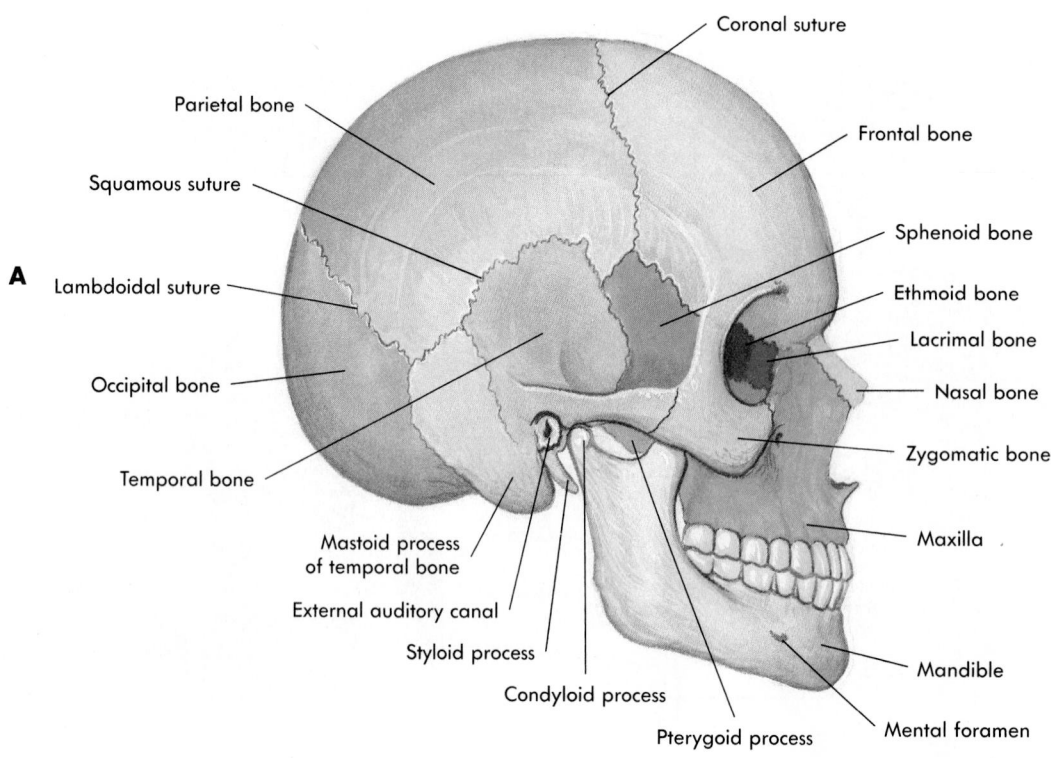

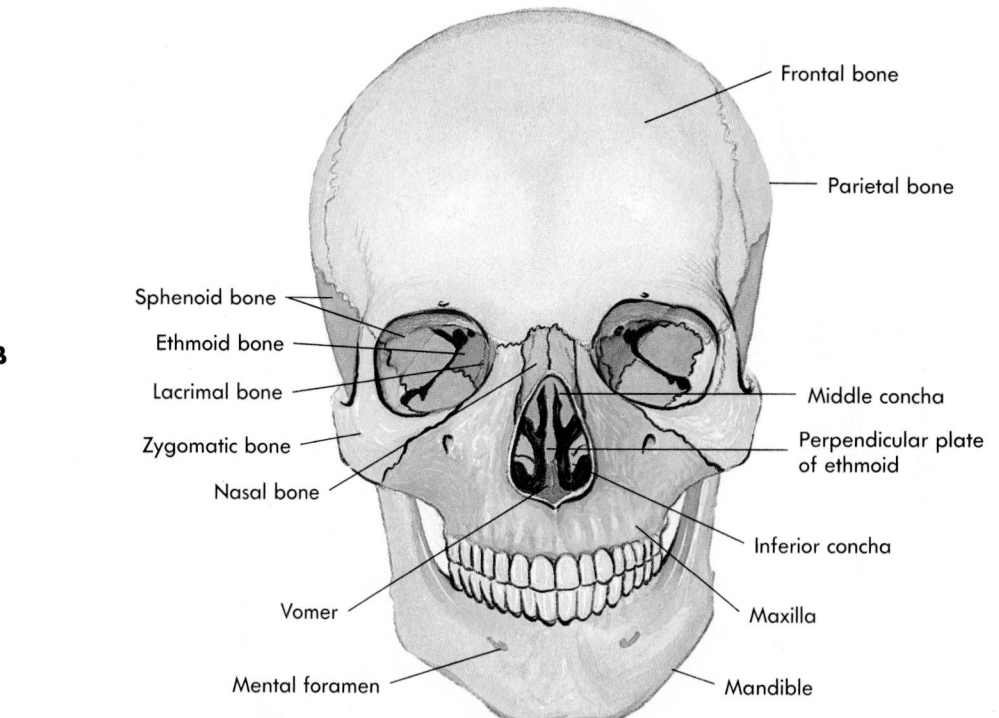

Fig. 10-10 Skull viewed from the right side **(A)** and the front **(B).**

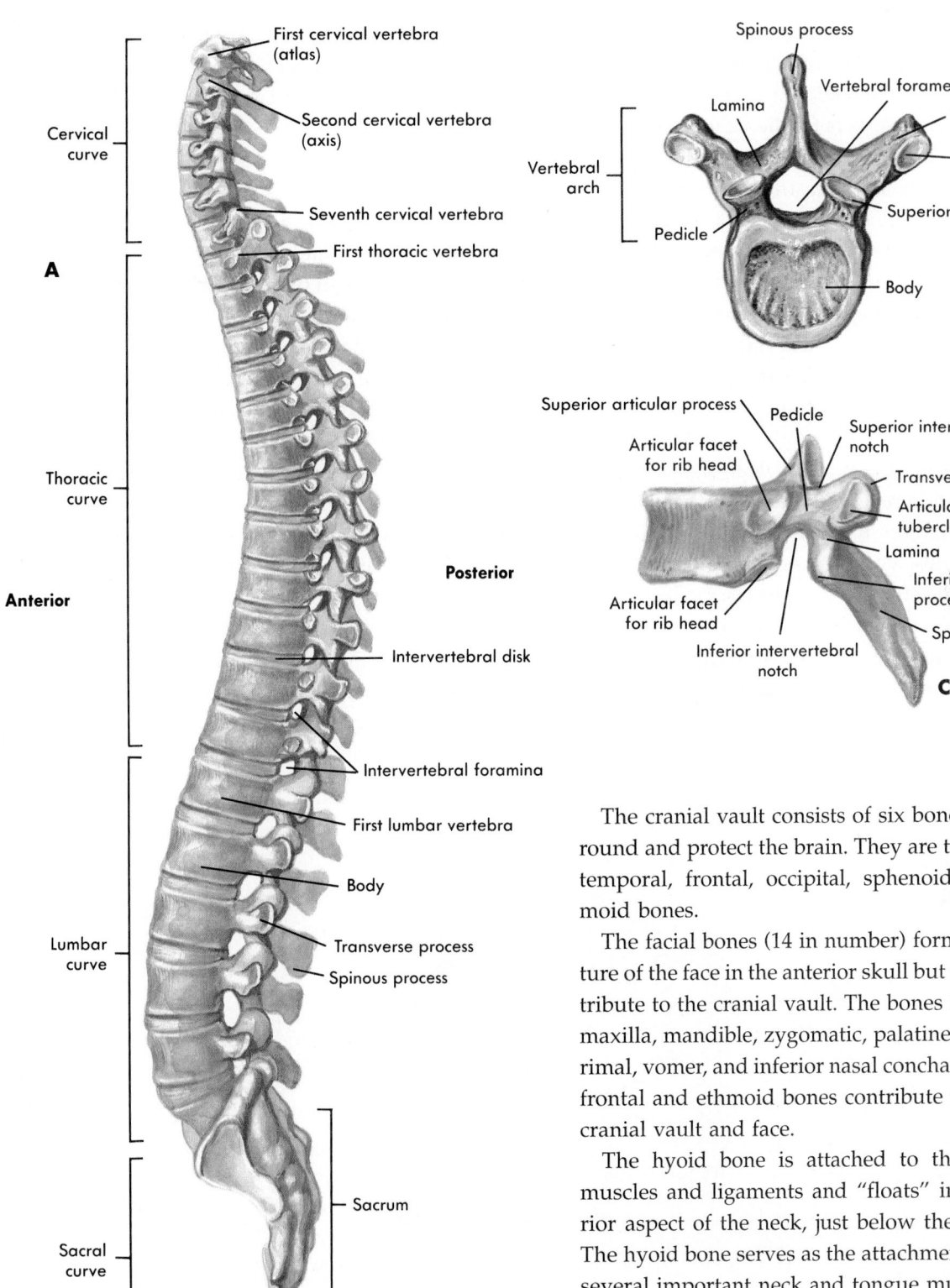

Fig. 10-11 A, Vertebral column viewed from the left side. **B,** Superior view of the vertebrae. **C,** Lateral view of the vertebrae.

The cranial vault consists of six bones that surround and protect the brain. They are the parietal, temporal, frontal, occipital, sphenoid, and ethmoid bones.

The facial bones (14 in number) form the structure of the face in the anterior skull but do not contribute to the cranial vault. The bones include the maxilla, mandible, zygomatic, palatine, nasal, lacrimal, vomer, and inferior nasal concha bones. The frontal and ethmoid bones contribute to both the cranial vault and face.

The hyoid bone is attached to the skull by muscles and ligaments and "floats" in the superior aspect of the neck, just below the mandible. The hyoid bone serves as the attachment point for several important neck and tongue muscles.

The vertebral column consists of 26 bones, which can be divided into five regions: 7 cervical vertebrae, 12 thoracic vertebrae, 5 lumbar vertebrae, 1 sacral bone, and 1 coccygeal bone (Fig. 10-11). A total of 34 vertebrae originally form during development, but the 5 sacral vertebrae fuse to form 1 bone, as do the 4 or 5 coccygeal bones.

The weight-bearing portion of the vertebrae is a bony disk called the *body.* Intervertebral disks, located between the bodies of adjacent vertebrae, serve as shock absorbers for the vertebral column, provide additional support for the body, and prevent the vertebral bodies from rubbing against each other. The spinal cord is protected by the vertebral arch and the dorsal portion of the body. A transverse process extends laterally from each side of the arch, and a single spinous process is present at the point of junction. Much vertebral movement is accomplished by the contraction of skeletal muscles attached to the transverse and spinous processes.

The thoracic cage protects vital organs within the thorax and prevents the collapse of the thorax during respiration. It consists of the thoracic vertebrae, the ribs with their associated costal cartilages, and the sternum (Fig. 10-12).

The 12 pairs of ribs can be divided into true and false ribs. The superior 7 (the true ribs) articulate with the thoracic vertebrae and attach directly through their costal cartilages to the sternum. The inferior 5 (the false ribs) articulate with the tho-

racic vertebrae but do not attach directly to the sternum. The eighth, ninth, and tenth ribs are joined to a common cartilage, which is attached in turn to the sternum. The eleventh and twelfth ribs are "floating" ribs that have no attachment to the sternum.

The sternum is divided into three parts: the manubrium, the body, and the xiphoid process. At the superior margin of the manubrium is the jugular notch, which can be easily palpated at the anterior base of the neck. The point at which the manubrium joins the body of the sternum is the sternal angle (also known as the *angle of Louis*). The second rib is found lateral to the sternal angle and is used clinically as a starting point for counting the other ribs.

The appendicular skeleton consists of the bones of the upper and lower extremities and their girdles, by which they are attached to the body.

The scapula and clavicle constitute the pectoral girdle, attaching the upper limbs to the axial skeleton. The direct point of attachment between the bones of the appendicular and axial skeleton occurs at the sternoclavicular joint between the

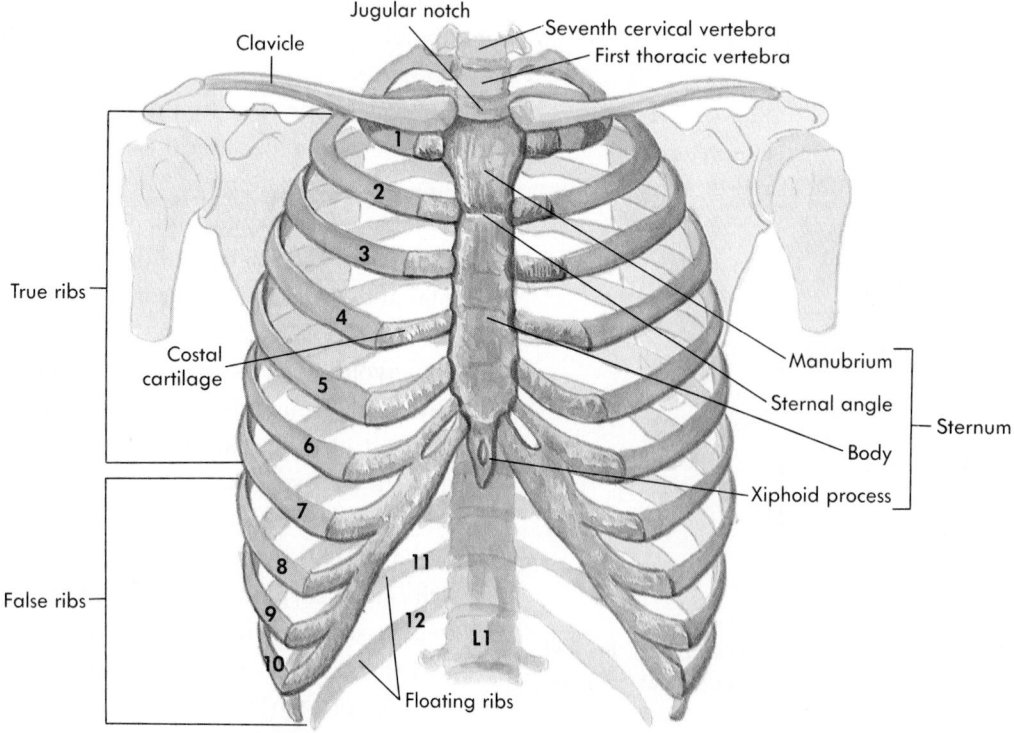

Fig. 10-12 Entire rib cage as seen from the front.

clavicle and the sternum. Fig. 10-13 illustrates the bones of the upper extremity.

The humerus is the second longest bone in the body. The head of the humerus articulates with the scapula. The greater and lesser tubercles are on the lateral and anterior surfaces of the proximal end of the humerus, where they function as sites of muscle attachments. The humerus articulates with the radius and ulna at its distal end. The capitulum (lateral aspect of the humerus) articulates with the head of the radius, and the trochlea (medial aspect of the humerus) articulates with the ulna. Proximal to the trochlea and capitulum are the medial and lateral epicondyles, respec-

tively, which function as muscle attachments for the muscles of the forearm.

The large bony process of the ulna (the olecranon process) can be felt at the point of the elbow. This process fits in a large depression on the posterior surface of the humerus known as the *olecranon fossa*. The structural relationship between these two processes makes movement of the joint possible. The distal end of the ulna has a small head that articulates with both the radius and the wrist bones. The posterior-medial side of the head has a small styloid process to which ligaments of the wrist are attached. The proximal end of the radius articulates with the humerus, and the medial surface of the head constitutes a smooth cylinder where the radius rotates against the radial notch of the ulna. Major anterior arm muscles (biceps brachii) are attached to the radial tuberosity.

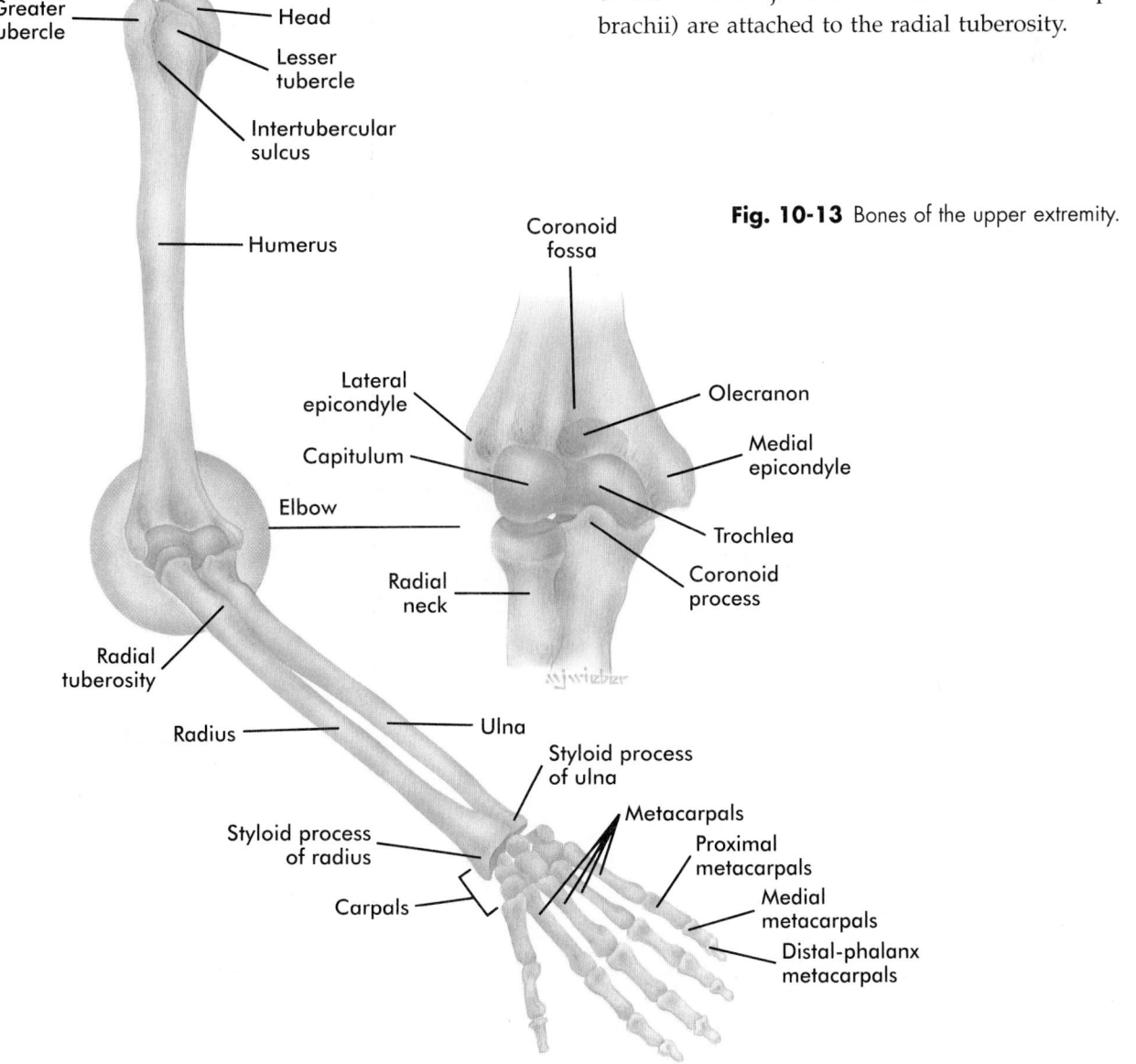

Fig. 10-13 Bones of the upper extremity.

Greater tubercle

Head

Lesser tubercle

Intertubercular sulcus

Humerus

Coronoid fossa

Lateral epicondyle

Capitulum

Elbow

Radial neck

Olecranon

Medial epicondyle

Trochlea

Coronoid process

Radial tuberosity

Radius

Ulna

Styloid process of ulna

Metacarpals

Proximal metacarpals

Medial metacarpals

Distal-phalanx metacarpals

Styloid process of radius

Carpals

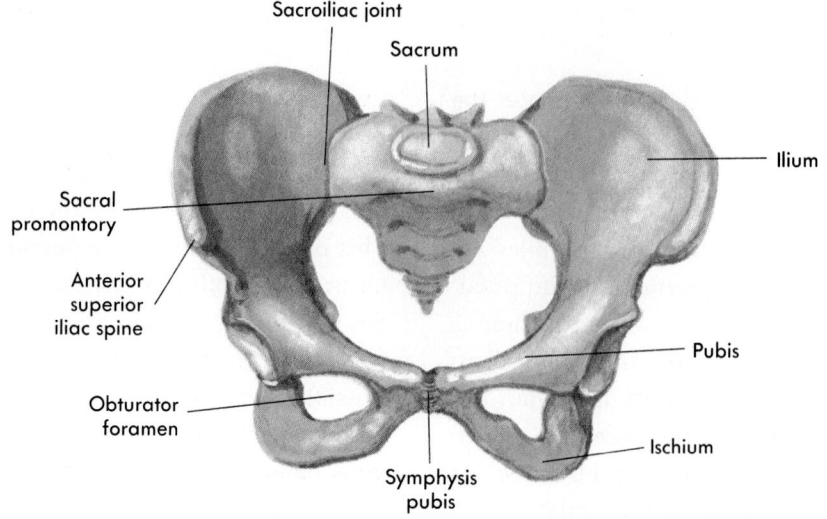

Fig. 10-14 Complete pelvic girdle, anterior view.

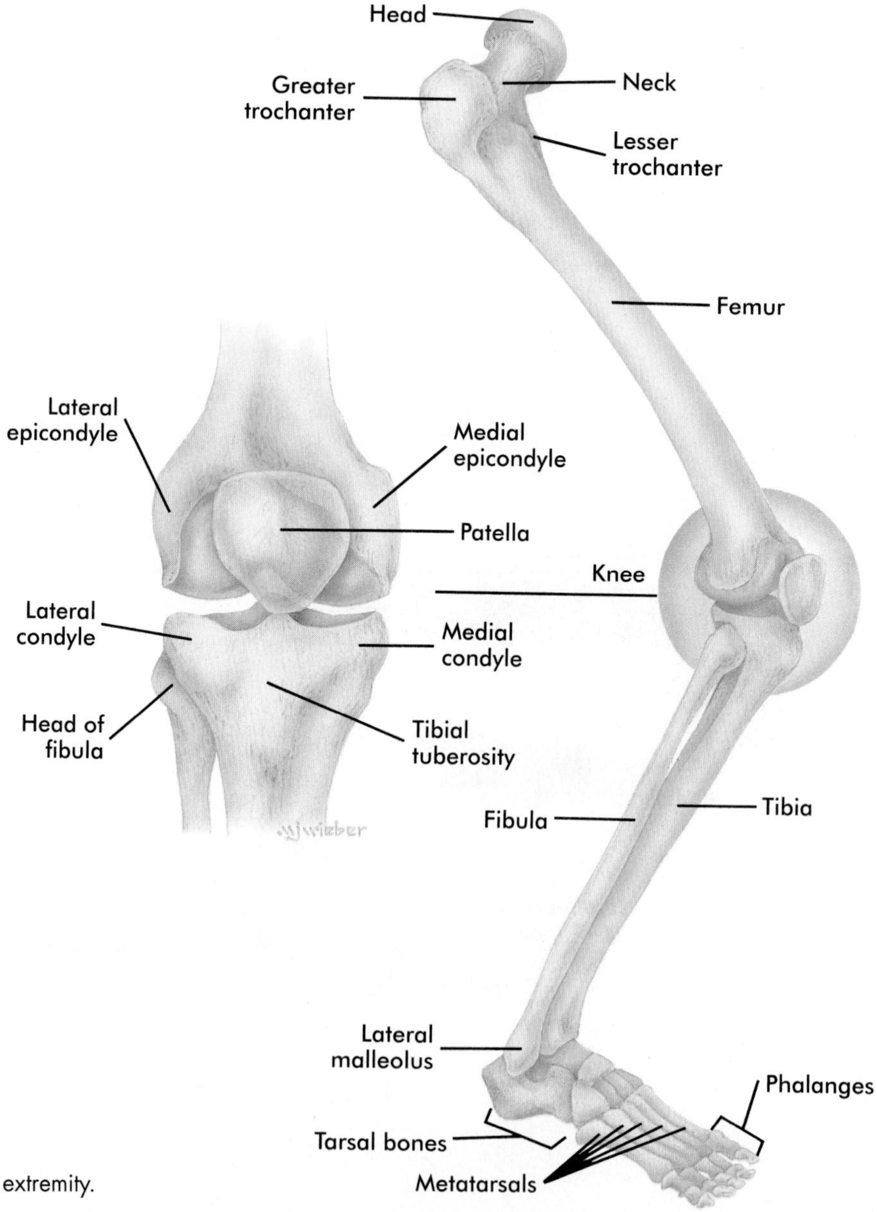

Sacroiliac joint

Sacrum

Sacral promontory

Anterior superior iliac spine

Obturator foramen

Symphysis pubis

Ilium

Pubis

Ischium

Head

Greater trochanter

Neck

Lesser trochanter

Femur

Lateral epicondyle

Medial epicondyle

Patella

Knee

Lateral condyle

Medial condyle

Head of fibula

Tibial tuberosity

Fibula

Tibia

Lateral malleolus

Phalanges

Tarsal bones

Metatarsals

mjwieber

Fig. 10-15 Bones of the lower extremity.

The wrist is composed of 8 carpal bones, which are arranged in two rows of 4 each. A total of 5 metacarpals are attached to the carpal bones and constitute the bony framework of the hand. A total of 28 phalanges make up the 10 digits of the hands. There are 2 phalanges for each thumb and 3 for each finger.

The pelvic girdle attaches the legs to the trunk (Fig. 10-14). The girdle consists of two coxae (hip bones), one located on each side of the pelvis. Each coxa surrounds a large obturator foramen through which muscles, nerves, and blood vessels pass to the leg. A fossa called the *acetabulum* is located on the lateral surface of each coxa and is the point of articulation of the lower limb with the girdle. During development, each coxa is formed by the fusion of three separate bones: the ilium, ischium, and pubis. The superior portion of the ilium is called the *iliac crest*. The crest ends anteriorly as the anterior-superior iliac spine and posteriorly as the posterior-superior iliac spine.

Fig. 10-15 illustrates the bones of the lower extremity. The femur is the longest bone in the body. It has a well-defined neck and a prominent rounded head that articulates with the acetabulum. The proximal shaft has two tuberosities: a greater trochanter lateral to the neck and a smaller or lesser trochanter inferior and posterior to the neck. Both trochanters are attachment sites for muscles that attach the hip to the thigh. The distal end of the femur has medial and lateral condyles that articulate with the tibia. Located laterally and proximally to the condyles are the medial and lateral epicondyles, which are sites of muscle and ligament attachment.

Distally, the femur also articulates with the patella, which is located in a major tendon of the thigh muscle. The patella allows the tendon to turn the corner over the knee.

The two bones of the leg are the tibia and the fibula. The tibia is the largest of the two and supports most of the weight of the leg. A tibial tuberosity can be seen and palpated just inferior to the patella. The proximal end of the tibia has flat medial and lateral condyles that articulate with the condyles of the femur. The distal end of the tibia forms the medial malleolus, which helps to form the medial side of the ankle joint.

The fibula does not articulate with the femur but does have a small proximal head that articulates with the tibia. The distal end of the fibula forms the lateral malleolus to create the lateral aspect of the ankle joint.

The foot consists of seven tarsal bones (Fig. 10-16). The talus articulates with the tibia and the

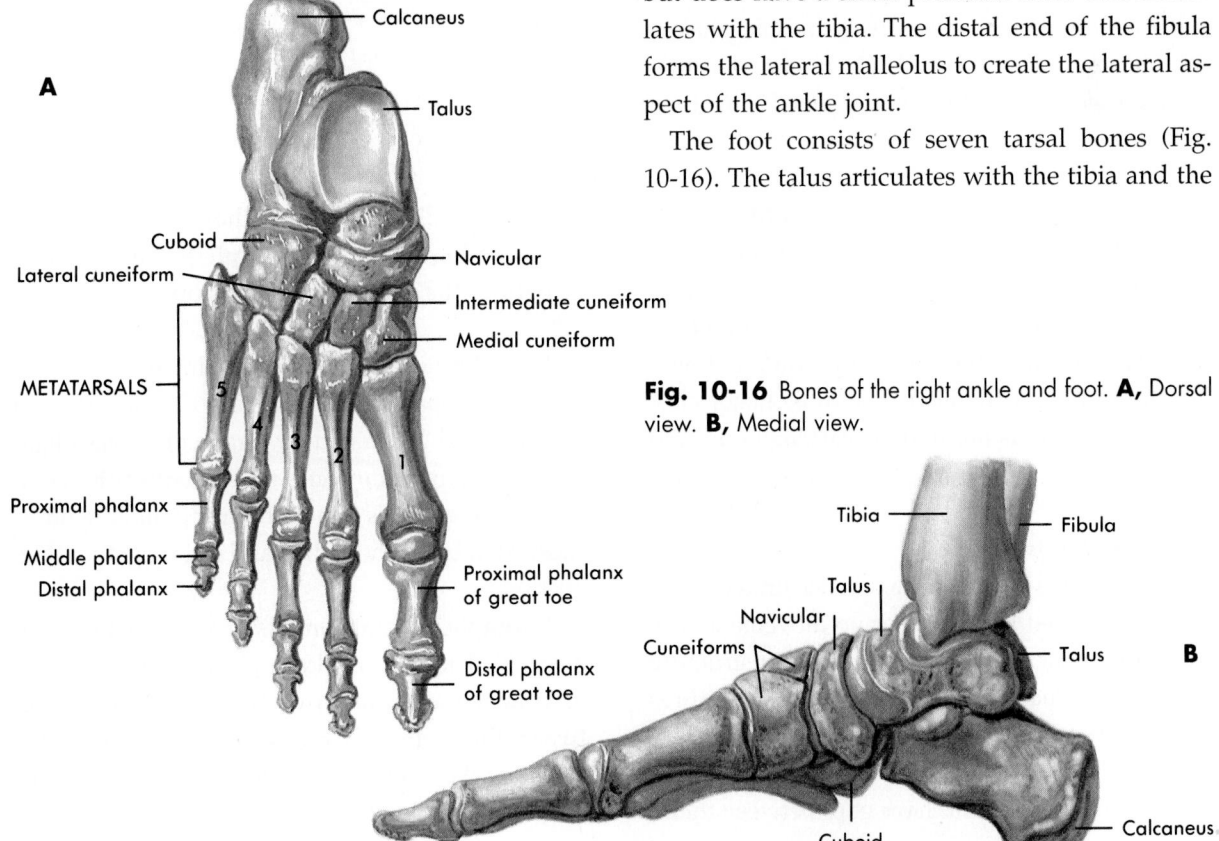

Fig. 10-16 Bones of the right ankle and foot. **A,** Dorsal view. **B,** Medial view.

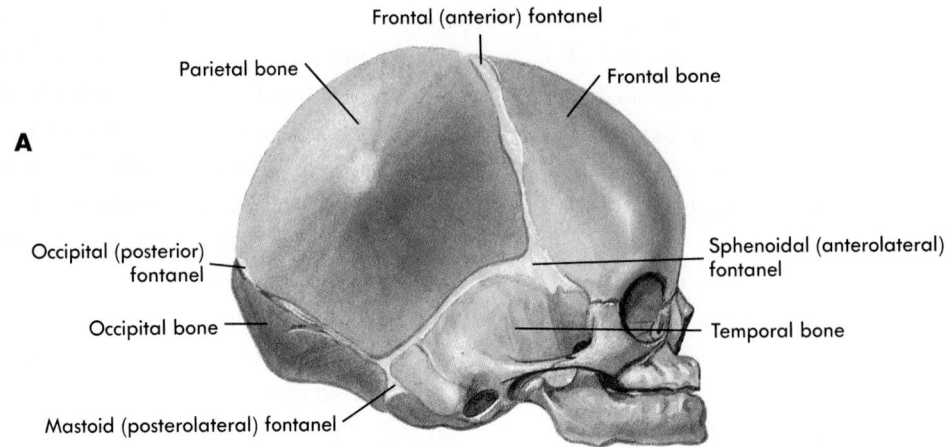

Fig. 10-17 Fetal skull showing fontanels. **A,** Lateral view. **B,** Superior view.

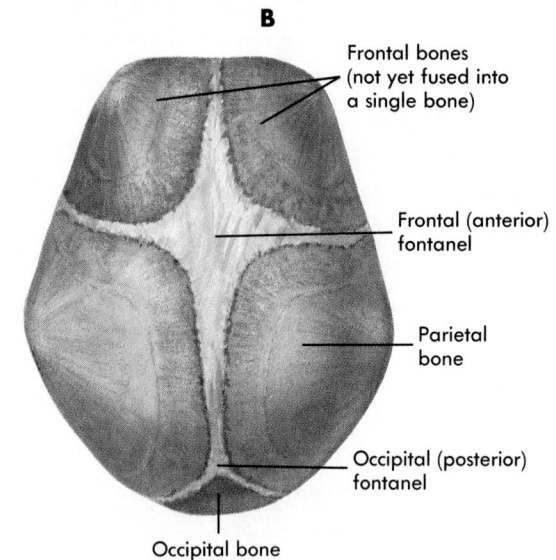

fibula to form the ankle joint. The calcaneus is located inferior and just lateral to the talus, supporting the bone. It protrudes posteriorly where the calf muscles attach to it and is easily identified as the heel. The foot consists of tarsals, metatarsals, and phalanges, which are arranged in a manner similar to the metacarpals and phalanges of the hand, the great toe being analogous to the thumb. The ball of the foot is the junction between the metatarsals and the phalanges. Strong ligaments and leg muscle tendons normally hold the foot bones firmly in their arched position.

Biomechanics of Body Movement

With the exception of the hyoid bone, every bone in the body connects to at least one other bone. The connections or joints are commonly named according to the bones or portions of bones that are united at the joint. The three major classifications of joints are fibrous, cartilaginous, and synovial.

Fibrous Joints

Fibrous joints consist of two bones united by fibrous tissue that have little or no movement. The joints are further divided on the basis of structure as sutures, syndesmoses, or gomphoses. Sutures (seams between flat bones) are located in the skull bones and may be completely immobile in adults. In newborns, the sutures have gaps between them,

which are called *fontanelles;* these gaps are fairly wide to allow "give" to the skull during birth and growth of the head during development (Fig. 10-17).

A syndesmosis is a fibrous joint in which the bones are separated by a greater distance than in a suture and are joined by ligaments. These ligaments may provide some movement of the joint. An example of this joint is the radioulnar syndesmosis that binds the radius and ulna together (Fig. 10-18).

A gomphosis joint consists of a peg that fits into a socket. The peg is held in place by fine bundles of collagenous connective tissue. The joints between the teeth and the sockets along the processes of the mandible and maxillae are examples of gomphoses joints.

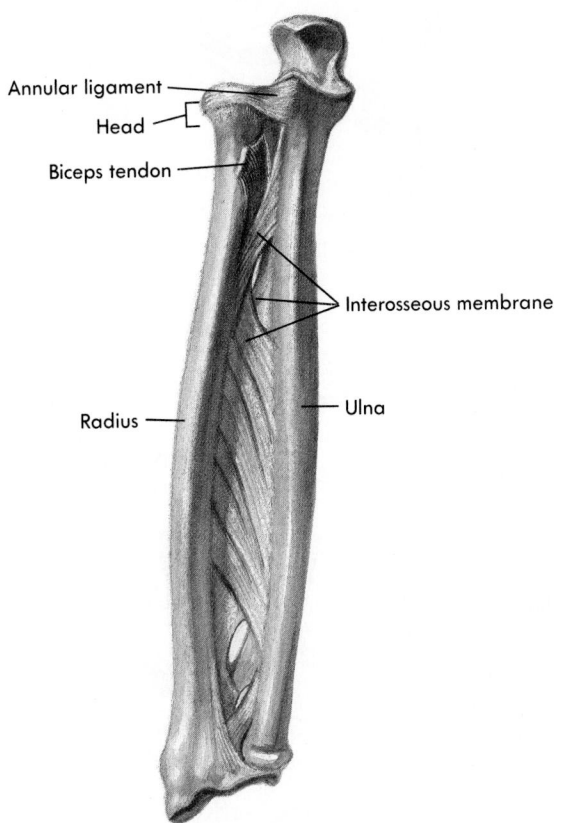

Fig. 10-18 Radioulnar syndesmosis of right forearm.

Labels: Annular ligament, Head, Biceps tendon, Interosseous membrane, Radius, Ulna

Cartilaginous Joints

Cartilaginous joints unite two bones by means of hyaline cartilage (synchondroses) or fibrocartilage (symphyses). A synchondrosis allows only slight movement at the joint. Common examples of this type of joint are the epiphyseal plate of a growing bone and the cartilage rod between most of the ribs and the sternum.

Symphysis joints are slightly moveable because of the flexible nature of the fibrocartilage. Symphyses include the junction between the manubrium and the body of the sternum in adults, the symphysis pubis of the coxae, and the intervertebral disks.

Synovial Joints

Synovial joints contain synovial fluid, a thin, lubricating film that allows considerable movement between articulating bones. Most joints that unite the bones of the appendicular skeleton are synovial. The articular surfaces of bones within synovial joints are covered with a thin layer of hyaline cartilage, which provides a smooth surface where the bones meet. The joint is enclosed by a joint capsule that consists of an outer fibrous capsule and an inner synovial membrane. The synovial membrane lines the joint and produces synovial fluid. Synovial joints are classified into six divisions according to the shape of the adjoining articular surfaces (Fig. 10-19):

1. Plane or gliding joints consist of two opposed flat surfaces that are approximately equal in size. Examples of these joints are the articular processes between vertebrae.

2. Saddle joints consist of two saddle-shaped articulating surfaces oriented at right angles to one another. Movement in these joints can occur in two planes. An example of a saddle joint is the carpometacarpal joint of the thumb.

3. Hinge joints consist of a convex cylinder in one bone applied to a corresponding concavity in another bone. These joints permit movement in one plane only. Examples of hinge joints are those of the elbow and knee.

4. Pivot joints consist of a relatively cylindrical bony process that rotates within a ring composed partly of bone and partly of ligament. An example of a pivot joint is the head of the radius articulating with the proximal end of the ulna.

5. Ball-and-socket joints consist of a ball (head) at the end of one bone and a socket into an adjacent bone into which a portion of the ball fits. These joints allow wide ranges of movement in almost any direction. Examples are the shoulder and hip joints.

6. Ellipsoid joints are modified ball-and-socket joints where the articular surfaces are ellipsoid rather than spherical in shape. The shape of the joint limits movement similar to hinge motion but in two planes. The atlantooccipital joint is an ellipsoid joint.

Types of Movement

Body movement may be described in relation to the anatomical position, that is, movement away from the anatomical position and movement toward it. Examples of each are listed in Table 10-3 (Figs. 10-20 through 10-24).

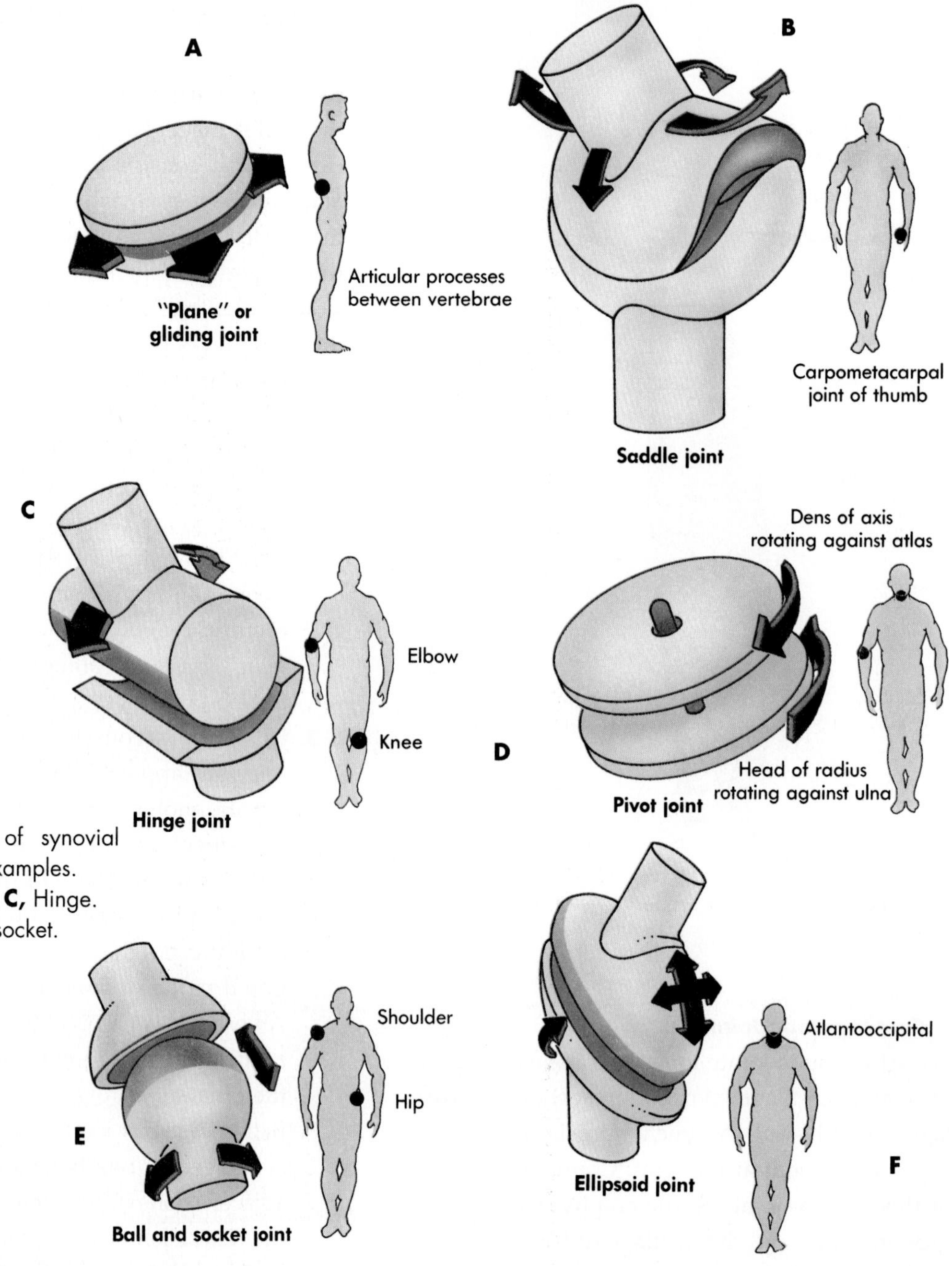

A

"Plane" or gliding joint

Articular processes between vertebrae

B

Saddle joint

Carpometacarpal joint of thumb

C

Hinge joint

Elbow

Knee

D

Dens of axis rotating against atlas

Pivot joint

Head of radius rotating against ulna

Fig. 10-19 Types of synovial joints and selected examples. **A,** Plane. **B,** Saddle. **C,** Hinge. **D,** Pivot. **E,** Ball-and-socket. **F,** Ellipsoid.

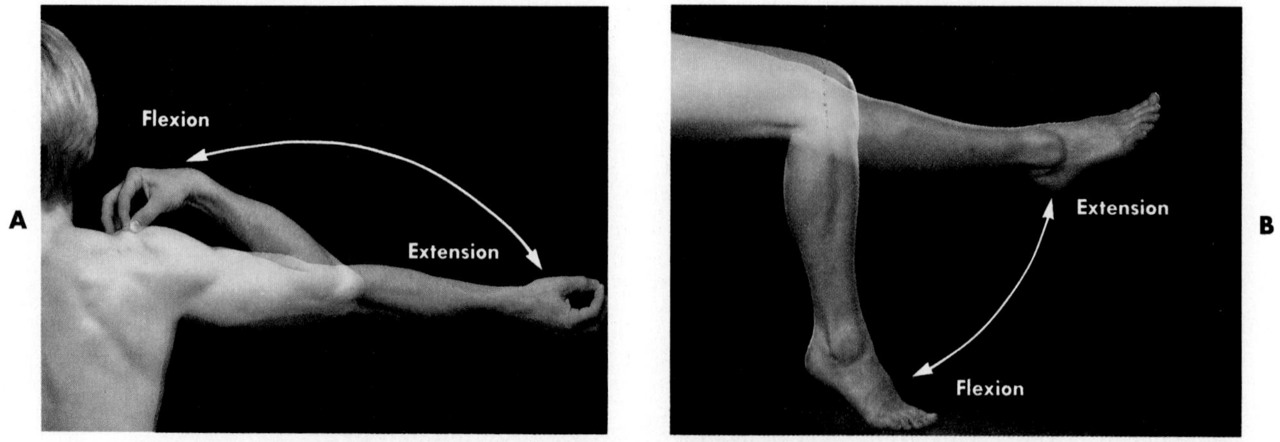

E

Ball and socket joint

Shoulder

Hip

F

Ellipsoid joint

Atlantooccipital

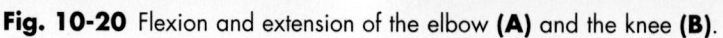

A Flexion / Extension

B Extension / Flexion

Fig. 10-20 Flexion and extension of the elbow **(A)** and the knee **(B)**.

TABLE 10-3 Body Movement Terminology

Term	Definition
Flexion	Bending
Extension	Stretching out
Protraction	Movement in the anterior direction
Retraction	Movement in the posterior direction
Abduction	Movement away from the midline
Adduction	Movement toward the midline
Inversion	Turning inward
Eversion	Turning outward
Excursion	Movement from side to side
Rotation	Movement of a structure about its axis
Circumduction	Movement in a circular motion
Pronation	Rotation of the forearm so that the anterior surface is down
Supination	Rotation of the forearm so that the anterior surface is up
Elevation	Movement of a structure in a superior direction
Depression	Movement of a structure in an inferior direction
Opposition	Movement of the thumb and little finger toward each other
Reposition	Movement of a structure to its original position

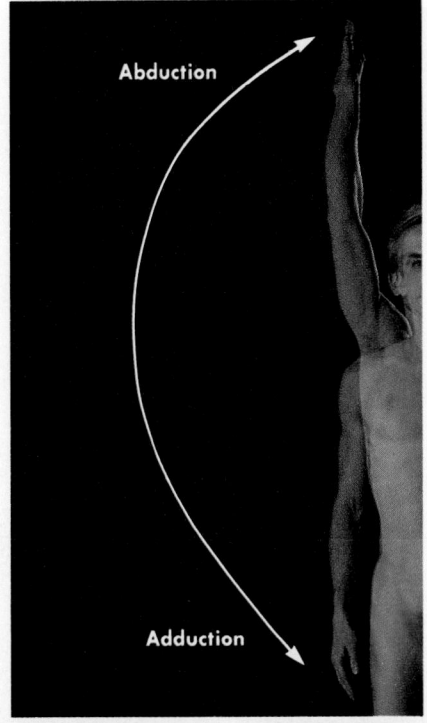

A

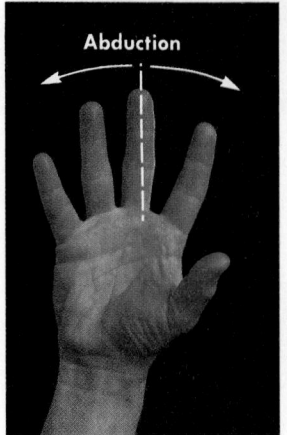 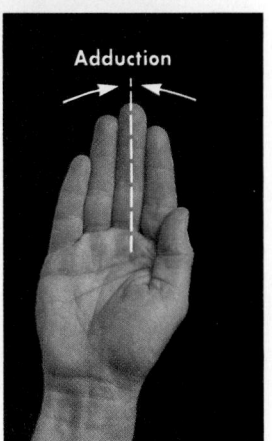

B

Fig. 10-21 Abduction and adduction of the upper extremity (**A**) and the fingers (**B**).

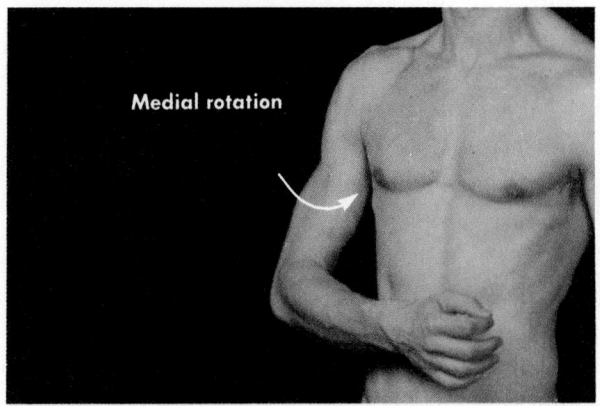 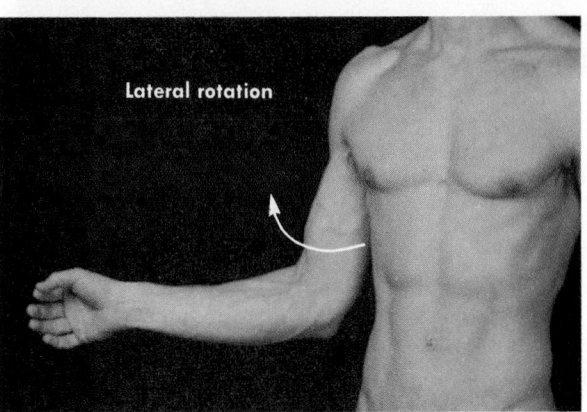

Fig. 10-22 Medial and lateral rotation of the humerus.

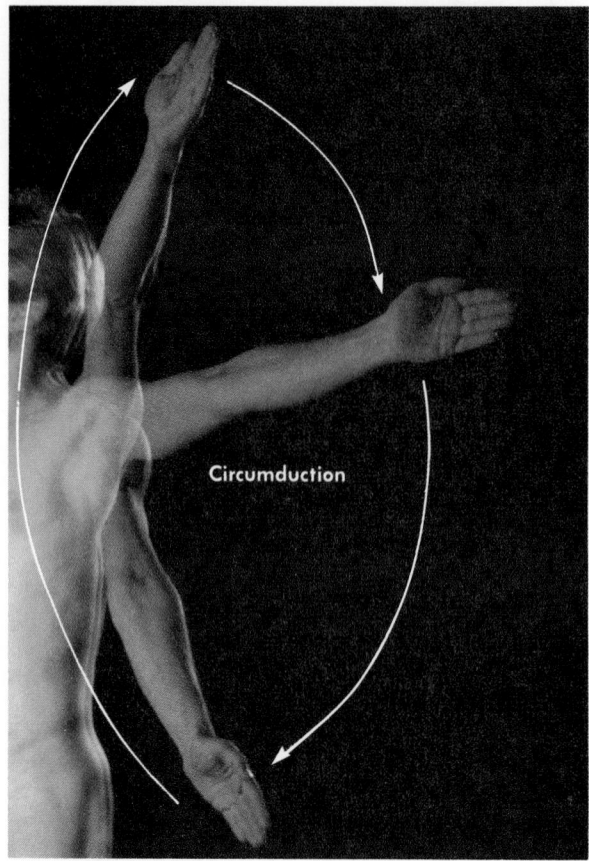

Fig. 10-23 Circumduction of the shoulder.

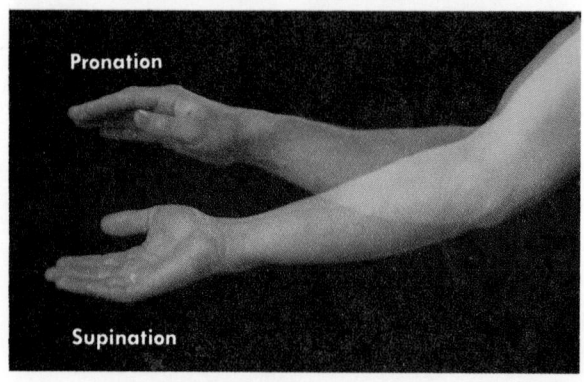

Fig. 10-24 Pronation and supination.

The Muscular System

The three primary functions of the muscular system are movement, postural maintenance, and heat production. As previously discussed, the major types of muscles are skeletal, cardiac, and smooth muscle. Skeletal muscle is far more com-

mon than other types of muscle in the body and will be the focus of this particular section. Cardiac and smooth muscle will be presented later in this text. These muscle types are compared in Table 10-4.

Physiology of Skeletal Muscle

Muscle tissue consists of specialized contractile cells or muscle fibers. Skeletal muscle contracts in response to electrochemical stimuli. Nerve cells regulate the function of skeletal muscle fibers by controlling the series of events that result in muscle contraction.

Each skeletal muscle fiber is filled with thick and thin myofilaments, which are fine, threadlike structures. The thick myofilaments are formed from the protein myosin, and the thin myofilaments are composed of the protein actin. The sarcomere is the contractile unit of skeletal muscle, containing thick and thin myofilaments. During the contraction process, energy obtained from ATP molecules enables the two types of myofilaments to slide toward each other and shorten the sarcomere and eventually the entire muscle.

The Neuromuscular Junction

A nervous impulse enters the muscle fiber through a specialized nerve known as a *motor neuron*. The point of contact between the nerve ending and the muscle fiber is the neuromuscular junction or synapse (Fig. 10-25). Each muscle fiber receives a branch of an axon, and each axon innervates more than a single muscle fiber. When a nerve impulse passes through this junction, specialized chemicals are released, causing the muscle to contract.

Skeletal Muscle Movement

Most muscles extend from one bone to another and cross at least one joint. Muscle contraction causes most body movements by pulling one of the bones toward the other across the moveable joint. The points of attachment of each muscle are the origin and insertion. The origin is the end of the muscle attached to the more stationary of the two bones. The insertion is the end of the muscle attached to the bone undergoing the greatest movement. Some muscles of the face are not at-

TABLE 10-4 Comparison of Muscle Types

Features	Skeletal Muscle	Cardiac Muscle	Smooth Muscle
Location	Attached to bones	Heart	Walls of hollow organs, blood vessels, eyes, glands, and skin
Cell shape	Very long and cylindrical (1-40 mm in length and may extend the entire length of a muscle, 10-100 μm in diameter)	Cylindrical and branched (100-500 μm in length, 100-200 μm in diameter)	Spindle-shaped (15-200 μm in length, 5-10 μm in diameter)
Nucleus	Multiple, peripherally located	Single, centrally located	Single, centrally located
Special features		Intercalated disks join the cells to each other	
Striations	Yes	Yes	No
Control	Voluntary	Involuntary	Involuntary
Capable of spontaneous contraction	No	Yes	Yes
Function	Body movement	Pumps blood	Food movement through the digestive tract, emptying of the urinary bladder, regulation of blood vessel diameter, change in pupil size, contraction of many gland ducts, movement of hair, and many other functions

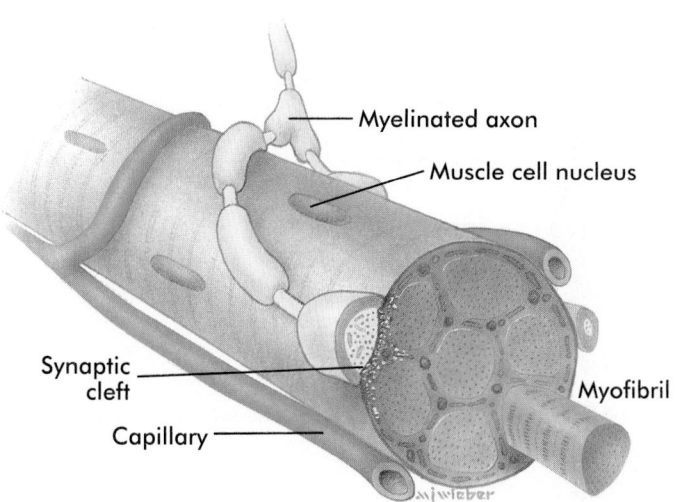

Fig. 10-25 Neuromuscular junction.

tached to bone at both ends but attach to the skin, which moves when muscles contract.

The contraction of some muscles with the simultaneous relaxation of others produces movement. Muscles that work in cooperation with one another to cause movement are synergists, and a muscle working in opposition to another muscle (moving the structure in an opposite direction) is an antagonist. The muscle that is primarily responsible for a particular movement is called the

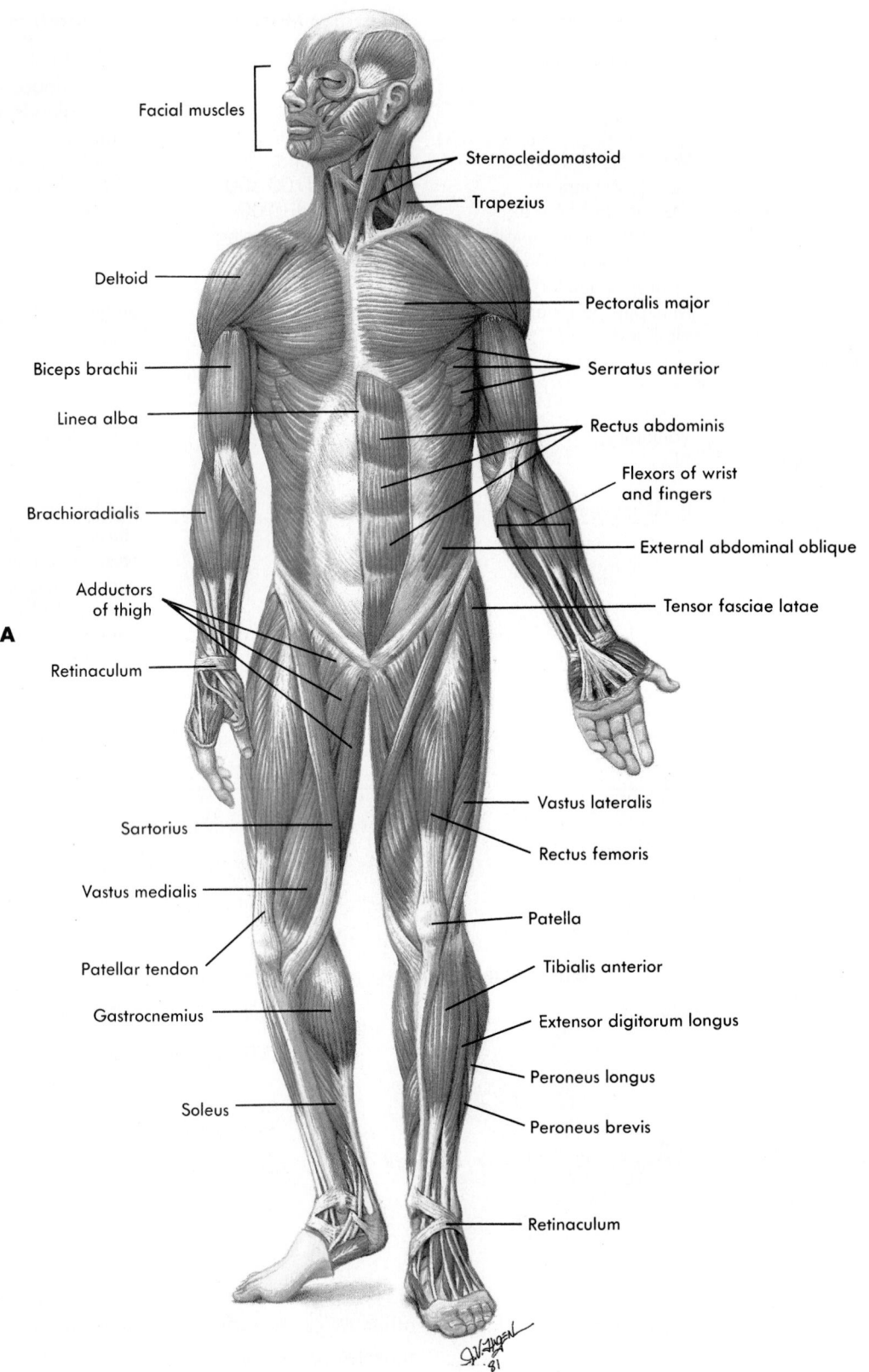

Facial muscles

Sternocleidomastoid

Trapezius

Deltoid

Pectoralis major

Biceps brachii

Serratus anterior

Linea alba

Rectus abdominis

Brachioradialis

Flexors of wrist and fingers

External abdominal oblique

Adductors of thigh

Tensor fasciae latae

Retinaculum

Vastus lateralis

Sartorius

Rectus femoris

Vastus medialis

Patella

Patellar tendon

Tibialis anterior

Gastrocnemius

Extensor digitorum longus

Peroneus longus

Soleus

Peroneus brevis

Retinaculum

A

Fig. 10-26 A, Anterior view of body musculature.

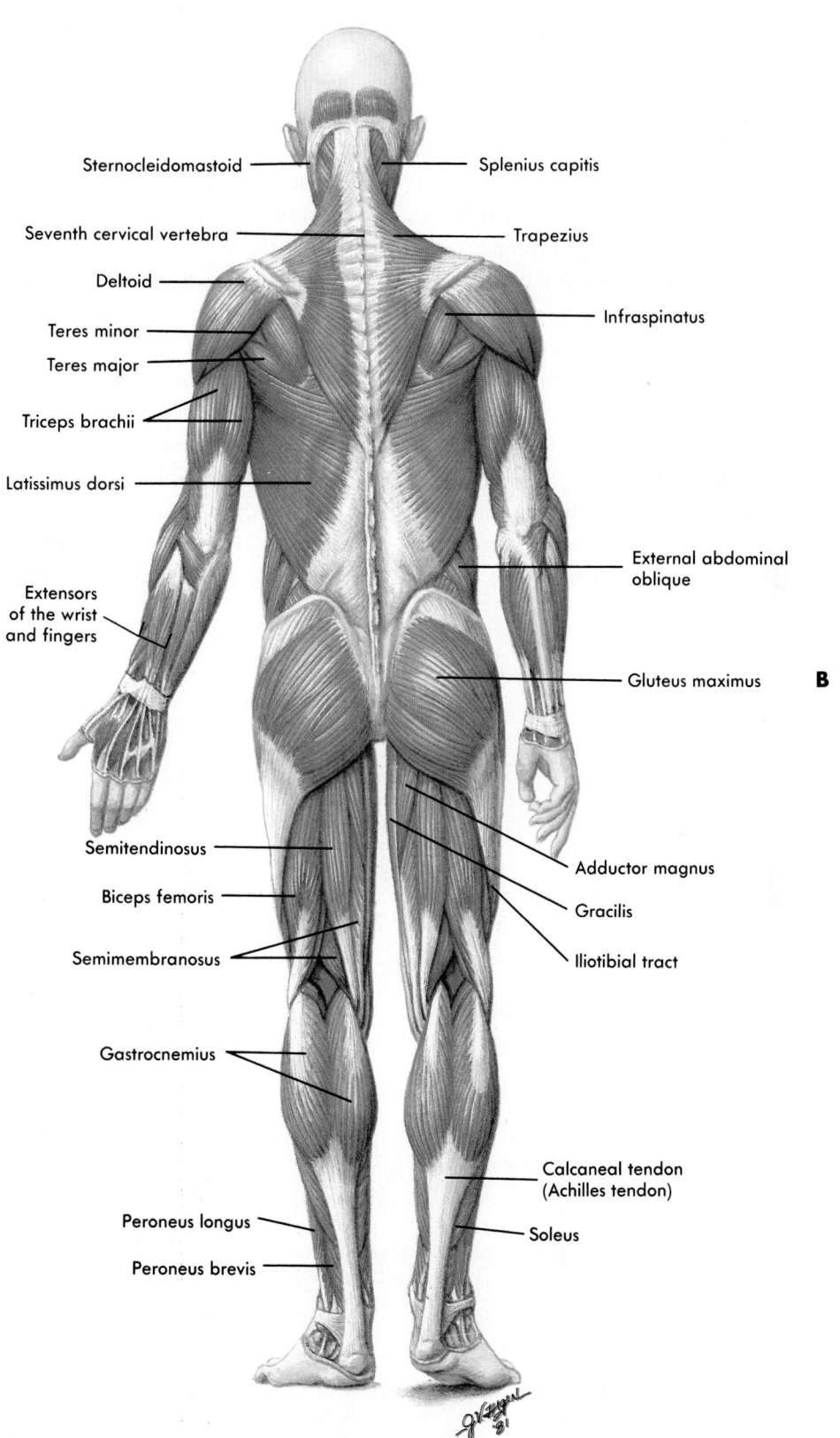

Sternocleidomastoid

Splenius capitis

Seventh cervical vertebra

Trapezius

Deltoid

Teres minor

Infraspinatus

Teres major

Triceps brachii

Latissimus dorsi

External abdominal oblique

Extensors of the wrist and fingers

Gluteus maximus

B

Semitendinosus

Adductor magnus

Biceps femoris

Gracilis

Semimembranosus

Iliotibial tract

Gastrocnemius

Calcaneal tendon (Achilles tendon)

Peroneus longus

Soleus

Peroneus brevis

Fig. 10-26 B, Posterior view of body musculature.

prime mover. For example, the biceps brachii, brachialis, and triceps brachii muscles are all involved in flexion and extension of the forearm at the elbow joint. The biceps brachii is the prime mover during flexion, and the brachialis is the synergistic muscle. When the biceps brachii and the brachialis muscles flex the forearm, the triceps brachii relaxes (antagonistic muscle). During extension of the forearm, the triceps brachii becomes the prime mover, and the biceps and brachialis become the antagonistic muscles. The combined and coordinated activity of synergists and antagonists is what makes muscular movement smooth and graceful (Fig. 10-26).

Types of Muscle Contraction

Muscle contractions are classified as either isometric or isotonic, depending on the type of contraction that predominates. In isometric contrac-

tions, the length of the muscle does not change, but the amount of tension increases during the contraction process. Isometric contractions are responsible for the constant length of the postural muscles of the body. During isotonic contractions, the amount of tension produced by the muscle is constant during contraction, but the length of the muscle changes. An example of isotonic contraction is the movement of the arms or fingers. Most muscle contractions are a combination of isometric and isotonic contractions.

Postural Maintenance

Postural maintenance is a result of muscle tone, the constant tension produced by muscles of the body for long periods. This tone is responsible for keeping the back and legs straight, the head in an upright position, and the abdomen from bulging. These positions balance the distribution of weight

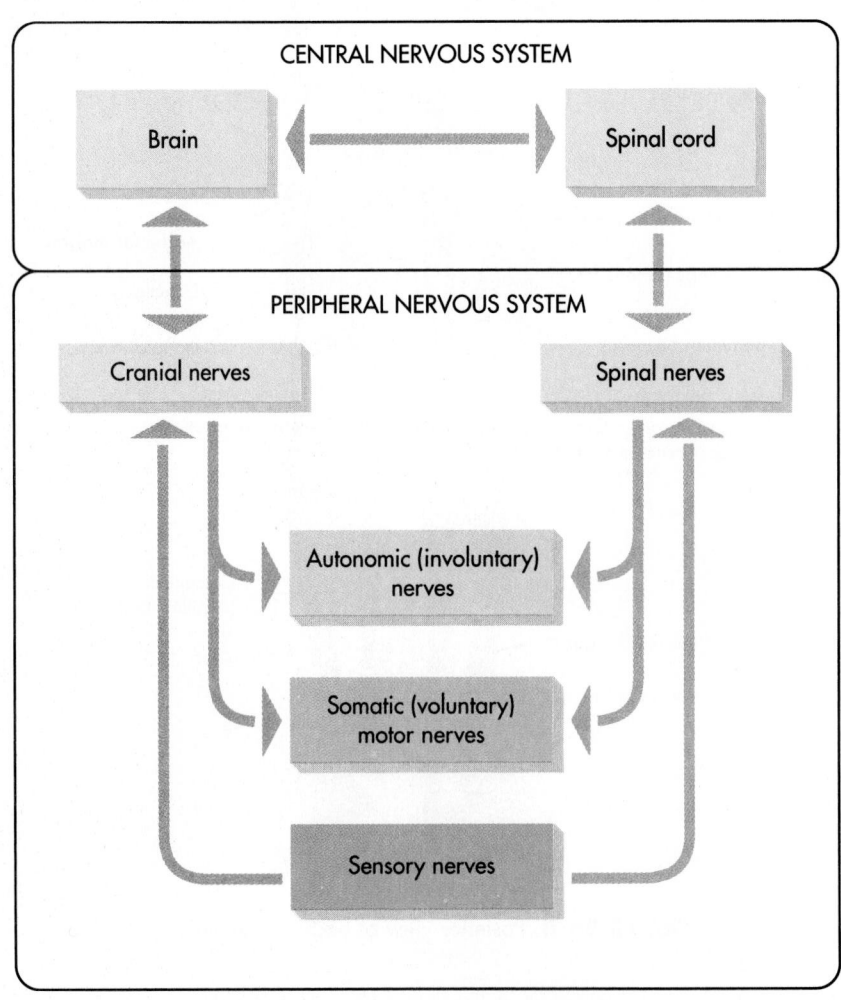

Fig. 10-27 Divisions of the nervous system.

and therefore put less strain on muscles, tendons, ligaments, and bones.

Heat Production

Energy required to produce muscle contraction is obtained from ATP. Most of the energy released in the breakdown of ATP during a muscular contraction is used to shorten the muscle fibers, but some energy is lost as heat during the chemical reaction. The normal body temperature results in large part from this metabolism in skeletal muscle.

If the body temperature declines below a certain level, the nervous system responds by inducing shivering. Shivering involves rapid contractions of skeletal muscle that produce shaking rather than coordinated movements. The muscle movement increases heat production up to 18 times that of resting levels. The heat produced during shivering can exceed that produced during moderate exercise, helping to raise the body temperature to its normal range.

The Nervous System

The nervous system and the endocrine system are the major regulatory and coordinating systems of the body. The nervous system rapidly transmits information by means of nerve impulses conducted from one body area to another. The endocrine system transmits information more slowly by means of chemicals secreted by ductless glands into the blood stream. These chemicals and hormones are then circulated to other parts of the body. The constancy of the internal environment of the body (homeostasis) is maintained to a large degree by these regulatory and coordinating activities.

Divisions of the Nervous System

The human body has a single nervous system, even though some of its subdivisions are referred to as separate systems. Each subdivision has structural and functional features that separate it from the other subdivisions (Fig. 10-27).

The **central nervous system (CNS)** consists of the brain and spinal cord, which are encased in and protected by bone. The brain and spinal cord are continuous with each other.

The **peripheral nervous system (PNS)** consists of the nerves and ganglia (collections of nerve cell bodies located outside the CNS). A total of 43 pairs of nerves originate from the CNS to form the PNS: 12 pairs, the cranial nerves, originate from the brain, and the remaining 31 pairs, the spinal nerves, originate from the spinal cord. The afferent division transmits action potentials from the sensory organs to the CNS. The efferent division transmits action potentials from the CNS to effector organs such as muscles and glands (Fig. 10-28).

The efferent division is further divided into the somatic nervous system and the autonomic ner-

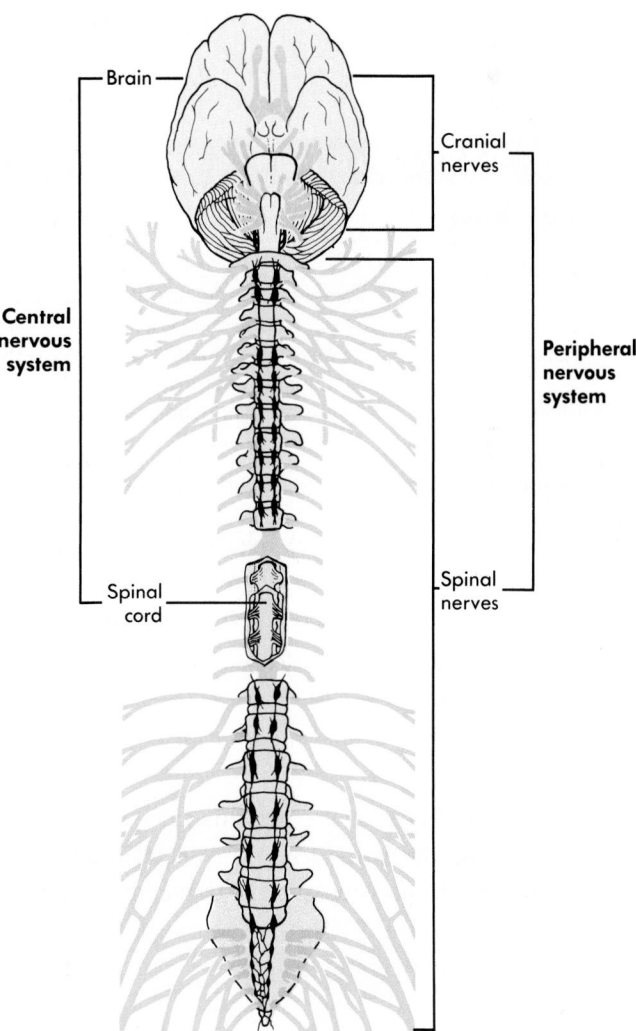

Fig. 10-28 The central nervous system consists of the brain and spinal cord. The peripheral nervous system consists of cranial nerves, which arise from the brain, and spinal nerves, which arise from the spinal cord.

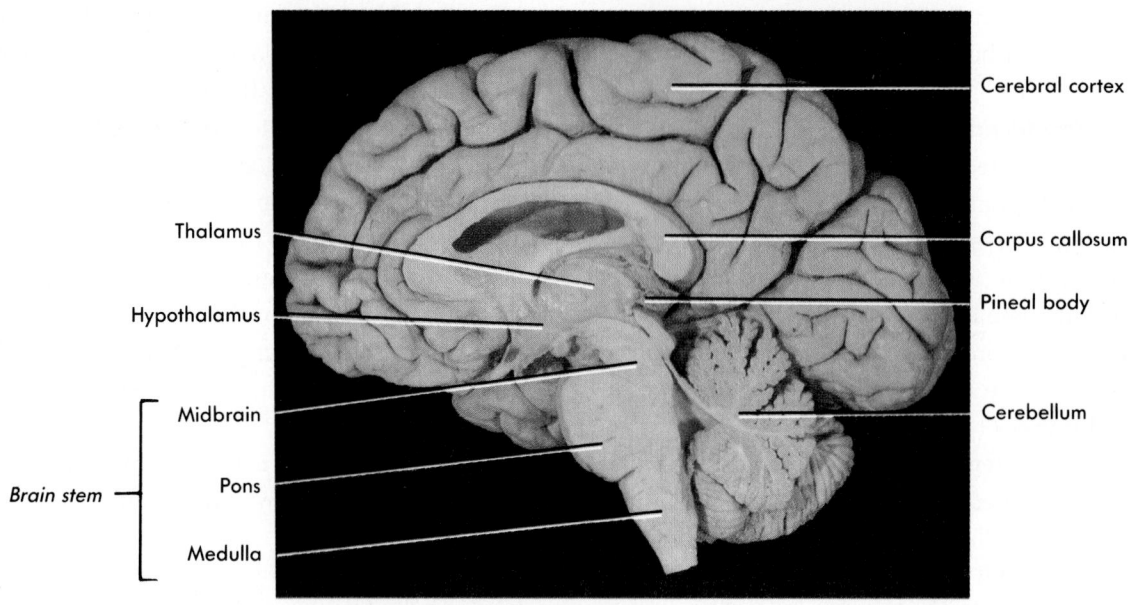

Fig. 10-29 Section of preserved brain.

TABLE 10-5 Functions of Major Divisions of the Brain

Brain Area	Function
Brain Stem	
Medulla	Two-way conduction pathway between the spinal cord and higher brain centers; cardiac, respiratory, and vasomotor control centers
Pons	Two-way conduction pathway between areas of the brain and other regions of the body; influences respiration
Midbrain	Two-way conduction pathway; relay point for visual and auditory impulses
Diencephalon	
Hypothalamus	Regulation of body temperature, water balance, sleep-cycle control, appetite, and sexual arousal
Thalamus	Sensory relay station from various body areas to cerebral cortex; emotions and alerting or arousal mechanisms
Cerebellum	Muscle coordination; maintenance of equilibrium and posture
Cerebrum	Sensory perception, emotions, willed movements, consciousness, and memory

vous system. The somatic nervous system transmits impulses from the CNS to skeletal muscle. The autonomic nervous system transmits action potentials from the CNS to smooth muscle, cardiac muscle, and certain glands.

The Central Nervous System

The CNS consists of the brain and spinal cord. The major regions of the adult brain are the brain stem (consisting of the medulla, pons, and midbrain), the diencephalon (which includes the thalamus and hypothalamus), the cerebrum, and the cerebellum (Fig. 10-29). The functions of these divisions are described in Table 10-5.

Brain stem

The medulla, pons, and midbrain constitute the brain stem. The brain stem connects the spinal cord to the remainder of the brain and is responsible for many essential functions. All but 2 of the 12 cranial nerves enter or exit the brain through the brain stem.

TABLE 10-6 Hypothalamic Functions

Function	Description
Autonomic	Helps control heart rate, urine release from the bladder, movement of food through the digestive tract, and blood vessel diameter
Endocrine	Helps regulate pituitary gland secretions and influences metabolism, ion balance, sexual development, and sexual functions
Muscle control	Controls muscles involved in swallowing and stimulates shivering in several muscles
Temperature regulation	Promotes heat loss when the hypothalamic temperature increases by increasing sweat production (anterior hypothalamus) and promotes heat production when the hypothalamic temperature decreases by promoting shivering (posterior hypothalamus)
Regulation of food and water intake	Hunger center promotes eating and satiety center inhibits eating; thirst center promotes water intake
Emotions	Large range of emotional influences over body functions; directly involved in stress-related and psychosomatic illnesses and with feelings of fear and rage
Regulation of the sleep-wake cycle	Coordinates responses to the sleep-wake cycle with other areas of the brain (for example, the reticular activating system)

The medulla, also known as the *medulla oblongata,* is the most inferior portion of the brain stem. It acts as a conduction pathway for both ascending and descending nerve tracts. Several body functions, such as regulation of heart rate, blood vessel diameter, breathing, swallowing, vomiting, coughing, and sneezing, are controlled by the medulla.

The pons contains ascending and descending nerve tracts and relays information from the cerebrum to the cerebellum. In addition, the pons houses the sleep center and respiratory center, which along with the medulla, help control breathing.

The midbrain, or mesencephalon, is the smallest region of the brain stem. It is involved in hearing through audio pathways in the CNS and in visual reflexes such as visual tracking of moving objects and turning of the eyes. Other parts of the midbrain help regulate the automatic functions that require no conscious thought (for example, the coordination of motor activities and muscle tone).

The reticular formation is a group of nuclei scattered throughout the brain stem that receives axons from a large number of sources, especially from the nerves that innervate the face. The reticular formation and its connections are known as the *reticular activating system.* This system is involved in the sleep-wake cycle and is important in arousing and maintaining consciousness. Coma after head injury results from damage to the reticular activating system.

Diencephalon

The diencephalon is the part of the brain between the brain stem and the cerebrum. Major components of this organ include the thalamus and hypothalamus.

The thalamus is the largest portion of the diencephalon. The thalamus receives sensory input from various sense organs of the body and relays these impulses to the cerebral cortex. The thalamus also has other functions, such as influencing mood and general body movements associated with strong emotions such as fear or rage.

The hypothalamus is a major controller in the brain. It serves as a "gatekeeper" to determine which information is passed along to the cerebrum and is an active participant in emotions, hormonal cycles, and sexuality. A summary of the various hypothalamic functions appears in Table 10-6.

Cerebrum

The cerebrum is the largest portion of the brain. It is divided into left and right hemispheres, and each cerebral hemisphere is divided into lobes

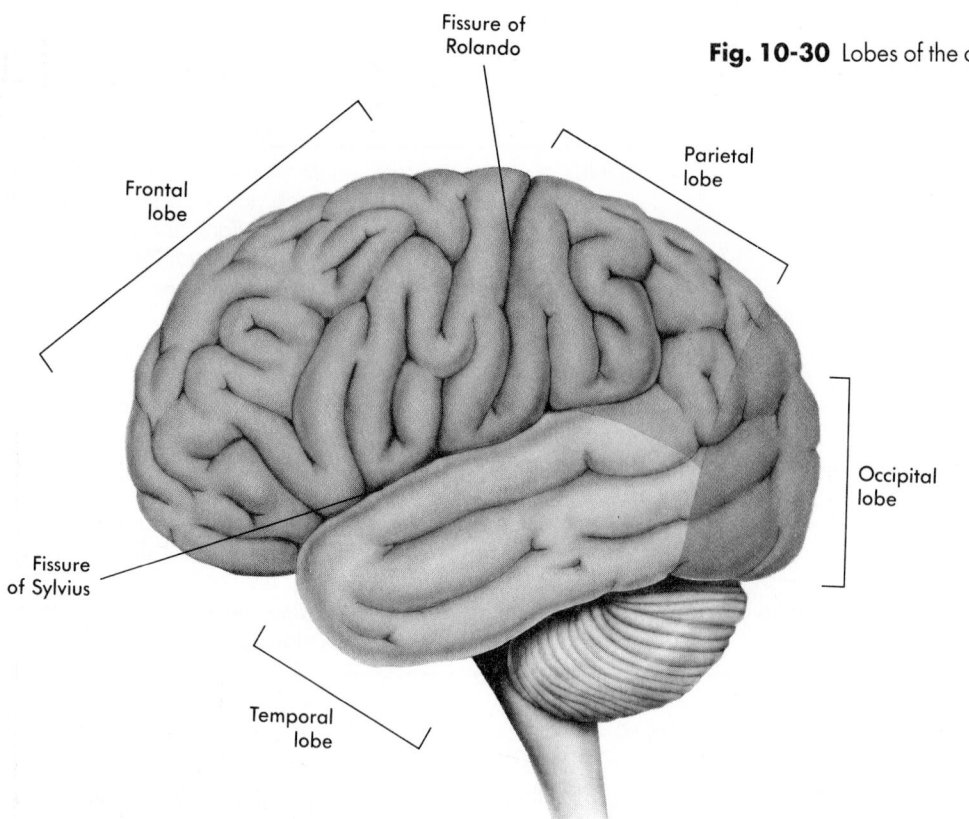

Fig. 10-30 Lobes of the cerebrum.

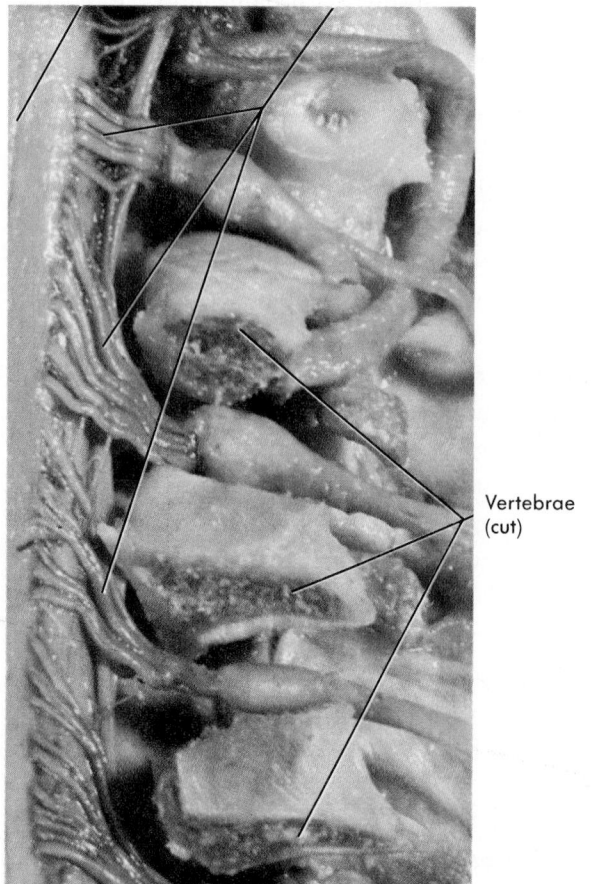

Fig. 10-31 Dissection of the cervical segment of the spinal cord.

named for the bones that lie over them (Fig. 10-30.

The frontal lobe is important in voluntary motor function, motivation, aggression, and mood. The parietal lobe is the major center for the reception and evaluation of most sensory information (excluding smell, hearing, and vision). The occipital lobe functions in the reception and integration of visual input and is not distinctly separate from other lobes. The temporal lobe receives and evaluates olfactory and auditory input and plays an important role in memory. A thin layer of gray matter made up of neuron dendrites and cell bodies composes the surface of the cerebrum (cerebral cortex).

The limbic system consists of portions of the cerebrum and diencephalon. It influences emotions, visceral responses to those emotions, motivation, mood, and sensations of pain and pleasure.

Cerebellum

The cerebellum is the second largest part of the human brain. It is involved in gross motor coordination, producing smooth, flowing movements.

A major function of the cerebellum is to compare impulses from the motor cortex with those from moving structures (for example, position of the body or body parts that innervate the joints and tendons of the structure being moved). The cerebellum compares the intended movement with the actual movement. If a difference is detected, the cerebellum sends impulses to the motor cortex and the spinal cord to correct the discrepancy. Loss of cerebellum functioning results in an inability to make precise movements.

The Spinal Cord

The spinal cord lies within the spinal column and extends from the occipital bone to the level of the second lumbar vertebrae. The spinal cord has a central gray portion and a peripheral white portion. The white matter consists of nerve tracts, and the gray matter consists of nerve cell bodies and dendrites. The dorsal root conveys afferent nerve processes to the cord, and the ventral route conveys efferent nerve processes away from the cord. Spinal ganglia, or dorsal root ganglia, contain the cell bodies of sensory neurons (Fig. 10-31).

The spinal cord is the primary reflex center of the body. Many of these reflexes are autonomic or visceral, for example, increased heart rate in response to decreased blood pressure. Other reflexes include the stretch reflex ("knee-jerk reflex") and withdrawal reflexes (removing a limb or other body part from a painful stimulus).

In addition to functioning as a primary reflex center, the spinal cord tracts carry impulses to the brain in afferent, ascending tracts, and carry motor impulses from the brain in efferent, descending tracts. Ascending and descending pathways are further addressed in Chapter 20.

The organs of the nervous system are surrounded by a tough, fluid-containing membrane known as the *meninges.* The meninges are surrounded by bone and have three connective tissue layers. The most superficial and thickest layer is the dura mater, consisting of two layers around the brain and one layer around the spinal cord. The two layers of the dura mater are fused around most of the brain but separate in several places. It is tightly attached and continuous with the periosteum of the cranial vault, whereas the dura mater of the spinal cord is separated from the periosteum of the vertebral canal by the epidural space.

The arachnoid layer is the second meningeal layer. The space between this layer and the dura mater is known as the *subdural space,* which contains a small amount of serous fluid.

The third meningeal layer is the pia mater. It lies external to a basement membrane formed by special cells termed the *glia limitans,* which completely invests the CNS. The space between the pia mater and the arachnoid layer is the subarachnoid space. This space is filled with blood vessels and cerebrospinal fluid (Fig. 10-32).

The cerebrospinal fluid is similar to plasma and interstitial fluid (fluid that occupies the space outside the blood vessels). It serves to bathe the brain and spinal cord and to act as a protective cushion

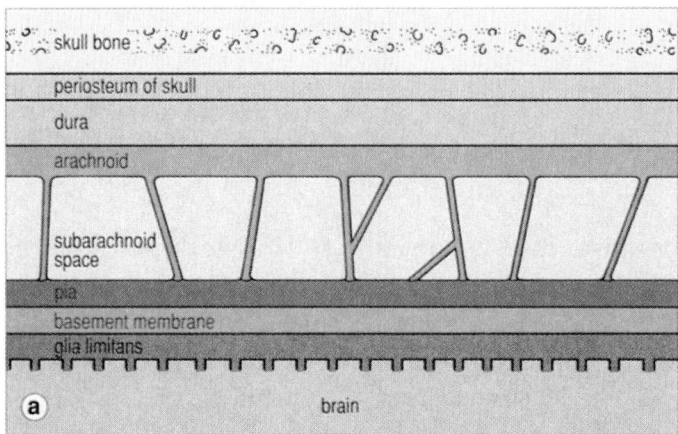

Fig. 10-32 Meningeal coverings of the brain and spinal cord.

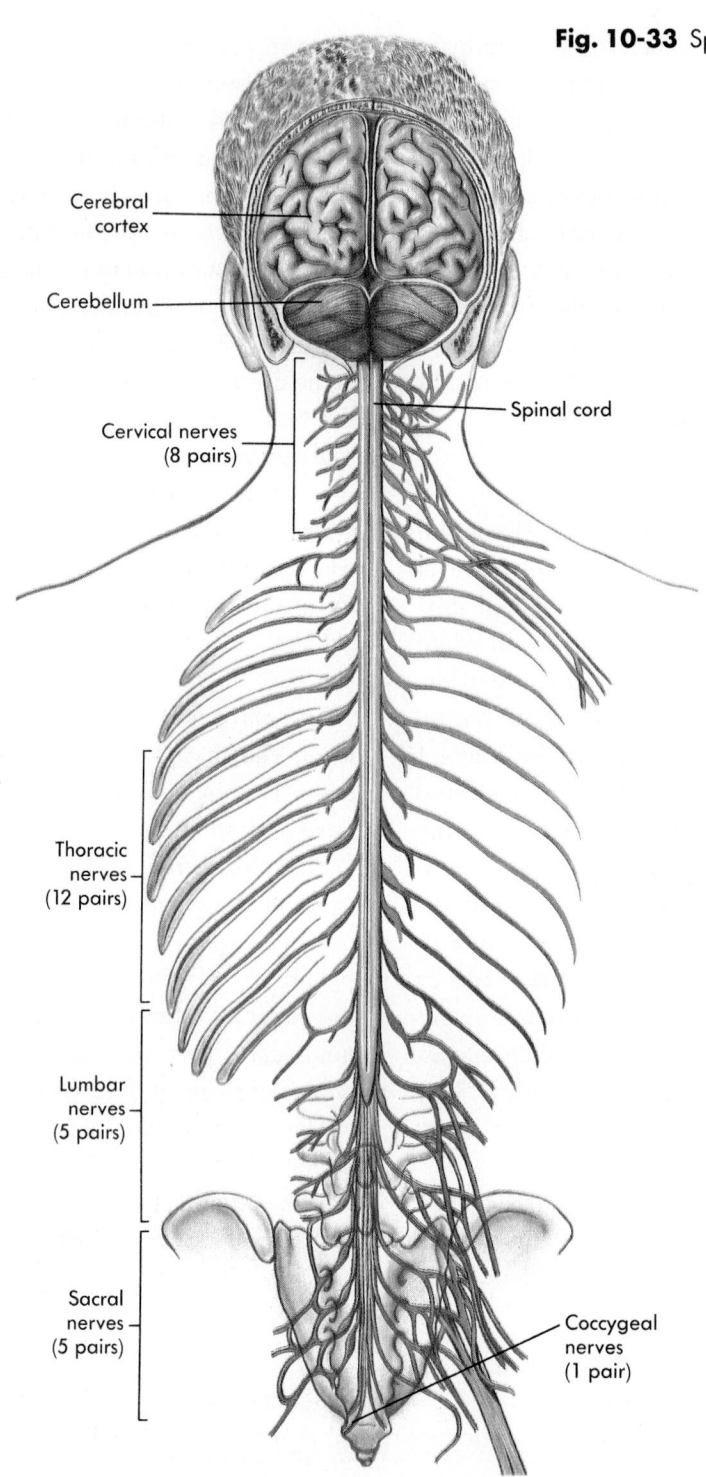

Fig. 10-33 Spinal cord and spinal nerves.

Cerebral cortex

Cerebellum

Spinal cord

Cervical nerves (8 pairs)

Thoracic nerves (12 pairs)

Lumbar nerves (5 pairs)

Sacral nerves (5 pairs)

Coccygeal nerves (1 pair)

around the CNS. Cerebrospinal fluid is formed continually from fluid filtering out of the blood in a network of brain capillaries and cells known collectively as the *choroid plexus*. This special fluid fills the ventricles of the brain, the subarachnoid space, and the central canal of the spinal cord.

The Peripheral Nervous System

The PNS collects information from numerous sources, from both inside the body and the body surface. This information is relayed by way of afferent fibers to the CNS, where it is evaluated. Efferent fibers in the PNS relay information from the CNS to various parts of the body, primarily to muscles and glands.

Spinal Nerves

The spinal nerves arise from numerous rootlets along the dorsal and ventral surfaces of the spinal cord. All of the 31 pairs of spinal nerves, except the first pair of spinal nerves and the spinal nerves in the sacrum, exit the vertebral column though adjacent vertebrae. The first pair of spinal nerves exits between the skull and the first cervical vertebrae. The spinal nerves in the sacrum exit through the bone. A total of 8 spinal nerve pairs exit the vertebral column in the cervical region, 12 in the thoracic region, 5 in the lumbar region, 5 in the sacral region, and 1 in the coccygeal region (Fig. 10-33).

Each spinal nerve except C1 has a specific cutaneous sensory distribution. Detailed mapping of the skin surface reveals a close relationship between the source on the cord of each spinal nerve and the level of the body it innervates. (An understanding of this relationship is important when examining a patient with spinal cord injury.) The skin surface areas supplied by a single spinal nerve are known as *dermatomes*. A dermatome "map" of the body is illustrated in Fig. 10-34.

Cranial Nerves

The 12 cranial nerves are divided into three general categories: sensory, somatomotor and proprioception, and parasympathetic. Sensory functions include the special senses, such as vision, and the more general senses, such as touch and pain. Somatomotor functions control the skeletal muscles through motor neurons, and proprioception provides the brain with information about position of the body and its various parts, including joints and muscles. Parasympathetic function involves the regulation of glands, smooth muscle, and cardiac muscle (functions of the autonomic nervous system). Some cranial nerves have only one of the three functions, whereas others have more than one (Table 10-7). Fig. 10-35 illustrates the origin of cranial nerves.

The Autonomic Nervous System

As previously stated, the PNS is composed of afferent and efferent neurons. Afferent neurons carry action potentials from the periphery to the CNS, and efferent neurons carry action potentials

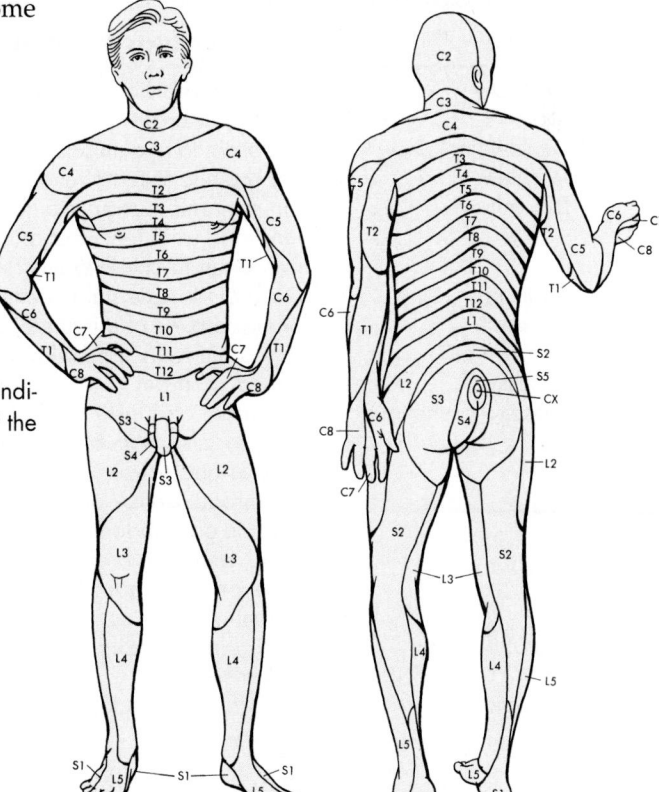

Fig. 10-34 Dermatome map. Letters and numbers indicate the spinal nerves innervating a given region of the skin.

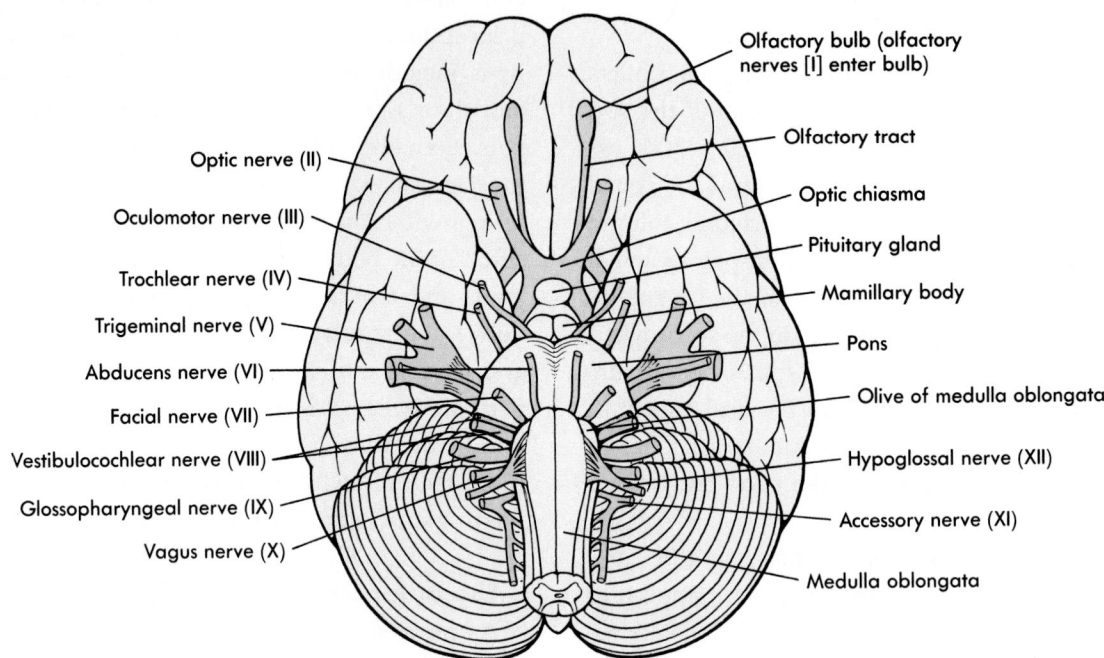

Fig. 10-35 Origin of cranial nerves.

TABLE 10-7 Cranial Nerves

	Nerve	Conducts Impulses	Functions
I	Olfactory	From nose to brain	Sense of smell
II	Optic	From eye to brain	Vision
III	Oculomotor	From brain to eye muscles	Eye movements
IV	Trochlear	From brain to external eye muscles	Eye movements
V	Trigeminal	From skin and mucous membranes of head and from teeth to brain; also from brain to chewing muscles	Sensations of face, scalp, and teeth; chewing movements
VI	Abducens	From brain to external eye muscles	Turning eyes outward
VII	Facial	From taste buds of tongue to brain; from brain to face muscles	Sense of taste; contraction of muscles of facial expressions
VIII	Acoustic	From ear to brain	Hearing; sense of balance
IX	Glossopharyngeal	From throat and taste buds of tongue to brain; also from brain to throat muscles and salivary glands	Sensation of throat, taste, swallowing movements; secretion of saliva
X	Vagus	From throat, larynx, and organs in thoracic and abdominal cavities to brain; also from brain to muscles of throat and to organs in thoracic and abdominal cavities	Sensations of throat and larynx and of thoracic and abdominal organs; swallowing, voice production, slowing of heartbeat, acceleration of peristalsis
XI	Spinal accessory	From brain to certain shoulder and neck muscles	Shoulder movements; turning movements of head
XII	Hypoglossal	From brain to muscles of tongue	Tongue movements

TABLE 10-8 Functions of the Autonomic Nervous System

Visceral Effectors	Sympathetic Control	Parasympathetic Control
Heart muscle	Accelerates heartbeat	Slows heartbeat
Smooth muscle		
Of most blood vessels	Constricts blood vessels	None
Of blood vessels in skeletal muscles	Dilates blood vessels	None
Of the digestive tract	Decreases peristalsis; inhibits defecation	Increases peristalsis
Of the anal sphincter	Stimulates—closes sphincter	Inhibits—opens sphincter for defecation
Of the urinary bladder	Inhibits—relaxes bladder	Stimulates—contracts bladder
Of the urinary sphincters	Stimulates—closes sphincter	Inhibits—opens sphincter for urination
Of the eye		
Iris	Stimulates radial fibers—dilation of pupil	Stimulates circular fibers—constriction of pupil
Ciliary	Inhibits—accommodation for far vision (flattening of lens)	Stimulates—accommodation for near vision (bulging of lens)
Of hairs (pilomotor muscles)	Stimulates—"goose pimples"	No parasympathetic fibers
Glands		
Adrenal medulla	Increases epinephrine secretion	None
Sweat glands	Increase sweat secretion	None
Digestive glands	Decrease secretion of digestive juices	Increase secretion of digestive juices

from the CNS to the periphery. Afferent neurons provide information to the CNS that may stimulate both somatomotor and autonomic reflexes. Therefore they cannot be easily divided into functional groups. In contrast, efferent neurons differ structurally and functionally. They can be clearly separated into either the somatomotor nervous system or the autonomic nervous system.

Somatomotor neurons innervate skeletal muscles and play an important role in locomotion, posture, and equilibrium. The movements controlled by the somatomotor nervous system are usually considered to be conscious movements. Their effect on skeletal muscle is always excitatory. Neurons of the autonomic nervous system innervate smooth muscle, cardiac muscle, and glands and are usually considered to be unconsciously controlled. The effect of autonomic neurons on their target tissue is either inhibitory or excitatory.

The autonomic nervous system is composed of sympathetic and parasympathetic divisions. Both of these divisions, in turn, consist of autonomic

ganglia and nerves. The action potentials in sympathetic neurons generally prepare an individual for physical activity, whereas parasympathetic stimulation activates vegetative functions such as digestion, defecation, and urination.

The functions of the autonomic nervous system serve to maintain or quickly restore homeostasis (Table 10-8). Many internal organs receive fibers from parasympathetic and sympathetic divisions. Therefore sympathetic and parasympathetic impulses continually bombard them, influencing their function in opposite or antagonistic ways. For example, the heart receives sympathetic impulses that increase the heart rate and parasympathetic impulses that decrease the heart rate. The ratio between these two forces determines the actual heart rate (Fig. 10-36).

The Endocrine System

The endocrine system is composed of glands that secrete hormones into the circulatory system (Fig. 10-37). The endocrine and nervous systems

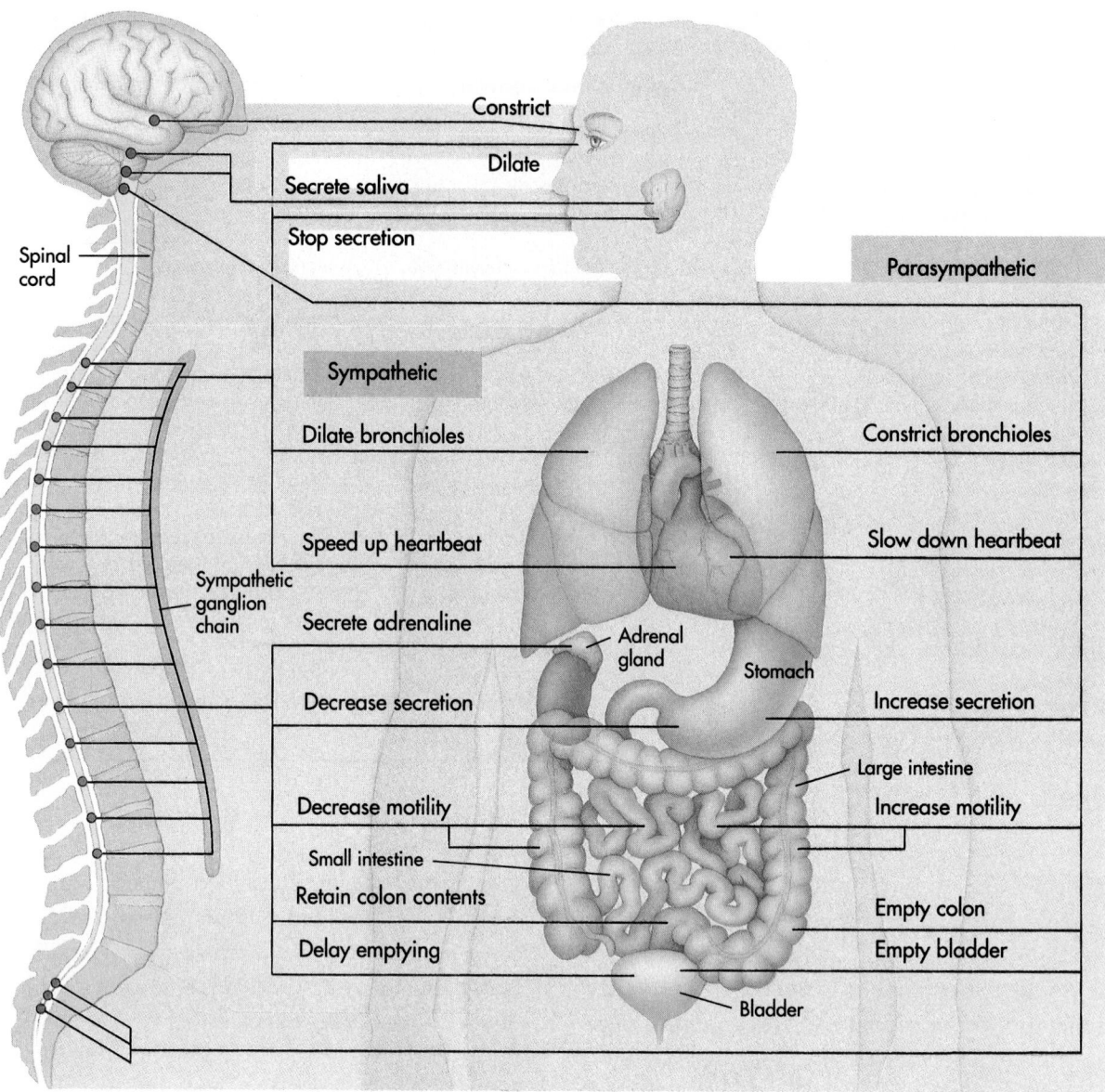

Fig. 10-36 Innervation of major target organs by the ANS. The sympathetic fibers are highlighted with red, and the parasympathetic are highlighted with blue.

have a significant amount of functional and anatomical overlap. Some neurons secrete regulatory chemicals (neurohormones) that function as hormones, such as antidiuretic hormone (ADH), into the circulatory system. Other neurons innervate endocrine glands and influence their secretory activity. Conversely, some hormones secreted by the endocrine glands affect the nervous system.

Hormones, including neurohormones, are classified as proteins, polypeptides, derivatives of amino acids, or lipids. Lipid hormones are either steroids or derivatives of fatty acids. Hormones are dissolved in blood plasma and are quickly distributed throughout the body. In general, the amount of hormone that reaches the target tissue directly correlates with the concentration of the hormone in the blood. (Table 10-9 lists endocrine glands, hormones, and their functions.)

Some hormones are present in relatively constant levels in the circulatory system; others

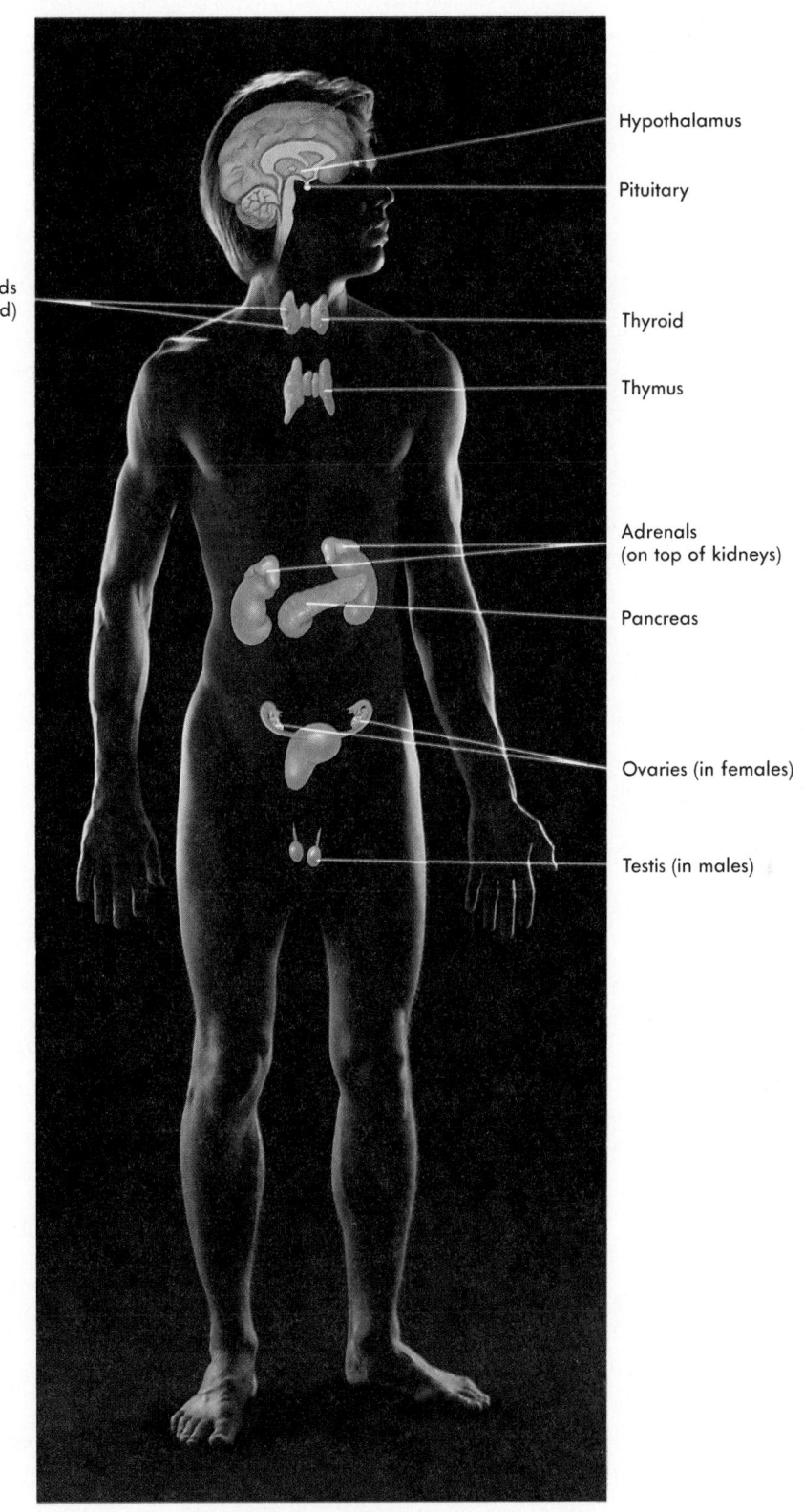

Hypothalamus

Pituitary

Parathyroids
(behind thyroid)

Thyroid

Thymus

Adrenals
(on top of kidneys)

Pancreas

Ovaries (in females)

Testis (in males)

Fig. 10-37 Endocrine system.

TABLE 10-9 Endocrine Glands, Hormones, and Their Functions	
Gland/Hormone	**Function**
Anterior Pituitary	
Thyroid-stimulating hormone (TSH)	Tropic hormone Stimulates secretion of thyroid hormones
Adrenocorticotropic hormone (ACTH)	Tropic hormone Stimulates secretion of adrenal cortex hormones
Follicle-stimulating hormone (FSH)	Tropic hormone *Female:* stimulates development of ovarian follicles and secretion of estrogens *Male:* stimulates seminiferous tubules of testes to grow and produce sperm
Luteinizing hormone (LH)	Tropic hormone *Female:* stimulates maturation of ovarian follicle and ovum; stimulates secretion of estrogen; triggers ovulation; stimulates development of corpus luteum (luteinization) *Male:* stimulates interstitial cells of the testes to secrete testosterone
Melanocyte-stimulating hormone (MSH)	Stimulates synthesis and dispersion of melanin pigment in the skin
Growth hormone (GH)	Stimulates growth in all organs; mobilizes food molecules, causing an increase in blood glucose concentration
Prolactin (lactogenic hormone)	Stimulates breast development during pregnancy and milk secretion after pregnancy
Posterior Pituitary*	
Antidiuretic hormone (ADH)	Stimulates retention of water by the kidneys
Oxytocin	Stimulates uterine contractions at the end of pregnancy; stimulates the release of milk into the breast ducts
Hypothalamus	
Releasing hormones (several)	Stimulate the anterior pituitary to release hormones
Inhibiting hormones (several)	Inhibit the anterior pituitary's secretion of hormones
Thyroid	
Thyroxine (T_4) and triiodothyronine (T_3)	Stimulate the energy metabolism of all cells
Calcitonin	Inhibits the breakdown of bone; causes a decrease in blood calcium concentration
Parathyroid	
Parathyroid hormone (PTH)	Stimulates the breakdown of bone; causes an increase in blood calcium concentration
Adrenal Cortex	
Mineralocorticoids: aldosterone	Regulate electrolyte and fluid homeostasis
Glucocorticoids: cortisol (hydrocortisone)	Stimulate gluconeogenesis, causing an increase in blood glucose concentration; also have antiinflammatory, antiimmunity, and antiallergy effects
Sex hormones (androgens)	Stimulate sexual drive in the female but have negligible effects in the male
Adrenal Medulla	
Epinephrine (adrenaline) and norepinephrine	Prolong and intensify the sympathetic nervous response during stress
Pancreatic Islets	
Glucagon	Stimulates liver glycogenolysis, causing an increase in blood glucose concentration
Insulin	Promotes glucose entry into all cells, causing a decrease in blood glucose concentration
Ovary	
Estrogens	Promotes development and maintenance of female sexual characteristics
Progesterone	Promotes conditions required for pregnancy

*Posterior pituitary hormones are synthesized in the hypothalamus but released from axon terminals in the posterior pituitary.

TABLE 10-9 Endocrine Glands, Hormones, and Their Functions—cont'd

Gland/Hormone	Function
Testis	
Testosterone	Promotes development and maintenance of male sexual characteristics
Thymus	
Thymosin	Promotes development of immune-system cells
Placenta	
Chorionic gonadotropin, estrogens, progesterone	Promote conditions required during early pregnancy
Pineal	
Melatonin	Inhibits tropic hormones that affect the ovaries; may be involved in the body's internal clock
Heart (atria)	
Atrial natriuretic hormone (ANH)	Regulates fluid and electrolyte homeostasis

change suddenly in response to certain stimuli, and others change in relatively constant cycles. For example, thyroid hormones in the blood vary within a small range of concentrations, so their concentration is chronically maintained. Epinephrine is released in large amounts in response to stress or physical exercise, so its concentration changes acutely. Reproductive hormones increase and decrease in cyclic fashion in women during their reproductive years.

The Circulatory System

Blood vessels extend throughout the body, carrying blood to and from all tissues. Blood transports nutrients and oxygen to tissues, carries carbon dioxide and waste products away from tissues, and carries hormones produced in endocrine glands to their target tissues. In addition, blood plays an important role in temperature regulation and fluid balance and protects the body from bacteria and foreign substances. These and other functions of blood help to maintain homeostasis.

Blood Components

Blood is a special form of connective tissue consisting of cells and cell fragments (formed elements) surrounded by a liquid intercellular matrix (plasma). Approximately 95% of the volume of formed elements consists of red blood cells (erythrocytes). The remaining 5% consists of white blood cells (leukocytes) and cell fragments called platelets.

Plasma

Plasma is a pale yellow fluid composed of approximately 92% water and 8% dissolved or suspended molecules. Plasma contains proteins such as albumin, globulins, and fibrinogen. When the proteins that produce clots are removed from the plasma, the remaining fluid is called *serum*.

Formed Elements

There are three formed elements of blood: erythrocytes, leukocytes, and platelets or thrombocytes (cell fragments) (Table 10-10). Formed elements are produced in the embryo and fetus and in tissues such as the liver, thymus, spleen, lymph nodes, and red bone marrow.

1. Erythrocytes are the most numerous of the formed elements. There are approximately 5.2 million erythrocytes in one drop of male blood and approximately 4.5 million in one drop of female blood. The major erythrocyte contents include lipids, ATP, and the enzyme carbonic anhydrase. The main component of

TABLE 10-10 Classes of Blood Cells

Blood Cell	Function
Erythrocyte	Oxygen and carbon dioxide transport
Neutrophil	Immune defenses (phagocytosis)
Eosinophil	Defense against parasites
Basophil	Inflammatory response
B lymphocyte	Antibody production (precursor of plasma cells)
T lymphocyte	Cellular immune response
Monocyte	Immune defenses (phagocytosis)
Platelet	Blood clotting

body against invading microorganisms and in removing dead cells and debris. Some leukocytes are classified according to their appearance, based on the presence or absence of cytoplasmic granules. This classification includes neutrophils, eosinophils, and basophils. Other types of leukocytes are nongranular and are named according to nuclear morphology and major site of proliferation. These include lymphocytes and monocytes.

Neutrophils are the most common type of leukocyte in the blood. These cells normally remain in the circulation for 10 to 12 hours, after which they move into tissue to seek out and destroy bacteria and other foreign matter (phagocytosis). They also secrete lysosomes that can destroy certain bacteria. Neutrophils usually survive for 1 to 2 days after leaving the circulation.

Eosinophils leave the circulation to enter the tissues during an inflammatory reaction. Their numbers are usually elevated in the blood of people who have allergies and certain parasitic infections. Although these cells have phagocytic properties, they are not thought to be as important in this function as neutrophils.

Basophils are the least common of all leukocytes. Like eosinophils, basophils leave the circulation and migrate through tissues to play a role in allergic and inflammatory reactions. They also release heparin, which inhibits blood clotting.

Lymphocytes are the smallest of all leukocytes and are capable of migrating through the cytoplasm of other cells. The many different types of lymphocytes play a major role in immunity, including antibody production. Lymphocytes originate in bone marrow and are most abundant in lymphoid tissues: the lymph nodes, spleen, tonsils, lymph nodules, and thymus.

Monocytes are the largest of the leukocytes. They remain in the circulation for approximately 3 days before transforming into macrophages, large "eating" cells that migrate through various tissues. An increase in the number of monocytes is common in patients with chronic infections.

erythrocytes is hemoglobin, the protein that gives blood its red color. The primary functions of erythrocytes are to transport oxygen from the lungs to the various tissues of the body and to transport carbon dioxide from the tissues to the lungs. Under normal conditions, approximately 2.5 million erythrocytes are destroyed and replaced by the body each second. The average erythrocyte circulates for 120 days.

2. Leukocytes are clear white blood cells that do not contain hemoglobin. There are several types; all are involved in protecting the

3. Platelets are produced within bone marrow and are 40 times as common in blood as leukocytes. Platelets play an important role in preventing blood loss by forming "plugs" that seal holes in small vessels and by forming clots that seal off larger wounds in the vessels.

The Cardiovascular System

The heart and cardiovascular system are responsible for circulating blood throughout the body. The cardiovascular system is discussed more thoroughly in Chapters 13 and 18.

Anatomy of the Heart

The heart is a muscular pump consisting of four chambers: two atria and two ventricles. The adult heart is shaped like a blunt cone and is approximately the size of a closed fist. It is located in the mediastinum of the thoracic cavity in the pericardial cavity. The blunt, rounded point of the heart is the apex, and the larger, flat portion at the opposite end is the base.

The heart lies obliquely in the mediastinum, with the base directed posteriorly and slightly superiorly. The apex is directed anteriorly and slightly inferiorly. Two thirds of the heart's mass lies to the left of the midline of the sternum (Figs. 10-38 and 10-39).

Pericardium

The pericardium, or the pericardial sac, has a fibrous outer layer (fibrous pericardium) and a thin inner layer (serous pericardium) that surrounds the heart. The portion of the serous pericardium that lines the fibrous pericardium is the parietal pericardium; the portion that covers the heart surface is the visceral pericardium or the epicardium. The cavity between the parietal pericardium and the visceral pericardium normally contains a small amount of pericardial fluid that reduces friction as the heart moves within the pericardial sac.

Coronary Vessels

Seven large veins normally carry blood to the heart: four pulmonary veins carry blood from the lungs to the left atrium, the superior and inferior venae cavae carry blood from the body to the right atrium, and the coronary sinus carries blood from the walls of the heart to the right atrium. Two arteries, the aorta and pulmonary trunk, exit the heart. The aorta carries blood from the left ventricle to the body, and the pulmonary trunk carries blood from the right ventricle to the lungs. The right and left coronary arteries exit the aorta near the point where the aorta leaves the heart and supply the heart muscle with oxygen and nutrients (Fig. 10-40).

Fig. 10-38 Location of the heart in the thorax.

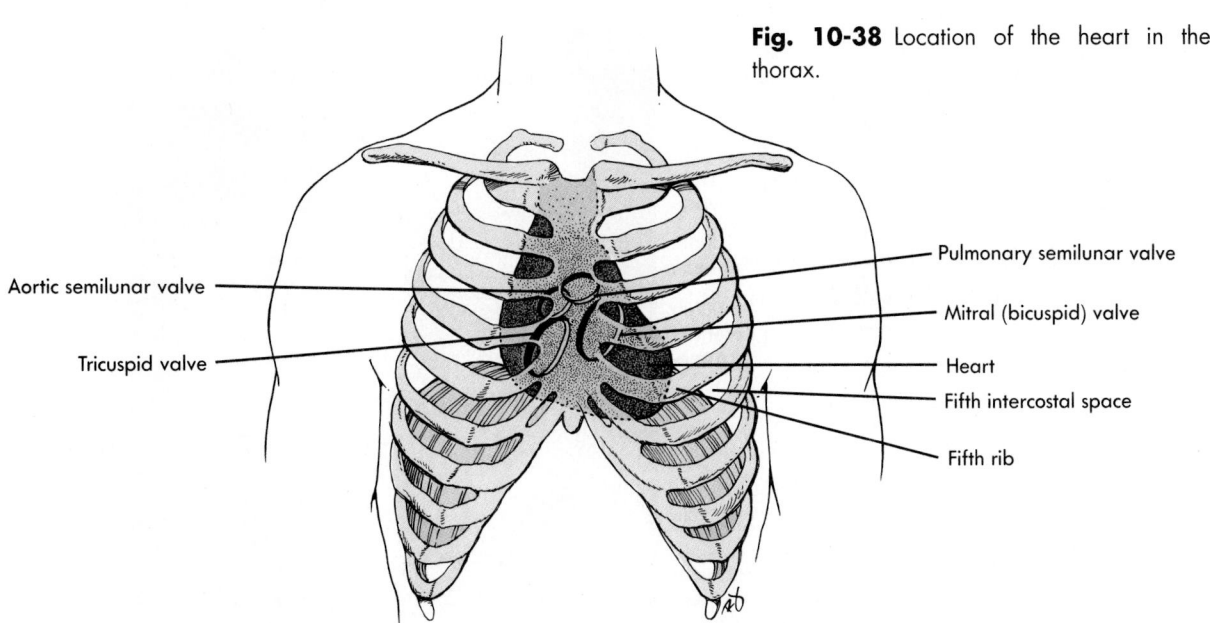

Aortic semilunar valve

Tricuspid valve

Pulmonary semilunar valve

Mitral (bicuspid) valve

Heart

Fifth intercostal space

Fifth rib

Fig. 10-39 Internal view of the heart.

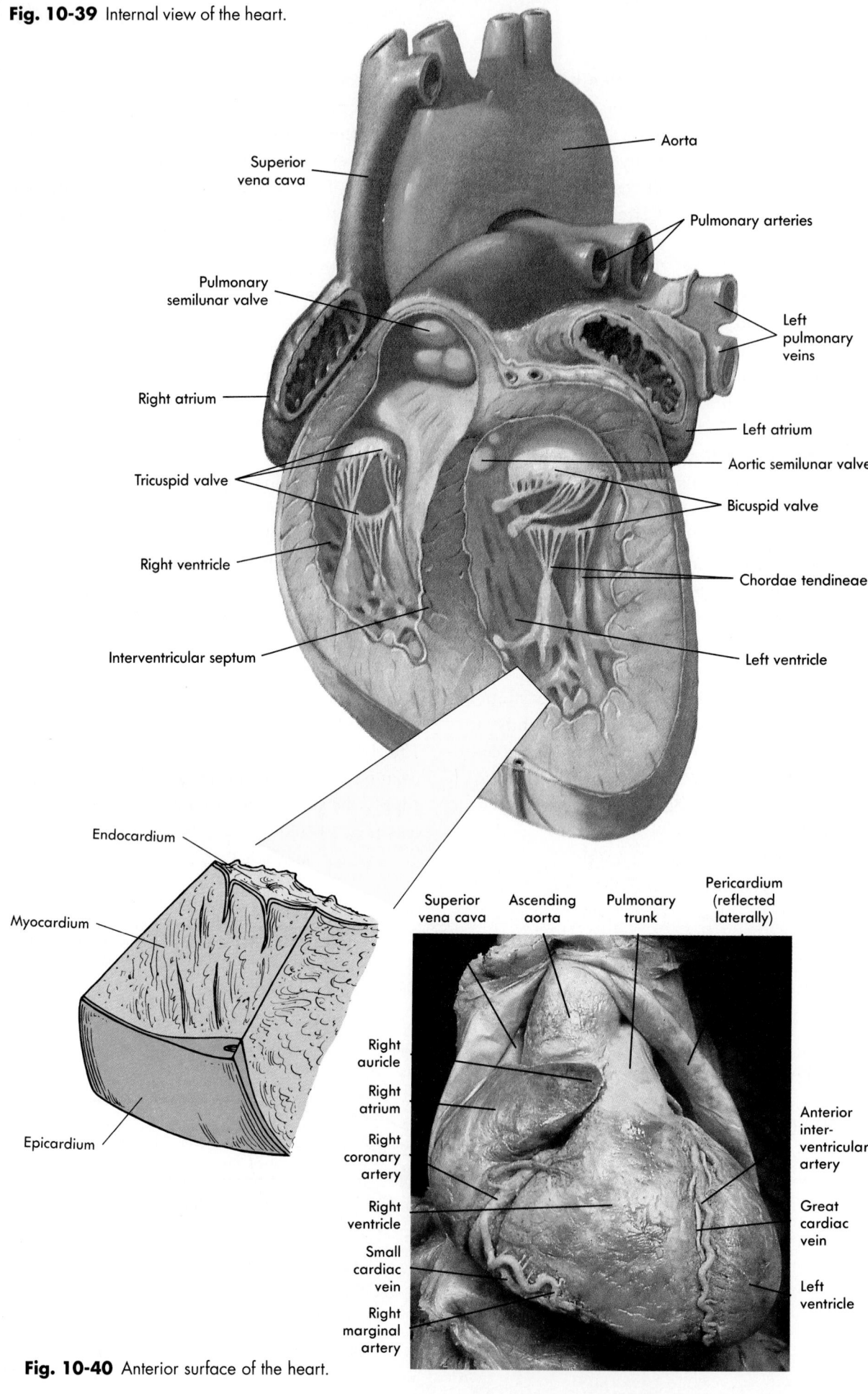

Superior vena cava

Aorta

Pulmonary arteries

Pulmonary semilunar valve

Left pulmonary veins

Right atrium

Left atrium

Aortic semilunar valve

Tricuspid valve

Bicuspid valve

Right ventricle

Chordae tendineae

Interventricular septum

Left ventricle

Endocardium

Myocardium

Epicardium

Superior vena cava

Ascending aorta

Pulmonary trunk

Pericardium (reflected laterally)

Right auricle

Right atrium

Right coronary artery

Right ventricle

Small cardiac vein

Right marginal artery

Anterior interventricular artery

Great cardiac vein

Left ventricle

Fig. 10-40 Anterior surface of the heart.

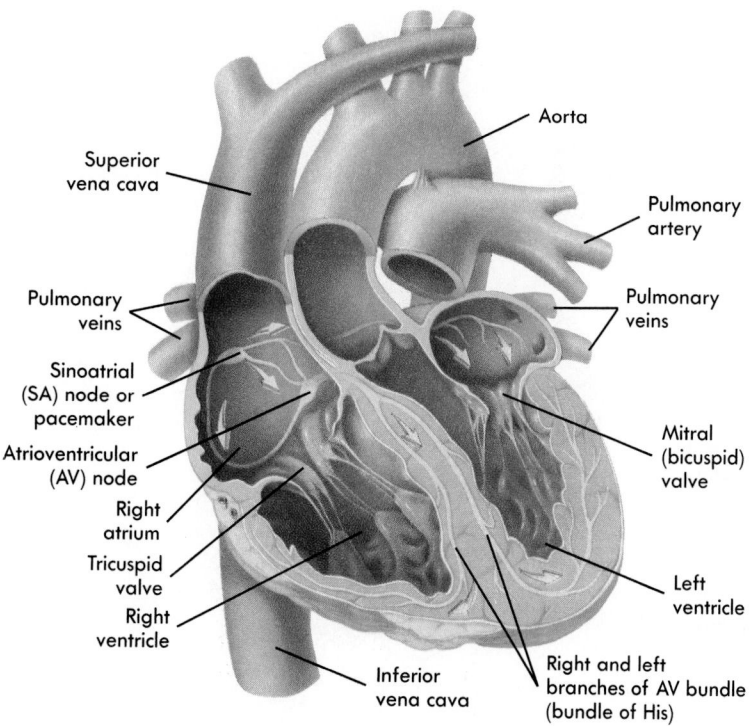

Superior
vena cava

Aorta

Pulmonary
artery

Pulmonary
veins

Pulmonary
veins

Sinoatrial
(SA) node or
pacemaker

Mitral
(bicuspid)
valve

Atrioventricular
(AV) node

Right
atrium

Tricuspid
valve

Left
ventricle

Right
ventricle

Inferior
vena cava

Right and left
branches of AV bundle
(bundle of His)

Fig. 10-41 Conduction system of the heart.

Heart Chambers and Valves

The right and left chambers of the heart are separated by a septum. The interatrial septum separates the right and left atria, and the interventricular septum separates the two ventricles. The atria open into the ventricles through the atrioventricular canals. An atrioventricular valve on each atrioventricular canal is composed of cusps or flaps. These valves allow blood to flow from the atria into the ventricles but prevent blood from flowing back into the atria. The atrioventricular valve between the right atrium and right ventricle has three cusps and is called the *tricuspid valve.* The atrioventricular valve between the left atrium and left ventricle has two cusps and is called the *bicuspid* or *mitral valve.*

The aorta and pulmonary trunk possess aortic and pulmonary semilunar valves, which meet in the center of the artery to block blood flow. Blood flowing out of the ventricles pushes against each valve, forcing it open, but when blood flows back from the aorta or pulmonary trunk toward the ventricles, the valves close.

Conduction System Of The Heart

The heart's specialized muscle tissue has the unique capability for spontaneous, rhythmic self-excitation by way of four specialized structures embedded in the wall of the heart. These structures are the sinoatrial node (SA node), the atrioventricular node (AV node), the bundle of His, and the Purkinje fibers.

An impulse conduction normally begins in the SA node. From there it spreads in all directions through both of the atria, causing an atrial contraction. As the electrical impulses reach the AV node, they are relayed to the ventricles through the bundle of His and the Purkinje fibers. This impulse conduction causes both of the ventricles to contract shortly after the atrial contraction (Fig. 10-41).

Route of Blood Flow Through the Heart

We present blood flow through the heart through a discussion of right heart and left heart circulation (Fig. 10-42). It is important to remember that both atria contract at the same time, fol-

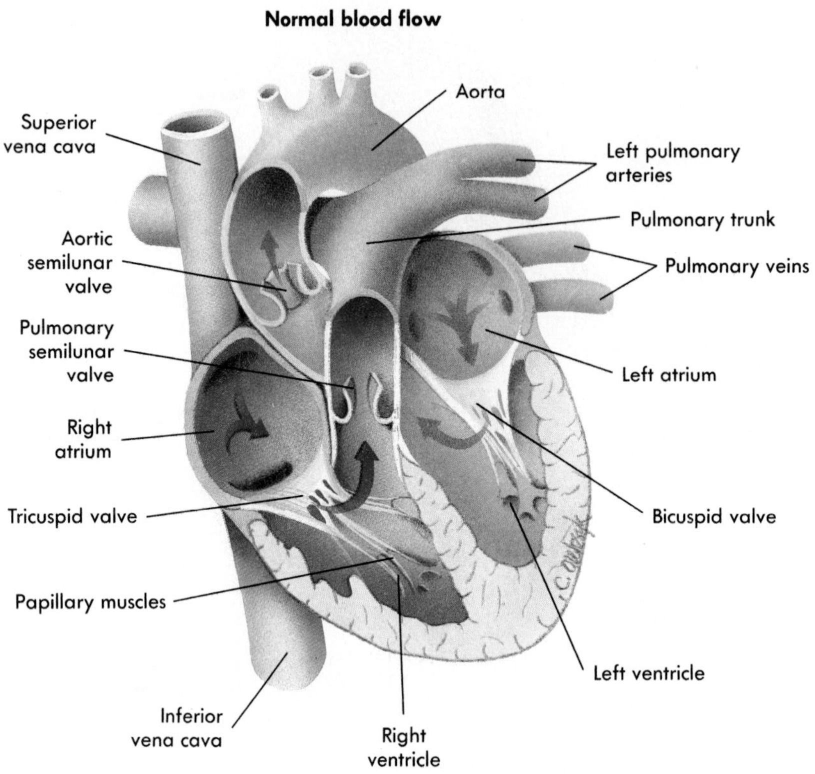

Normal blood flow

Fig. 10-42 Frontal section of the heart revealing the four chambers and direction of blood flow through the heart.

lowed shortly thereafter by essentially simultaneous contraction of both ventricles, to clearly understand electrical impulses of the heart, pressure changes, and heart sounds, which are discussed in other chapters.

Blood enters the right atrium from the systemic circulation via the inferior and superior venae cavae and from the heart via the coronary sinus. Most of this blood passes into the right ventricle as the ventricle relaxes after the previous contraction. When the right atrium contracts, the blood remaining in the atrium is pushed into the ventricle. The contraction of the right ventricle pushes blood against the tricuspid valve, forcing it closed, and against the pulmonary semilunar valve, forcing it open. This flow allows blood to enter the pulmonary trunk. The pulmonary trunk divides into left and right pulmonary arteries that carry blood to the lungs, where carbon dioxide is released and oxygen is picked up.

Blood returning from the lungs enters the left atrium through four pulmonary veins. The blood passing from the left atrium to the relaxed left ventricle opens the bicuspid valve. The contraction of the left atrium completes the filling of the left ventricle.

Contraction of the left ventricle pushes blood against the bicuspid valve, closing it. The pressure of the blood against the aortic semilunar valve causes it to open, allowing blood to enter the aorta. Blood flowing through the aorta is distributed to all parts of the body, except for the pulmonary vessels in the lungs.

The Peripheral Circulation

Blood is pumped from the ventricles of the heart into large elastic arteries, which branch repeatedly to form many progressively smaller arteries. As these vessels become smaller, the amount of elastic tissue in the arterial wall decreases and the amount of smooth muscle increases.

Blood flows from the arterioles into capillaries and from capillaries into the venous system. Compared with artery walls, vein walls are thinner and contain less elastic tissue and fewer smooth

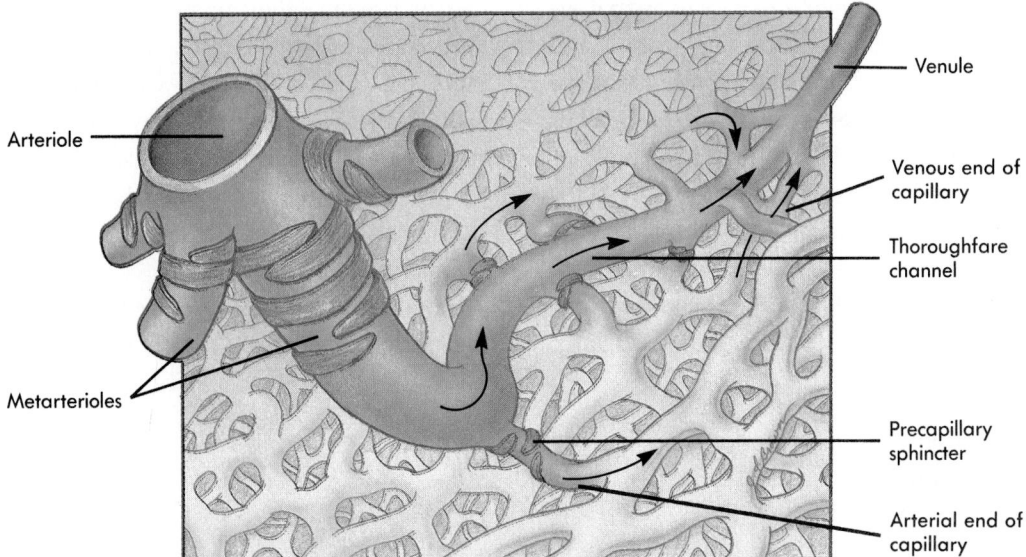

Arteriole

Metarterioles

Venule

Venous end of capillary

Thoroughfare channel

Precapillary sphincter

Arterial end of capillary

Fig. 10-43 Capillary network. The metarteriole, giving rise to the network, feeds directly from the arteriole into the thoroughfare channel, which feeds into the venule. The network forms numerous branches that transport blood from the thoroughfare channel and may return to the thoroughfare channel.

muscle cells. As veins approach the heart, the walls increase in diameter and thickness.

The Capillary Network

Arterioles supply blood to each capillary network (Fig. 10-43). Blood flows through this network and into the venules. The ends of the capillaries closest to arterioles are arterial capillaries; the ends closest to venules are venous capillaries.

Blood flow through arterioles may continue through metarterioles and into a thoroughfare channel to a venule in a relatively constant way or may enter the capillary circulation. Flow in the capillaries is regulated by smooth muscle cells known as *precapillary sphincters*. Nutrient and product waste exchange is the major function of capillaries.

Arteries and Veins

With the exception of capillaries and venules, blood vessel walls are composed of three distinct layers (tunics) of elastic tissue and smooth muscle: the tunica intima (inner layer), the tunica media (middle layer), and the tunica adventitia (outer layer). The thickness and composition of each layer vary with the type and diameter of the blood vessel.

Large elastic arteries are often called *conducting arteries* because they are the largest-diameter arteries. These vessels have more elastic tissue and less smooth muscle than other arteries. Medium-sized and small arteries have relatively thick muscular walls and well-developed elastic membranes. These vessels are called *distributing arteries* because the smooth muscle allows these vessels to partially regulate blood supply to various body regions by constriction or dilation. Arterioles are the smallest arteries in which the three tunics can be identified. Like small arteries, arterioles are capable of vasodilation and vasoconstriction.

Venules have only a few isolated smooth muscle cells and are very similar in structure to the capillaries. Venules collect blood from the capillaries and transport it to small veins, which in turn transport the blood to the medium-sized veins. Nutrient exchange occurs across the walls of the venules, but as the small veins increase in thickness, the degree of nutrient exchange decreases.

As venules increase in diameter, the vessels become veins, whose walls are a continuous layer of smooth muscle cells. Medium-sized and large veins collect blood from small veins and deliver it to the large venous trunks. Large veins transport blood from the medium-sized veins to the heart.

Veins with large diameters have valves that allow blood to flow to but not from the heart. There are many valves in medium-sized veins, and more in the veins of the lower extremities than of the upper extremities. They help prevent backflow of blood, especially in dependent tissues.

Arteriovenous anastomoses (AV shunts) allow blood to flow from arteries to veins without passing through capillaries. Natural AV shunts occur in large numbers in the sole of the foot, palm, and nail bed, where they regulate body temperature. Pathological shunts can result from injury or tumors and cause a direct flow of blood from arteries to veins. Severe shunts may lead to "high output" heart failure from increased venous return to the heart and demand on cardiac output.

Pulmonary Circulation

Blood from the right ventricle is pumped into the pulmonary trunk, which bifurcates into the

Fig. 10-44 Principal arteries of the body.

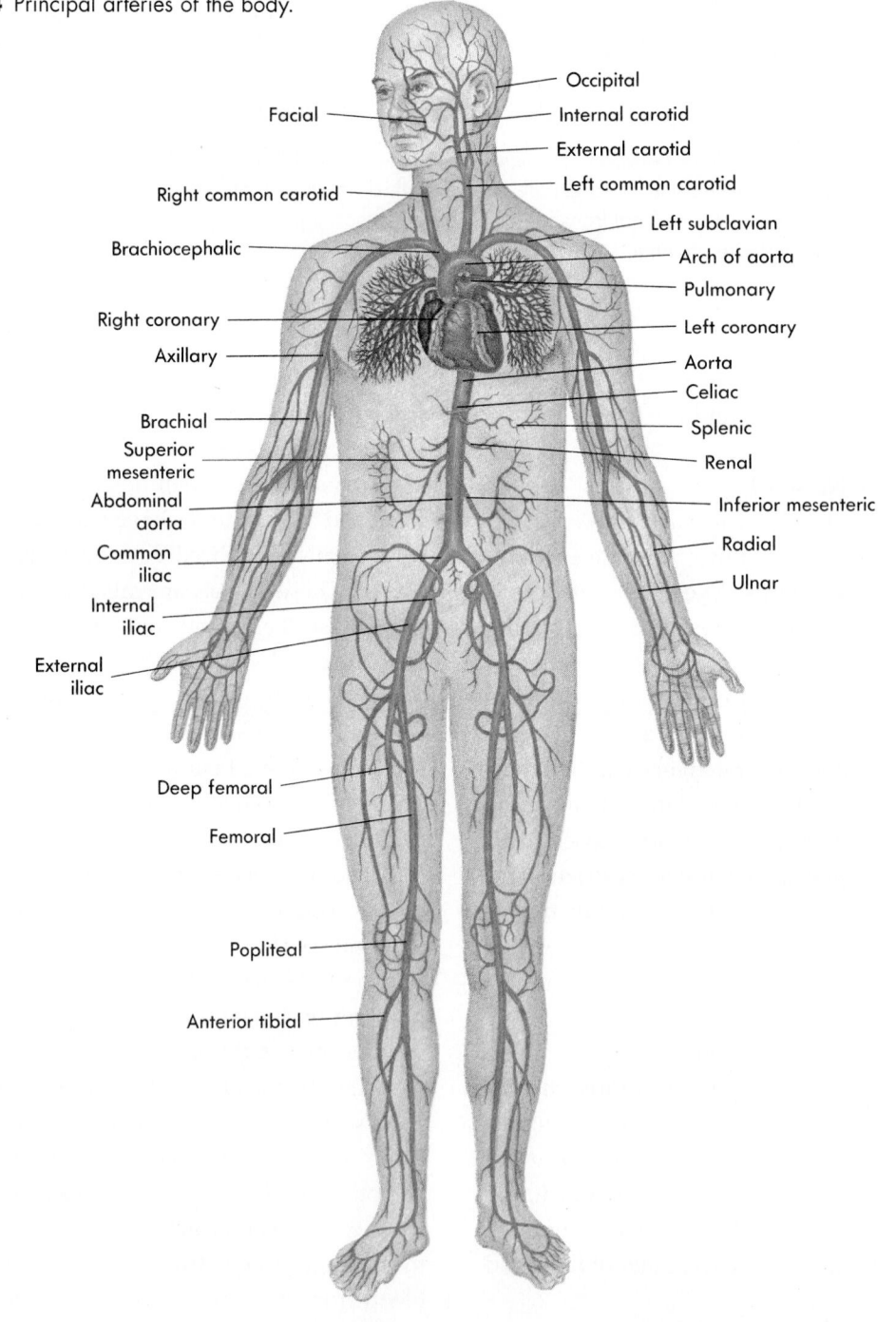

right and left pulmonary arteries (which transport blood to the respective lungs). After the exchange of oxygen and carbon dioxide, two pulmonary veins exit each lung and enter the left atrium.

Systemic Circulation

Oxygenated blood enters the heart from the pulmonary veins, passing through the left atrium into the left ventricle and from the left ventricle into the aorta. From the aorta, blood is distributed to all parts of the body. The arteries of systemic circulation include the aorta, coronary arteries, arteries to the head and neck, arteries of the upper and lower limbs, the thoracic aorta and its branches, the abdominal aorta and its branches, and arteries of the pelvis.

The veins of systemic circulation include coronary veins, veins of the head and neck, veins of the upper and lower limbs, veins of the thorax, veins of the abdomen and pelvis, and the hepatic portal system, which transports blood from the digestive tract to the liver (Figs. 10-44 and 10-45).

Fig. 10-45 Principal veins of the body.

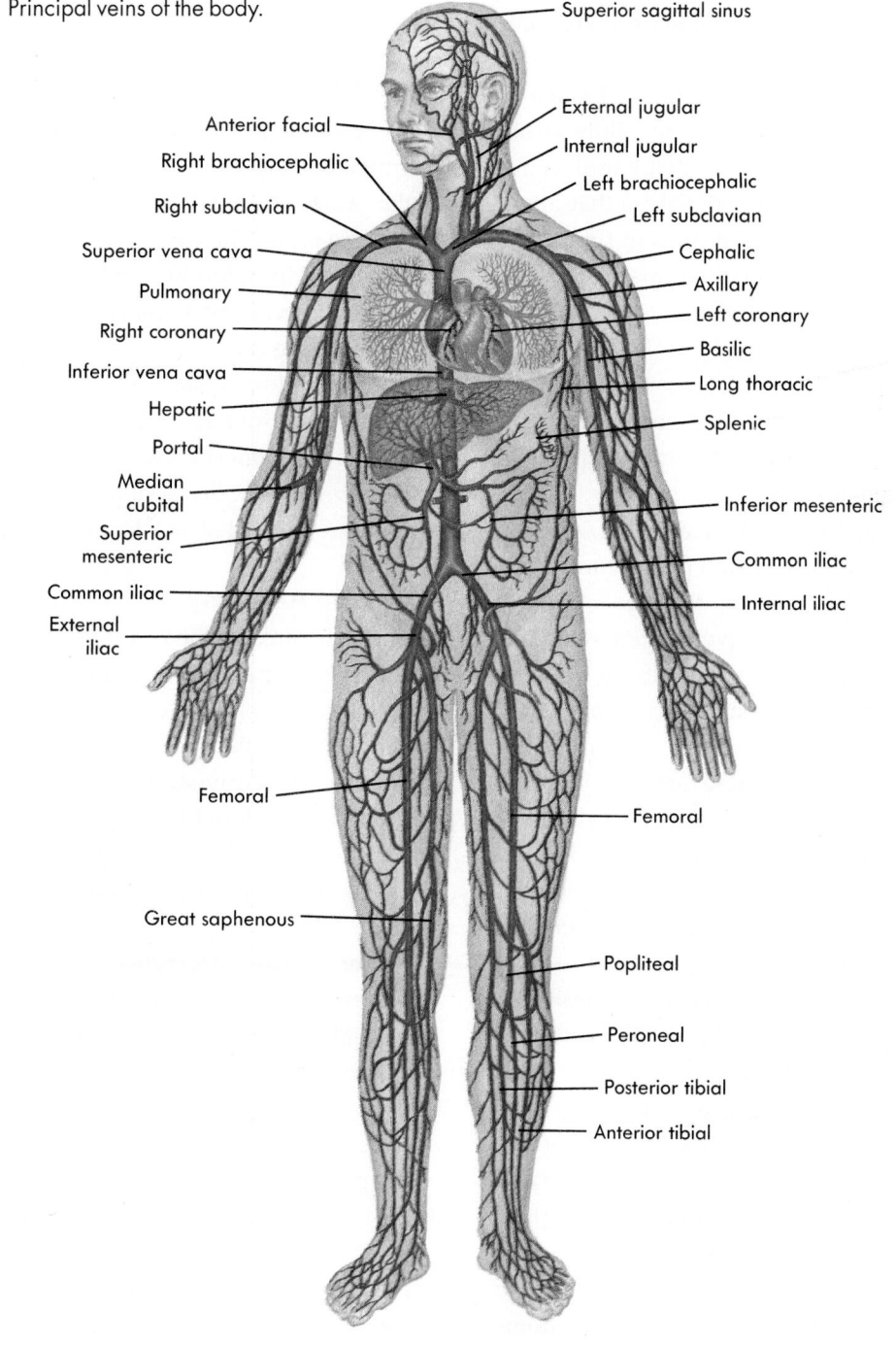

The Lymphatic System

The lymphatic system is considered part of the circulatory system because it consists of a moving fluid that comes from the body and returns to the blood. Unlike the circulatory system, the lymphatic system only carries fluid away from the tissues.

The lymphatic system includes lymph, lymphocytes, lymph nodes, tonsils, spleen, and thymus gland. The three basic functions of the lymphatic system are to help maintain fluid balance in tissues, to absorb fats and other substances from the digestive tract, and to play a role in the body's immune defense system.

The lymphatic system begins in the tissues as lymph capillaries. Lymph capillaries differ structurally from blood capillaries in that lymph capillaries have a series of one-way valves that allow fluid to enter the capillary but prevent fluid from passing back into the interstitial spaces. Lymph capillaries are present in almost all tissues of the body with the exception of the CNS, bone marrow, and tissues without blood vessels (for example, cartilage, epidermis, and cornea). Lymph capillaries join to form larger lymph capillaries that resemble small veins.

Lymph nodes are distributed along various lymph vessels, and most lymph passes through at least one node before entering the blood. Passing through the node filters the lymph, removing microorganisms or foreign substances to prevent them from entering the general circulation. Three major collections of lymph nodes are located on each side of the body. These are the inguinal nodes, the axillary nodes, and the cervical nodes. If a part of the body is inflamed or otherwise diseased, the nearby lymph nodes become swollen and tender as they limit the spread of microorganisms or foreign substances.

After passing through lymph nodes, lymph vessels converge toward either the right or left subclavian vein. Vessels from the upper right limb and the right side of the head enter the right lymphatic duct. Lymph vessels from the rest of the body enter the larger thoracic duct. The right lymphatic duct drains the right thorax, right upper limb, and right side of the head and neck and opens into the right subclavian vein. The thoracic duct drains the left thorax, the left upper extrem-

ity, and the left side of the head and neck. The duct ends by entering the left subclavian vein. Thus all fluid drained from the tissue spaces eventually returns to the venous circulation.

Lymph serves a unique transport function by returning tissue fluid, proteins, fats, and other substances to the general circulation. The lymphatic system does not form a closed ring or circuit like the "true" circulatory system. Once lymph is formed, it flows only once through its system of lymphatic vessels before draining into the right and left subclavian veins.

The Respiratory System

Oxygen is an essential requirement for normal cell metabolism, from which carbon dioxide is a major waste product. The organs of the respiratory system and the cardiovascular system transport oxygen to individual cells and transport carbon dioxide from individual cells to where it is released into the air.

The respiratory system is a very complex component of the human body. The purpose of this section is to familiarize the reader with respiratory anatomy. Further discussions of the respiratory system are presented in Chapters 12 and 17.

Airway Anatomy

The structures of the respiratory system are divided into upper airway and lower airway by their locations relative to the glottic opening (the vocal cords and the space between them). For our purposes, all airway structures located above the glottis are considered to be upper airway, and all structures located below the glottis are considered to be lower airway (Fig. 10-46).

Upper Airway Structures

The entrance to the respiratory tract begins with the nasal cavity and includes the nasopharynx, oropharynx, laryngopharynx, and larynx.

Nasopharynx

Air passes into the nasal cavity through the nostrils or nares. The right and left nasal cavities are separated by the nasal septum, a bony partition covered with a mucous membrane. This membrane has a rich blood supply that warms and humidifies the nasal lining and the inspired air as it passes through the nose. Inside each nostril, a slight enlargement known as the *vestibule* is lined with coarse hairs that trap foreign substances carried into the nasal cavity with inspired air. The floor of the nasal cavity is composed of the hard palate; the lateral walls are formed by bony ridges coated with respiratory mucosa. These ridges are known as *conchae* or *turbinates*.

Two patches of yellow-gray tissue lie just beneath the bridge of the nose and compose the olfactory membranes. Located in the roof of the nasal cavity, these membranes contain the receptors for the sense of smell. The nasal cavities also connect to the middle-ear cavities through the auditory or eustachian tubes.

Sinuses are cavities in the bones of the skull that connect to the nasal cavities by small channels (Fig. 10-47). There are four groups of sinuses, each

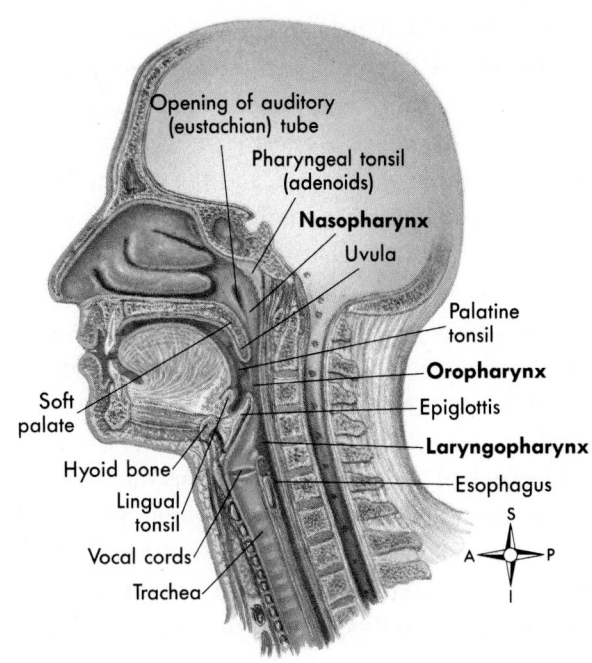

Fig. 10-46 Airway structures.

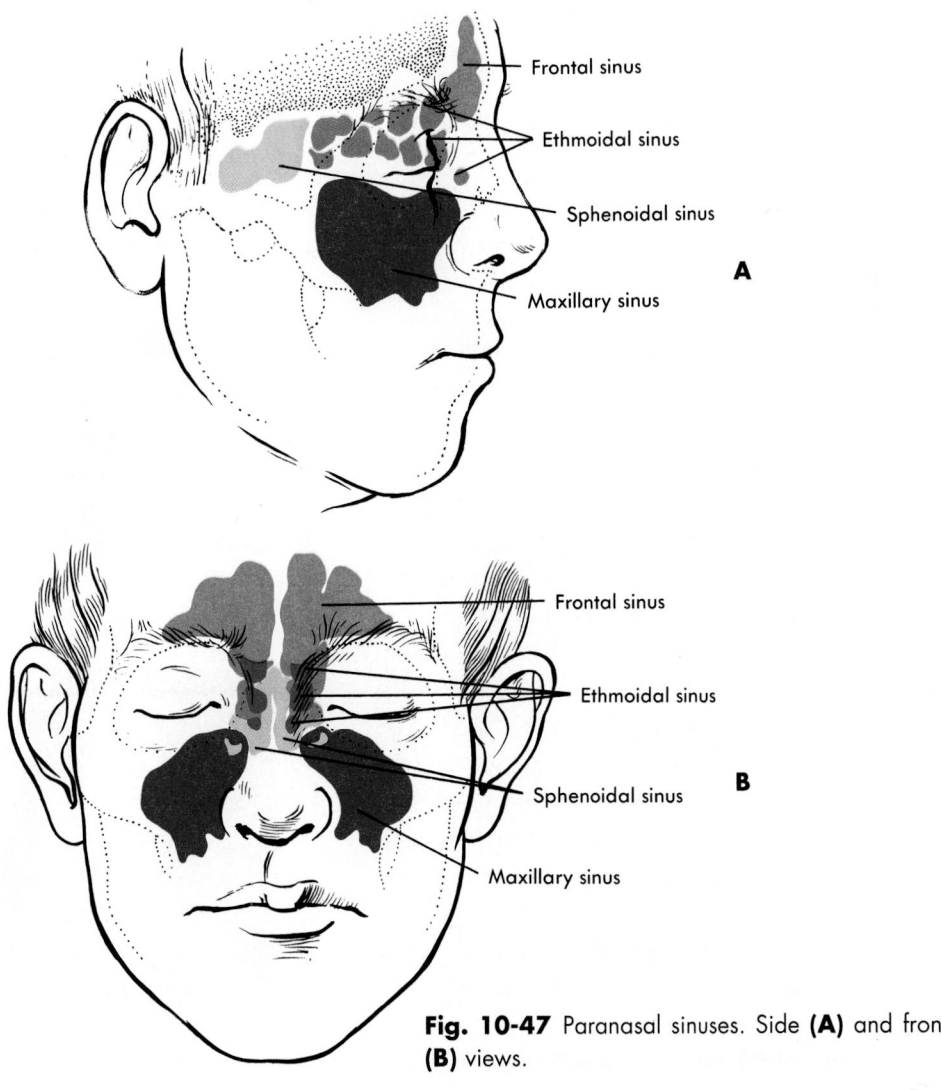

Fig. 10-47 Paranasal sinuses. Side **(A)** and front **(B)** views.

named for the skull bone in which it lies. The frontal sinuses are located above the eyebrows. Maxillary sinuses (the largest sinuses) are in the cheekbones. Others, called *ethmoid sinuses,* lie just behind the bridge of the nose, and the sphenoid sinuses lie in a bone that cradles the brain, slightly anterior to the pituitary gland. These hollow chambers are lined with mucous membranes that secrete mucus into the nasal cavities. They are thought to aid in two other functions: adding resonance to voice and decreasing the weight of the skull.

The back of each nasal cavity opens into the nasopharynx, the superior part of the pharynx, which extends from the internal nares to the level of the uvula. Like the nasal cavity, the nasopharynx is lined with mucous membrane.

Oropharynx

At the level of the uvula, the nasopharynx ends and the oropharynx begins, extending downward to the level of the epiglottis. Anteriorly, the oropharynx opens into the oral cavity, which contains the lips, cheeks, teeth, tongue (which is attached to the mandible), hard and soft palates, and palatine tonsils. The palatine tonsils and the pharyngeal tonsils (located in the roof and posterior wall of the nasopharynx) form a partial ring of lymphoid tissue surrounding the respiratory tract. This ring is completed by the lingual tonsils, which lie on the floor of the oropharyngeal passageway at the base of the tongue.

Laryngopharynx

The laryngopharynx extends from the tip of the epiglottis to the glottis and the esophagus. The laryngopharynx is lined with mucous membrane that protects internal surfaces from abrasion.

Larynx

The laryngopharynx opens into the larynx, which lies in the anterior neck (Fig. 10-48). The lar-

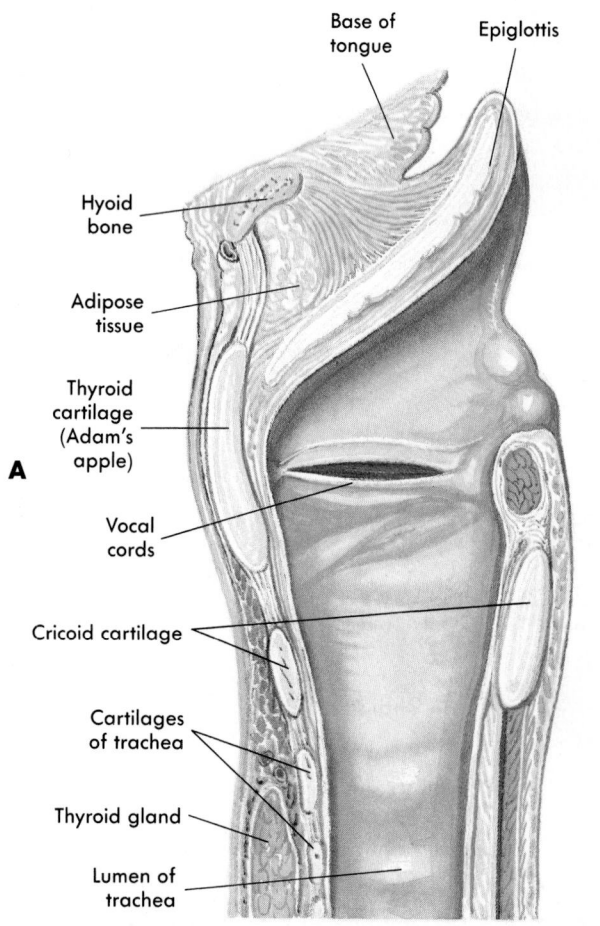

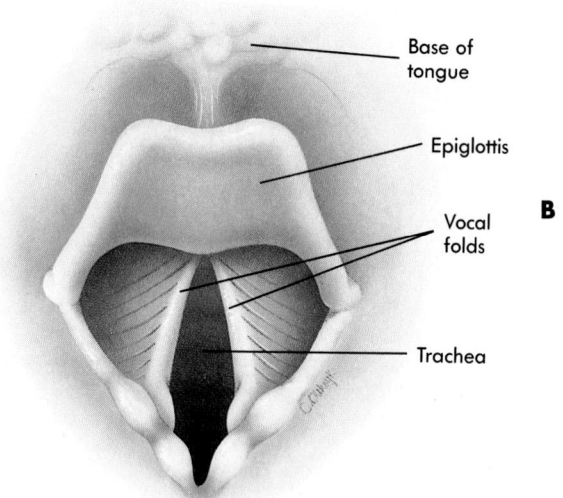

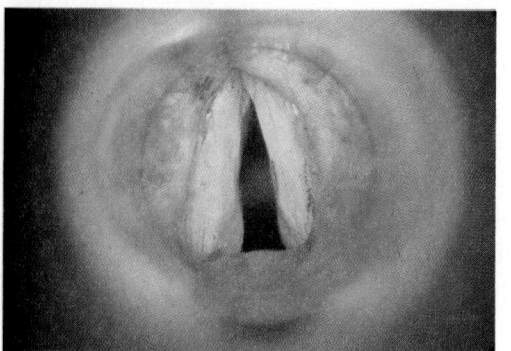

Fig. 10-48 Larynx. **A,** Sagittal section. **B,** Superior view. **C,** Photograph taken with an endoscope.

ynx serves three main functions: it is the air passageway between the pharynx and the lungs, it is a protective sphincter to prevent solids and liquids from passing into the respiratory tree, and it is involved in producing speech.

The larynx consists of an outer casing of nine cartilages connected to each other by muscles and ligaments. Six of the nine cartilages are paired, and three are unpaired. The largest and most superior of the cartilages is the unpaired thyroid cartilage, or Adam's apple. This prominence is hardly visible in children or adult females but is marked in males after puberty.

The most inferior cartilage of the larynx is the unpaired cricoid cartilage (the only complete cartilaginous ring in the larynx). This cartilage forms the base of the larynx on which all other cartilages rest. The third unpaired cartilage is the epiglottis.

The six paired cartilages are stacked in two pillars between the cricoid cartilage and the thyroid cartilage. The largest inferior cartilages are ladle shaped and are known as the *arytenoid cartilages.* The middle pair are horn shaped and are known as *corniculate cartilages.* The smallest, most superior cartilages are wedge shaped and are known as *cuneiform cartilages.*

The U-shaped hyoid bone is tucked beneath the mandible. As previously mentioned, it is the only bone of the human body that does not articulate with another bone. The hyoid bone helps to suspend the airway by anchoring the muscles (particularly those of the tongue) to the jaw. The fibrous membrane that joins the hyoid and the thyroid cartilage is the thyroid membrane. The membrane joining the thyroid and cricoid cartilages is the cricothyroid membrane.

Two pairs of ligaments extend from the anterior surface of the arytenoid to the posterior surface of the thyroid cartilage. The superior pair forms the vestibular folds or false vocal cords. (False vocal cords are not directly involved in the production of voice sounds.) The inferior pair of ligaments composes the vocal cords or true vocal cords, which participate directly in producing voice sounds. In talking, air expelled from the lungs rushes up the throat to the larynx. There, the air creates sound by vibrating the vocal cords. Muscles tighten the folds of the cords to produce the high-pitched tones and relax the cords to pro-

duce the deeper tones. The lip, the tongue, and the jaw further modify the sounds into intelligible words.

Lower Airway Structures

Below the glottis are the structures of the lower airway and lungs. These structures include the trachea, the bronchial tree (primary bronchi, secondary bronchi, and bronchioles), the alveoli, and the lungs (Fig. 10-49).

Trachea

The trachea is the air passage from the larynx to the lungs. It is composed of dense connective tissue and smooth muscle reinforced with 15 to 20 C-shaped pieces of cartilage that form an incomplete ring. This ring protects the trachea and maintains an open passage for air. The adult trachea is approximately 1.4 to 1.6 cm in diameter and 9 to 15 cm in length. The trachea is located anterior to the esophagus and extends from the larynx to the fifth thoracic vertebrae.

The trachea is lined with ciliated epithelium that contains many goblet cells. These cilia protect the lower airway by sweeping mucus, bacteria, and other small particles toward the larynx. There, they may be expelled through coughing or enter the esophagus, where they are swallowed and digested. Constant exposure to some irritants (for example, cigarette smoke) may produce a tracheal epithelium that lacks cilia and goblet cells. When this protective mechanism is disrupted, the mucus and bacteria may contribute to disease.

Bronchial Tree

The lower airway may be thought of as an inverted tree; the many subdivisions become narrower and shorter until they terminate at the alveoli. The large branches are primary bronchi; they divide into smaller secondary bronchi and bronchioles.

The trachea divides into the right and left primary bronchi at the level of the angle of Louis (the sternomanubrial joint). The point of bifurcation of the trachea into the right and left mainstem bronchi is called the *carina.* The right primary bronchus is shorter, wider, and more vertical. Like the trachea, the primary bronchi are lined with ciliated epithelium and are supported by C-shaped carti-

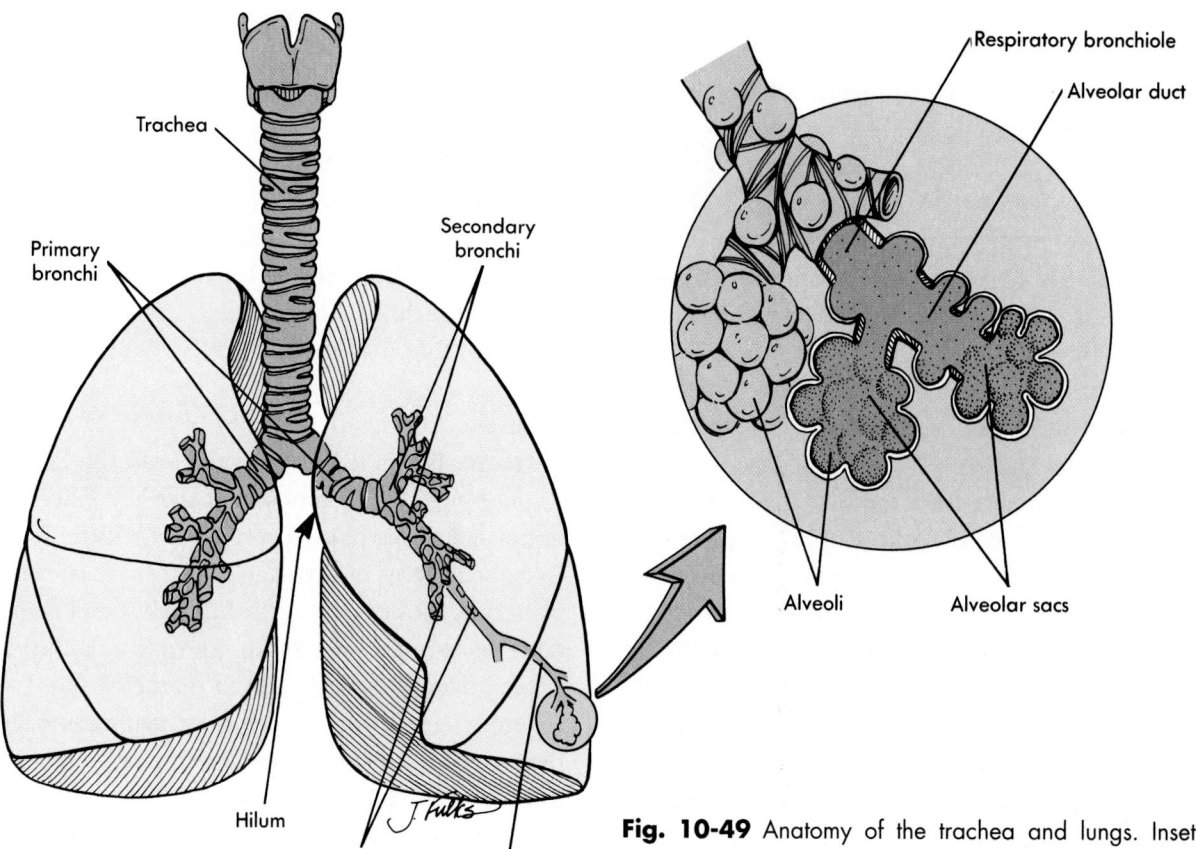

Fig. 10-49 Anatomy of the trachea and lungs. Inset shows enlargement of a terminal bronchiole and its associated alveoli.

lage rings. As the bronchi sequentially branch into smaller subdivisions, the amount of cartilage decreases and the bronchi become increasingly muscular until there is no cartilage. The primary bronchi extend from the mediastinum to the lungs.

The primary bronchi divide into the secondary bronchi as they enter the right and left lungs. Two secondary lobar bronchi in the left lung conduct air to its two lobes; three in the right lung conduct air to its three lobes. From there, the secondary bronchi divide into the tertiary segmental bronchi, of which there are 10 in the right lung and 9 in the left. The tertiary bronchi extend to the individual segments of each lobe of the lung (lobule). The bronchial tree continues to branch several times. As the cartilage continues to decrease and the diameter is reduced to approximately 1 mm, the bronchi become bronchioles.

The bronchiole walls are devoid of cartilage, and their muscles are sensitive to certain circulating hormones, such as epinephrine. Contraction and relaxation of these muscles alter resistance to air flow. The bronchioles can constrict if the smooth muscle contracts forcefully. (An example of this phenomenon is an asthma attack.) Bronchioles continue to divide, eventually becoming terminal bronchioles and finally respiratory bronchioles. Each respiratory bronchiole divides to form alveolar ducts. These ducts end as grapelike clusters of tiny, hollow air sacs called *alveoli*. It is here that the majority of respiratory gas exchange takes place.

Alveoli

The alveoli are the functional units of the respiratory system and are the prominent constituent of lung tissue. There are some 300 million alveoli in the two lungs. The wall of an alveolus consists of a single layer of epithelial cells and elastic fibers that permit it to stretch and contract during breathing. The exchange of oxygen and carbon dioxide in the lungs takes place in the alveoli.

Each alveolus is surrounded by a fine network of blood capillaries arranged so that air within the

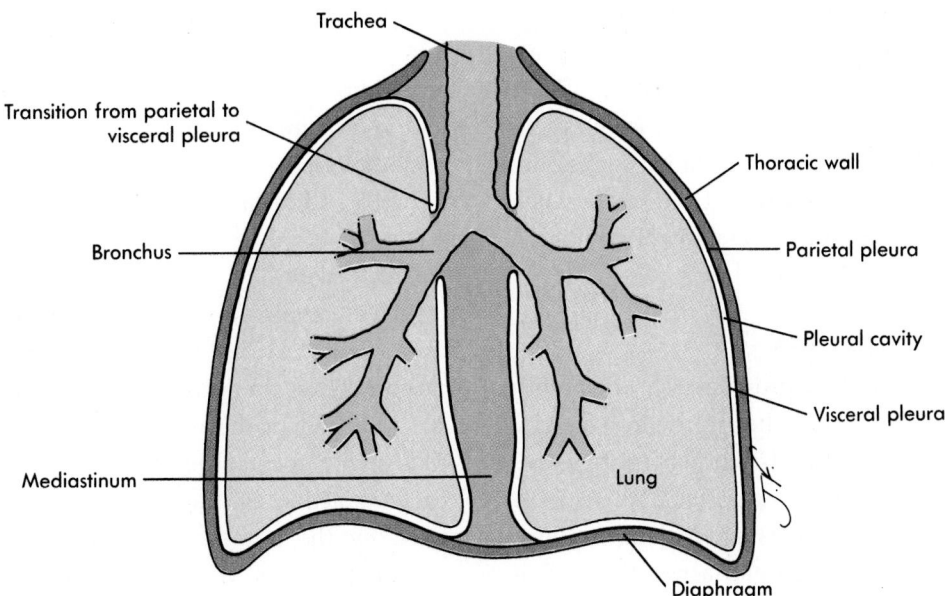

Fig. 10-50 Lungs surrounded by pleural cavities.

alveolus is separated from the blood contained within the alveolar capillaries by a thin respiratory membrane. The large surface area of the respiratory membrane may be decreased by respiratory diseases such as emphysema and lung cancer, significantly restricting the exchange of oxygen and carbon dioxide.

Alveoli are coated with pulmonary surfactant, a thin film produced by type II alveolar cells. This fluid prevents the alveoli from collapsing. In addition, there are pores in the alveolar membrane that allow for a limited flow of air between alveoli. This collateral ventilation provides some protection for the alveolus that is occluded by disease.

Lungs

The lungs are large, paired, spongy organs whose principal function is respiration. Although there is smooth muscle in the bronchioles of the lungs, the lungs expand and contract during the respiratory cycle as a result of the expansion of the thoracic cavity during inspiration and elastic recoil during expiration. The lungs are attached to the heart by the pulmonary artery and veins. The two lungs are separated by the mediastinum and its contents (the heart, blood vessels, trachea, esophagus, lymphatic tissues, and vessels). The point of entry for the bronchi, vessels, and nerves of each lung is known as the *hilum,* or root, of each

lung. At birth, the color of the lungs is rose pink. However, by adulthood, the color of the lungs changes to slate gray with dark patches as particulate matter is inhaled and deposited in the tissues. An adult lung weighs less than 2 pounds.

Each lung is conical in shape, with its base resting on the diaphragm and its apex extending to a point about 2.5 cm superior to each clavicle. The right lung is divided into three lobes. The left lung is slightly smaller than the right and is divided into two lobes. Each lobe is divided into lobules separated by connective tissue. Major blood vessels and bronchi do not cross this connective tissue, allowing for a diseased lobule to be surgically removed, leaving the remaining lung relatively intact. There are 9 lobules in the left lung and 10 lobules in the right lung.

Both lungs are surrounded by a separate pleural cavity and are attached to each other only at the point of entry of the bronchi, vessels, and nerves of each lung (Fig. 10-50). The two layers of pleura (visceral and parietal) are so close that they are virtually in contact with each other. They are separated by a thin lubricating fluid known as *pleural fluid*. The pleural fluid acts as a lubricant to allow the pleural membranes to slide past each other during respiration.

Between the two pleurae there is a potential space known as the *pleural space*. When there is significant chest wall injury or pulmonary pathology, the pleural space may become filled with air (pneumothorax) or blood (hemothorax). Other fluid collections that may accumulate in the pleural space include transudates, most commonly from congestive heart failure and exudates, which can result from infectious or malignant etiologies.

The Digestive System

The digestive system provides the body with water, electrolytes, and other nutrients used by cells. To accomplish this function, the digestive system is specialized to ingest food, propel the food through the gastrointestinal (GI) tract (digestive tract), and absorb nutrients across the wall of the lumen of the GI tract.

The GI tract is an irregular-shaped tube associated with accessory organs (primarily glands) that secrete fluid into the digestive tract. The first section of the digestive tract is the oral cavity. The salivary glands and tonsils are accessory organs of the oral cavity. The oral cavity opens posteriorly into the pharynx and inferiorly into the esophagus. The esophagus opens inferiorly into the stomach (through the muscular cardiac sphincter), where small glands secrete acids and enzymes to assist with digestion. The cardiac sphincter prevents food from reentering the esophagus when the stomach contracts.

The stomach opens into the duodenum, the first section of the small intestine. Important accessory structures in this segment of the GI tract are the liver, the gallbladder, and the pancreas. The jejunum, the major site of absorption, is the next segment of the small intestine. The last segment of the small intestine is the ileum. It is similar in function to the jejunum but has fewer digestive enzymes and provides less absorption.

The last section of the digestive tract is the large intestine, whose major functions are to absorb water and salts and to concentrate undigested food into feces. Its major accessory glands secrete mucus. The first segment of the large intestine is the cecum with its attached appendix. The cecum is followed by the ascending, transverse, descending, and sigmoid portions of the colon and the rectum. The rectum joins the anal canal, which ends at the anus.

Functions of the Digestive System

As food moves through the digestive system, secretions are added to liquify and digest the food and to provide lubrication. The processes of secretion, movement, and absorption are regulated by nervous and hormonal mechanisms.

Oral Cavity

Saliva contains a digestive enzyme called *salivary amylase* that begins the chemical digestion of carbohydrates. In addition, saliva prevents bacterial infection in the mouth by washing the oral cavity with substances that provide a weak antibacterial action. Salivary gland secretion is stimulated by the parasympathetic and sympathetic nervous systems, with the parasympathetic controlling salivation in the relaxed state.

Food taken into the mouth is chewed (masticated) by the teeth to physically break it up to facilitate swallowing and processing. Food is then swallowed by voluntary and involuntary mechanisms. The pharynx elevates to receive the food from the mouth. As the pharyngeal muscles contract, the upper esophageal sphincter relaxes, the esophagus opens, and food is pushed into the esophagus. During this phase of swallowing, the vocal folds are moved medially and the epiglottis is tipped posteriorly to close the entrance of the airway and to prevent aspiration.

Muscular contractions in the esophagus occur in peristaltic waves, pushing the food through the esophagus toward the stomach. These contractions cause relaxation of the cardiac sphincter (also known as the *lower esophageal sphincter*) and allow food to enter the stomach.

Stomach

The stomach functions primarily as a storage area and mixing chamber for ingested food. Although some digestion and absorption occur in the stomach, these are not its major functions. The stomach secretes mucus to protect the surface of the stomach wall and duodenum. It is lined by mucous membranes that contain thousands of microscopic gastric glands. These gastric glands secrete hydrochloric acid, intrinsic factor, gastrin, and pepsinogen.

Approximately 2 to 3 L of gastric secretions are produced by the stomach each day; the pro-

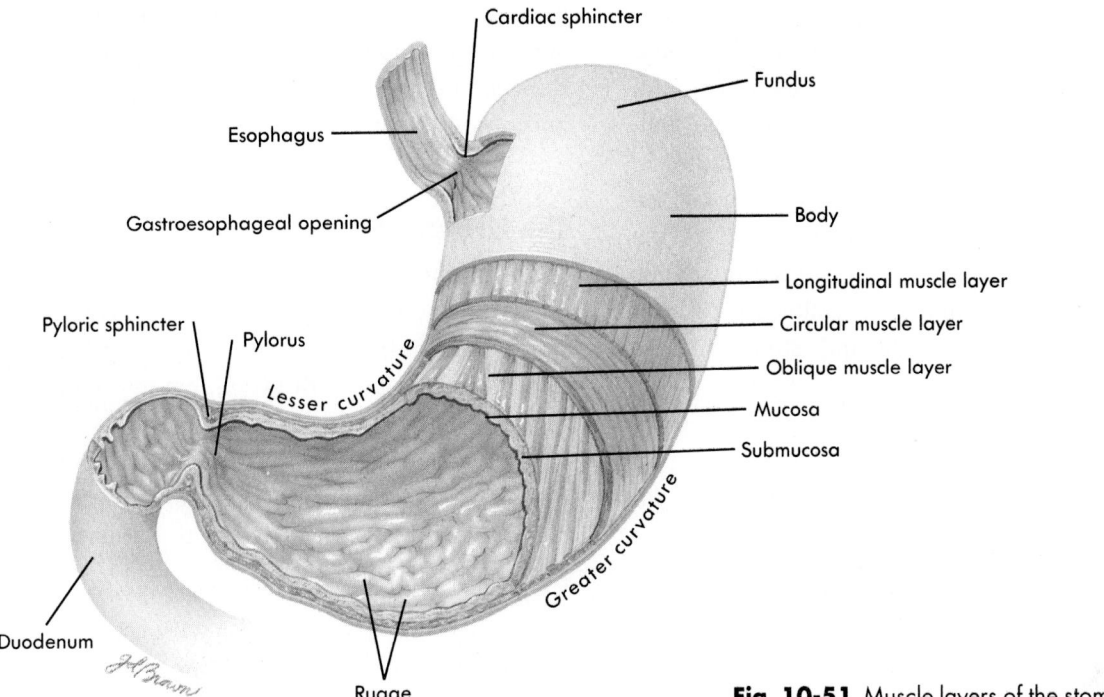

Fig. 10-51 Muscle layers of the stomach wall.

cess is regulated by nervous and hormonal mechanisms. The ingested food is thoroughly mixed with the secretions of the stomach glands to produce a semisolid mixture called *chyme.* Movements resembling peristalsis slowly force chyme toward the pyloric sphincter, through the pyloric opening, and into the duodenum (Fig. 10-51).

Small Intestine

The mucosa of the small intestine produces secretions that contain mucus, electrolytes, and water. These substances lubricate and protect the intestinal wall from the acidic chyme and digestive enzymes. In addition, secretions of the liver and pancreas enter the small intestine to aid in the digestive process.

Mixing and propulsion of chyme along with absorption of fluid and nutrients are the primary mechanical functions of the small intestine. Peristaltic contractions move the chyme through the small intestine toward the ileocecal sphincter, where the chyme enters the cecum. When the cecum distends from the chyme, the sphincter closes. This closure slows the rate of movement of chyme from the small intestine into the large intestine and prevents material from returning to the ileum from the cecum.

Liver

The liver is the largest internal organ and serves a myriad of biochemical functions. It lies just under the diaphragm in the upper regions of the abdominal cavity. It is a very vascular organ that receives a blood supply from two sources, the hepatic artery and the portal vein. The liver plays a major role in iron metabolism, plasma-protein production, detoxification of drugs and other substances circulating in plasma, and numerous other biochemical pathways.

Approximately 600 to 1000 ml of bile are secreted by the liver each day. Bile contains no digestive enzymes, but it dilutes stomach acid and emulsifies fats. Most bile salts are reabsorbed in the ileum and carried back to the liver in the blood. Other bile salts are lost through the feces.

In addition to secreting bile, the liver performs other functions necessary for healthy survival. It plays a major role in the metabolism of certain foods and helps maintain a normal blood glucose concentration. The liver is also a line of defense against many by-products of metabolism that are toxic if accumulated in the body. Blood proteins, for example, albumin, fibrinogen, globulins, and clotting factors, are also produced and released into the circulation by the liver.

Gallbladder

Bile is continuously secreted by the liver and stored in the gallbladder. When chyme containing lipid or fat enters the duodenum, the gallbladder is stimulated by the hormones cholecystokinin and secretin, which are secreted by the intestinal mucosa. This stimulation causes the gallbladder to contract, forcing concentrated bile into the small intestine. The gallbladder's only function is to concentrate and store the bile produced by the liver.

Pancreas

The pancreas is both an exocrine gland that secretes pancreatic juice and an endocrine gland that secretes hormones (for example, insulin) into the blood. Pancreatic juice is the most important digestive juice. It contains digestive enzymes, sodium bicarbonate, and alkaline substances that neutralize the hydrochloric acid in the digestive juices entering the small intestine. Pancreatic juice also contains amylase, which continues digestion initiated in the oral cavity.

Large Intestine

Chyme moves through the small intestine in 3 to 5 hours, but passage through the large intestine takes 18 to 24 hours. Processes involving the absorption of water and salts, the secretion of mucus, the action of microorganisms, and the conversion of chyme produce feces. Feces remains in the colon until it is eliminated through defecation.

The contents of the large intestine are propelled toward the anus by peristaltic contractions 3 to 4 times each day. During movement through the large intestine, material that escaped digestion in the small intestine is acted on by bacteria. As a result of this bacterial action, additional nutrients may be released and absorbed. Some of the bacteria also synthesize vitamin K, which is needed for normal blood clotting to produce the B-complex vitamins. Once formed, these vitamins are absorbed from the large intestine, where they enter the blood.

Distention of the rectal wall by feces initiates the defecation reflex, causing weak contractions and relaxations of the internal anal sphincter. The external anal sphincter (under conscious cerebral control) prevents the movement of feces out of the rectum until it is relaxed. During defecation, pressure in the abdominal cavity increases and forces the contents of the colon through the anal canal and out of the anus.

The Urinary System

The urinary system works with other body systems to maintain homeostasis by removing waste products from the blood and by helping to maintain a constant body fluid volume and composition. The kidneys are also involved in the control of red blood cell production and in vitamin D metabolism. The contents of the urinary system include two kidneys, two ureters, the urinary bladder, and the urethra.

Kidneys

The kidneys, each shaped very much like a kidney bean, lie on the posterior abdominal wall behind the peritoneum. They are located on either side of the vertebral column near the lateral border of the psoas muscles. The superior pole of each kidney is protected by the rib cage. The right kidney is slightly lower than the left because of the superior position of the liver. A fibrous renal capsule surrounds each kidney, as does a dense deposit of adipose tissue that protects the kidney from injury.

The kidney is divided into an outer cortex and an inner medulla. The medulla consists of a number of triangular divisions called the *renal pyramids* that extend into the cortex (Fig. 10-52). The papilla is the innermost end of a pyramid. Several large urinary tubes (calyces) extend to the renal pelvis from the kidney tissue.

The basic functional unit of the kidney is the nephron. The nephron consists of a large terminal end called a *renal corpuscle,* a proximal convoluted tubule, the loop of Henle, and a distal convoluted tubule. The distal convoluted tubule empties into a collecting duct, which carries the urine from the cortex of the kidney to the calyces. The terminal end of the nephron is enlarged to form Bowman's capsule. The wall of Bowman's capsule is indented to form a double-walled chamber occupied by a network of blood capillaries known as the *glomerulus.* Together, the glomerulus and Bowman's capsule form the renal corpuscle.

Fig. 10-52 Magnified wedge cut from a renal pyramid.

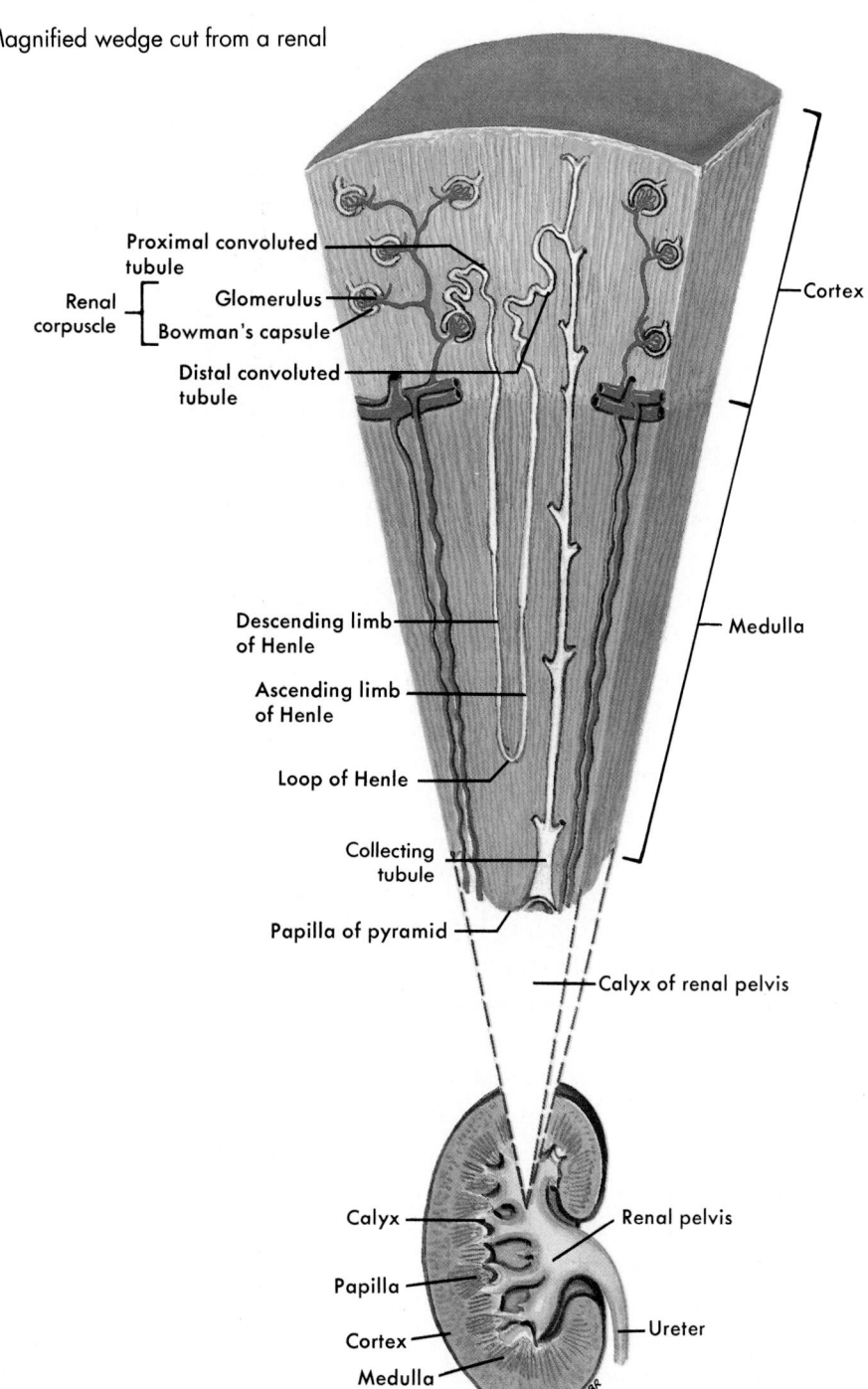

Proximal convoluted tubule

Renal corpuscle

Glomerulus

Bowman's capsule

Distal convoluted tubule

Cortex

Descending limb of Henle

Ascending limb of Henle

Loop of Henle

Collecting tubule

Papilla of pyramid

Medulla

Calyx of renal pelvis

Calyx

Renal pelvis

Papilla

Cortex

Medulla

Ureter

AFTER NBR

Ureters, Urinary Bladder, and Urethra

The ureters extend from the renal pelvis to the urinary bladder. The triangular area of the bladder wall between the two ureters and the urethra is called the *trigone.* (Fig. 10-53 depicts the male urinary bladder.) This region differs from the rest of the bladder wall in that it does not expand during bladder filling.

The urinary bladder is a hollow, muscular organ that lies in the pelvic cavity just posterior to the pubic symphysis. The size of the bladder depends on the volume of urine.

At the junction of the urethra with the urinary bladder, smooth muscle of the bladder forms the internal urinary sphincter. The external urinary sphincter surrounds the urethra as the urethra ex-

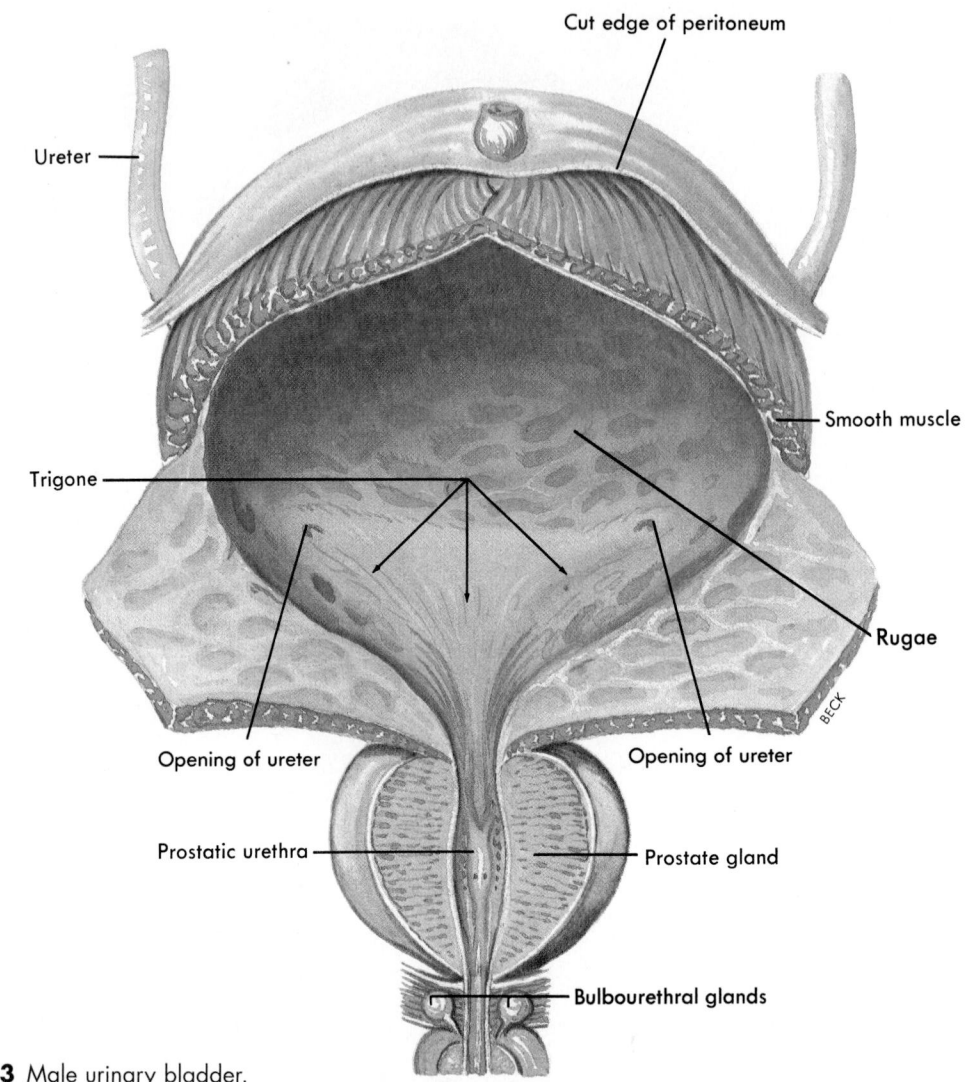

Fig. 10-53 Male urinary bladder.

tends through the pelvic floor. These sphincters control the flow of urine through the urethra. In the male, the urethra extends to the end of the penis, where it opens to the outside (see Fig. 10-53). The female urethra is much shorter than the male urethra and opens into the vestibule anterior to the vaginal opening.

Urine Production

Nephrons are the structural components of the kidney and are where urine is produced. The more than two million nephrons form urine in a three-step process that includes filtration, reabsorption, and secretion.

1. The first step of urine formation is the passage of fluid from the glomerular capillaries into Bowman's capsule. Blood flowing through the glomeruli exerts pressure, and this glomerular blood pressure pushes water and small molecular dissolved substances out of the glomeruli into the Bowman's capsule. Simply stated, glomerular blood pressure causes filtration through the glomerular capillaries. Glomerular filtration normally occurs at the rate of 125 ml/min or 180 L/day (glomerular filtration rate), of which 90% is reabsorbed. Healthy people produce 1 to 2 L of urine each day.

2. The filtrate leaves the renal capsule and flows through the proximal convoluted tubule, the loop of Henle, the distal convoluted tubule, and then into the collecting duct. During this process, many substances in the filtrate are reabsorbed by the blood capillar-

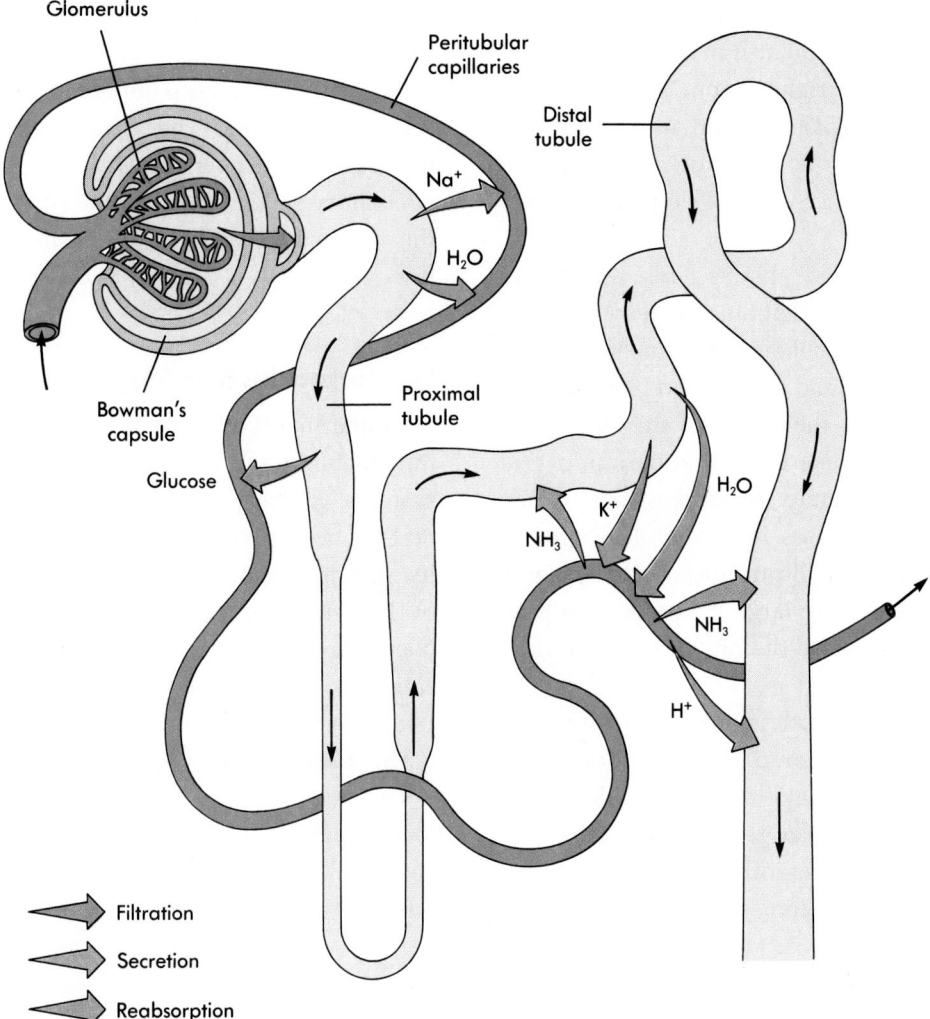

Glomerulus

Peritubular capillaries

Distal tubule

Na^+

H_2O

Bowman's capsule

Proximal tubule

Glucose

NH_3

K^+

H_2O

NH_3

H^+

Filtration

Secretion

Reabsorption

Fig. 10-54 Formation of urine. Steps in urine formation in successive parts of a nephron: filtration, reabsorption, and secretion.

ies around the tubules (peritubular capillaries) and reenter the general circulation. Substances reabsorbed include water, glucose and other nutrients, and most of the sodium and other ions.

3. Secretion is the process by which substances move into urine in the distal convoluted tubule and collecting duct from blood in the capillaries around these structures. Unlike reabsorption, which moves substances out of the urine and into the blood, secretion moves substances out of the blood and into the urine. Secreted substances include hydrogen ions, potassium ions, ammonia, and certain drugs. Fig. 10-54 depicts the formation of urine.

Urine Regulation

The body can usually control both the amount and composition of urine it secretes. This involves hormonal mechanisms, autoregulation, and sympathetic nervous system stimulation.

Aldosterone is a steroid hormone secreted by the adrenal gland. The hormone passes through the circulatory system from the adrenal gland to the kidney and stimulates the tubules to reabsorb sodium salts and water.

ADH secreted by the posterior pituitary gland tends to decrease the amount of urine produced by making distal and collecting tubules permeable to water, thus increasing water reabsorption. As a result, water is retained by the body in the presence of ADH.

Atrial natriuretic factor is a hormone secreted from the cells in the right atrium of the heart when the pressure in the right atrium increases. This hormone inhibits ADH secretion and reduces the ability of the kidney to concentrate urine. As a result, the body produces a large volume of dilute urine.

Prostaglandins and kinins are substances formed in the kidneys that affect kidney function. These substances are believed to influence the rate of filtrate formation and sodium ion reabsorption.

Autoregulation is the ability of the kidneys to regulate a stable glomerular filtration rate over a wide range of systemic blood pressures. When there are small increases in glomerular capillary pressure, the rate of filtrate formation increases substantially. Therefore large increases in arterial blood pressure increase the rate of urine production.

Conversely, when arterial blood pressure decreases, urine production decreases. Through autoregulation, the kidneys change the degree of constriction or dilation of the arterioles in the renal capsule to maintain glomerular capillary pressure and urine production within normal limits over a rather wide range of arterial blood pressures.

Sympathetic neurons innervate the blood vessels of the kidney. The sympathetic stimulation in response to severe stress, intense exercise, or circulatory shock constricts the small arteries and the afferent arterioles, decreasing renal blood flow.

The Reproductive System

Unlike many other organs and systems of the human body, the male and female reproductive systems are very different. The purpose of the male reproductive system is to produce and transfer spermatozoa to the female, and the purposes of the female reproductive system are to produce oocytes and to receive the spermatozoa for fertilization, conception, gestation, and birth.

The Male Reproductive System

The male reproductive system consists of the testes, epididymis, ductus deferens, urethra, seminal vesicles, prostate gland, bulbourethral glands, scrotum, and penis (Fig. 10-55).

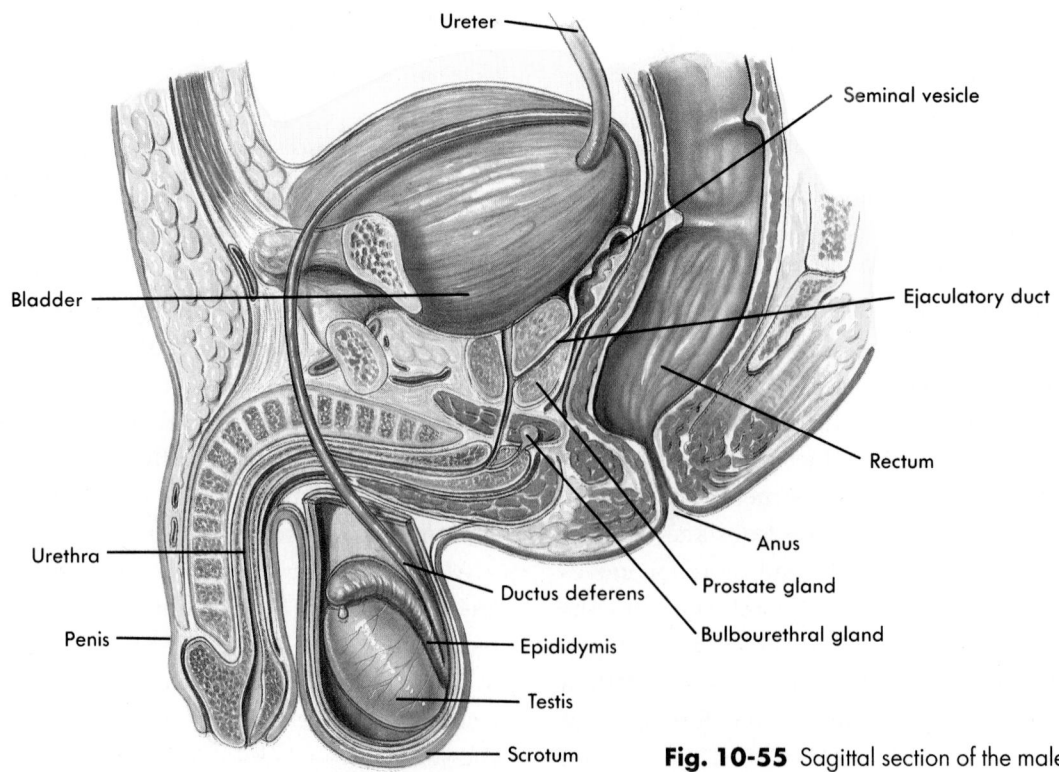

Fig. 10-55 Sagittal section of the male pelvis.

The testes are ovoid organs within the scrotum that develop as retroperitoneal organs in the abdominopelvic cavity. They move from the abdominal cavity to the scrotum by way of the inguinal canal, a canal common to both men and women. Normally the inguinal canal is closed, but it represents a weak spot in the abdominal wall as the testes pass through it. If the inguinal canal weakens or ruptures, an inguinal hernia may result. Interstitial cells of the testes secrete the male hormone testosterone. Before puberty (12 to 14 years of age), the testes remain relatively simple and unchanged. At the time of puberty, however, the interstitial cells increase in number and size, and spermatozoa production begins. The testes contribute approximately 5% of the seminal fluid (semen).

The final maturation of spermatozoa occurs within the epididymis, a convoluted comma-shaped structure on the posterior side of the testis. Infection or injury can block one epididymis or both, resulting in infertility.

The ductus deferens, or vas deferens, emerges from the tail of the epididymis and ascends to the seminal vesicle, finally associating with the blood vessels and nerves that supply the testis. These structures and their coverings constitute the spermatic cord. The ductus deferens and the spermatic cord structures ascend and pass through the inguinal canal to enter the abdominal cavity. The ductus deferens crosses the lateral wall of the cavity, travels over the ureter, and loops over the posterior surface of the urinary bladder to approach the prostate gland. The ductus deferens is surrounded by smooth muscle that helps to propel sperm through this duct.

The urethra is a passageway for both urine and male reproductive fluids. The urethra can be divided into three portions: the prostatic portion (the part of the urethra that passes through the prostate gland), the membranous portion (extending from the prostatic urethra through the muscular floor of the pelvis), and the spongy portion (extending the length of the penis).

The seminal vesicle is a sac-shaped gland that lies adjacent to each ductus deferens. A short duct from the seminal vesicle joins the ductus deferens to form the ejaculatory duct. These ducts project into the prostate gland and end by opening into the urethra. Seminal vesicles produce approximately 60% of seminal fluid.

The prostate gland consists of both glandular and muscular tissue and is approximately the size and shape of a walnut. It is located dorsal to the symphysis pubis at the base of the bladder, surrounding the prostatic urethra and the two ejaculatory ducts. A total of 20 to 30 small prostatic ducts secrete prostatic fluid into the prostatic urethra. The prostate gland contributes approximately 30% of seminal fluid.

The bulbourethral glands are a pair of small glands located near the membranous portion of the urethra. In young adults, they are each about the size of a pea but decrease in size with age. The gland is a compound mucous gland with small ducts that unite to form a single duct from each gland. The two bulbourethral glands enter the spongy urethra at the base of the penis. The bulbourethral glands add secretions to semen, contributing approximately 5% of seminal fluid.

The scrotum is divided into two internal compartments by a connective tissue septum. Beneath the skin of the scrotum are a layer of superficial fascia (loose connective tissue) and a layer of cutaneous muscle called the *dartos muscle*. The dartos and the cremaster muscles of the abdomen are important for regulating temperature in the testes (as required for spermatogenesis). They pull the testes near the body in cold temperatures and allow the testes to descend away from the body in warm temperatures and during exercise.

The penis consists of three columns of erectile tissue. Engorgement of this tissue with blood causes the penis to enlarge and become firm, producing an erection. The penis is the male organ of copulation and functions in the transfer of spermatozoa from the male to the female.

The Female Reproductive System

The female reproductive organs consist of the ovaries, uterine (or fallopian) tubes, uterus, vagina, external genital organs, and mammary glands. The internal reproductive organs lie within the pelvis between the urinary bladder and the rectum and are held in place by a group of ligaments (Fig. 10-56).

The small ovaries are attached to the posterior of the broad ligament called the *mesovarium*. Two

Fig. 10-56 Sagittal section of the female pelvis.

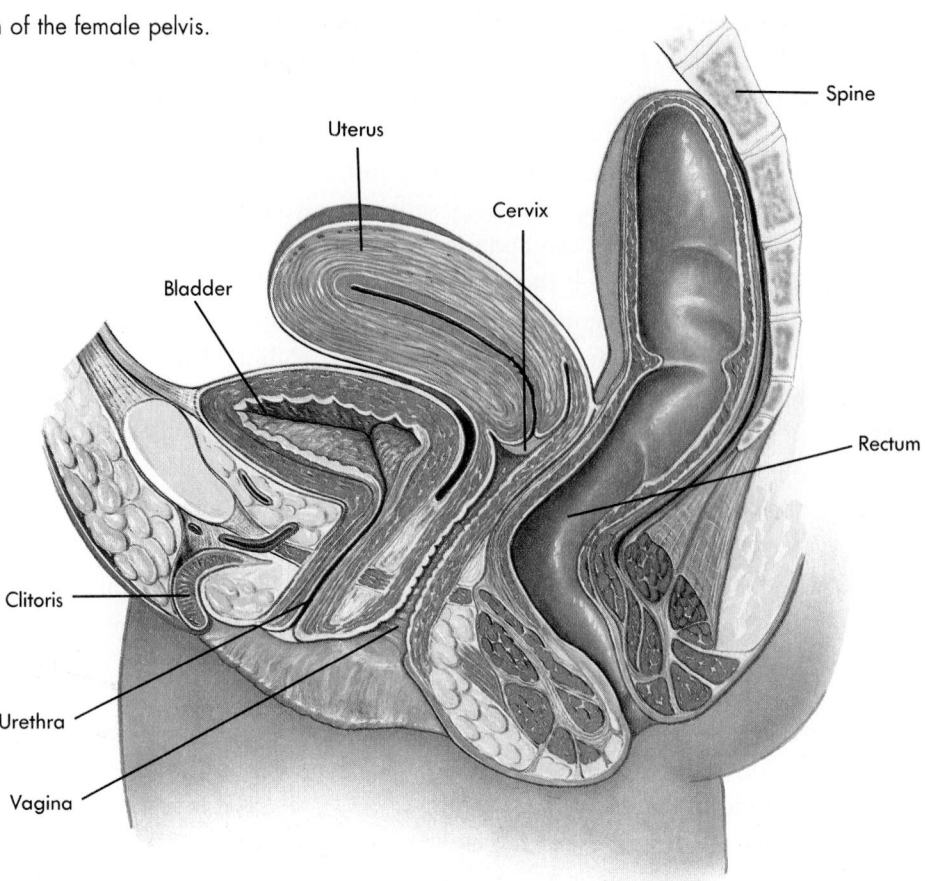

other ligaments associated with the ovary are the suspensory ligament and the ovarian ligament. The ovarian arteries, veins, and nerves traverse the suspensory ligament and enter the ovary through the mesovarium. Each ovary consists of a dense outer portion called the *cortex* and a looser inner portion called the *medulla*. Numerous small vesicles called *ovarian follicles* (each of which contains an oocyte) are distributed throughout the cortex.

The uterine tubes are ducts for the ovaries. Each tube is located along the superior margin of the broad ligament and opens directly into the peritoneal cavity to receive the oocyte. Once inside the uterine tube, of the oocyte is transported by cilia and peristaltic contractions of the smooth muscle in the uterine tube.

The uterus is the size and shape of a medium-sized pear. It is oriented in the pelvic cavity with the larger rounded portion (the fundus) directed superiorly. The narrower portion (the cervix) is directed inferiorly. The main portion of the uterus (the body) is positioned between the fundus and the cervix. The major ligaments holding the uterus in place are the broad ligament, round ligaments, and uterosacral ligaments (Fig. 10-57).

The vagina is the female organ of copulation and functions to receive the penis during intercourse. It extends from the uterus to the outside of the body and provides a passage for menstrual flow and childbirth. The smooth muscle layer of the vagina allows the organ to increase in size to accommodate the penis during intercourse and to greatly stretch during delivery. The vaginal orifice is covered by a thin mucus membrane called the *hymen*. The openings in the hymen are usually enlarged during the first sexual intercourse but may also be perforated or torn during strenuous exercise.

The external genitalia, referred to as the *vulva*, consists of the vestibule and its surrounding structures (Fig. 10-58). The vestibule is the space into which the vagina and urethra open. It is bordered by a pair of thin, longitudinal skin folds called the *labia minora*. A small erectile structure, the clitoris, is located in the anterior margin of the vesti-

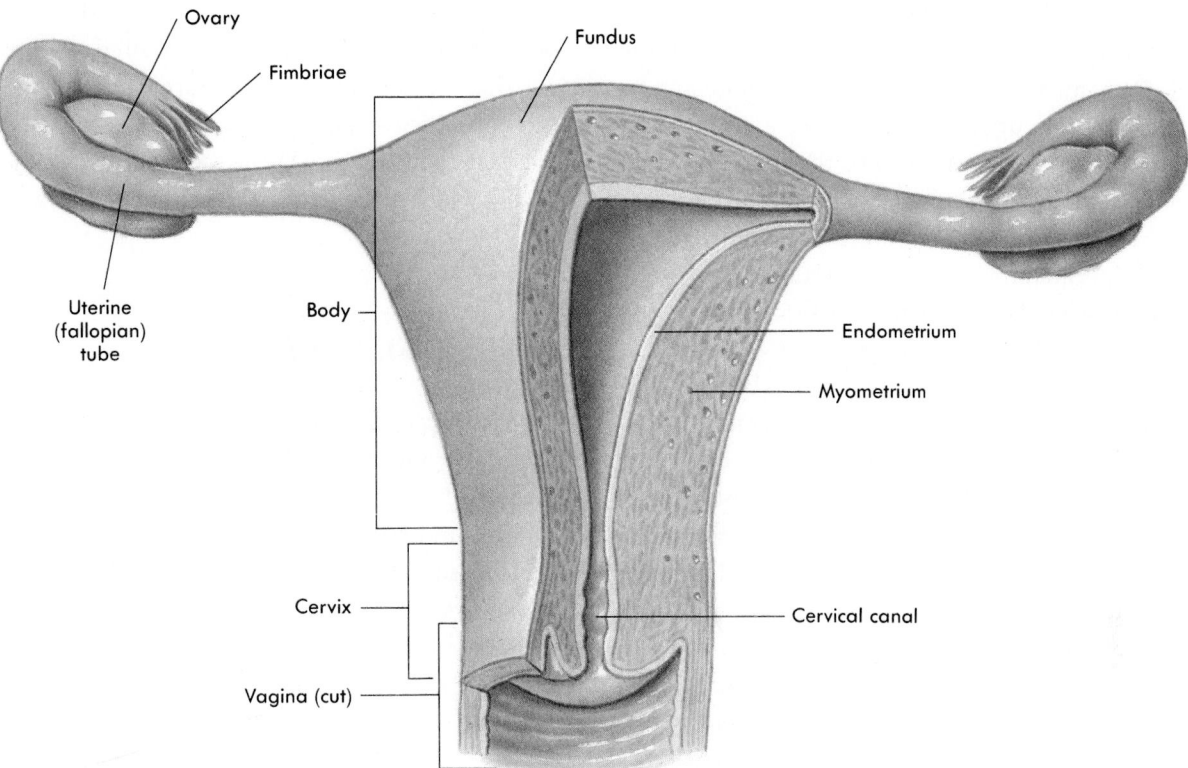

Fig. 10-57 Internal anatomy of the female pelvis.

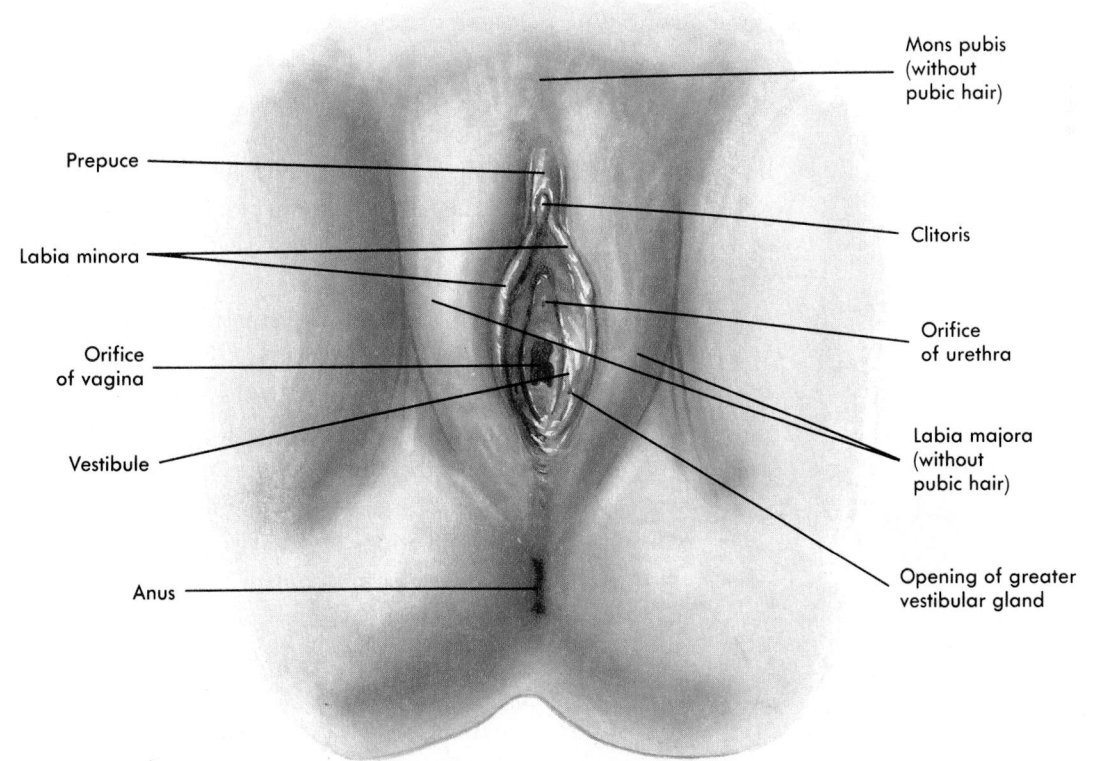

Fig. 10-58 Female external genitalia.

bule. The two labia minora unite over the clitoris to form a fold of skin known as the *prepuce*. Lateral to the labia minora are two prominent folds of skin called the *labia majora,* which unite anteriorly in an elevation over the pubic symphysis to form the mons pubis. Most of the time, the labia majora are in contact with each other, concealing the deeper structures within the vestibule.

The perineum is divided into triangles by perineal muscles. The urogenital triangle contains the external genitalia, and the posterior anal triangle contains the anal opening. The region between the vagina and the anus is called the *clinical perineum* (an area that sometimes tears during childbirth).

The mammary glands are the organs of milk production located within the breasts or mammae. Externally, the breasts of both males and females have a raised nipple surrounded by a circular pigmented areola. Nipples are very sensitive to tactile stimulation and may become erect in response to sexual arousal. The areolae normally have a slightly bumpy surface because of the presence of areolar glands just below their surface. Secretions from these glands protect the nipple and areolar from chafing during nursing.

The female breasts begin to enlarge during puberty under the influence of estrogen and proges-

terone. Each adult female mammary gland consists of 15 to 20 glandular lobes covered by adipose tissue. Each lobe possesses a single lactiferous duct, which subdivides to form smaller ducts, each of which supplies a lobule. These ducts expand at their ends to form secretory sacs called *alveoli,* which secrete milk during nursing (Fig. 10-59).

● SPECIAL SENSES

Senses provide the brain with information about the outside world. Four senses are recognized as "special senses": smell, taste, sight, and hearing and balance. (The sense of touch is now considered to be a "general sense," which consists of several types of nerve endings scattered throughout the body and not localized to a specific area.)

Olfactory Sense Organs

The receptors for the fibers of the olfactory or first cranial nerves lie in the mucosa of the upper part of the nasal cavity (Fig. 10-60). Most of the nasal cavity is involved with respiration, and only a small portion is devoted to olfaction (olfactory recess).

The dendrites of olfactory neurons extend to the epithelial surface of the nasal cavity, where they form vesicles. These vesicles possess extremely long cilia that lie in a thin, mucous film on the epithelial surface. When olfactory cells are stimulated by airborne molecules, the resulting nerve impulses travel through the olfactory nerves in the olfactory bulb and olfactory tract. There they enter the thalamic and olfactory centers of the brain, where the nervous impulses are interpreted as specific odors.

The exact mechanism of olfactory stimulation is not clearly understood. It is generally believed that the variety of detectable smells are actually combinations of a smaller number of seven primary odors: (1) camphoraceous, (2) musky, (3) floral, (4) pepperminty, (5) ethereal, (6), pungent, and (7) putrid. Although olfactory receptors are extremely sensitive (even to slight odors), they are also easily fatigued. The olfactory system quickly

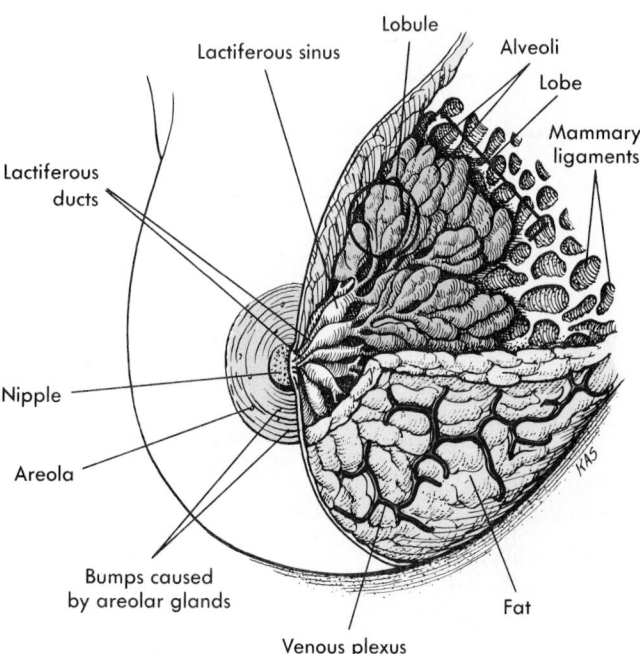

Fig. 10-59 Blood supply, mammary glands, and duct system of the right mamma.

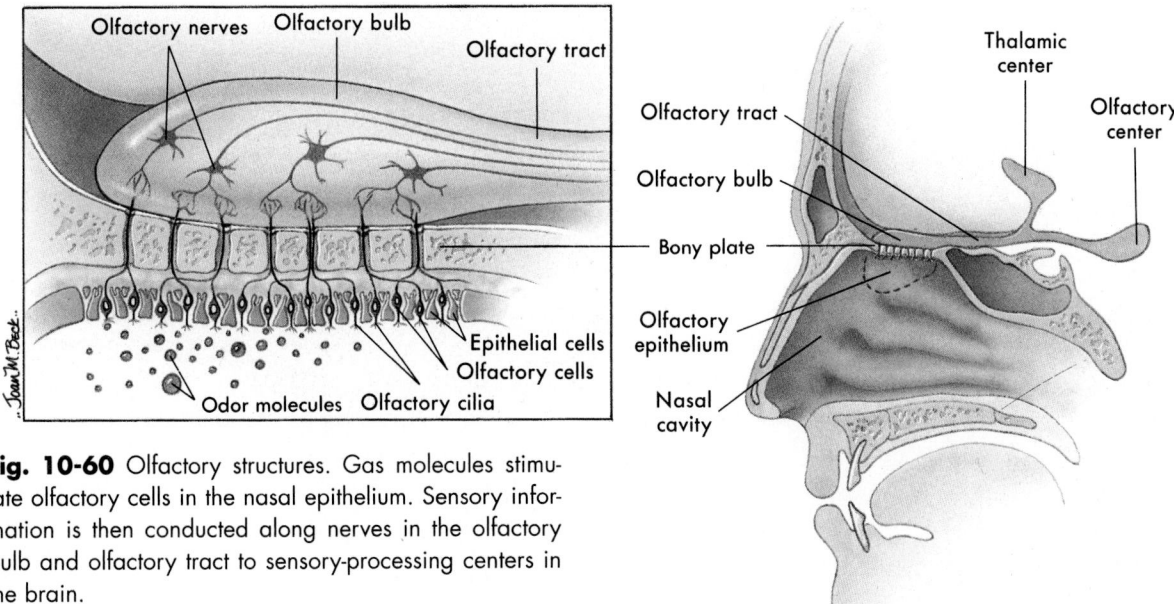

Fig. 10-60 Olfactory structures. Gas molecules stimulate olfactory cells in the nasal epithelium. Sensory information is then conducted along nerves in the olfactory bulb and olfactory tract to sensory-processing centers in the brain.

adapts to continued stimulation, and a particular odor may cease to be noticed in a short time. This is an important factor to consider when dealing with hazardous materials incidents.

Taste

The sensory structures that detect taste stimuli are the taste buds, and the receptors for the taste nerve fibers are in the seventh and ninth cranial nerves. Most taste buds are associated with specialized portions of the tongue. However, taste buds are also located on other areas of the tongue, palate, lips, and throat.

Taste detected by taste buds can be divided into four basic types: bitter, sour, salty, and sweet. The tip of the tongue reacts more strongly to sweet and salty tastes, the back of the tongue to bitter taste, and the sides of the tongue to sour taste (Fig. 10-61). All the other taste sensations result from a combination of taste bud and olfactory receptor stimulation.

Visual System

The visual system includes the eyes, the accessory structures (eyelids, eyebrows, eyelashes, and tear glands), and the optic nerve, tracts, and path-

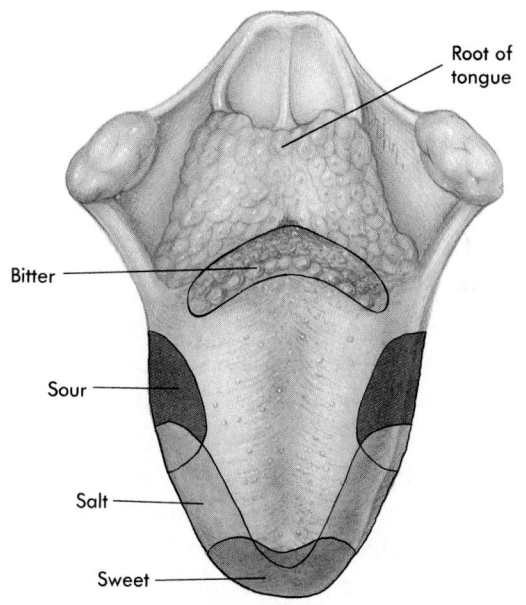

Fig. 10-61 Tongue. Dorsal surface and regions sensitive to various tastes.

ways. The second cranial nerve (optic nerve) conducts impulses from the eye to the brain, where these impulses produce the sensation of vision. The third cranial nerve (oculomotor nerve) conducts impulses from the brain to muscles of the eye, where they cause contractions that move the eye.

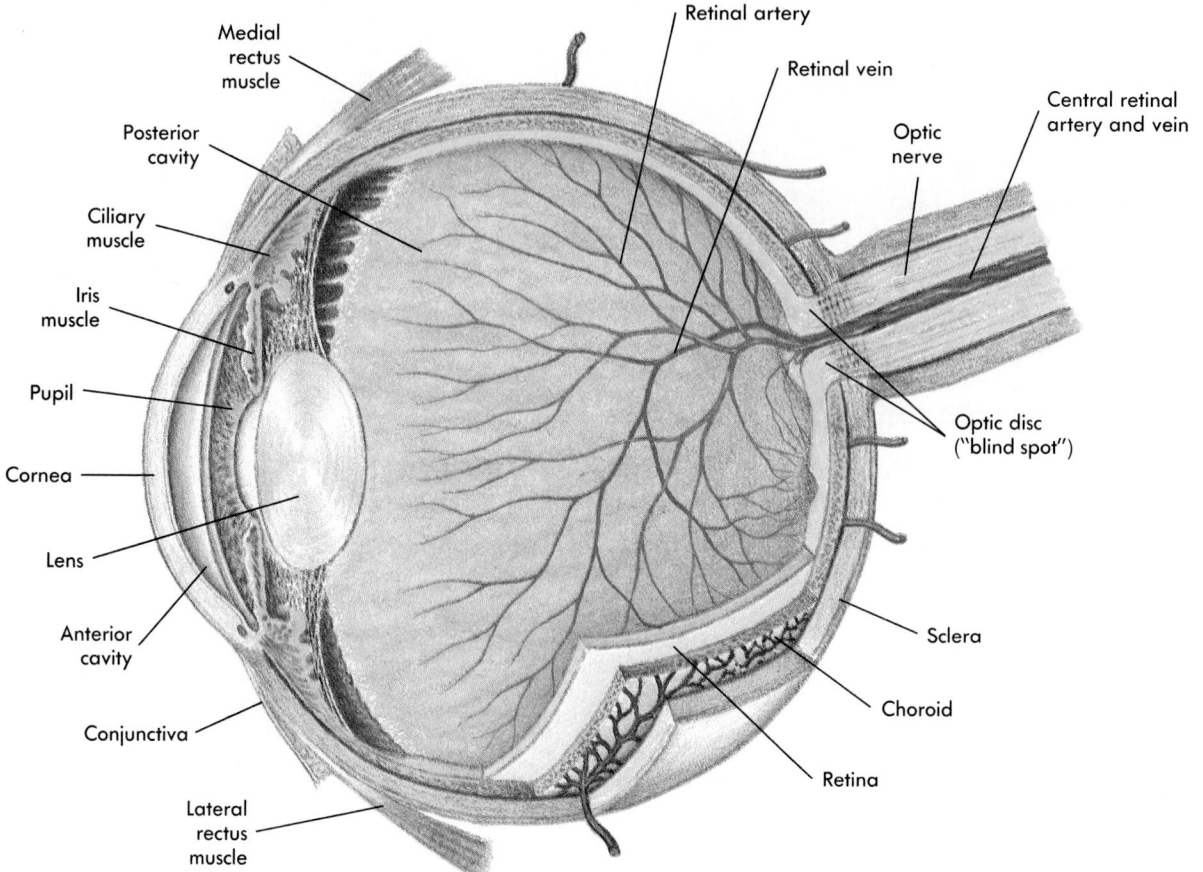

Fig. 10-62 Horizontal section through the left eyeball. The eye is viewed from above.

Anatomy of the Eye

The eye is composed of three layers: the fibrous tunic, consisting of the sclera and cornea; the vascular tunic, consisting of the choroid, ciliary body, and iris; and the nervous tunic, consisting of the retina (Fig. 10-62).

1. The sclera is the firm, opaque, white outer layer of the eye. The sclera helps to maintain the shape of the eye, protects the internal structures of the eye, and provides an attachment point for the muscles that move the eye. The sclera is continuous with the meningeal layers of the brain that extend along the optic nerve.

   The cornea is continuous with the sclera. It is an avascular and transparent structure that permits light to enter the eye. The cornea also bends and refracts entering light.

2. The vascular tunic contains most of the blood vessels of the eyeball. The part of this layer associated with the sclera is the choroid. Anteriorly, the vascular tunic consists of the ciliary body and the iris. The ciliary body consists of ciliary muscles that can change the shape of the lens and of complex capillaries involved in producing aqueous humor.

   The iris is the colored part of the eye. It consists mainly of smooth muscle that surrounds the pupil. Light enters through the pupil, and the iris regulates the amount of light by controlling the size of the pupil.

3. The retina consists of an outer pigmented retina and an inner sensory layer, which responds to light. The sensory retina contains photoreceptor cells, called *rods* and *cones*, and numerous relay neurons. (Rods are the receptors for night vision, and cones are the receptors for daytime and color vision.)

Compartments of the Eye

There are two compartments of the eye that are separated by a lens suspended between the two eye compartments by ligaments. These two compartments are known as the *anterior* and *posterior chambers*. The anterior chamber is filled with aqueous humor, which helps maintain intraocular pressure (pressure within the eye that keeps the eye inflated), refract light, and provide nutrition for the anterior chamber.

The posterior chamber of the eye is almost completely surrounded by the retina. It is filled with a transparent, jellylike substance called *vitreous humor.* Like aqueous humor, the vitreous humor helps maintain intraocular pressure. In addition, it helps to hold the retina in place and functions in the refraction of light in the eye.

Accessory Structures

The eye's accessory structures protect, lubricate, move, and aid in the function of the eye. These structures include the eyebrows, eyelids, conjunctiva, and lacrimal gland.

Eyebrows protect the eyes by providing shade from direct sunlight and by preventing perspiration from running into the eyes.

Eyelids protect the eyes from foreign objects. Blinking, which normally occurs approximately 25 times per minute, helps to lubricate the eyes by spreading tears over their surfaces. Eyelids also help to regulate the amount of light entering the eyes.

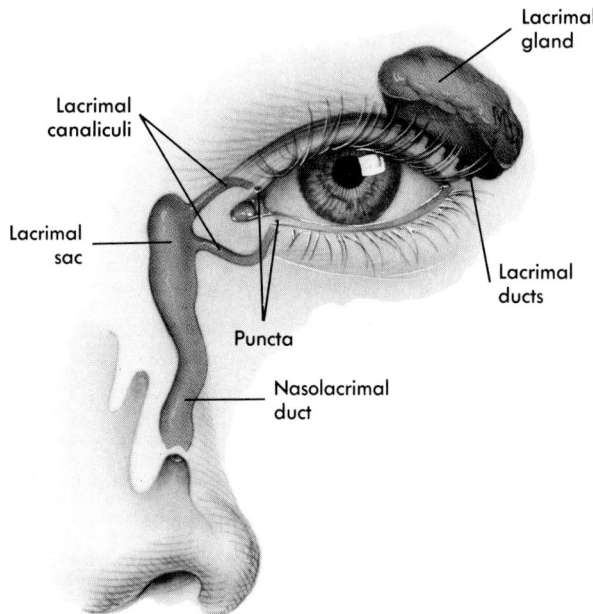

Fig. 10-63 Lacrimal structures of the eye.

The conjunctiva is a thin, transparent mucous membrane that covers the inner surface of the eyelids, as well as the outer surface of the sclera.

The lacrimal gland produces lacrimal fluid (tears) that leaves the gland through several ducts, passing over the anterior surface of the eyeball. The gland is situated in the superolateral corner of the orbit. Tears are constantly produced by this gland to moisten the surface of the eye, lubricate the eyelids, and wash away foreign objects. Tears also contain lysosomes that destroy some forms of bacteria.

Most tears evaporate from the surface of the eye. Excess fluid is collected in the medial corner of the eye by the lacrimal canals through a punctum (the opening of each canal). The lacrimal canals open into a lacrimal sac, which in turn continues into the nasolacrimal duct (Fig. 10-63).

Hearing and Balance

The organs of hearing can be divided into three portions: external, middle, and inner ear (Fig. 10-64). The external and middle ear are involved in hearing only, and the inner ear functions in both hearing and balance. The special senses of hearing and balance are both transmitted by the vestibulocochlear nerve (eighth cranial nerve).

The external ear includes the auricle, or pinna, and the external auditory meatus, which opens into the external auditory canal. The external auditory canal is lined by hairs and ceruminous glands that produce cerumen. It terminates medially at the eardrum, or tympanic membrane. The middle ear is an air-filled space within the temporal bone, which contains the auditory ossicles.

The inner ear contains the sensory organs for hearing and balance. It consists of interconnecting tunnels and chambers within the bony labyrinth. Inside the bony labyrinth is another set of membranous tunnels and chambers called the *membranous labyrinth*, which is filled with a clear fluid called *endolymph*. The space between the membranous and bony labyrinth is filled with a fluid called *perilymph*. These fluids are similar to cerebrospinal fluid.

The auricle is shaped to collect sound waves and direct them toward the external auditory meatus. From the external auditory meatus, sound

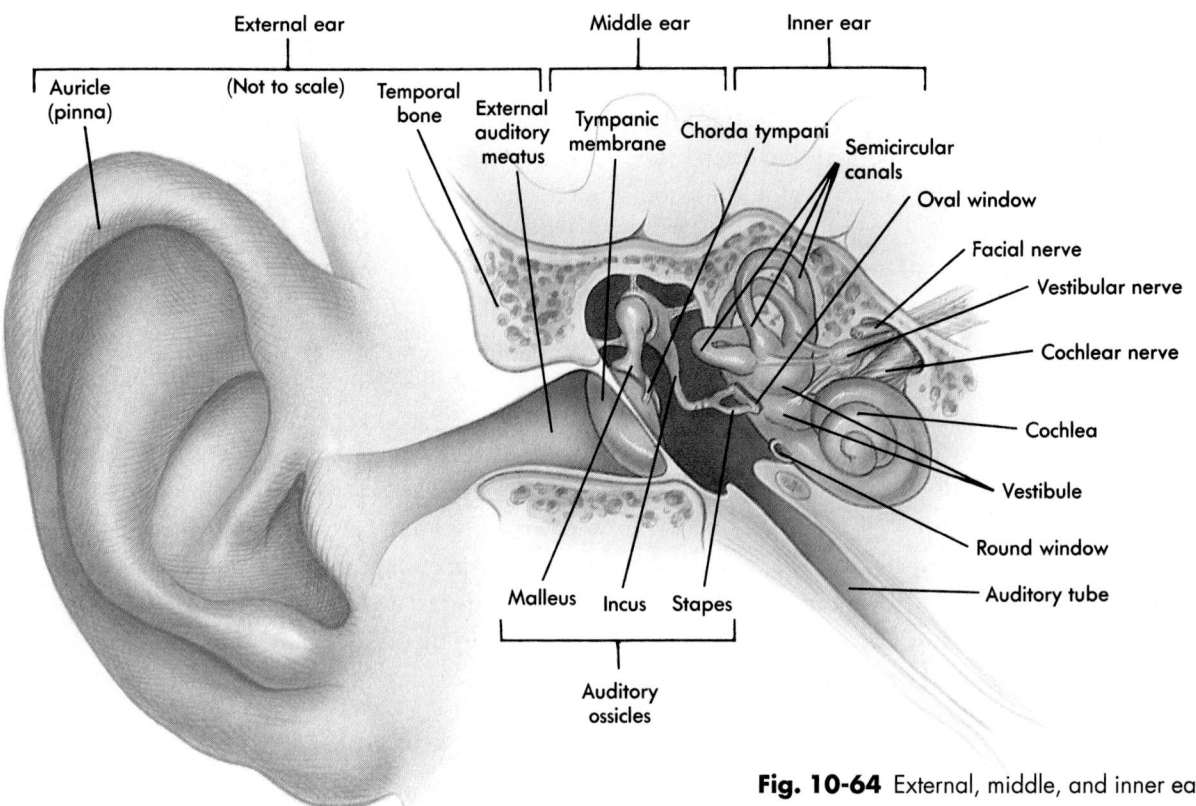

Fig. 10-64 External, middle, and inner ear.

waves travel through the auditory canal to the tympanic membrane, causing the membrane to vibrate.

The middle ear is connected to the inner ear by two membrane-covered openings, the round and oval windows. Two other openings that are not covered by membranes provide a passage for air from the middle ear. One opens into the mastoid air cells. The second opening, the auditory, or eustachian, tube, opens into the pharynx and permits the equalization of air pressure between the outside air and middle ear cavity. (The shorter eustachian tubes in children make it easier for bacteria to travel from infected areas in the throat to the middle ear. This anatomical difference between children and adults is responsible for the increased frequency of pediatric earaches and infections). The auditory ossicles of the middle ear (the malleus, incus, and stapes) transmit vibrations from the tympanic membrane to the oval window.

The bony labyrinth of the inner ear is divided into three regions: vestibule, cochlea, and semicircular canals. The vestibule and semicircular canals are involved primarily in balance, and the cochlea is involved in hearing. The hearing sense organ, which lies inside the cochlea, is called the *organ of Corti*. In young, healthy people, the frequencies that can be detected by the ear range (over octaves) from 20 to 20,000 cycles per second.

Summary

Understanding the function and structure of the human body is important in providing emergency care. Although most patient care encounters are focused on a particular injury or illness, a thorough patient assessment should include a consideration of the body's complex systems and the many ways in which they interrelate.

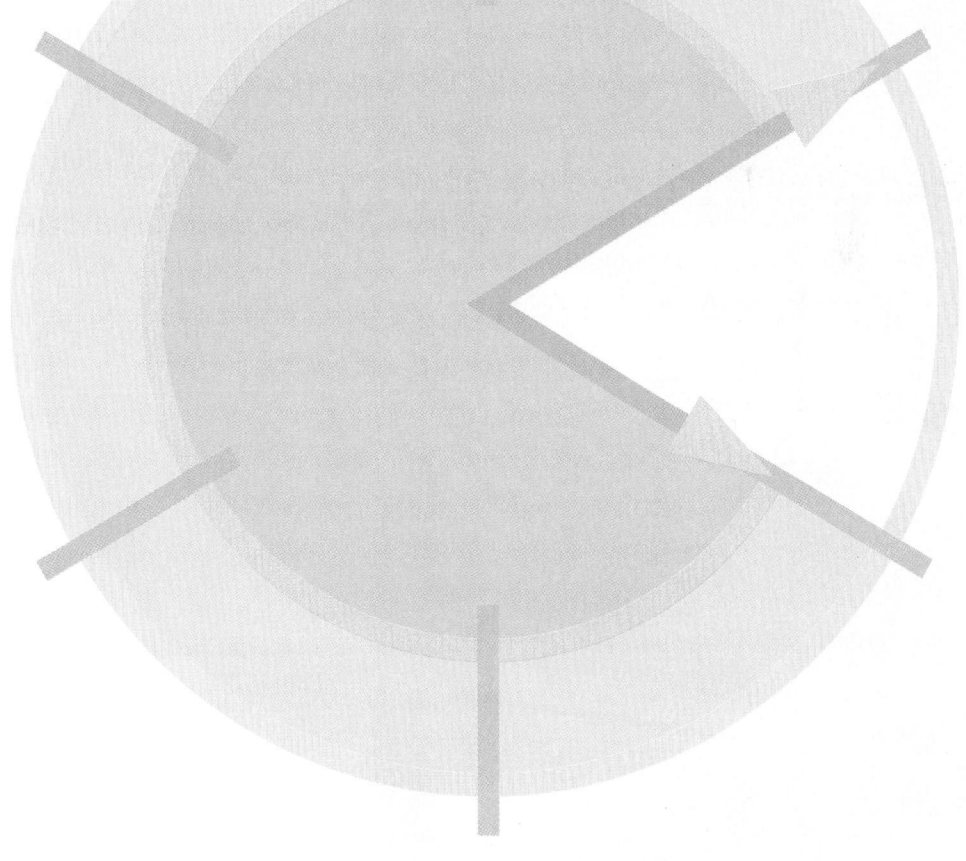

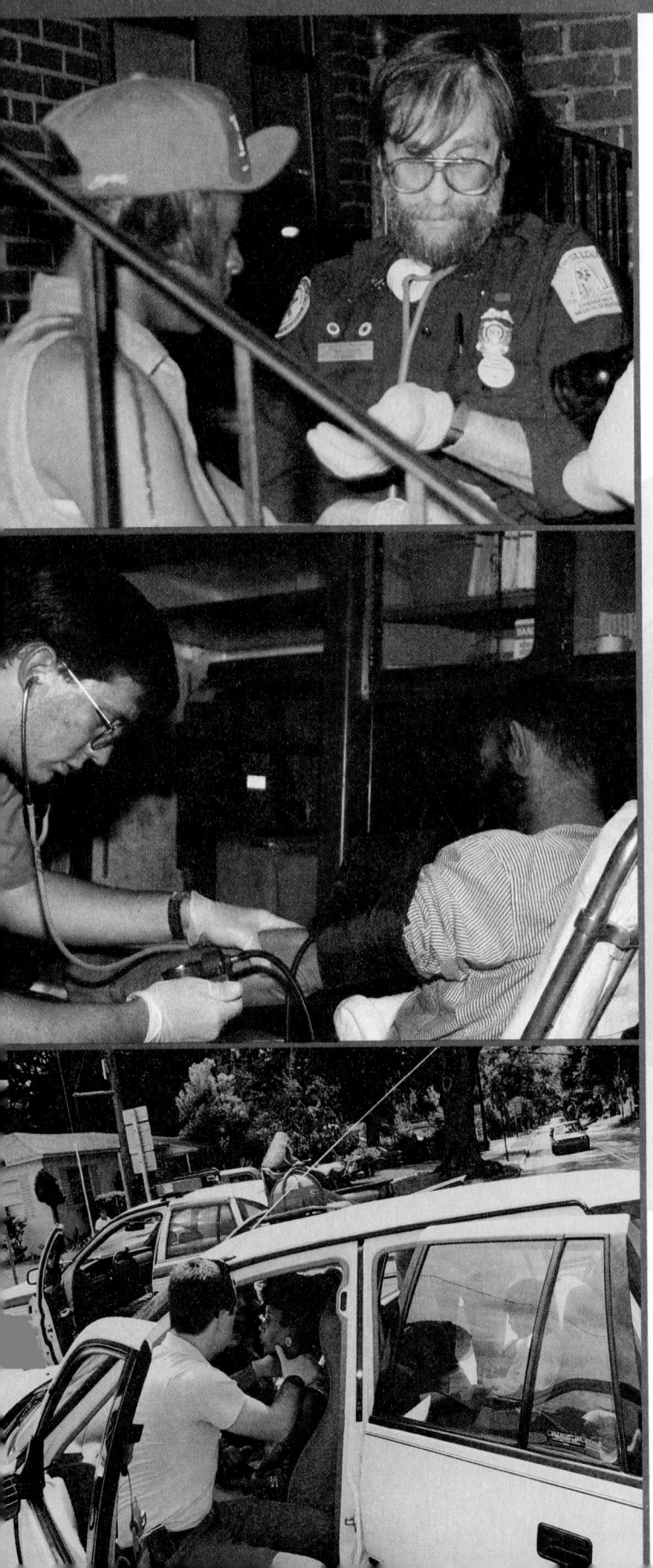

The prehospital environment usually lacks on-scene emergency physicians and diagnostic services. Therefore priorities of care must be established based on patient assessment. These priorities include scene safety, recognition and stabilization of life-threatening conditions, and identification of patients who require rapid stabilization and transport for definitive care.

As a paramedic, you should be able to:

1. Establish priorities of care based on life-threatening conditions.
2. Distinguish between patient assessment and patient management.
3. Explain the purpose of the primary and secondary surveys.
4. Detail in the correct order the assessment of each component of the primary survey.
5. Identify potentially life-threatening conditions that can be discovered in the primary survey.
6. Discuss patient management techniques that may be used if abnormalities are found in the primary survey.
7. Differentiate between resuscitation procedures for medical patients and trauma patients.
8. Describe the examination techniques for inspection, palpation, and auscultation.
9. Explain in detail the physical examination for each component of the secondary survey.
10. Apply effective patient-interviewing techniques to given scenarios.
11. Describe the essential elements of the patient history.
12. Describe the process of patient reevaluation.
13. Describe special considerations in assessing pediatric, geriatric, disabled, and non-English-speaking patients.

● INITIAL SCENE ASSESSMENT

In any EMS response, needs and hazards that may endanger the rescuer or the patient must be assessed. For example, law enforcement, fire service, or back-up ambulances may be needed to provide additional man power. Other important elements that may affect scene safety, personal protection, and patient protection include environmental conditions (fire or the risk of fire, electrical hazards), the physical environment of the scene (terrain, vehicle, building), inclement weather (rain, snow, heat, cold), special equipment needs (self-contained breathing apparatus [SCBA], extrication, rescue), and the potential for hostile situations (perpetrators, unruly crowds).

KEY TERMS

auscultation: Listening for sounds within the body to evaluate the condition of the heart, lungs, pleura, intestines, or other organs or to detect fetal heart sound.

capillary refill test: A test used to evaluate the rate of blood flow through peripheral capillary beds.

crackles: Fine, bubbling sounds heard on auscultation of the lung; produced by air entering distal airways and alveoli that contain serous secretions.

inspection: Visual assessment of the patient and patient surroundings.

palpation: A technique used in physical examination in which the examiner feels the texture, size, consistency, and location of certain parts of the body with the hands.

rhonchi: Abnormal sounds heard on auscultation of a respiratory airway obstructed by thick secretions, muscular spasm, neoplasm, or external pressure.

wheezes: A form of rhonchus characterized by a high-pitched, musical quality; caused by high-velocity airflow through narrowed airways.

> **NOTE:**
> The Centers for Disease Control and the Occupational Safety and Health Administration have recommended that all health care workers wear gloves "when handling blood-soiled items, body fluids, excretions and secretions, as well as surfaces, materials, and objects exposed to them."[1] This text assumes that all emergency personnel are gloved during patient care activities. Personal protective measures are listed on the inside cover of this text and are further addressed in Chapter 24.

● PATIENT ASSESSMENT PRIORITIES

After determining that the scene is safe and that necessary resources are available or have been requested, the emergency team can begin patient assessment. See Fig. 11-1 for components of a patient assessment. Patient assessment entails the following six priorities[2]:

1. Primary survey: to recognize and manage all immediate life-threatening conditions
2. Resuscitation: to provide lifesaving intervention in critical patient conditions identified in the primary survey
3. Secondary survey: to obtain vital signs, reassess changes in the patient's condition, and perform appropriate physical examination
4. History: to determine the chief complaint, history of present illness or injury, and significant past medical history
5. Field management procedures: to prepare the patient for transportation to an appropriate medical facility, which includes communications with medical control
6. Reevaluation: to continue monitoring patient status en route and to provide treatment as necessary

● PRIMARY SURVEY

The primary survey (Box 11-1) is used for both trauma and medical patients to establish priorities of care based on potentially life-threatening conditions. The primary survey entails assessing the patient's level of consciousness. This is followed by the A-B-C-D-E steps of emergency care, in which the paramedic systematically evaluates the *airway* (and cervical spine immobilization), *breathing,* and *circulation* (including control of severe hemorrhage); assesses the patient for *disability* (a brief neurological examination); and *exposes the body for examination.*

Level of Consciousness

The first step with any patient is to assess the patient's level of consciousness. This can usually be accomplished by a cordial exchange with the patient (for example, "I'm a paramedic, how can I help you?") If the patient appears to be unconscious, gentle tactile stimulation along with questions such as "Are you okay?" and "Can you hear me?" may elicit a response.

Management

The next step is to assess the patient's airway. If the patient is unconscious or if spinal injury is suspected, the patient's cervical spine should be immobilized.

Airway

Assess the airway for patency by determining if the patient can speak, noting signs of airway obstruction or respiratory insufficiency (stridor, gurgling), and by inspecting the oral cavity for for-

> **BOX 11-1**
>
> ### Elements of the Primary Survey
>
> Level of consciousness (responsiveness)
> Airway (includes cervical spine immobilization)
> Breathing
> Circulation
> Disability (brief neurological examination)
> Expose

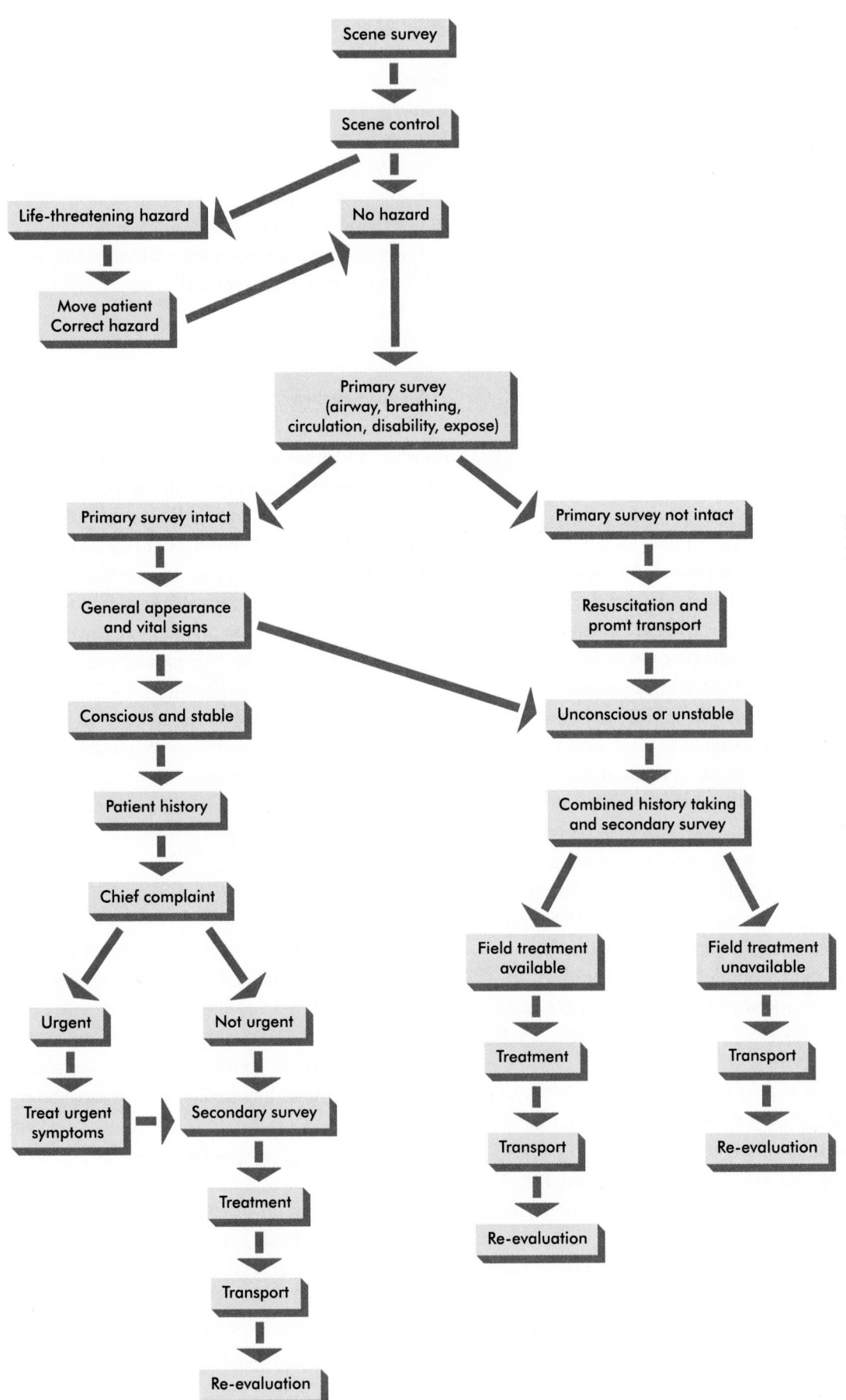

Fig. 11-1 Components of patient assessment.

eign objects. Any condition that compromises the delivery of oxygen to body tissues is potentially life threatening and must be managed immediately. Factors that may compromise the airway include the following:

- Tongue obstructing the airway in an unconscious patient
- Loose teeth or foreign objects in the patient's airway
- Epiglottitis
- Upper airway obstruction from any cause
- Facial and oral bleeding
- Vomitus
- Soft-tissue trauma to the patient's face and neck
- Facial fractures

Management

A compromised airway must be secured manually or with adjunct equipment (for example, using modified jaw thrust, chin lift, oral or nasal airways, suction, or endotracheal (ET) or esophageal intubation). In an airway procedure for patients who may have cervical spine injury, manipulation of the cervical spine should be minimal, and the head and neck should be stabilized in a neutral position. All patients must have an airway established and maintained in the primary survey.

Manage any patient whose airway is obstructed by a foreign object as currently recommended by the American Heart Association and the American Red Cross. If these maneuvers fail, medical control may recommend direct laryngoscopy or cricothyrotomy. The techniques for basic and advanced airway procedures are addressed in Chapter 12.

Breathing

The respiratory status of the patient is assessed by evaluating the rate, depth, and symmetry of chest movement. Expose the chest wall and palpate for structural integrity, tenderness, and crepitus. Observe for accessory respiratory use of the muscles of the neck, chest, and abdomen, and auscultate for the presence of bilateral breath sounds. Listen to the patient talk. A patient who has difficulty speaking without pain or who cannot talk

without gasping for air may need ventilatory support. Other respiratory abnormalities discoverable on physical examination that may indicate a potentially life-threatening condition include the following:

- Cyanosis
- Respiratory distress with dyspnea or hypoxia
- Asymmetrical chest wall movement
- Chest injury (tension pneumothorax, flail segment, open chest wound)
- Tracheal deviation
- Distended neck veins

Management

Ill or injured patients with ineffective respirations need ventilatory support supplemented with high-concentration oxygen. If the respiratory rate of a critically ill or injured patient is less than 10 or greater than 28 per minute, ventilations may require assistance. Assisted ventilations may be synchronized with the patient's respiratory efforts or interspersed as needed to maintain adequate oxygenation. Depending on the patient's condition, ET intubation may be indicated.

If respirations are absent, initiate rescue breathing followed by positive-pressure ventilation via bag-valve device or demand valve and ET intubation. Consider spinal precautions and barrier protection in all airway procedures.

Circulation

After airway and breathing, the patient's circulatory status is evaluated. For trauma patients, this includes a quick head-to-toe visual survey to note and control severe bleeding. Quickly assess the patient's skin color, moisture, and temperature. Evaluate the pulse for quality, rate, and regularity.

Pulse

A quick evaluation of the patient's pulse may reveal a normal heart rate of 60 to 80 beats per minute, a rapid heart rate (defined as tachycardia if greater than 100 beats per minute), a slow heart rate (defined as bradycardia if less than 60 beats per minute), or an irregular heart rate. The location of an obtainable pulse may also indicate the

TABLE 11-1 Pulse Site and Blood Pressure Estimates

Pulse Site	Estimated Minimal Systolic Blood Pressure
Radial	80 mm Hg
Femoral	70 mm Hg
Carotid	60 mm Hg

BOX 11-2

AVPU Scale of Level of Consciousness

A—Alert
V—Responds to verbal stimulus
P—Responds to painful stimulus
U—Unresponsive

patient's systolic blood pressure. If the carotid pulse is present but the radial pulse is not palpable, for example, it is generally believed that the systolic blood pressure is between 60 and 80 mm Hg. See Table 11-1 for pulse sites and corresponding blood pressure estimates.

Capillary Refill

Capillary filling time (the **capillary refill test**) may also provide information about the patient's cardiovascular status. This test is performed by blanching the patient's nail bed or the fleshy eminence at the base of the thumb and observing how long it takes for normal color to return. A filling time greater than 2 seconds caused by shunting and capillary closure to peripheral capillary beds indicates inadequate circulation and impaired cardiovascular function. Note that capillary filling time may be affected by the patient's age, gender, and environmental factors and should only be used as a possible indicator of circulatory status. Other signs and symptoms include:

- Altered or decreased level of consciousness
- Distended neck veins
- Pale, cool, diaphoretic skin
- Distant heart sounds
- Restlessness
- Thirst

Management

When an unconscious person lacks a carotid pulse, chest compressions and cardiac arrest protocols should be implemented. In cases of severe external hemorrhage, control the bleeding with direct pressure, elevation, and use of pressure points. In most cases, these procedures stabilize the patient during transportation. Regardless of the cause, all patients with circulatory compromise need rapid stabilization, which may include intravenous (IV) fluids, other medications, and transportation to an appropriate medical facility.

Disability

The brief neurological examination is used to determine a baseline level of consciousness and discuss any obvious central nervous system (CNS) dysfunction. The patient's level of consciousness can be quickly assessed by using the mnemonic evaluation *AVPU* (Box 11-2).

Many EMS services classify the patient as being alert and oriented to person, place, and date or time of day. A patient who is aware of his or her name, location, and the date or time is said to be *alert and oriented times three*. A patient who is confused or unsure of his or her name or surroundings is said to be *disoriented*. Change in level of consciousness is a very important indicator of CNS dysfunction. Altered levels of consciousness may be associated with traumatic injury and numerous medical conditions, such as hypoxia, hypoglycemia, shock, and drug misuse or abuse.

Evaluate the patient's ability to understand and respond appropriately to verbal commands. A patient who is able to move a particular body part when requested, for example, demonstrates a level of consciousness that is important when documenting baseline data. The patient's ability to respond to painful stimulus with purposeful movement should also be documented. Providing these baseline evaluations helps others involved in the patient's care to determine whether the patient's status is improving or deteriorating. Avoid vague terms such as *stuporous, obtunded,* and *semiconscious* when describing the patient's mental status. Describing the patient's reactions and verbal and motor responses is better patient information.

Management

A patient who has an abnormal disability evaluation or suspected neurological trauma, as indicated by the mechanism of injury, should receive a rigid cervical collar and full spinal immobilization (see Chapter 15). Head and spinal injuries cannot be adequately assessed in the prehospital setting and require physician evaluation.

Exposing and Examining

Exposing the patient's body surfaces is important in caring for the critically ill or injured. In the medical patient, removing clothing may reveal medical alert tags, implanted pacemakers, edematous tissue, and other significant findings. For the trauma patient, exposing body surfaces may reveal injured areas that would otherwise go unnoticed. Examples include fractures, gunshot wounds, and stab wounds that may be covered by heavy clothing. Remove restrictive clothing that might impair patient movement, respirations, or distal circulation.

Management

During the "expose and examine" phase of the primary survey, carefully maintain the patient's body temperature by covering him or her with a blanket or sheet after each body region is examined. If the patient is lying on pavement or ground, place a blanket underneath him or her. Exposing body surfaces may embarrass some patients or cause them to be ill at ease. Respect the patient's right to privacy and remove only enough clothing to determine the presence or absence of a condition or injury.

● RESUSCITATION

The resuscitation phase of patient assessment is done simultaneously with the primary survey.

The paramedic begins resuscitative measures such as airway maintenance, ventilatory assistance, and cardiopulmonary resuscitation (CPR) immediately after recognizing the life-threatening condition that necessitates each respective maneuver.

A number of emergency care procedures are generally initiated in situations involving seriously ill or injured patients. Nearly all medical and trauma patients, for example, need some form of supplemental oxygen. Other resuscitation procedures for medical and trauma patients are listed below:

Resuscitation Procedures for Medical Patients
- Oxygen and airway control
- Inserting an IV lifeline to administer drugs or volume-expanding fluid
- Taking blood samples for laboratory analysis (for example, blood glucose levels)
- Administering resuscitation medications
- Applying a pneumatic antishock garment (PASG) if appropriate
- Administering electrical therapy (defibrillation, cardioversion, external pacing)

Resuscitation Procedures for Trauma Patients
- Oxygen and airway control
- Cervical spine immobilization
- Inserting IV lifelines for volume-expanding fluid
- Administering resuscitation medications
- Applying a PASG, if appropriate

Care of Medical versus Trauma Patients

Much of the definitive care for medical patients can be initiated in the prehospital setting. For some cardiac patients and patients with respiratory difficulties and other medical emergencies, appropriate care can be instituted by paramedic crews. With medical patients, then, the scene time may be longer.

In contrast, most trauma patients can receive definitive care only when rapidly stabilized and transported to an appropriate medical facility. Patients with internal bleeding, major fractures, head injury, and multiple-systems trauma need lifesaving care that can only be provided by specially trained physicians and support staff. Minimal time should be spent at the scene with these patients. Emergencies that require immediate transport to an appropriate medical facility include the following:

- Airway obstruction that cannot be quickly relieved
- Trauma-related cardiorespiratory arrest
- Massive hemothorax
- Tension pneumothorax
- Pericardial tamponade
- Penetrating wounds of the chest or the abdomen
- Head injury with rapidly deteriorating neurological status

Most trauma life-support training programs recommend that patients requiring immediate transport be stabilized and packaged within 10 minutes after EMS arrival. Field management should be limited to airway control, spinal immobilization, and major fracture stabilization. IV fluid therapy, if initiated, should be done en route to the hospital. (Trauma management is further addressed in Chapter 15.)

● SECONDARY SURVEY

After the primary survey and management of life-threatening situations, the patient is assessed more thoroughly. This assessment may reveal potentially dangerous patient conditions that were not recognized initially. The secondary survey includes assessment of vital signs and a systematic head-to-toe examination using a "look, listen, feel, and smell" approach. Depending on the patient's condition, the secondary survey may be done at the scene or en route to the hospital. Note that the purpose of the secondary survey is to discover medical conditions or injuries that are not immediately life threatening but may become so if left untreated.

Vital Sign Assessment

Determining the presence of vital signs is part of the primary survey; vital signs are usually evaluated as the first step of the secondary survey. Vital signs are generally considered to include the following five parameters:

1. *Pulse:* A normal resting pulse rate is usually between 60 and 80 beats per minute; it may be affected by the patient's age and physical condition. A child's pulse rate may be 80 to 100 beats per minute, for example, and a well-trained athlete's pulse rate may be 50 to 60 beats per minute. Factors such as pregnancy, anxiety, and fear may also produce a higher-than-normal pulse rate in healthy individuals.

Pulse rates may be obtained at the carotid artery in the neck or at any pulse site where the artery lies close to the skin surface. To evaluate the radial pulse, the pads of the examiner's index and middle fingers are placed at the distal end of the patient's wrist, just medial to the radius. If pulsations are regular, they should be counted for 15 seconds and multiplied by 4 to determine the number of beats per minute. In addition to the number of times the heart beats per minute, the *regularity* and *strength* of the pulse should be assessed. For example, the pulse can be characterized as regular or irregular or weak or strong. Application of an electrocardiographic (ECG) monitor may also be useful in evaluating cardiovascular status after initial assessment of the pulse.

2. *Blood pressure:* The systolic blood pressure is the reading that identifies the amount of pressure exerted against the arterial walls when the heart contracts. Diastolic pressure reflects the amount of pressure exerted against the arterial walls during relaxation of the heart. Normal systolic blood pressure is considered to be 100 plus the patient's age up to 140 mm Hg (minus 8 to 10 mm Hg for women and children). Normal diastolic pressure should be between 65 and 90 mm Hg.

Blood pressure is best measured by auscultation. Place the sphygmomanometer on the patient's arm with the lower end of the cuff positioned 1 to 2 inches above the antecubital space. Inflate the cuff to a point approximately 30 mm Hg above where the brachial pulse can no longer be palpated. Place the stethoscope over the brachial artery and slowly deflate the cuff at a rate of 2 to 3 mm Hg per second. As the pressure falls, observe the gauge and note where the first sound or pulsation is heard. This is the patient's systolic pressure. As the cuff continues to deflate, note at what point the sounds change in quality or become muffled. This reading is the patient's diastolic pressure.

> **NOTE:**
> Determining accurate diastolic pressure is sometimes difficult. The difference between the point of muffled tones and the complete disappearance of pulsations varies by individual. In some persons the difference is a few mm Hg; at the opposite end of the range are people whose pulsations never totally disappear. The ability to measure accurate diastolic pressures develops from experience and requires careful listening in a quiet environment.

Blood pressure may be estimated by palpation when vascular sounds are difficult to hear with a stethoscope because of environmental noise, but this method is less accurate than measuring blood pressure by auscultation. To estimate blood pressure by palpation, locate the brachial or radial pulse and apply the sphygmomanometer as previously described. Maintain finger contact at the pulse location as the cuff slowly deflates. When the pulse becomes palpable, observe the gauge and record the systolic blood pressure. As the cuff continues to deflate, observe the gauge to note where the pulse changes from bounding to weak.

Sphygmomanometers are available in a number of sizes. Adult widths should be one third to one half the circumference of the limb. For children, the width should cover approximately two thirds of the upper arm or thigh. As a rule, blood pressure cuffs that are too wide give a false low reading, and cuffs that are too narrow give a false high reading. Like pulse rates, a patient's blood pressure may be unusually high because of fear or anxiety. Other factors, such as a patient's age and normal level of physical activity, may be responsible for unusual blood pressure readings.

3. *Respirations:* The normal respiratory rate for adults is between 12 and 20 breaths per minute. (See Table 11-2 for average vital signs by age.) The respiratory rate is obtained by watching the patient breathe, feeling for chest movement, or by auscultating. Count the patient's respirations for 30 seconds and multiply by two to determine breaths per minute. Assess the rhythm and depth of respirations through visualization and auscul-

tation of the thorax. Abnormal findings include shallow, rapid, noisy, or deep breathing; asymmetrical chest wall movement; accessory respiratory muscle involvement; or congested, unequal, or diminished breath sounds.

4. *Skin:* Skin color, temperature, and moisture provide additional information on the patient's status. The patient's skin color may of course be normal. Red indicates heat-related illness or injury, fever, vasodilation, or possible carbon monoxide poisoning (a late finding). Yellow or jaundice indicates liver dysfunction. Pale skin indicates vasoconstriction, which may result from hemodynamic abnormalities, fright, and cold-related illness or injury. Blue, or *cyanotic*, skin indicates poor tissue oxygenation. Mottled skin may indicate an allergic reaction, vascular compromise to an extremity, or clinical death.

In darkly pigmented patients, assess skin color by noting the color of the mucous membranes of the mouth and by examining the fingernail beds for color changes. When evaluating the patient's skin, be alert to the presence of abnormal findings such as ulcers, rashes, or lesions that would suggest systemic illness or possible allergic reactions.

Skin temperature may be normal (warm), hot, or cold. Skin that is hot to the touch indicates a possible fever or heat-related illness or injury. Cold skin may indicate decreased tissue perfusion and cold-related illness or injury. The dorsal surface of the hand is more sensitive than the palmar surface and should be used to estimate body temperature. Body temperature can be measured more accurately by applying plastic heat-sensitive tape to the patient's skin or by using standard mercury

TABLE 11-2 Average Vital Signs by Age			
Age	**Pulse**	**Respirations**	**Blood Pressure**
Newborn	120-160	40-60	80/40
1 year	80-140	30-40	82/44
3 years	80-120	25-30	86/50
5 years	70-115	20-25	90/52
7 years	70-115	20-25	94/54
10 years	70-115	15-20	100/60
15 years	70-90	15-20	110/64
Adult	60-80	12-20	120/80

clinical thermometers, electronic thermometers, or tympanic membrane thermometers. Evaluations of body temperature may have specific applications in emergencies, such as febrile seizures and hyperthermic and hypothermic emergencies.

When a standard thermometer is used, a patient's body temperature may be evaluated by oral, axillary, or rectal means. (Rectal readings provide the most accurate assessment, but rectal tissue is easily damaged, and this route is often impractical for prehospital use). Temperature readings are obtained by placing the thermometer under the conscious patient's tongue for 4 to 6 minutes, under the patient's armpit for 10 minutes, or in the patient's rectum for 5 to 8 minutes. Normal body temperature is 37° C (98.6° F). Standard clinical thermometers record body temperatures from 34.4° C (94° F) to 40° C (106° F).

Skin moisture is usually classified as dry (normal) or wet (clammy or diaphoretic). Diaphoretic skin may indicate a hemodynamic deficit, such as hypovolemia, or another illness or injury that results in decreased tissue perfusion or increased sweat gland activity. Examples are cardiovascular and heat-related emergencies, respectively.

5. Pupils: Examining the pupils for response to light may yield information on the neurological status of some patients. Normally, the pupils are equal and constrict when exposed to light. (The acronym *PERRL* indicates that the *p*upils are *e*qual, *r*ound, and *r*eact to *l*ight.) When testing the pupils for light response, shine a penlight directly into one eye. The normal reaction is for the pupil exposed to the light to constrict with a consensual constriction of the opposite eye. Abnormal pupillary reactions and possible causes are given in Table 11-3.

The Head-To-Toe Survey

The head-to-toe examination should be systematic and organized by body region. Focus the examination on patient conditions that are manageable in the prehospital setting, and always be alert to findings that may alter priorities in patient care activities.

The physical examination requires many special skills, including a thorough understanding of the

TABLE 11-3 Abnormal Pupil Reactions

Pupil Size	Possible Causes
Equal Dilated or unresponsive	Cardiac arrest, CNS injury, hypoxia or anoxia, drug use (LSD, atropine, amphetamines)
Constricted or unresponsive	CNS injury or disease, narcotic drug use (heroin, morphine), eye medications
Unequal One dilated or unresponsive	Cerebrovascular accident (CVA), head injury, direct trauma to the eye, eye medications

human body, an aptitude for personal communication and compassion, and the ability to perform a hands-on assessment of the patient. These skills are obtained through experience and exposure to many patient care situations. Each patient contact should be viewed as a learning experience that can enhance clinical assessment skills.

Examination Techniques

The examination techniques commonly used in patient assessment are inspection, palpation, and auscultation. These terms are referred to frequently throughout this text as they relate to the evaluation of specific body systems. Depending on the situation, these examination techniques may be the sole method available for patient evaluation (for example, assessment of an unconscious trauma patient) or may be integrated with history taking and other patient care procedures. If time permits, explain each examination technique to the patient before initiating it.

Inspection

Inspection is visual assessment of the patient and the surroundings, which may alert the EMS crew to the patient's mental status and possible injury or underlying illness. For example, patient hygiene, clothing, eye gaze, body language, body position, skin color, and odor may be significant. If the emergency response was to the patient's home, be alert to findings such as cleanliness, prescription medicines, illegal drug paraphernalia,

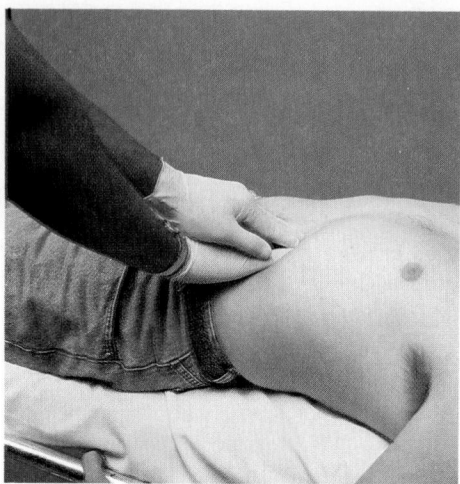

Fig. 11-2 Deep bimanual palpation.

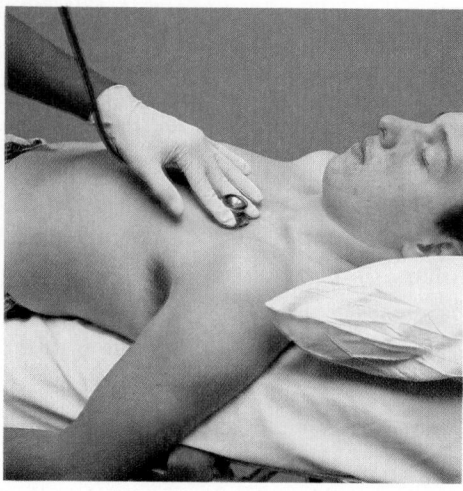

Fig. 11-3 Position of the stethoscope between the index and middle fingers.

and signs of alcohol use. These and other observations may play an important role in determining emergency patient care activities.

Palpation

Palpation is a technique in which the examiner uses the hands and fingers to gather information by touch. Generally, the palmar surface of the fingers and finger pads are used to palpate for texture, masses, fluid, and crepitus (Fig. 11-2). Palpation may either be superficial or deep; the applications for each are addressed throughout this text. Examining a patient by palpation is a form of invasion of the patient's body, so the approach should be gentle and initiated with respect.

Auscultation

Auscultation requires the use of a stethoscope and is employed to assess body sounds produced by the movement of various fluids or gases in the patient's organs or tissues. Perform this examination technique in a relatively quiet environment where attention can be focused on each body sound being assessed. Isolate a particular area to note characteristics of intensity, pitch, duration, and quality. In the prehospital setting, auscultation is usually performed to assess blood pressure and evaluate breath sounds, heart sounds, and bowel sounds.

To auscultate, press the diaphragm of the stethoscope firmly against the patient's skin for stabilization (Fig. 11-3). If a bell endpiece is used, position it lightly on the body surface, making sure that there is skin contact around the entire edge of the bell. This prevents the damping of vibrations.

NOTE:

Any patient examination must be tailored to the presenting situation and available subjective data. A medical patient who is conscious and complaining of abdominal pain, for example, would not be expected to have a cervical spine injury or cerebral spinal fluid in the ears or nose, so minimal assessment of the patient's head would be performed. In contrast, in evaluating a trauma patient involved in a motor vehicle crash, head and spine assessment would be much more extensive. The following descriptions of body region examinations are intended to provide a foundation for *general* techniques in patient assessment. Examination techniques specific to a particular injury or illness are addressed throughout this text by subject matter.

● PATIENT ASSESSMENT

The Head and Neck

To examine the head, inspect the skull for shape and symmetry, keeping in mind that hair can hide abnormalities. Perform a systematic palpation, moving from front to back, noting any swelling, tenderness, indentations, or depressions. (Take care when palpating over any abnormal findings.) The scalp should move freely over the skull, and the patient should not complain of pain or discomfort during the examination. Inspect the facial area for symmetry. The cavities of the facial skull include the eyes, ears, nose, and mouth.

Examining the Eyes

Verify that both eyes can see by soliciting the patient's history regarding visual disturbances or by asking the patient to demonstrate visual acuity (for example, counting fingers with one eye closed). Observe the orbital area for edema and puffiness. The scleras should be white and may be observed by gently pulling the lower eyelids down. The cornea and the iris should be clearly visible, and the pupils should be of equal size, round, and reactive to light. Both eyes should move equally well in all four directions (up, down, right, left). Palpate the lower orbital rim to determine structural integrity; be alert to the presence of contact lenses and ocular prostheses.

Examining the Ears

Inspect the external ear and surrounding tissues for signs of bruising, deformity, or discoloration. There should be no discharge from either ear canal. Pulling gently on the ear lobes (lobules) should not produce pain or discomfort. Palpate the skull and facial bones surrounding the ear for tenderness and swelling. An alert, hearing patient who speaks the same language as the paramedic should be able to respond to questions without excessive requests for repetition. Be alert to the presence of hearing-aid devices.

Examining the Nose

Inspect the patient's nose for shape, size, color, and stability. The column of the nose should be midline with the face, and the nares should be symmetrically positioned. Palpate the column of the nose and surrounding soft tissues for pain, tenderness, or deformity. The frontal and maxillary sinuses may be inspected for the presence of swelling and palpated for tenderness along the bony brow on each side of the nose and the zygomatic processes.

Discharge from the nose can have a number of causes. For example, cerebral spinal fluid may be present as a result of head trauma; a bloody discharge (epistaxis) may result from trauma, mucosal erosions involving blood vessels, hypertension, or bleeding disorders; and a mucous discharge commonly results from allergy, upper respiratory tract infection, or cold exposure. Describe and document any discharge on the prehospital care report.

Examining the Mouth

Inspect the lips for symmetry, color, edema, and skin surface irregularities. The lips should be pink. Pallor of the lips is associated with anemia; cyanosis is associated with cardiorespiratory insufficiency; red is occasionally a late finding in carbon monoxide poisoning. There should be no swelling, deformity, or pain on palpation.

Healthy gums in the oral cavity are pink and free of lesions and swelling. Patchy areas of pigmentation in the mouths of African Americans are not uncommon. Enlarged gums may indicate pregnancy, leukemia, poor oral hygiene, puberty, or use of some medications (for example, phenytoin [Dilantin]), a commonly prescribed drug for patients with seizure disorders.) The mouth should be free of loose or broken teeth. (Dental emergencies are further addressed in Chapter 15.) Be alert to the presence of dental appliances.

Inspect the tongue for size and color. It should be positioned in the midline of the oral cavity and appear nonswollen, dull red, moist, and glistening. When inspecting the oropharynx, use a tongue blade to depress the tongue. If the area is reddened or covered with exudate, an infection may be present. Be alert for the presence of breath odors that may indicate alcohol or drug consumption or illness such as diabetes mellitus.

Examining the Neck

Inspect the neck in the patient's normal anatomical position. If trauma is suspected, use spinal precautions. The trachea should be midline, and there should be no use of accessory muscles or tracheal tugging during respirations. To palpate the neck, place both thumbs along the sides of the distal trachea and systematically move toward the head (Fig. 11-4). Care should be taken not to apply bilateral pressure to the carotid arteries.

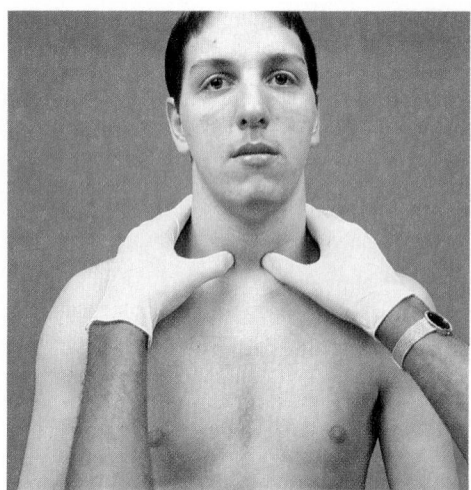

Fig. 11-4 Position of the thumbs to evaluate the midline position of the trachea.

The thyroid and cricoid cartilages should be nontender and move when the patient swallows. Bubbling or crackling sensations that can be palpated in the soft tissues of the neck may indicate the presence of subcutaneous emphysema. Distended neck veins or prominent carotid arteries should be noted.

The Thorax

A thorough knowledge of the structure of the thoracic cage is required to perform an adequate respiratory and cardiac assessment. In addition to protecting the vital organs within the thorax, the ribs provide support for respiratory movements of the diaphragm and intercostal muscles. A loss of thoracic structural integrity (for example, a flail segment) prevents or limits respiratory function. The ribs of the thorax are also used as anatomical landmarks in locating specific areas for examination. Fig. 11-5 shows the topographical landmarks of the chest.

The thoracic cage is composed of 12 pairs of ribs, the sternum, and the 12 thoracic vertebrae. The superior 7 ribs (true ribs) articulate with the thoracic vertebrae and attach directly to the sternum by their costal cartilages. Ribs 8, 9, and 10 (false ribs) do not attach directly to the sternum

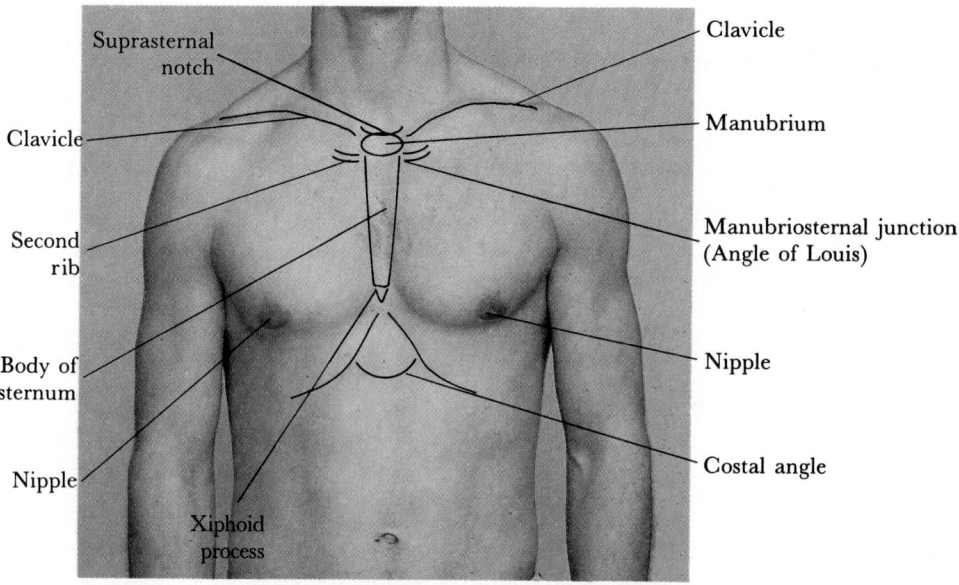

Fig. 11-5 Topographical landmarks of the chest.

but are joined to common cartilage attached to the sternum. Ribs 11 and 12 (floating ribs) have no attachment to the sternum.

The sternum is approximately 7.78 cm long and is divided into three parts: the manubrium, the body, and the xiphoid process. The superior margin of the manubrium has a jugular notch (suprasternal notch) that can easily be felt at the anterior base of the neck. The sternal angle (manubriosternal junction) is the point at which the manubrium joins the body of the sternum and is also the location of the second rib. When examining the thorax, use the sternal angle as a starting point for counting other ribs.

The thorax can be evaluated by using imaginary lines to focus on physical examination findings (Fig. 11-6).

Inspection

Inspect the chest wall for symmetry on both the anterior and posterior surfaces. Although the thorax is not completely symmetrical, a visual inspection of one side should offer a reasonable comparison for the other. Chest wall diameter is often increased in patients with obstructive pulmonary disease, resulting in a barrel-shaped appearance of the thorax. Inspect the skin and nipples for cyanosis and pallor, and be alert to the presence of

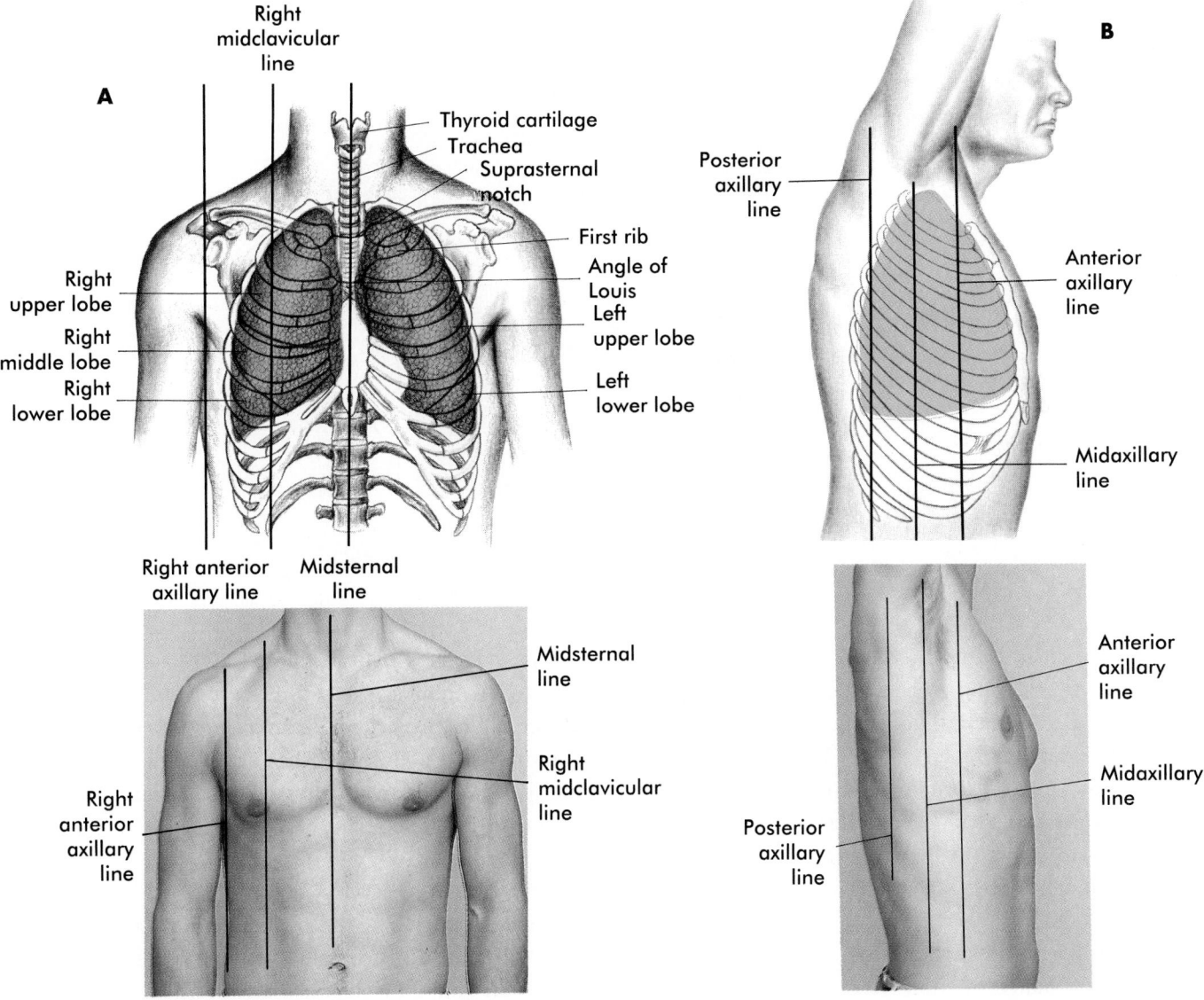

Fig. 11-6 Thoracic landmarks. **A,** Anterior thorax. **B,** Right lateral thorax. *Continued.*

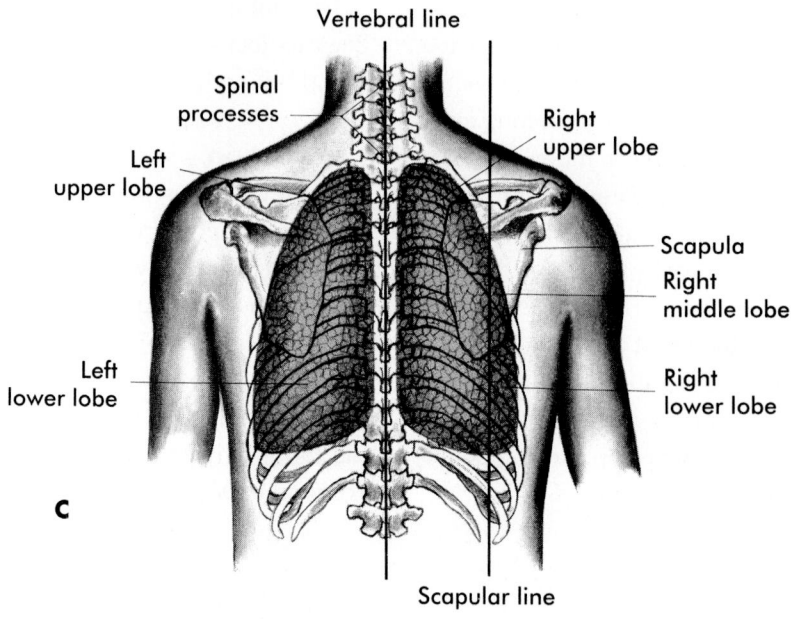

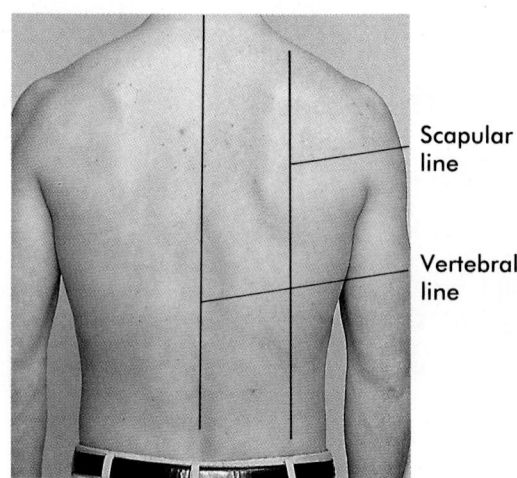

Fig. 11-6, cont'd **C,** Posterior thorax.

suture lines from chest wall surgery and skin pockets enclosing implanted pacemaker devices or implanted central venous lines.

Evaluate respiratory status by inspection, palpation, and auscultation. Note the pattern or rhythm of respirations and observe for use of accessory respiratory muscles (for example, intercostal or supraclavicular retractions, or both).

Patterns of Respiration
A normal respiratory rate for an adult is between 12 and 20 breaths per minute. The breath-

ing process should be comfortable, regular, and initiated without distress. Any variations should be noted; they may help determine appropriate intervention. Box 11-3 describes abnormal respiratory patterns that may help evaluate ill or injured patients (Fig. 11-7).

Palpation
Palpate the thorax for pulsations, tenderness, bulges, depressions, crepitus, subcutaneous emphysema, and unusual movement and position. Begin the examination by noting the position of

BOX 11-3

Abnormal Respiratory Patterns

Ataxic: A type of cluster or irregular breathing pattern characterized by a series of inspirations and expirations. Ataxic respiration is usually associated with a structural or compressive lesion in the medullary respiratory centers.

Biot's: A respiratory pattern involving irregular respirations varying in depth and interrupted by intervals of apnea (absence of breathing). Although similar to Cheyne-Stokes, this pattern lacks the repetitiveness and is often irregular. Biot's respiration is usually seen in patients with head injuries who have increased intracranial pressure. Unlike Cheyne-Stokes, Biot's ataxic pattern frequently produces ventilatory failure and may lead to apnea.

Bradypnea: A persistent respiratory rate slower than 12 breaths per minute. This abnormal rate may be a result of the patient "guarding" against respiratory discomfort caused by chest wall injury, respiratory failure, CVA, pulmonary infection, or narcotic poisoning. However, bradypnea is more commonly caused by respiratory drive depression secondary to neurological disturbances.

Cheyne-Stokes: A regular, periodic pattern of breathing with equal intervals of apnea followed by a crescendo-decrescendo sequence of respirations. Cheyne-Stokes respirations are thought to represent a level of cortical dysfunction of the brain. Although some children and older adults breathe in this pattern during sleep, it is usually seen in patients who are seriously ill or injured.

Hyperventilation: A persistent, rapid, and deep respiration that often results in hyperpnea. Compared with tachypnea, hyperpnea is usually slower and much deeper. It causes include exercise, anxiety, metabolic disturbances (such as diabetic ketoacidosis), and CNS illness.

Kussmaul: An abnormally deep, very rapid sighing respiratory pattern characteristic of diabetic ketoacidosis or other metabolic acidosis.

Tachypnea: A persistent respiratory rate that exceeds 20 breaths per minute. It may be common in patients who are in pain, frightened, or anxious. There are many other causes of tachypnea, including fractured ribs, pneumonia, pneumothorax, pulmonary embolus, and pleurisy.

---

the trachea, which should be midline and directly above the sternal notch. Starting with the patient's clavicles, firmly palpate both sides of the patient's chest wall simultaneously—front to back and right side to left side. The examination should proceed systematically, without pain or discomfort.

To evaluate the anterior chest wall for equal expansion during inspiration, place both thumbs along the patient's costal margin and the xiphoid process, with palms lying flat on the chest wall. Equal movement should be noted as the patient inhales and exhales. To evaluate the posterior chest wall for symmetrical respiratory movement, the thumbs are placed along the spinous processes at the level of the tenth rib (Fig. 11-8).

Auscultation

The thorax is best auscultated with the patient sitting upright (if possible) and breathing deeply and slowly through an open mouth during the examination. Be alert to the possibility of resulting hyperventilation and fatigue, which may occur in ill and older patients.

Use the diaphragm of the stethoscope to auscultate the high-pitched sounds of the patient's chest wall. Hold the stethoscope firmly on the patient's skin and listen carefully as the patient inhales and exhales. The chest auscultation should be systematic as well as thorough, evaluating both the anterior and the posterior lung fields (Fig. 11-9).

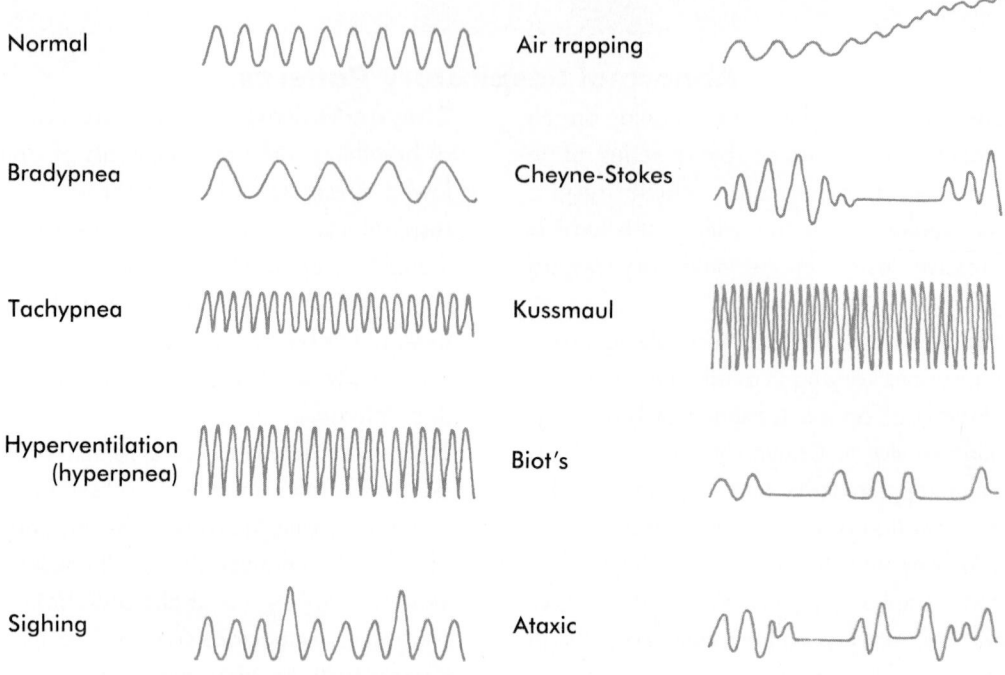

Normal

Bradypnea

Tachypnea

Hyperventilation (hyperpnea)

Sighing

Air trapping

Cheyne-Stokes

Kussmaul

Biot's

Ataxic

Some influences on the rate and depth of breathing
The rate and depth of breathing will

Increase with
Acidosis
  (metabolic)
Anxiety
Aspirin poisoning
Oxygen need
  (hypoxemia)
Pain
Central nervous system
  lesions (pons)

Decrease with
Alkalosis
  (metabolic)
Central nervous system
  lesions (cerebrum)
Myasthenia gravis
Narcotic overdoses
Obesity (extreme)

Fig. 11-7 Patterns of respiration. Horizontal axis indicates relative rate; vertical swings indicate relative depth.

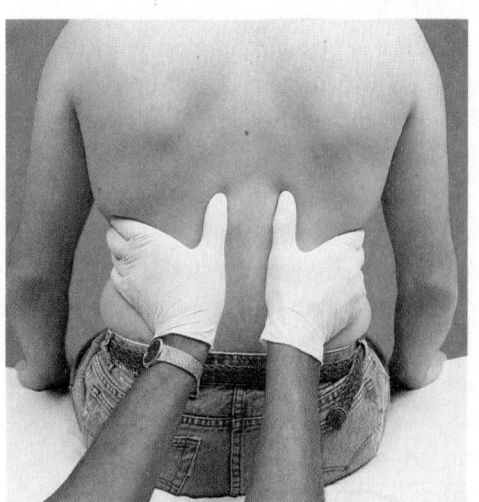

Fig. 11-8 Palpating the thoracic expansion. The thumbs are at the level of the tenth ribs.

Breath Sounds

Air movement creates turbulence as it passes through the respiratory tree and produces breath sounds during inhalation and exhalation. During inhalation, air moves first into the trachea and major bronchi and then into progressively smaller airways to its final destination, the alveoli. During exhalation, the air flows from small airways to larger ones, which creates less turbulence. Therefore normal breath sounds are generally louder during inspiration.

Normal Breath Sounds

Normal breath sounds are classified as vesicular, bronchovesicular, and bronchial. Vesicular breath sounds are heard over most of the lung

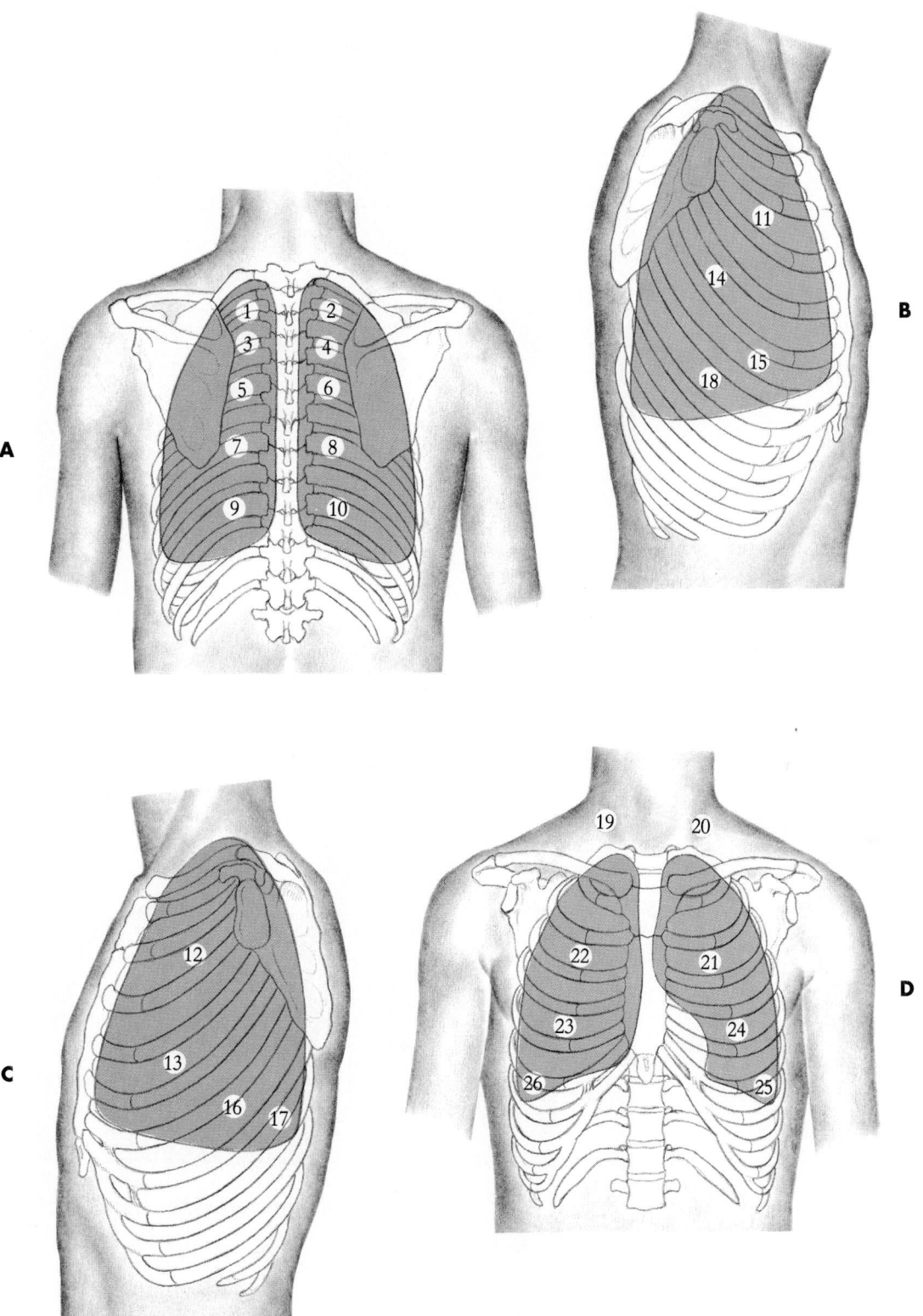

Fig. 11-9 Suggested sequence for systematic auscultation of the thorax. **A,** Posterior thorax. **B,** Right lateral thorax. **C,** Left lateral thorax. **D,** Anterior thorax.

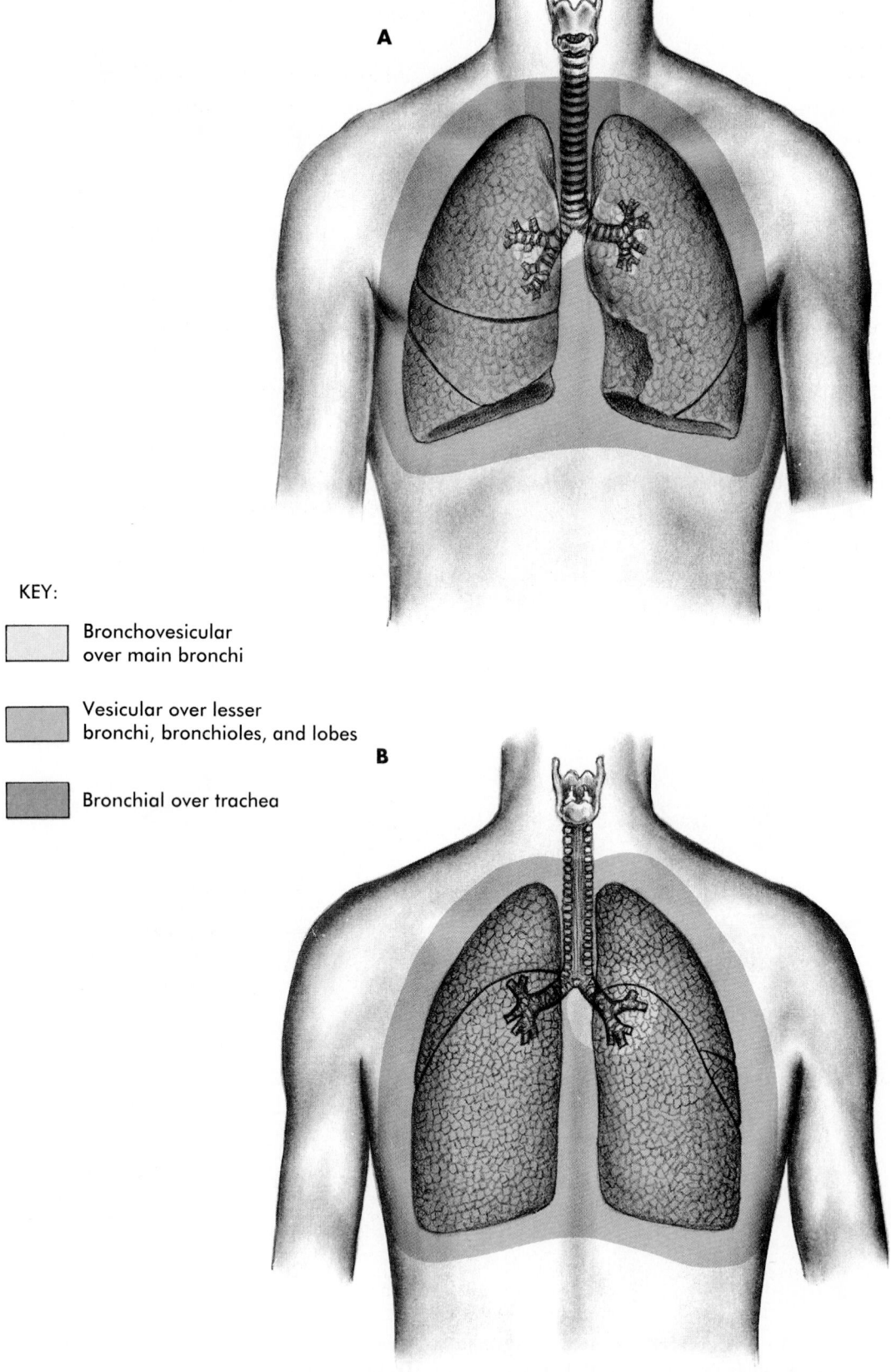

KEY:

■ Bronchovesicular over main bronchi

■ Vesicular over lesser bronchi, bronchioles, and lobes

■ Bronchial over trachea

Fig. 11-10 Normal auscultatory sounds on the anterior (**A**) and posterior (**B**) chest wall.

fields and are the major normal breath sound. Lungs considered "clear" make normal vesicular breath sounds. These sounds are low pitched and soft and have a long inspiratory phase and a shorter expiratory phase (Fig. 11-10).

Vesicular breath sounds are further classified as harsh or diminished. Harsh vesicular sounds may result from vigorous exercise in which ventilations are rapid and deep. They also occur in children who have thin and elastic chest walls in which breath sounds are more easily audible. Vesicular breath sounds may be diminished in older people, who have less ventilation volume, and in obese or very muscular persons whose additional overlying tissue muffles the sound.

Bronchovesicular breath sounds are heard over the major bronchi and over the upper right posterior lung field. They are louder and harsher than vesicular breath sounds and are considered to be of medium pitch. Bronchovesicular breath sounds have equal inspiration and expiration phases and are heard throughout respiration.

Bronchial breath sounds are heard only over the trachea and are the highest in pitch. They are coarse, harsh, loud sounds with a short inspiratory phase and a long expiration. A bronchial sound heard anywhere but over the trachea is considered an abnormal breath sound.

Abnormal Breath Sounds

Abnormal breath sounds are classified as absent, diminished, and incorrectly located bronchial sounds and adventitious breath sounds. (See Fig. 11-11 for a schema of breath sounds.) Absent breath sounds may indicate total cessation of the breathing process (for example, complete airway obstruction), or they may only be absent in a specific area. Causes of localized absent breath sounds include endotracheal tube misplacement, pneumothorax, and hemothorax.

Diminished breath sounds may result from any condition that lessens the airflow. Examples include ET tube misplacement, pneumothorax, partial airway obstruction, and pulmonary disease. Although some airflow is present, diminished breath sounds usually indicate that some portion of the alveolar tissue is not being ventilated.

Bronchial breath sounds auscultated in the peripheral lung field indicate the presence of fluid

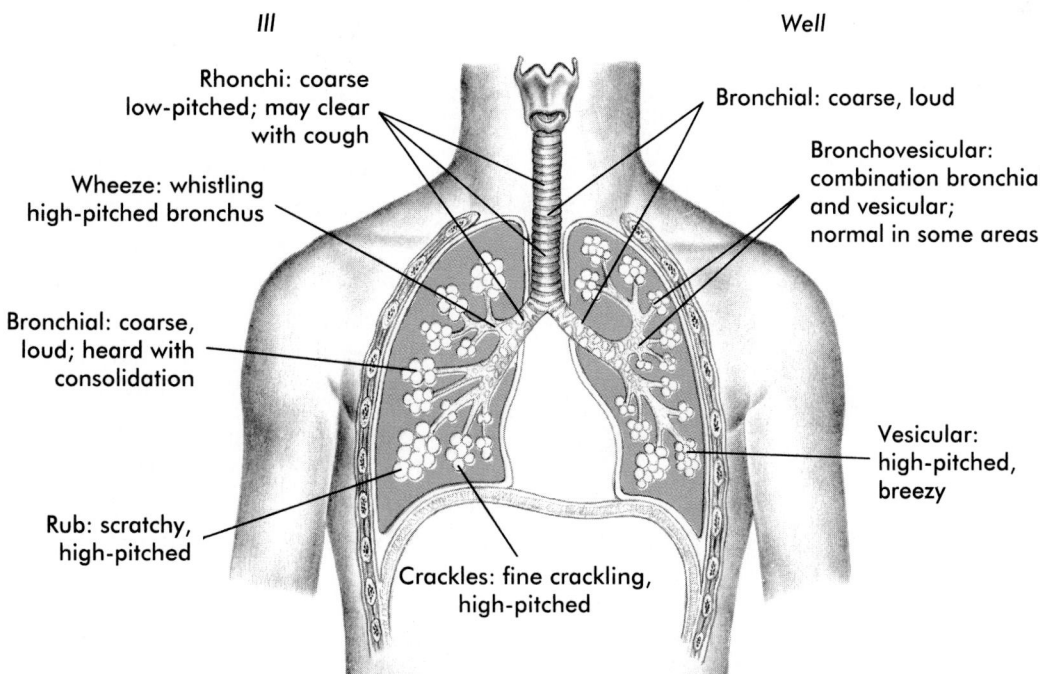

Fig. 11-11 Schema of breath sounds in ill and well patients.

or exudate in the alveoli, either of which may block airflow. Diseases that contribute to this condition are tumors, pneumonia, and pulmonary edema.

Adventitious Breath Sounds

Adventitious breath sounds are abnormal sounds that are heard in addition to normal breath sounds. They may be divided into two categories: discontinuous and continuous, based on acoustical recordings and lung sound analysis. Adventitious breath sounds result from obstruction of either the large or small airways and are most commonly heard during inspiration. Adventitious breath sounds are classified as **crackles** (formerly known as *rales*), **wheezes,** and **rhonchi** (Fig. 11-12).

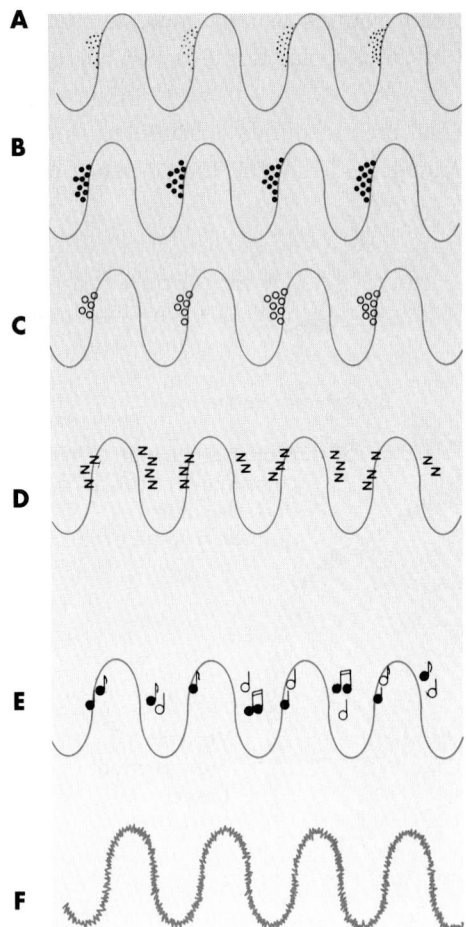

Fig. 11-12 Adventitious breath sounds. **A**, Fine crackles. **B**, Medium crackles. **C**, Coarse crackles. **D**, Rhonchi. **E**, Wheeze. **F**, Pleural friction rub.

Discontinuous Breath Sounds

Crackles are the high-pitched, discontinuous sounds (similar to the sound of hair being rubbed between the fingers) that are usually heard during the end of inspiration. They indicate disease of the small airways, alveoli, or both and may be heard anywhere in the peripheral lung field. There is some debate about the etiology of crackles. Some experts believe that the alveoli become filled with fluid, mucus, or pus and tend to close on expiration. With inspiration, the air forces the alveoli open again, producing a "popping" sound. Others contend that the popping sound is produced by air movement through the fluid.

The most typical causes of crackles are pulmonary edema and pneumonia in its early stages. Because gravity draws fluid downward, they often start in the bases of the lungs. Crackles may be further classified as coarse crackles (wet, low-pitched sounds) and fine crackles (dry, high-pitched sounds). Crackles are discrete and sometimes difficult to hear and may be overridden by louder respiratory sounds. If crackles are suspected when auscultating the chest, ask the patient to cough. A cough may clear secretions and make crackles more easily audible.

Continuous Breath Sounds

Wheezes (also known as *sibilant wheezes*) are high-pitched, "musical" noises that are usually louder during expiration. They are caused by high-velocity air traveling through narrowed airways and may occur because of asthma and other constrictive diseases as well as congestive heart failure. When wheezing occurs in a localized area, a foreign body obstruction, tumor, or mucous plug should be suspected. Wheezes are classified as mild, moderate, and severe and should be described as occurring on inspiration, expiration, or both.

Rhonchi (also known as *sonorous wheezes*) are continuous, low-pitched, rumbling sounds usually heard on expiration. Although rhonchi sound similar to wheezes, they do not involve the small airways. They are less discrete than crackles and are easily auscultated. Rhonchi are caused by the passage of air through an airway obstructed by thick secretions, muscular spasm, new tissue growth, or external pressure collapsing the airway lumen. They may result from any condition that increases secretions. Examples are pneumonia, drug overdose, intralumenal or extralumenal growth, and long-term postoperative recovery.

Stridor is usually an inspiratory, crowing-type sound that can be heard without the aid of a stethoscope. It indicates significant narrowing or obstruction of the larynx or trachea and may be caused by epiglottitis, viral croup, foreign body aspiration, or a combination of these factors. Stridor is heard best over the site of origin, usually the larynx or trachea. Stridor often indicates a life-threatening problem, especially in children, and its presence requires careful observation for ventilatory failure and hypoxia.

Pleural Friction Rub

Although it occurs outside the respiratory tree, a pleural friction rub may also be considered an adventitious breath sound. It is a low-pitched, dry, rubbing, or grating sound caused by the movement of inflamed pleural surfaces as they slide on one another during breathing. The friction rub may be auscultated on both inspiration and expiration and is usually loudest over the lower lateral anterior surface of the chest wall. Presence of a pleural friction rub may indicate pleurisy, viral infection, tuberculosis, or pulmonary embolism.

The Heart

In the prehospital setting, the heart must be examined indirectly. However, information about the size and effectiveness of pumping action is obtained through a skilled assessment that includes palpation and auscultation.

Palpation

The apical impulse is the visible and palpable force produced by the contraction of the left ventricle. Palpating this impulse may be useful in the prehospital setting to compare the relationship of other pulses with the ventricular cycle. The hearts of some patients with cardiac irregularities, for example, do not always produce a peripheral pulse with every ventricular contraction. By palpating the apical impulse and the carotid pulse simulta-

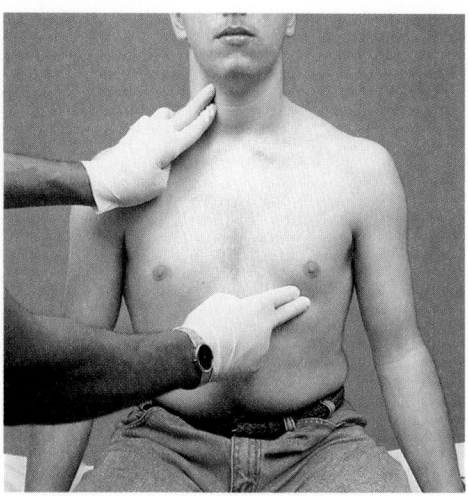

Fig. 11-13 Simultaneous palpation of the carotid artery and apical impulse.

neously, these pulse deficits can be noted (Fig. 11-13). Factors such as obesity, large breasts, and muscularity may make this landmark difficult to see or palpate.

Auscultation

Heart sounds may be auscultated for frequency (pitch), intensity (loudness), duration, and timing in the cardiac cycle. A thorough evaluation of heart sounds requires a high level of skill and experience, a quiet environment, and sufficient time to listen closely. Two basic heart sounds, however, may be assessed relatively quickly and improve understanding of the patient's condition. These are the basic heart sounds, S_1 and S_2, which are normal heart sounds that occur when the myocardium contracts. They are best heard toward the apex of the heart at the fifth intercostal space. For evaluation of heart sounds, the patient should be sitting up and leaning slightly forward (Fig. 11-14, *A*), supine (Fig. 11-14, *B*), or in a left lateral recumbent position (Fig. 11-14, *C*). These positions bring the heart closer to the left anterior chest wall. To listen for S_1, instruct the patient to breathe normally and hold the breath in expiration. To listen for S_2, have the patient breathe normally again and hold the breath in inspiration.

Heart sounds may be muffled or diminished by obesity or obstructive lung disease and by the

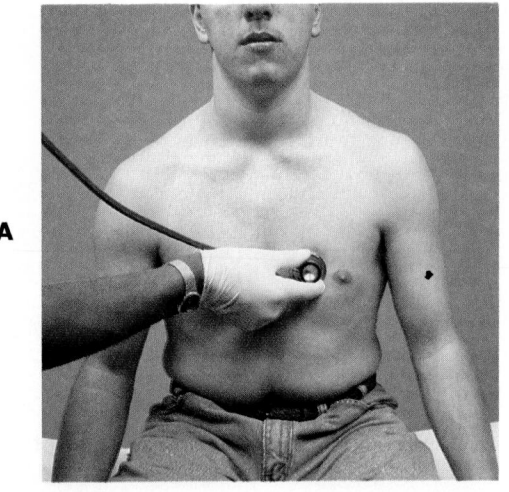

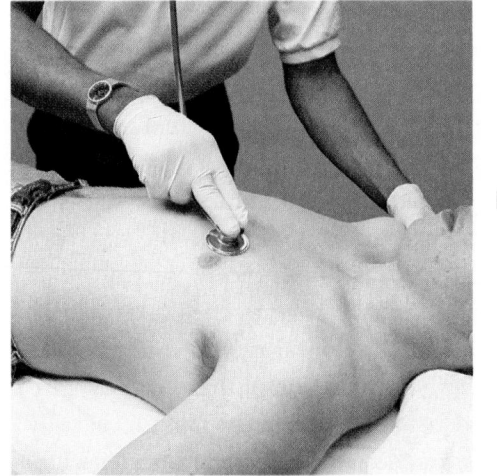

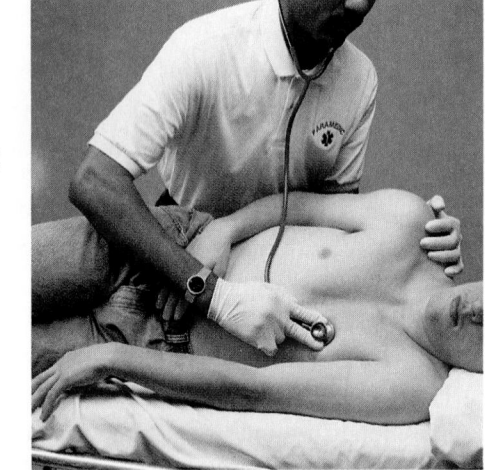

Fig. 11-14 Patient positions for auscultation. **A,** Sitting up, leaning slightly forward. **B,** Supine. **C,** Left lateral recumbent.

presence of fluid in the pericardial sac surrounding the heart muscle. This is usually the result of penetrating or severe blunt chest trauma, cardiac tamponade, or cardiac rupture and is considered a true emergency. (See Chapters 15 and 18 for further discussion of abnormal heart sounds.)

Inflammation of the pericardial sac may produce a rubbing sound audible with a stethoscope. This is a pericardial friction rub, which may result from infectious pericarditis, myocardial infarction, uremia, trauma, and autoimmune pericarditis. These rubs have a scratching, grating, or squeaking quality and tend to be louder on inspiration. They can be differentiated from pleural friction rubs by their continued presence when the patient holds the breath.

The Abdomen

The abdomen is divided by two imaginary lines that separate the abdominal region into four quadrants: upper right, lower right, upper left, and lower left (Fig. 11-15). These quadrants and their contents provide the basis for inspection, palpation, and auscultation (Box 11-4).

Inspection

Visually inspect the abdomen for signs of cyanosis, pallor, jaundice, bruising, discoloration, swelling, masses, aortic pulsations, and penetrating trauma. Be alert to the presence of surgical scars and implanted devices such as automatic implanted cardioverter defibrillators (AICDs). The abdomen should be evenly round and symmetrical. Symmetrical distention of the abdomen may result from obesity, enlarged organs, fluid, or gas. Asymmetrical distention may result from hernias, tumors, bowel obstructions, or enlarged abdominal organs. A flat abdomen is common in athletic adults, and convex abdomens are common in children and in adults with poor exercise

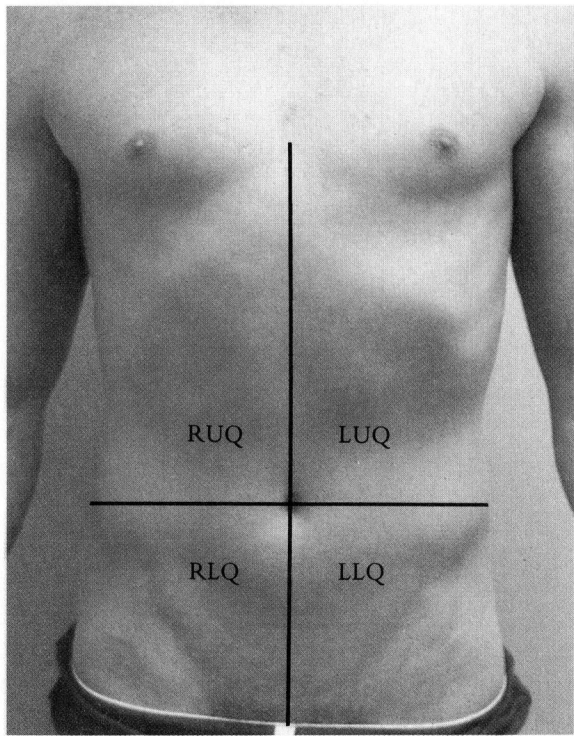

Fig. 11-15 Four quadrants of the abdomen.

habits. The umbilicus should be free of swelling, bulges, and signs of inflammation. The normal umbilicus is usually inverted, or it may protrude slightly.

Abdominal movement during respiration should be smooth and even. As a rule, males have more abdominal involvement than females during respiration, so limited abdominal movement in the symptomatic male may indicate abdominal pathology. Visible pulsations in the upper abdomen may be normal in thin adults, but marked pulsations may indicate an abdominal aortic aneurysm.

Auscultation

Noting the presence or absence of bowel sounds to assess motility and to discover vascular sounds has limited value in the prehospital setting because it does not affect or determine the approach to patient care. In addition, the time required for thorough bowel sound assessment (approximately 5 minutes per quadrant) far exceeds the justifiable scene time for most patients. If auscultation is to be performed, however, it should always precede palpation, since the latter maneuvers may alter the intensity of bowel sounds.

BOX 11-4

Abdominal Quadrants

Right Upper Quadrant
Liver and gallbladder
Pylorus
Duodenum
Head of pancreas
Right adrenal gland
Portion of right kidney
Hepatic flexure of colon
Portions of ascending and transverse colon

Right Lower Quadrant
Lower pole of right kidney
Cecum and appendix
Portion of ascending colon
Appendix
Bladder (if distended)
Ovary and salpinx
Uterus (if enlarged)
Right ureter

Left Upper Quadrant
Left lobe of liver
Spleen
Stomach
Body of pancreas
Left adrenal gland
Portion of left kidney
Splenic flexure of colon
Portions of transverse and descending colon

Left Lower Quadrant
Lower pole of left kidney
Sigmoid colon
Portion of descending colon
Bladder (if distended)
Ovary and salpinx
Uterus (if enlarged)
Left ureter

To auscultate bowel sounds, hold the diaphragm of the stethoscope on the abdomen with light pressure. If bowel sounds are present, they are usually heard as rumblings or gurgles that occur irregularly, ranging in frequency from 5 to 35 per minute. Auscultation should be done in all four quadrants, and a minimum of 5 minutes per quadrant is required to determine that normal bowel sounds are absent. Increased bowel sounds may indicate gastroenteritis or intestinal obstruction. Decreased or absent bowel sounds may indicate peritonitis (inflammation of the lining of the abdominal cavity).

Palpation

Palpating the abdomen may be useful to detect the presence of fluid, air, and solid masses. Employ a systematic approach, moving either from side to side or in a clockwise direction, noting any rigidity, tenderness, or abnormal skin temperature or color. Observe the patient's face for signs of pain or discomfort. If the patient is complaining of abdominal pain, examine the painful quadrant last so that the patient will not unnecessarily tighten or "guard" the abdominal area. Begin the abdominal assessment with a light palpation, using an even pressing motion. For patient comfort, the hands should be warm and sharp, and quick jabs should be avoided.

The Pelvis

In cases of abdominal or pelvic trauma, perform an initial examination to verify the structural integrity of the pelvis bones. To palpate the iliac crest and the symphysis pubis, place both hands on each anterior iliac crest, pressing downward and outward. Then place the heel of the hand on the symphysis pubis, pressing downward to determine stability (Fig. 11-16).

Deformity and point tenderness of the pelvis may be signs of fracture, masking major structural and vascular injuries. In addition, be alert to the possible presence of a ruptured bladder and large amounts of blood loss from hemorrhage or hematoma formation. Evaluate femoral pulses for strength and regularity. If inspection of the genitalia is indicated, prehospital examination should include only the external genitalia.

Assessing the genital area can make patients anxious. If the external genitalia must be visualized because of trauma, pregnancy, or illness, make every effort to ensure patient privacy. When possible, provide draping so that exposure of the

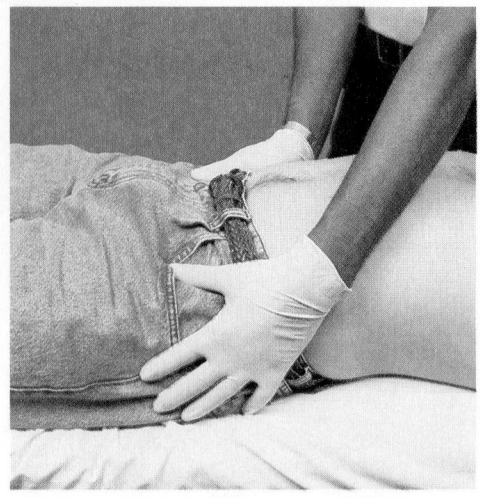

Fig. 11-16 Palpating the pelvis for stability.

patient's body is minimal. Maintain eye contact with the patient before, during, and after the examination as a comforting measure.

When examining the female external genitalia, first perform a visual inspection to note any swelling, redness, discharge, bleeding, or evidence of trauma. Discoloration or tenderness may be the result of traumatic bruising. Ulcers, vesicles, and discharge (with or without pain) indicate sexually transmitted diseases. If it is necessary to touch the anal area, gloves should be changed so as not to introduce bacteria into the vaginal area.

When examining the male external genitalia, visually inspect the genital area for bleeding and signs of trauma. The shaft of the penis should be nontender and flaccid. Patients with leukemia, sickle cell disease, and spinal injury may have a persistent painful erection (priapism, a rare condition). The urethral opening should be free of blood (a possible result of pelvic trauma) or discharge (a sign of sexually transmitted disease). The scrotum should be nontender and slightly asymmetrical. A swollen or painful scrotum may result from infection, herniation, testicular torsion, or trauma.

The Musculoskeletal System

Examination of the musculoskeletal system begins with a visual inspection of the patient's physical characteristics. For example, the way a patient walks, stands from a sitting position, and follows directions provides clues as to structural stability, muscular strength, and joint function.

Visually assess the overall appearance of immobile or unconscious patients. Fractures or deformities may be obvious, and the position of the patient may indicate the nature of the physical injury or illness. Be alert to the presence of crutches, walkers, and other personal items that may indicate physical impairment.

Examining the Upper and Lower Extremities

Systematically inspect both upper and lower extremities. Assess the skin and tissue overlying the muscles, cartilage, bones, and joints for soft tissue injury, discoloration, swelling, and masses. The upper and lower extremities should be reasonably symmetrical in both structure and muscularity. Evaluate the circulatory status of each extremity during the assessment by determining capillary refill time, skin color, temperature, sensation, and the presence of distal pulses.

Palpation

Assess the bones, joints, and surrounding tissues of the extremities for structural integrity and continuity. The examination includes evaluating swelling, tenderness, soft tissue injury, and crepitus. Muscle tone should be firm and nontender.

Range of Motion

A joint is assessed for function by instructing the patient to move each joint through its full range of motion. A normal range of motion occurs without pain, deformity, limitation, or instability.

> **NOTE:**
> In trauma patients with potential joint injury or in cases in which an injury may be exacerbated by movement, this assessment should be deferred until arrival at the emergency department.

Muscle Strength

Evaluating muscle strength is important for patients with spinal injury, head injury, or CVA.

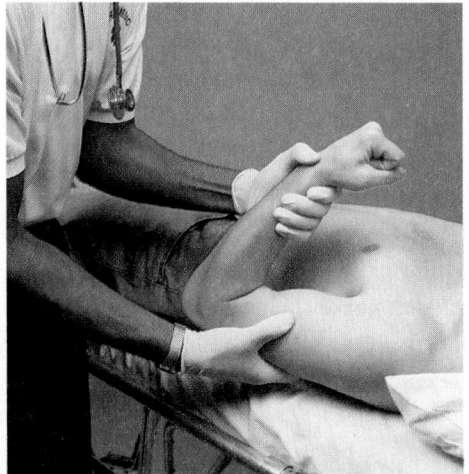

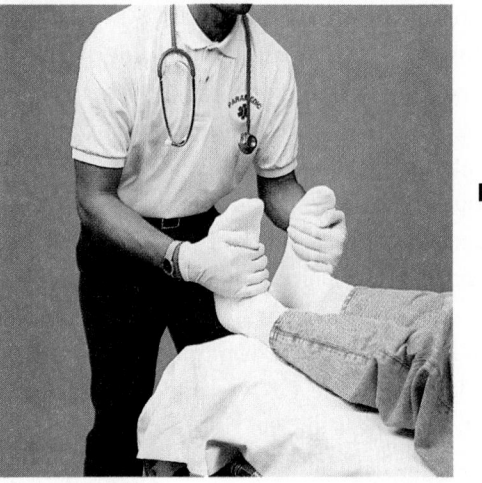

Fig. 11-17 Evaluating muscle strength of the upper **(A)** and lower **(B)** extremities.

Muscle strength should be bilaterally symmetrical, and the patient should be able to provide reasonable resistance to opposition. One method to evaluate muscle strength in the upper extremities is to instruct the patient to flex his or her elbow and to pull it toward the chest while using opposing resistance (Fig. 11-17, *A*).

Muscle strength in the lower extremities is evaluated by requesting the patient to push the soles of his or her feet against the paramedic's palms. Next, direct the patient to pull his or her toes toward the head while providing opposing resistance (Fig. 11-17, *B*). These and other methods offer some indication of the patient's bilateral muscle strength.

Evaluating Specific Joints

The joints of the shoulders, elbows, hands and wrists, hips, knees, feet, and ankles should be evaluated as part of a systematic, thorough assessment of the extremities. An underlying fracture is typified by marked local bony tenderness directly over the fracture site. All patients with possible bony injuries require stabilization of neurovascular status distal to the possible fracture and examination for occult injury to nerves or blood vessels at the fracture site. In addition, palpate joints above and below the suspected fracture to detect occult fracture. The focus of the examination is based on the particular patient situation or suspected mechanism of injury.

Inspect and palpate the shoulders for symmetry and integrity of the clavicles, scapulae, and humeri. Pain, tenderness, or asymmetric contour indicates a fracture or dislocation. The patient should be able to shrug shoulders and raise and extend both arms without pain or discomfort.

Inspect and palpate the elbows in both flexed and extended positions. Request the patient to rotate his or her hands from palm up to palm down to determine the elbow's range of motion. Pain and tenderness should not be present.

Inspect both hands for contour and positional alignment. Palpate the wrists, hands, and joints of each finger for tenderness, swelling, or deformity. To determine range of motion, request the patient to flex and extend the wrists, make a fist, and touch the thumb to each fingertip. All movements should be performed without pain or discomfort.

Inspect and palpate the hips for instability, tenderness, and crepitus. Evaluate the supine or unconscious patient by assessing the structural integrity of the iliac crest as previously described. Injuries involving the head or, more commonly, the neck of the femur may be obvious from the position of the patient's lower extremities. Generally, a fracture of the neck of the femur causes the affected extremity to appear shortened and externally rotated. In contrast, dislocation of the head of the femur from the hip generally causes the affected extremity to turn inward. A mobile patient should be able to walk without discomfort. A supine patient should be able to raise the legs and knees and rotate the legs inward and outward.

Inspect and palpate the knees for swelling and tenderness. The patella should be smooth, firm, nontender, and midline in position. The patient should be able to bend and straighten each knee without pain.

Inspect the feet and ankles for contour, position, and size. Tenderness, swelling, and deformity are abnormal findings on palpation. The toes should be straight and aligned with each other. Determine range of motion by requesting the patient to bend his or her toes, point his or her toes, and rotate his or her feet both inward and outward from the ankle. These movements should be possible without pain or discomfort.

The Back

A thorough physical examination includes assessment of the patient's posterior body surfaces. If a supine patient has been traumatized or spinal injury is suspected, carefully log-roll the patient with in-line spinal immobilization. (This maneuver and evaluation is performed as the patient is moved to a long spine board for immobilization and transportation.)

Cervical Spine

Inspect the patient's neck for midline position. If the patient is alert and denies neck pain, palpate the posterior aspect for point tenderness and swelling. The only palpable landmark should be the spinous process of the seventh cervical vertebrae at the base of the neck. In the absence of suspected injury, test range of motion by directing the patient to bend the head forward, backward, and from side to side. These movements should be performed without pain or discomfort.

Immobilize the cervical spine in all trauma patients with neck pain or a decreased level of consciousness, and do not attempt to palpate or perform range-of-motion evaluation in these patients.

> **NOTE:**
> Never attempt to move an individual's neck to test range of motion in patients who are unconscious or who are unable or unwilling to do so on their own.

As a rule, the cervical spine should be immobilized whenever the following five criteria cannot be completely ruled out:

1. Supraclavicular trauma
2. Mechanism of injury or evidence of mechanism (for example, shattered windshield) compatible with cervical spine injury
3. Drug or alcohol intoxication
4. Altered consciousness resulting from trauma (including a seizure or fall)
5. Neck pain on palpation or passive or active range-of-motion testing

Thoracic and Lumbar Spine

Inspect the thoracic and lumbar areas for signs of injury, swelling, and discoloration. Begin palpation at the first thoracic vertebrae and move downward to the sacrum. Under normal conditions, the spine is nontender to palpation. If point tenderness is present or the patient provides a recent history of trauma, full spinal precautions should be employed.

Evaluate range of motion by requesting the patient to bend at the waist, forward and backward and to each side and also to rotate the upper trunk from side to side in a circular motion. Trauma patients who complain of back pain with point tenderness or evidence of neurological involvement such as numbness, tingling, or weakness of the legs should not be evaluated for range of motion.

● THE PATIENT INTERVIEW

Obtaining an adequate history of the patient's chief complaint, recent illnesses, and significant past medical history may be as important as physical assessment skills. The information gathered during the patient interview often determines the direction of the physical examination and may indicate possible causes of the patient complaint that are not readily observable. Although we present this discussion separately, the patient interview should be integrated early in the patient encounter and continue throughout the examination.

Because of the nature of emergency medical care, EMS personnel often think in terms of specific illness and injury, grouping patients into general classifications such as *trauma* or *medical* cases. However, good emergency care involves viewing each patient as a total individual and attending to patient needs in a caring, concerned, and receptive manner.

Communication with a patient begins as the EMS crew arrives at the scene. The patient's first impression of the paramedic's appearance, professional approach, and sincerity often sets the tone of the emergency environment. Improved scene control and better patient cooperation result if the patient, family members, loved ones, and bystanders perceive the event as being attended to by professional emergency care providers.

Approach the conscious patient and make a personal introduction by name and title: "Hello. My name is [name], and I am a paramedic with [name of EMS agency]. What's your name?" A verbal exchange with the patient provides information on the patient's level of consciousness, sensorium, any hearing or speech impediments, and language barriers. During the introduction, take a position that allows eye contact with the patient. Eye contact is a type of nonverbal communication that can work to express gentleness, sincerity, and authority and can help make the patient feel safe and secure.

Nonverbal communication may also convey negative feelings or the insecurities of both the patient and paramedic. Voice inflection, facial expression, and body position, for example, may reflect feelings of anger, fear, or impatience. Similarly, initiating IV therapy with trembling, sweaty hands will make the patient question the paramedic's skills. Be aware of nonverbal communication to gain the trust and cooperation required to effectively care for the patient.

Touch is another form of communication that conveys compassion and reassurance to the patient. Small gestures such as holding a patient's hand, squeezing a shoulder, or wiping tears from the eyes do much to comfort an individual in distress. Experience and familiarity with patient care activities help to determine the appropriateness of these gestures.

Be aware of the patient's "private space." This space is culturally defined and delineates a personal comfort zone for contact with other people.

For example, studies have shown that the average comfort zone for Americans is 45.72 cm to 1.219 m from their bodies.[3] Anyone entering this space usually causes the individual to back away. Although this zone is a form of subconscious personal protection and varies by individual, some patients are very protective of their space and may become defensive if this space is invaded.

Conversing with a patient includes the communication skill of listening—not only hearing what is said but interpreting what is said. The patient may say, for example, that he or she feels fine, but his or her appearance and the tone in his or her voice may indicate that he or she is ill and afraid. If you are unsure of the message in a patient's response, pursue a line of questioning to better understand what the patient is trying to communicate.

Most patients do not converse in medical terminology, and many have only a vague understanding of their bodies. The patient interview should accordingly consist of common words and phrases that can be clearly understood. Guide and direct the patient interview without manipulating the patient's response, and avoid leading questions or questions that can only be answered with "yes" or "no." Employ open-ended questions that allow a free-form response, such as "When did this pain begin?" rather than "Did this pain begin this morning?"

Ask the patient only one question at a time, and give the patient ample time to answer the question before asking another. If the patient responds with something that does not appear relevant to the question, clarify the response. Be flexible, and do not discount the patient's experiences or information he or she may provide.

Make every effort to answer all questions. This does not mean that a full explanation is required of each inquiry but that a sensitive response that addresses the question is in order. Be very careful in choosing an answer and attempt to avoid any response that increases the patient's anxiety.

Chief Complaint

The chief complaint is usually the problem that initiated the EMS response. The complaint may be verbal, such as a patient complaining of chest pain, or nonverbal, as when a bystander reports a vehicle crash with injuries. Most chief complaints are characterized by pain, abnormal function, a change in the patient's normal state, or an unusual observation made by the patient, such as hematuria or heart palpitations. Be alert to the possibility that a problem more serious than the patient's chief complaint may be present. For example, the patient who has fallen down a flight of steps may complain of an injured ankle, but physical examination may reveal suspected internal injuries.

After determining the chief complaint and stabilizing any life-threatening situations, begin the patient interview. Depending on the situation, this interview may precede or occur simultaneously with the secondary assessment. As previously mentioned, the patient interview should be conducted early in the patient encounter. This interview should include a history of the present illness and any significant past medical history.

History of Present Illness

Obtaining a thorough history of the patient's illness requires skill both in asking appropriate questions related to the chief complaint and in interpreting the patient's response to those questions. For example, the patient complains of low back pain that suggests a muscle strain. During the interview, he or she reveals that he or she has had a burning sensation with urination and a low-grade fever for the past several days, suggesting a urinary tract infection or renal stones. Thus the history of the present illness may be more important than the obvious chief complaint. The mnemonic *PQRST* helps define the patient's complaint by focusing on essential elements of assessment (Box 11-5). Using this memory device may help lead the patient through a thorough sequence of questions and answers to better understand the chief complaint.

Significant Past Medical History

After gaining a clear understanding of the patient's chief complaint, gather other significant past medical history that may offer additional insight into the patient's current problem. For ex-

---

BOX 11-5

PQRST Mnemonic

P (Provokes): What provokes the symptoms?

Q (Quality): What makes the symptom better? What makes it worse?

R (Region): Where is the symptom? Where does it go? Is it in one spot or more than one spot?

S (Severity): On a scale of 1 to 10, with 1 being the least and 10 being the worst, what number would you assign your pain or discomfort?

T (Time): How long have you had this symptom? When did it start? When did it end? How long did it last?

BOX 11-6

Elements of the AMPLE Survey

A: Allergies

M: Medications

P: Past medical history

L: Last meal or oral intake

E: Events before the emergency

---

ample, information on a history of renal disease, cardiac problems, respiratory disease, diabetes, or epilepsy may well direct patient care activities. Other history, such as recent surgery or hospitalization, may also be important. For example, a patient complains of severe, sharp chest pain and difficulty breathing. The initial presentation indicates a possible myocardial infarction. When questioned, the patient reveals that he or she had a recent surgery for a fractured lower leg. Based on this information, the possibility of a pulmonary embolism must be considered. A variety of mnemonics or memory devices are used to remember relevant questions for gathering medical history. One example is the *AMPLE* Survey (Box 11-6).

Although the depth and focus of the patient interview are based on the particular scenario, gather as much information as possible at the scene and during transport to the hospital. Regardless of the method used to obtain medical history, a series of questions should be used to gather information.

Allergies

Very few emergency medications produce an allergic reaction, but information on allergies is important and useful to others involved in the patient's care. For example, the patient may be

sensitive to tetanus prophylaxis, antibiotics, radiographical contrast mediums, and other medications administered during the course of patient care.

Allergies to food and other substances may also offer valuable information on the patient's condition, as when a patient with food allergies becomes ill after eating or a patient with difficulty breathing is allergic to cat hair. If the patient is unconscious or unable to converse, look for medical alert information and question family members or friends for allergy information.

Medications

Ascertain if the patient takes any medications on a regular basis and, if so, for what reasons. In addition, the patient's medication compliance (taking the medication as directed) should be ascertained. The medication history may provide clues as to the chief complaint. For example, a diabetic patient may have administered his or her insulin but have eaten irregularly. Other examples include a patient with chest pain who takes various cardiac medications, an irrational patient who takes prescribed sedatives, and a trauma patient who takes blood-thinning medications.

The patient's medication history may not always be relevant to the present problem, but it can indicate potential problems that may be encountered during patient care. For example, if the patient advises the paramedic that he or she takes seizure medication, the possibility of a seizure should be considered.

Last Oral Intake

The time of the patient's last meal or fluid consumption is important when considering potential airway problems in a patient who loses consciousness or begins to deteriorate. This information also helps determine the appropriateness of surgery. Surgery for a patient who has consumed food or drink within the previous 6 to 8 hours is generally delayed if possible because stomach contents may be aspirated during induction of anesthesia.

Determining the patient's last oral intake may also help rule out problems such as food poisoning and food allergies. Symptoms of food poisoning, for example, do not usually appear for several hours after ingestion. Therefore if the patient complains of severe abdominal cramping and vomiting shortly after eating, it is probably unrelated to the contents of that meal. In contrast, patients who are sensitive to certain food substances, such as peanut oil or shellfish, would be expected to develop the allergic reaction immediately after eating.

Last Menstrual Period

Obtain a menstrual history when dealing with a female patient between the ages of 12 and 55 years who has abdominal pain. This line of questioning may prompt the patient to discuss other significant symptoms such as vaginal discharge, bleeding, and pregnancy history. The patient's response should determine the need to pursue additional questions regarding contraceptive use, venereal disease, urinary tract infection, and ectopic pregnancy.

Last Bowel Movement

Question the patient regarding bowel habits to determine if they have been normal or abnormal. If a patient with abdominal pain gives a recent history of diarrhea, constipation, or bloody bowel movements, this information will be important to the receiving physician as the patient is assessed for bowel obstruction, dehydration, or lower gastrointestinal bleeding. During this time, discuss with the patient any symptoms of abnormal urinary function, such as blood in the urine, urethral discharge, pain or burning with urination, frequent urination, and the inability to void.

Family History

Family history of illness or disease may be relevant to the patient complaint. Establish whether there is a family history of heart disease, high blood pressure, cancer, tuberculosis, stroke, diabetes, kidney disease, and other ailments. The presence or absence of hereditary diseases such as hemophilia or sickle cell anemia should also be established during the patient interview.

Personal and Social History

The patient's personal and social history may reveal information on the patient's overall health. Depending on the situation, include the following topics as part of a thorough patient interview. Much of this information can be gathered during transport and should not prolong scene time.

- Personal status: home environment, marital status, hobbies, interests
- Habits: special diets, eating and sleeping habits, exercise, use of coffee, tea, tobacco, alcohol, and illicit drugs
- Home conditions: housing, economic condition, pets and their health
- Occupation: description of past and present work, exposure to heat, cold, and industrial toxins
- Environment: travel, exposure to contagious diseases, residence in tropics, water and milk supply, and other possible sources of infection
- Military record: geographical areas, exposure to chemicals
- Religious preference: special beliefs regarding medical care

Events Before the Emergency

Important information may be obtained by questioning the patient, bystanders, or both regarding actions or events that occurred before the emergency. For example, was a syncopal episode preceded by exertion or straining? Did a loss of consciousness occur before or after a fall? The paramedic should attempt to correlate any event with the beginning or progression of an illness or injury.

● THE RADIO REPORT

After an appropriate physical assessment and patient interview, contact medical direction with significant findings. As discussed in Chapter 4, radio use should be kept to a minimum, and the radio report should only include pertinent information on patient status and the request for specific patient care orders (IV lines, medications).

● FIELD MANAGEMENT PROCEDURES

Before transporting a patient for physician evaluation, a variety of field management procedures are indicated. Depending on the situation, preparing the patient for transportation may include the following:
- Airway control
- Ventilation support
- Spinal immobilization
- Hemorrhage control
- Extrication
- Maintenance of body temperature
- Vital sign determination
- Cardiac monitoring
- Medication therapy
- Venipuncture for blood samples
- IV fluid administration
- PASG application
- Fracture stabilization
- Bandaging

Patient Loading and Transportation

After the patient has been prepared for transport, he or she is stabilized on an ambulance stretcher and loaded into the emergency vehicle. The choice of medical facilities for hospital evaluation may be determined by EMS service protocols, the patient's preference, or a facility's capacity for specialized care. If possible, advise family members or friends of the patient's destination.

Patients who cannot be stabilized in the prehospital setting require rapid delivery to a medical facility and should be transported expeditiously. Other patients, such as those with chest pain, may best be served by a less hurried and stressful environment. These patients should be transported in comfort, often without the use of lights and sirens, which may add to their anxiety. Many experts recommend a "scoop and run" approach for

seriously injured patients but recommend attempting resuscitation at the scene for patients in cardiac arrest. If it is not possible to perform field resuscitation, rapid transport is indicated.

Reevaluation

After the patient has been stabilized and packaged for transport to an appropriate medical facility, continually evaluate the patient's status en route to the receiving hospital. Update medical direction about significant changes in the patient's condition. Rapid changes such as deteriorating vital signs, blood loss, and airway compromise may alter the priorities of patient care activities.

In most cases, EMS transportation allows time for the paramedic crew to continue with patient assessment. Injuries or other significant findings overlooked at the scene because of life-threatening problems or a poor evaluation environment may become apparent during transport and patient reevaluation. Continuous reassessment should focus on the following:
- Airway
- Ventilation
- Oxygenation
- Lung sounds
- Pulse
- Skin color
- Blood pressure
- ECG monitoring
- Neurological status
- Circulation distal to a fracture
- IV fluid administration

● SPECIAL CONSIDERATIONS IN PEDIATRIC ASSESSMENT

Examining the ill or injured child requires special assessment skills. The child differs physiologically, psychologically, and anatomically from the adult, so pediatric patient assessment must take age and development into account.

Approaching the Pediatric Patient

The assessment and management objectives in caring for critically ill or injured children are similar to those for any other patient encounter. The approach to the pediatric patient must differ, however. The initial encounter with the sick or injured child sets the tone for the entire patient care episode, so consider the patient's age and be sensitive to how the child perceives the emergency environment. The following six guidelines should be considered when approaching the pediatric patient[4]:

1. Remain calm and confident. The parent's anxiety is infectious. Stay under control and take charge of the situation in a gentle but firm manner.

2. Do not separate the child from the parent unless absolutely necessary. In fact, once parents are reassured, encourage them to touch, hold, or cuddle the child when such actions are practical. This comforts the parents as well as the child.

3. Establish rapport with the parents as well as the child. Much of a child's fear and anxiety reflects the parent's behavior. When the family is calm, the child is reassured and is less fearful.

4. Be honest with both child and parent. In simple, direct, nonmedical language, explain to both the parent and the child what is happening as it occurs. When a procedure is going to hurt, inform the child. Never lie. Do not give the impression that there are options when none exist. For example, do not say, "Would you like to go for a ride in the ambulance?" The child may answer "No."

5. Whenever possible, assign one emergency care-giver to stay with the child. This person should obtain the history and be the primary person to initiate therapy. Even in a few moments, one person who remains on the child's level can establish a trusting relationship.

6. Observe the patient before the physical examination. When possible, the alert child should be initially assessed without touching the patient. After the physical examination begins, the child's behavior may drastically change, making it difficult to assess whether the behavior is a reaction to a physical state or to the perceived intrusion. The patient's general appearance, skin signs, level of consciousness, respiratory rate, and behavior can usually be assessed easily before approaching the patient. During this observation, also note any particular area of the body that appears painful. Avoid manipulating this area until the end of the examination and inform the child that you will give warning before you have to touch the area.

The Patient's General Appearance

As previously stated, a child's general appearance is best assessed from a distance. While the patient is in safe, familiar surroundings (for example, a parent's arms), visually assess the child's level of consciousness, spontaneous movement, respiratory effort, and skin color. The child's body position can also provide helpful information; for example, the child may be lying limp or sitting upright to facilitate breathing. Other clues (for example, crying, eye contact, concentration, distractibility) may help determine the child's willingness to cooperate during the physical examination.

A visual inspection of the child's general appearance is a fairly reliable indicator of the patient's need for emergency care. A child who is seriously ill or injured does not usually attempt to disguise or hide his or her condition and generally exhibit behaviors that reflect the severity of the situation. Therefore the patient's general appearance is a valuable assessment tool for the paramedic. Table 11-4 gives the components of general appearance important in initial assessment of the pediatric patient.

The Physical Examination

A hands-on examination is best conducted through an age-related evaluation. The following guidelines will vary according to the child's development but may be used as a reference for examination procedures. Parents and family members may also be a source of information during the examination. Questions regarding "normal" behavior and activity levels may be directed to the parents.

TABLE 11-4 Components of General Appearance for Assessing Pediatric Patients	
Assessment Finding	**Evaluation Considerations**
Alertness	How perceptive is the child, and how responsive to the presence of a stranger or other aspects of the environment?
Distractibility	How readily does a person, object, or sound draw the child's attention? For example, drawing a child's attention to a toy when the child initially appeared disinterested in the surroundings is a positive sign.
Consolability	Can a distressed child be comforted? For example, stopping a child from crying by speaking softly or offering a pacifier or a toy is an encouraging sign.
Speech or cry	Is the speech or cry strong and spontaneous? Weak and muffled? Hoarse? Absent unless stimulated? Absent altogether?
Spontaneous activity	Does the child appear flaccid? Do the extremities move only in response to stimuli, or are there spontaneous movements?
Color	Is there pallor, a flushed appearance, cyanosis, or mottling? Does the skin coloring of the trunk differ from that of the extremities?
Respiratory efforts	Are there intercostal, supraclavicular, or suprasternal retractions in the resting state? Nasal flaring also indicates respiratory difficulty.
Eye contact	Does the child appear to gaze aimlessly, or does he or she maintain eye contact with objects or people? Even very small infants, when well, preferentially fix their gaze on a face rather than other objects.

Birth to 6 Months

Children under 6 months of age are not typically frightened by the approach of a stranger, and the physical examination is relatively easy. During the examination, give special consideration to maintaining the child's body temperature.

Healthy and alert infants are usually in constant motion and may have a lusty cry. If the patient is under 3 months of age, poor head control is normal. Infants are "abdominal breathers," which causes the stomach to protrude and the infant's chest wall to retract during inspiration. This diaphragmatic involvement may give the impression of labored breathing. Skin color, nasal flaring, and intercostal muscle retraction are the best indicators of respiratory insufficiency.

In the infant, it is particularly important to assess the fontanelles. These sutures between the flat bones of the skull are fairly wide to allow a "give" in the skull during the birth process. (The anterior fontanelle, known as the *soft spot*, is usually present up to the age of 18 months.) The anterior fontanelle should be level with the skull or slightly depressed and soft. It usually bulges during crying and may feel firm if the child is lying down. In the absence of injury, the fontanelle is best examined with the child in an upright position. A sunken fontanelle may indicate dehydration, and a bulging fontanelle in the noncrying upright infant may indicate an increase in intracranial pressure.

7 Months to 3 Years

These patients are often difficult to evaluate. They have little capacity to understand the emergency event and are likely to experience emotional problems as a result of illness, injury, or hospitalization. Children of this age fear strangers and may show separation anxiety. If possible, parents should be present and be allowed to hold the child during the examination. Approach the child with a quiet, reassuring voice, and if time permits, allow the patient to become accustomed to the examination environment.

During the physical assessment, explain each activity in short, simple sentences, even though it may not improve cooperation. Be gentle and firm, and complete the examination as quickly as possible. If physical restraint is necessary and if patient care activities will not be hindered, the child should be restrained with hands rather than mechanical devices (for example, backboards).

4 to 10 Years

Children in this age group are developing a capacity for rational thought and may be very cooperative during the physical examination. Depending on the child's age and the emergency scenario, they may be able to provide a limited history of the event. These children may also experience separation anxiety and may view their illness or injury as punishment. Therefore approach the child slowly, and speak in quiet and reassuring tones. Questions should be simple and direct.

During the examination, allow the child to participate by holding the stethoscope, penlight, or other pieces of equipment. This "helping" activity may lessen the child's fear and improve the paramedic-patient relationship. Children of this age group have a limited understanding of their bodies and are reluctant to allow the examiner to see or touch their "private parts." All examination procedures should be explained simply and completely, and the child should be advised of any expected pain or discomfort.

Adolescents

Adolescents generally understand what is happening and are usually calm, mature, and helpful. These patients are more adult than child and should be treated as such. Adolescents are preoccupied with their bodies and are usually very concerned about modesty, disfigurement, pain, disability, and death. If appropriate, provide reassurance about these concerns during the examination.

During the patient interview, be sensitive to the patient's need for privacy. Some adolescents may be hesitant to reveal pertinent history in the presence of family and friends. If the adolescent gives incomplete answers or appears uncomfortable during the interview, interview the patient privately. Be alert to the possibility of alcohol or drug use.

● SPECIAL CONSIDERATIONS IN EXAMINING THE OLDER ADULT

As in pediatric patients, age-related physiological and psychological variations in older adults may create special challenges in patient assess-

ment. However, do not assume that all older adults are victims of age-related disorders. Individual differences in knowledge, mental reasoning, experience, and personality influence how these patients respond to examination.

Communicating with the Older Adult

Some older adults have sensory losses that make communication more difficult. Hearing and visual impairments, for example, are not uncommon. In addition, many older adults experience some memory loss and may become easily confused. Extra time may be needed to communicate effectively with these patients.

During the interview, remain close to the patient. The older adult generally perceives a reassuring voice and gentle touch as comforting. Use short, simple questions. It may be necessary to speak more loudly than usual, and questions may have to be repeated. Be patient and careful not to patronize or offend the patient by assuming that he or she has a hearing impairment or cannot understand a particular line of questioning.

The Patient History

Older patients often have multiple health problems that may present simultaneously. The patient may be vague and nonspecific when describing his or her chief complaint, making it difficult to isolate a nonapparent injury or illness. In addition, normal signs and symptoms of illness or injury may be absent because of decreased sensory function in some older adult patients.

Older adult patients with multiple health problems often take several medications, which increases the risk of illness from medication use and misuse. Attempt to gather a complete medication history, and be alert to the relationship among drug interactions, disease, and the aging process.

As part of the history, assess the patient's functional abilities and any recent changes in daily activities. Many older adults attribute these changes to age and will not mention them unless asked. This information may help indicate patient conditions that are not readily observable and may reveal the need for other pertinent lines of questioning. Examples of functional activities to be discussed with the patient include the following:

- Walking
- Getting out of bed
- Dressing
- Driving a car
- Using public transportation
- Preparing meals
- Taking medications
- Sleeping habits
- Bathroom habits

The Physical Examination

When examining the older adult patient, try to ensure patient comfort. Clearly explain examination procedures and sensitively answer all questions. Remember that many older patients with chronic illness may have lived with pain or discomfort for quite some time. Therefore their perception of what is painful may be quite different from that of other patients. Observe for signs such as grimacing or wincing during the physical examination, which may indicate pain or a possible injury site. If the situation permits, perform the examination slowly and gently and be considerate of the patient's feelings and needs.

Many older adults believe they will die in a hospital, so if transportation is necessary, the patient may become fearful and anxious. Be sensitive to these concerns, and if appropriate, reassure the patient that his or her condition is not serious. Attempt to calm the patient and advise him or her that he or she will be well cared for in the hospital.

● SPECIAL CONSIDERATIONS IN EXAMINING PATIENTS WITH DISABILITIES

Disabilities may take the form of physical or emotional disorders. For example, the patient may be deaf, blind, brain injured, or developmentally or emotionally disabled or have some combination of these conditions. Dealing with patients who have disabilities can pose special problems in communication and patient care. Regardless of the nature of the disability, be courteous and sensitive to the special needs of each patient. (The evaluation of emotionally disabled patients is addressed in Chapter 30.)

Hearing Impaired and Deaf Patients

Hearing impairments should be considered whenever an uncommunicative patient is encountered. If the patient is suspected to be hearing impaired or deaf, try to gain the patient's attention by gentle touch, by waving your hands in front of the patient, by speaking a little louder, or if necessary, by speaking directly into the patient's ear if no hearing aid is present. Many deaf people read and write, and some read lips if one speaks slowly and enunciates each word clearly. Use short phrases versus lengthy sentences when conversing with these patients.

When communicating with the hearing impaired and deaf, stay in full view of the patient at all times. If the patient is to be transported to a medical facility, advise the emergency department staff as soon as possible so that they can arrange for personnel to aid in communication. Finger-spelling and simple sign language are easily learned and may help in the prehospital setting.

Blind Patients

When approaching a blind patient, ascertain if the patient has a hearing impairment as well (although it is unusual for sightless people to also be deaf). Identify yourself in a normal voice and answer any questions the patient may have about the emergency scene and the surroundings. Explain all examination and treatment procedures in detail before beginning the assessment. Most patients who have disabilities are very independent and may resent unsolicited assistance.

If a sightless person has a guide dog and the situation permits, try not to separate them. If the dog has been injured during the emergency event, immediately advise dispatch to make special arrangements to care for the dog.

Patients with Brain Injuries and Developmental Disabilities

If possible, allow time for the patient to become familiar with the EMS crew before beginning the patient examination. Friendly conversation can provide a baseline on the patient's intellectual ability. Once this has been established, begin the interview at a level that the patient can clearly understand.

When conducting the interview, allow extra time for questions to be answered and do not be patronizing or condescending. Evaluate the patient's understanding of the questions, and reword them if necessary. Families and friends are often available to help communicate with these patients and interpret examination findings as normal or abnormal.

Depending on the patient's level of intellectual functioning, the physical examination may need to be performed in a manner similar to that used to assess a child. Patients with higher intellectual function can receive an adult assessment. Explain all procedures in advance so that the patient knows what to expect. Answer all questions posed by the patient to the extent that the patient is capable of understanding. Take extra care in listening to these patients and reassuring them about their concerns.

● COMMUNICATING WITH NON-ENGLISH-SPEAKING PATIENTS

Emergencies involving non-English-speaking patients are common events. Attempt to communicate in English first to determine whether the patient understands or speaks some English words and phrases. Many medical terms have roots in other languages, and the patient may recognize certain terms if they are spoken slowly and clearly. Bystanders, co-workers, or family members may also be available to provide some assistance. If the patient does not speak or understand English, attempt to communicate with signs and gestures.

If time permits, perform all assessment procedures slowly, pointing to the part of the body that needs to be examined before touching the patient. Advise medical direction of the situation as soon as possible to prepare for an interpreter to assist with patient care activities in the emergency department.

REFERENCES

1. Centers for Disease Control: *Curriculum guide for public-safety and emergency-response workers: prevention of transmission of human immunodeficiency virus and hepatitis B virus*, Atlanta, 1989, US Government Printing Office.
2. *E.M.T. paramedic national standard curriculum*, Washington, DC, 1986, US Government Printing Office.
3. Seidel J, Henderson D, editors: *Prehospital care of pediatric patients*, California EMSC Project, Los Angeles, 1987, American Academy of Pediatrics.
4. Rathus S: *Psychology*, ed 3, New York, 1987, Holt, Rinehart & Winston.

Summary

The paramedic must have a wide spectrum of knowledge and skills to perform a thorough patient assessment and to make effective patient care determinations in the prehospital setting. In each emergency response, the scene must be evaluated, life-threatening conditions must be recognized and stabilized, and priorities of care based on these assessments must be established.

12 AIRWAY AND VENTILATION

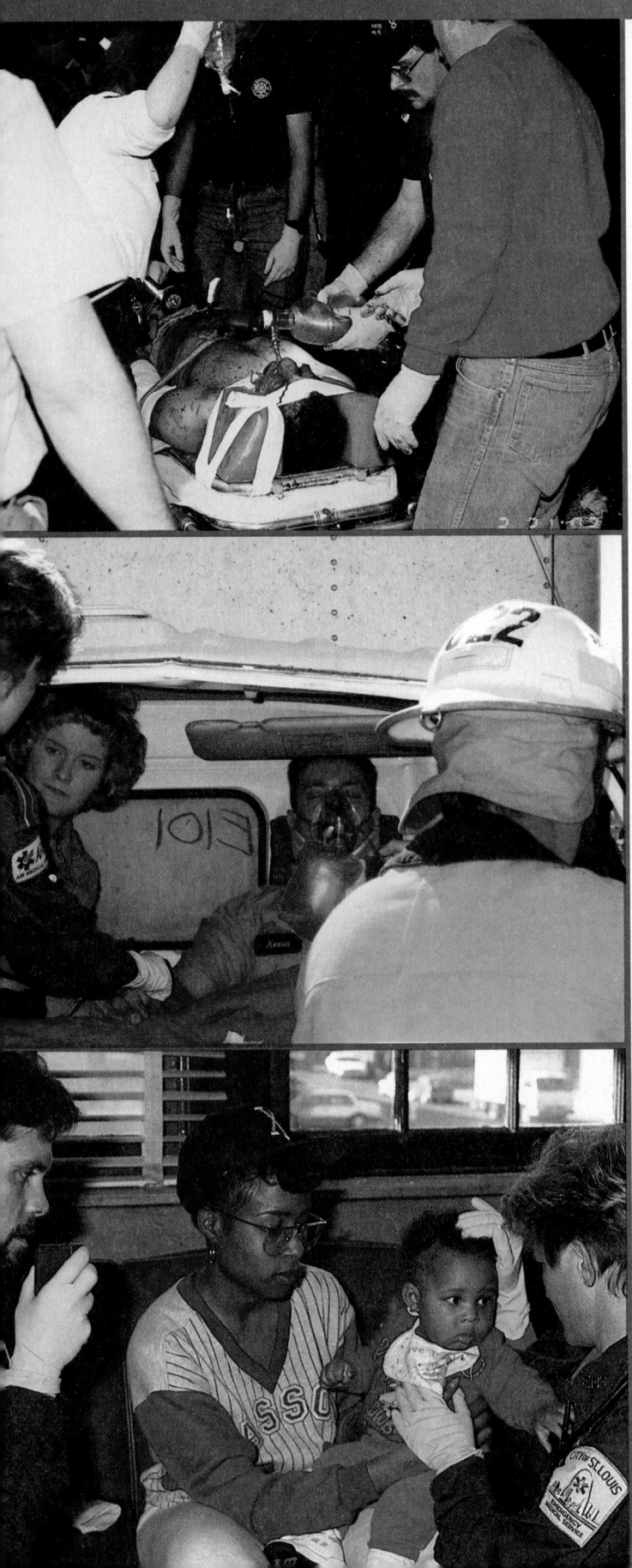

The absence of an adequate airway and ineffective ventilation are major causes of preventable death and cardiopulmonary complications in both medical and trauma patients. A thorough understanding of the respiratory system and mastery of airway management and ventilation are important aspects of emergency care.

As a paramedic, you should be able to:

1. Describe the function and location of the anatomical structures of the upper and lower airways.
2. Explain the mechanics of respiration.
3. Relate the partial pressures of gases in the blood and lungs to atmospheric gas pressures.
4. Describe pulmonary circulation.
5. Explain the process of exchange and transport of gases in the body.
6. Describe voluntary, chemical, and nervous regulation of respiration.
7. Discuss the assessment and management of medical or traumatic obstruction of the airway.
8. Describe preventative measures, assessment, and management for aspiration by inhalation.
9. Describe the use of manual airway maneuvers and mechanical airway adjuncts based on knowledge of their indications, contraindications, potential complications, and techniques.
10. Describe assessment techniques and devices used to ensure adequate oxygenation and elimination of carbon dioxide.
11. Discuss methods for patient ventilation based on knowledge of their indications, contraindications, potential complications, and use.
12. Explain variations in assessment and management of airway problems in pediatric and older patients.
13. Describe the use of oxygen regulators.
14. Given a patient scenario, select the correct oxygen delivery device based on a knowledge of proper indications and contraindications.

Section One
Anatomy and Physiology

● AIRWAY ANATOMY

The upper and lower respiratory system were described in Chapter 10. Readers are encouraged to refer to that chapter for a review.

KEY TERMS

anaerobic metabolism: Metabolism that occurs in the absence of oxygen.

atmospheric pressure: The pressure exerted by the weight of the atmosphere. At sea level this pressure is 760 mm Hg.

compliance: A measure of the distensibility of lung volume produced by a unit pressure change.

intrapulmonic pressure: The pressure of the gas within the alveoli; varies slightly above and below 760 mm Hg.

intrathoracic pressure: The pressure in the pleural space; usually 751 to 754 mm Hg.

minute volume: Tidal volume multiplied by respiratory rate, or the amount of gas inhaled or exhaled in 1 minute.

partial pressure: The pressure exerted by a single gas; denoted by a P.

pH: A scale representing the relative acidity or alkalinity of a solution.

pulmonary ventilation: Movement of air in and out of lungs, moving oxygen in and carbon dioxide out.

respiration: The process of molecular exchange of oxygen and carbon dioxide within the body's tissues.

tidal volume: The volume of air inspired or expired in a single, resting breath.

● THE MECHANICS OF RESPIRATION

Respiration is the exchange of oxygen and carbon dioxide between an organism and the environment. For this gas exchange to occur, air must move freely in and out of the lungs, bringing oxygen to the lungs and removing carbon dioxide **(pulmonary ventilation).** The two phases of respiration are as follows:

1. External respiration: the transfer of oxygen and carbon dioxide between the inspired air and pulmonary capillaries

2. Internal respiration: the transfer of oxygen and carbon dioxide between the peripheral blood capillaries and the tissue cells

Pressure Changes and Ventilation

Gas flows from an area of higher pressure or concentration to an area of lower pressure or concentration. For gas to flow into the lungs, a pressure gradient is required. This pressure gradient is produced by differences in atmospheric pressure, intrapulmonic pressure, and intrapleural or intrathoracic pressure.

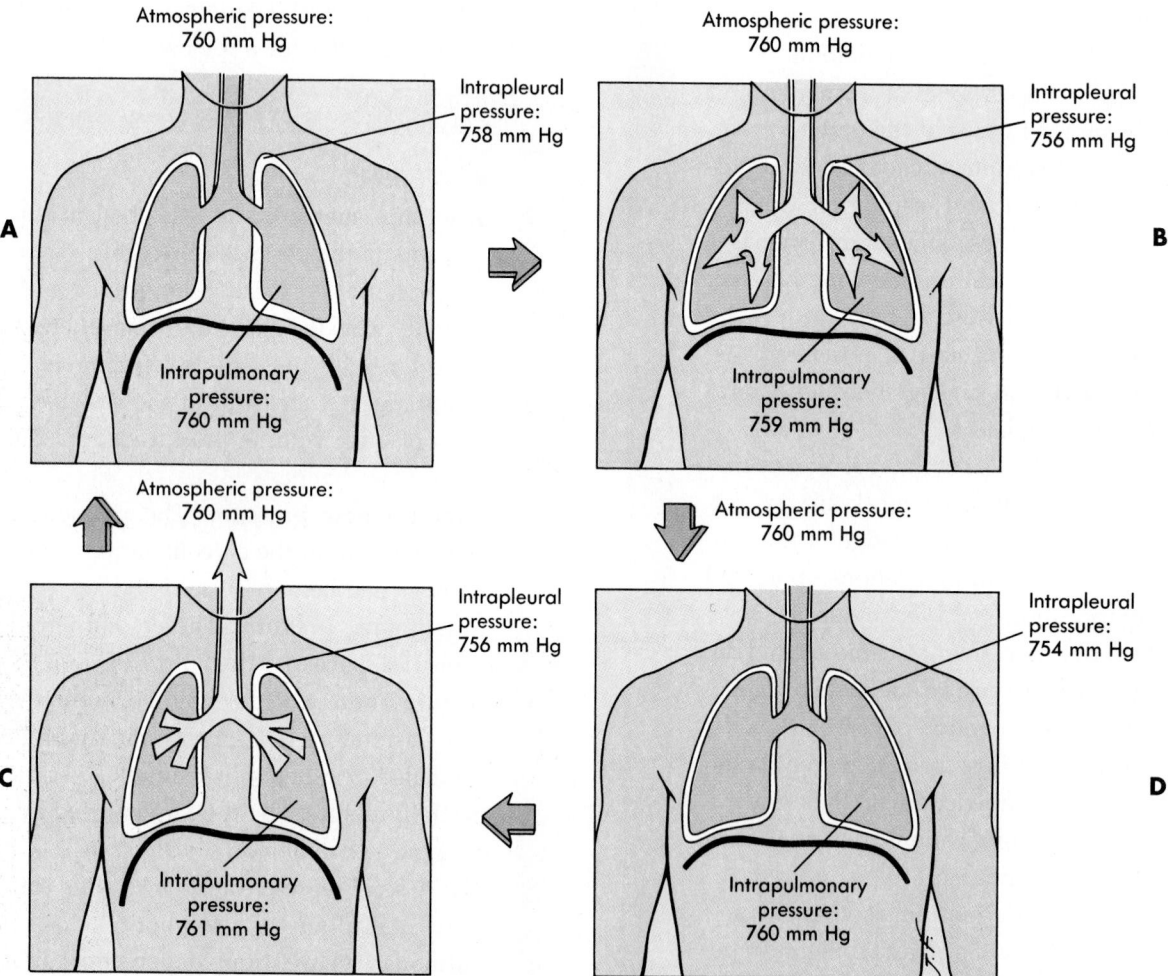

Fig. 12-1 Pressure changes during inspiration and expiration. **A,** At the end of expiration, intrapulmonary pressure equals atmospheric pressure, and there is no movement of air. **B,** During inspiration, the volume of the pleural space increases, causing the pressure in the intrapulmonary spaces (alveoli) to decrease. Air then flows from the outside of the body, where the pressure is greater (760 mm Hg), into the alveoli, where the pressure is lower (759 mm Hg). **C,** At the end of inspiration, intrapulmonary pressure again equals atmospheric pressure, and there is no movement of air. **D,** During expiration, the volume of the pleural spaces decreases, causing the intrapressure to increase. Because the intrapulmonary pressure exceeds the atmospheric pressure, air flows out of the body.

Atmospheric pressure is the pressure of the gas around us. It varies with differences in altitude, but at sea level it is 760 mm Hg. **Intrapulmonic pressure** is the pressure of the gas within the alveoli. Depending on the size of the thorax, this pressure varies slightly above and below 760 mm Hg, depending on whether it is measured during inspiration or expiration. Intrapleural or **intrathoracic pressure** is the pressure in the pleural space. It is normally less than atmospheric pressure (usually 751 to 754 mm Hg), but it may exceed atmospheric pressure during coughing and the straining associated with bowel movements.

During inspiration, the chest wall expands, which increases the size of the thoracic cavity and expands the lungs. The expansion results from muscle movement and negative intrapleural pressure in the pleural space. As the thorax expands, the lung space increases, causing a drop in intrapulmonic pressure of about 1 mm Hg below atmospheric pressure. The pressure gradient results in gas flow into the lungs. At end inspiration, the thorax stops expanding, the alveoli stop expanding, intrapulmonic pressure becomes equal to atmospheric pressure, and gas no longer moves into the lungs.

As the chest wall relaxes during expiration, the respiratory muscles are essentially at rest, and the process of inspiration reverses. Elastic recoil causes the thorax and lung space to decrease in size, which increases intrapulmonic pressure. The pressure gradient created in the thoracic cavity produces a decrease in alveolar volume and increases intrapulmonic pressure about 1 mm Hg over atmospheric pressure. The pressure gradient results in gas flow out of the lungs. At end expiration, the opposing forces and pressures equilibrate, and thoracic volume no longer decreases. Intrapulmonic pressure becomes equal to atmospheric pressure, and gas movement out of the lungs ceases (Fig. 12-1).

Muscles of Respiration

The expansion of the lungs and thorax during volume changes in intrapulmonic pressure is made possible by the movement of the diaphragm and the internal and external intercostal muscles (Fig. 12-2). During inspiration, the diaphragm contracts and the dome of the diaphragm flattens. This increases the superior-inferior dimension of the chest cavity. The internal and external intercostal muscles also contract, raising the ribs and increasing in the anterior-posterior and side-to-side dimensions of the chest cavity.

During expiration (a passive motion), relaxation of the diaphragm and external intercostal muscles allows the elastic recoil properties of the lungs to decrease the size (or volume) of the thoracic cavity. The ability of the lungs and thorax to expand

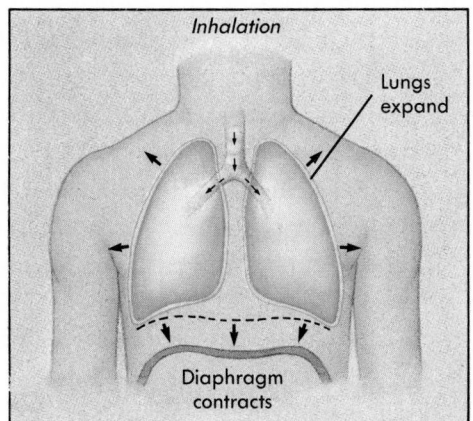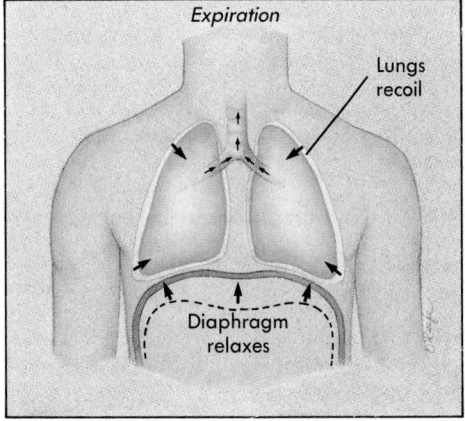

Fig. 12-2 Mechanics of breathing. During inhalation, the diaphragm contracts, increasing the volume of the thoracic cavity. The increase in volume results in a decrease in pressure, which causes air to rush into the lungs. During expiration, the diaphragm returns to an upward position, reducing the volume in the thoracic cavity. Air pressure increases and forces air out of the lungs.

during volume changes is referred to as **compliance.** The greater the compliance, the easier the expansion. Diseases that decrease compliance (for example, asthma, emphysema, bronchitis, pulmonary edema) increase the energy required for breathing.

The Work of Breathing

The energy required for normal, quiet breathing is approximately 3% of the total body expenditure in healthy individuals. Factors that increase the amount of energy needed for respiration are loss of pulmonary surfactant, an increase in airway resistance, and a decrease in pulmonary compliance, which together can increase the energy required for respiration up to one third of the total body expenditure.

The pulmonary alveoli have a natural tendency to collapse. This is a result of recoil caused by the elastic fibers in the alveolar walls and of surface tension, which results from the attractive forces between the water molecules in the alveolar membrane. Pulmonary surfactant lowers the surface tension by interspersing with the water molecules to reduce the cohesive force, which helps prevent collapsing of the alveolus at the end of expiration.

Surfactant is continuously replenished by certain alveolar cells, and its production is thought to be stimulated by normal ventilation. If surfactant production decreases (for example, in pneumonia), extremely high pressures may be required to maintain lung expansion.

Although elastic forces of the lung oppose lung expansion, viscous and frictional forces impede airflow into and out of the lungs. Much of the resistance to airflow is provided by the upper airways of the respiratory tract. The nasal passages cause about 50% of the total airway resistance during nose breathing. The mouth, pharynx, larynx, and trachea account for approximately 20% to 30% of airway resistance during quiet mouth breathing; this may increase to approximately 50% during periods of increased ventilation (for example, strenuous exercise).

Airway resistance falls dramatically as the bronchial tree continues to branch toward the alveoli because of the large increase in the total cross-sectional diameter of the airways. However, the presence of airway secretions or bronchiolar constriction can lead to increased airway resistance. These factors may occur separately but more commonly occur together (for example, in asthma). When resistance to airflow increases, the usual pressure gradient required for ventilation does not suffice, and muscular effort is required to create a larger pressure gradient.

Structural changes in the lung or thorax resulting from trauma or disease may also increase the amount of work required for effective ventilation. This increased work of ventilation is usually evident from the use of accessory muscles during labored breathing. These accessory muscles include the scalenes and sternocleidomastoid (deep muscles of the neck and thorax), posterior neck and back muscles, and the abdominal muscles (Fig. 12-3).

Lung Volumes and Capacities

At rest, the average adult male breathes approximately 10 to 12 times per minute. One fifth of this inspired air fills the upper respiratory tract and lower nonrespiratory bronchioles, never reaching the alveoli for gas exchange. This area is referred to as *anatomical dead space. Physiological dead space* refers to the anatomical dead space plus the volume of any nonfunctional alveoli. Normally, the anatomical and physiological dead space are nearly equal. However, in patients with respiratory diseases such as emphysema, the alveolar walls begin to degenerate. The destruction of alveolar walls can increase the size of the physiological dead space up to 10 times that of anatomical dead space (Fig. 12-4).

The lungs can hold approximately 8 times the amount of air contained in a normal, resting inhalation. From the first breath of life, the lungs are never completely emptied. A total of 16 breaths or more are required to renew this "residual volume" of air in the lungs.

Tidal volume is the volume of gas inhaled or exhaled during a normal breath. The average adult male tidal volume is approximately 500 to 600 ml. Of this, 150 ml remain in the anatomical dead space (the bronchi, bronchioles, and other

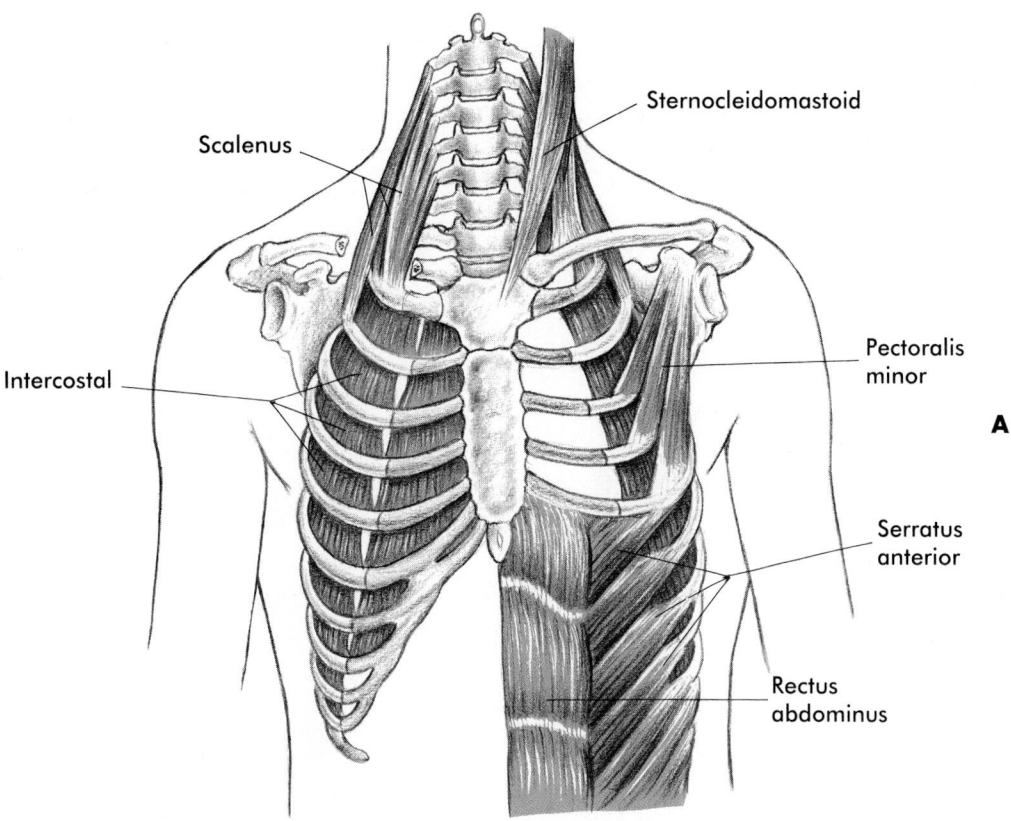

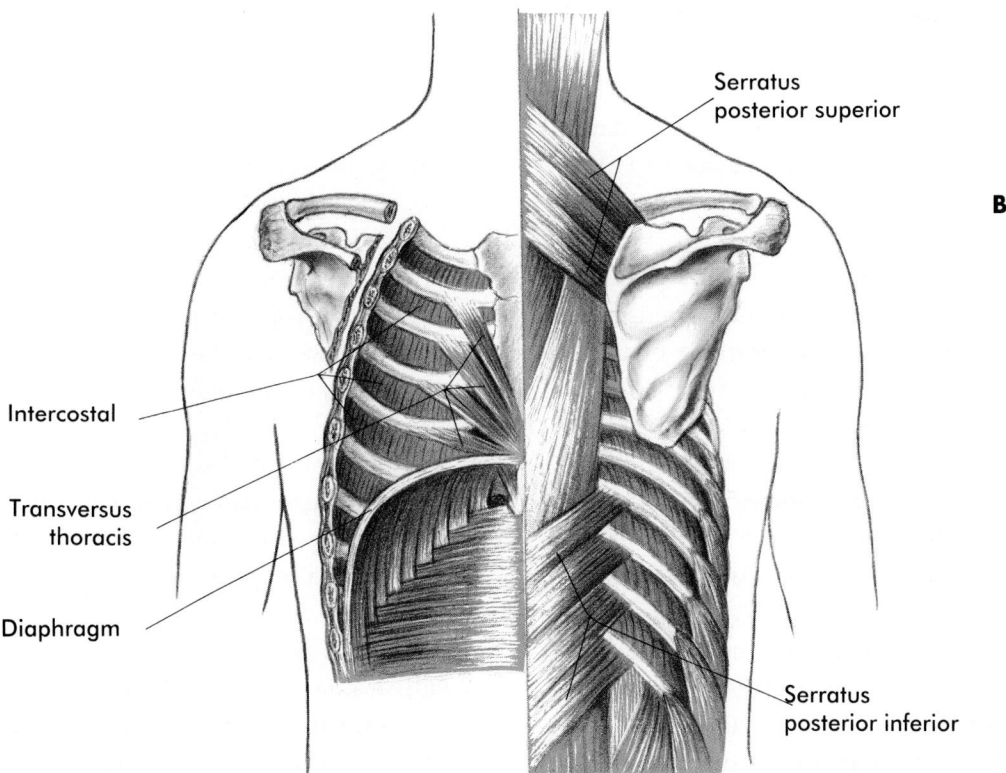

Fig. 12-3 Muscles of ventilation. **A,** Anterior view. **B,** Posterior view.

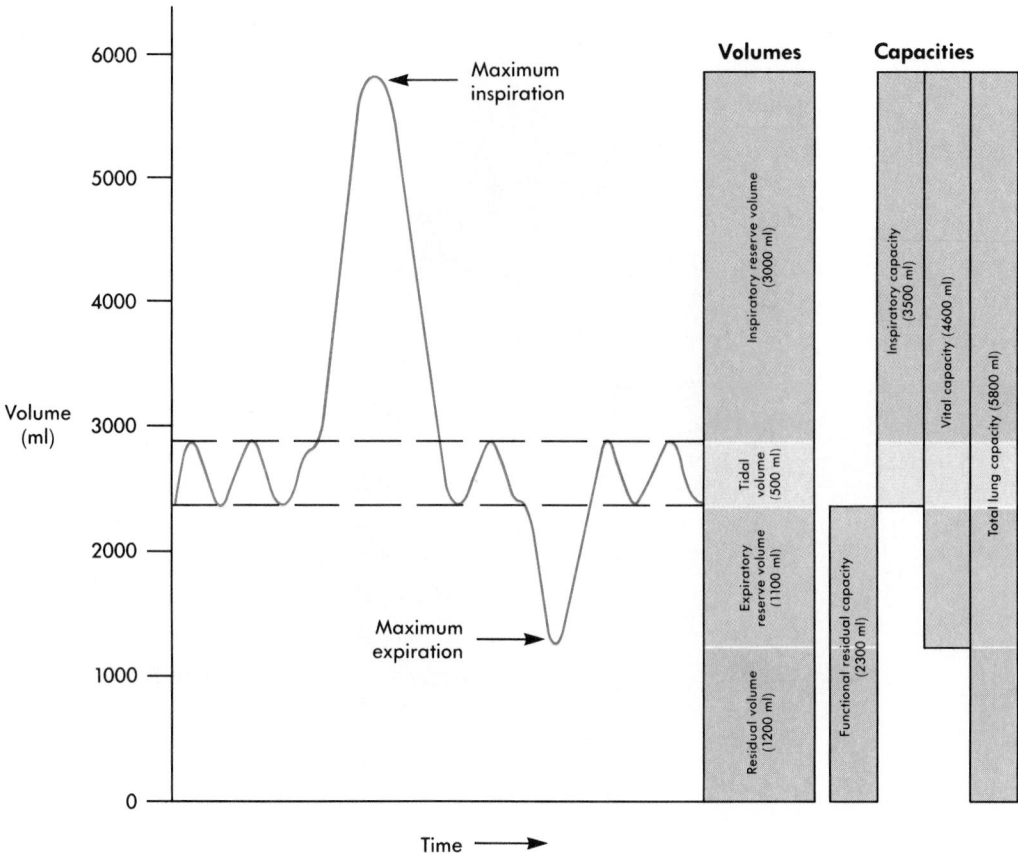

Fig. 12-4 Lung volumes and capacities. Tidal volume during resting conditions.

prealveolar structures) until it is exhaled during the following respiratory cycle. Therefore 150 ml of the atmospheric gas entering the respiratory system during each inspiration never reach the alveoli but are merely moved in and out of the airways. A paramedic observing the rise and fall of a patient's chest is indirectly observing tidal volume.

The inspiratory reserve volume is the amount of gas that can be forcefully inspired after inspiration of the normal tidal volume. This amount is usually 2000 to 3000 ml.

The expiratory reserve volume is the amount of gas that can be forcefully expired after expiration of the normal tidal volume. The normal expiratory reserve volume is usually less than the inspiratory reserve volume (approximately 1200 ml).

The residual volume is the gas that remains in the respiratory system after forced expiration. The normal residual volume is usually 1000 to 1200 ml.

The combined measurements of tidal volume, inspiratory reserve volume, expiratory reserve volume, and residual volume all constitute the maximum volume to which the lungs can be expanded.

Pulmonary capacities are the sum of two or more pulmonary volumes. The more common pulmonary capacities follow:

- Inspiratory capacity: Inspiratory capacity is the tidal volume plus the inspiratory reserve volume. This capacity reflects the amount of gas that a person can inspire maximally after a normal expiration (approximately 3500 ml).

- Functional residual capacity: Functional residual capacity is the expiratory reserve volume plus the residual volume. This capacity reflects the amount of gas remaining in the lungs at the end of a normal expiration (approximately 2300 ml).

- Vital capacity: Vital capacity is the volume of gas moved on deepest inspiration and expiration or the sum of the inspiratory reserve volume, the tidal volume, and the expiratory reserve volume. This capacity is approximately 4600 ml.
- Total lung capacity: Total lung capacity is the sum of the inspiratory and expiratory reserve volumes plus the tidal volume and the residual volume (approximately 5800 ml).

Minute Volume and Minute Alveolar Ventilation

The **minute volume** is the tidal volume multiplied by the respiratory rate, or the amount of gas inhaled or exhaled in 1 minute. If, for example, the patient's respiratory rate is 10 per minute and the resting tidal volume is 500 ml, the average minute volume is 5 L per minute.

Since much of the gas inspired during respiration fills the anatomical dead space before reaching the alveoli, that amount of air is unavailable for gas exchange. The amount of inspired gas that is available for gas exchange during 1 minute is referred to as the *minute alveolar ventilation.*

The minute alveolar ventilation is calculated by subtracting the amount of dead space from the tidal volume and then multiplying this figure by the respiratory rate

$$\text{Minute alveolar ventilation} =$$
$$\text{Tidal volume} - \text{Dead space} \times$$
$$\text{Respiratory rate}$$

If the tidal volume, the respiratory rate, or both, increase, the minute volume also increases. Conversely, the minute volume decreases if the tidal volume, respiratory rate, or both, decrease. The paramedic must note the depth of respiration (tidal volume) and the rate of ventilation to determine if the patient's respiratory status is adequate.

● THE MEASUREMENT OF GASES

In any mixture of gases, the combination of the pressures exerted by all the gases is referred to as the *total pressure*, and the pressure exerted by a single gas is referred to as the **partial pressure.** Partial pressure is measured in millimeters of mercury or torr. (One torr equals 1 mm Hg.) The partial pressure of a gas in a mixture is denoted by a P preceding the gas (for example, P_{O_2}).

The mixture of gases that compose the atmosphere exerts a combined partial pressure of 760 mm Hg at sea level. Nitrogen composes 79% of the volume of dry atmospheric gas at sea level. The partial pressure resulting from nitrogen is calculated by multiplying 79% by 760 mm Hg, which equals 600.2 mm Hg, or a P_{N_2} of 600 torr. Oxygen composes 21% of the volume of atmospheric gas. The partial pressure resulting from oxygen is 21% multiplied by 760 mm Hg, or 159.5 mm Hg (a P_{O_2} of 160 torr). Another partial pressure can be measured when gas comes into contact with water. The water molecules convert into a gas, evaporate, and exert a partial pressure known as *water vapor pressure* (P_{H_2O}).

The composition of alveolar gas and dry atmospheric gas are not the same. This is a result of several factors: the air entering the respiratory system being humidified by the body, the exchange of oxygen and carbon dioxide between the alveoli and the blood, and the incomplete emptying of the alveoli with expiration.

● PULMONARY CIRCULATION

The process of gas exchange in the lungs is opposite to that occurring in the tissues throughout the rest of the body. As inspired gas enters the lungs, the respiratory system brings oxygen to the blood and removes carbon dioxide. Blood low in oxygen converges on the heart from all parts of the body. Passing through the right side of the heart, the blood flows into either lung through the pulmonary artery. From there it flows into the smaller pulmonary arterioles and then into capillaries that surround each of the hundreds of millions of alveoli inside the lungs (Fig. 12-5).

The alveoli, now filled with a high concentration of oxygen molecules and a low concentration of carbon dioxide from inhaled air, have the pressure gradient required for gas exchange. Oxygen molecules move into the surrounding capillaries

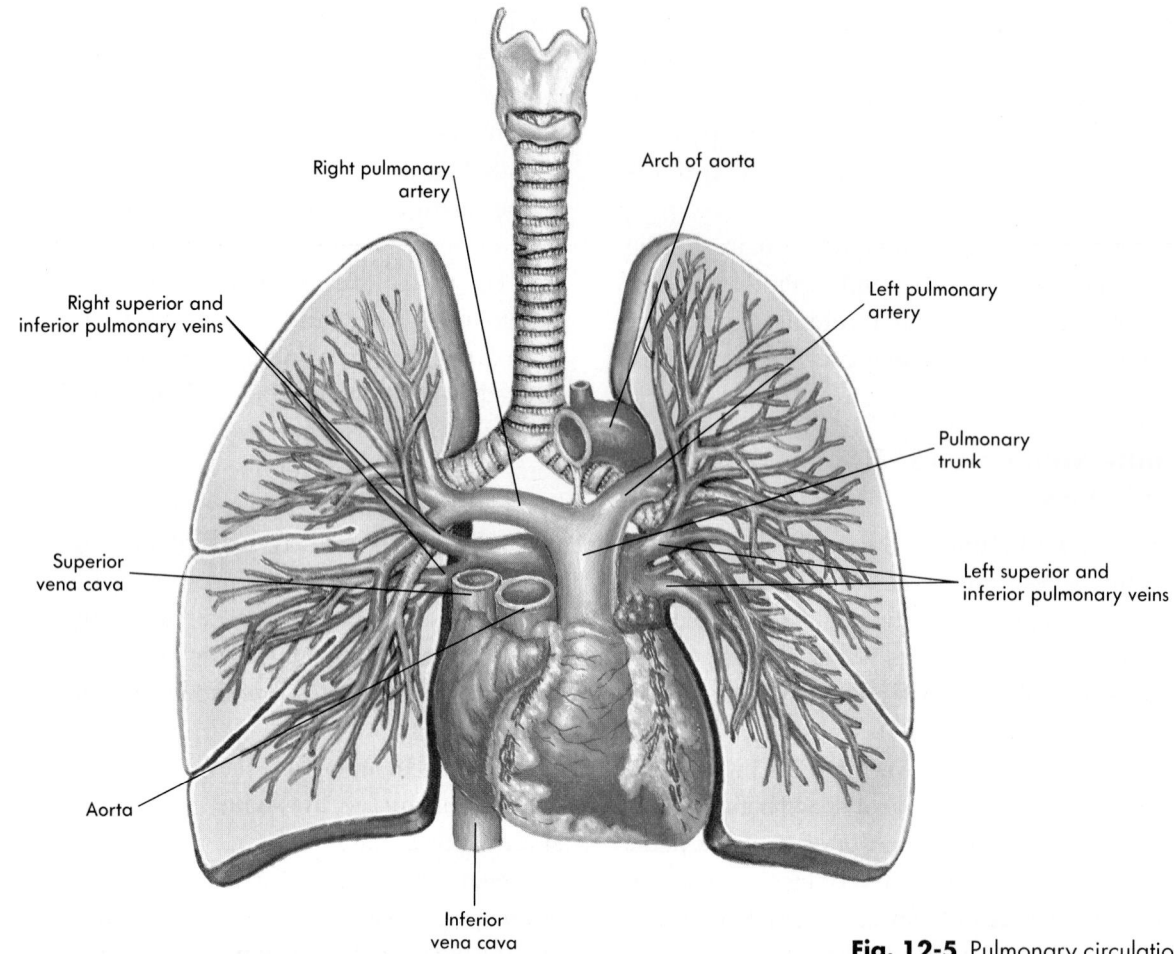

Fig. 12-5 Pulmonary circulation.

at the same time that carbon dioxide molecules move into the alveoli to be exhaled. The blood, now rich in oxygen, flows through the pulmonary venules into the pulmonary veins, then through the left side of the heart, and back out through the aorta to the body's tissues. To supply enough oxygen to the body tissues, an alveolus fills and empties more than 15,000 times in a day of normal breathing.

● EXCHANGE AND TRANSPORT OF GASES IN THE BODY

The volume of oxygen taken up in the lungs may be calculated from the difference in the amount of oxygen in the inspired and expired air. The volume of carbon dioxide that is eliminated may be determined in a similar fashion.

As described in Chapter 10, the metabolism is the total of all the chemical changes that occur in the body. In a healthy body with a constant metabolism, the relationship between tissue carbon dioxide production and oxygen consumption is fixed. Ordinarily, the amount of oxygen taken up by the capillary blood is greater than the amount of carbon dioxide released by the blood to the alveolar gas. Therefore the expired volume is slightly less than the inspired volume.

At rest, the combined consumption of all of the body cells is approximately 200 ml of oxygen each minute, with approximately the same amount of carbon dioxide being produced. Because approximately 20% of atmospheric gas is oxygen, the total oxygen inspired is 20% multiplied by 5 L, or approximately 1 L of oxygen per minute. Of this 200 ml cross the alveoli into the pulmonary capillaries, and the remaining 800 ml are exhaled. The

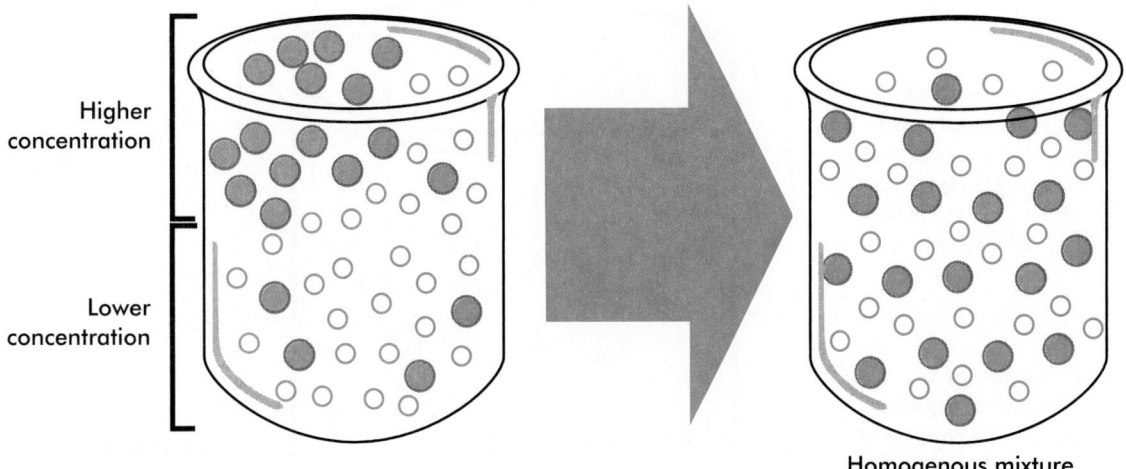

Higher concentration

Lower concentration

Homogenous mixture

Fig. 12-6 Random movement of gas is from a higher concentration to a lower concentration until a homogenous mixture of gases is achieved.

200 ml of oxygen are added to the quantity of oxygen already in the pulmonary capillaries and are then transported to the body tissues by the circulatory system. After the body cells use the necessary oxygen, the oxygen remaining in the blood returns to the heart and lungs. This exchange of oxygen and carbon dioxide is accomplished by a passive process known as *diffusion,* which is the tendency for molecules in solution to move from an area of higher concentration to an area of lower concentration.

Diffusion

Molecules of gases are in constant, random motion, which is fueled by collisions with other molecules. If the blood is divided by a permeable barrier, such as a capillary wall or cell membrane, many gas molecules will come into contact with and cross the barrier. There will be a much greater likelihood that highly concentrated molecules will strike and cross the membrane than less concentrated molecules. Thus the concentration of molecules across a permeable membrane tends to equilibrate (Fig. 12-6).

The diffusion of gases through liquid is determined by the pressure of the gases and the solubility of the gases in liquid (Fig. 12-7). When a free gas comes into contact with liquid, the number of gas molecules that dissolve in the liquid is directly

proportional to the pressure of the gas. When the free gas pressure is higher than the pressure of the gas in the liquid, enough molecules dissolve in the liquid for the free gas pressure to equal the dissolved gas pressure.

Conversely, if a liquid containing a dissolved gas at a high pressure is exposed to a free gas at a lower pressure, gas molecules leave the liquid and enter the free gas until the pressures become equal (the general gas law). This is the underlying theme of the exchange of gases between the cells and the capillary blood throughout the body. The free gas (P_{O_2}) in the lungs is greater than that in the blood stream, so oxygen diffuses from the lungs to the blood. The partial pressure of oxygen in the blood is higher than that in the peripheral tissues, so oxygen diffuses from the blood into the tissues.

In addition to the pressure of gases, the solubility of the gases in a liquid affects the behavior of the gases. The ease with which gases dissolve determines the absolute number of gas molecules that diffuse through the liquid at a given pressure. For example, if a liquid is exposed to two different gases at the same pressure, the number of molecules of each gas that will diffuse may not be identical because of the differing solubilities of the two gases.

Blood entering the pulmonary capillaries is systemic venous blood that has been circulated to the

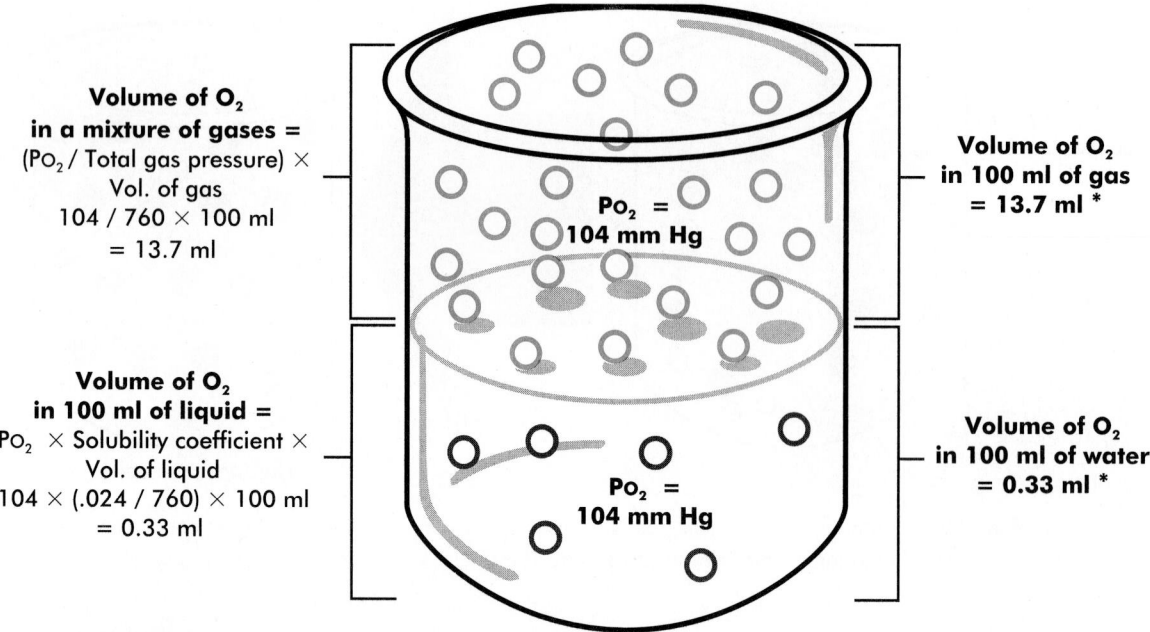

Volume of O₂ in a mixture of gases =
(Po₂ / Total gas pressure) × Vol. of gas
104 / 760 × 100 ml
= 13.7 ml

$$\text{Volume of O}_2 \text{ in a mixture of gases} = (\text{Po}_2 / \text{Total gas pressure}) \times \text{Vol. of gas}$$
$$104 / 760 \times 100 \text{ ml} = 13.7 \text{ ml}$$

Volume of O₂ in 100 ml of liquid =
Po₂ × Solubility coefficient × Vol. of liquid
104 × (.024 / 760) × 100 ml
= 0.33 ml

$$\text{Volume of O}_2 \text{ in 100 ml of liquid} = \text{Po}_2 \times \text{Solubility coefficient} \times \text{Vol. of liquid}$$
$$104 \times (.024 / 760) \times 100 \text{ ml} = 0.33 \text{ ml}$$

$\text{Po}_2 = 104 \text{ mm Hg}$

$\text{Po}_2 = 104 \text{ mm Hg}$

Volume of O₂ in 100 ml of gas = 13.7 ml *

Volume of O₂ in 100 ml of water = 0.33 ml *

Fig. 12-7 At equilibrium, the concentration of a gas in liquid is determined by its partial pressure in the gas and by its solubility in the liquid. *At atmospheric pressure (760 mm Hg) and 37° C.

lungs via the pulmonary arteries. This blood is relatively high in Pco_2 and low in Po_2. Because the alveoli contain a greater concentration of oxygen than the blood entering the pulmonary capillaries, oxygen molecules diffuse from the alveoli into the blood. Carbon dioxide moves from the blood, where it is more concentrated, to the alveoli, where it is less concentrated (Fig. 12-8).

The blood flowing through the pulmonary capillaries is separated from the alveolar air by a thin layer of tissue known as the *respiratory membrane.* This membrane is composed of the alveolar wall (surfactant, epithelial cells, and basement membrane), interstitial fluid, and the wall of the pulmonary capillary (basement membrane and endothelial cells). The differences in the partial pressures of oxygen and carbon dioxide on the two sides of the respiratory membrane result in the diffusion of oxygen into the blood and of carbon dioxide into the alveoli. With this diffusion, the capillary blood Po_2 rises, and the Pco_2 falls. The diffusion of these gases ceases when alveolar and capillary partial pressures become equal. In healthy individuals, this process of gas exchange is so rapid that the blood leaving the lungs to be pumped through the arteries has nearly the same

Po_2 (80 to 100 mm Hg) and Pco_2 (35 to 40 mm Hg) as alveolar air.

The diffusion of gases at the capillary-alveolar level may be affected in several ways. Some respiratory diseases (for example, emphysema) cause destruction and collapse of the alveolar walls (atelectasis), with the formation of fewer but larger alveoli. This degeneration results in a reduction of the total area available for diffusion. The alveolar capillary membrane may also become thickened or less permeable in some disease states, forcing gas molecules to travel farther and thereby decreasing the rate of diffusion. An example is pulmonary edema, in which fluid accumulates in the alveoli and pulmonary interstitial space and the gases must diffuse through a thicker-than-normal layer of fluid and tissue.

Acid-Base Balance

Acids and bases are produced by the body through normal metabolism. For physiological functioning (including respiration), a balance of these acids and bases must be maintained in a narrow range. Acids are substances that release, or donate, hydrogen ions (protons with a positive

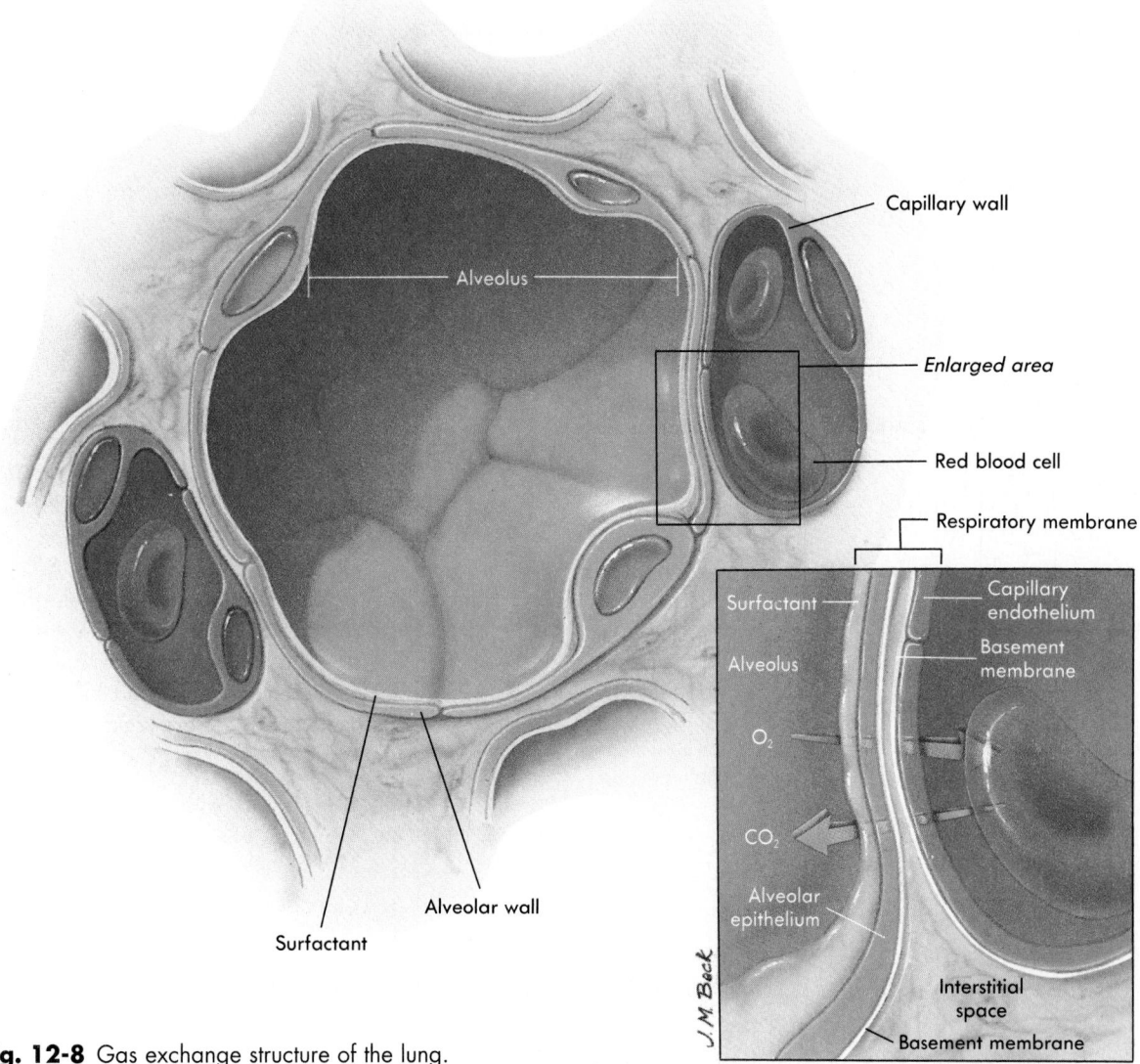

Fig. 12-8 Gas exchange structure of the lung.

charge); bases receive, or absorb, hydrogen ions. A solution increases in acidity as the hydrogen ion concentration increases and increases in alkalinity (basicity) when the hydrogen ion concentration falls.

Hydrogen ion concentration (moles/liter) is expressed by the term **pH,** which is the negative logarithm (base 10) of the concentration of hydrogen ions. A mole (in chemistry) is 6.023 multiplied by 10^{23} molecules (Avogadro's number). Although there is no need to grasp the meaning of a number this large in real terms, it is necessary to understand the significance of a small change in pH: *the strength of an acid or base changes by 10 times with each unit change of pH* (Fig. 12-9 and Box 12-1).

BOX 12-1

pH

A solution of pH 1 is 1,000,000 times as acidic as a solution of pH 7.

pH 2 is 100,000 times as acidic as pH 7.

pH 3 is 10,000 times as acidic pH 7.

pH 4 is 1000 times as acidic as pH 7.

pH 5 is 100 times as acidic as pH 7.

pH 6 is 10 times as acidic as pH 7.

A pH of 7 is neutral (distilled water).

A pH of 8 is 1/10 as acidic as a pH of 7, or 10 times as alkaline.

pH 9 is 1/100 as acidic and 100 times as alkaline as pH 7.

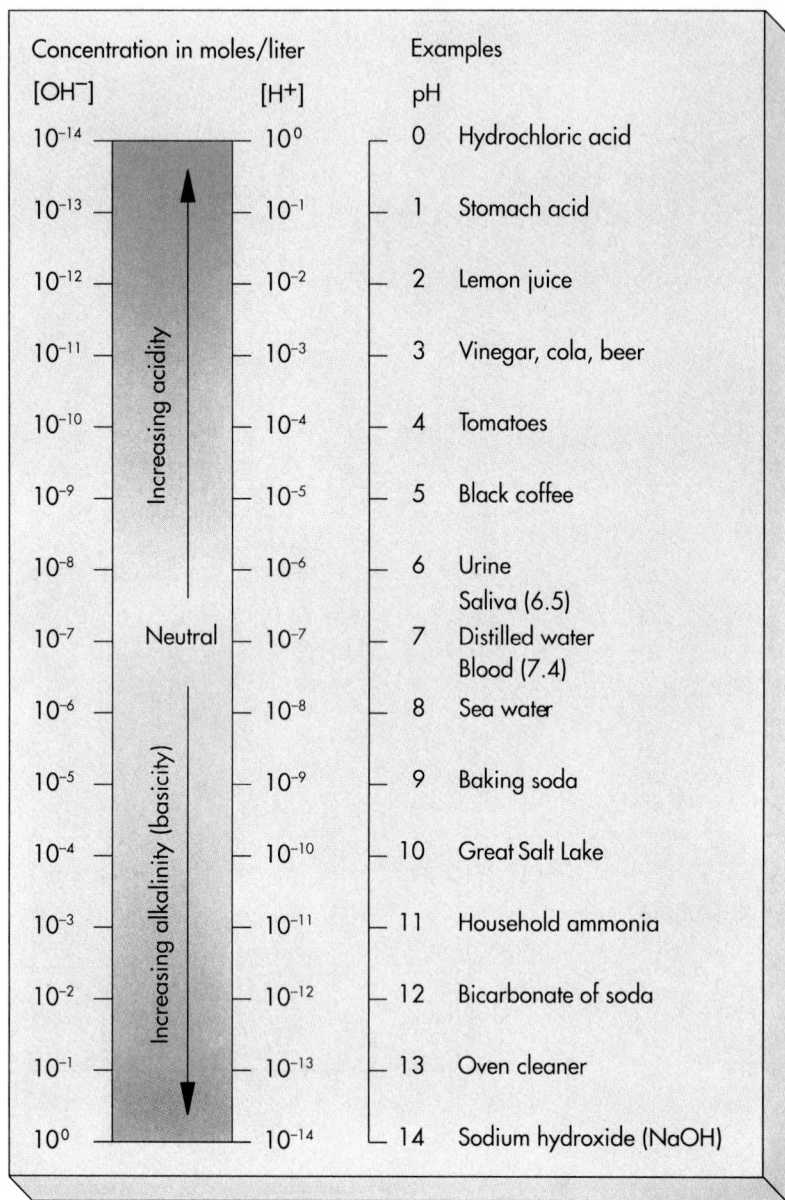

Concentration in moles/liter		Examples	
[OH⁻]	[H⁺]	pH	
10^{-14}	10^{0}	0	Hydrochloric acid
10^{-13}	10^{-1}	1	Stomach acid
10^{-12}	10^{-2}	2	Lemon juice
10^{-11}	10^{-3}	3	Vinegar, cola, beer
10^{-10}	10^{-4}	4	Tomatoes
10^{-9}	10^{-5}	5	Black coffee
10^{-8}	10^{-6}	6	Urine / Saliva (6.5)
10^{-7}	10^{-7}	7	Distilled water / Blood (7.4)
10^{-6}	10^{-8}	8	Sea water
10^{-5}	10^{-9}	9	Baking soda
10^{-4}	10^{-10}	10	Great Salt Lake
10^{-3}	10^{-11}	11	Household ammonia
10^{-2}	10^{-12}	12	Bicarbonate of soda
10^{-1}	10^{-13}	13	Oven cleaner
10^{0}	10^{-14}	14	Sodium hydroxide (NaOH)

(Increasing acidity / Neutral / Increasing alkalinity (basicity))

Fig. 12-9 pH scale. A pH of 7 is considered neutral. Values less than 7 are acidic (the lower the number, the more acidic the substance). Values greater than 7 are basic (the higher the number, the more basic the substance). Representative fluids and their approximate pH values are listed.

The acid-base balance of the body is maintained by several compensatory mechanisms that protect the body against rapid or severe changes in pH. The principal mechanism for providing stabilization is the bicarbonate buffer system. Bicarbonate (HCO_3^-) arises from the transport of carbon dioxide in the blood. Carbon dioxide dissolves in the water of blood and reacts with water in red blood cells to form carbonic acid (H_2CO_3). Carbonic acid breaks down into hydrogen and bicarbonate ions. At a physiological pH of 7.4, the normal ratio of carbonic acid to bicarbonate is 1:20, respectively, and is summarized by the chemical equation: $CO_2 + H_2O \rightleftharpoons H_2CO_3 \rightleftharpoons H + HCO_3^-$.

The direction in which this reaction proceeds depends in part on the presence of specific substrates. For example, inadequate ventilation with carbon dioxide retention causes the reaction to proceed to the right in an effort to balance the system. Conversely, if the system becomes acidic from an increase in hydrogen ions, the reaction would proceed to the left.

Oxygen Content of Blood

Oxygen is present in the blood in two forms: (1) physically dissolved in the blood and (2) chemically bound to hemoglobin (Hb) molecules. Compared with carbon dioxide and nitrogen, oxygen is relatively insoluble in water. Only 3 ml of oxygen can be dissolved in 1 L of blood at the normal alveolar and arterial P_{O_2} of 100 mm Hg. In contrast, 197 ml of oxygen (approximately 98%) are carried in red blood cells where it is chemically bound to hemoglobin (oxyhemoglobin). Hemoglobin can unload carbon dioxide and absorb oxygen 60 times faster than blood plasma.

Each hemoglobin molecule, when completely converted to oxyhemoglobin (HbO_2), can carry four molecules of oxygen and is said to be *fully saturated*. Hemoglobin nears full saturation at a P_{O_2} of 80 to 100 mm Hg.

The extent to which hemoglobin combines with oxygen increases rapidly when the P_{O_2} is 10 to 60 mm Hg. (Approximately 90% of total hemoglobin is combined with oxygen when the P_{O_2} is 60 mm Hg.) Further increases in P_{O_2} produce only small increases in oxygen binding to hemoglobin. Understanding this adaptive plateau at higher P_{O_2} values is important when dealing with patient situations involving high altitudes, excessive exercise, and cardiac and pulmonary disease. If P_{O_2} falls moderately, the amount of oxyhemoglobin decreases only slightly, still providing adequate oxygenation to tissues.

The partial pressure of oxygen in the blood plasma is the most important factor in determining the extent to which oxygen combines with hemoglobin. Oxyhemoglobin, however, does not contribute to the P_{O_2} of the blood. Only the physically dissolved oxygen molecules can create gas pressure. This oxygen uptake by hemoglobin molecules removes dissolved oxygen from blood plasma and maintains a low P_{O_2}, allowing diffusion to continue (Fig. 12-10).

Venous blood entering the lungs has a P_{O_2} of 40 mm Hg and a hemoglobin saturation of 75%. Oxygen diffuses from the alveoli (because of its higher P_{O_2} of 100 mm Hg) into the plasma. This diffusion raises plasma P_{O_2}, producing an increase in the uptake of oxygen by the hemoglobin molecules. In the tissue capillaries, this process is reversed. As the blood enters the capillaries, plasma P_{O_2} is greater than the P_{O_2} in the fluid surrounding the capillaries, causing diffusion across the capillary membranes to the cells of the tissues.

Carbon Dioxide Content of Blood

The amount of carbon dioxide produced by the body is relatively constant and is determined by the body's rate and type of metabolism. If the metabolic rate increases (for example, during exercise), more carbon dioxide is produced. Conversely, as the metabolic rate decreases (for example, during sleep), so does the production of carbon dioxide. Certain types of metabolic processes also result in increased carbon dioxide production. Examples include metabolism that occurs in the absence of oxygen **(anaerobic metabolism)** and the body's production of ketoacids in the absence of insulin (ketoacidosis).

Carbon dioxide is transported in the blood in three major forms: plasma, blood proteins, and bicarbonate ions. As with oxygen, the solubility of carbon dioxide in water is quite small, accounting for 8% of the carbon dioxide carried in plasma. Approximately 20% of the carbon dioxide is present in blood proteins (including hemoglobin), and approximately 72% is in the form of bicarbonate ions. When arterial blood flows through tissue capillaries, oxyhemoglobin gives up oxygen to the tissues, and carbon dioxide diffuses from the tissues into the blood. This results in a small amount of the carbon dioxide dissolving in the plasma.

Oxygen-free hemoglobin binds more readily to carbon dioxide than does hemoglobin bound with oxygen. Therefore some of the carbon dioxide that diffuses into red blood cells binds to hemoglobin to form carbaminohemoglobin (HbNHCOOH). The remainder of the carbon dioxide reacts with water to form carbonic acid. Bicarbonate, in contrast to carbon dioxide, is extremely soluble in water. Venous blood rich in carbon dioxide is returned to the lungs. Because the blood P_{CO_2} is greater than that in the alveoli, carbon dioxide from the blood diffuses into the alveoli. From

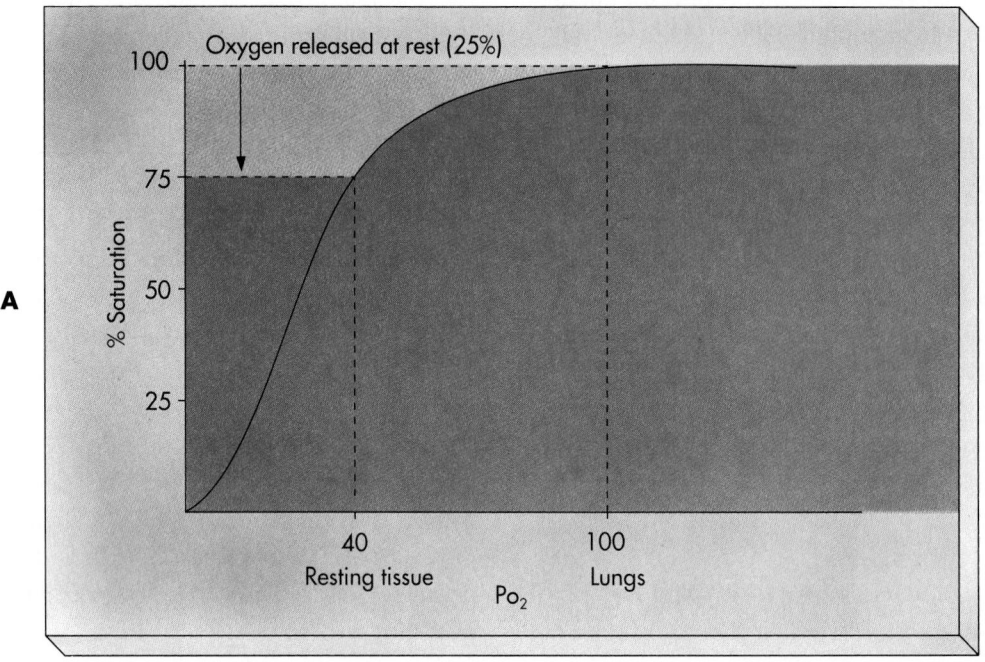

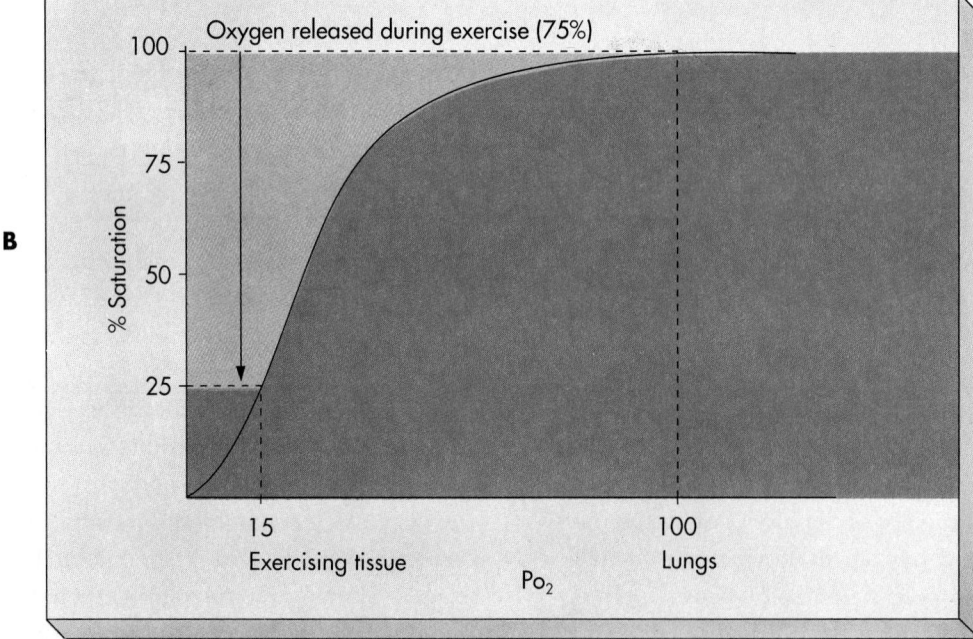

Fig. 12-10 Oxygen-hemoglobin dissociation curves. The graphs indicate the percentage of the hemoglobin saturated with oxygen as the partial pressure of oxygen increases. **A,** At the Po_2 in the lungs, hemoglobin is 100% saturated. At the Po_2 of resting tissues, hemoglobin is 75% saturated. Consequently, 25% of the oxygen picked up in the lungs is released to the tissues. **B,** In exercising tissues the percent saturation of hemoglobin can decrease to 25%, resulting in the release of 75% of the transported oxygen.

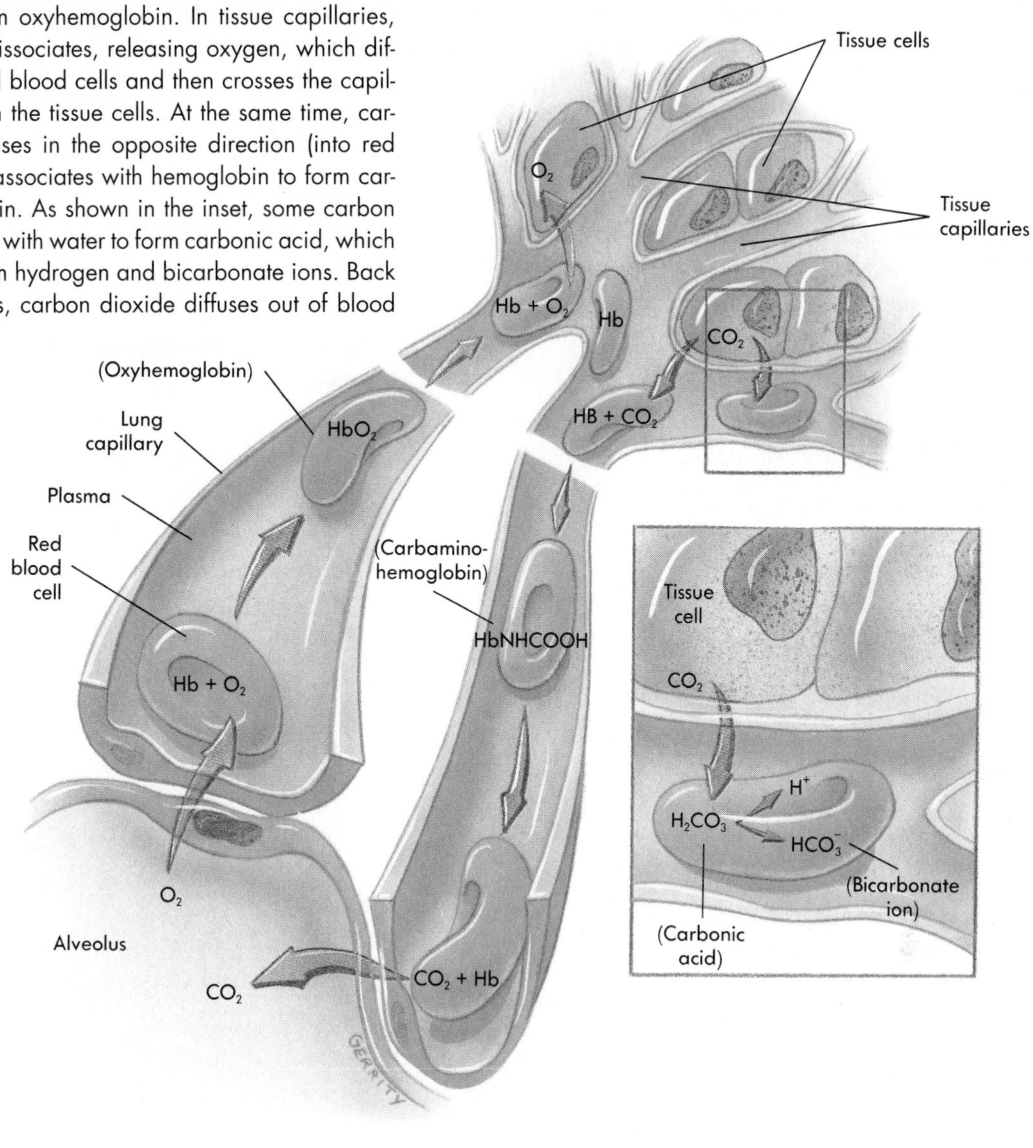

Fig. 12-11 Exchange of gases in lung and tissue capillaries. The diagram shows oxygen diffusing out of alveolar air into blood and associating with hemoglobin in lung capillaries to form oxyhemoglobin. In tissue capillaries, oxyhemoglobin dissociates, releasing oxygen, which diffuses from the red blood cells and then crosses the capillary wall to reach the tissue cells. At the same time, carbon dioxide diffuses in the opposite direction (into red blood cells) and associates with hemoglobin to form carbaminohemoglobin. As shown in the inset, some carbon dioxide combines with water to form carbonic acid, which dissociates to form hydrogen and bicarbonate ions. Back in lung capillaries, carbon dioxide diffuses out of blood into alveolar air.

there it is expired and eliminated from the body (Fig. 12-11).

Factors That Influence Blood Oxygenation

In healthy individuals, the breathing process allows blood to become fully oxygenated at the alveolus-capillary level and for carbon dioxide to be eliminated. (See Box 12-2 for abnormal conditions that can affect adequate blood oxygenation.)

● REGULATION OF RESPIRATION

Respiration is controlled at any instant by several factors. When evaluating any patient, it is important to consider the various mechanisms responsible for rhythmic ventilation, as well as the rate and depth of breathing.

Voluntary Control of Respiration

Breathing is primarily an involuntary process, but within limits, the pattern of respiration can be

---

BOX 12-2

Abnormal Conditions that Can Affect Blood Oxygenation

Depressed Respiratory Drive

Head injury

Central nervous system depressants (anesthetics, narcotics, sedatives)

Paralysis of Respiratory Muscles

Spinal injury

Inhalation injury

Neuromuscular diseases

Increased Resistance in the Respiratory Airways

Asthma

Bronchitis

Emphysema

Congestion

Decreased Compliance of the Lungs and Thoracic Wall

Interstitial lung disease as a result of inhalation of toxic substances

Infection (pneumonia, tuberculosis)

Lung cancer

Connective tissue diseases

Chronic pulmonary hypertension

Chest Wall Abnormalities

Chest wall injury (flail chest)

Scoliosis

Eschar (full-thickness burn contractions)

Decreased Surface Area for Gas Exchange

Emphysema

Tuberculosis

Pneumonia

Pulmonary edema

Atelectasis

Increased Thickness of Respiratory Membrane

Pulmonary edema (caused by heart failure, pneumonia, infections)

Intersitital fibrosis

Ventilation and Perfusion Mismatching*

Asthma

Pneumonia

Pulmonary embolus

Pulmonary edema

Myocardial infarction

Respiratory distress syndrome

Shock

Reduced Capacity of the Blood to Transport Oxygen

Anemias

Hemoglobin alterations

Carbon monoxide poisoning

Methemoglobinemia

*Ventilated alveoli that are not perfused or perfused alveoli that are not ventilated.

---

consciously altered. For example, voluntary hyperventilation can lead to a decrease in blood P_{CO_2}, vasodilation of the peripheral blood vessels, a decrease in blood pressure, or a combination. Hyperventilation causes excessive loss of exhaled carbon dioxide, which produces hypocarbia, resulting in cerebral vascular constriction, reduced cerebral perfusion, paresthesias, dizziness, or even feelings of euphoria.

Breathing can also be affected by voluntary apnea (for example, when a child holds his or her breath). When this occurs, the arterial blood P_{CO_2} level increases while the P_{O_2} level decreases. As the apneic period continues, the abnormal levels of P_{CO_2} and P_{O_2} trigger the respiratory centers and override the individual's conscious influence. If a loss of consciousness occurs, the respiratory center resumes normal function.

Fig. 12-12 Respiratory center and its control in the regulation of respiration.

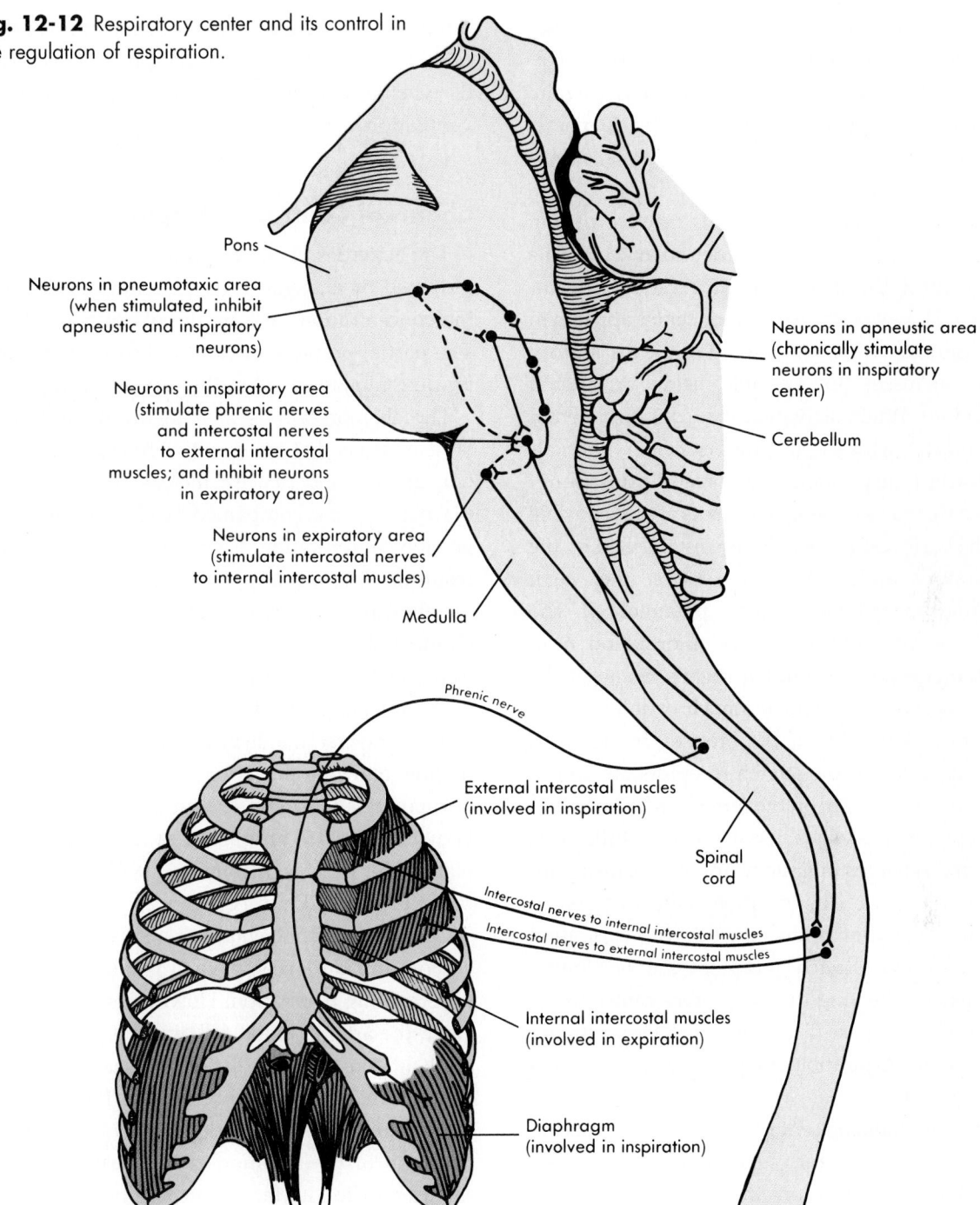

Pons

Neurons in pneumotaxic area (when stimulated, inhibit apneustic and inspiratory neurons)

Neurons in inspiratory area (stimulate phrenic nerves and intercostal nerves to external intercostal muscles; and inhibit neurons in expiratory area)

Neurons in expiratory area (stimulate intercostal nerves to internal intercostal muscles)

Medulla

Neurons in apneustic area (chronically stimulate neurons in inspiratory center)

Cerebellum

Phrenic nerve

External intercostal muscles (involved in inspiration)

Spinal cord

Intercostal nerves to internal intercostal muscles

Intercostal nerves to external intercostal muscles

Internal intercostal muscles (involved in expiration)

Diaphragm (involved in inspiration)

Nervous Control of Respiration

The inspiratory muscles (the diaphragm and intercostal muscles) are composed of skeletal muscle and cannot contract unless they are stimulated by nerve impulses. The two phrenic nerves responsible for moving the diaphragm originate from the third, fourth, and fifth cervical spinal nerves. The 11 pairs of intercostal nerves are formed from the first to the eleventh thoracic spinal nerves. The nerve impulses responsible for controlling these respiratory muscles originate within neurons of the medulla. This respiratory center is bilateral, with each lateral area composed of two groups of neurons (the inspiratory and expiratory centers) that are responsible for the basic rhythm of respiration (Fig. 12-12).

The inspiratory center neurons are spontaneously active and exhibit a pattern of activity, followed by fatigue and spontaneous activity again. When active, they send impulses along the spinal cord to the phrenic and intercostal nerves, stimulating the muscles of inspiration.

The expiratory center remains inactive during quiet respiration. The exact neural mechanisms that control the activity of this center are unknown. However, the expiratory center appears to be stimulated when the activity of the inspiratory center increases (for example, heavy or labored breathing). When activated, the expiratory center reciprocates with the inspiratory center, alternating forceful inspiration with forceful expiration.

Two distinct neural mechanisms are responsible for the basic respiratory rhythm established by the inspiratory and expiratory centers: the vagal (Hering-Breuer reflex) and the pneumotaxic. The vagus nerve conveys sensory information from the thoracic and abdominal organs. Some of the vagus nerve fibers end in stretch or inflation receptors in the walls of the bronchi, bronchioles, and lungs. When the stretch receptors are stimulated by expansion of the lungs, information is conveyed by the vagus nerve to the medulla. This in turn discharges inhibitory impulses, causing inspiration to cease. The cessation of breathing is followed by deflation of the lungs. As this expiration continues, the stretch receptors are no longer stimulated, allowing the inspiratory center to become active again. Therefore the Hering-Breuer reflex limits inspiration and prevents overinflation of the lungs.

The pneumotaxic center located in the pons superior to the respiratory center of the medulla has an inhibitory effect on the inspiratory center. When the activity of the inspiratory center ceases, inhibitory impulses no longer flow from the pneumotaxic center, and the inspiratory center discharges impulses to initiate inspiration. The pneumotaxic center appears to be active only in labored breathing. In quiet breathing, the stretch receptors are the primary control mechanisms for rhythmic breathing.

The apneustic center is located in the lower portion of the pons. Nerve impulses from this area stimulate the inspiratory center. The apneustic center neurons are constantly active at a baseline rate but are overridden by the pneumotaxic center when it is stimulated by demand for increased ventilation.

Chemical Control of Respiration

The activities of the respiratory centers are determined by changes in oxygen and carbon dioxide concentrations and by the pH of body fluids. The partial pressure of carbon dioxide is the major determinant in controlling respiration.

The chemoreceptive area in the medulla contains neurons that are sensitive to changes in carbon dioxide and pH. An increase or decrease in plasma P_{CO_2} is accompanied by changes in hydrogen ion concentration. An increase in P_{CO_2} and the resulting decrease in pH adversely affect cellular metabolism. Thus excess carbon dioxide must be eliminated to return the pH to normal limits. For example, the body responds to an increase in P_{CO_2} of 5 mm Hg with an increase in ventilation of 100%. Conversely, a decrease in P_{CO_2} inhibits ventilation, allowing the carbon dioxide produced by normal metabolism to accumulate and return the P_{CO_2} to normal. Through these adaptive mechanisms, the P_{CO_2} is maintained within a normal range of 35 to 45 mm Hg.

Compared with the body's sensitivity to pH and carbon dioxide levels, oxygen plays a small part in regulating respiration. However, if the P_{O_2} levels in the arterial blood fall and the pH and P_{CO_2} are held constant, ventilation increases.

Chemoreceptors monitor arterial P_{O_2}. They are located in the medulla and, peripherally, in the bifurcation of the common carotid arteries and in the arch of the aorta. These peripheral receptors are known as the *carotid* and *aortic bodies*. The carotid and aortic bodies are in intimate contact with the arterial blood of the great vessels. Therefore their blood supply is greater than their use of oxygen, and the P_{O_2} of their tissues is very close to that of arterial blood. The nerve fibers from these bodies enter the brain stem, where they synapse with the neurons of the medulla and initiate a respiratory response.

Although carbon dioxide and hydrogen ion concentrations are the most important regulators of respiration, reduced P_{O_2} in the arterial blood may also play an important stimulatory role. In conditions of shock in which the patient is hypotensive, for example, the P_{O_2} in the arterial blood may fall to levels low enough to stimulate the sensory receptors of the carotid and aortic bodies, leading to an increased rate and depth of ventilation. This can occur without a significant change in the blood P_{CO_2}, although it is usually accompanied by metabolic acidosis secondary to anaerobic metabolism.

A situation in which P_{O_2} clearly plays a role in respiratory regulation occurs at high altitudes where the barometric pressure is low. The low barometric pressure causes the P_{O_2} in the arterial blood to fall low enough to stimulate the carotid and aortic bodies. Even though the arterial P_{O_2} is reduced, the body's ability to eliminate carbon dioxide is not greatly affected by lowered barometric pressure. The blood carbon dioxide levels become lower than normal because of the increased ventilations initiated in response to the lowered arterial P_{O_2}.

Patients with severe emphysema or chronic bronchitis have chronically elevated P_{CO_2} and may rely on the low P_{O_2} as the main drive for ventilation (hypoxic drive). In diseases with chronic P_{CO_2} elevation, the chemoreceptors become less sensitive to a high carbon dioxide level and fail to be stimulated by it. Over time, hypoxia becomes the only remaining respiratory drive.

Control of Respiration by Other Factors

Several other factors may contribute to the control of respiration. These include body temperature, drugs and medications, pain, emotion, and sleep.

An increase in body temperature caused by febrile illness or physical activity can affect the respiratory center neurons, causing an increase in ventilation. Conversely, significant decreases in body temperature can lower the ventilation rate. An extreme example of this phenomenon is hypothermia.

Some medications, such as epinephrine, stimulate respiration by unknown mechanisms. The re-

lease of epinephrine increases ventilation by promoting cellular metabolism during stressful events and strenuous exercise. Diazepam and morphine used in prehospital care may decrease respirations. Patients taking an overdose of narcotics or barbiturates can become apneic.

Painful stimulation anywhere in the body may produce a reflex stimulation of ventilation. Examples include the previous practice of spanking a newborn and stepping into a cold shower.

The movement of air into and out of the lungs is required during expressions of emotions such as laughing or crying. Stimulation of ventilation (rapid breathing) also occurs in situations involving fear and anger.

As the body's metabolism slows, so do the impulses for stimulation of the respiratory centers. Therefore during periods of decreased activity, ventilation decreases.

Modified Forms of Respiration

The cough reflex and the sneeze reflex are protective mechanisms with the function of dislodging foreign matter or irritants from the respiratory passages. Coughing is generally preceded by an inspiration of greater amplitude than normal (approximately 2.5 L of gas). The glottis then closes, and the muscles of the thorax contract forcibly, causing an increase in intrapulmonic pressure. The pressure change in the lungs increases to approximately 100 mm Hg. When this pressure is reached, the vocal cords part, and air escapes from the lungs at a high velocity, carrying foreign particles and substances.

Sneezing is a violent expulsion of gas that is forced or directed through the nasal cavity. It may occur as a result of nasal irritants, stimulation of the fifth cranial (trigeminal) nerve in the nose, or exposure to bright lights. During the sneeze reflex, the uvula and the soft palate are depressed to direct air through both the nasal passages and the oral cavity.

Other forms of modified respiration include the sigh and the hiccough (rarely, these are chronic disorders). Sighing is a slow, deep inspiration followed by a prolonged expiration. This modified respiratory effort is thought to be a protective reflex to hyperinflate the lungs and to reexpand alveoli that might have been collapsed (atelectasis).

The hiccough results from a spasmodic contraction of the diaphragm with the sudden inspiration cut short by the closure of the glottis. Hiccoughs serve no known useful physiological purpose and usually pass with time.

Section Two
Pathophysiology

A common cause of inadequate ventilation is upper airway obstruction and aspiration by inhalation. Establishing and maintaining a patent airway in any patient who has respiratory compromise from any cause is the most important lifesaving maneuver and should always be a first-order priority of patient care.

● FOREIGN BODY AIRWAY OBSTRUCTION

According to the National Safety Council, there were approximately 3600 deaths in 1988 from foreign body obstruction of the airway.[1] Immediate removal of the obstruction might have prevented the resulting hypoxemia, unconsciousness, or cardiopulmonary arrest that caused these deaths.

Airway Obstruction in the Conscious Patient

Meat is the most common cause of foreign body airway obstruction in conscious adults (although a variety of other foods and foreign objects are also responsible for obstruction in children and in some adults).[2] Factors associated with choking include large, poorly chewed pieces of food; elevated blood alcohol level; and poor-fitting dentures. Often, the patient is middle-aged or older.

Foreign bodies may cause either partial or complete airway obstruction. Patients with partially obstructed airways can usually speak (phonation) and can produce a forceful cough in an effort to expel the object. If air exchange is adequate, no rescuer intervention is recommended in these situations.[2] The patient should be encouraged to persist with monitored, spontaneous coughing and breathing efforts. If the obstruction persists or air exchange becomes inadequate (evidenced by a weak, ineffective cough; wheezing; increased respiratory difficulty; decreased air movement; and cyanosis), the patient should be managed as though a complete airway obstruction exists.

Patients with complete airway obstruction cannot speak, exchange air, or cough. Often, these patients grasp their neck between their thumbs and fingers (a universal sign of choking). These patients require immediate rescuer intervention. In addition to the threat of hypoxemia from complete airway obstruction, anoxia may precipitate an acute myocardial infarction in patients with concurrent atherosclerotic cardiovascular disease, leading inevitably to cardiac arrest in all patients if not corrected within minutes. Guidelines for managing the obstructed airway in conscious adult and pediatric patients are given in Fig. 12-13.[3]

Airway Obstruction in the Unconscious Patient

Although upper airway obstruction may lead to unconsciousness and cardiopulmonary arrest, more often the obstruction is caused by unconsciousness and cardiopulmonary arrest.[2] The primary source of upper airway obstruction in the unconscious patient is the tongue.

The tongue is attached to the mandible by the muscles that form the floor of the mouth. The normal tone of these muscles allows for air exchange through a patent posterior pharynx. If a patient is unconscious or has a neuromuscular dysfunction, laxity of these muscles may cause airway occlusion by the tongue. Some causes of airway obstruction by the tongue are the following:

- Cardiac arrest
- Trauma
- Stroke
- Intoxication with alcohol, barbiturates, or other psychotropic drugs
- Paralysis resulting from muscle relaxants

	OBJECTIVES	ACTIONS		
		Adult (over 8 yrs)	Child (1 to 8 yrs)	Infant (under 1 yr)
Conscious victim	1. Assessment: Determine airway obstruction.	Ask, "Are you choking?" Determine if victim can cough or speak.		Observe breathing difficulty.
	2. Act to relieve obstruction.	Perform five subdiaphragmatic abdominal thrusts (Heimlich maneuver).		Give up to five back blows. Give five chest thrusts.
	3. Be persistent.	Repeat Step 2 until obstruction is relieved or victim becomes unconscious.		
Victim who becomes unconscious	4. Position victim.	Turn on back as unit, supporting head and neck, face up, arms by sides.		
	5. Check for foreign body.	Perform tongue-jaw lift and finger sweep.	Perform tongue-jaw lift. Remove foreign object only if visible.	
	6. Give rescue breaths.	Open airway with head-tilt/chin-lift. Attempt rescue breathing. If first ventilation attempt is unsuccessful, reposition head and reattempt ventilation.		
	7. Act to relieve obstruction.	Perform five subdiaphragmatic abdominal thrusts (Heimlich maneuver).		Give up to five back blows. Give five chest thrusts.
	8. Check for foreign body.	Perform tongue-jaw lift and finger sweep.	Perform tongue-jaw lift. Remove foreign object only if visible.	
	9. Attempt rescue breathing.	Open airway with head-tilt/chin-lift. Attempt rescue breathing (slow ventilations 1½-2 sec each for adult and 1-1½ sec each for child or infant).		
	10. Be persistent.	Repeat Steps 6-8 until obstruction is relieved.		
Unconscious victim	1. Assessment: Determine unresponsiveness.	Tap or gently shake shoulder. Shout, "Are you okay?"		Tap or gently shake shoulder.
	2. Position victim.	Turn on back as unit, supporting head and neck, face up, arms by sides.		
	3. Open airway.	Open airway with head-tilt/chin-lift.		Open airway with head-tilt/chin-lift without hyper-extension.
	4. Assessment: Determine breathlessness.	Maintain an open airway. Place ear over mouth; observe chest. Look, listen, feel for breathing (3-5 sec).		
	5. Give rescue breaths.	Seal mouth-to-mouth with barrier device or bag-valve device.		Seal mouth-to-nose/mouth with barrier device.
		Attempt rescue breathing (slow ventilations 1½-2 sec each for adult and 1-1½ sec each for child or infant). If first ventilation is unsuccessful, reposition head and reattempt ventilation.		
	6. Act to relieve obstruction.	Perform five subdiaphragmatic abdominal thrusts (Heimlich maneuver).		Give up to five back blows. Give five chest thrusts.
	7. Check for foreign body.	Perform tongue-jaw lift and finger sweep.	Perform tongue-jaw lift. Remove foreign object only if visible.	
	8. Provide rescue breathing.	Open airway with head-tilt/chin-lift. Attempt rescue breathing (slow ventilations 1½-2 sec each for adult and 1-1½ sec each for child or infant).		
	9. Be persistent.	Repeat Steps 6-8 until obstruction is relieved.		

Fig. 12-13 Foreign body airway obstruction management.

• Myasthenia gravis
• Fractured facial and nasal bones

Guidelines for managing obstructed airways in both adult and pediatric patients who are unconscious are also described in Fig. 12-13.[3]

Laryngeal Edema

Swelling of the glottic and subglottic tissues of the airway can lead to laryngeal closure. The formation of edema may result from inflammatory or mechanical causes such as epiglottitis, croup, allergic reaction, thermal injuries, strangulation, blunt trauma, or drowning. Associated swelling may partially or completely obstruct the airway, making aggressive airway management mandatory for patient survival.

Fractured Larynx

The most common cause of external trauma to the larynx is motor-vehicle accidents. If a trauma patient has localized laryngeal pain, stridor, hoarseness, difficulty with speech, or hemoptysis, a fracture of the larynx should be suspected. Larynx injury can result in nonsupport of the vocal cords, causing them to collapse into the tracheal-laryngeal lumen and obstruct the airway. Subcutaneous emphysema, dysphagia, and throat discomfort that increases with coughing or swallowing indicate the possibility of an impending respiratory arrest. The paramedic should remain alert to the possibility of laryngeal fracture because laryngeal edema can rapidly occlude the airway.

Certain types of injury, such as clothesline injury and blunt trauma to the neck, are relatively likely to cause laryngeal fracture. Rapid intervention is needed to obtain a patent airway before complete occlusion is caused by laryngeal edema and hemorrhage.

Tracheal Trauma

Trauma to the trachea is rare but serious. The most common site for tracheal injury is in the area bordered by the cricoid cartilage and the third tracheal ring. This injury seldom occurs as an isolated event and is often associated with other injuries to the surrounding esophagus and cervical spine. In addition, there is usually central nervous system injury and abdominal and thoracic trauma.

● ASPIRATION BY INHALATION

Aspiration is the active inhalation of food, a foreign body, or fluid (vomitus, saliva, blood, neutral liquids) into the airway. Depending on the type of aspiration, the syndrome may precipitate spasm, mucus production, atelectasis, pH change (if the aspirant is acidic), or cough. The primary means of preventing aspiration is to control and maintain the airway; prevention is far superior to any known treatment. The paramedic should always be prepared for the possibility of aspiration in patients with a decreased level of consciousness.

Large food particles and other foreign bodies can occlude the airway and cause hypoventilation of distal lung segments. The size of the particle determines which airway is obstructed and to what extent.

Some 80% of the approximate 3600 deaths each year from foreign body aspiration occur in children.[1] Running with food or other objects in the mouth, seizures, and forced feeding are among the risk factors in this age group. Hot dogs and peanuts are foodstuffs children commonly aspirate. In adults, obstruction may result from dental or nasal surgery, unconsciousness, swallowing poorly chewed food, and alcohol intoxication.

Some 60% of foreign bodies are found in the right bronchus, 19% in the left and 21% at the larynx or vocal cords.[4] (The left mainstem bronchus branches from the trachea at a 45- to 60-degree angle, so foreign body occlusion of this bronchus is less likely than of the right mainstem bronchus, which is shorter, wider, and more vertical.) When the larynx or trachea is completely obstructed, the victim can die from asphyxiation within minutes.

The average adult stomach has a capacity of 1.4 L and manufactures an additional 1.4 L of gastric juices in each 24-hour period. Hydrochloric acid is manufactured by special cells in the gastric mucosa. With the assistance of a protein-dissolving enzyme (pepsin), this acid helps break down large pieces of food into smaller ones. Vomitus contains not only partially digested food particles but also acidic gastric fluid.

Saliva is a watery, slightly alkaline fluid secreted in the mouth by the major salivary glands and the smaller salivary glands in the mucous membranes that line the mouth. Saliva contains the digestive enzyme amylase, which helps break down carbohydrates. In addition to this enzyme, saliva contains minerals such as sodium, calcium, and chloride; proteins; mucin (the principal constituent of mucus); urea; white blood cells; and debris from the lining of the mouth.

Approximately half the volume of blood consists of cells (erythrocytes, leukocytes, and platelets). The remainder is plasma, a watery solution that contains dissolved proteins, sugars, fats, and minerals.

The consequences of aspiration of neutral liquids (liquids that are not acidic or basic) are easier to reverse with supportive therapy than the consequences of aspiration of other fluids. Nonetheless, aspiration of a large volume of neutral liquids is associated with a high mortality rate.

Pathophysiology of Aspiration

The predisposing conditions associated with high risk of aspiration are reduced level of consciousness and mechanical disturbances of the airway and gastrointestinal tract.

A reduced level of consciousness may be caused by trauma, alcohol and drug intoxication, a seizure disorder, cardiopulmonary arrest, a cerebrovascular accident, and central nervous system dysfunction. The common element of these conditions is depression or loss of the gag reflex, with or without the presence of a full stomach.

A common type of mechanical disturbance is iatrogenic (caused by medical procedures) and involves the use of various devices to control upper airway problems. Examples include removal of an esophageal obturator airway (risk of vomiting on removal), placement of a nasogastric tube (the artificial opening through the esophageal sphincter increases the risk of regurgitation and aspiration), and intubation, which requires an adequate seal at the tracheal orifice to prevent aspiration. These mechanical airway devices are discussed later in this section.

Other mechanical disturbances that may lead to a high risk of aspiration include tracheostomy and esophageal motility disorders such as hiatal hernia and esophageal reflux. (Up to 70% of patients with permanent tracheostomies have mild forms of aspiration.[5]) Other patients at risk include those with either an ileus or a mechanical bowel obstruction.

The potential for aspiration increases whenever vomiting occurs. Vomiting follows stimulation of the vomiting center of the medulla. This stimulation can result from irritation anywhere along the gastrointestinal tract, from information passed to the medulla from the frontal lobes of the brain, or from disturbances in the balance mechanism of the inner ear. Once this center is stimulated, the following seven events occur:

1. A deep breath is taken.
2. The hyoid bone and larynx are elevated, opening the preesophageal sphincter.
3. The opening of the larynx is closed.
4. The soft palate is elevated, closing the posterior nares.
5. The diaphragm and the abdominal muscles are forcefully contracted, compressing the stomach and increasing the intragastric pressure.
6. The lower esophageal sphincter is relaxed, and stomach contents are propelled into the lower esophagus.
7. If the patient is unconscious or unable to protect his or her airway, pulmonary aspiration may occur.

Effects of Pulmonary Aspiration

The following statistics show the significance of pulmonary aspiration to the prehospital provider[5]:

- Aspiration is the chief cause of death after head injury and cerebrovascular accident.
- Patients who had an episode of aspiration are hospitalized on average 21 days longer than those who did not.
- Mortality from massive aspiration of gastric contents ranges from 70% to 90%.

The severity of pulmonary aspiration depends on the pH of the aspirated material, the volume of the aspirate, and the presence in the aspirate of particulate matter such as food and bacterial contamination. It is generally accepted that when the pH level of an aspirate is 2.5 or less, a severe pulmonary response occurs. When the pH is below 1.5, the patient usually dies. The mortality among patients who aspirate material grossly contaminated, as in bowel obstruction, approaches 100%.

The toxic effects of gastric acid (with a pH of less than 2.5) on the lungs can be equated with those of chemical burns. These are severe injuries that produce pulmonary changes such as destruction of surfactant-producing alveolar cells, alveolar collapse and destruction, and destruction of pulmonary capillaries. The permeability of the capillaries increases with massive flooding of the alveoli and bronchi with fluid. The resulting pulmonary edema creates areas of hypoventilation, shunting, and severe hypoxemia. The massive fluid shift from the intravascular compartment to the lungs may also produce hypovolemia severe enough to require volume replacement.

Management

The risk of pulmonary aspiration can be minimized by continuously monitoring the patient's mental status, properly positioning the patient to allow for drainage of secretions, limiting ventilation pressures to avoid gastric distention, and using suction devices and esophageal or endotracheal (ET) intubation. Sellick's maneuver (cricoid cartilage pressure directed posteriorly to compress the trachea against the cervical vertebra, thus occluding the esophagus) is useful to limit risk of aspiration during intubation. Airway protection should be provided when there is a risk of aspiration or promptly after an aspiration episode.

Section Three
Airway Management

Science and technology have produced numerous adjuncts for providing airway management.

BOX 12-3
Personal Protective Equipment

The Centers for Disease Control recommend that health care workers, in addition to taking the normal precautions for personal protection from communicable diseases, use masks, eyewear (for example, safety glasses and face shields), and gowns in situations where splashes of blood or other body fluids are likely. Because of the possibility during airway management procedures of patient reactions such as vomiting and coughing and the potential for exposure to blood and other body fluids, the paramedic should take barrier precautions.

However, the paramedic must not neglect basic airway management in favor of a procedure that is technically more difficult than necessary to secure a safe and functional airway. Airway management should progress rapidly from the least to the most invasive modality.

For a discussion of personal protective equipment, see Box 12-3.

SPECIAL CONSIDERATIONS IN AIRWAY MANAGEMENT

Because unconscious patients lack the muscular tone and control to maintain a patent airway, *the airways of all unconscious patients must be established and maintained in the primary survey.* The paramedic should also remember that any injury severe enough to produce a loss of consciousness is severe enough to produce spinal injury. *Spinal precautions should be considered in all trauma patients who need airway management or ventilatory support.*

MANUAL TECHNIQUES FOR AIRWAY MANAGEMENT

Manual techniques for airway management have been described by the American Heart As-

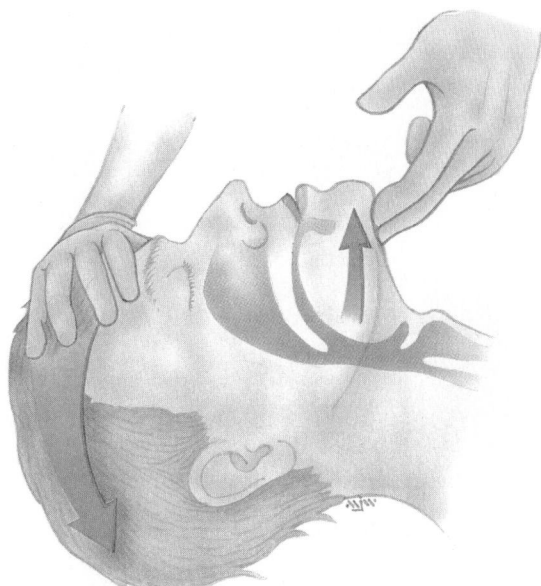

Fig. 12-14 Head-tilt/chin-lift maneuver.

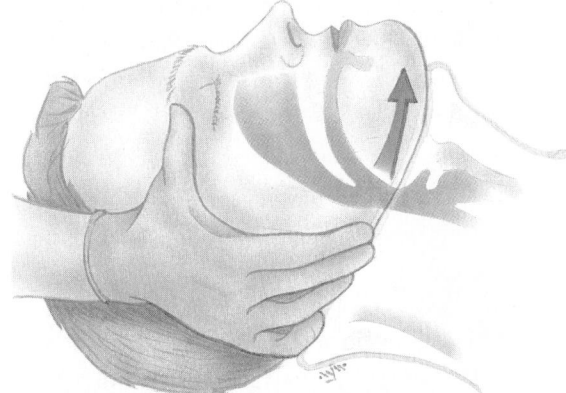

Fig. 12-16 Jaw-thrust without head-tilt maneuver.

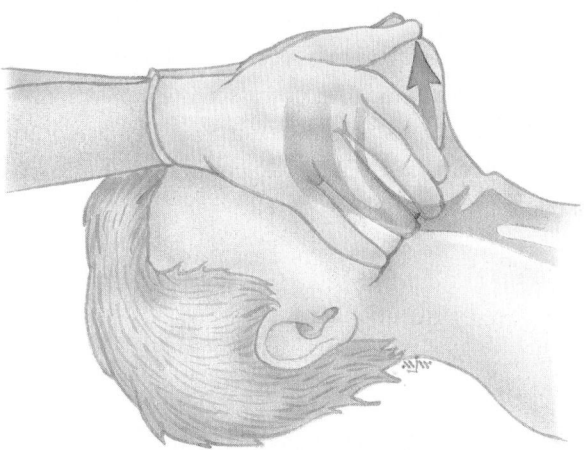

Fig. 12-15 Jaw-thrust maneuver.

sociation and the American Red Cross. These include the head-tilt chin-lift method, the jaw-thrust, and the jaw-thrust without head-tilt.

The head-tilt chin-lift method (Fig. 12-14) is preferred for opening the airway when spinal injury is not suspected. The head-tilt is accomplished by placing one hand on the victim's forehead and applying firm backward pressure with the palm to tilt the head back. Then the fingers of the other hand are placed under the bony part of the lower jaw (near the chin) and lifted to bring the chin forward, supporting the jaw and helping to maintain the head-tilt position.

In the absence of suspected spinal injury, the jaw-thrust maneuver (Fig. 12-15) may be used to gain additional forward displacement of the mandible. This is accomplished by grasping the angles of the patient's lower jaw and lifting with both hands, one on each side, displacing the mandible forward while tilting the head back.

If spinal injury is suspected, the jaw-thrust without head-tilt (Fig. 12-16) should be used to open the airway. During this maneuver, the patient's head should be stabilized and the cervical spine immobilized with neutral, in-line stabilization. The jaw-thrust maneuver should then proceed without extending the neck.

● MECHANICAL ADJUNCTS IN AIRWAY MANAGEMENT

The use of mechanical devices in airway management should never delay the opening of a compromised airway. These devices should be used only after efforts have been made to open the airway manually.

Nasopharyngeal Airway (Nasal Airway)

The nasal airway is used to maintain an airway in a semiconscious or unconscious patient (Fig. 12-17). Insertion of a nasal airway may also be a useful temporizing maneuver to control the airway in patients with seizures or possible cervical spine

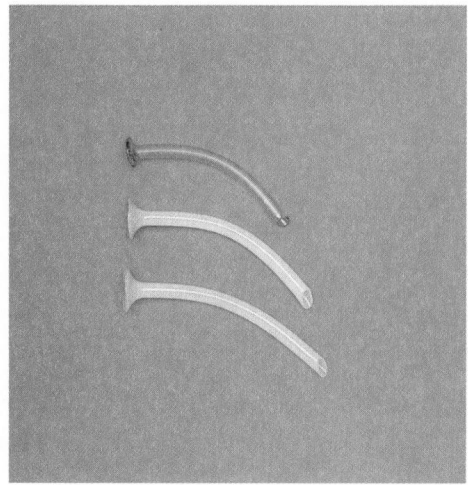

Fig. 12-17 Nasal airways.

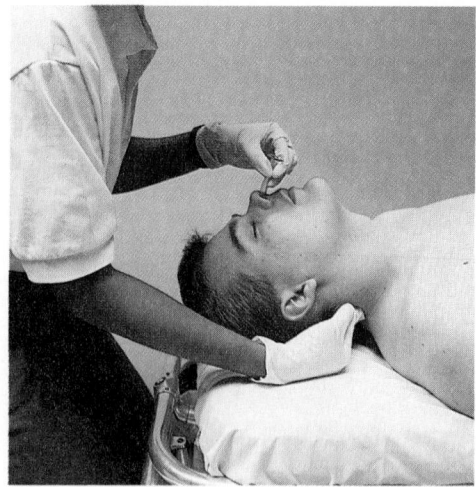

Fig. 12-19 Insertion of a nasal airway.

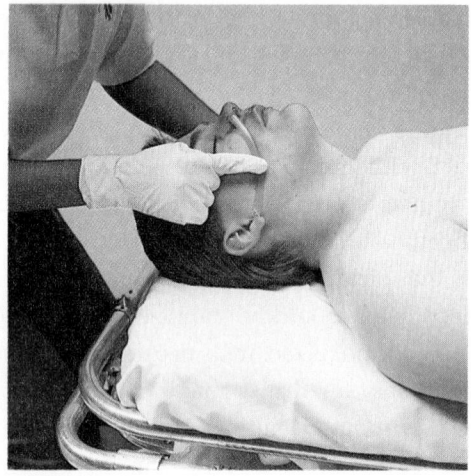

Fig. 12-18 Measuring a nasal airway.

injury and also before nasotracheal intubation. In addition, this adjunct may serve as a guide for inserting a nasogastric tube.

Description

The nasal airway is soft and pliable. It has a gentle curve, and the outer end is flared. Nasal airways are available in a variety of sizes to accommodate infants and adults. They vary from 17 to 20 cm in length and 12 to 36 French. (As with most other catheters, the French Scale System is used to indicate internal diameter [i.d.]. Each unit of the scale equals approximately ⅓ mm. A 21-French catheter, for example, is 7 mm in diameter.)

To determine the correct size, the paramedic should choose an airway that has a tube length equal to the distance between the tip of the patient's nose and the tragus of the ear, which is the cartilaginous area anterior to the external auditory canal (Fig. 12-18). Recommended sizes of nasopharyngeal airways follow:

- Large adult: 8.0-9.0 mm i.d. (24-27 French)
- Medium adult: 7.0-8.0 mm i.d. (21-24 French)
- Small adult: 6.0-7.0 mm i.d. (18-21 French)

Insertion

The nasal airway should be lubricated with a water-soluble lubricant to minimize resistance in the nasal cavity. The device is placed in the nostril with the beveled tip (designed to protect nasal structures) directed toward the nasal septum. The airway is gently passed close to the midline, along the floor of the nostril, following the natural curvature of the nasal passage. The insertion should be made perpendicular to the coronal plane of the face. The airway should not be forced. If resistance is encountered, rotating the tube slightly may help, or insertion can be attempted through the other nostril (Fig. 12-19).

After insertion, the nasal airway rests in the posterior pharynx behind the tongue. If the patient begins to gag after the airway is inserted, the tube may be stimulating the posterior pharynx. Removal, withdrawing the airway 0.5 to 1 cm, and reinsertion may be indicated. The paramedic should remember to maintain displacement of the mandible by head-tilt chin-lift or by jaw-thrust without head-tilt when using this airway.

> **NOTE:**
> Nasopharyngeal airways are contraindicated in patients who have fractures to the basal skull or facial bones because inadvertent intracranial placement is a potential complication.

Advantages

- It is well tolerated by conscious and semiconscious patients with gag reflex.
- It may be inserted rapidly.
- It may be used when insertion of an oropharyngeal airway is contraindicated or difficult because of facial trauma or soft tissue injury.

Potential Complications

- Long nasal airways may enter the esophagus.
- It may precipitate laryngospasm and vomiting in patients with a gag reflex.
- It may injure nasal mucosa, producing bleeding and possible airway obstruction.
- Small-diameter airways may become obstructed by mucus, blood, vomitus, and soft tissues of the pharynx.
- It does not protect lower airway from aspiration.
- It is difficult to suction through it.

Oropharyngeal Airway (Oral Airway)

Description

The oral airway is a semicircular device designed to hold the tongue away from the posterior wall of the pharynx. It should be used only in patients who are unconscious or semiconscious and without a gag reflex. Most oropharyngeal airways are made of disposable plastic. The two types of airways most frequently used are the Guedel, distinguished by its tubular design, and the Berman, distinguished by airway channels along each side (Fig. 12-20)

Like nasopharyngeal airways, oral airways are available in a variety of sizes, from infant to adult.

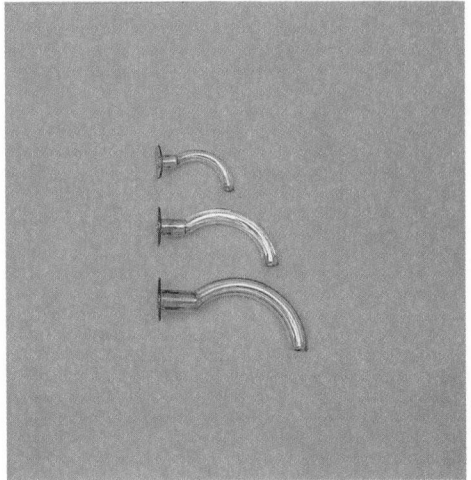

Fig. 12-20 Oral airways.

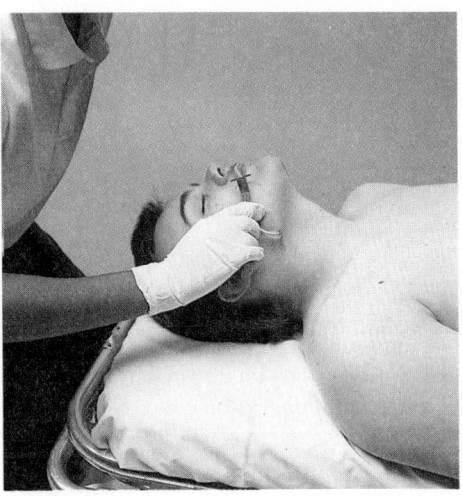

Fig. 12-21 Measuring an oral airway.

The size is based on the distance in millimeters from the flange to the distal tip. The proper size for the patient may be determined by placing the airway next to the face so that the flange is at the level of the patient's central incisors and the bite block segment is parallel to the patient's hard palate. The airway should extend from the corner of the mouth to the tip of the ear lobe at the angle of the jaw (Fig. 12-21). The following sizes are recommended[6]:

- Large adult: 100 mm (Guedel size 5)
- Medium adult: 90 mm (Guedel size 4)
- Small adult: 80 mm (Guedel size 3)

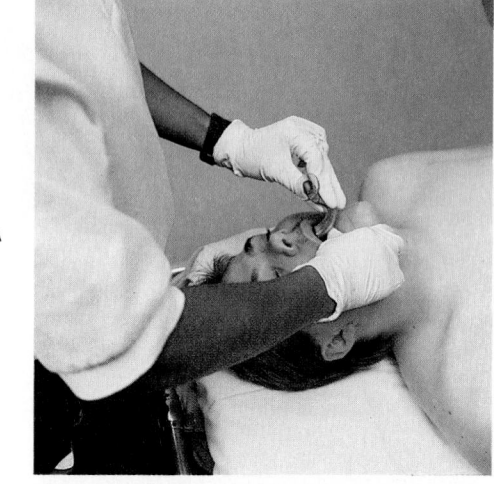

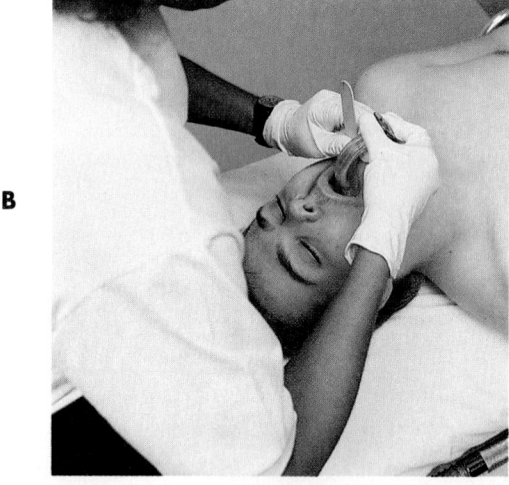

Fig. 12-22 A, Inserting an airway upside down. **B,** Alternative method of inserting an oral airway.

Insertion

Before insertion of any oral airway, the mouth and pharynx should be cleared of all secretions, blood, or vomitus. In the adult or older child the oral airway may be inserted upside-down or at a 90-degree angle to avoid catching the tongue during insertion (Fig. 12-22, *A*). As the oral airway passes the crest of the tongue, it is rotated into the proper position so that it is situated against the posterior wall of the oropharynx. Another method of insertion, recommended for pediatric patients and usable in adult patients, is to use a tongue blade to displace the tongue inferiorly and anteriorly. The airway is then inserted and moved posteriorly toward the back of the oropharynx, following the normal curvature of the oral cavity (Fig. 12-22, *B*). Regardless of the method of inser-

tion, trauma to the face and oral cavity should be avoided. In addition, the paramedic should be sure that the patient's lips and tongue are not caught between the teeth and the airway.

Proper placement of the airway is confirmed by the presence of observable chest wall expansion and good breath sounds on auscultation of the lungs during ventilation. The paramedic should remember that even with the oral airway in place, proper head position of the patient must be maintained to help ensure a patent airway.

Advantages

- It secures the tongue forward and down, away from the posterior pharynx.
- It provides easy access for airway suction.
- It serves as a bite block to protect an ET tube and in the event of convulsions.

Potential Complications

- Small airways may fall back into the oral cavity, occluding the airway.
- Long airways may press the epiglottis against the entrance of the trachea, producing a complete airway obstruction.
- It may stimulate vomiting and laryngospasm in the patient with a gag reflex.
- It does not protect the lower airway from aspiration.
- It may push the tongue back and obstruct the airway if improperly inserted

NOTE:
All advanced airway procedures presented in this text require special training. Before initiating any advanced procedure, paramedics should have direct authorization from medical direction or be operating under protocols that have been developed and approved by medical direction and the paramedic's EMS agency. The paramedic should also be aware that long-term complications may result from advanced airway procedures, even when properly performed. These include aspiration, tracheal stenosis, infection, transient dysphagia, and voice changes.

● ADVANCED AIRWAY PROCEDURES

Esophageal Intubation Devices

Esophageal intubation devices were introduced to the medical community in the early 1970s. They were designed to be used as an alternative to conventional bag-valve mask ventilation in patients who were in respiratory arrest or when tracheal intubation was not technically desirable or possible (for example, when equipment was unavailable or inoperable or personnel were untrained). The best-known esophageal intubation device is the esophageal obturator airway (EOA). Several other similar devices have been developed, including the esophageal gastric tube airway, esophageal pharyngeal airway, laryngeal mask airway, tracheal-esophageal airway, and Berman intubating-pharyngeal airway.

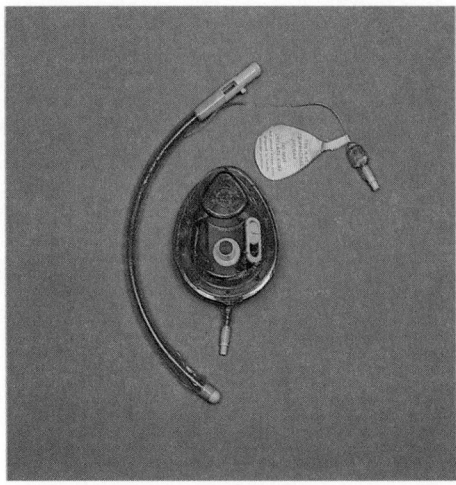

Fig. 12-23 EOA.

> ### NOTE:
> This text will describe the EOA as representative of all esophageal intubation devices. The paramedic is encouraged to become familiar with other similar devices authorized for use by medical control and local EMS protocol.

Description

The EOA is a large-bore, flexible tube approximately 37 cm long (Fig. 12-23). The airway has a high-volume cuff close to the distal end that, when inflated after insertion into the esophagus, prevents regurgitation and gastric insufflation during use. The EOA has multiple openings at the level of the pharynx through which air or oxygen is delivered, usually by bag-valve-mask (BVM). The tube is mounted to a clear, detachable face mask that, when properly seated against the patient's face, prevents air from leaking around and through the nose.

Necessary Equipment

- 35-ml syringe
- Water-soluble lubricant
- BVM
- Oxygen source with oxygen tubing
- Suction equipment
- Stethoscope
- Oropharyngeal airway

Insertion

While preparing for insertion, the paramedic should maintain the patient's airway by manual or adjunctive means and provide adequate ventilatory support. The tube should be attached to the mask and the cuff tested for leaks. The EOA is then lubricated with a water-soluble jelly and prepared for insertion. Immediately before insertion, the patient's lungs should be hyperventilated with 100% oxygen for at least 2 minutes.

With the patient's head in midposition or slight flexion, the tongue and jaw are elevated with one hand while the tube is inserted into the mouth and esophagus. The tube is then advanced until the mask is seated tightly on the face. When the mask is in this position, the cuff should be in the proper location, just below the level of the carina. If the cuff is above the carina, it may compress the posterior membranous portion of the trachea, causing tracheal obstruction. Fig. 12-24 illustrates the steps of EOA insertion.

Ventilations should be delivered via BVM or demand valve before balloon inflation to ensure that the tube did not enter the trachea. The chest should be inspected for rise and fall, and the lungs and abdomen should be auscultated to verify placement. If the chest rises and the lungs have

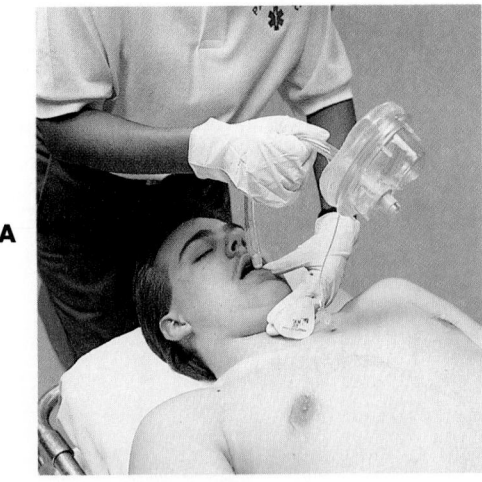

Fig. 12-24 A, After hyperventilation with 100% oxygen, insert the EOA into the patient's mouth and esophagus. Advance the tube until the mask is sealed tightly on the face. **B,** After EOA insertion, verify correct placement and inflate the cuff with 35 cc of air. **C,** After inflation of the cuff, confirm the presence of bilateral breath sounds. Ventilate the patient's lungs via a bag-valve device or demand-valve device.

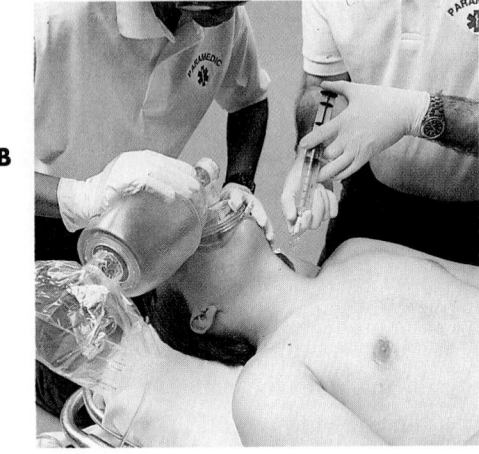

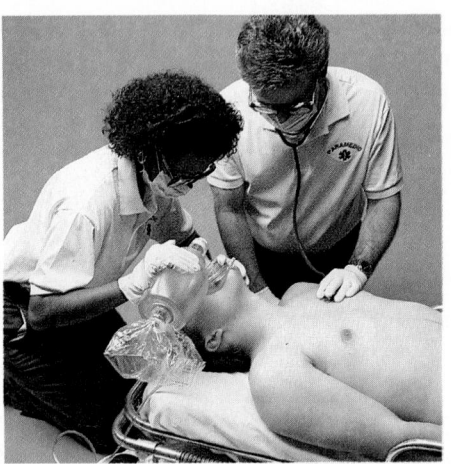

adequate breath sounds with ventilation, it may be assumed that the tube has entered the esophagus, and the cuff should then be inflated with 35 ml of air. After inflation of the cuff, auscultation in the midaxillary line should be repeated to confirm the presence of bilateral breath sounds. The patient should then be ventilated via BVM or demand-valve device. After successful intubation of the esophagus, the patient can be ventilated until the trachea is intubated. The EOA may be removed after tracheal intubation, but removal is not immediately necessary unless extreme gastric distention has occurred.

Gurgling sounds heard over the epigastric area and poor breath sounds on auscultation of the lungs or increasing abdominal size with ventilation indicate that the EOA is improperly placed in the trachea. If this occurs or if there is difficulty during insertion, the tube should be withdrawn, and the patient should be well ventilated by other means before reinsertion is attempted.

> **NOTE:**
> The time required for esophageal or ET intubation should not exceed 30 seconds (that is, the patient should not go without ventilatory support for more than 30 seconds). If the intubation procedure takes more than 30 seconds, the intubation should be stopped and the patient's lungs well ventilated with 100% oxygen before further attempts are made.

Method of Removal

The EOA should only be removed in the prehospital setting if severe gastric distention is present after intubation or if the patient regains consciousness or develops a gag reflex. The procedure for removal is as follows:

1. Have suction available.
2. Turn the patient on his or her side if not endotracheally intubated. Use spinal precautions as indicated.
3. Detach the mask from the tube.
4. Deflate the cuff.
5. Gently and quickly remove the tube.
6. Be prepared for vomiting. (Suction should be on and a tonsil suction catheter attached.) Use Sellick's maneuver to control the egress of vomiting if necessary.
7. Assess the patient's respiratory status.
8. Provide supplemental oxygen to the patient.

Advantages

- Visualization of the lower airway is not required for insertion.
- It requires less technical training than ET intubation.
- It can usually be inserted more easily and quickly than an ET tube.

Potential Complications

- There is difficulty maintaining an adequate seal between the mask and the patient's face, thereby producing inadequate ventilatory volumes.
- Inadvertent tracheal intubation may occur.
- Tracheal compression may occur.
- Esophageal injury (such as esophageal pressure necrosis or rupture) may occur.
- Laryngospasm may occur.
- Vomiting and aspiration may occur.

To minimize complications, the paramedic should use the following precautions[7]:

- The EOA should be used only by trained individuals.
- It should not be used in individuals with esophageal disease (for example, esophageal varices, strictures, diverticuli) or in patients who have swallowed caustic material.
- It should not be used in patients younger than 16 years of age or in patients who are under 5 feet tall or over 7 feet tall.
- It should not be used in conscious patients or those who are breathing spontaneously.

- It should be left in place no longer than 2 hours. (This reduces the incidence of necrosis of the esophageal mucosa secondary to ischemia in the area of the cuff.)
- Force should not be used during insertion.
- Suction should be immediately available during insertion and removal.

There is much debate in the medical community as to the efficacy of esophageal intubation devices; experience to date has demonstrated that they present an increased risk of complications compared with ET intubation.[3] In 1992, the American Heart Association classified all esophageal intubation devices as Class IIb: "a therapeutic option that is not well established by evidence but may be helpful and probably is not harmful."[3] Intubation of the trachea, performed by qualified personnel, is the preferred choice for securing an airway in a compromised patient.

Esophageal Gastric Tube Airway

The esophageal gastric tube airway (EGTA) is a modification of the EOA. It includes a gastric tube that can be passed through the lumen of the airway to decompress the stomach. Ventilation is carried out by way of an additional port in the mask (Fig. 12-25).

The technique for inserting the EGTA is the same as for the EOA except for measuring and placing the gastric tube. The tubing should be extended from the tip of the nose to the ear lobe and then to the xiphoid process to measure the gastric tube for insertion after the esophagus has been intubated. It is then passed through the lu-

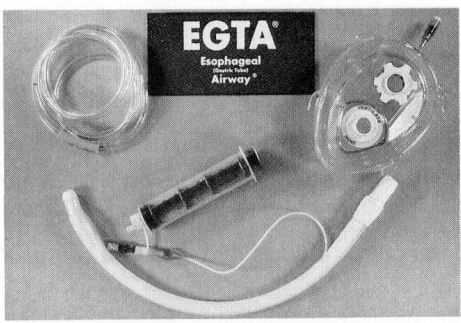

Fig. 12-25 EGTA.

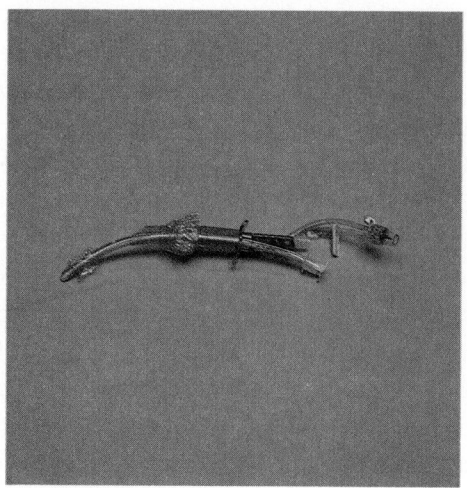

Fig. 12-26 PtL airway.

men of the airway into the stomach. Gastric suction can then be carried out. This benefits the patient by reducing abdominal distention and emptying stomach contents, both of which may reduce the risk of aspiration. The indications, complications, and contraindications associated with use of the EGTA are the same as those for the EOA.

Pharyngeal Tracheal Multiple Balloon System

Description

In 1985, an airway device known as the *pharyngeal tracheal lumen (PtL)* airway was introduced that allowed for either esophageal or tracheal insertion (Fig. 12-26). This airway and others similar in design (for example, the Esophageal Tracheal Combitube) use a plastic tube with twin lumens separated by a partition wall. One tube resembles an ET tube and has an open distal end. The second tube resembles an EOA and is blocked by an obturator at the distal end. Both tubes use low-pressure balloons that provide a seal for either the trachea or esophagus, depending on placement. The PtL airway uses an additional balloon to occlude the oropharynx. This helps obviate the need for a good seal with a face mask and prevents blood or other secretions from being aspirated or swallowed.

NOTE:
Multiple-balloon-system airways are relatively new to prehospital care, and the efficacy of their use in the prehospital setting is currently under study. Paramedics should consult with medical direction and local EMS protocol regarding their use.

Insertion

Balloon-system airways are inserted by gently guiding the device into the esophagus or trachea. This insertion is accomplished much like insertion of the EOA, without hyperextension or flexion of the patient's head and without visualization of the glottic opening. The balloons are inflated, and ventilation is initially provided through the "esophageal" lumen. (This lumen is chosen first because of the high probability of esophageal placement after blind insertion.) In this position, air passes through the perforations of the esophageal lumen into the pharynx and beyond the glottis into the trachea. Placement is confirmed by auscultation of bilateral breath sounds and visualization of chest excursions. Fig. 12-27 illustrates placement of the PtL airway in the esophagus and trachea.

In the absence of breath sounds and chest movement with ventilation through the esophageal lumen, ventilation should be performed through the "tracheal" lumen without changing the position of the airway. Air passes through this lumen directly into the trachea. Placement is confirmed in the manner described for the EOA.

Necessary Equipment
- Water-soluble lubricant
- BVM or demand valve
- Oxygen source and connecting tubing
- Suction equipment
- Stethoscope

With the various kinds of balloon-system devices available, it is beyond the scope of this text to list the advantages, disadvantages, and contraindications of each specific airway. However, common elements are shared among the different devices.

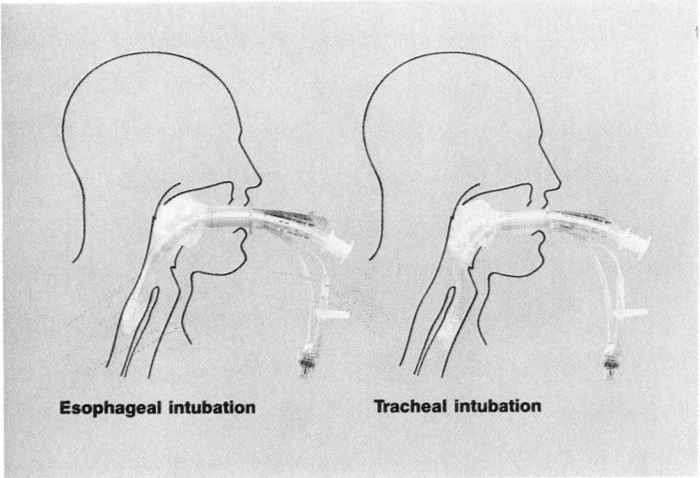

Fig. 12-27 Esophageal and tracheal placement of PtL airway.

Common Advantages
- Airways cannot be improperly placed.
- It requires little skill training or maintenance.
- It requires minimal spinal movement for insertion.
- It suctions easily.

Common Disadvantages
- The patient must be unresponsive without a gag reflex.
- It must be removed when the patient becomes responsive or agitated.
- Proper identification of tube location may be difficult, leading to ventilations through the wrong lumen.
- It should be replaced with an ET tube as soon as possible.

Common Contraindications
- Patients under 5 feet tall or younger than 14 years of age
- Caustic ingestion
- Esophageal disease
- Presence of a gag reflex

Endotracheal Intubation
Tracheal intubation is the preferred technique for airway control in patients who are unable to maintain a patent airway. Indications for tracheal intubation include the following situations:
- When the rescuer is unable to ventilate an unconscious patient with conventional methods (mouth-to-mask, BVM)
- When the patient cannot protect his or her own airway (coma, respiratory and cardiac arrest)
- When prolonged artificial ventilation is needed

In addition, tracheal intubation provides the following advantages:
- Isolates the airway, preventing aspiration of material into the lower airway
- Facilitates ventilation and oxygenation
- Facilitates suctioning of the trachea and bronchi
- Prevents wasted ventilation and gastric insufflation during positive-pressure ventilation
- Provides a route for the administration of some medications (*epinephrine, atropine, lidocaine,* and *naloxone*)

Description
The common ET tube is a flexible tube that is open at both ends (Fig. 12-28). The proximal end has a standard 15-mm adapter that connects to various oxygen-delivery devices for positive-pressure ventilation. The distal end of the tube is

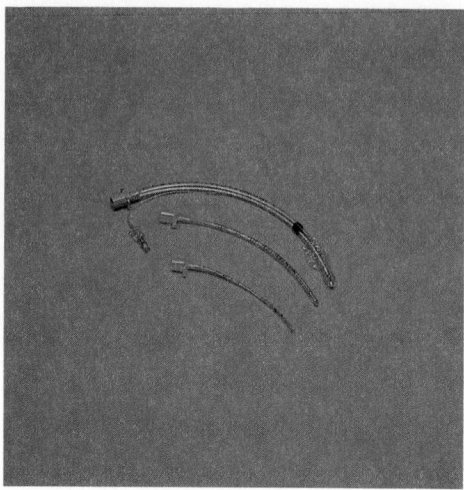

Fig. 12-28 ET tube.

TABLE 12-1 Suggested Sizes for ET Tubes	

Age	Internal Diameter of Tube in mm
Newborn	3.0
6 months	3.5
18 months	4.0
3 years	4.5
5 years	5.0
6 years	5.5
8 years	6.0
12 years	6.5
16 years	7.0

beveled to facilitate placement between the vocal cords and has a balloon cuff that occludes the remainder of the tracheal lumen. This cuff prevents aspiration around the tube and minimizes air leaks during ventilation. The cuff is attached by the inflating tube to a one-way inflating valve with an inlet port designed to accept a syringe for inflation. A properly positioned ET tube with its cuff inflated permits administration of high concentrations of oxygen at controlled pressures. In addition to the common ET tube, specialized variations are available. They include the following:

- Armored or anode tubes that have an inner spiral of flat metal to prevent kinking or compression
- "Trigger" tubes that have a thin cord running down the anterior wall of the tube, to which a ring is attached proximally. (Pulling on the ring with a finger or thumb increases the curvature. This ring may help maneuver the tube anteriorly without a stylet.)
- Some ET tubes have medication ports for ET drug administration.

Endotracheal Tube Sizes
The markings on the ET tube indicate the tube's i.d. in millimeters. (The tubes are available in graduated sizes from 3.0 to 9.0 mm.) The length of the tube from the distal end is indicated in centi-

meters at several levels. Recommended ET tube sizes for the adult are as follows[3]:

- Adult females: 7.5 to 8.0 i.d.
- Adult males: 8.0 to 8.5 i.d.

Infant and pediatric ET tubes are available with and without balloon cuffs. Cuffed ET tubes are indicated only for children over the age of 8 years. Children less than 8 years of age have a circular narrowing at the level of the cricoid cartilages. This narrowing serves as a functional cuff, allowing minimal air leakage at the cricoid ring. Accordingly, uncuffed ET tubes are recommended for this age group. Various methods may be used to determine the correct ET tube size for infants and children. One such method recommended by the American Heart Association is to choose an ET tube with an outside diameter equal to the diameter of the child's little finger. Regardless of the method used, appropriate ET tube selection is more reliably based on the patient's size than age. Suggested sizes for ET tubes are listed in Table 12-1.[3]

Necessary Equipment
A laryngoscope is required for visualizing the glottis during tracheal intubation. Although there are various makes, all have several features in common. The standard laryngoscope includes a handle made of stainless steel. The handle contains the batteries for the light source and attaches to a stainless steel blade with a bulb placed in the

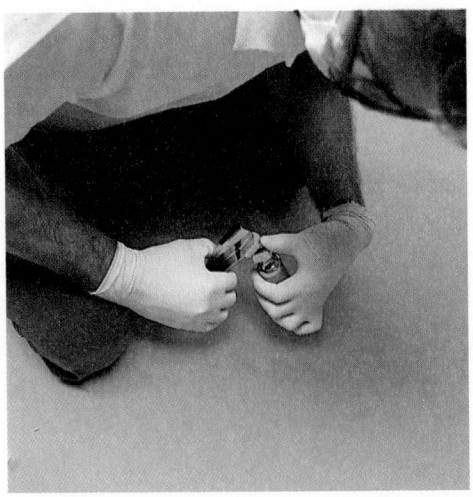

Fig. 12-29 Attaching blade to laryngoscope handle.

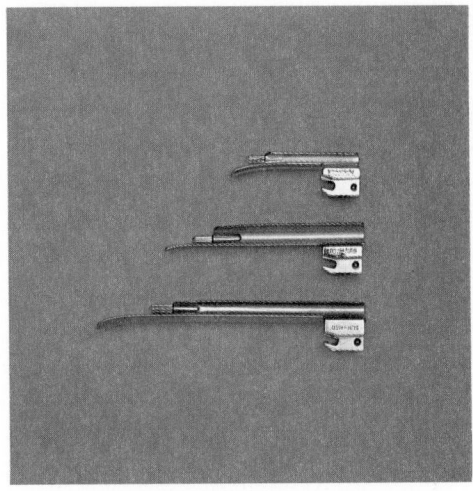

Fig. 12-30 Straight blades.

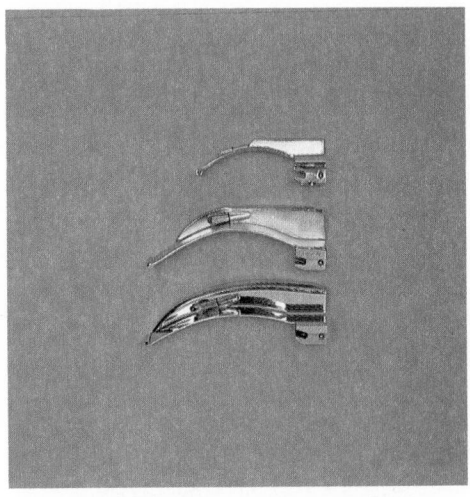

Fig. 12-31 Curved blades.

distal third. The electrical contact between the blade and the handle is made at a connection point called the *fitting*. The indentation of the blade is attached to the bar of the handle. When the blade is elevated to a right angle with the laryngoscope handle, the blade snaps into place and the bulb lights (Fig. 12-29). (The bulb's failure to light may result from a loose connection between the bulb and the bulb socket, a damaged bulb, or faulty batteries.) Other necessary equipment includes a 10-ml syringe for cuff inflation, water-soluble lubricant, and suction equipment.

Two types of blades (available in various sizes) are used with the laryngoscope: a straight blade, such as the Miller, Wisconsin, or Flagg (Fig. 12-30), and a curved blade, such as a MacIntosh (Fig. 12-31). The tip of a straight blade is applied directly to the epiglottis to expose the vocal cords. Advocates of the straight blade claim it provides more exposure of the glottis and less need for a stylet. A straight blade is usually recommended for infant intubation because it provides greater displacement of the tongue into the floor of the mouth and better visualization of the glottic structures.

The curved blade design is intended to displace the tongue to the left and to elevate the epiglottis without touching it. Advocates of the curved blade claim it reduces the chance of dental trauma and provides more room for passage of the ET

tube. The choice of blade is a matter of personal preference. Paramedics should acquire expertise in using both curved and straight blades because some patients can be intubated more easily with one type than the other. Occasions may also arise when only one type of blade is available. Versatility with both curved and straight blades may enhance patient survival.

A malleable stylet (preferably plastic coated) may be inserted through the ET tube before intubation (Fig. 12-32). The stylet will conform to any desired configuration and may facilitate proper placement of the ET tube. If used, the stylet must

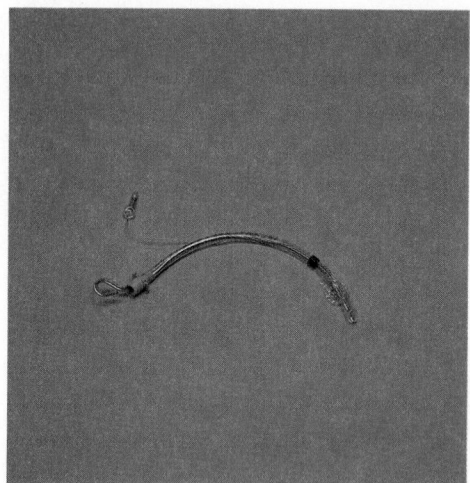

Fig. 12-32 ET tube with malleable stylet.

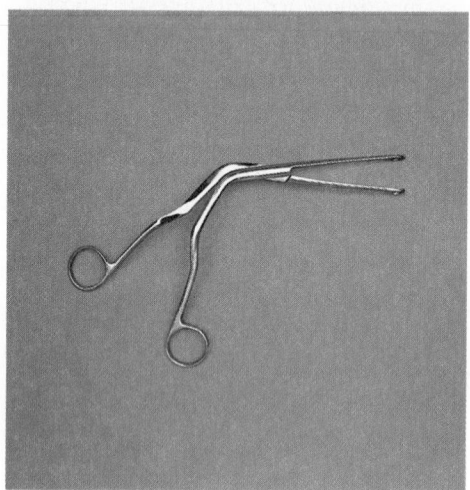

Fig. 12-33 Magill forceps.

ET tube into the larynx during intubation. Use of this device requires special training and authorization from medical direction.

> **NOTE:**
> Patient ventilation should be established by other means before intubation (for example, mouth-to-mask, BVM). The adequacy of ventilation should be assessed by observing of chest rise and fall during ventilation, by auscultating for breath sounds, and by noting the patient's skin color. When preparing for intubation, the paramedic should remember that the patient's lungs should first be hyperventilated with 100% oxygen for at least 2 minutes. In addition, the time required for intubation (that is, the time lapse without ventilating the patient's lungs) should not exceed 30 seconds. If intubation is not completed within this time, the procedure should be stopped and the patient's lungs ventilated by other means before attempting intubation again.

Preparing for Intubation

Before intubation, all equipment should be examined and tested for defects. The cuff of the ET tube should be checked for integrity by inflating the balloon with 5 to 8 ml of air and checking for leaks in the cuff or inlet port. The laryngoscope blade should be snapped into place to examine the light bulb. The bulb should be secure in its socket and checked for brightness.

Anatomical Considerations

The ET tube may be passed into the trachea through the mouth (orotracheal) or through the nose (nasotracheal). The orotracheal method is most commonly used and is performed under direct visualization of the glottic opening. The nasotracheal route is essentially a "blind" technique. The following anatomical structures are important landmarks during intubation:

- The trachea is in the midline of the neck and has its superior entry at the level of the glottic opening. In orotracheal intubation, the vo-

be lubricated with a water-soluble jelly to ensure easy removal and must be recessed at least 1.27 cm from the distal end of the ET tube to prevent patient injury. Recession of the stylet tip is maintained by bending the proximal end of the stylet over the proximal rim of the adapter so that it does not advance through the lumen with manipulation of the ET tube. If the stylet is allowed to extend beyond the distal end of the tube, the mucosal surface or vocal cords may be damaged.

Some physicians also authorize the use of Magill forceps, a scissor-style clamp that has circular tips (Fig. 12-33), to help direct the tip of the cal cords should be visualized while passing the tube to ensure passage into the trachea.

- The uvula is suspended from the midline of the soft palate and is used as a guide in placing the laryngoscope properly.
- The epiglottis is attached to the base of the tongue and should be visualized and elevated to expose the glottis and vocal cords. Pressure on the solid ring of the cricoid (Sellick's maneuver) can occlude the esophagus, reducing the risk of regurgitation during the intubation attempt. It may also help better visualize the entrance of the trachea by pushing it slightly posteriorly.
- The trachea extends to the level of the second intercostal space anteriorly, at which point it bifurcates into left and right mainstem bronchi. The right main bronchus branches off at a very slight angle to the trachea, whereas the left branches at a 45- to 60-degree angle.

NOTE:
Because of this anatomical configuration, it is more common for an ET tube that has been advanced too far to enter the right main bronchus, bypassing and occluding the origin of the left main bronchus. If this occurs, atelectasis and pulmonary insufficiency of the left lung may result. It is therefore important for the paramedic to evaluate ET tube placement by auscultation of both lungs. With proper ET tube placement, breath sounds should be of almost equal intensity over both lung fields. Certain pathological conditions (such as pneumothorax, hemothorax, or surgical removal of a lung) may result in unequal breath sounds even when an ET tube is in the proper position.

Orotracheal Intubation

In preparation for orotracheal insertion, the nontrauma patient should be placed in the sniffing position (Fig. 12-34) so that the neck is flexed at the fifth and sixth and the head extended at the first and second cervical vertebrae. This allows the

Removal of Foreign Bodies by Direct Laryngoscopy

Direct laryngoscopy and use of McGill forceps to remove foreign bodies should only be attempted after manual techniques of clearing the airway have been unsuccessful. The steps in removing a foreign body from the airway by direct laryngoscopy are as follows:

1. Assemble the necessary laryngoscopy equipment. (Have suction ready for immediate use in case of vomiting.)
2. Place the supine patient in the sniffing position (Fig. 12-34) with the head extended.
3. Hyperventilate the patient with supplemental oxygen, if possible.
4. Insert the laryngoscope, visualizing the glottic opening and surrounding structures.
5. If foreign matter is visualized, grasp the foreign matter with McGill forceps or a Kelly clamp and remove it from the airway.

NOTE: Forceps removal of foreign matter should only be attempted with direct visualization of the obstruction. Even then, caution must be exercised to avoid soft tissue damage from the teeth of the forceps.

6. If spontaneous respirations resume within 5 seconds, remove the laryngoscope blade and monitor the patient.
7. If spontaneous respirations do not resume, insert an ET tube, administer 100% oxygen, and assess the patient's circulatory status.

If complete foreign body obstruction of the upper airway cannot be relieved, needle cricothyrotomy or transtracheal jet insufflation may be warranted (described later in this section). These advanced airway procedures provide oxygenation until tracheal intubation or tracheostomy can be performed in a controlled setting.

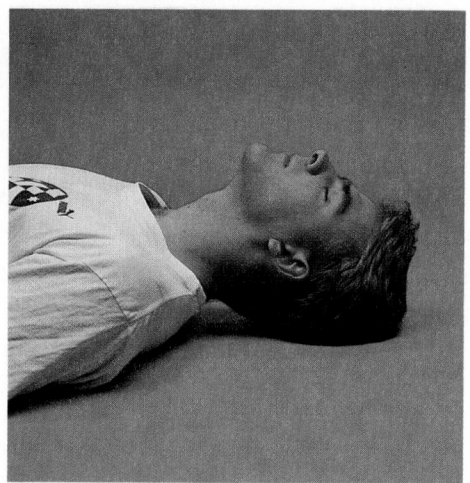

Fig. 12-34 Sniffing position.

three axes of the mouth, pharynx, and trachea (oropharyngeolaryngeal axis) to be aligned for direct visualization of the larynx. (It may be helpful to place several layers of toweling under the patient's head for elevation.)

The tube should be lubricated, and a stethoscope, stylet, and suction equipment (with large-bore catheters) should be readily available. As in all advanced airway procedures, the patient's lungs should be hyperventilated with 100% oxygen for at least 2 minutes before intubation. The orotracheal intubation procedure is as follows (Fig. 12-35):

1. Position yourself at the patient's head.
2. Inspect the oral cavity for secretions and foreign material. Suction the mouth and pharynx if needed.
3. Open the patient's mouth with the fingers of the right hand. Retract the patient's lips on the teeth or gums to prevent pinching them in the blade. The "crossed-finger technique" may also be useful in opening the patient's mouth. To perform this procedure, cross the right thumb and index finger to form an X. Place the thumb on the patient's lower incisors and the index finger on the patient's upper incisors, and apply crossed-finger pressure to open the patient's mouth.

> **NOTE:**
> It is unwise to place fingers in the mouth of any patient who is either conscious or seizing unless a bite block is used.

4. Grasp the lower jaw with the right hand, and draw it forward and upward. Remove any dentures.
5. Holding the laryngoscope in the left hand, insert the blade in the right side of the mouth, displacing the tongue to the left. Move the blade toward the midline and the base of the tongue, and identify the uvula. Gentleness and the avoidance of pressure on the lips and teeth are essential.
6. When using a curved blade, advance the tip of the blade into the vallecula, the space between the base of the tongue and the pharyngeal surface of the epiglottis (Fig. 12-36). When using a straight blade, insert the tip under the epiglottis (Fig. 12-37). The glottic opening is exposed by exerting upward traction on the handle. *Never use a prying motion with the handle, and do not use the teeth as a fulcrum.*
7. Advance the ET tube through the right corner of the mouth and, under direct vision, through the vocal cords (Fig. 12-38). If a stylet has been used, it should be removed from the tube after the tube passes through the cords into the trachea.
8. After viewing the vocal cords, ensure that the proximal end of the cuffed tube has advanced between the cords approximately 1 to 2.5 cm (½ to 1 inch) (Fig. 12-39). The tip of the tube should then be halfway between the vocal cords and the carina. This position causes some displacement of the tube tip during flexion or extension of the patient's neck without extubation or movement of the tip into the mainstem bronchus. (In the average adult, the distance from teeth to carina is 27 cm. The paramedic should observe the depth markings on the ET tube during intubation. In the average adult, the tube is properly positioned when the

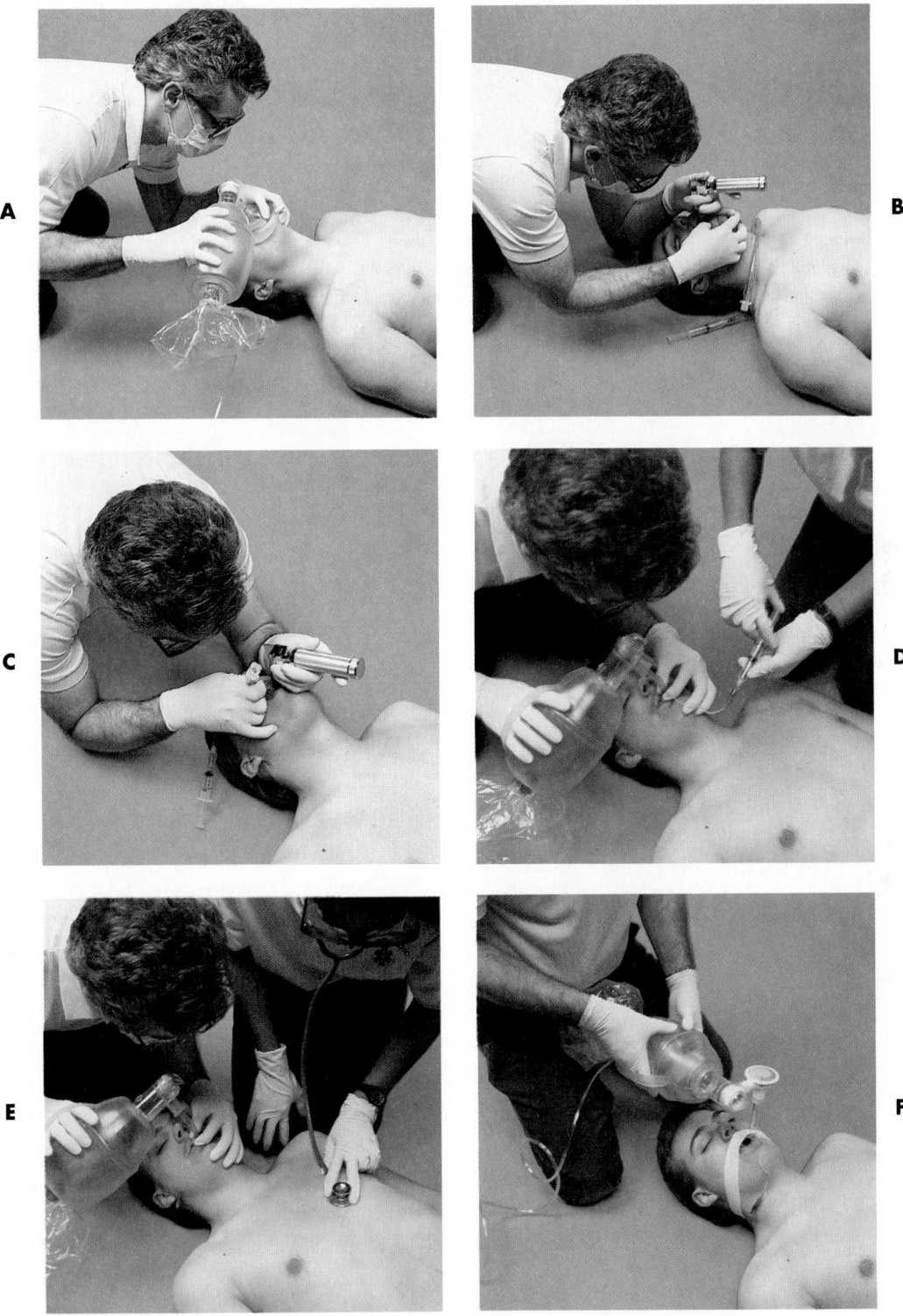

Fig. 12-35 A, Before intubation, hyperventilate the patient's lungs with 100% oxygen for at least 2 minutes. **B,** With the laryngoscope held in the left hand, insert the blade in the right side of the mouth, displacing the tongue to the left. **C,** Advance the ET tube through the right corner of the mouth and, under direct vision, through the vocal cords. **D,** Inflate the cuff with 5 to 8 cc of air, and ventilate the patient's lungs with a mechanical airway device. **E,** Confirm ET placement by auscultation of the abdomen and chest during ventilation. **F,** Secure the ET tube to the patient's head and face, and provide ventilatory support with supplemental oxygen.

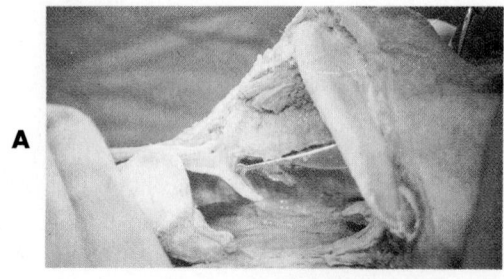
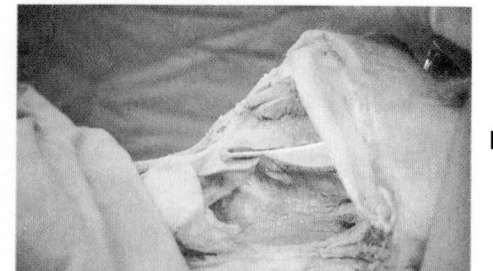

Fig. 12-36 A, The tip of the blade is inserted into the vallecula. **B,** Pressure is directed caudally and anteriorly, lifting to expose the vocal cords.

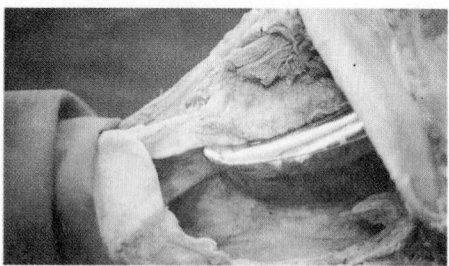

Fig. 12-37 The blade is used to lift the epiglottis directly, exposing the vocal cords.

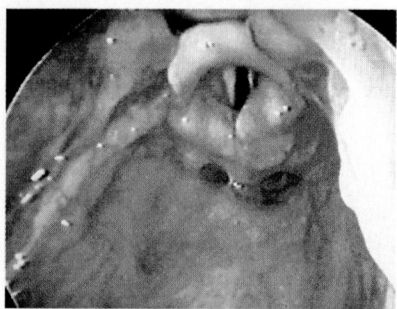

Fig. 12-38 View of the vocal cords.

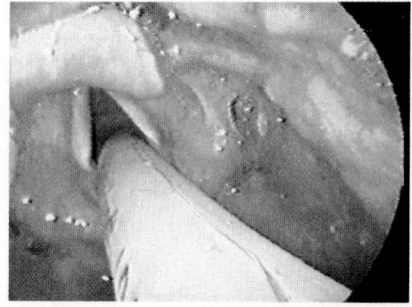

Fig. 12-39 ET tube passing through the vocal cords.

patient's teeth are between the 19- and 23-cm marks on the tube, placing the tip of the tube 2 to 3 cm above the carina.)

> **NOTE:**
> Patients who have spontaneous respirations or intact gag reflexes may have closed vocal cords. These cords open during inspiration.

9. Inflate the cuff with 5 to 8 ml of air to prevent any air leaks around the tracheal-cuff seal.
10. Attach the tube to a mechanical airway device such as a BVM. Begin to ventilate and oxygenate the patient.
11. During ventilation, confirm ET placement by first auscultating the abdomen while visualizing chest expansion. Then auscultate the lateral aspect of the chest at the midaxillary line bilaterally. If breath sounds are decreased or absent in the left lung, the tube may have passed into the right main-stem bronchus, effectively bypassing the origin of the left main bronchus. If this is the case, the cuff should be deflated and the tube withdrawn 1 to 2 cm; then the cuff should be reinflated. All resources should be used to assess proper ET placement, including direct observation of tube passage, auscultation of bilateral breath sounds equal in all fields, visualization of equal chest excursion on the right and left sides, absent or diminished

epigastric sounds with auscultation, positive clear tracheal sounds with auscultation, vapor formation on the tube, absence of air leak around the cuff on bag-valve inflation of the lungs, improvement in patient color or level of consciousness, a feeling of compliance (recognizable with experience), and confirmation with end-tidal carbon dioxide detectors. Increasing abdominal distention frequently indicates esophageal ET tube placement.

12. After successful intubation, insert an oropharyngeal airway in the unconscious patient to prevent biting the ET tube, and note and record the tube marker at the front of the teeth.

13. Secure the ET tube to the head and face by tape or a commercially available device designed for this use. (The cuff of the tube is intended to provide an effective air seal. It is not intended to secure the tube.) Evaluate the lung sounds after taping to ensure that the tube was not inadvertently repositioned.

Fiberoptic Intubation

Fiberoptic technology has led to the development of new equipment to aid in intubation. Fiberoptic strands are slender, flexible, light-conductive fibers that can be bound in bundles. The bundles conduct enough light to convey an image. These bundles are usually protected by a sheath of flexible, woven metal (or a rigid, metal casing for some instruments). A high-intensity light source is conducted to the tip of the instrument by one bundle, and the image is returned via another (Fig. 12-40).

Malleable fiberoptic stylets, or "light wands" (Fig. 12-41), have a high-intensity light at the distal end, powered by a small battery housing at the operator end. This method has the advantage of not requiring manipulation of the patient's head and neck, since visualization of the vocal cords is not required or attempted. These stylets are 6 mm in diameter and are therefore too large for pediatric use.

The procedure for fiberoptic intubation is as follows:

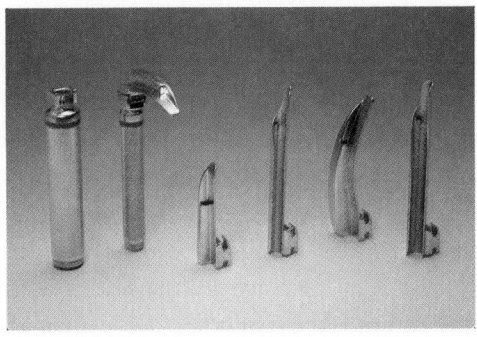

Fig. 12-40 Various fiberoptic blades.

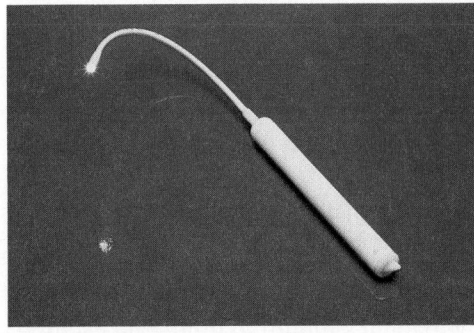

Fig. 12-41 Light wand for fiberoptic intubation.

1. Be positioned at the side of the patient's head. Maintain in-line spinal immobilization by a second rescuer if spinal injury is suspected.

2. Ensure hyperventilation with 100% oxygen for at least 2 minutes before intubation of the patient.

3. Lift the patient's tongue and mandible anteriorly by hand to position the epiglottis.

4. Advance the ET tube in combination with the lighted stylet through the oropharynx and the glottis. Transillumination of the skin of the neck will cause the airway structures to become more distinct. When the thyroid and cricoid cartilages are illuminated by a bright circle of light, the stylet should be held stationary and the ET tube advanced 1 to 2 cm.

5. Inflate the cuff and remove the stylet. Verify proper tube placement in the usual manner.

If the illumination produces a dim, indistinct light, the esophagus has probably been intubated.

If this occurs, the ET tube should be removed, and the patient's lungs should be hyperventilated with 100% oxygen before reattempting the intubation. A disadvantage to this method is that ambient light may make it difficult to see illumination produced by the stylet. This problem can be minimized by darkening the work area during intubation or by placing several layers of dark blankets around the patient's neck during the procedure.

Fiberoptic stylets can also be used to help verify placement after intubation by other methods. Once the cuff has been inflated and lung sounds auscultated, the stylet is advanced through the ET tube. A bright light inferior to the thyroid cartilage indicates proper placement. In addition, the list of indicators of proper ET positioning should be applied to evaluate correct placement.

Digital or Blind Intubation

Before the advent of laryngoscopes, intubation was performed by inserting the intubator's fingers into the patient's mouth to guide the ET tube into the trachea. Although this is not a common prehospital procedure, digital intubation may be necessary in cases of patient entrapment, in patients who have their airway blocked from view by large amounts of blood or other secretions, or if equipment fails. Digital intubation may also be applied in certain disaster situations in which victims are widespread and equipment is in short supply. The procedure for digital intubation is as follows:

1. Be positioned at the patient's left side. In-line spinal immobilization should be maintained by a second rescuer if spinal injury is suspected.
2. Ensure hyperventilation with 100% oxygen for at least 2 minutes before intubation.
3. Use a dental clamp, bite-stick, or other device to hold the patient's mouth open to protect the rescuer's fingers.
4. Bend the tube and stylet combination into a J or hockey-stick configuration.
5. Insert the gloved left middle and index fingers into the patient's mouth. Alternating fingers, "walk" down the patient's tongue, pulling the tongue and epiglottis away from the glottic opening.

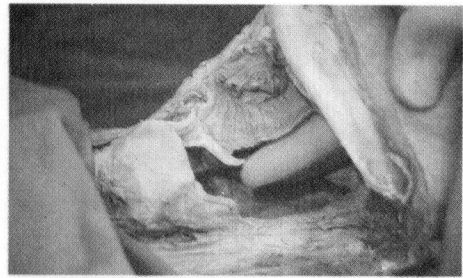
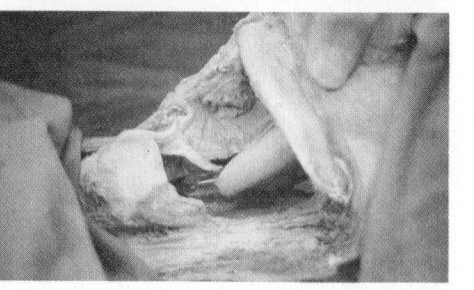

Fig. 12-42 A, Locate the epiglottis with the tips of the fingers of one hand. **B,** Using the palpated epiglottis as a landmark, guide an ET tube into the larynx.

6. When a flap of cartilage covered by mucous membrane is felt with the middle finger, the epiglottis has been located (Fig. 12-42, *A*). Maintain contact and advance the ET tube with the right hand, using the index finger of the left hand as a guide (Fig. 12-42, *B*). The index finger maintains the tube position against the middle finger, leading the tip of the tube into the glottic opening. It may be helpful for a second rescuer to perform Sellick's maneuver to occlude the esophagus and to help prevent aspiration.
7. Once the cuff of the ET tube passes the tips of the paramedic's fingers, inflate the cuff, remove the stylet, and verify placement in the usual manner.

Potential Complications

- Trauma may occur during intubation.
  - Lacerated lips or tongue
  - Dental trauma from laryngoscope
  - Lacerated pharyngeal or tracheal mucosa
  - Tracheal rupture
  - Avulsion of an arytenoid cartilage
  - Vocal cord injury
  - Vomiting and aspiration of stomach contents

- Intubation may produce significant releases of epinephrine and norepinephrine, leading to hypertension, tachycardia, or cardiac rhythm disturbances.
- Intubation may lead to vagal stimulation (particularly in infants and children), resulting in bradycardia and hypotension.
- Intubation may increase intracranial pressure in patients with head injury.
- The esophagus may be accidentally intubated.
- A bronchus may be accidentally intubated.
- Rupture of the cuff, inflation port malfunction, or severance or kinking of the inflation tube may cause cuff malfunction and air leak.

Nasotracheal Intubation

Nasotracheal intubation may be the airway procedure of choice in patients who have spontaneous respirations when laryngoscopy is difficult or the motion of the cervical spine must be limited. Examples include the following:

- Medication overdose
- Asthma
- Chronic obstructive pulmonary disease
- Cerebral vascular accident
- Seizure (status epilepticus with constant seizure activity)
- Altered mental status

These and other situations may make it difficult to align the oropharyngolaryngeal axis, precluding successful orotracheal intubation. It should be recognized that nasotracheal intubation is a "blind" procedure and carries a significant risk of improper tube placement because the paramedic cannot directly visualize the vocal cords.

Generally, conscious patients tolerate a nasotracheal tube better than an orotracheal tube. In addition, a nasotracheal tube usually causes less recurrent trauma to the tracheal mucosa because there is less intratracheal tube movement with head motion with a nasotracheal tube. When time permits, the patient should be prepared by use of a vasoconstrictor spray (for example, phenylephrine) and topical anesthetic (for example, *lidocaine* jelly). These measures make the patient more comfortable and less susceptible to nasal hemorrhage secondary to the procedure. If time

permits, placement of a soft nasopharyngeal airway before the procedure may indicate which nostril is more passable and may compress the mucosa to allow a less traumatic placement.

> **NOTE:**
> Nasotracheal intubation is contraindicated in patients who are apneic, who have midfacial fractures or suspected basal skull fractures, and who have bleeding disorders. Other contraindications include severe nasal trauma, pharyngeal hemorrhage, acute epiglottitis, and suspected laryngeal fracture.

Insertion

1. Choose a cuffed ET that is 1 mm in size smaller than optimal for oral intubation. (Most ET tubes are designed for both orotracheal and nasotracheal intubation procedures.) Prepare and check all necessary equipment (balloon cuff, syringe, suction, stethoscope). Stylets are not to be used in nasotracheal intubation because of the risk of injury during blind insertion.
2. Ensure that the patient's lungs are well oxygenated and hyperventilated for at least 2 minutes before insertion.
3. Lubricate the ET tube with a water-soluble jelly.
4. Advance the tube along the nasal floor of the nostril that is clearest and most direct. If both nares appear open, advance through the largest nostril first. If the chosen nostril is impassable, try the other nostril before selecting an ET tube that is 0.5 mm smaller in diameter.
5. Stand on the side of the patient with one hand on the tube and the thumb and index finger of the other hand palpating the larynx. The curve of the tube should follow the natural curvature of the airway. Gently advance the tube while rotating it medially 15 to 30 degrees until maximal airflow is heard through the tube. Gently and swiftly advance the tube during early inspiration. Voluntary tongue extrusion in cooperative patients is

helpful, or the tongue can be wrapped with gauze and pulled forward. Flexion of the neck (in the absence of suspected spinal instability) as well as posterior pressure on the thyroid cartilage may help position the larynx.

6. Externally observe the advancement of the tube toward the carina. "Misting" or condensation on the tube should be evident as the tube approaches tracheal placement. This phenomenon occurs because the patient's exhaled breath has a high concentration of water vapor, which promptly condenses on exposure to cooler room air.

7. On completion of intubation, auscultate lung and epigastric sounds bilaterally to verify proper tube placement. Inflate the cuff with 5 to 8 ml of air, and secure the tube in place. Ventilations may then be assisted with supplemental oxygen or the patient's lungs can be ventilated by mechanical means.

8. If intubation fails, withdraw the tube and redirect it after ventilation and oxygenation of the patient. It may be possible to recognize tube misplacement by inspecting and palpating the neck for bulges.

Potential Complications
- Epistaxis
- Injury to the nasal septum or turbinates
- Retropharyngeal laceration
- Vocal cord injury

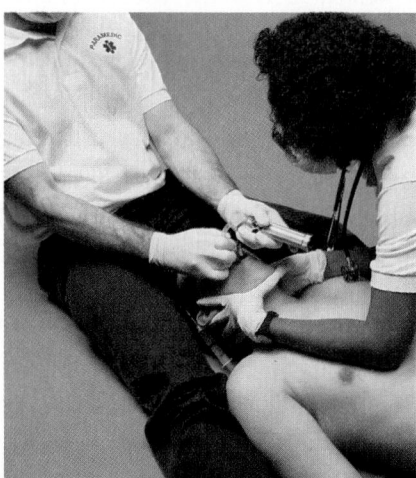

Fig. 12-43 Intubation in a sitting position.

- Avulsion of an arytenoid cartilage
- Esophageal intubation
- Intracranial tube placement if the patient has a basilar skull fracture

Intubation with Spinal Precautions
Nasal or oral intubation may be performed in patients with suspected spinal injury.

> **NOTE:**
> Intubation of patients with suspected spinal injury is controversial[8] and should be authorized by medical direction. Any type of airway manipulation may be dangerous. If the paramedic and the medical control agency elect to intubate the lungs of a patient with suspected spinal injury, the following procedure should be used to maintain in-line stabilization. Two trained rescuers are required.

1. Auscultate for bilateral breath sounds while manual or mechanical ventilations are in progress. This provides a baseline.

2. A second person should apply manual in-line stabilization from the patient's side. The second individual places his or her hands over the patient's ears. The little fingers should be under the occipital skull and the thumbs on the face over the maxillary sinuses. Stabilization (without distraction) should be maintained in a neutral position throughout the procedure. Thin padding under the patient's head may be necessary to maintain neutral, in-line positioning.

3. In one method of intubation, the paramedic is positioned at the patient's head. The legs straddle the patient's shoulders and arms, and the patient's head is secured between the paramedic's thighs. The grip of both rescuers keeps the head from moving during the intubation. In this position, it may be necessary for the paramedic to lean back to visualize the vocal cords (Fig. 12-43).

4. Another method is for the paramedic to lie prone at the patient's head. When using this technique, the second rescuer maintains the in-line position alone (Fig. 12-44).

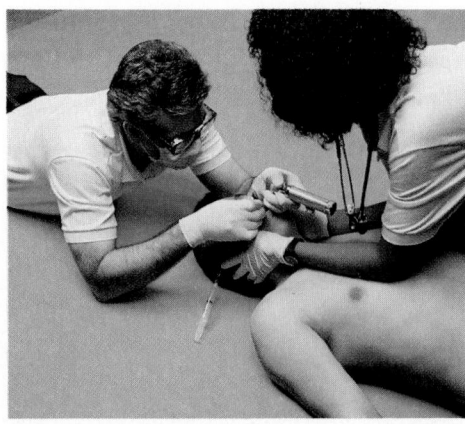

Fig. 12-44 Intubation in a prone position.

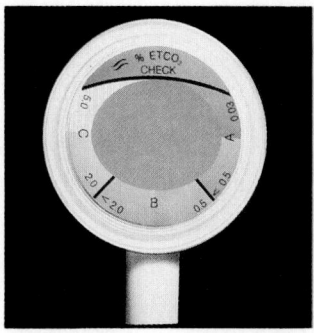

Fig. 12-45 FEF end-tidal carbon dioxide detector.

Extubation

Removal of the ET tube is not usually indicated in the prehospital setting. However, if the patient develops intolerance to the tube, medical control may recommend extubation. If time permits, the patient's lungs should be hyperventilated with 100% oxygen before the procedure. To remove the ET tube, the paramedic should do the following:

1. Have suction available. (The oral cavity and the area above the cuff should be suctioned before extubation.)
2. Deflate the cuff completely.
3. Swiftly withdraw the tube on inspiration while ventilating the tube.
4. Assess respiratory status.
5. Provide high-concentration oxygen and assist ventilations as needed.

Advantages of ET Intubation

- It provides complete airway control.
- It helps prevent aspiration.
- Positive-pressure ventilation can be delivered.
- Tracheal suctioning is possible.
- It prevents gastric distention.
- High concentrations of oxygen and large volumes of ventilation can be delivered.
- It may provide a route for some medications.
- Tube may be placed alongside an esophageal obturator airway

Potential Complications

- Possible soft tissue damage or tracheal perforation

- Possible esophageal intubation
- Laryngospasm

End-Tidal Carbon Dioxide Detectors

In 1988, end-tidal carbon dioxide detectors were made available for prehospital use. They were designed to help verify ET placement and to recognize inadvertent esophageal intubation. They can also provide a noninvasive estimate of alveolar ventilation, carbon dioxide production, and arterial carbon dioxide content. Their use as an adjunct to assessment of ET tube placement is strongly encouraged.[3]

End-tidal carbon dioxide devices are made of a white plastic and contain a chemical indicator in the upper part that is sensitive to carbon dioxide gas. When the detector is attached to an ET tube, the color of the indicator changes with elevated carbon dioxide concentrations, such as would be expected in the tracheal but not esophageal environment (Fig. 12-45). Any color change indicates tracheal placement; no color change indicates esophageal intubation. The device may be useful as an indicator of circulation during cardiac arrest situations, since end-tidal carbon dioxide concentrations seem to be related to perfusion during external chest compression.[9]

> **NOTE:**
> With very low cardiac output during cardiopulmonary resuscitation, there may be no color change of the carbon dioxide detector even though the ET tube is in the trachea.

Percutaneous Transtracheal Ventilation

Description

Percutaneous transtracheal ventilation (also known as *needle cricothyrotomy*) may be valuable in the initial stabilization of a patient whose airway cannot be managed by manual measures, and in patients who cannot be intubated by oral or nasal means. It is a temporary procedure to provide oxygenation when the airway is obstructed as a result of edema of the glottis, fracture of the larynx, or severe oropharyngeal hemorrhage. The percutaneous transtracheal ventilation procedure requires special training and authorization from medical direction.

Necessary Equipment

- A 12- or 14-gauge over-the-needle catheter with a 5- or 10-ml syringe
- Alcohol or povidone-iodine swabs
- Adhesive tape or appropriate ties
- Pressure-regulating valve and pressure gauge attached to a high-pressure (30 to 60 psi) oxygen supply (Most oxygen tanks and regulators can provide 50 psi at 15 L/min or when opened to flush.)

> **NOTE:**
> Demand-valve devices are limited to 50-cm water pressure (70-cm water pressure equals 1 psi) and will not provide enough tidal volume through 12- or 14-gauge catheters. Thus demand valves should not be used for transtracheal ventilation.

- High-pressure tubing connecting the high-pressure regulating valve to a hand-operated release valve (Five-foot tubing is recommended.)
- A release valve connected by tubing to the catheter. (This may be provided through a Y

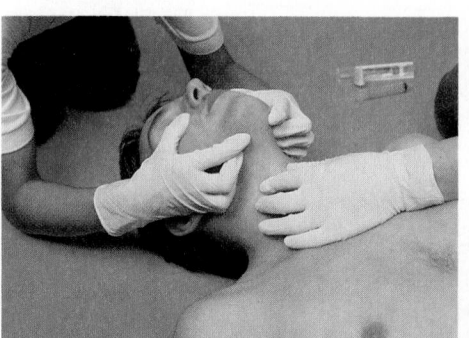
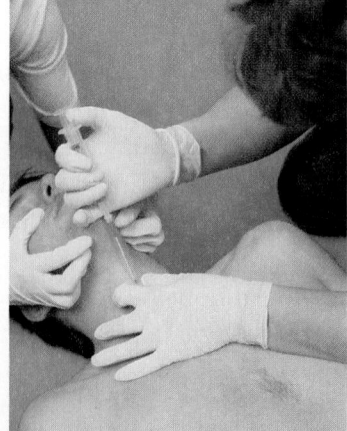
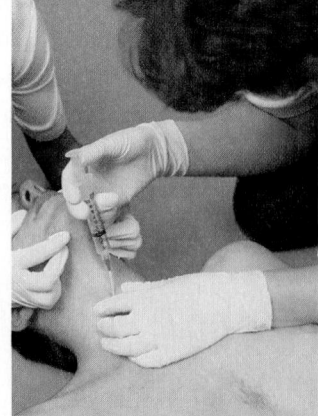
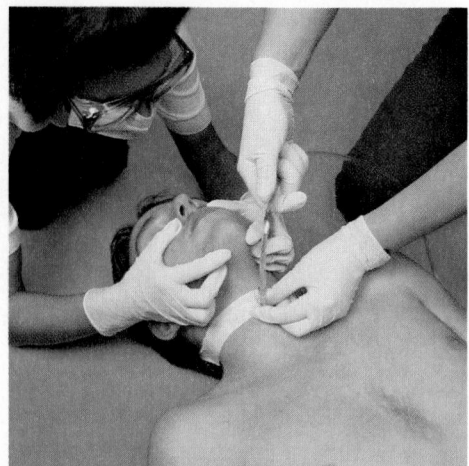

Fig. 12-46 A, Stabilize the larynx and identify the cricothyroid membrane. **B,** Insert the needle of the syringe downward through the midline of the membrane toward the carina. **C,** During insertion, apply negative pressure to the syringe. The entrance of air into the syringe indicates that the needle is in the trachea. **D,** After removing the needle and syringe, stabilize the catheter and connect the end of the oxygen tubing from the hub of the cannula to the oxygen regulator. Provide for a release valve.

or T connector, through a three-way stopcock directly attached to the high-pressure tubing, or by cutting a hole in the oxygen line to provide a "whistle-stop" effect.)

Technique

The following steps in transtracheal ventilation should be followed (Fig. 12-46):

1. Ensure that the patient is supine and the cricothyroid membrane is identified. (If spinal injury is suspected, in-line stabilization may be provided as for nasal and tracheal intubation.)
2. Stabilize the larynx using the thumb and middle finger of one hand. With the other hand, palpate the small depression below the thyroid cartilage (the "Adam's apple"), sliding the index finger down to locate the cricothyroid membrane.
3. Insert the needle of the syringe downward through the midline of the membrane at a 45- to 60-degree angle toward the patient's carina, applying negative pressure to the syringe during insertion (Fig. 12-47, *A*). The entrance of air into the syringe indicates that the needle is in the trachea.
4. Advance the catheter over the needle toward the carina, and remove the needle and syringe (Fig. 12-47, *B*). Care must be taken not to kink the polytef (Teflon) catheter when removing the needle and syringe.
5. Hold the hub of the catheter to prevent accidental dislodgment during the time required

to provide ventilation. Connect the end of the oxygen tubing from the hub of the cannula to the oxygen regulator. Provide for a release valve as previously described.

When the release valve is closed, oxygen under pressure is introduced into the trachea. The pressure is adjusted to a level that allows adequate lung expansion. The patient's chest must be observed carefully and the release valve opened to allow for exhalation. The correct ratio of inflation to deflation varies, depending on whether upper airway obstruction is present. For an open upper airway, an inspiratory-to-expiratory ratio of 1 to 4 seconds is adequate. Ratios of approximately 1 to 8 seconds are needed to prevent barotrauma (injuries caused from excessive pressures [for example, pneumothorax]) when the upper airway is obstructed.[10]

> **NOTE:**
> Should the chest remain inflated during the period of exhalation, a proximal complete airway obstruction may be present, and a longer expiratory time should be used. If this does not produce adequate deflation, a second large-bore catheter may be inserted through the cricothyroid membrane next to the first one. If the chest continues to remain distended, a cricothyrotomy should be performed.

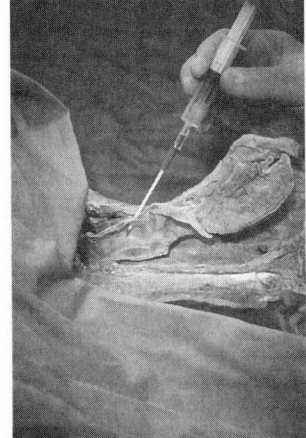

A

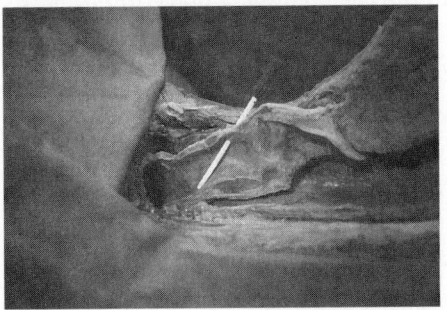

B

Fig. 12-47 Needle cricothyrotomy. **A,** Insert a large-bore catheter through the cricothyroid membrane, directing it caudally. Aspirate on the syringe as it is passed; when air is aspirated, the airway has been entered. **B,** Slide the catheter off the stylet into the larynx.

Advantages

- It is simple, inexpensive, and effective when properly performed.
- It requires minimal spinal manipulation.
- It is the least invasive of surgical procedures.
- It may be initiated quickly.

Disadvantages

- It is an invasive procedure.
- It requires constant monitoring.
- It does not protect the airway.
- It does not allow for efficient elimination of carbon dioxide.
- It may adequately ventilate the patient's lungs for only 30 to 45 minutes.

Potential Complications

- High pressure during ventilation and air entrapment may produce pneumothorax.
- Hemorrhage may occur at the insertion site, and the thyroid and esophagus can be perforated if the needle is advanced too far.
- It does not allow direct suctioning of secretions.
- Subcutaneous emphysema may occur.

Method of Removal

Because transtracheal ventilation is a temporary emergency procedure to allow time for other airway management techniques, removal should only follow successful orotracheal or nasotracheal intubation or commencement of a more definitive surgical airway, such as cricothyrotomy or tracheostomy. Removal entails withdrawing the catheter and dressing the wound.

Cricothyrotomy

Description

Cricothyrotomy is a surgical procedure that allows rapid entrance to the airway for ventilation and oxygenation for patients in whom airway control is not possible by other means. It should not be performed on patients who can be orally or nasally intubated. Although few situations require this surgical procedure, relative indications for cricothyrotomy include severe facial or nasal injuries that preclude oral or nasal intubations, massive midfacial trauma, possible spinal trauma, anaphylaxis, and chemical inhalation injuries. Like percutaneous transtracheal ventilation, cricothyrotomy requires special training and authorization from medical control.

Necessary Equipment

Commercially prepared cricothyrotomy kits are available through a number of manufacturers. In the absence of such kits, the following equipment is required:

- Scalpel blade
- 6.0 or 7.0 ET tube
- Antiseptic solution
- Oxygen source
- Bag-valve device

Technique

In patients with suspected spinal injury, in-line stabilization should be maintained throughout the procedure. If possible, the neck should be cleaned with alcohol or another antiseptic solution. The technique for performing the surgical procedure follows (Fig. 12-48):

1. Locate the anatomical landmarks of the neck, and identify the cricothyroid membrane.
2. Make a 2-cm horizontal incision with the scalpel at the level of the cricothyroid membrane. (Some physicians may recommend a vertical skin incision rather than a horizontal one.)
3. Open the incision of the cricothyroid membrane by inserting the scalpel handle. Rotate it 90 degrees to allow placement of a 6.0 or 7.0 ET tube that does not damage the larynx. The cuff should be inflated and the tube securely tied.
4. Provide ventilation by a bag-valve device with the highest available oxygen concentration.
5. Determine adequacy of ventilation through bilateral auscultation and observation of rise and fall of the chest.

Potential Complications

- Prolonged execution time
- Hemorrhage
- Aspiration
- Possible misplacement
- False passage

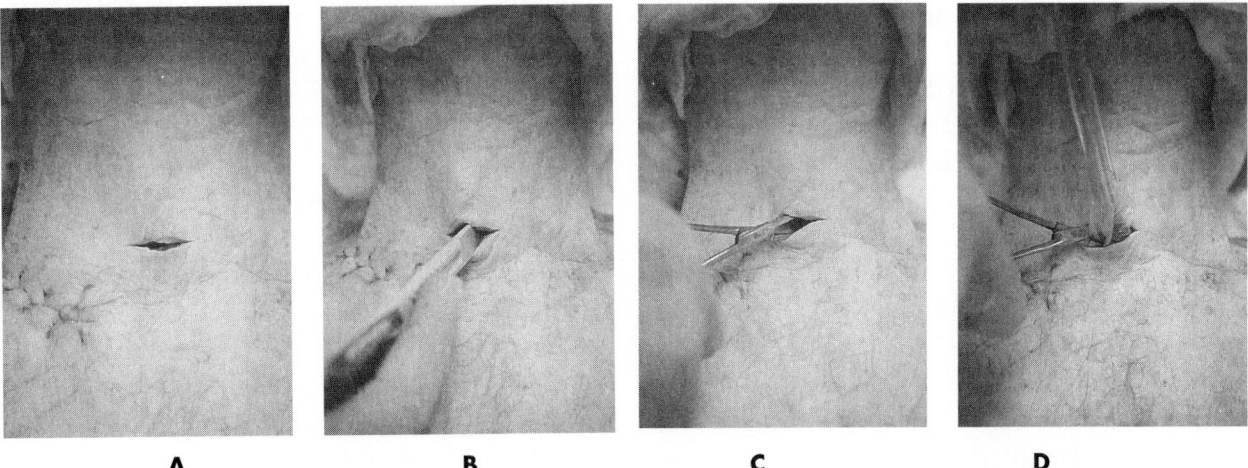

A   **B**   **C**   **D**

Fig. 12-48 A, Make an incision through the cricothyroid membrane. **B,** Open the hole by twisting the handle of a scalpel in it or **C,** by opening it with a clamp. **D,** Insert the ET tube.

- Perforation of the esophagus
- Injury to the vocal cords and carotid and jugular vessels lateral to the incision (The patient must be immobilized.)
- Subcutaneous emphysema

Contraindications
- Acute laryngeal disease caused by trauma or infection

- Small children under 10 years of age (In these patients, inserting a 12- to 14-gauge catheter over the needle may be safer than a cricothyrotomy.)

Method of Removal
The removal of adjuncts used during an emergency cricothyrotomy should not be attempted in the prehospital setting.

NOTE:

A position paper, developed by the American Heart Association (AHA) Emergency Cardiac Care Committee in cooperation with the American Red Cross, reports that there are no known cases of transmission of serious chronic diseases during rescue breathing. According to the report, "The probability of a rescuer becoming infected with HBV (hepatitis) or HIV (AIDS) as a result of performing CPR is minimal. To date, transmission of HBV or HIV infection during mouth-to-mouth resuscitation has not been documented."[11] This position is supported by research conducted by the Centers for Disease Control (CDC). According to the CDC, blood remains the only documented source of HIV infection for health workers. However, authorities believe that there is a *theoretical* risk of disease transmission, which providers should note:

"If a victim's saliva became contaminated by blood during ventilation . . . and the rescuer suffered a similar injury, such as a lip laceration," according to Joseph P. Ornato, M.D., this would provide "a theoretical route for blood-to-blood transmission of the virus."[12] The AHA advises that health care providers with a duty to respond to patients have access to mechanical ventilation or barrier devices. The AHA further recommends that health care workers with infections that may be transmitted by blood or saliva not perform mouth-to-mouth ventilation if other ventilation devices are available.

● METHODS OF VENTILATION

There are several methods by which patient ventilation can be provided in the prehospital setting. These methods include rescue breathing (mouth-to-mouth, mouth-to-nose, mouth-to-stoma), mouth-to-mask, use of bag-valve devices, and oxygen-powered, manually triggered devices

Rescue Breathing

As previously discussed, inspired air has an oxygen concentration of 21%. Of this 21%, approximately 4% is used by the body, and the remaining 17% is exhaled. Rescue breathing ventilation can accordingly provide adequate oxygenation to a patient with respiratory insufficiency.

The advantages of rescue breathing are that it requires no equipment and it is immediately available. The disadvantages are the limitation of the vital capacity of the rescuer (approximately 800 to 1200 cc are needed to effectively ventilate the adult patient) and the low concentration of oxygen in expired air compared with other methods of ventilation with supplemental oxygen delivery. It may also be difficult for the rescuer to force air past obstructions in the airway. There is the theoretical risk of disease transmission.

Mouth-to-Mouth

The following guidelines should be observed when delivering ventilations mouth-to-mouth:

1. In the absence of suspected spinal injury, position the patient with optimal head-tilt and chin-lift. (If spinal injury is suspected, maintain in-line stabilization and maintain an open airway through the jaw-thrust without head-tilt technique.) If necessary, clear the airway of vomitus, body fluids, and foreign objects.
2. Pinch the patient's nostrils closed.
3. Inhale a deep breath.
4. Seal your mouth over the patient's mouth, which should be slightly open.
5. Exhale into the patient's mouth until the chest rises and resistance is produced by the patient's lung expansion.
6. Break contact with the patient's mouth to allow for passive exhalation.

7. Repeat the process, providing a full ventilation of 800 to 1200 cc (1.5 to 2 seconds in duration) every 5 to 6 seconds as needed.

Mouth-to-Nose

Mouth-to-nose ventilation is very similar to the technique described for mouth-to-mouth rescue breathing. The differences in the mouth-to-nose method are as follows:

- In the absence of suspected spinal injury, one hand must be kept on the patient's forehead to maintain an open airway while the rescuer's other hand is used to close the patient's mouth. (If spinal injury is suspected, the jaw-thrust-without-head-tilt technique should be used, and the rescuer's cheek is used to seal the patient's mouth.)
- The patient's nose is left open.
- The rescuer's mouth is placed over the patient's nose with as tight a seal as possible.
- During passive exhalation by the patient, the rescuer's mouth is removed from the patient's nose, and the patient's mouth is opened for exhalation. The head-tilt position must be maintained to ensure an open airway.

Mouth-to-nose ventilation may be appropriate in the following patient situations:

- Injuries to the mouth and lower jaw
- A patient with missing teeth or dentures (making a tight seal around the mouth difficult)
- As an alternative to mouth-to-mouth contact with a patient

Mouth-to-Stoma

A stoma is a temporary or permanent surgical opening in the neck of a patient who has had a laryngectomy or tracheostomy (Fig. 12-49). The airway of such a patient has been surgically interrupted, and the larynx is no longer connected to the trachea.

The postlaryngectomy stoma is large and round, and the edge of the tracheal lining can be seen attached to the skin. The stoma in tracheostomy patients is usually no more than several millimeters in diameter and contains one or two concentric tubes made of plastic or metal. The method of ventilating these patients is the same, regardless of the type of stoma.

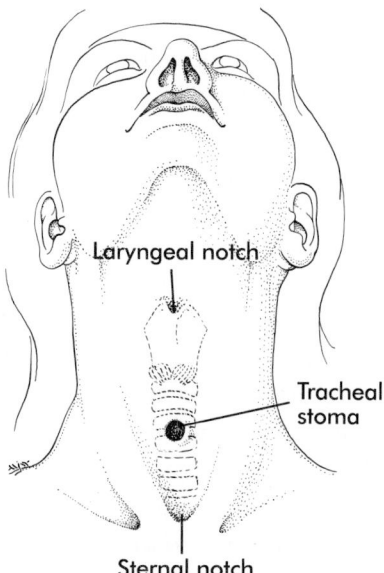

Fig. 12-49 Stoma.

> **NOTE:**
> Stomas and breathing tubes may become clogged with secretions, encrusted mucus, and foreign matter, leading to inadequate ventilation.

If cleaning is necessary, wipe the neck opening with gauze. If the breathing tubes are clogged, they can be removed or suctioned. The tracheostomy tube or stoma is suctioned by passing a sterile suction catheter through the external opening and into the trachea. *Do not insert the catheter more than 3 to 5 inches into the trachea.* Once the airway is partially open, begin ventilations by mouth-to-stoma (mouth-to-stoma ventilation is bacteriologically cleaner than the mouth-to-mouth method) by using a pediatric-size pocket mask over the top of the stoma, or by securing the airway with an ET tube placed through the stoma.

The technique for stoma ventilation is basically the same as that for other methods of artificial ventilation. However, the patient's head should be kept straight (rather than tilted back), with slight elevation of the patient's shoulders. This position permits more effective ventilation. If the patient's chest does not rise or air is heard to escape through the patient's upper airway, the patient may be a partial neck breather. These patients are able to inhale and exhale some air through their nose and mouth. Should this occur, it will be nec-

essary to pinch the patient's nostrils closed and seal the mouth with the palm of one hand during ventilation.

Ventilating Infants and Children

To provide ventilations to infants and children, the paramedic should use the mouth-to-mouth-and-nose technique as described below:

> **NOTE:**
> The AHA defines an infant as less than 1 year of age and a child as 1 to 8 years of age.

1. Position the patient with a *slight* head-tilt and chin-lift sufficient to open the airway. Hyperextension of the pediatric patient's neck may occlude the airway. (If spinal injury is suspected, use spinal precautions as previously described.)
2. When ventilating, the rescuer's mouth should cover both the mouth and the nose of the infant or small child.
3. Use smaller breaths than are needed for an adult patient yet large enough to make the chest rise.
4. When allowing for passive exhalation, break contact with the patient's mouth and nose.
5. Provide slow ventilations (1 to 1.5 seconds in duration) every 3 seconds for the infant and every 4 seconds for the child.

Mouth-To-Mask

Mouth-to-mask devices have become popular as an alternative to mouth-to-mouth methods of ventilation. These masks are of a clear, flexible construction and are available with one-way valves and ports for supplemental oxygen delivery (Fig. 12-50). They are produced by a number of manufacturers and are available in a variety of sizes. The mouth-to-mask technique offers several advantages:

- It eliminates direct contact with the patient's mouth and nose.
- Supplemental oxygen delivery is possible.
- The one-way valve eliminates exposure to exhaled gases and sputum.

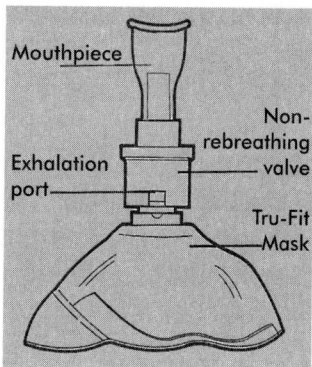

Fig. 12-50 LSP mask and airflow schematic.

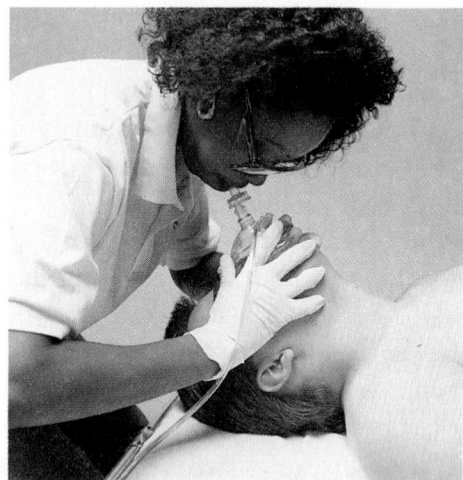

Fig. 12-51 Mouth-to-mask ventilation technique.

- It is easy to apply.
- It may provide more effective ventilation than mouth-to-mouth or BVM.
- It is aesthetically more acceptable than mouth-to-mouth ventilation.

Technique

The mask device can be used in patients with or without spontaneous respirations. If immediately available, mouth-to-mask is the preferred method of initial ventilation (Fig. 12-51). To apply the mask, follow these steps:

1. In the absence of suspected spinal injury, position the patient with optimal head-tilt and chin-lift. The use of an oropharyngeal or na-sopharyngeal airway is indicated in unconscious patients. (If spinal injury is suspected, the spinal precautions previously described should be used.)

2. Connect the one-way valve to the mask. Oxygen tubing should be connected to the inlet port with an oxygen flow rate of 10 to 15 L/min. Using supplemental oxygen provides a higher concentration of oxygen in the inspired air. An oxygen flow rate of 10 L/min, combined with rescuer ventilations, can supply an oxygen concentration of 50%. An oxygen flow rate of 15 L/min provides an inspired oxygen concentration of approximately 80%.

3. Position yourself at the patient's head. If necessary, clear the airway of secretion, vomitus, and foreign objects. Place the mask on the patient's face, providing an airtight seal. With the thumb side of the palm of both hands, apply pressure to the sides of the mask. Apply upward pressure to the mandible just in front of the ear lobes, using the index, middle, and ring fingers of both hands while maintaining head-tilt.

4. Blow into the opening of the mask, observing chest rise and fall. If available, a second rescuer should apply cricoid pressure to help prevent gastric inflation during positive pressure ventilation and to reduce the possibility of regurgitation and aspiration.

5. Break contact with the mask to allow for passive exhalation.

Bag-Valve Devices

Bag-valve devices consist of a self-inflating bag and a nonrebreathing valve (Fig. 12-52). They may be used with a mask, an ET tube, or another invasive airway device. An adequate bag-valve unit should have (1) a self-refilling bag that is disposable or easily cleaned or sterilized, (2) a nonjam valve system allowing a minimum oxygen inlet flow of 15 L/min, (3) a non-pop-off valve, (4) standard 15-mm and 22-mm fittings, (5) a system for delivering high-concentration oxygen through an inlet port at the back of the bag or by an oxygen reservoir, and (6) a nonrebreathing valve. Further-

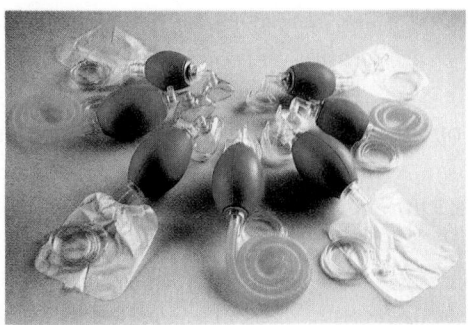

Fig. 12-52 Disposable and reusable adult and pediatric bag-valve devices.

more, it should perform under all common environmental conditions and extremes of temperature and be available in both the adult and the pediatric sizes.[3]

When the bag-valve device is compressed, air is delivered to the patient through a one-way valve. The air inlet to the bag is closed during delivery. When the bag is released, the patient's expired gas passes through an exhalation valve into the atmosphere, preventing the patient's gas from reentering the bag-valve device. As the patient exhales, atmospheric air and supplemental oxygen from the reservoir refill the bag.

Use of the bag-valve device with a mask is difficult. This is because of the problem of providing an effective mask seal on the patient's face while maintaining an open airway. Therefore a BVM should only be used by well-trained and experienced personnel. It has been recommended that two rescuers use the BVM, one holding the mask and maintaining the airway while the second compresses the bag with two hands.

When properly used, the bag-valve device has many benefits. The rescuer can provide a wide range of inspiratory pressures and volumes to adequately ventilate patients of varying sizes and underlying pathological conditions: It can be used to assist patients with shallow respirations, it performs adequately in extremes of environmental temperatures, and oxygen concentrations ranging from 21% (room air concentration) to nearly 100% (using supplemental oxygen and a reservoir) can be achieved. In addition, manual compression of the bag can give the rescuer a sense of the patient's

lung compliance, which is an advantage over mechanical methods of ventilation (for example, the demand-valve).

Technique

Ventilation with the bag-valve device is best accomplished when the patient is intubated. In the absence of intubation, the bag-valve device may be used with a mask. The following technique is recommended for use with the BVM:

1. The rescuer is positioned at the top of the patient's head.
2. In the absence of suspected spinal injury, the patient should be in the optimal head-tilt chin-lift position, and the patient's head should be elevated in extension. If spinal injury is suspected, spinal precautions as previously described should be used.
3. If necessary, the airway should be cleared of secretions, vomitus, and foreign objects. If the patient is unconscious, an oropharyngeal or nasopharyngeal airway should be inserted. The patient's mouth should remain open under the mask.
4. An oxygen source is connected with a reservoir and flushed with high-concentration oxygen.
5. The mask is placed on the patient's face, making a tight seal. This can be accomplished by placing the thumb on the nose area, placing an index finger on the chin, and spreading the remaining fingers along the mandible. The anterior displacement of the mandible must be maintained.
6. To compress the bag, the rescuer's other hand presses the bag against his or her body (for example, the thigh), or another rescuer compresses the bag as recommended by the AHA. The bag should be compressed quickly and smoothly, delivering 500 to 800 ml of air every 5 to 6 seconds for the adult patient.

Pediatric Considerations

Smaller bag-valve devices are needed for infants and children to reduce the chances of overinflation and subsequent barotrauma. Bag-valve devices are used primarily to provide ventilatory support in pediatric patients who are in respiratory arrest. BVM devices equipped with a fish-mouth– or leaf-flap–operated outlet valve cannot be used to provide supplemental oxygen to the spontaneously breathing infant or child because the child receives only the exhaled gases contained within the mask itself if the valve fails to open during inspiration. For this reason, bag-valve devices for ventilation of full-term neonates, infants, and children should have a minimum volume of 450 ml.[3] At least 10 to 15 L/min of oxygen flow are required to maintain an adequate oxygen volume in the reservoir of a pediatric bag.

Oxygen-Powered, Manually Triggered Devices

Oxygen-powered, manually triggered devices (Fig. 12-53) allow for positive-pressure ventilation, delivering nearly 100% oxygen with a tight mask seal. These devices consist of high-pressure tubing that connects to an oxygen supply (under pressure of 50 psi). They are easily connected to a mask, tracheostomy tube, esophageal obturator, or ET tube. A valve on the device is activated by a lever or push button, allowing oxygen to flow to the patient.

Oxygen-powered, manually triggered devices should provide (1) a constant flow rate of 100% oxygen at less than 40 L/min, (2) an inspiratory pressure relief valve that opens at 60 to 80 cm of water and vents any remaining volume to the atmosphere or ceases gas flow, (3) an audible alarm that sounds whenever the relief valve pressure is exceeded to alert the rescuer that the patient requires high inflation pressures and may not be receiving adequate ventilatory volumes, (4) satisfactory operation under environmental extremes, and (5) a demand flow system that does not impose additional work.

When using these devices, *the paramedic must be alert for adequate rise and fall of the patient's chest,* making sure not to deliver too much or too little ventilatory volume. Gastric distention is common because of the high inspiratory flow rates. Therefore the paramedic must carefully observe the patient for signs of a distended abdomen, which could lead to regurgitation and aspiration. Many oxygen-powered breathing devices have restricted flow rates of 40 L/min and require unacceptably high triggering pressures in the demand mode and should not be used for spontaneously breathing patients. In addition, these devices are not to be used on pediatric patients.

Automatic Transport Ventilators

There are several time-cycled, gas-powered automatic transport ventilators (ATVs) for field use or intrahospital transport when caring for patients who require ventilatory support (Fig. 12-54). Most of these ventilators consist of a plastic control module connected by tubing to any 50-psi gas source (such as air or different concentrations of oxygen, including 100% oxygen). The exit valve of the control module is connected by two tubes to the patient valve assembly to deliver selected tidal volumes (400 to 1200 ml for adults, 200 to 600 ml

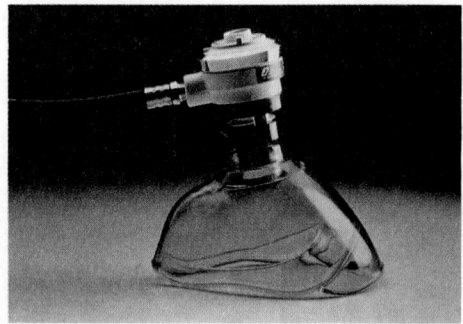

Fig. 12-53 Oxygen-powered, manually triggered (demand-valve) device.

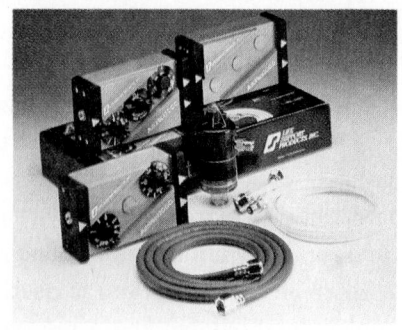

Fig. 12-54 Autovent 1000, 2000, and 3000.

for children). Another control selects respiratory rates from 8 to 22 breaths per minute for adults and 8 to 30 breaths per minute for children. (ATVs are not to be used in children under 5 years old.) Most units provide a 40 L/min flow of oxygen, which remains constant regardless of changes in the patient's airway or lung compliance.

The volume of gas delivered by the automatic ventilator is determined by the length of time the manual trigger is depressed or by the inspiratory effort of the spontaneously breathing patient. Most units are designed to limit the inspiratory pressure to 60 to 80 cm of water. When this pressure is reached, an audible alarm sounds, and gas flow from the unit stops, preventing possible lung damage. ATVs allow the paramedic to use both hands to obtain a tight mask seal in the nonintubated patient and to perform other tasks when the ventilator is used with ET intubation.

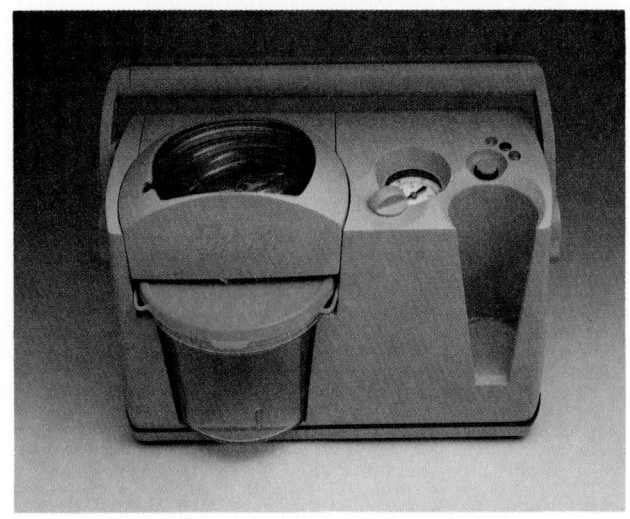

Fig. 12-55 Fixed suction unit.

Suction

Suction can be used to remove vomitus, saliva, blood, food, and other foreign objects that might occlude the airway or increase the likelihood of pulmonary aspiration by inhalation. There are many predisposing factors to aspiration, so every patient should be regarded as a potential aspiration victim.

Suction Devices

Fixed and portable mechanical suction devices are available through a number of manufacturers. Fixed suction devices (Fig. 12-55) are mounted in patient care areas of hospitals and nursing homes and in many emergency vehicles. These systems are electrically operated by vacuum pumps or powered by the vacuum produced by a vehicle engine manifold. Fixed suction devices furnish an air intake of at least 30 L per minute and provide a vacuum of more than 300 mm Hg when the tube is clamped.

Portable suction devices (Fig. 12-56) may be oxygen or air powered, electrically powered, or manually powered. These devices should furnish an air intake of no less than 20 L per minute to operate effectively.

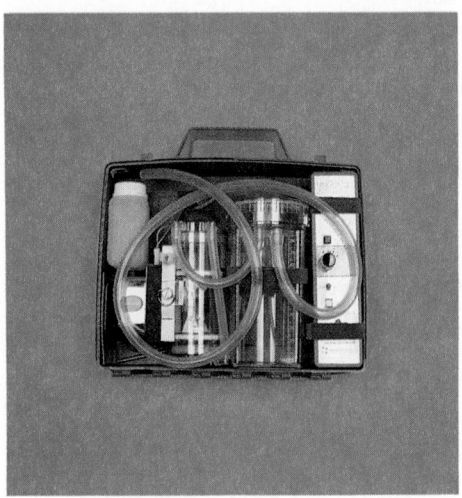

Fig. 12-56 Portable suction units.

Suction Catheters

Suction catheters are used to clear the air passages of secretions and debris. The two broad classifications of catheters are the whistle-tip suction catheter and the tonsil-tip suction catheter.

The whistle-tip catheter is a narrow, flexible tube used primarily for tracheobronchial suctioning to clear secretions through either an ET tube or the nasopharynx (Fig. 12-57). This catheter is designed with molded ends and side holes to produce minimal trauma to the mucosa. In the proxi-

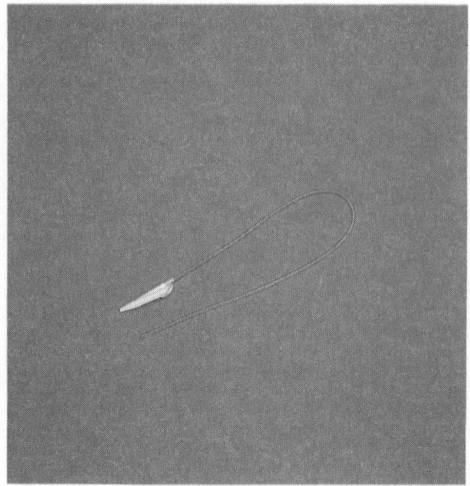

Fig. 12-57 Soft suction catheters.

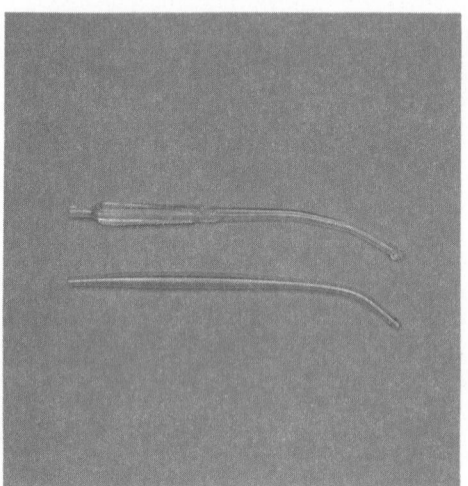

Fig. 12-58 Rigid suction catheter.

mal end it has a side opening that is covered with the thumb to produce suction. Using sterile technique, the catheter is advanced to the desired location, and suction is applied intermittently as the catheter is withdrawn.

The tonsil-tip suction catheter is a rigid pharyngeal catheter used to clear secretions, blood clots, and other foreign material from the mouth and pharynx (Fig. 12-58). It is carefully inserted into the oral cavity under direct visualization and slowly withdrawn while suction is activated.

Before any suctioning procedure is initiated, all equipment should be checked and the suction set between 80 and 120 mm Hg. The patient's lungs should be oxygenated with 100% oxygen for at least 2 minutes before suction is initiated, if possible. *Suction should never be applied for more than 10 seconds.* If additional suctioning is warranted, the patient's lungs should be reoxygenated before repeating the procedure. Potential complications from suctioning include the following:

- Sudden hypoxemia secondary to decreased lung volume during the suction application
- Severe hypoxemia that may lead to cardiac rhythm disturbances and cardiac arrest
- Airway stimulation that may increase arterial pressure and cardiac rhythm disturbances
- Coughing that may result in increased intracranial pressure with reduced blood flow to the brain and increased risk of **herniation** in patients with head injury
- Soft-tissue damage to the respiratory tract

● SPECIAL CONSIDERATIONS FOR PEDIATRIC PATIENTS

In addition to the differences in airway and ventilation procedures for pediatric patients, the anatomical differences of the pediatric airway must be considered.[12]

The infant's upper airway is relatively small, and the tongue is disproportionately large. Therefore posterior displacement of the tongue easily obstructs the airway. In addition, the larger tongue of the pediatric patient tends to make laryngoscopy more difficult.

The epiglottis is omega shaped and is narrower and longer in children than in the adult. Because of this, the epiglottis is more difficult to control with a laryngoscope blade. The larynx lies more anteriorly in relation to the base of the tongue than in the adult, and it is also elevated under the base of the tongue, making visualization more difficult. The glottic opening is at the third cervical vertebra in premature neonates, the third to fourth cervical vertebra in term neonates, and the fourth to fifth cervical vertebra in adults.

During the first few months of life, the vocal cords of the infant slope from back to front, frequently causing the ET tube to "hang up" in the angle formed by the cords. This problem can be minimized by rotating the ET tube or by having a second rescuer perform the Sellick maneuver during intubation.

The cricoid cartilage is the narrowest part of the airway in the infant and young child. Therefore an ET tube that is too large may pass through the cords and then meet resistance at the cricoid cartilage. As the child reaches 8 years of age, the vocal cords become the narrowest part, and this position is maintained into adulthood.

The distance from the vocal cords to the carina varies and can be correlated with the patient's height. This distance is approximately 4 to 5 cm at birth and 6 to 7 cm at age 6. During placement of the ET tube, it is recommended that the tube be advanced until breath sounds are lost unilaterally (usually on the left side). It should then be slowly withdrawn until breath sounds return, indicating that the tube tip is at the carina. After the return of breath sounds, the tube should be withdrawn 2 to 3 cm farther, placing it at a safe distance above the carina and below the cords. The tube should then be secured with tape.

Children use their diaphragm as the major muscle for ventilation and require full diaphragmatic excursion to breathe. Gastric distention caused by swallowing air or artificial ventilation can inhibit the child's respiratory efforts. Infants are nasal breathers until 3 to 5 months of age.

Deciduous teeth begin to develop at approximately 6 months and are lost between 6 and 8 years. They may become dislodged during airway procedures such as intubation and oral airway insertion and by the child biting on the airway.

During any airway procedure, the paramedic should remember that the airway structures of the pediatric patient are very fragile and easily damaged. Therefore great caution must be exercised so as not to injure these patients.

increase in ventilation-perfusion mismatching, which leads to a gradually lowered P_{O_2}.

The changes in pulmonary physiology include:
- Alterations in lung and chest wall compliance:
  - Increased thoracic rigidity
  - Decreased elastic recoil (Total lung capacity remains unchanged because of opposing loss of chest wall compliance and weakened respiratory muscles.)
- Enlarged alveolar ducts and sacs:
  - Fewer alveoli
  - Less alveolar surface for gas exchange

The aging process also changes the body's ventilatory control mechanisms. As the patient grows older, for example, the body's arterial P_{O_2} falls, although there is no significant change in arterial P_{CO_2}. (This is thought to be a result of airway closure during exhalation rather than age-related changes in perfusion capacity.) Several methods have been developed to calculate expected P_{O_2} in older patients. One method is to remember that a patient who is 70 years old is expected to have a P_{O_2} of 70 mm Hg. Using this value as a baseline, allow a 1 mm Hg decrease in P_{O_2} for every year above 70, or a 1 mm Hg increase in P_{O_2} for every year below 70. A patient who is 65 years old, for example, would be expected to have a P_{O_2} of 75 mm Hg, and a 75-year-old patient would be expected to have a P_{O_2} of 65 mm Hg.

The function of the body's chemoreceptors also declines with age. This results in a diminished ventilatory response to hypoxia, hypercapnia, and similar conditions and may predispose the older patient to respiratory failure. It is therefore important that older patients who have respiratory compromise from any cause receive immediate intervention, oxygenation, and ventilatory support.

● SPECIAL CONSIDERATIONS FOR OLDER PATIENTS

Respiratory disorders pose special problems for the older patient, whose respiratory function may be compromised as a result of the aging process. Pulmonary changes that occur as a result of aging decrease vital capacity and increase physiological dead space. There also tends to be an

> ### Section Four
> ### Oxygen Equipment and Delivery Devices

Oxygen equipment and delivery devices are used to provide emergency care at basic and advanced levels. These devices are briefly described.

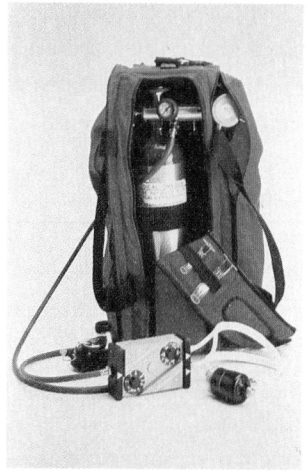

Fig. 12-59 Portable resuscitators.

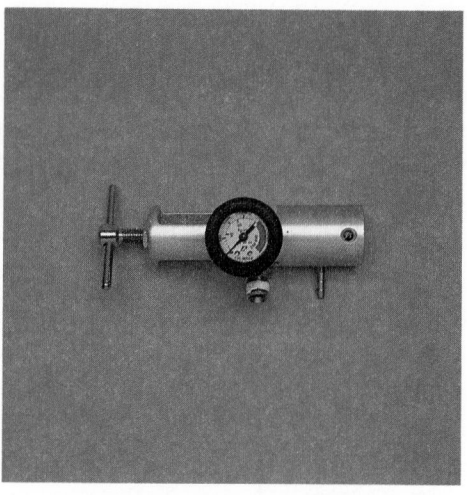

Fig. 12-60 Pressure regulator.

● OXYGEN AND OXYGEN EQUIPMENT

The most common form of oxygen used in the prehospital setting is pure oxygen gas. This gas is stored under pressure in stainless steel or lightweight alloy cylinders (Fig. 12-59). These cylinders have been color coded by United States Pharmacopeia to distinguish various compressed gases. Steel green and white cylinders have been assigned to all grades of oxygen. Stainless steel and aluminum cylinders are not painted. Oxygen cylinders are filled under a pressure of 2000 to 2200 psi. Therefore safety is of prime importance when handling this equipment. Common sizes used in emergency care are as follows:

- D cylinders (350 L of oxygen)
- E cylinders (625 L of oxygen)
- M cylinders (3000 L of oxygen)
- G cylinders (5300 L of oxygen)
- H cylinders (6900 L of oxygen)

The pressure in oxygen cylinders must be reduced for safe administration. This is accomplished by a pressure regulator that reduces the pressure from 70 psi to 30 psi (Fig. 12-60). The regulators are attached to smaller oxygen cylinders by a yoke assembly with a pin index safety system (Fig. 12-61). This system protects the user from using a regulator with the wrong type of gas. It requires that the yoke pins match the corre-

> ### BOX 12-4
>
> #### Liquid Oxygen
>
> Liquid oxygen (LOX) is used by hospitals and some air medical services and other EMS agencies when weight and the space that an oxygen system occupies must be considered. Its main advantage is its lighter weight and smaller volume. Disadvantages of prehospital use of liquid oxygen are the cost (LOX is more expensive than pressurized oxygen) and smaller system volumes, which require frequent replenishing.

sponding holes in the valve assembly for oxygen to be delivered. Larger oxygen cylinders have valve assemblies with a threaded outlet specific to medical oxygen (Box 12-4).

Flowmeters control the amount of oxygen delivered to the patient (Fig. 12-62). These devices are connected to the pressure regulator and adjusted to deliver oxygen in a certain number of liters per minute. Some EMS agencies attach disposable humidifiers to the flowmeter to provide moisture to the dry oxygen coming from the supply cylinder.

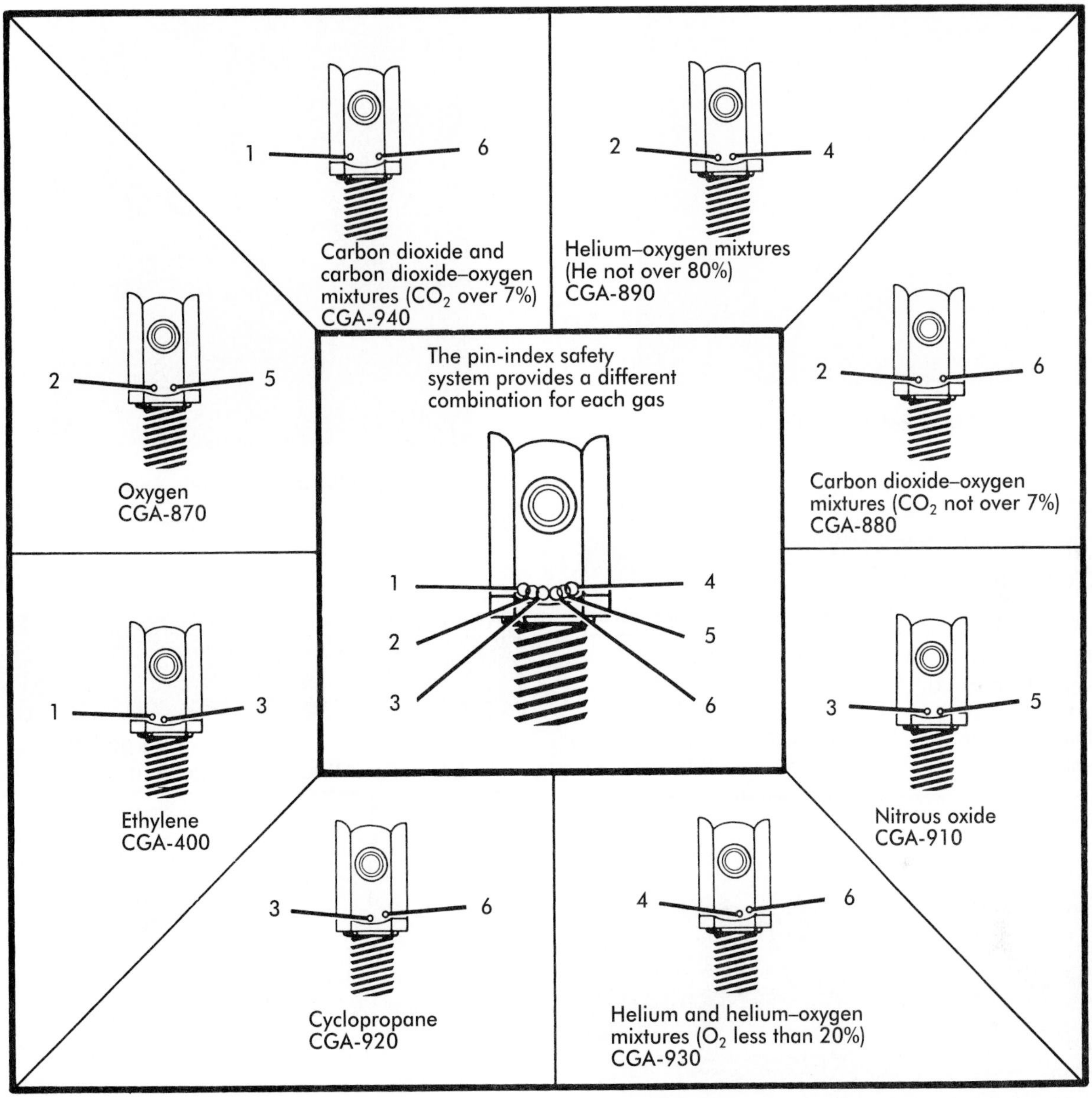
1
6
Carbon dioxide and
carbon dioxide–oxygen
mixtures (CO2 over 7%)
CGA-940
2
4
Helium–oxygen mixtures
(He not over 80%)
CGA-890
2
5
Oxygen
CGA-870
The pin-index safety
system provides a different
combination for each gas
1
2
3
4
5
6
2
6
Carbon dioxide–oxygen
mixtures (CO2 not over 7%)
CGA-880
1
3
Ethylene
CGA-400
3
5
Nitrous oxide
CGA-910
3
6
Cyclopropane
CGA-920
4
6
Helium and helium–oxygen
mixtures (O2 less than 20%)
CGA-930

Fig. 12-61 Pin index safety system.

● OXYGEN-DELIVERY DEVICES

Five oxygen-delivery devices can be used to provide supplemental oxygen to prehospital patients who have spontaneous respirations. They are the nasal cannula, simple face mask, partial rebreather mask, nonrebreather mask, and Venturi mask (Table 12-2).

The nasal cannula (Fig. 12-63) delivers low-concentration oxygen to patients by way of two small plastic prongs placed into the nostrils. The

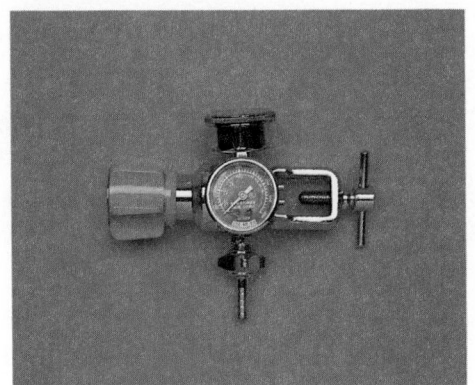

Fig. 12-62 Flowmeter.

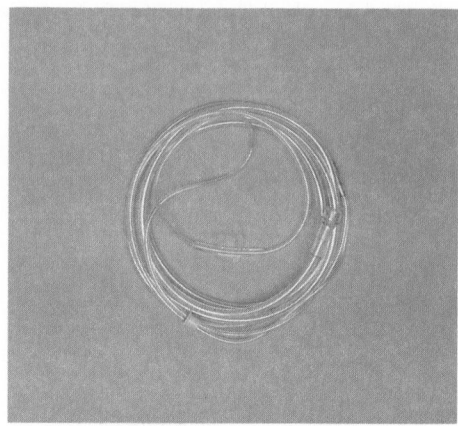

Fig. 12-63 Nasal cannula.

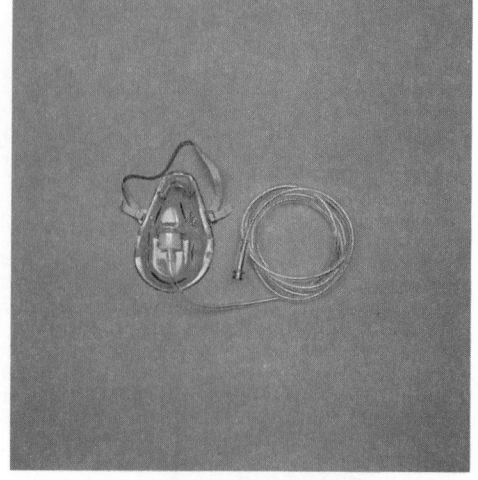

Fig. 12-64 Simple face mask.

TABLE 12-2 Oxygen Delivery Devices

Device	Flow Rate	O_2% Delivered
Nasal cannula	1-6 L/min	24%-44%
Simple face mask	6-15 L/min	35%-60%
Partial rebreather	6-10 L/min	35%-60%
Nonrebreather	10-15 L/min	80%-95%
Venturi	4-8 L/min	24%-50%

TABLE 12-3 Approximate Oxygen Concentration to Liter Per Minute Flow

Liters Per Minute	Oxygen Concentration
1	24%
2	28%
3	32%
4	36%
5	40%
6	44%

NOTE:

It is difficult to obtain oxygen concentrations greater than 30% to 35% via nasal cannula. This is a result of the mouth breathing that occurs during oxygen administration, which decreases the concentration of inspired oxygen. Therefore nasal cannula use is limited to patients who would benefit from low-concentration oxygen delivery (for example, some patients with chest pain and patients who have chronic obstructive pulmonary disease). The device is also ineffective if the patient's nares are occluded by blood or mucus.

relationship of approximate oxygen concentrations to liter per minute flow is listed in Table 12-3.

The simple face mask (Fig. 12-64) is a soft, clear plastic mask that conforms to the patient's face. Small perforations in the mask allow for atmospheric gas to be mixed with oxygen during inhalation and permit the patient's exhaled air to escape. Oxygen concentrations of 35% to 60% can be delivered through this device with a flow rate of 6 to 8 L/min. Flow rates of less than 6 L/min can produce an accumulation of carbon dioxide in the mask, so oxygen delivery through *any* face mask should always exceed this minimum.

The partial rebreather mask (Fig. 12-65) has an attached oxygen reservoir bag that should be filled before patient use. This device allows a portion of the patient's exhaled gas that filled the anatomical dead space to enter the reservoir bag and be reused. The remainder of the carbon dioxide–loaded gas escapes to the atmosphere. Oxygen concentrations of 35% to 60% can be delivered

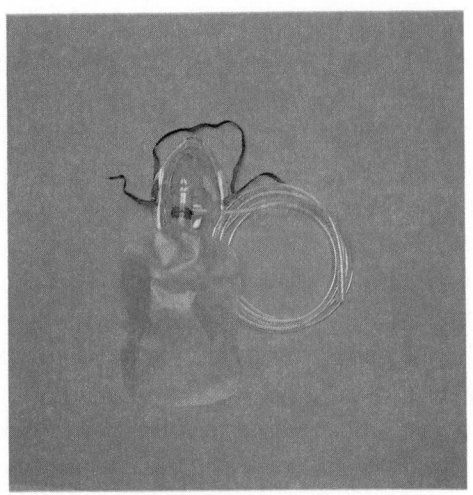

Fig. 12-65 Partial rebreather mask.

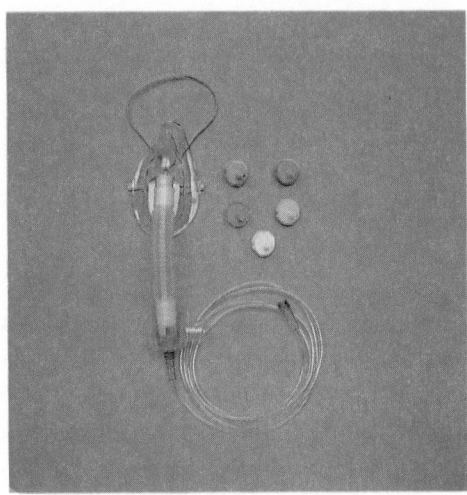

Fig. 12-67 Venturi mask.

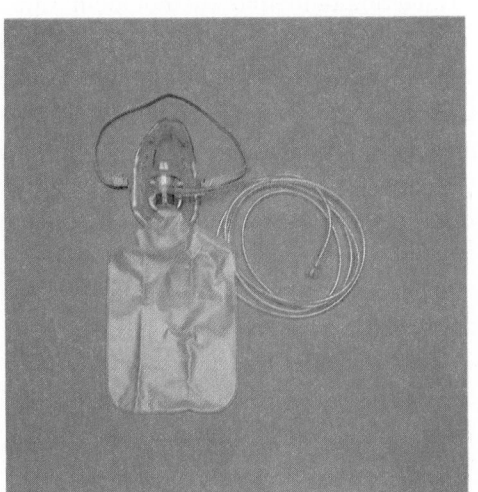

Fig. 12-66 Nonrebreather mask.

with a flow rate that prevents the reservoir bag from collapsing completely on inspiration. Partial rebreather masks must be well fitted to the patient's face for optimal benefit.

The nonrebreather mask (Fig. 12-66) is similar in design to the partial nonrebreather. However, a flutter valve assembly in the face piece prevents the patient's exhaled air from returning to the reservoir bag. This device delivers oxygen concentrations ranging above 95% with an adequate flow rate that keeps the reservoir bag partially inflated during inspiration. The paramedic should ensure

that the mask is seated firmly over the patient's mouth and nose and that the reservoir bag is never less than two-thirds full. This device is most commonly used in patients who require high-concentration oxygen delivery (10 to 15 L/min).

The Venturi mask (Fig. 12-67) is a high-air-flow oxygen entrainment delivery device that delivers a precise fraction of inspired oxygen (Fio_2) at typically low concentrations. The device was originally designed to deliver 30% to 40% concentrations but has since been adapted to deliver higher oxygen percentages. The Venturi mask uses "jet mixing" of atmospheric gas and oxygen to achieve the desired mixture.

Various sized color-coded adapters are attached to the mask to control the oxygen flow rate. (Standard sizes are 3-, 4-, and 6-L/min adapters.) The color codes and adapters state the exact liter flow to use to obtain the precise Fio_2. Choosing a different liter flow drastically alters the Fio_2 delivered. The various Venturi masks deliver 24% to 50% oxygen and are recommended for patients who rely on a hypoxic respiratory drive (for example, those with chronic obstructive pulmonary disease). The main benefit to the Venturi mask is that it allows precise regulation of Fio_2. In addition, its use permits the paramedic to titrate oxygen to the patient with chronic obstructive pulmonary disease so as not to exceed the patient's hypoxic drive while allowing enrichment of supplemental oxygen. Care must be taken to match the appropriate Fio_2 to the correct flow rate or the mask will not deliver the indicated Fio_2.

● PULSE OXIMETERS

Pulse oximeters (Fig. 12-68) are used as an adjunct in determining effective patient oxygenation by measuring the transmission of red and near-infrared light through arterial beds. Hemoglobin absorbs red and infrared light waves differently when it is bound with oxygen (oxyhemoglobin) and when it is not (reduced hemoglobin). Oxyhemoglobin absorbs more infrared than red light, and reduced hemoglobin absorbs more red than infrared light. Pulse oximetry reveals arterial saturation by measuring this difference.

The oximeter probe is placed on a thin tissue, such as a finger, toe, or ear lobe. One side of the probe emits wavelengths of light into the arterial bed. The other side detects the presence of red or infrared light. Using this balance of red and infrared colors, the oximeter calculates the oxygen saturation of the blood and displays it on the monitor screen.

The percentage of hemoglobin saturated with oxygen is denoted as Sao_2 and depends on a number of factors, including Pco_2, pH, temperature, and whether the hemoglobin is normal or altered. Normal Sao_2 is between 93% and 95%. When the Sao_2 falls below 90%, there is a rapid decline in oxygen content.

Because difficulties and inaccuracies may result from the use of pulse oximeters, paramedics should consider their use as only another tool to assist in patient monitoring. Circumstances that may produce false readings include the following[13]:

- Dyshemoglobinemia (hemoglobin saturated with compounds other than oxygen [for example, carbon monoxide, methemoglobinemia])
- Excessive ambient light (sunlight, fluorescent lights) on the oximeter's sensor probe

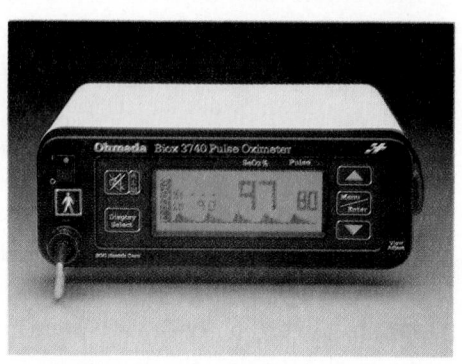

Fig. 12-68 Pulse oximeter.

- Patient movement
- Hypotension
- Hypothermia
- Patient use of vasoconstrictive drugs
- Patient use of nail polish
- Jaundice

REFERENCES

1. National Safety Council: *Accident facts,* Chicago, 1991, The Council.
2. American Heart Association. *Health care provider's manual,* Dallas, 1988, The Association.
3. American Heart Association: *Guidelines for cardiopulmonary resuscitation and emergency cardiac care, JAMA* 268(16):2172, 1992.
4. Tintinalli J et al, editors: *Emergency medicine: a comprehensive study guide,* ed 2, New York, 1988, McGraw-Hill.
5. Rothstein R, editor: Respiratory emergencies. II. *Top Emerg Med* 2(2):45, 1980.
6. Gorback M: *Emergency airway management,* Philadelphia, 1990, BC Decker.
7. American Heart Association: *Textbook of advanced cardiac life support,* Dallas, 1987, The Association.
8. American College of Surgeons: *Upper airway management: advanced trauma life support,* Chicago, 1985, The College.
9. Garnet R et al: End-tidal carbon dioxide monitoring during cardiopulmonary resuscitation, *JAMA* 257(4):1379, 1987.
10. Stothert J et al: High pressure percutaneous transtracheal ventilation: the use of large gauge intravenous-type catheters in the totally obstructed airway, *Am J Emerg Med* 8:184, 1990.
11. Risk of infection during CPR training and rescue: supplemental guidelines, *JAMA* 262(19):2714, 1989.
12. Ornato J: Providing CPR and emergency care during the AIDS epidemic, *Emerg Med Serv* 18(4):45, 1989.
13. Mackreth B: Assessing pulse oximetry in the field, *JEMS* 15(6):56, 1990.

Summary

Effective airway management is the first priority of patient care in any emergency response. The skilled paramedic can quickly recognize the signs and symptoms of airway compromise and is equipped to provide life saving measures in airway maintenance and ventilatory support.

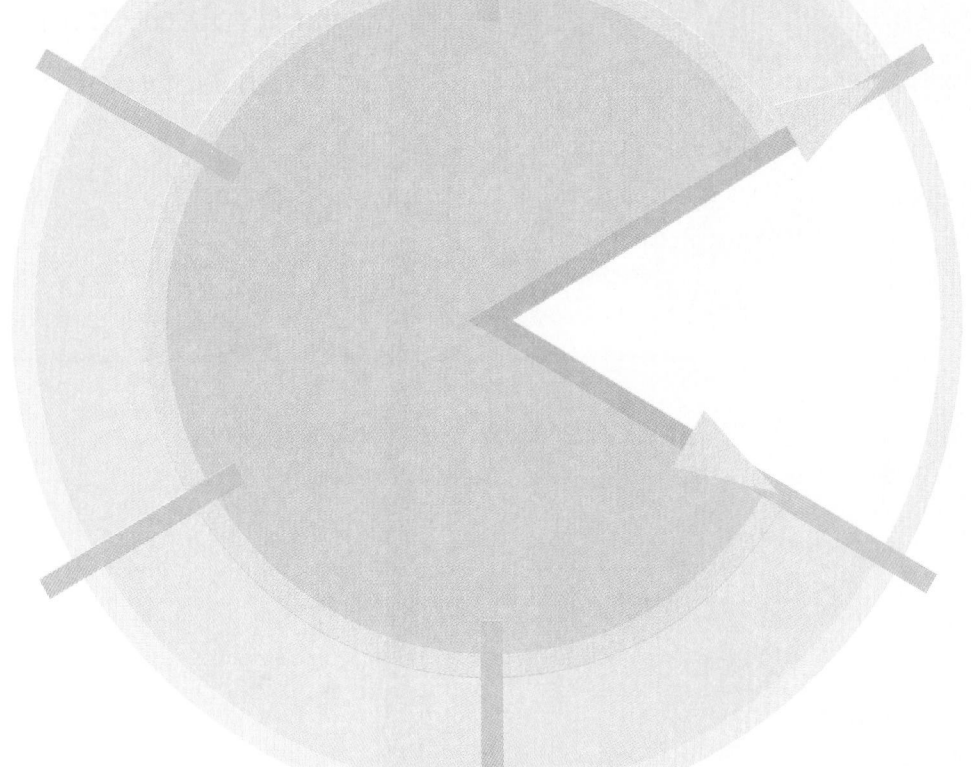

13 SHOCK

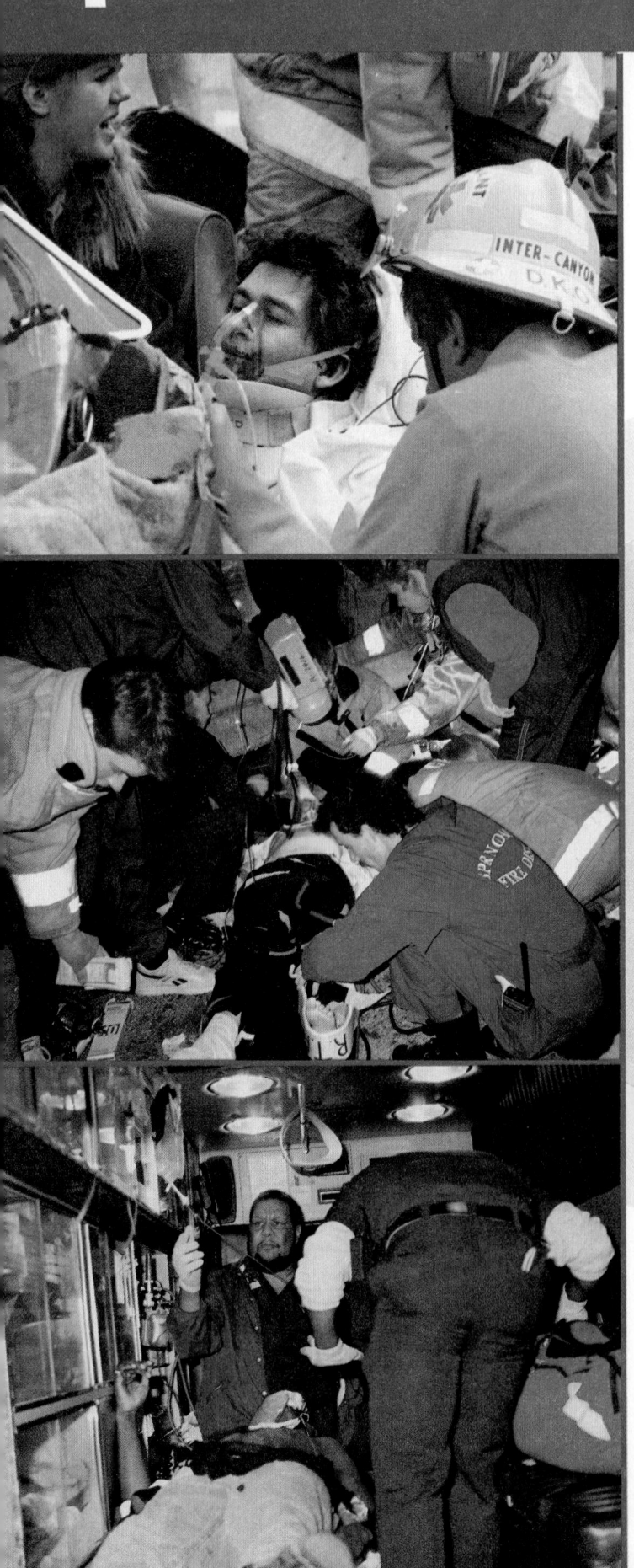

Severe medical illnesses and traumatic events threaten the human body's internal environment. During these events, the protective systems of the body attempt to compensate in an effort to maintain cellular oxygenation. Decreased tissue perfusion is the first stage of shock. For a successful outcome, the paramedic must understand shock and early management of the syndrome and rapidly transport the patient to an appropriate medical facility.

OBJECTIVES

As a paramedic, you should be able to:

1. Differentiate aerobic from anaerobic metabolism.
2. Describe the role of the heart, vasculature, and lungs in tissue perfusion.
3. Describe the constituents of blood and their functions.
4. Distinguish among the fluid compartments of the body.
5. Explain the various mechanisms for moving fluid and electrolytes among the body fluid compartments.
6. Describe the assessment and management of a patient with an imbalance of fluids, electrolytes, or both.
7. Discuss prehospital interventions for acid-base imbalances not corrected by the body's compensatory mechanisms.
8. Describe the role of negative feedback mechanisms in maintaining normal tissue perfusion.
9. Discuss the factors that influence microcirculation.
10. Recognize the stages in the progression of shock from vasoconstriction to death.
11. Differentiate the etiologies, signs, symptoms, and management of each classification of shock.
12. Describe the body's response to shock during the compensated, uncompensated, and irreversible stages of the syndrome.
13. Discuss factors that influence an individual's physiological response to shock.
14. Outline the physical examination of a patient in shock.
15. Discuss the indications, contraindications, complications, and techniques of intervention for shock.

Section One
Physiology of Perfusion

● THE DEFINITION OF SHOCK

Shock was defined by Gross in 1850 as "a rude unhinging of the machinery of life"[1] and has since

KEY TERMS

anaphylactic shock: Shock that occurs when the body is exposed to a substance that produces a severe allergic reaction.

anion: An ion with a negative charge.

cardiac output: The volume of blood pumped by the heart per minute. Also known as *minute volume.*

cardiogenic shock: Shock that results when cardiac action cannot deliver a circulating blood volume adequate for tissue perfusion.

cation: An ion with a positive charge.

Fick principle: Principle that the amount of oxygen uptake of each unit of blood as it passes through the lungs equals the oxygen concentration difference between arterial and mixed venous blood; used to determine cardiac output.

hypovolemic shock: Shock caused most often by hemorrhage or dehydration.

osmotic pressure: The force required to prevent the movement of water across a selectively permeable membrane.

peripheral vascular resistance: The total resistance against which blood must be pumped. Also known as *afterload.*

preload: The amount of blood returning to the ventricle.

septic shock: Shock that often results from a serious systemic bacterial infection.

been redefined by many others. Robert M. Hardaway, professor of surgery at Texas Tech University School of Medicine in El Paso, defines *shock* in this way[2]:

> I believe that the best definition of shock is inadequate capillary perfusion. As a corollary of this broad definition, almost anyone who dies, except one who is instantly destroyed, must go through a stage of shock—a momentary pause in the act of death.

Shock is not a single entity with a specific cause and treatment but rather a complex group of physiological abnormalities that can result from a variety of disease states and injuries. Because of the many complexities involved in shock, it is not adequately defined by pulse rate, blood pressure, or cardiac function, and it cannot be reduced to hypovolemia or loss of systemic vascular resistance. The entire organism may be affected, or it can occur at a tissue or cellular level, even with normal hemodynamics. An understanding of cellular physiology is necessary to recognize subtle aspects of shock and to properly assess the severity of various stages of shock.

● TISSUE OXYGENATION

To achieve adequate oxygenation of tissue cells (perfusion), three distinct components of the cardiovascular system must function properly: the heart, the vasculature, and the lungs. When any one of these malfunctions, cellular oxygenation can occur.

The Myocardium

The pumping action of the heart produces pressure changes that circulate blood throughout the body. This repetitive pumping action is referred to as the *cardiac cycle.*

Cardiac output (minute volume) is the total amount of blood separately pumped by each ventricle per minute, usually expressed in liters per minute. It is determined by multiplying the heart rate by the volume of blood ejected by each ventricle during each beat (stroke volume). For example, if each ventricle contracts 72 times per minute and ejects 70 ml of blood with each contraction, the cardiac output would be 72 beats per minute multiplied by 70 ml per beat, or 5.01 L/min.

Cardiac output is a crucial determinant of organ perfusion and depends on several factors. These include the strength of contraction, rate of contraction, and amount of venous return available to the ventricle **(preload).**

In 1870, Adolph Fick developed the first method for measuring cardiac output in healthy animals and people. The basis for this method, called the **Fick principle,** derives from the quantity of oxygen delivered to an organ being equal to the amount of oxygen consumed by that organ plus the amount of oxygen carried away from the organ. The Fick principle is frequently used to estimate perfusion either to an organ or to the whole body when oxygen content of both the arterial and venous blood is known and oxygen consumption is assumed to remain fixed (Box 13-1).

The Vasculature

The entire vascular system is lined with smooth, low-friction endothelial cells. All vessels larger than capillaries have layers of tissue surrounding the endothelium. These layers of tissue, or tunics, provide supporting connective tissue to counter the pressure of blood contained in the vascular system, elastic properties to dampen pressure pulsations and minimize flow variations throughout the cardiac cycle, and muscle fibers to control the vessel diameter. The vascular system maintains blood flow by changes in pressure and **peripheral vascular resistance.**

Fluid flows through a tube in response to pressure gradients between the two ends of the tube. It is not the absolute pressure in the tube that determines flow but the difference in pressure between the two ends. In many animals, including humans, the two ends are the aorta and the vena cavae.

The systemic pressure (left-sided pressure) and pulmonic pressure (right-sided pressure) are measurements of pressure in the vascular system. Sys-

The Fick Principle

1. An adequate amount of oxygen must be available to red blood cells through the alveolar membrane in the lungs to ensure hemoglobin saturation with oxygen. This requires adequate ventilation of the lungs through the patient's airway, a high partial pressure of oxygen in inspired air (FiO_2), and minimal obstruction to the diffusion of oxygen across the alveolar capillary membrane.

2. The red blood cells must be circulated to the tissue cells. This requires adequate cardiac function, an adequate volume of blood flow, and proper routing of blood through the vascular channels.

3. The red blood cells must be able to adequately load oxygen in the pulmonary capillaries and unload the oxygen at the site of peripheral tissue cells. This requires normal hemoglobin levels, circulation of the oxygenated red blood cells to the tissues in need, close approximation of the tissue cells to the capillaries to allow for diffusion of oxygen, and ideal conditions of pH, temperature, and other factors. Fick principle (Tissue oxygenation) = (Arterial oxygen content − Venous oxygen content) × Perfusion

temic pressure, like pulmonic pressure, has two phases: systolic and diastolic. The difference between these two pressures is the pulse pressure. Pressure is greatest at its origin (the heart) and least at its terminating point (the vena cava). This pressure gradient changes significantly at the arteriole as a result of peripheral vascular resistance.

The peripheral vascular resistance (afterload) is the total resistance against which blood must be pumped. It is essentially a measure of friction between the vessel walls and fluid and between the molecules of the fluid themselves (viscosity), both of which oppose flow. When the resistance to flow increases and the flow remains constant, blood pressure increases. Resistance to blood flow depends on fluid viscosity, vessel length, and vessel diameter.

Viscosity is the physical property of a liquid characterized by the degree of friction between its component molecules (for example, between the blood cells and between the plasma proteins). Viscosity normally plays a minor role in blood flow regulation because it remains fairly constant in healthy individuals. Vessel length in the human body also remains constant. Vessel diameter is the primary factor affecting the resistance to blood flow.

Major arteries are large and offer little resistance to flow. Arterioles have a much smaller diameter than arteries and offer the major resistance to blood flow. The smooth muscle in the arteriole walls can relax or contract, changing the diameter of the inside of the arteriole as much as fivefold. Arterial blood pressure is thus regulated primarily by the vasoconstriction or vasodilation of these vessels.

The Lungs

Adequate oxygenation of tissue cells requires that adequate oxygen be made available to the red blood cells at the capillary membrane in the lungs (the first component of the Fick principle). This is made possible by the high partial pressure of oxygen in inspired air, adequate depth and rate of ventilation, and matching of pulmonary ventilation and perfusion.

● THE BODY AS A CONTAINER

The healthy body may be viewed as a smooth-flowing fluid delivery system inside a container. The container must be filled to achieve adequate preload and tissue oxygenation. Though the size of the container of any particular human body is relatively constant, the volume of the container is directly related to the diameter of the resistance vessels, which may change rapidly. Any change in the diameter of the vessels changes the volume of fluid the container holds, thereby affecting preload.

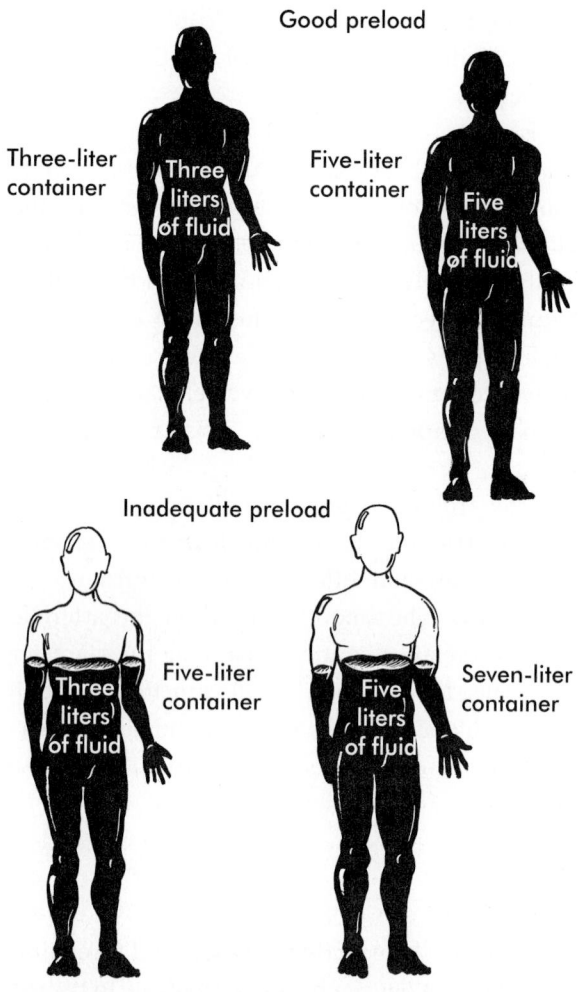

Good preload

Three-liter container — Three liters of fluid

Five-liter container — Five liters of fluid

Inadequate preload

Three liters of fluid — Five-liter container

Five liters of fluid — Seven-liter container

Fig. 13-1 Fluid versus container volume.

An example of this principle is a 5-L container, the normal container size for a 70-kg adult male (Fig. 13-1). If the fluid volume is 5 L, preload is adequate. With a strong myocardium, cardiac output and perfusion are also adequate. If 2 L of this fluid have been lost, either externally or internally, the remaining 3 L are inadequate to supply an effective preload. Since cardiac output depends on preload, a decrease in preload significantly decreases cardiac output.

If the patient is hypovolemic and the 5-L container has remained the same size despite the 3-L volume, the patient becomes hypotensive because of decreased cardiac output. However, if the container is reduced to 3 L by compensatory mechanisms (for example, vasoconstriction), the 3-L container can provide adequate preload to the heart with the 3 L of available fluid. (This is obviously

at the expense of certain tissues that are not perfused in this constricted state.)

If fluid is adequate for a 5-L container but the container size has been enlarged to 7 L by illness or injury that results in vasodilation, the 5 L of fluid do not provide adequate preload for the container (relative hypovolemia). Other factors that are occasionally responsible for vasodilation include cardiac and blood pressure medications, allergic reaction, heat- and cold-related injuries, and alcohol and drug use.

● BLOOD AND ITS COMPONENTS

The average adult male has a blood volume of 7% of total body weight, and the average adult female, 6.5% of total body weight (70 ml multiplied by kg body weight). Normal adult blood volume is 4.5 to 5 L. This amount remains fairly constant in the healthy body.

Plasma is approximately 92% water and is the blood's solvent (the liquid portion of blood). It is through plasma that salts, minerals, sugars, fats, and proteins are circulated in the body.

Plasma contains three major proteins: albumin, globulin, and fibrinogen. Albumin is the most plentiful plasma protein. It is similar in consistency to egg white and gives blood its gummy texture. This large protein helps keep the water concentration of blood low enough to allow water to diffuse readily from tissues into blood. Globulins (alpha, beta, and gamma) serve two main functions: alpha and beta globulins transport other proteins, and gamma globulins give people immunity to disease. Fibrinogen aids in blood clotting by forming a web of protein fibers that binds blood cells together.

In addition to helping the body maintain its blood supply, plasma proteins serve several purposes. Should blood acidity change, the proteins can act together as an acid or base to correct it. If the body runs short of food, plasma protein can also temporarily meet the nutritional needs of the body.

Although oxygen dissolves in plasma, it can only carry about 1% of the oxygen the body demands. Red blood cells (erythrocytes) transport

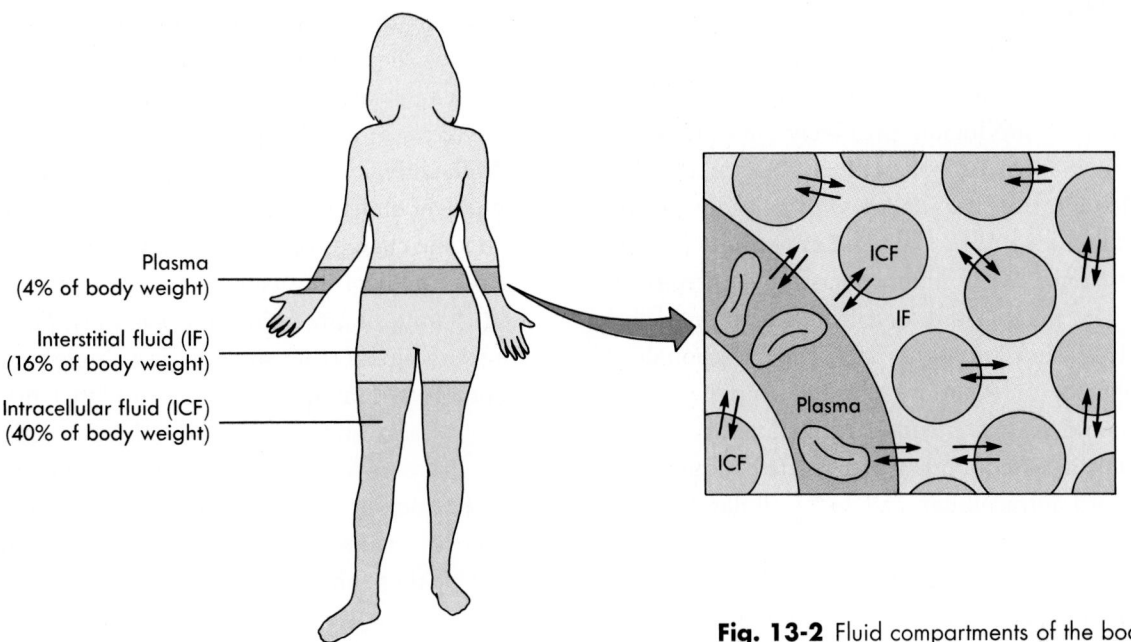

Plasma
(4% of body weight)

Interstitial fluid (IF)
(16% of body weight)

Intracellular fluid (ICF)
(40% of body weight)

Fig. 13-2 Fluid compartments of the body.

the other 99%. Red blood cells make up approximately 45% of the blood and are the most abundant cells in the body. Red blood cells provide oxygen to tissues and remove carbon dioxide. Each red blood cell contains approximately 270 million hemoglobin molecules. These molecules allow erythrocytes to pick up oxygen in the lungs and release it to body tissues.

White blood cells (leukocytes) defend the body against various pathogens (bacteria, viruses, fungi, and parasites). The bone marrow and lymph glands constantly produce and maintain a reserve of white blood cells, but not many are present in a healthy blood stream. (White cells are outnumbered by red cells 600 to 1.) When a pathogen invades the body, the leukocyte reserves are released.

Another part of the body's defense mechanism is platelets, which help to stop escaping blood. Platelets are formed in the red bone marrow and work by swelling and adhering together to form sticky plugs, thereby initiating the clotting phenomenon.

● FLUIDS AND ELECTROLYTES

Water is the main component of body mass, accounting for 50% to 60% of body weight in adults.

The importance of body water is highlighted by two facts: it is the medium in which all metabolic reactions occur, and the precise regulation of the volume and composition of body fluid is essential to health. (A 20% to 25% loss of body water usually results in death.) The human body can be viewed as containing two fluid compartments: the extracellular fluid and the intracellular fluid (Fig. 13-2).

Extracellular Fluid

Extracellular fluid is the water found outside the cells and includes the intravascular and interstitial compartments. This fluid accounts for approximately 20% of total body weight, the intravascular component comprising approximately one third of this. Interstitial fluid is the extracellular fluid between the cells and outside the vascular bed. This category also includes special fluids, such as cerebrospinal fluid and intraocular fluid, and accounts for 15% to 16% of total body weight.

Intracellular Fluid

Intracellular fluid is the fluid found in all of the body cells. It accounts for 40% of total body weight.

Electrolytes

Electrolytes are salt substances whose molecules dissociate into charged components when in water, producing positively and negatively charged ions. An ion with a positive charge is called a **cation,** and an ion with a negative charge is called an **anion.** The most important cations in body fluid are sodium, potassium, calcium, hydrogen, magnesium, and iron. Important anions include chloride, phosphate, and bicarbonate. In physiological solutions, the total number of cations and anions is equal and maintains electrical neutrality. Predominant electrolyte concentrations of both intracellular and extracellular fluid are listed in Table 13-1.

In addition to electrolytes, the body also contains nonelectrolytes (substances with no electrical charge). Examples include glucose and urea.

Particles and Solutions

A solution is either a liquid or a gas that contains one or more solutes. The liquid or gas in which solutes are dissolved is called a *solvent.* Any water solution that contains charged particles conducts electricity and can be referred to as an *electrolyte solution.* Because atoms of different chemicals have different molecular weights, the number of ions formed when 1 g of sodium chloride is dissolved in water differs from the number of ions formed when 1 g of potassium phosphate is dissolved.

Chemical reactions depend more on the number of charges on a particle than on the particle's molecular weight. The concept of equivalent weight (the molecular weight divided by the

charges on the ion) was developed to facilitate calculations. To make the calculations easier to work with, values are expressed as thousandths of an equivalent, or a milliequivalent (mEq).

Milliequivalents represent the chemical combining power of the ion based on the number of available ionic charges of an electrolyte solution. A total of 1 mEq of any cation can react completely with 1 mEq of any anion. For example, Na^+ is a singly charged cation, and Cl^- is a singly charged anion. Thus 1 mEq of Na^+ reacts with 1 mEq of Cl^- to form sodium chloride (NaCl). Calcium (Ca^{++}) has two positive charges, and therefore 1 mEq of calcium requires 2 mEq of a single charged anion to combine. These examples are summarized by these chemical equations:

$$1\ Na^{++} + 1\ Cl^- \leftrightharpoons 1\ NaCl$$
$$1\ Ca^{++} + 2\ Cl^- \leftrightharpoons 1\ CaCl_2$$

Proteins

Proteins account for about 50% of the organic material in the body. They are components of most body structures and have roles in the chemical reactions that occur within the body. Specialized proteins are responsible for immune responses, coagulation, digestion of foodstuffs, metabolism of nutrients, and many other functions.

● MOVEMENT OF BODY FLUIDS

Body fluids constantly move from one compartment to another. In healthy individuals, the volume of fluid in each compartment remains approximately the same. To keep the volume stable, the body uses osmosis, diffusion, and mediated transport mechanisms.

Osmosis

The movement of molecules within a cell or across cell membranes is essential for normal body functioning. Fluid compartments are separated by membranes, most of which allow water to pass freely but regulate or restrict the flow of solutes on the basis of their size, shape, electrical charge, or other chemical properties. These membranes are referred to as *semipermeable membranes.* Chan-

TABLE 13-1 Electrolyte Concentrations of Intracellular and Extracellular Fluid	
Predominant Cations	
Intracellular	Potassium (K^+)
	Calcium (Ca^{++})
	Magnesium (Mg^{++})
Extracellular	Sodium (Na^+)
Predominant Anions	
Intracellular	Phosphate (PO_4^{3-})
Extracellular	Chloride (Cl^-)
	Bicarbonate (HCO_3^-)

nels in membranes permit passage of solutes; they may be open at all times to specific solutes, or closed at times, depending on the physiology of the cell. The ability of the cell membrane to selectively regulate solute transition enables the cell to maintain homeostasis.

Osmosis is functionally defined as the flow of fluid across a semipermeable membrane from a lower solute concentration to a higher solute concentration (Fig. 13-3). With gases, the driving force of osmosis **(osmotic pressure)** is the pressure produced by the partial pressure of the dissolved gases. These include oxygen, nitrogen, carbon dioxide, and water, which has a vapor pressure around 47 mm Hg at body temperature and 1 atm. With nongaseous particles, osmotic pressure depends on the number and molecular weights of particles on each side of the membrane and the permeability of the membrane of these electrolytes.

When a living cell is placed in a solution that has a higher solute concentration (and thus a lower water concentration) than that inside the cell, the solution is referred to as *hypertonic* with respect to the cell. The osmotic pressure exerted on the cell produces a net movement of water molecules out of the cell. This net movement causes the cell to dehydrate, shrink (crenate), and perhaps die.

When a living cell is placed in a solution that has a lower solute concentration (and thus a higher water concentration) than that inside the cell, the solution is referred to as *hypotonic* with respect to the cell. In this situation, osmotic pressure draws water molecules from the surrounding solution into the cell. The net movement of water molecules into the cell causes it to swell and perhaps burst, or lyse.

When a living cell is placed in a solution in which the solute concentration (and water concentration) is the same as the solution inside the cell, the solution is referred to as *isotonic*. There is no

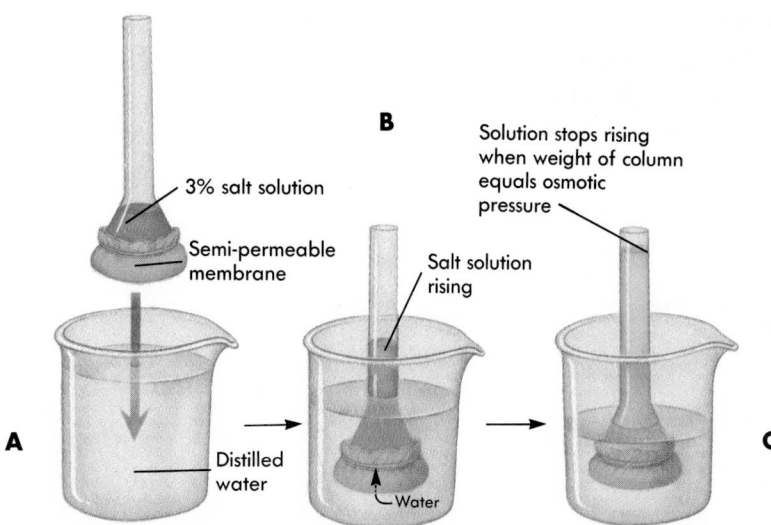

Fig. 13-3 Osmosis. **A,** The end of a tube containing a 3% salt solution is closed at one end with a semipermeable membrane that allows water molecules to pass through it but retains the salt molecules within the tube. **B,** The tube is immersed in distilled water. Because the tube contains salt and water molecules, the tube has proportionately less water than the beaker, which contains only water. The water molecules diffuse with their concentration gradient into the tube. Because the salt molecules cannot leave the tube, the total fluid volume inside the tube increases, and fluid moves up the glass tube as a result of osmosis. **C,** Water continues to move into the tube until the weight of the column of the water in the tube (hydrostatic pressure) exerts a downward force equal to the osmotic force moving water molecules into the tube. The hydrostatic pressure that prevents net movement of water into the tube is called the *osmotic pressure* of the solution in the tube.

Fluid Replacement Therapy

Intravenous therapy is based on hypertonic, hypotonic, and isotonic properties.

Hypertonic Solutions

A hypertonic solution has a higher concentration of solute molecules than that inside normal cells. When this solution is infused into a normally hydrated patient, it draws water from the cells into the vascular space. Examples of hypertonic solutions are mannitol (Osmitrol), sodium bicarbonate, and 50% dextrose (D_{50}).

These solutions are often used to treat cerebral edema (mannitol), metabolic acidosis (bicarbonate), and profound hypoglycemia (50% dextrose). In addition, recent studies have suggested the use of some hypertonic solutions (for example, dextran, hetastarch, and NaCl [3%, 5%, and 7.5%]), for volume restoration after trauma.[3] By drawing tissue fluid into the vascular space, hypertonic solutions may reduce the volume of infusion and postresuscitation pulmonary problems.

Hypotonic Solutions

A hypotonic solution has a solute concentration lower than that of the cells. When this solution is infused into a normally hydrated patient, water moves from the solution into the cells. These solutions supply calories and replenish salt and water and are used to hydrate patients or to prevent dehydration. Examples of hypotonic solutions include 2.5% dextrose in water and 0.45% normal saline (½NS). Although technically isotonic, D_5W acts physiologically as a hypotonic solution because the solute (glucose) is actively transported into cells, leaving excess free water behind.

Isotonic Solutions

In an isotonic solution, the concentration of solute molecules equals that inside most normal cells. When this solution is infused into a normally hydrated patient, it neither draws water out of the cells nor moves water into the cells but rather stays in the vascular space. Isotonic solutions are usually prescribed to replace extracellular fluid lost from blood loss, severe vomiting, or any situation in which the chloride loss equals or exceeds the sodium loss. Examples of isotonic solutions are 0.9% normal saline and lactated Ringer's solution.

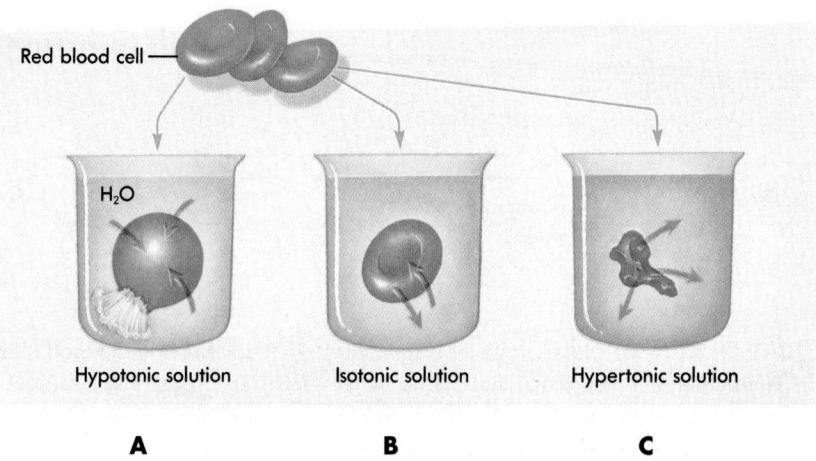

Fig. 13-4 Effects of hypotonic, isotonic, and hypertonic solutions on red blood cells. **A,** Hypotonic solutions with low ion concentrations result in swelling and lysis of cells. **B,** Isotonic solutions with normal ion concentrations result in normal-shaped cells. **C,** Hypertonic solutions with high ion concentrations result in shrinkage (crenation) of the cell.

net movement of water molecules in isotonic solutions (Fig. 13-4).

Diffusion

Diffusion results from the constant, random motion of all the atoms, molecules, or ions in a solution. This passive process moves molecules or ions from an area of higher concentration to an area of lower concentration (Fig. 13-5). Because there are more solute particles in an area of high concentration than in an area of low concentration and because the particles move randomly, more solute particles move from the higher to the lower concentration than in the opposite direction. At equilibrium, in contrast, the net movement of solute stops. The random molecular motion continues, but the movement of solutes in one direction is balanced by equal movement in the opposite direction.

If a solute concentration is greater at one point than at another point in the solvent, a concentration gradient exists. Solutes diffuse down their concentration gradients from high to low concentration until equilibrium is achieved. Some nutrients enter and some waste products leave the cell by diffusion. The maintenance of appropriate intracellular concentrations of certain substances depends on this process.

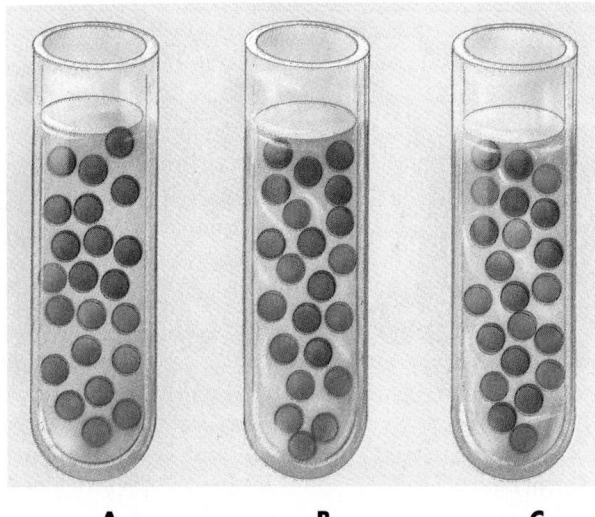

Fig. 13-5 Diffusion. **A,** One solution (*red,* representing one type of molecule) is layered onto a second solution (*blue,* representing a second type of molecule). A concentration gradient for the red molecules from the red solution into the blue solution exists because there are no red molecules in the blue solution. A concentration gradient for the blue molecules from the blue solution into the red solution also exists because there are no blue molecules in the red solution. **B,** Red molecules move with their concentration gradient into the blue solution, and the blue molecules move with their concentration gradient into the red solution. **C,** Red and blue molecules are distributed evenly throughout the solution. Even though the red and blue molecues continue to move randomly and equilibrium exists, no net movement occurs because no concentration gradient exists.

Mediated Transport Mechanisms

A number of essential molecules (for example, glucose) cannot enter most cells by diffusion, and a number of products (for example, some proteins) cannot exit most cells by diffusion. To move large water-soluble molecules or electrically charged molecules across the cell membranes, mediated transport mechanisms are necessary. These transport mechanisms use carrier molecules, proteins that combine with solutes on one side of a membrane and transport the solute to the other side (Fig. 13-6). There are two kinds of mediated transport: active transport and facilitated diffusion.

Active transport is a carrier-mediated process that can move substances against a concentration gradient from areas of lower concentration to areas of higher concentration. To work against this concentration gradient, energy is expended by the cell. Active transport occurs at a faster rate than diffusion.

Facilitated diffusion is a carrier-mediated process that moves substances into and out of cells from a high to a low concentration. For these substances, the direction of movement is *with* the concentration gradient, but like active transport, the movement is faster than ordinary diffusion can account for. Facilitated diffusion is distinguished from active transport in that it does not require an expenditure of energy. Its moving force is a downhill concentration gradient.

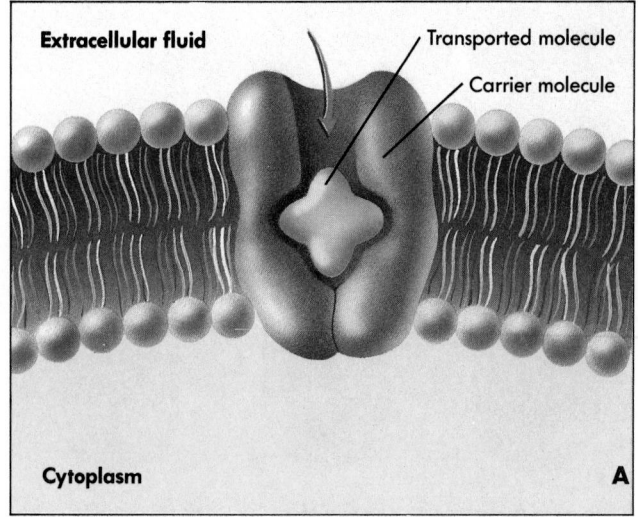

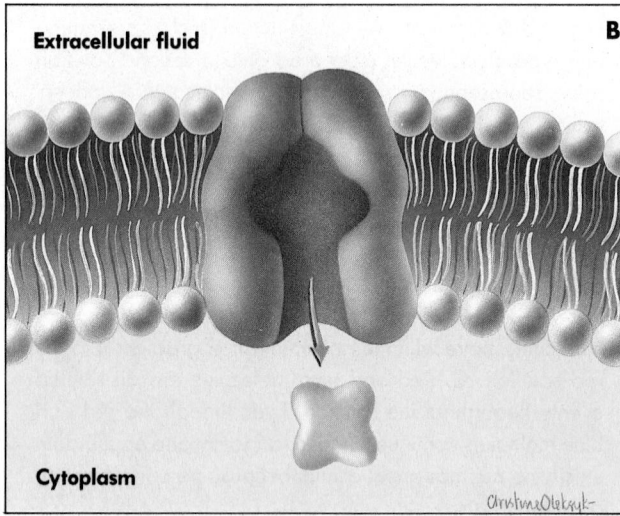

Fig. 13-6 Mediated transport by a carrier molecule. **A,** The carrier molecule binds with a molecule on one side of the plasma membrane and changes shape. **B,** The molecule is released on the other side of the plasma membrane.

● BODY FLUIDS AND FLUID IMBALANCES

In the healthy body, homeostatic mechanisms maintain a constant balance between intake and excretion of water. The water gained each day approximately equals the water lost. The body gains water primarily by drinking fluids, by ingesting food containing moisture, and by forming water through the oxidation of hydrogen in food during the metabolic process. The body loses water through the kidneys as urine, through the feces, through the skin as perspiration, through exhaled air as vapor, and by the excretion of tears and saliva. Two abnormal states of body-fluid balance can occur. If the water gained exceeds the water lost, there is a water excess or overhydration. If the water lost exceeds the water gained, there is a water deficit or dehydration.

Dehydration

Dehydration may be classified as isotonic (excessive loss of sodium and water in equal amounts), hypernatremic (loss of water in excess of sodium), and hyponatremic (loss of sodium in excess of water).

Isotonic Dehydration
- Causes:
  - Usually, severe or long-term vomiting or diarrhea
  - Systemic infection
  - Intestinal obstruction
- Signs and symptoms:
  - Dry skin and mucous membranes
  - Poor skin turgor
  - Longitudinal wrinkles or furrows of the tongue
  - Oliguria (low urinary output—100 to 400 ml/24 hours)
  - Anuria (reduced urinary output—100 ml or less in 24 hours)
  - Acute weight loss
  - Depressed or sunken fontanelles in infants
- Treatment: intravenous infusion of an isotonic solution that has a solute concentration equal to that of blood

Hypernatremic Dehydration
- Possible causes:
  - Excessive use or misuse of diuretics
  - Continued administration of sodium in the absence of water intake
  - Excessive loss of water with little loss of salt
  - Profuse, watery diarrhea
  - Inhalation or ingestion of saltwater (for example, near-drowning), which may cause hypernatremia without dehydration

- Signs and symptoms:
  - Dry, sticky mucous membranes
  - Flushed skin
  - Intense thirst
  - Oliguria or anuria
  - Increased body temperature
  - Altered mental status
- Treatment: volume replacement with isotonic or occasionally hypotonic solutions (based on serum sodium levels and the clinical condition of the patient)

Hyponatremic Dehydration

- Possible causes:
  - Use of diuretics
  - Excessive perspiration (heat-related illness)
  - Salt-losing renal disorders
  - Increased water intake (for example, excessive use of water enemas)
  - Inhalation or ingestion of fresh water (for example, near-drowning) and compulsive water drinking, which may cause hyponatremia without dehydration
- Signs and symptoms:
  - Abdominal or muscle cramps
  - Seizures
  - Rapid, thready pulse
  - Diaphoresis
  - Cyanosis
- Treatment: intravenous fluid replacement with normal saline or lactated Ringer's solution; occasionally, hypertonic saline (for example, in seizures caused by hyponatremia)

Overhydration

Overhydration is an increase in body water with a decrease in solute concentration. This water excess may result from parenteral administration of excessive fluids, impaired cardiac function, impaired renal function, or some endocrine dysfunctions. Signs and symptoms of overhydration include the following:

- Shortness of breath
- Puffy eyelids
- Edema
- Polyuria (voiding a large volume of urine in a given time)
- Moist crackles
- Acute weight gain

The treatment of overhydration depends on the cause. For excessive water administration and certain endocrine problems, water restriction is the primary treatment. For patients with cardiac or renal impairment, a diuretic may be indicated. When profound hyponatremia is associated with overhydration (serum sodium level less than 120 mEq/L and associated seizures or altered consciousness), administration of saline may be indicated.

● ELECTROLYTE IMBALANCES

In addition to the possibility of fluid imbalances, disturbances in the balance of electrolytes (other than sodium) may occur. These include potassium, calcium, and magnesium.

Potassium

Potassium is the major positively charged ion in intracellular fluid. The body must maintain a narrow range of normal values (serum level of 3.5 to 5 mEq/L) for normal nerve, cardiac, and skeletal muscle function. Obligate potassium losses (those that cannot be avoided) are usually minimal and are replenished through dietary intake. Excess potassium is usually readily excreted by the kidneys. Potassium plays an important role in muscle contraction, enzyme action, nerve impulses, and cell membrane function. Potassium imbalances interfere with neuromuscular function and may cause cardiac rhythm disturbances (including sudden death).

Hypokalemia (potassium deficit) can be caused by reduced dietary intake (rare), poor potassium absorption by the body, loss of gastrointestinal secretions as a result of vomiting or diarrhea, renal disease, infusion of solutions poor in potassium, and medications (most commonly diuretics, but steroids, theophylline, and others have also been implicated). Signs and symptoms of hypokalemia include the following:

- Malaise
- Skeletal muscle weakness
- Decreased reflexes

- Weak pulse
- Faint or distant heart sounds
- Shallow respiration
- Low blood pressure
- Gastrointestinal tract
  ◦ Anorexia
  ◦ Vomiting
  ◦ Gaseous distention
- Excessive thirst

In-hospital treatment of hypokalemia is intravenous or oral potassium replacement. Caution must be exercised when using intravenous potassium, since rapid administration can lead to fatal potassium excess.

Hyperkalemia results from increased potassium levels. This condition may be caused by acute or chronic renal failure, burns, crush injuries, severe infections in which large amounts of potassium are released, excessive use of potassium salts, and a shift of potassium from the cells into the extracellular fluid. Signs and symptoms of hyperkalemia include the following:

- Irritability
- Abdominal distention
- Nausea
- Diarrhea
- Oliguria
- Weakness and paralysis (severe hyperkalemia)

In-hospital treatment for hyperkalemia involves restricting potassium and administering a cation exchange resin, either orally or by a nasogastric tube. In emergencies, intravenous administration of glucose and insulin (1 amp D_{50} and 10 units regular insulin) helps lower serum potassium levels by forcing potassium intracellularly along with the glucose. Sodium bicarbonate also causes potassium to shift intracellularly. Calcium may be used intravenously as an antagonist to the cardiac effects of high potassium levels.

Calcium

Calcium, a bivalent cation (an ion with two positive charges), is essential for a variety of body functions, including neuromuscular transmission, cell membrane permeability, hormone secretion, growth and ossification of bones, and muscle con-

traction (including smooth, cardiac, and skeletal muscle). Calcium intake in a balanced diet is sufficient for normal body needs. Calcium is excreted through urine, feces, and perspiration.

A decrease in serum calcium (hypocalcemia) may result from endocrine (mostly parathyroid) dysfunction, renal insufficiency, decreased intake or malabsorption of calcium, or deficiency, malabsorption, or inability to activate vitamin D. Signs and symptoms of hypocalcemia include the following:

- Paresthesia
- Tetany
- Abdominal cramps
- Muscle cramps
- Neural excitability
  ◦ Personality changes
  ◦ Abnormal behavior
  ◦ Convulsions

In-hospital treatment for hypocalcemia is intravenous administration of calcium ions. Calcium salt and vitamin D may be given orally for maintenance.

Hypercalcemia may be caused by various neoplasms (tumors). Other common causes include parathyroid dysfunction, thyroid dysfunction, diuretic therapy, and excessive administration of vitamin D (as in the treatment of osteoporosis). Calcium can be deposited in various body tissues, including many organ systems. Examples include the gastrointestinal system, central nervous system, renal system, neuromuscular system, and the cardiovascular system. Signs and symptoms of hypercalcemia include the following:

- Hypotonicity of the muscles (decreased muscle tone or tension)
- Renal stones
- Altered mental status
- Deep bone pain

The treatment of hypercalcemia is aimed at controlling the underlying disease, hydration, and occasionally, drug therapy to lower calcium. In-hospital therapy for severe hypercalcemia may include forced diuresis with normal saline and furosemide, as well as the administration of calcium-lowering drugs such as thyrocalcitonin, steroids (glucocorticoids), and plicamycin (a cytotoxic drug that inhibits bone reabsorption).

Magnesium

Magnesium is a bivalent cation that activates many enzymes. Approximately 50% of the body's magnesium exists in an insoluble state in bone, 45% as an intracellular cation, and 5% in extracellular solution. Magnesium is excreted by the kidneys and has physiological effects on the nervous system similar to those seen with calcium.

Magnesium deficit (hypomagnesemia) may be encountered in alcoholism, malabsorption, starvation, diarrhea, diuresis, and diseases causing hypocalcemia and hypokalemia. The condition is characterized by increased irritability of the nervous system. Signs and symptoms of hypomagnesemia include the following:

- Tremors
- Nausea or vomiting
- Diarrhea
- Hyperactive deep reflexes
- Confusion (including hallucinations)
- Seizures or myoclonus
- Cardiac dysrhythmias

In-hospital treatment for significant symptomatic hypomagnesemia is intravenous fluid administration of a solution that contains magnesium, most commonly magnesium sulfate.

Magnesium excess (hypermagnesemia) occurs primarily in patients with chronic renal insufficiency. It can also occur in patients ingesting large amounts of magnesium-containing compounds such as cathartics (magnesium citrate, magnesium sulfate) or antacids (for example, magnesium hydroxide). Hypermagnesemia causes central nervous system depression, profound muscular weakness, and areflexia; it also causes cardiac rhythm disturbances, which may lead to sudden death. Signs and symptoms include:

- Sedation
- Confusion
- Muscle weakness
- Respiratory paralysis

The most effective treatment for hypermagnesemia is hemodialysis, which can return blood levels to normal in approximately 4 hours. In addition, calcium salts that act as an antagonist to magnesium may be given parenterally. Administration of intravenous glucose and insulin may also drive magnesium back into the cells and can be used in emergencies when respiratory depression or cardiac conduction defects are present.

● ACID-BASE BALANCE

As explained in Chapter 12, the body constantly produces acids and bases, which are characterized by their tendency to release or absorb hydrogen ions. The following discussion serves as a review.

Ions balance themselves much like a seesaw: Solutions turn acid when the concentration of their hydrogen ion rises and turn basic when it falls. The concentration of hydrogen ions is measured in terms of pH. The pH of a neutral solution, such as water, is 7.0. Low pH indicates an acid (acidosis), and high pH indicates a base (alkalosis). The normal pH of blood is 7.4, and it only varies by 0.05 (a very narrow range) when compensatory mechanisms function. When the pH is less than 7.35, the patient's blood is considered acidotic; when it is greater than 7.4, it is considered alkalemic.

Compensatory Mechanisms

The healthy body is sensitive to changes in the concentration of hydrogen ions and tries to maintain the pH of extracellular fluid at 7.4. This is accomplished through three interrelated compensatory mechanisms: the bicarbonate–carbonic acid buffer system in the plasma, the lungs, and the kidneys. These compensatory mechanisms are stimulated by changes in pH and require normal organ function to be effective in maintaining acid-base balance.

1. Buffers: Bicarbonate, carbon dioxide, and carbonic acid are always present in a dynamic balance in the blood. Carbonic acid is formed in the extracellular fluid when carbon dioxide unites with water. When the cations sodium, potassium, calcium, or magnesium unite with the anion bicarbonate, they form base bicarbonate, summarized by the chemical equation:

$$\overset{\text{Carbonic anhydrase}}{CO_2 + H_2O \leftrightarrows H_2CO_3 \leftrightarrows H^+ + HCO_3^-}$$

Carbon + Water ⇆ Carbonic ⇆ Hydrogen + Bicarbonate
dioxide   acid   Ion   Ion

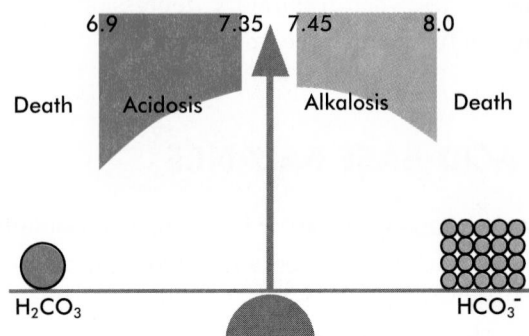

Fig. 13-7 Bicarbonate buffer system. When body fluids are in acid-base balance, the ratio of HCO_3 to H_2CO_3 is normally 20:1, and the pH is between 7.35 and 7.45.

It is the ratio of carbonic acid to base bicarbonate that determines the concentration of hydrogen ions. As long as there is 1 mEq of carbonic acid for each 20 mEq of base bicarbonate in the extracellular fluid, the hydrogen ion concentration stays within normal limits.

Although other buffer pairs are present in blood plasma, the concentration of bicarbonate and carbon dioxide is primarily responsible for holding the pH within normal limits. This compensatory mechanism occurs immediately in response to changes in pH (Fig. 13-7).

2. The lungs. After releasing oxygen in the peripheral tissues, hemoglobin binds with carbon dioxide and hydrogen ions. As the blood reaches the lungs, these actions reverse themselves. Hemoglobin binds with oxygen, releasing carbon dioxide and hydrogen ions. The hydrogen ions released combine with bicarbonate ions, forming carbonic acid. The carbonic acid breaks down into carbon dioxide and water, and the lungs expel the carbon dioxide. Therefore in normal circumstances, respirations help maintain pH.

Because the respiratory centers are more responsive to pH changes than P_{O_2}, it is the amount of carbon dioxide (and hence the pH) in the blood, rather than the need for oxygen in the tissues, that controls the rate of breathing in healthy individuals. Increasing alveolar ventilation to lower P_{CO_2} occurs within minutes in response to decreases in pH.

3. The kidneys. The kidneys help maintain acid-base balance through three mechanisms. The first is recovery of bicarbonate, which is filtered into the tubules. The second is excretion of hydrogen ions against a gradient to acidify the urine. (Normally, the kidney can acidify urine to a pH of approximately 5.0.) The third is excretion of ammonium ions (NH_4^+), each of which carries a hydrogen ion with it. The renal system compensates for acid-base imbalances slowly in comparison with the respiratory and bicarbonate buffer systems. The kidneys can take from several hours to days to restore the pH to within the normal biological range.

Any condition that increases the carbonic acid or decreases the base bicarbonate causes acidosis. Any condition that increases base bicarbonate or decreases carbonic acid causes alkalosis. Metabolic disturbances tend to affect the bicarbonate side of the equation, whereas respiratory disturbances tend to affect the carbonic acid side.

Respiratory Acidosis

Respiratory acidosis is caused by the retention of carbon dioxide, leading to an increase in P_{CO_2}. This state is usually caused by an imbalance in the production of carbon dioxide and its elimination through alveolar ventilation (Fig. 13-8). Respiratory acidosis can be summarized by the chemical equation:

$$\downarrow Respiration = \uparrow CO_2 + H_2 \rightarrow \uparrow H_2CO_3 \rightarrow \uparrow H^+ + HCO_3^-$$

Reductions in alveolar ventilation may occur as a result of the following:
- Respiratory depression
  - Respiratory arrest
  - Cardiac arrest
  - Neuromuscular impairment
  - Medications (sedatives, hypnotics)

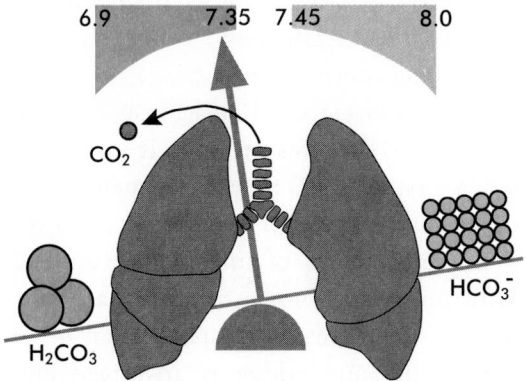

Fig. 13-8 Respiratory acidosis. An excess of carbon dioxide in the body results in acidosis.

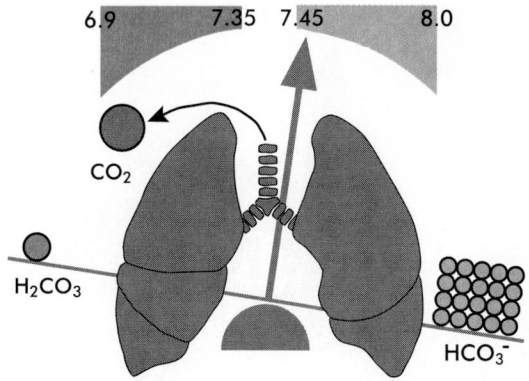

Fig. 13-9 Respiratory alkalosis. A deficit of carbon dioxide results in alkalosis.

- Chest wall injury
  - Flail chest
  - Pneumothorax
- Pulmonary processes
  - Obstructed airway
  - Chronic obstructive pulmonary disease
  - Pulmonary edema

When the respiratory system cannot continue as a compensatory mechanism to correct the acidosis, the body's renal system must conserve bicarbonate and excrete more hydrogen ions to help bring the pH into normal limits. Because the kidneys take some time to restore pH, the patient in respiratory acidosis should be treated by improving ventilation to quickly eliminate carbon dioxide. This may be accomplished by assisting ventilations to decrease P_{CO_2}. Supplemental oxygen should also be administered to help correct any accompanying hypoxemia (which can itself lead to acidosis).

Respiratory Alkalosis

Hyperventilation may produce respiratory alkalosis by decreasing P_{CO_2} (Fig. 13-9). Hyperventilation is common in patients who are acutely ill and is frequently seen in the early stages of sepsis, peritonitis, shock, and respiratory ailments. Respiratory alkalosis can summarized by the chemical equation:

$$\uparrow\text{Respiration}=\downarrow CO_2+H_2O\rightarrow\downarrow H_2CO_3\rightarrow\downarrow H^++HCO_3^-$$

When carbonic acid is lacking because of excessive carbon dioxide elimination, the blood pH rises. Therefore the kidneys must excrete bicarbonate ions and retain hydrogen ions in an effort to return the pH to normal. The treatment for respiratory alkalosis is directed at treating the underlying cause of the hyperventilation.

Metabolic Acidosis

Metabolic acidosis results from an accumulation of acid or a loss of base. When excessive acid is produced by the body, the acid spills into the extracellular fluid, consuming some bicarbonate buffers. This results in an increase in acid and a decrease in available base (Fig. 13-10). Metabolic acidosis can be summarized by the equation:

$$\uparrow H^++HCO_3^-\rightarrow\uparrow H_2CO_3\rightarrow H_2O+\uparrow CO_2$$

The healthy respiratory system immediately attempts to compensate for the acidosis by increasing the rate and depth of ventilation to reduce carbon dioxide. As the carbon dioxide level falls, so does the concentration of carbonic acid, returning pH toward normal. In addition, the kidneys excrete more hydrogen ion to equilibrate the excess acid in the extracellular fluid.

The four most common forms of metabolic acidosis encountered in the prehospital setting are lactic acidosis, diabetic ketoacidosis, acidosis re-

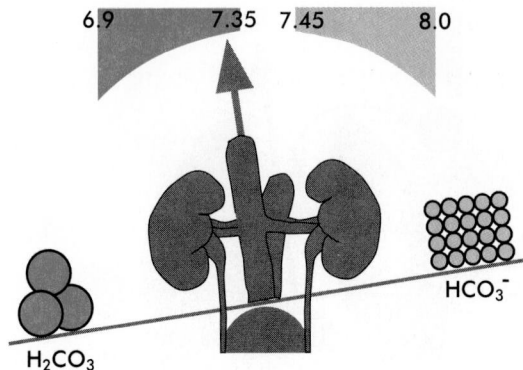

6.9   7.35 7.45   8.0

H₂CO₃   HCO₃⁻

Fig. 13-10 Metabolic acidosis. An excess of metabolic acids consume bicarbonate and liberate hydrogen ions, resulting in acidosis.

sulting from renal failure, and acidosis from ingestion of toxins.

1. Lactic acidosis. Lactic acid is produced when large muscle beds are inadequately perfused, resulting in a shift from aerobic to anaerobic metabolism. The end product of anaerobic metabolism is lactic acid, which releases hydrogen ions, creating systemic acidosis. Normally, lactate is converted by the liver back to glucose or is oxidized to carbon dioxide and water. When the rate of lactic acid production exceeds the rate of its metabolism, lactic acidosis occurs. The most common causes of lactic acidosis are circulatory failure and shock. Specific complications associated with lactic acidosis are thought to include the following:

   a. Decreased force of cardiac contraction

   b. Decreased peripheral response to catecholamines

   c. Hypotension and shock

   d. Cardiac muscle that is refractory to defibrillation

   The treatment for lactic acidosis is to reestablish tissue perfusion and cardiac output. This permits the liver to regenerate bicarbonate by metabolizing lactate to carbon dioxide and water. Medical direction may recommend hyperventilation to induce respiratory alkalosis, vigorous rehydration to support circulation, and intravenous administration of bicarbonate for immediate compensation.

Correction of lactic acidosis frequently depend on identification and correction of the underlying cause.

2. Diabetic ketoacidosis. Ketoacidosis is a complication of diabetes mellitus. It may result when a patient fails to take adequate insulin or when the need for insulin increases (for example, in cases of infection or trauma). With impaired glucose use, fatty acid metabolism increases, as do production of ketone bodies and release of hydrogen ions. Large quantities of ketone bodies exceed the ability of the body's buffering system, resulting in acidosis and a decrease in blood pH. The pathophysiology of this disorder is further addressed in Chapter 19.

3. Renal failure. The kidneys help maintain acid-base balance by reabsorbing or secreting either bicarbonate or hydrogen ions as needed to keep the pH constant. Renal failure affects the compensatory mechanisms of the kidneys to varying degrees. Patients with moderate-to-severe renal failure frequently have mild-to-moderate acidosis.

4. Ingestion of toxins. The ingestion of some toxins, such as ethylene glycol, methanol, and salicylate, can cause metabolic acidosis. These and other toxins lead to the production of toxic metabolites and may result in acid-base disorders characterized by metabolic acidosis and compensatory respiratory alkalosis. Treatment for various toxic ingestions frequently includes gastrointestinal decontamination but may also entail hemodialysis, diuresis, hydration to promote excretion, and specific antagonistic or antidotal therapy.

Metabolic Alkalosis

Metabolic alkalosis most often results from loss of hydrogen ions (primarily from the stomach), ingestion of large amounts of absorbable base sodium bicarbonate (baking soda) or calcium carbonate (Tums, other antacids), or excessive intravenous administration of alkali (for example, intravenous injection of sodium bicarbonate). Diuretic use may also contribute to development

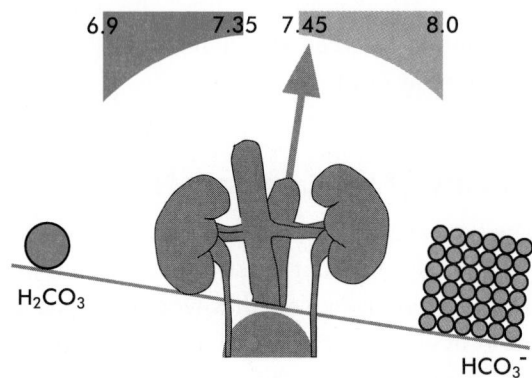

Fig. 13-11 Metabolic alkalosis. An excess of bicarbonate results in alkalosis.

of metabolic alkalosis (Fig. 13-11). Metabolic alkalosis can be summarized by the chemical equation:

$$\downarrow H^+ + HCO_3^- \rightarrow \downarrow H_2CO_3 \rightarrow H_2O + \downarrow CO_2$$

Loss of hydrogen ions is the initial cause of metabolic alkalosis. This may result from vomiting (hydrochloric acid loss), gastric suction, or increased renal excretion of hydrogen ion in urine. When vomiting occurs, not only is gastric acid lost but volume is depleted.

Chronic diuretic use can result in volume depletion. The loss of sodium chloride and potassium causes a relative increase in bicarbonate. (The kidney defends against volume depletion by increasing its reabsorption of sodium.) When sodium is reabsorbed, either potassium or hydrogen ions must be excreted to maintain electrical neutrality. Excretion of hydrogen ions can lead to a net increase in bicarbonate and subsequent metabolic alkalosis.

Initially, the respiratory system tries to compensate by retaining carbon dioxide. However, this compensatory mechanism is limited by the development of hypoxemia (the rise in Pco_2 and decrease in Po_2 as a result of hypoventilation stimulate respiration). The treatment for metabolic alkalosis is directed at correcting the underlying condition. Volume depletion, if present, should be corrected with isotonic solutions, and hypokalemia may require correction with potassium replacement.

Mixed Acid-Base Disturbances

The various forms of shock may produce abnormalities of acid-base regulation. In these patients, simultaneous respiratory and metabolic alterations are commonly seen because of compromised compensatory mechanisms. Examples of mixed acid-base disturbances include the following:

- Combined respiratory and metabolic acidosis
- Metabolic acidosis and respiratory alkalosis
- Respiratory acidosis and metabolic alkalosis
- Combined respiratory and metabolic alkalosis

Blood Gas Analysis

Blood gases are obtained for two reasons: to determine if the patient is well oxygenated and to determine the patient's acid-base status. Most often, blood gases are measured on arterial blood obtained from the patient in a heparinized syringe (Box 13-2). Arterial samples are more commonly obtained than venous samples because arterial samples give more direct information about the lung's ability to oxygenate blood and remove carbon dioxide.

TABLE 13-2 Simple Acid-Base Disturbances			
Acid-Base Disturbance	**HCO_3^-**	**Pco_2**	**pH**
Metabolic acidosis	↓	↓	↓
Respiratory acidosis	↓	↑	↓
Metabolic alkalosis	↑	↑	↑
Respiratory alkalosis	↑	↓	↑

The acid-base status of a patient is assessed by measuring arterial Pco_2 and pH level. The pH level indicates whether an acid or base state is present. The Pco_2 level indicates whether there is a respiratory component to the acidosis or alkalosis (that is, whether there is alveolar hypoventilation or hyperventilation). Table 13-2 summarizes the abnormalities that occur in the partially compensated, simple acid-base disturbances.

Acid-Base Determinants and Other Laboratory Studies

At present, determining pH by blood gas analysis is not considered part of the duty of paramedics in the prehospital setting. The use of pulse oximetry provides a continuous reading of arterial oxygen saturation without invasive procedures. (Under normal circumstances, a saturation of 90% correlates with a Po_2 of 60 mm Hg.)

Section Two
Pathophysiology of Shock

● THE CAPILLARY-CELLULAR RELATIONSHIP

There are approximately 10 billion capillaries in the human body, and few functional cells of the body are more than 5/1000 of an inch (20 to 30 microns) away from one. To understand the capillary-cellular relationship in shock, one must understand the factors that affect the transfer of fluid volume between the circulating blood and the interstitial fluid.

Anatomy of the Capillary Network

The typical capillary is a thin-walled tube of endothelial cells without elastic tissue, connective tissue, or smooth muscle that would impede the transfer of water and solutes. Blood enters the capillary network from the arterioles and flows through the capillary network into the venules. The ends of the capillaries closest to the arterioles are called *arteriolar capillaries,* and the ends closest to the venules are called *venous capillaries.*

The arterioles give rise directly to capillaries or in some tissues to metarterioles, which then give rise to capillaries. Most tissues appear to have two distinct types of capillaries: true capillaries and thoroughfare channels. From a metarteriole, blood may flow into a thoroughfare channel that connects arterioles and venules directly, bypassing the true capillaries. Blood flow through thoroughfare channels is relatively constant. From these thoroughfare channels, fluid commonly exits and reenters the network of true capillaries, where the exchange of nutrients and metabolic end products takes place. (Refer to illustrations in Chapter 10.)

The capillaries of some tissues contain small cuffs of smooth muscle that encircle their proximal and distal portions, known as the *capillary sphincters.* The sphincter at the arterial end is known as the *precapillary sphincter,* and that at the venous end is known as the *postcapillary sphincter.* These sphincters control capillary blood flow by opening and closing the entrance and exit to the capillary. Blood flow in true capillaries is not uniform and depends on the contractile state of the arterioles and the precapillary and postcapillary sphincters (if present).

The blood flow through the capillaries that provides the exchange of gases and solutes between blood and tissue is referred to as *nutritional flow.* Blood that bypasses the capillaries in traveling from the arterial to the venous side of the circulation is known as *nonnutritional* or *shunt flow.* True arteriovenous anastomoses (AV shunts), which occur naturally in the sole of the foot, the palm of the hand, the terminal phalanges, and the nail bed, are important in regulating body temperature. Some evidence also suggests the presence of AV shunts upstream from the capillary sphincters.

Sympathetic fibers innervate all blood vessels of the body except the capillaries, capillary sphincters, and most metarterioles. Sympathetic innervation of blood vessels includes both vasoconstrictor and vasodilator (vasomotor) fibers. However, the sympathetic vasoconstrictor fibers are the most important in regulating blood flow. During normal circulation in the healthy body when arterial blood pressure is adequate, arterioles are open (though with some vasomotor tone), AV shunts are closed, and approximately 20% of the capillaries are open at any given time (Fig. 13-12).

Diffusion Across the Capillary Wall

Tissue cells do not exchange material directly with blood. The interstitial fluid always acts as a middleman. Nutrients must diffuse across the capillary wall into the interstitial fluid to enter cells, and metabolic end products must first move across cell membranes into interstitial fluid to diffuse into the plasma.

At the arteriole end of the capillary, the forces moving fluid out of the capillary are greater than the forces attracting fluid into it. At the venous end, these forces are reversed, so more fluid is attracted into the capillary. Hydrostatic and osmotic pressure are the two forces responsible for this movement of fluid. The osmotic pressure, which results from the presence of plasma proteins (mostly albumin) too large to pass through the wall of the capillary, is referred to as *blood colloid osmotic pressure* or *oncotic pressure*.

At the venous end of the capillary, the hydrostatic pressure is lower. The concentration of proteins in the capillary increases slightly because of the movement of fluid out of the arteriolar end, resulting in a greater plasma protein concentration and a greater colloid osmotic pressure.

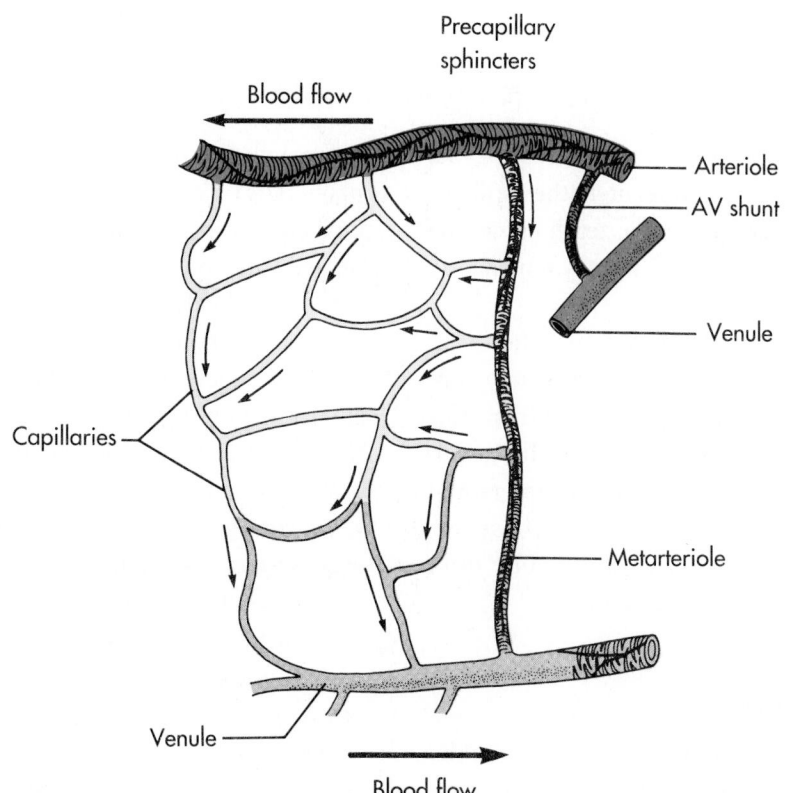

Fig. 13-12 Microcirculation. The circular structures on the arteriole and venule represent smooth muscle fibers; branching solid lines represent sympathetic nerve fibers. The arrows indicate the direction of blood flow.

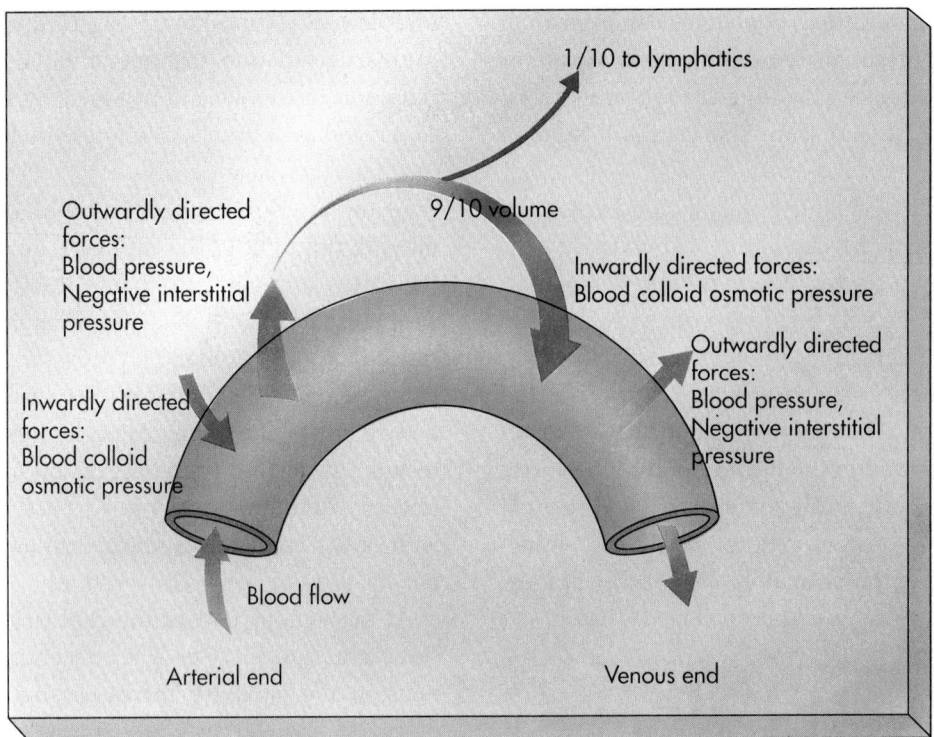

Fig. 13-13 Total pressure differences between the inside and the outside of the capillary at its arteriolar and venous ends. At the arteriolar end, the sum of the forces causes fluid to move from the capillaries into the tissues. At the venous end, the sum of the forces attracts fluid into the capillary.

As a result, nine tenths of the fluid that leaves the capillary at its arteriolar end reenters the capillary at its venous end. The remaining tenth enters the lymphatic capillaries and is eventually returned to the general circulation.

Fluid may also be exchanged across the capillary wall as a result of the cyclic dilation and constriction of the capillary sphincter. When this sphincter dilates, the pressure rises in the capillary, forcing fluid to move into the interstitial spaces. When the capillary sphincter constricts, the pressure in the capillary drops, and fluid moves into the capillary (Fig. 13-13).

Energy Production

Virtually all cellular activities on which life depends require energy. The cell membrane requires a substantial percentage of the cell's energy production to maintain normal fluid and electrolyte composition within the cell. Adenosine triphosphate (ATP) and other high-energy phosphate molecules provide the fuel for all of the energy-related functions of the cell. Most cellular metabolism in the healthy body is accomplished through aerobic metabolism. Anaerobic metabolism occurs in the absence of oxygen but can supply only a small fraction of the energy produced by aerobic metabolism and cannot meet the body's energy requirements alone.

Glucose is an important fuel for producing energy and is essentially the only fuel that can be used anaerobically under conditions of cellular hypoxia (as occurs in a state of shock). Under these conditions, glucose is metabolized to lactate and pyruvate, producing a net sum of two ATP molecules. If oxygen is present (aerobic metabolism), pyruvate enters the Krebs cycle, a sequence of reactions that breaks down a molecule of pyruvic acid into molecules of carbon dioxide and water.

The Krebs cycle, which is 18 times more efficient in producing ATP than glycolysis (the breakdown of glucose to lactate), cannot occur in the absence of oxygen. Because anaerobic ATP production is so inefficient, the rate of glycolysis must be greatly increased to meet the body's energy requirements. This leads to an increase in production of lactic acid and a resultant metabolic acidosis.

As tissue metabolites continue to accumulate, they stimulate vasodilation. This vasodilation opposes the constriction of the precapillary sphincters, which helps continue tissue perfusion by maintaining the proper container size. (The postcapillary sphincters are more resistant to the vasodilatory effects of tissue metabolites and stay constricted long after the precapillary sphincters dilate.) This in turn increases the capillary hydrostatic pressure, causing a fluid loss from the vascular space into the interstitial space. In addition, the insufficient energy production from anaerobic metabolism affects the cells' ability to maintain a normal sodium-potassium differential across the cell membrane. Intracellular potassium leaks into the extracellular space, and sodium leaks into the cell, producing alterations in the membrane potential. Energy production is further impaired until finally the cells are irreversibly damaged.

Microcirculation

The body's microcirculation can be divided into pulmonary microcirculation and peripheral microcirculation. Pressure in each of these divisions is produced by separate pumps: the right and left heart, respectively.

At any given moment, approximately 5% of the total circulating blood is flowing through the capillaries. It is this 5% that is performing the ultimate function of exchanging nutrients and metabolic end products. The muscular arterioles, which are the major resistance vessels, regulate regional blood flow to the capillary beds. The venules and veins serve as collecting channels and storage (capacitance) vessels. The various mechanisms controlling blood flow to the tissues fall into two general categories: (1) local control of blood flow by the tissues and (2) nervous control of blood flow.

Local Control of Blood Flow by the Tissues

Blood usually does not flow at a continuous rate through capillaries but rather intermittently. This is a result of two features of circulation: the pulsatile manner of blood flow resulting from cardiac pumping action and vasomotion, the intermittent constriction and dilation of the arterioles, metarterioles, and precapillary sphincters.

Vasomotion is regulated primarily by the concentration of oxygen in the tissues, although a number of other mediators also play a substantial role. When the oxygen concentration in tissues is low, the cells lining and adjacent to the closed capillary secrete histamine (a substance thought to be responsible for arteriolar smooth muscle relaxation and subsequent vasodilation), causing the capillary to open. The histamine is quickly destroyed in the blood and does not enter the general circulation. As these cells become reoxygenated, they stop the histamine secretion and the capillary closes. Therefore a decrease in oxygen concentration leads to local release of vasodilating substances, which allows blood flow to increase. This in turn increases the delivery of oxygen and restores aerobic metabolism.

Blood flow is much greater to some organs than to others, and the need for blood to any given organ may vary considerably. For example, the heart, skeletal muscle, and other muscular organs have an increased blood flow whenever their metabolic activity increases. This phenomenon is known as *reactive hyperemia* and is the direct result of arteriolar dilation within the more active organ.

Vasodilation from active hyperemia does not depend on the presence of nerves or hormones. It is a locally mediated response that results from local chemical changes produced by increased cellular activity. Several chemicals, including carbon dioxide, lactic acid, adenosine, adenosine monophosphate, adenosine diphosphate, potassium ions, and hydrogen ions, cause vasodilation. These molecules are breakdown products of metabolism, and their concentration in the extracellular fluid rises as the increase in metabolism of a given tissue outstrips its perfusion. The resultant

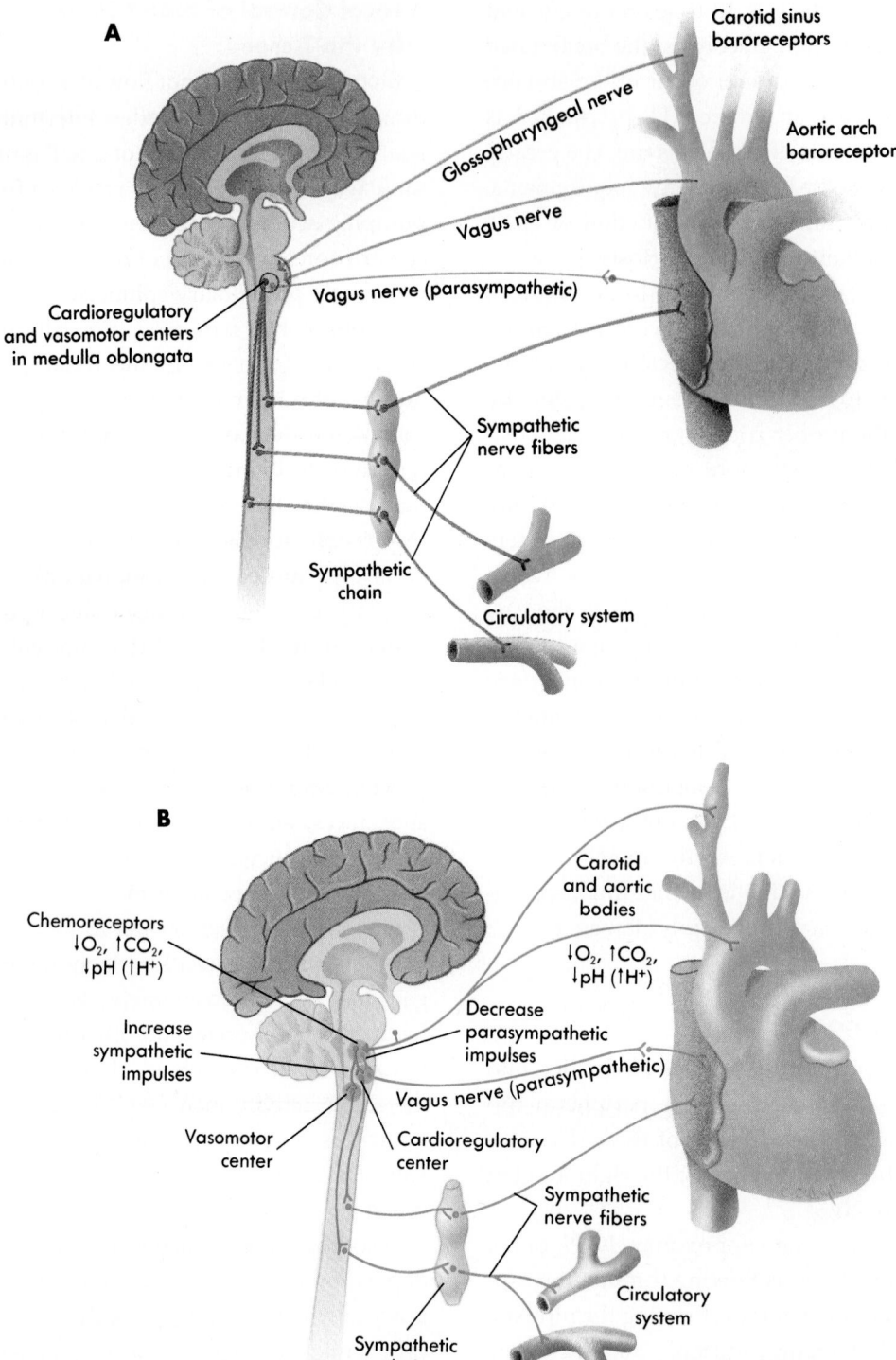

Fig. 13-14 A, Baroreceptor reflexes. Baroreceptors located in the carotid sinuses and the aortic arch detect changes in blood pressure. Impulses are conducted to the cardioregulatory and vasomotor centers. The heart rate can be decreased by the parasympthetic system; the heart rate and stroke volume can be increased by the sympathetic system. The sympathetic system can also constrict or dilate blood vessels. **B,** Chemoreceptor reflexes. Chemoreceptors located in the medulla and carotid and aortic bodies detect changes in blood oxygen, carbon dioxide, or pH levels. Impulses are conducted to the medulla. In response, the vasomotor center can cause vasoconstriction or dilation of blood vessels by the sympathetic system, and the cardioregulatory center can cause changes in the pumping activity of the heart through the parasympathetic and sympathetic system.

vasodilation leads to an increase in perfusion and, ideally, restores balance between the tissues' requirements for energy substrates and the circulation's supply.

Reactive hyperemia may also produce arteriolar dilation after a period of ischemia. For example, if a tourniquet has been applied around the upper arm and tightened to occlude arterial flow, the tissues of the arm are deprived of blood. The concentrations of carbon dioxide, hydrogen ions, and metabolites increase because they are not removed by the blood as quickly as they are produced. When the tourniquet is released, the arm becomes red and very warm as a result of increased blood flow. The value of reactive hyperemia is that a tissue that suffers ischemia (for example, an extremity with partial arterial occlusion) can maintain an adequate blood supply by local arteriolar dilation.

Nervous Control of Blood Flow

Nervous control of circulation is accomplished by a number of negative feedback mechanisms (any mechanism that tends to balance a change in a system). Negative feedback mechanisms important in maintaining tissue perfusion are baroreceptor reflexes, chemoreceptor reflexes, central nervous system ischemia responses, hormonal mechanisms, and reabsorption of tissue fluids.

Baroreceptor Reflexes

High in the neck, each carotid artery divides into external and internal carotid arteries. At this bifurcation, the wall of the artery is thinner than usual and contains a large number of vinelike nerve endings. This small portion of the artery is called the *carotid sinus*. The nerve endings in this area are sensitive to stretch or distortion and serve as pressure receptors or baroreceptors. An area functionally similar to the carotid sinus is found in the arch of the aorta, which serves as a second important arterial baroreceptor. Other portions of the vascular tree (namely large arteries, the large veins, and the walls of the myocardium) also contain baroreceptors that play a less important role in maintaining homeostasis (Fig. 13-14, *A*).

Baroreceptors help maintain blood pressure in two ways (both of which are negative feedback

mechanisms): (1) by lowering blood pressure in response to increased arterial pressure and (2) by increasing blood pressure in response to decreased arterial pressure. Normal blood pressure partially stretches the arterial walls so that the baroreceptors produce a constant, low-frequency stimulation. This stimulation increases progressively from a lower pressure limit of 60 mm Hg, reaching a maximum at 180 to 200 mm Hg. Impulses from the baroreceptors inhibit the vasoconstrictor center of the medulla and excite the vagal center. These impulses result in vasodilation in the peripheral circulatory system and a decrease in the heart rate and strength of contraction. The combined effect is a decrease in arterial pressure. (Baroreceptors adapt in 1 to 3 days to whatever pressure level they are exposed). Therefore they do not change the average blood pressure on a long-term basis. This adaptation is common in people who have chronic hypertension.)

Baroreceptors are not stimulated by pressures between 0 and 60 mm Hg. When baroreceptor stimulation ceases because of a fall in arterial pressure, the negative feedback mechanism evokes several cardiovascular responses (Box 13-3). Vagal stimulation is reduced and sympathetic response is increased. The increase in sympathetic impulses results in increased peripheral resistance and an increase in heart rate and stroke volume. Sympathetic discharges also produce generalized arteriolar vasoconstriction, which decreases the container size. Constricting capacitance vessels shift

---

BOX 13-3

Baroreceptor Responses to Low Blood Pressure: Sympathetic Nervous System

Cardiac Effects

Increased strength of contraction

Increased rate of contraction

Peripheral Effects

Arteriolar constriction

Decreased container size

Increased peripheral resistance

blood into the central circulation. This, coupled with the constriction of blood vessels in skin, muscles, and viscera, helps maintain perfusion of the central organs. The vasoconstriction in these peripheral vascular beds results in the characteristic pale, cold skin of patients suffering from hypovolemic shock.

Chemoreceptor Reflexes

Low arterial pressure (if it leads to hypoxemia, acidosis, or both) may also stimulate peripheral chemoreceptor cells that lie within the carotid and aortic bodies. Because of the location of these bodies, the chemoreceptor cells have an abundant blood supply. When oxygen or pH decreases, these cells stimulate the vasomotor center of the medulla. At the same time, the rate and depth of ventilation are increased to help eliminate excess carbon dioxide and maintain acid-base balance. Chemoreceptors are more involved in regulation of respiration than in cardiovascular effects. During profound hypotension or acidosis, however, they can and do lead to vasoconstriction. This vasomotor stimulation results in enhanced peripheral vasoconstriction, which is initiated by the baroreceptors (Fig. 13-14, *B*).

Central Nervous System Ischemia Response

When blood flow to the vasomotor center of the medulla is decreased enough to cause ischemia, the neurons in the vasomotor center become excited, raising arterial pressure. This is known as the *central nervous system ischemic response*. The degree of sympathetic vasoconstriction can be so intense that it elevates arterial pressure for as long as 10 minutes, sometimes to above 200 mm Hg. If the ischemia lasts longer than a few minutes, the vagal centers are activated, resulting in vasodilation in the periphery and bradycardia. Like the chemoreceptor reflex, the cerebral ischemia response functions only in emergency situations and does not become active until blood pressure falls below 50 mm Hg.

Hormonal Mechanisms

Several hormonal mechanisms also help control arterial pressure through negative feedback. These include the adrenal medullary mechanism, the renin-angiotensin-aldosterone mechanism, and the vasopressin mechanism (Fig. 13-15).[4]

Adrenal Medullary Mechanism

When sympathetic stimulation of the heart and blood vessels increases, stimulation of the adrenal medulla also increases. The hormones secreted by the adrenal medulla, epinephrine and norepinephrine, affect the cardiovascular system in a way very similar to the sympathetic nervous system. There is a resultant increase in heart rate, stroke volume, and vasoconstriction.

Renin-Angiotensin-Aldosterone Mechanism

Renin is an enzyme released by the kidneys into the circulatory system. Renin acts on a plasma protein called *angiotensinogen* by altering its structure to produce angiotensin I, which is in turn cleaved by angiotensin-converting enzyme (mostly in the lungs) to angiotensin II (active angiotensin).

Angiotensin II causes vasoconstriction in arterioles and to a lesser degree in veins. This vasoconstriction results in increased peripheral resistance, increased venous return to the heart, and a resultant increase in blood pressure. In addition, angiotensin II stimulates the release of aldosterone, which acts on the kidneys to conserve sodium and water. Angiotensin II may also be partially responsible for stimulating thirst.

The renin-angiotensin-aldosterone mechanism is an important regulatory loop to increase blood pressure in circulatory shock. It requires approximately 20 minutes to become effective in hypovolemia caused by hemorrhage and remains active for approximately 1 hour.

Vasopressin Mechanism

When the blood pressure drops or the concentration of solutes in the plasma increases (increased serum osmolality), the hypothalamic neurons are stimulated. This stimulation causes the anterior pituitary to increase its secretion of vasopressin, or antidiuretic hormone (ADH). ADH acts directly on the blood vessels, causing vasoconstriction within minutes after a rapid fall in the

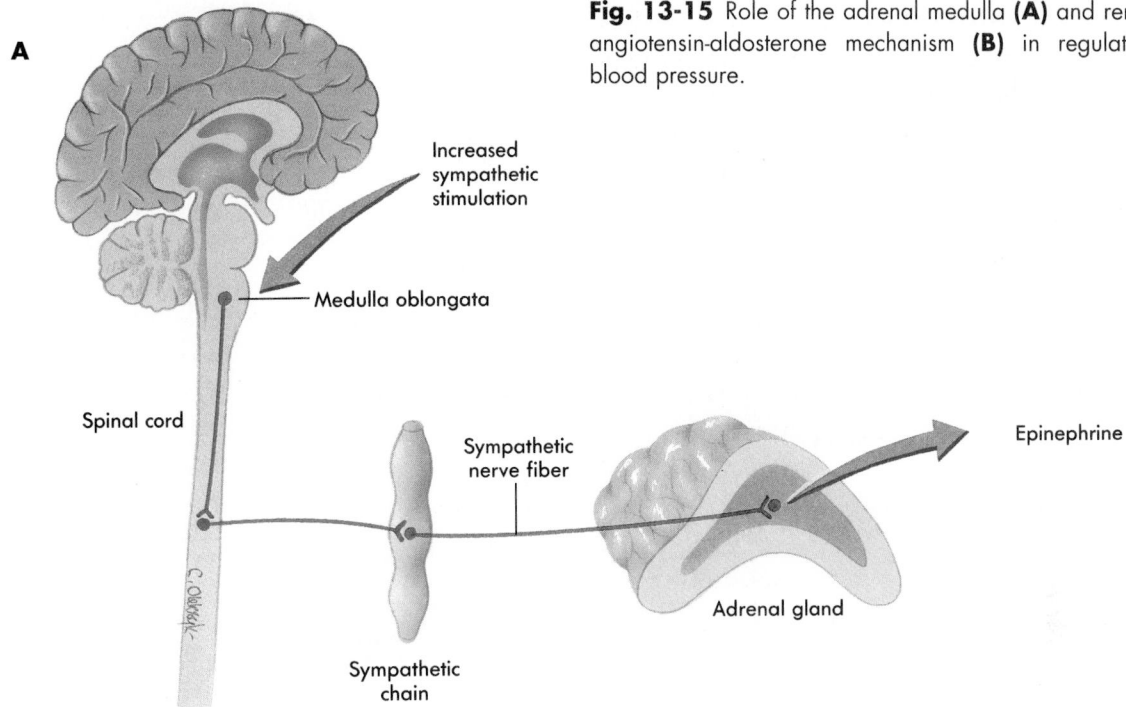

Fig. 13-15 Role of the adrenal medulla **(A)** and renin-angiotensin-aldosterone mechanism **(B)** in regulating blood pressure.

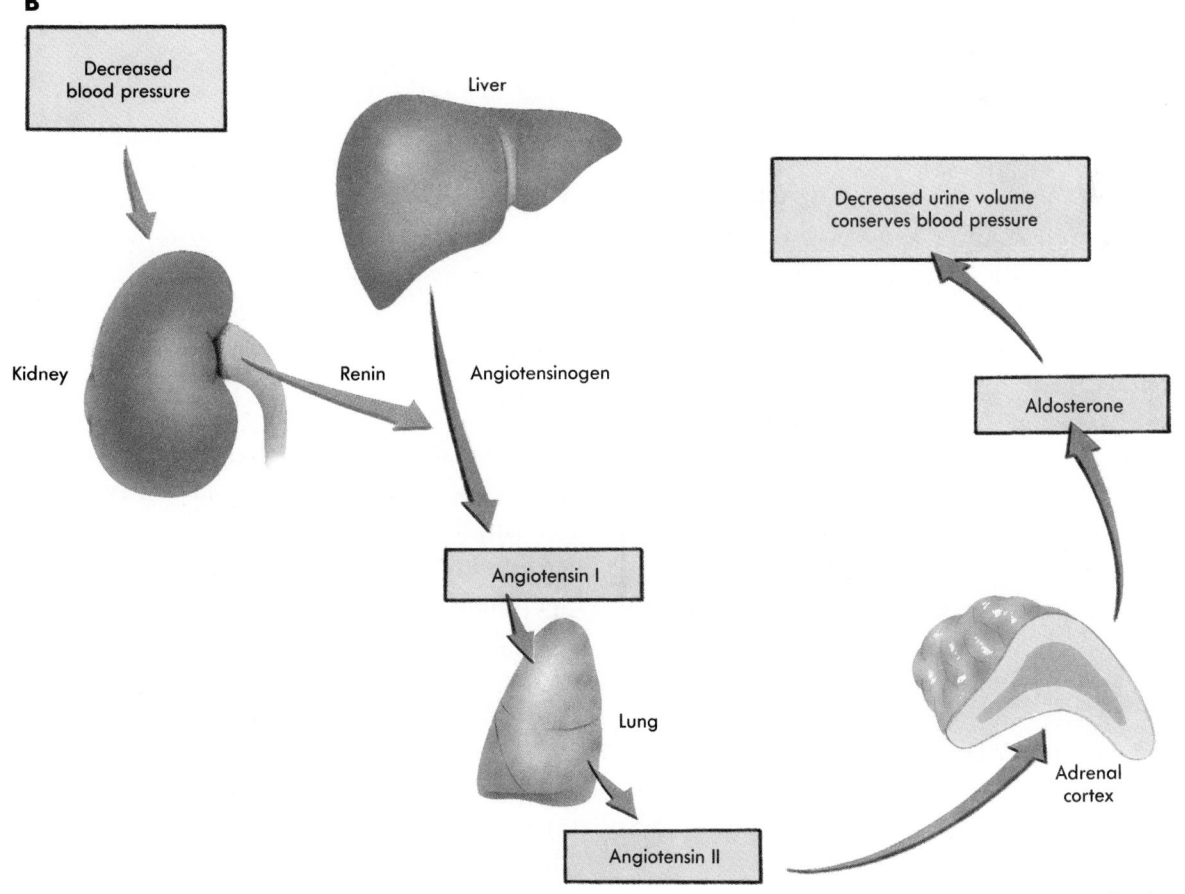

Continued.

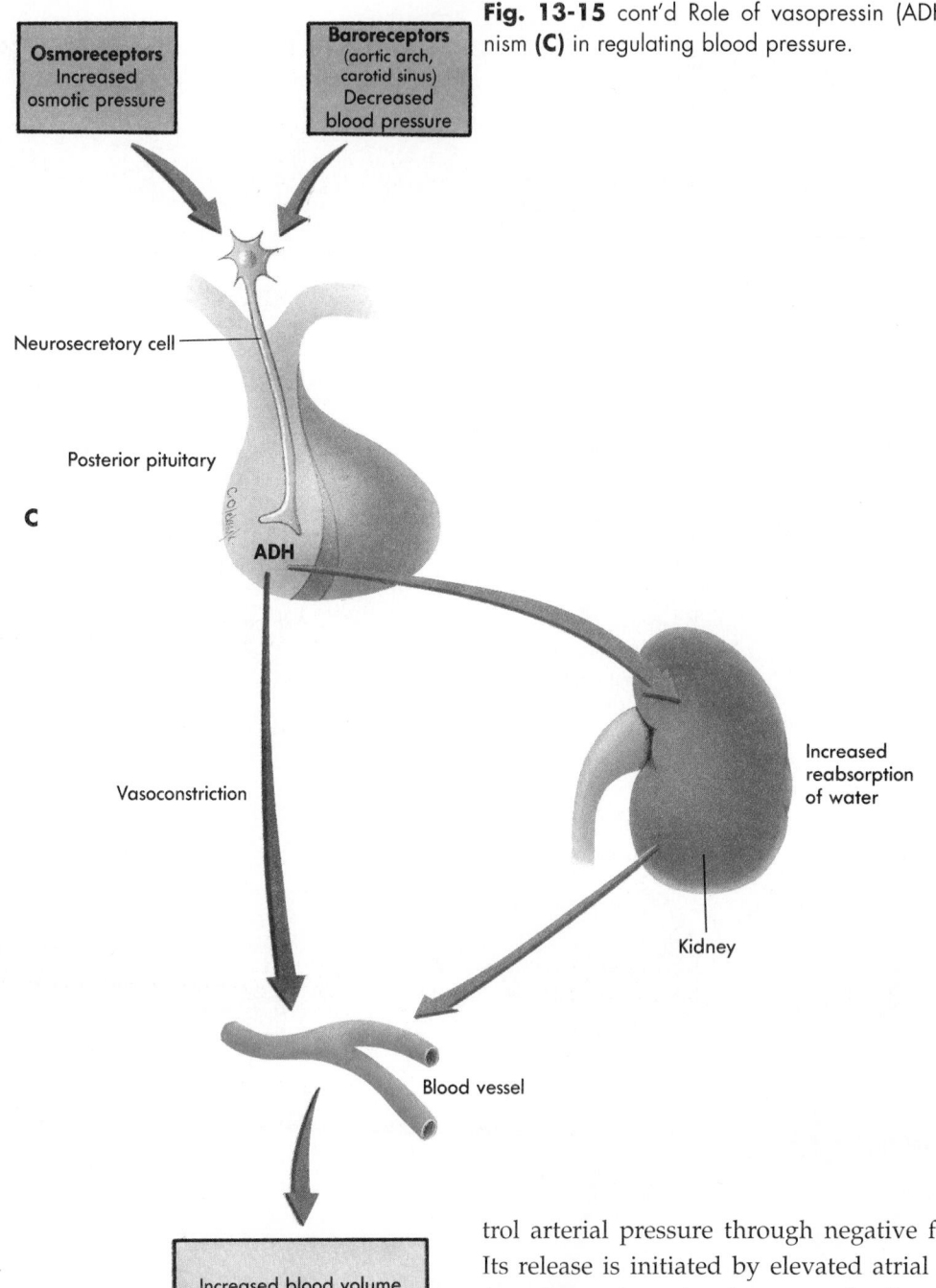

Fig. 13-15 cont'd Role of vasopressin (ADH) mechanism **(C)** in regulating blood pressure.

trol arterial pressure through negative feedback. Its release is initiated by elevated atrial pressure (usually a sign of volume overload), and it increases in the rate of urine production. Loss of water through the urine decreases blood volume, thus decreasing the atrial pressure.

Reabsorption of Tissue Fluids

Arterial hypotension, arteriolar constriction, and reduced venous pressure during hypovolemia lower the blood pressure in the capillaries (hydrostatic pressure). This decrease promotes reabsorption of interstitial fluid into the vascular compartment. Considerable quantities of fluid

blood pressure. ADH also decreases the rate of urine production (by enhancing reabsorption of water), helping maintain the blood volume and the blood pressure.

The atrial natriuretic factor, a substance released from the atrial cells of the heart, also helps con-

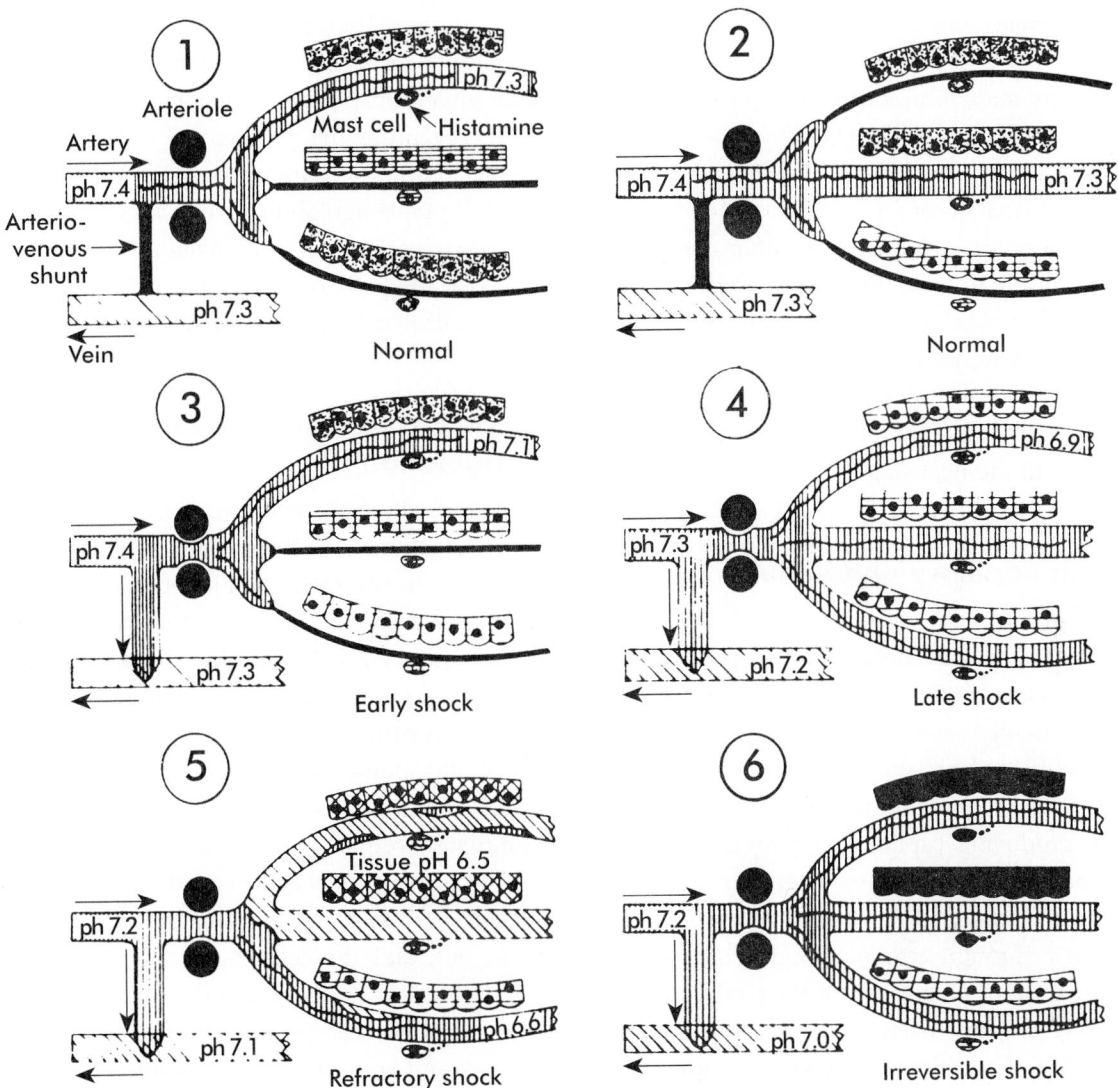

Fig. 13-16 Diagram of the microcirculation in shock, progressing from normal *(1, 2)* to vasoconstriction stage *(3)* to capillary and venule opening *(4)* to DIC *(5)* to tissue death *(6)*.

may be drawn into the circulation during hemorrhage. It has been estimated that approximately 0.25 ml/min/kg of body weight, or 1 L/hr in the adult male, can be autoinfused from the interstitial spaces after acute blood loss.

● CAPILLARY-CELLULAR RELATIONSHIP IN SHOCK

The progression of shock in the microcirculation follows a sequence of stages related to changes in capillary perfusion and cellular necrosis (Fig. 13-16).[2]

Stage 1: Vasoconstriction

Vasoconstriction begins as minimal perfusion to the capillaries continues. Oxygen and substrate delivery to the cells supplied by these capillaries decreases; anaerobic metabolism replaces aerobic metabolism and production of lactate and hydrogen ions increases. Shortly thereafter, the lining of the capillaries may begin to lose its ability to retain large molecular structures within its walls, permitting protein-containing fluid to leak into the interstitial spaces. This is known as the *leaky capillary syndrome.*

AV shunts open, particularly in the skin, kidneys, and gastrointestinal tract, causing less flow to the arterioles and therefore less flow through the capillaries. Sympathetic stimulation produces pale, sweaty skin; a rapid, thready pulse (caused by hypovolemia and vasoconstriction); and an elevation in blood glucose level. The release of epinephrine dilates coronary, cerebral, and skeletal muscle arterioles and constricts other arterioles. As a result, blood is shunted to the heart, brain, and skeletal muscle, and capillary flow to the kidneys and abdominal viscera decreases. If the vasoconstriction stage of shock is not treated by prompt restoration of circulatory volume, shock progresses to the next stage.

Stage 2: Capillary and Venule Opening

As the syndrome continues, the precapillary sphincter relaxes, with some resultant expansion of the vascular space. Because postcapillary sphincters resist local effects, they remain closed, causing blood to pool or stagnate in the capillary system, producing capillary engorgement. Arterial hypotension, secondary arteriolar vasoconstriction, and opening of AV shunts result in less blood flow through arterioles and contribute to the stagnation of blood flow in the capillaries.

As increasing hypoxemia and acidosis lead to the opening of additional venules and capillaries, the vascular space expands greatly. When this occurs, even normal blood volume may be inadequate to fill the container. The capillary and venule capacity may become great enough to reduce the volume of available blood for the great veins and vena cava, resulting in decreased venous return and a fall in cardiac output. In addition, the viscera (lung, liver, kidneys, and gastrointestinal mucosa) may become congested. The low arterial blood pressure, extremely restricted arterioles, presence of AV shunts, and many open capillaries result in stagnant capillary flow.

Sluggish blood flow and the reduced delivery of oxygen result in increased anaerobic metabolism and the production of lactic acid. The respiratory system attempts to compensate for the acidosis by increasing ventilation to blow off carbon dioxide, producing a partially compensated metabolic acidosis. As the acidosis increases and pH

falls, the red blood cells may cluster together (Rouleaux formation). This halts perfusion in the vital visceral capillaries, affecting nutritional flow and preventing the removal of cellular metabolites. Clotting mechanisms are also affected, leading to hypercoagulability. This stage of shock often progresses to the third stage if fluid resuscitation is inadequate or delayed or if the shock state is complicated by trauma or sepsis.

Stage 3: Disseminated Intravascular Coagulation

Stage 3 shock is resistant to treatment (refractory shock) but is still reversible. Blood begins to coagulate in the microcirculation, clogging capillaries. The capillaries become occluded by clumps of red blood cells. This occlusion decreases capillary perfusion and prevents removal of metabolites. As a result, distal tissue cells use anaerobic metabolism, and lactic acid production increases.

As this stage of shock continues, lactic acid accumulates around the cell. The cell membranes no longer have the energy needed to maintain homeostasis. Water and sodium leak in, potassium leaks out, and the cells swell and die. Microinfarcts develop in the viscera. Microthrombi produce capillary congestion, fluid leaks, and even rupture and hemorrhage. The pulmonary capillaries become permeable, leading to pulmonary edema, which decreases the absorption of oxygen and results in possible alterations in carbon dioxide elimination. This may lead to acute respiratory failure or adult respiratory distress syndrome, described in Chapter 17. If shock and disseminated intravascular coagulation continue, the patient progresses to multiple organ failure.

Stage 4: Multiple Organ Failure

The amount of cellular necrosis required to produce organ failure varies with each organ as well as the underlying condition of the organ. Usually hepatic failure occurs, followed by renal failure and then heart failure. However, if capillary occlusion persists for more than 1 to 2 hours, the cells nourished by that capillary undergo changes that rapidly become irreversible. In this stage of shock, blood pressure falls dramatically. The cells can no longer use oxygen, and metabolism stops.

If a critical amount of the vital organ is damaged by cellular necrosis, the organ soon fails. Failure of the liver and kidneys is common and often presents early in this stage. Capillary blockage may cause heart failure. Gastrointestinal bleeding and sepsis may result from gastrointestinal mucosal necrosis; pancreatic necrosis may lead to further clotting disorders and severe pancreatitis. Pulmonary thrombosis may produce hemorrhage and fluid loss into the alveoli, leading to death from respiratory failure.

● CLASSIFICATIONS OF SHOCK

There are many classifications of shock; more than 100 types have been discussed in the medical literature. A common classification of shock for use in emergency care is to describe the syndrome based on the initiating cause (Box 13-4). Although these classifications are separate and distinct, two or more types are often combined. For example, hypovolemia may occur in septic shock, or elements of cardiogenic shock may occur in hypovolemic shock. Regardless of the classification, the underlying defect is inadequate tissue perfusion.

Hypovolemic shock is most frequently caused by hemorrhage but also by dehydration. In either case, there is a loss of circulating volume. Scenarios that may lead to hypovolemic shock include hemorrhage, burns, severe or prolonged diarrhea, vomiting, and internal third space loss, as in peritonitis. In addition to loss of circulating volume, tissue injury resulting from trauma may exacerbate shock by causing microemboli and further activating the inflammatory and coagulation systems.

Cardiogenic shock results when cardiac action cannot deliver a circulating blood volume adequate for tissue perfusion. The patient in cardiogenic shock usually suffers from an acute myocardial infarction, a serious cardiac rhythm disturbance, cardiac tamponade, cardiac contusion, severe valvular heart disease, cardiomyopathy, pulmonary embolism, or dissecting aortic aneurysm. Cardiogenic shock has been estimated to occur in 5% to 10% of patients hospitalized for myocardial infarction. The associated mortality rate in these patients is greater than 80%.

Neurogenic or spinal-cord shock results from vasomotor paralysis below the level of injury. Normal vasomotor tone through sympathetic control is lost, and there is a resultant decrease in peripheral vascular resistance. The loss of sympathetic impulses and resultant vasodilation increases the size of the container, so even normal intravascular volume is insufficient to fill the vascular compartment and nourish the tissues. Because of the nature of the injuries responsible for this syndrome, respiratory insufficiency, head injury, or both may also be present.

Anaphylactic shock occurs when the body is exposed to a substance that produces a severe allergic reaction. Common causes include antibiotic agents (especially penicillins), venoms, and insect stings. Physiological responses result from the release of histamine and other mediators, which act on receptors in both the systemic and pulmonic microcirculation, as well as on bronchial smooth muscle. Histamine causes arterioles and capillaries to dilate and increases capillary membrane permeability. Intravascular fluid leaks into the interstitial space, resulting in a decrease in blood volume. In addition, many of the mediators released cause constriction of both the upper and lower airways, with the potential for complete airway obstruction (see Chapter 22).

Septic shock most often results from a serious systemic bacterial infection. It is thought to be mediated through toxins that are either a part of the microorganism (endotoxin—gram-negative sep

---

BOX 13-4

Common Etiological Classification of Shock

Hypovolemic shock
Cardiogenic shock
Neurogenic shock
Anaphylactic shock
Septic shock

sis) or are released by the organism (exotoxin— toxic shock). These toxins stimulate the release of complex vasoactive agents that affect arterioles, capillaries, and venules, altering microcirculatory pressure and capillary permeability. Septic shock may result from staphylococcal and streptococcal infections, pneumonia, postoperative infections, and infections resulting from indwelling urinary catheters. Between 40,000 and 100,000 people develop septic shock each year. It is most often seen in older adults (particularly nursing home residents), alcoholics, and neonates.

● STAGES OF SHOCK

Hypoperfusion and its associated anaerobic metabolism may be categorized by stages of the body's response to the shock syndrome. The three component stages are compensated shock, uncompensated shock, and irreversible shock.[5] Table 13-3 lists the stages of shock and the signs and symptoms of each.

Compensated Shock

Compensated shock (Fig. 13-17) entails some decreased tissue perfusion, but the body's compensatory responses are sufficient to overcome the decrease in available fluid. Cardiac output and a normal systolic blood pressure are maintained by increasing catecholamine production.

The decrease in perfusion and subsequent increase in acidosis lead to a chemoreceptor response that increases the rate and depth of ventilation (to decrease acidosis by decreasing P_{CO_2}). Sympathetic stimulation increases heart rate and contractility, creates bronchodilation, leads to increases in peripheral vascular resistance, and decreases capillary flow. The patient may exhibit delayed capillary refill and cool skin as the blood is shunted to the vital organs. In spite of maintaining normal blood pressure, some patients may exhibit signs of decreased central nervous system perfusion (lethargy, confusion, combativeness), even at this stage. If the underlying cause of shock is untreated, the compensatory mechanisms collapse.

Uncompensated Shock

Uncompensated shock (Fig. 13-18) occurs when the body is no longer able to maintain systolic pressure. Both the systolic and diastolic pressures begin to drop. The pulse pressure may be narrowed to such an extent that it is not detectable with a blood pressure cuff.

As the body's compensatory mechanisms begin to fail, cerebral blood flow decreases. P_{O_2} may drop, but P_{CO_2} usually remains normal or low unless the patient has a head or chest injury that leads to hypoventilation. The clinical signs of uncompensated shock include hypotension as well as tachycardia, tachypnea, and delayed capillary refill. Shunting of blood and tissue hypoxia may cause the patient to have cold extremities and cyanosis. Effects on the cardiovascular system include a decreased preload and an increased rate of contraction secondary to catecholamine stimulation. Although myocardial contractions may initially be stronger as a result of catecholamine release, in the

Signs and Symptoms	Compensated Shock	Uncompensated Shock	Irreversible Shock
Heart rate	Mild tachycardia	Moderate tachycardia	Bradycardia, severe dysrhythmias
Level of consciousness	Lethargy, confusion, combativeness	Confusion, unconsciousness	Coma
Skin	Delayed capillary refill, cool skin	Delayed capillary refill, cold extremities, cyanosis	Pale, cold, clammy skin
Blood pressure	Normal or slightly elevated measurement	Decreased systolic and diastolic pressure	Frank hypotension

TABLE 13-3 Stages of Shock

latter phases of uncompensated shock, myocardial strength can decrease as a result of the following factors:

1. Ischemia secondary to a reduction of circulating red blood cells, a lower oxygen saturation (Po_2), and decreased coronary perfusion secondary to hypotension (especially diastolic hypotension)

2. Necrosis of myocardium (essentially simulating myocardial infarction) from the same causes associated with ischemia

3. Decreased preload leading to decreased contractility

4. Acidosis possibly leading to decreased contractility

5. Cardiac rhythm disturbances secondary to hypoxia

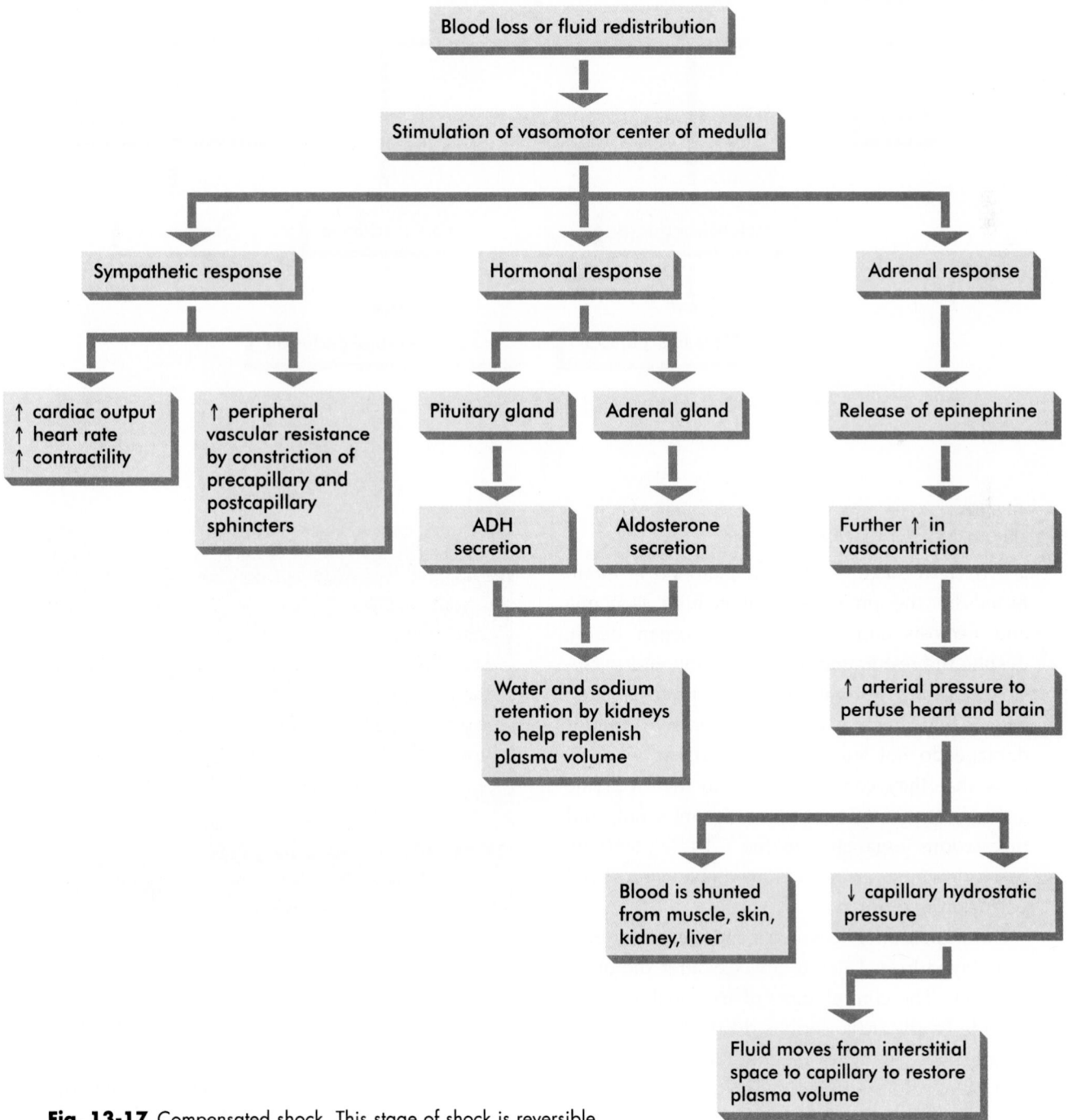

Fig. 13-17 Compensated shock. This stage of shock is reversible.

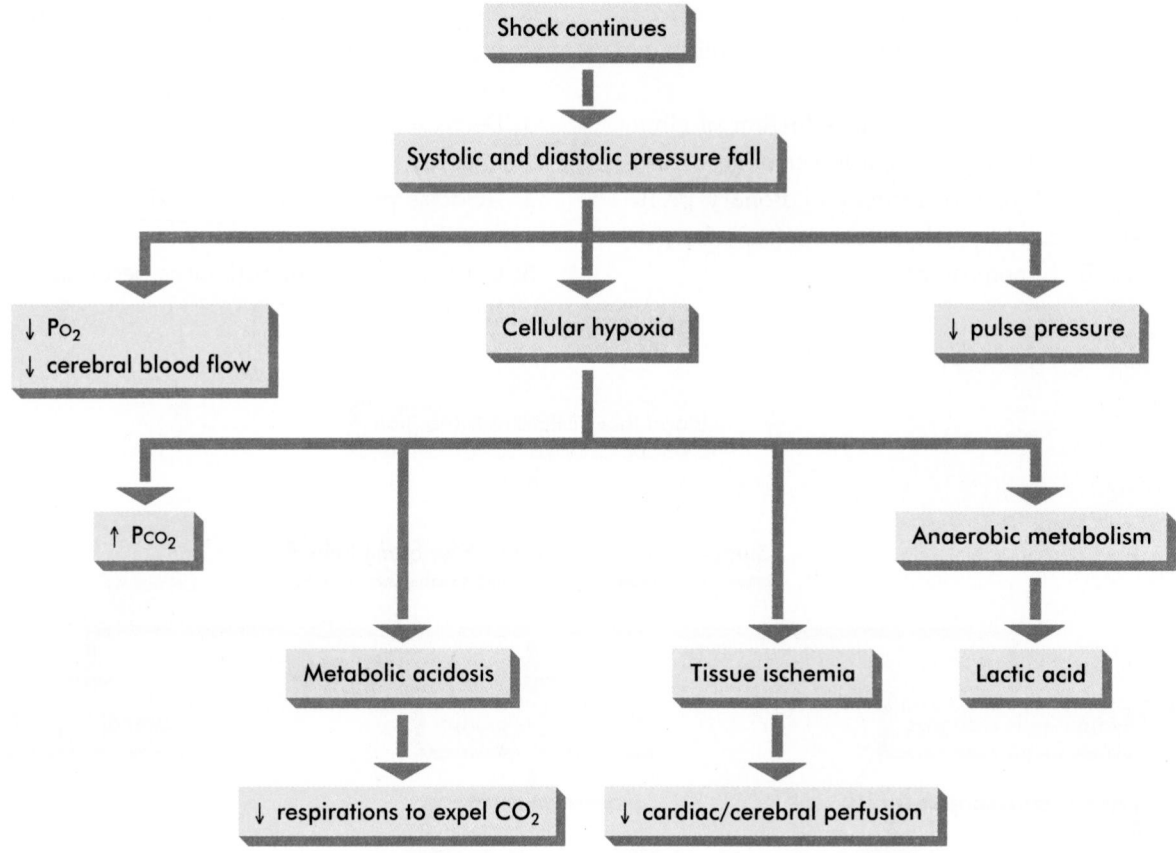

Fig. 13-18 Uncompensated shock. This stage of shock is reversible.

Irreversible Shock

The third stage of shock (Fig. 13-19) is manifested by the progression of cellular ischemia and necrosis and by subsequent organ death, despite the restoration of oxygenation and perfusion. Despite normal perfusion, patients with irreversible shock as a result of massive cellular damage do not survive. Cells and the vital organs that they comprise begin to die from the lack of energy. The membrane pumps fail, and the various organelles in the cells sequentially break down, so necrosis is inevitable even if cell perfusion is restored.

Decompensation may occur suddenly, or it may be delayed from 1 day to 3 weeks after the onset of shock. The clinical signs of irreversible shock include bradycardia, serious dysrhythmias, frank hypotension, evidence of multiple organ failure, and pale, cold, and clammy skin. Cardiopulmonary collapse is usually imminent in these patients.

> **NOTE:**
> During the prehospital management of shock, it is impossible to distinguish between uncompensated and irreversible shock. Prehospital management of the shock victim should always be directed at resuscitation, especially since irreversible shock is more a function of time than degree. Rapid resuscitation and transportation to an appropriate medical facility may abort the irreversible stage of shock in many situations.

Variations in Physiological Response to Shock

Many variations in physiological response occur among patients in shock. Determining factors include the following:

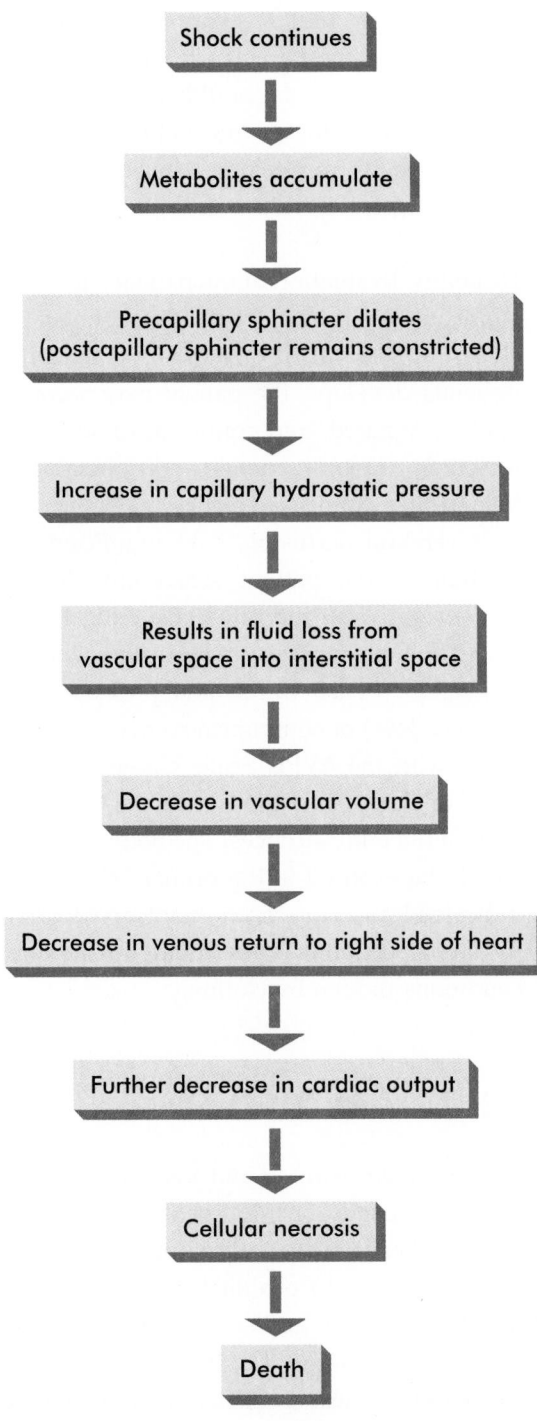

Fig. 13-19 Irreversible shock. Regardless of fluid replacement and an initial favorable response in blood pressure, death will ensue within 1 day to 3 weeks.

- Age and relative health
  - General physical condition
  - Preexisting disease
- Ability to activate compensatory mechanisms
  - Older adults (less able to compensate)
  - Children (compensate longer and deteriorate faster)
  - Medications (some may interfere with compensatory mechanisms)
- Specific organ system affected

Section Three
Evaluation and Resuscitation of the Shock Patient

Evaluation of the patient in shock must be directed at assessing oxygenation and perfusion of the various body organs. The goals of prehospital management of shock are to ensure a patent airway, to provide adequate oxygenation and ventilation, and to restore perfusion.

● PRIMARY SURVEY

Each step of the primary survey can help identify the adequacy of cellular perfusion. The following five-step description of the primary survey focuses on evaluating the shock victim, but the paramedic should be aware of common objectives in evaluating any patient with other types of serious illness or injury (see Chapter 11):

1. Airway. The airway must be opened and patency maintained to ensure adequate air movement.
2. Breathing. The respiratory pattern often reflects the adequacy of ventilation and may offer clues to the presence of shock. If the patient is acidotic, for example, the rate and depth of ventilation increase in an attempt to reduce carbon dioxide content of the blood and compensate for the metabolic acidosis.
3. Circulation. Evaluation of the patient's circulatory status should begin by assessing the patient for any uncontrolled arterial bleeding. In cases of external hemorrhage, control can almost always be obtained by applying direct pressure. This usually suffices until the patient can be transported to the emergency department for definitive care. Pressure

dressings (bandages, pneumatic antishock garments [PASG]) may be applied to control hemorrhage. If internal bleeding is suspected, rapid transportation to an appropriate medical facility is the highest priority after securing an airway and ensuring adequate ventilation. Internal bleeding is suspected in any trauma patient with signs of shock who has evidence of external blood loss. It may become even more obvious on observation or palpation of the abdomen or pelvis. Treatment for internal hemorrhage includes fluid replacement, PASG (per protocol), and rapid transportation to an appropriate medical facility. However, transportation should not be delayed to begin intravenous or PASG therapy.

As part of the circulatory assessment, the rate, character, and location of the patient's pulse should be evaluated. Pulse rates increase fairly early in shock to help maintain an adequate output. The strength of contraction may also increase, but this is often negated by the decrease in preload. This response normally occurs when the patient has suffered a 10% to 15% volume depletion (relative to container size) as a result of blood loss or an increase in container size. The character of the pulse may be strong or weak, which permits estimation of the effectiveness of the filling volume of the artery being palpated and an indirect measurement of systolic pressure. The location of the palpable pulse can also be used as an indirect measure of systolic pressure.

Tissue perfusion can sometimes be extimated by evaluating the skin's color, moisture, and temperature. These guidelines may be unreliable in patients exposed to extremes of temperature and in those suffering from septicemia and shock caused by neurological injury. Evaluation of the fingers and toes is important, since these areas may be the first to indicate inadequate tissue perfusion. The fingers and toes are the most distal points of circulation. If ambient temperatures are moderate and tissue perfusion is adequate, these areas will be pink, warm, and dry.

The capillary refill test may offer useful information on the patient's tissue perfusion. (These measurements should be used only as a guide because the accuracy of this test may be affected by the patient's general health, age, and gender and by environmental extremes.)

4. Disability. Evaluation of the patient's level of consciousness is an important component in assessing cerebral oxygenation. As cerebral ischemia develops, the patient may become restless, agitated, and confused. In addition to shock, cerebral edema and intracranial hemorrhage from head injury may compromise cerebral perfusion. Any significant alteration in the patient sensorium should be considered an indicator of a critical perfusion deficit, whether it be from shock or from an increase in intracranial pressure. The patient's level of consciousness may be measured with the AVPU Scale, Glasgow coma scale, or other evaluation methods.

5. Expose the body surfaces. The body surfaces should be exposed in the primary survey as indicated by scenario or mechanism of injury. Visual inspection may reveal life-threatening conditions hidden by clothing.

● SECONDARY SURVEY

After the primary survey and treatment of any life-threatening conditions, the patient should be evaluated further. A systematic secondary survey provides the means to evaluate potentially life-threatening conditions and to further assess the patient's perfusion status. This survey should begin with baseline measurements of the patient's vital signs and evaluation of the patient's electrocardiogram.

The paramedic should expect the pulse rate to increase above normal limits after a fluid deficit of 10% to 15%. Some patients, however, continue to have normal pulse rates even though a volume deficit of this magnitude exists. Therefore the patient's pulse rate should only be considered one factor in evaluating the patient's level of perfusion.

Bradycardia, which may result from hypoxemia, concomitant neurological injury, increased vagal tone, preexisting illness, or prior medication use, can also indicate severe myocardial ischemia (a primary cause of cardiogenic shock). Bradycardic rhythms frequently occur just before cardiac arrest. Immediately after a bradycardic rhythm is noted, oxygenation should be improved by assisting ventilations and increasing Fio_2.

As peripheral vascular resistance increases with increased vascular tone, the diastolic pressure initially rises. This decreases the container size and selectively shunts blood away from certain portions of the body. When the heart can no longer pump blood to keep the container full on the arterial side, the diastolic pressure begins to drop. This should be expected when the deficit in fluid-to-container-size ratio is greater than 15% to 20%.

When the heart can no longer pump enough blood to fill the container at the end of cardiac contraction, the systolic pressure falls. Systolic pressure is usually more sensitive to volume depletion than is diastolic pressure and therefore drops first. As the fluid deficit approaches 25%, however, systolic and diastolic pressure both begin to drop.

The evaluation of orthostatic vital signs should be considered in conscious patients suspected of being volume depleted, provided that spinal injury or another condition precluding this assessment is not suspected. A sudden rise from a recumbent position to a sitting or standing position associated with a fall in systolic pressure of 10 to 15 mm Hg and a concurrent rise in pulse rate of 10 to 15 beats per minute indicates a significant volume depletion (postural hypotension).

Even after the systolic pressure returns to normal after fluid replacement, a fluid deficit may still exist. Therefore fluid replacement initiated in the prehospital setting should continue until indicators of adequate tissue perfusion are present (for example, capillary refill less than 2 seconds, normal pulse oximetry readings).

● RESUSCITATION

Resuscitation of the shock victim is aimed at restoring adequate peripheral tissue oxygenation as quickly as possible. As previously stated, this is accomplished by ensuring adequate oxygenation, maintaining an effective ratio of volume to container size, and rapidly transporting the victim to an appropriate medical facility.

Red Blood Cell Oxygenation

Adequate oxygenation of red blood cells is the first requirement for adequate tissue oxygenation, as described by the Fick principle. For red blood cell oxygenation to be adequate, the patient must have a patent airway, and ventilation must be supported with a high Fio_2. If necessary, ventilation should be assisted with positive pressure. In addition, any abnormality that interferes with adequate ventilation (for example, obstructed airway, pneumothorax, hemothorax, open chest wound, unstable chest wall) should be corrected (see Chapter 15).

Ratio of Volume to Container Size

The second component of the Fick principle (adequate oxygen-carrying capacity) requires that the container be full of fluid. This may be accomplished by decreasing the size of the container through the use of a PSAG, through fluid replacement, or both. In addition, vasoactive medications may be used to manage some types of patient shock when reduction of container size is the primary concern.

NOTE:
The benefits of PASG have been questioned by the scientific community. To date, the outcome regarding long-term survival is not clear. Research is underway to better understand the efficacy of PASG use in patients who are victims of blunt trauma or pelvic fracture and in those who have prolonged transport times. The paramedic should follow the recommendations of medical direction regarding use of this device.

Pneumatic Antishock Garment

The PASG (Fig. 13-20) is thought by some to be effective in managing shock through the following mechanisms:

- Increased tissue pressure. As external force is applied to soft tissues, systemic vascular resistance increases. With this increase in tissue pressure, there is a potential for a net volume flow into the vascular space.
- Reduced vessel capacity. Reduced volume capacity in the lower body permits increased volume capacity to be circulated in the upper body, with an increase in central circulation. The PASG reduces vessel diameter and artificially increases peripheral resistance in the tissues beneath the PASG, which maintains perfusion pressure to the patient's other vital organs.
- Arrest of hemorrhage. The PASG may act to tamponade any bleeding vessels in the abdomen, pelvis, or lower extremities.
- Stabilization of pelvic and lower-extremity fractures. The PASG may help stabilize fractures when inflated, thus decreasing movement and subsequent blood loss.

Although decisions on the use of the PASG are left to local protocol, pulmonary edema, cardiogenic shock, and hemorrhage within the chest are generally considered contraindications for PASG.[2,6] Some medical control authorities feel that use of PASG is also contraindicated in the following situations:

- Impaled objects in the abdomen (precluding inflation of the abdominal section of the garment)
- Pregnancy (third trimester pregnancy precludes inflation of the abdominal compartment)
- Evisceration

Garment Application

PASG garments are made by a number of manufacturers and are available in adult and pediatric sizes. At present, there are three basic types, all of which have similar functions. One garment uses three gauges that measure the pressure in each of the three chambers (right leg, left leg, and abdomen). The second is a single-gauge garment that monitors the inflation pressures of each chamber separately or as a unit when all three chambers are inflated to the same pressure. The third type is designed to be used without gauges and contains "pop-off" valves that prevent overinflation (pressures above 104 mm Hg).

A number of methods may be used in applying the PASG. Regardless of the method chosen, two rescuers are required, and spinal precautions should be taken when indicated by the patient's condition or mechanism of injury.

Trouser Method

1. The PASG is assembled with Velcro straps loosely attached.
2. The first rescuer puts the hands and arms into the PASG from the lower leg openings, up through the abdominal opening, and grasps the patient's feet or ankles (Fig. 13-21, *A*).
3. The second rescuer pulls the PASG up onto the patient as if pulling on trousers (Fig. 13-21, *B*).
4. The Velcro straps are securely fastened.

NOTE:
This method should not be used if spinal injury is suspected.

Log-Roll Method

1. Position the unfolded PASG on a full backboard, patient side up (Fig. 13-22, *A*).
2. Log-roll the patient onto the backboard (Fig. 13-22, *B*).

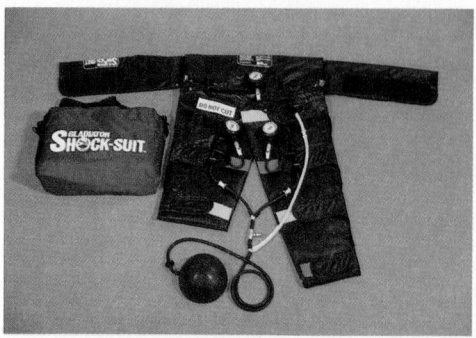

Fig. 13-20 JOBST Gladiator Shock Suit.

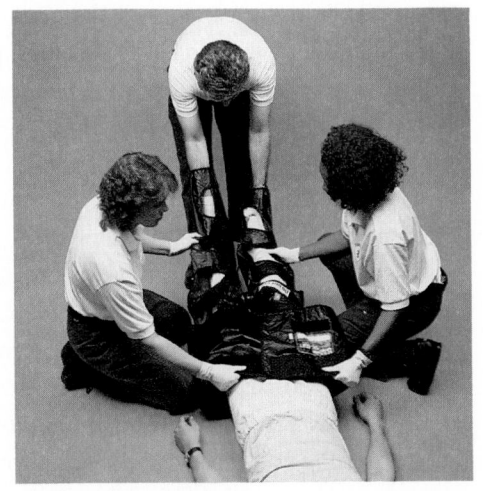 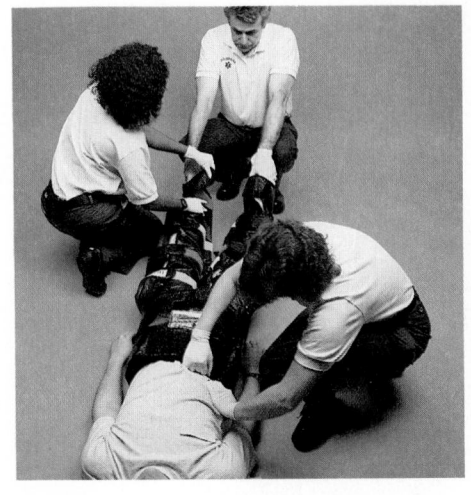

Fig. 13-21 A, The first rescuer puts hands and arms through the PASG from the lower leg openings, up through the abdominal opening, and grasps the patient's feet or ankles. **B,** The second rescuer pulls PASG up onto the patient as if pulling on trousers.

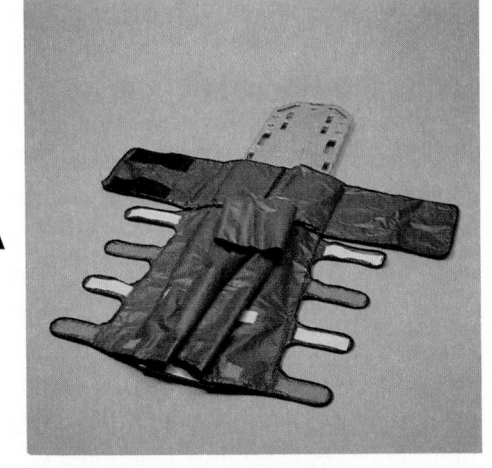

Fig. 13-22 A, The PASG is positioned unfolded on a long backboard, patient side up. **B,** The patient is log-rolled onto the backboard. **C,** After PASG positioning, the Velcro straps are securely fastened.

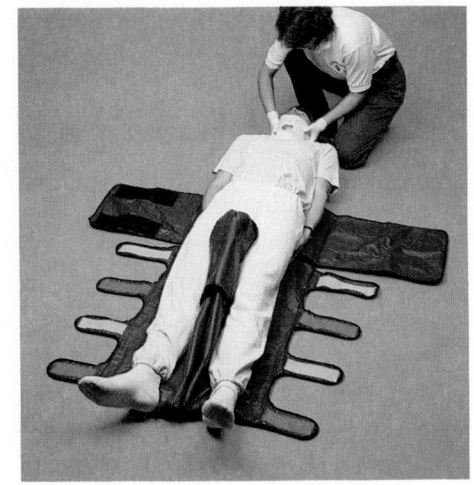 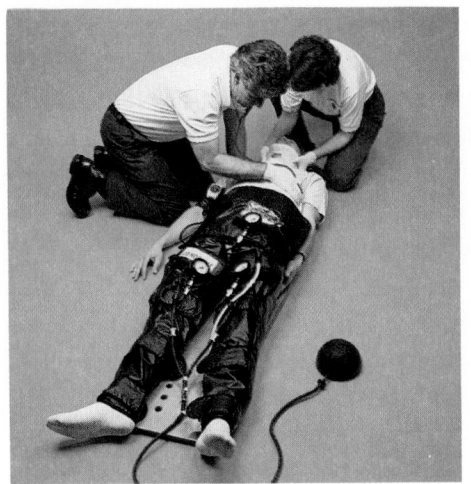

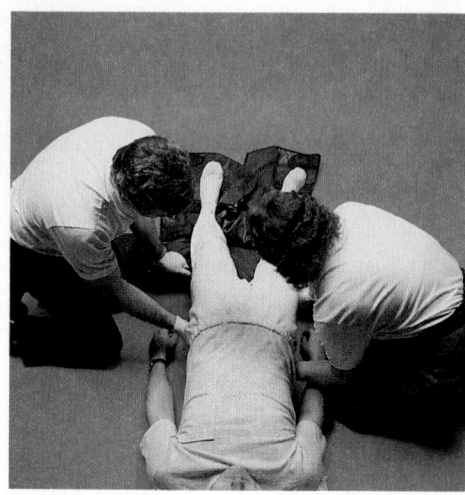

Fig. 13-23 PASG application by the diaper method.

3. Wrap the chambers around the appropriate body part, and secure the Velcro straps (Fig. 13-22, *C*).

Diaper Method
1. Lay the PASG flat, patient side up.
2. Roll the inner edges and the anterior abdominal section toward the center of the garment.
3. Two rescuers slide the PASG under the patient, with the rolled sections between the patient's legs (Fig. 13-23).
4. After PASG positioning, unroll the sections and secure the Velcro straps.

Garment Inflation with Pop-Off Valves
The left extremity, abdominal area, and right extremity compartments of the garment are secured with Velcro fasteners. The valves are opened, and all compartments are simultaneously inflated with the foot pump until the systolic blood pressure level reaches 100 mm Hg or the Velcro begins to crackle. An alternative method of inflation is a two-stage process whereby the leg compartments are inflated before the abdomen.

Garment Inflation Using Gauges
Each gauge is attached by a color-coded hose to each individual compartment of the PASG. The garment is inflated as previously described until the patient improves or until the gauges reveal a pressure of 60 to 80 mm Hg in each compartment.[7] Improvement of the patient is a better indicator of the effectiveness of the PASG than the gauge pressure in each compartment.

General PASG Guidelines
The PASG should be applied when indicated after the lower extremities and abdomen have been inspected for major wounds. The garment must always be positioned below the level of the patient's lowest rib, and the patient's blood pressure and lung sounds should be monitored before, during, and after inflation. Inflation should be stopped when an adequate blood pressure has been obtained. The leg compartments must be inflated before or with the abdominal compartment. *The abdominal compartment should never be inflated before the leg compartments.* Doing so may cause the abdominal compartment to act as a constrictive band that reduces venous return from the legs.

After PASG inflation, the garment should seldom if ever be deflated in the prehospital setting and only with a physician's direction. The abdominal compartment is deflated before the leg compartments. The patient should be closely monitored during the deflation process because removal of the garment before fluid replacement commonly results in a rapid fall of blood pressure and cardiac output and possibly cardiac arrest.

Changes in environmental temperature and atmospheric pressure may cause a significant fluctuation in the pressure within the PASG. The patient should be constantly monitored when moved from a cold environment to a warm one or when transported by air. The relationship among temperature, atmospheric pressure, and pressure within the PASG is as follows:
- A rise in temperature raises the pressure within the PASG, and a fall in temperature decreases the pressure.
- A fall in atmospheric pressure causes an increase in PASG pressure, and a rise in atmospheric pressure produces a decrease in garment pressure.

The PASG is not without complications even with appropriate use. Continued inflation of the garment for more than 1 to 2 hours can lead to decreased tissue perfusion, ischemia of the underlying tissues (including the development of compartment syndrome[8]), and loss of the limb, even without underlying fracture.

Fluid Resuscitation in Shock

Almost every shock victim (with the exception of patients in cardiogenic shock) requires volume expanders as part of resuscitation. The selection of intravenous fluids for initial volume replacement varies according to medical control. In prehospital care, the most common emergency requiring fluid replacement is volume depletion secondary to hemorrhage or dehydration. The type of fluid replacement needed depends on the nature and extent of the volume loss (Box 13-5). The two main categories of fluids used in resuscitation are crystalloids and colloids.

Crystalloids

Crystalloid solutions are created by dissolving crystals such as salts and sugars in water. These solutions do not have as much osmotic pressure as colloid solutions and can be expected to equilibrate more quickly between the vascular and extravascular spaces. (Two thirds of the infused crystalloid fluid leaves the vascular space within 1 hour, so 3 ml of a crystalloid solution is needed to replace 1 ml of blood.) Examples of crystalloid solutions are lactated Ringer's solution, normal saline, and glucose solutions in water.

Hypertonic solutions have higher osmotic pressure than that of body cells and include 5% dextrose in 0.9% sodium chloride and 5% dextrose in 0.45% sodium chloride. Hypotonic solutions have a lower osmotic pressure than that of body cells (for example, distilled water and 0.45% sodium chloride [0.45% NaCl]).

Lactated Ringer's solution is generally considered the fluid of choice for resuscitating patients in shock. It is a well-balanced solution containing many of the chemicals found in human blood. Lactated Ringer's solution contains sodium chloride, small amounts of potassium and calcium, and 28 mEq of lactate, which may act as a buffer

---

BOX 13-5

Fluid Resuscitation in Shock

Crystalloids
- Hypertonic sodium chloride
- Hypotonic sodium chloride
- Balanced salt solutions (isotonic)
  - Lactated Ringer's solution
  - Normal saline
- Glucose-containing solutions
  - D_5W

Colloids
- Blood
  - Typed and crossmatched
  - Type-specific
  - Packed red blood cells
- Plasma
- Plasma substitutes
  - Dextran
  - Hetastarch (Hespan)
  - Plasma protein fraction (Plasmanate)

---

when metabolized by the liver. (Ringer's solution is also available without added lactate, which may be preferred by some physicians.) One third of the infused solution remains in the vascular space after 1 hour.

Normal saline contains 154 mEq/L of sodium and has no buffering capabilities. Although preferred by some physicians, the higher chloride content of normal saline is generally considered less desirable than the more balanced lactated Ringer's solution. As in lactated Ringer's, nearly one third of the infused normal saline remains in the vascular space after 1 hour, making it an equally effective volume expander.

Glucose-containing solutions have immediate volume expansion effects, but the glucose leaves the intravascular compartment rapidly with a resultant free water increase. The volume-replacement benefits of glucose solutions may only last 5 to 10 minutes while the glucose is metabolized, so its use as a replacement fluid in vol-

Blood Types

In the early 1900s, it was found that there were individual differences in human blood. When a donor's blood was separated into plasma and red blood cell components and mixed with separated blood samples from another donor, two reactions were noted: When combined with foreign plasma, the red cells either clumped together (agglutinated) or did not. It was also discovered that two distinct agglutinins (substances on the red blood cells acting as antigens) were responsible for the clumping. Based on possible combinations of these antigens, four types of human blood were identified: A, B, AB, and O (Fig. 13-24).

Type A blood has anti-B antibodies in the plasma and would therefore clump Type B blood. Type B blood has anti-A antibodies and would clump Type A blood. Type AB blood has neither antibody and can therefore receive any of the four types of blood (universal recipient). Type O blood has both anti-A and anti-B antibodies, so it cannot receive any type of blood other than Type O. Type O blood has neither antigen, however, and can therefore be given to patients with any blood type. Type O blood has become known as the *universal donor*.

Rh Factor

In the late 1940s, another determinant in human blood was discovered: the Rh factor. (*Rh* was taken from the word *rhesus,* the monkey species used for the research.) It was found that when the blood of a rhesus monkey was injected into a rabbit, the rabbit's immune system developed antibodies; when a sample of the rabbit's plasma was mixed with a sample of human red blood cells, the human cells usually clumped (Rh positive). Approximately 85% percent of Americans have Rh-positive blood. The percentages in the population of ABO and Rh blood groups (based on population averages of American Red Cross blood service regions) are as follows[9]:

O positive 38.4%	B positive 9.4%
O negative 7.7%	B negative 1.7%
A positive 32.3%	AB positive 3.2%
A negative 6.5%	AB negative 0.7%

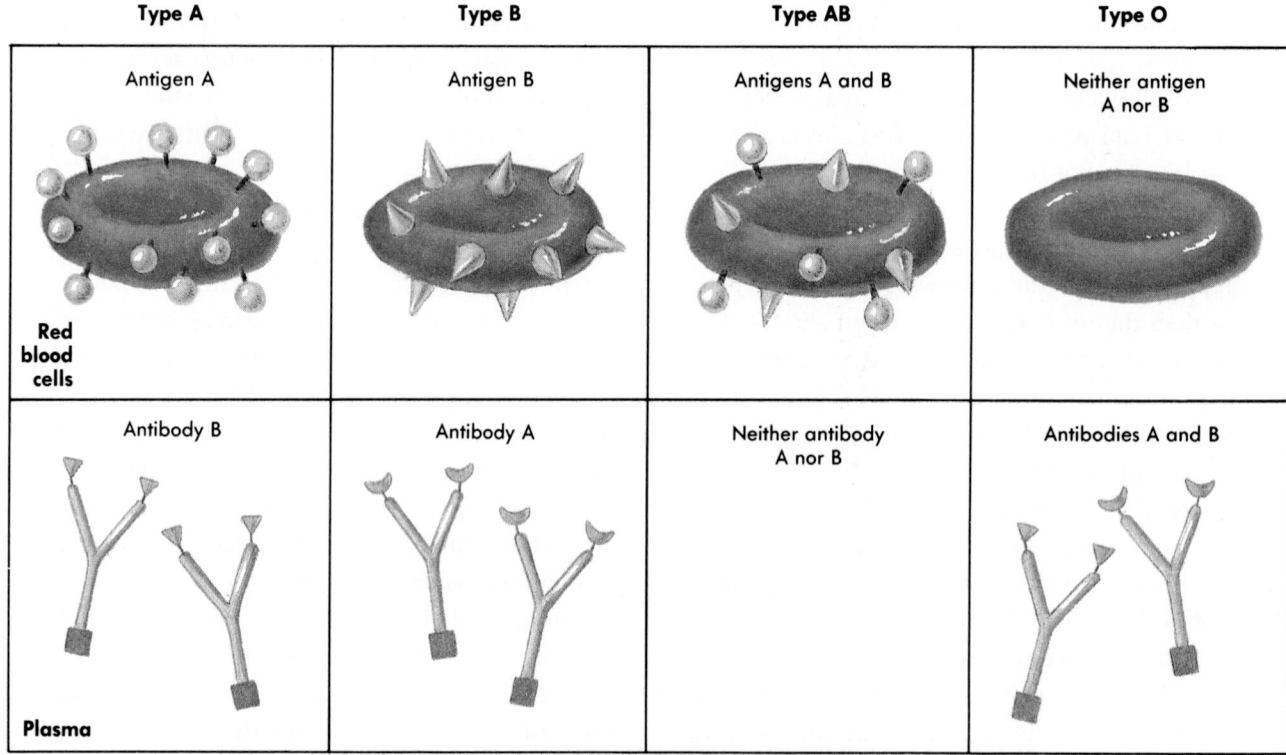

Type A	**Type B**	**Type AB**	**Type O**
Antigen A	Antigen B	Antigens A and B	Neither antigen A nor B
Antibody B	Antibody A	Neither antibody A nor B	Antibodies A and B

Red blood cells

Plasma

Fig. 13-24 ABO blood groups. Type A blood has red blood cells with type A surface antigens and plasma with type B antibodies. Type B blood has type B surface antigens and plasma with type A antibodies. Type AB blood has types A and B surface antigens and no plasma antibodies. Type O blood has no ABO surface antigens but A and B plasma antibodies.

ume deficits is inappropriate. Glucose solutions are most often used to maintain vascular access for administration of intravenous medications.

Colloids

Colloid solutions are those that contain molecules (usually protein) that are too large to pass through the capillary membrane. These solutions exhibit osmotic pressure and remain within the vascular compartment for a considerable time. Examples of colloid solutions are whole blood, plasma, packed red blood cells, and plasma substitutes. Whole blood, packed red cells, and plasma are generally reserved for in-hospital use.

Whole blood replacement is sometimes indicated after initial fluid resuscitation with a crystalloid solution in patients who have had a major loss of blood. Whole blood is drawn in a citrate solution to prevent clotting and is refrigerated until needed. According to blood bank regulations, the blood may be stored up to 3 weeks, but clotting factors and platelets deplete progressively. A type and crossmatch should be obtained (when possible) before a patient is given blood to determine the patient's ABO group and Rh type. The patient's blood must also be tested for red cell antibodies.

Packed red blood cells have been separated from the plasma component of blood by centrifugation. Like whole blood, packed red cells must be typed and crossmatched and may be refrigerated for up to 3 weeks. The advantage of packed red blood cells over whole blood is that the volume of hemoglobin per unit is almost twice that of whole blood. In addition, because there is no plasma, circulatory overload is less likely, transfusion reactions are less frequent, and transfusion hepatitis is less common.

Blood plasma is procured by separating the blood cells from the whole citrated blood. Blood plasma, which may be given without concern for ABO compatibility, contains fibrinogen, albumin, gamma globulins, hemoagglutinins (an agglutinin that clumps red blood corpuscles), prothrombin (a chemical that is part of the clotting cascade, the precursor of thrombin), other clotting factors, sugar, and salts. Blood plasma is sometimes used to restore effective blood volume in circulatory failure associated with burns, traumatic shock,

and hemorrhage. It is also used to correct clotting deficiencies.

Although plasma substitutes do not replace red blood cells or plasma protein, they are used to restore circulating blood volume as an emergency treatment for hypovolemia caused by blood loss. Plasma substitutes such as dextran, plasma protein fraction, and hetastarch have osmotic properties similar to those of plasma. Plasma substitutes do not carry the human immunodeficiency virus (HIV) or hepatitis viruses, do not require type and crossmatching before administration, and are readily available. Accordingly, their use is appealing, particularly in mass casualty situations when blood products are scarce. They do have adverse effects, however, most notably increasing bleeding tendencies and immune suppression. Plasma substitutes may be carried on emergency vehicles, but expense and storage problems make them impractical for general use in the prehospital setting.

> **NOTE:**
> Several types of blood transfusion reactions may occur during or up to 96 hours after infusion. Symptoms may range from mild fever to life-threatening shock. If a reaction is suspected, the transfusion should be stopped, and medical direction should be contacted.

Key Principles in Managing Shock

1. Establish and maintain an open airway.
2. Administer high-concentration oxygen, and assist ventilation as needed.
3. Control external bleeding (if present).
4. By order of medical control or per protocol, initiate intravenous fluid replacement if appropriate. It is usually recommended that two large-bore intravnous lines of a volume-expanding fluid be established in cases of hypovolemia. *The administration of intravenous fluids in the prehospital setting should not delay patient transport,* since crystalloid solutions cannot restore the oxygen-carrying capacity of blood. Generally, the patient is best served

by rapid assessment, airway stabilization, immobilization, and rapid transportation to an appropriate medical facility. Many EMS authorities recommend that intravenous therapy for shock resuscitation be initiated en route to the hospital.

5. Consider use of PASG (per protocol), especially if transport time is long or a patient is deteriorating after intravenous therapy has been initiated.
6. Maintain the patient's normal body temperature. Patients in shock are often unable to conserve body heat and easily become hypothermic.
7. In the absence of spinal or head injury, position the patient in the modified Trendelenburg position (legs elevated 15 to 18 inches).
8. Monitor cardiac rhythm.
9. Frequently assess vital signs en route to the emergency department.

Management of Specific Forms of Shock

In addition to the general management appropriate to all victims of shock, there are certain management guidelines specific to each etiological classification.

Hypovolemic Shock

The treatment of hypovolemic shock is not considered complete until the circulatory deficit and its cause or causes are corrected. This may include crystalloid fluid replacement in cases of simple dehydration or volume replacement resulting from hemorrhage, definitive surgery, critical care support, and postoperative rehabilitation.

Cardiogenic Shock

The treatment of cardiogenic shock is directed toward improving the pumping action of the heart and managing cardiac rhythm irregularities. Fluid resuscitation in the adult should be initiated with a fluid challenge of 100 to 200 ml of a volume-expanding fluid. If the patient improves, fluid therapy should continue until the blood pressure stabilizes and the pulse decreases. Lung sounds should be assessed frequently. If the patient shows signs of increased lung congestion, the rate of infusion should be adjusted to keep the vein open.

Drug therapy for cardiogenic shock varies according to cause and may include vasopressors, inotropic drugs, and antidysrhythmics (see Chapters 14 and 18).

Neurogenic Shock

The treatment of neurogenic shock is similar to the treatment for hypovolemia. However, care must be taken during fluid therapy to avoid circulatory overload. Throughout the resuscitation phase, the patient's lung sounds should be closely monitored for signs of pulmonary congestion. In addition, patients in neurogenic shock may respond to the administration of vasopressors.

Anaphylactic Shock

Subcutaneous administration of epinephrine is the treatment of choice in acute anaphylactic reactions. Depending on the severity of reaction, other treatment modalities may include oral, intravenous, or intramuscular administration of antihistamines. Bronchodilators may also be indicated to treat bronchospasm, and steroids may be given to reduce the inflammatory response.

Crystalloid volume replacement is also indicated to compensate for the increased container size caused by vasodilation that results from histamine release during an anaphylactic reaction. Paramedics should anticipate the need for aggressive airway management in any allergic reaction (see Chapter 22).

Septic Shock

The treatment of septic shock in the prehospital setting may include the management of hypovolemia (if present) and the correction of metabolic acid-base imbalance. Depending on the patient's response to the infection, prehospital care may involve fluid resuscitation, respiratory support, and the administration of cardiac medications to improve cardiac output. If possible, the paramedic should obtain a thorough patient history to help identify the septic focus. There is an increased risk of septic shock in any immunocompromised group such as those with HIV infection, some cancer patients receiving chemotherapy, and patients with indwelling urinary or vascular catheters.

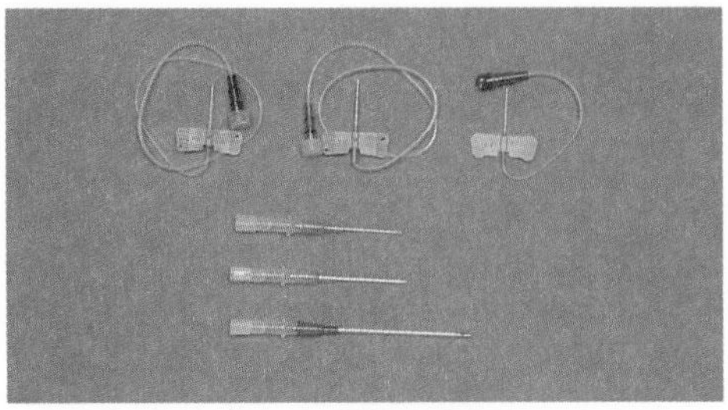

Fig. 13-25 Various types of IV catheters.

TABLE 13-4 Needle Gauges and Maximum Fluid Flow	
Needle Gauge (i.d.)	**Maximum Fluid Flow**
18 gauge	4.81 L/hr or 80 cc/min
16 gauge	7.45 L/hr or 124 cc/min
14 gauge	9.67 L/hr or 161 cc/min

Section Four
Techniques of Intravenous Therapy

Intravenous cannulation is used to gain access to the body's circulation. Intravenous cannulation is indicated (1) to administer fluids, (2) to obtain specimens for laboratory determinations, and (3) to administer drug therapy.

● ROUTE OF ADMINISTRATION

The route of choice for fluid replacement in the prehospital setting is through a peripheral vein in an extremity. Provided that the arms have no major injury, upper extremity veins should be used. (Some EMS services advise avoiding upper extremity sites when a major injury to the neck or upper thorax has occurred on that side.) When upper extremity sites are inappropriate, lower extremity sites may be used.

● CHOICE OF INTRAVENOUS CATHETERS

There are three main types of intravenous catheters: (1) hollow needles ("butterfly" type), (2) indwelling plastic catheters *over* a hollow needle (for example, Medicut), and (3) indwelling plastic catheters inserted *through* a hollow needle (for example, Intracath; seldom used in the prehospital setting) (Fig. 13-25).

Hollow needles are not recommended for intravenous fluid replacement in the prehospital setting because of the difficulty in stabilizing the needle. Occasionally, the paramedic chooses the "butterfly" type needle for the pediatric patient if adequate stabilization can be maintained through the use of armboards or other immobilization devices.

The over-the-needle catheter is generally preferred for use in the prehospital setting. It is easily secured and more comfortable for the patient.

● THEORY OF FLUID FLOW

The flow of fluid through a catheter is directly related to its diameter (to the fourth power) and inversely related to its length. Therefore a catheter with a large diameter has a much greater flow than a catheter with a small diameter; short catheters provide somewhat higher flow rates than longer catheters of equal diameter. Other factors that affect the flow of fluid include the diameter and length of the tubing, the size of the vein, and the viscosity and temperature of the intravenous fluid. (Viscosity is affected by temperature; warm fluids generally flow better than cold ones.) Pressure bags are available that pressurize the intravenous system to 300 mm Hg to maximize the rate of fluid administration.

Table 13-4 lists the maximum rate of fluid flow for various gauges of 2-inch Medicut catheters without pressure on the bag at a height of 1 m above the patient.[10]

To maximize the speed at which volume can be administered, the paramedic should remember the following guidelines:
- Use short, large-diameter catheters.
- Use warm fluids of low viscosity (if possible).
- Keep the tubing short and pressurize the intravenous system.

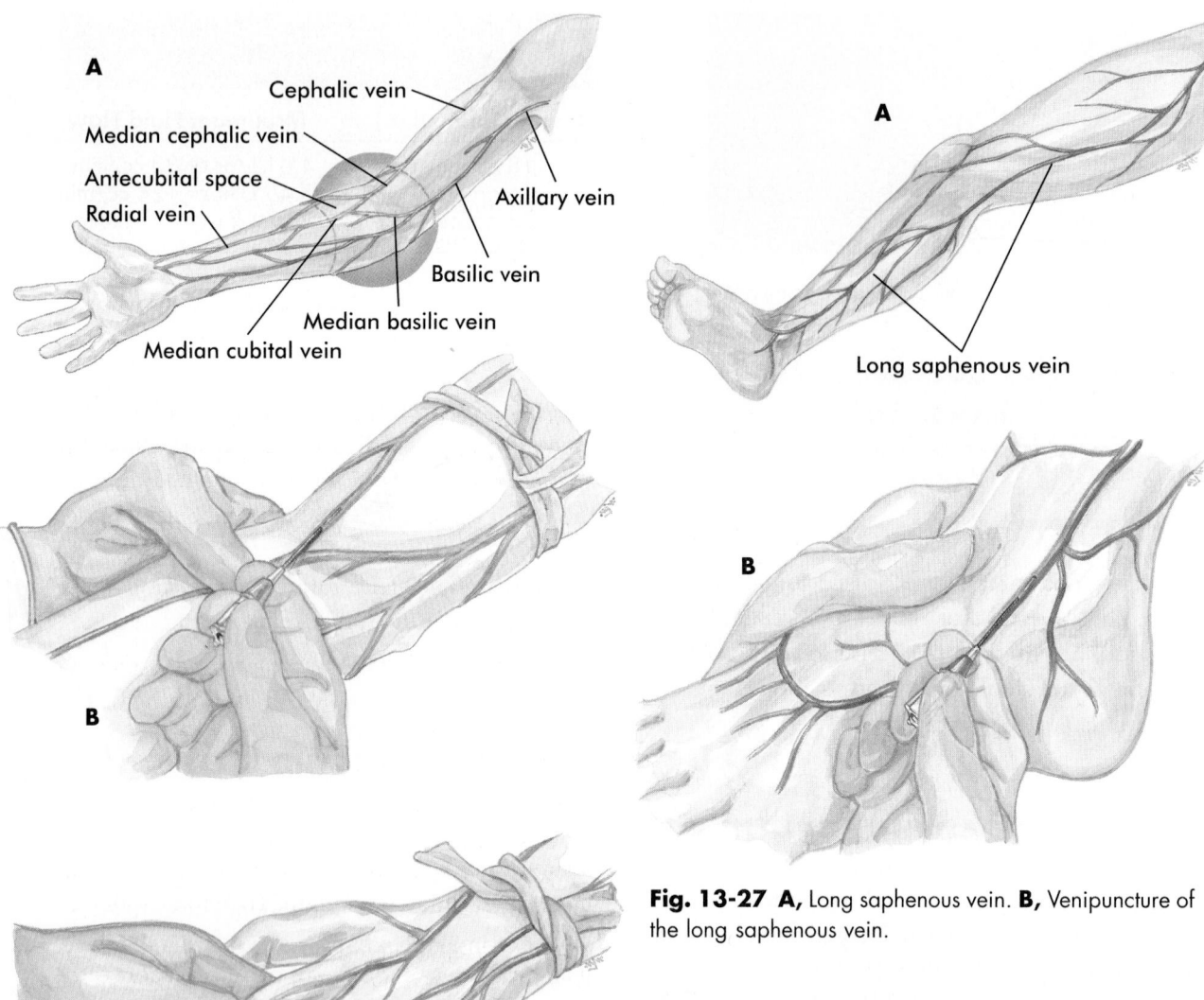

Fig. 13-26 A, Veins of the upper extremity. **B,** Antecubital venipuncture. **C,** Dorsal hand venipuncture.

Fig. 13-27 A, Long saphenous vein. **B,** Venipuncture of the long saphenous vein.

● PERIPHERAL INTRAVENOUS INSERTION

Because of the marked difference in fluid administration rates between small and large catheters, 14- or 16-gauge catheters are usually preferred for rapid fluid replacement. Common areas used for peripheral intravenous therapy are the hands and arms, including the antecubital fossae (AC space). Alternative sites include the long saphenous veins and the external jugular veins. However, the incidence of embolism and infection is higher at these alternative sites. Figs. 13-26 through 13-28 illustrate sites and techniques for peripheral cannulation.

Another consideration in choosing a puncture site for intravenous therapy is the clinical status of the patient. Injuries or diseases involving an extremity interfere with the use of veins in the affected area for venipuncture or venous cannulation. Examples include trauma, dialysis fistula, and a history of mastectomy.

Steps

1. If the patient is conscious, explain the procedure. This explanation should include why intravenous therapy is necessary and what the procedure entails.

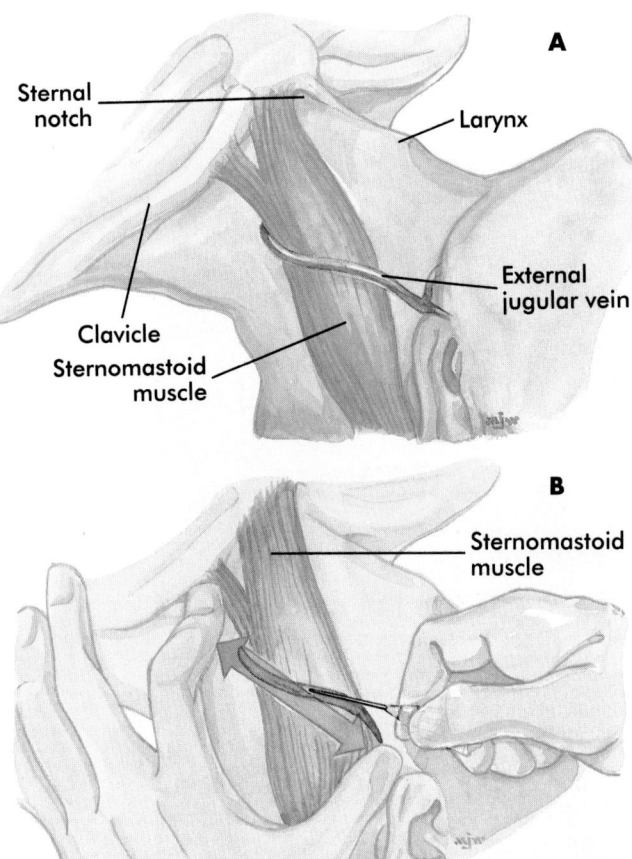

Sternal notch

Larynx

Clavicle

Sternomastoid muscle

External jugular vein

A

Sternomastoid muscle

B

Fig. 13-28 A, Anatomy of the external jugular vein. **B,** External jugular venipuncture.

2. Assemble the necessary equipment.
   a. Inspect the prescribed fluid for contamination, appearance, and expiration date. Never use fluids that are cloudy, outdated, or in any other way suspected of contamination.
   b. Prepare the microdrip or macrodrip infusion set, and attach the infusion set to the bag of solution. Infusion sets are commonly calibrated to deliver 10, 12, 15, 20, 50, or 60 drops/ml of fluid. (The drip factor for any particular infusion set can be found on the package in which it is supplied. Many hospitals and EMS services use only two sizes of infusion sets to minimize confusion (for example, a macrodrip that delivers 10 drops/ml and a microdrip that delivers 60 drops/ml). In addition, some EMS services use tubing extensions and blood tubing to avoid

changing the tubing after the patient arrives in the emergency department.)

3. Clamp the tubing and squeeze the reservoir on the infusion set until it fills half way. Then open the clamp, and flush the air from the tubing. Close the clamp.

4. Select the catheter. Large-bore tubing (14 to 16 gauge) should be used for fluid replacement, and smaller-bore tubing (18 to 20 gauge) should be used for "keep open" lines.

5. Prepare other equipment:
   a. Alcohol or iodine wipes to cleanse the skin
   b. Antibiotic ointment or cream
   c. Sterile dressings or 4 × 4 gauze pads
   d. Adhesive tape, torn or cut into several strips
   e. Syringes and vacutainers for blood samples
   f. Tourniquet (rubber tubing or blood pressure cuff may be used)

6. Apply gloves for personal and patient protection.

7. Select the puncture site. If using an upper extremity, allow the patient's arm to hang dependent, and apply the tourniquet above the acromioclavicular space. (The tourniquet should be just tight enough to tamponade venous vessels but not occlude arterial flow.) When selecting a suitable vein, begin by looking at the dorsum of the hand and forearm. Choose a vein that is fairly straight and easily accessible. The forearm is better than the hand because it allows hand movement and is more easily secured after cannulation. If a second puncture attempt is necessary, the second puncture should always be *proximal* to the first puncture. Therefore the vein selected for initial cannulation should be the most suitable *distal* vein. Avoid veins near joints, where immobilization will be difficult, and veins near injured areas. If the long saphenous vein is chosen, begin site selection near the medial malleolus of the foot. To locate the external jugular vein, place the patient in a supine head-down position, and turn the patient's head toward the opposite side.

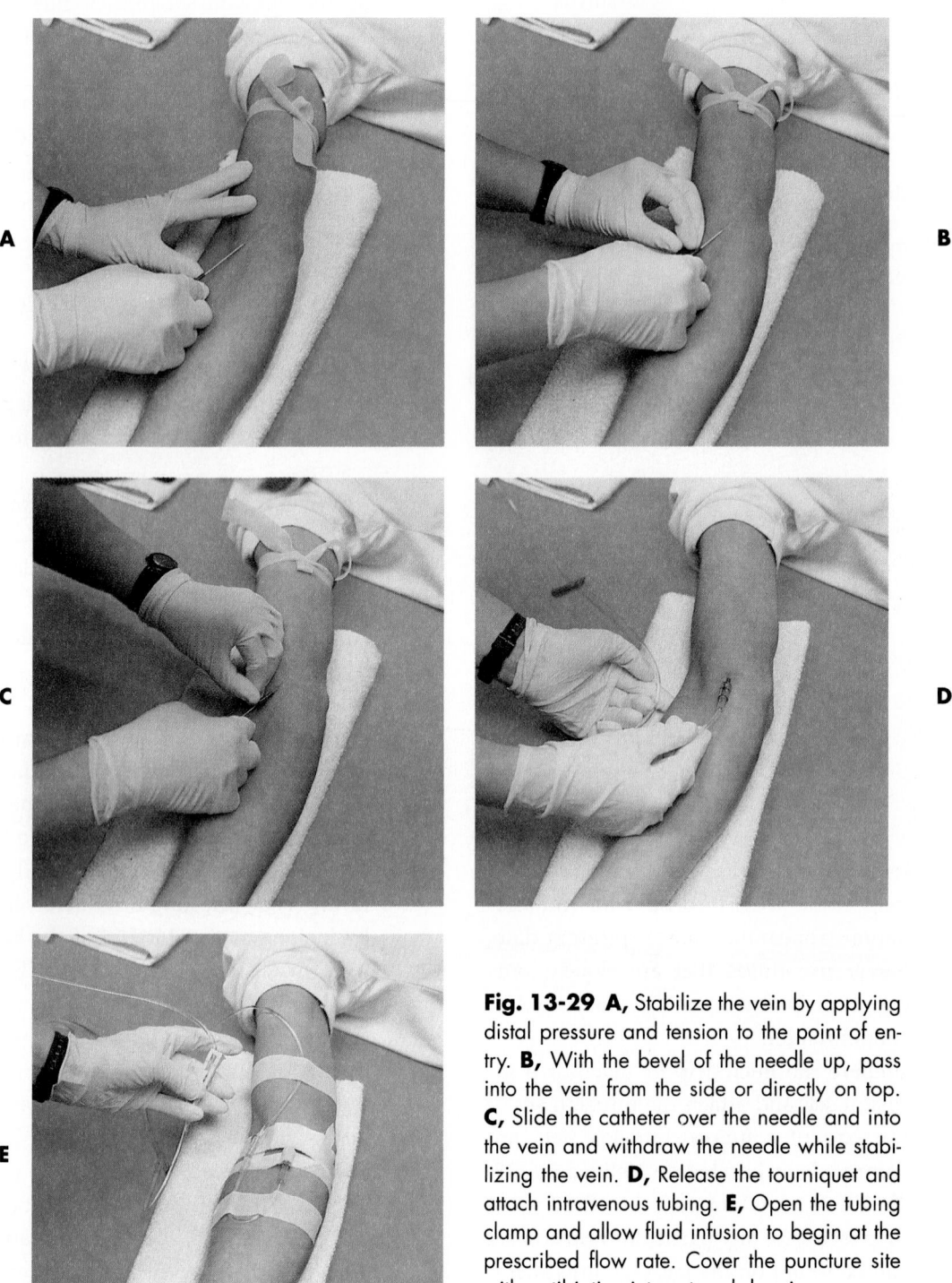

Fig. 13-29 A, Stabilize the vein by applying distal pressure and tension to the point of entry. **B,** With the bevel of the needle up, pass into the vein from the side or directly on top. **C,** Slide the catheter over the needle and into the vein and withdraw the needle while stabilizing the vein. **D,** Release the tourniquet and attach intravenous tubing. **E,** Open the tubing clamp and allow fluid infusion to begin at the prescribed flow rate. Cover the puncture site with antibiotic ointment and dressing.

8. Prepare the puncture site. Cleanse the area with alcohol or iodine wipes:
    a. Thoroughly clean the site with alcohol to remove dirt, dead skin, blood, and other surface contaminants.
    b. Disinfect the site with overlapping concentric circles, moving outward.
9. Stabilize the vein by applying distal pressure and tension to the point of entry (Fig. 13-29, *A*). With the bevel of the needle up, pass into the vein from the side or directly on top. Advance the needle and catheter approximately 2 mm beyond the point where blood return in the hub of the needle was first encountered. Slide the catheter over the needle and into the vein (Fig. 13-29, *B*). Withdraw the needle while stabilizing the catheter (Fig. 13-29, *C*). Apply pressure on the proximal end of the catheter to stop escaping blood. Obtain blood samples, if needed, with a syringe.
10. Release the tourniquet and attach tubing (Fig. 13-29, *D*). Open the tubing clamp, and allow fluid infusion to begin at the prescribed flow rate (Fig. 13-29, *E*).
11. Cover the puncture site with antibiotic ointment and dressing if time permits. Anchor the tubing, and secure the catheter. Catheter movement can increase the risk of phlebitis and cause migration of pathogens along the cannula into the vein.
12. Document the infusion procedure.

Advantages
- Rapid insertion
- Minimal equipment
- Fact that it can be accomplished during other patient activities
- Easy access

Disadvantages
- Difficulty in locating vessels in severe volume depletion
- Collapsed peripheral veins
- Instability (rolling veins)

● CENTRAL VENOUS CANNULATION

Central venous cannulation may be within the scope of paramedic practice in some advanced life-support systems. However, central venous infusion should never be considered as a means of rapid fluid replacement in the prehospital setting. Sites for central venous cannulation include the femoral vein, internal jugular vein, and subclavian vein. Figs. 13-30 through 13-32 illustrate sites and techniques for central venous cannualtion.

Steps

Preparation for cannulation of the central vessels is the same as for peripheral veins. The patient's body position and the paramedic's

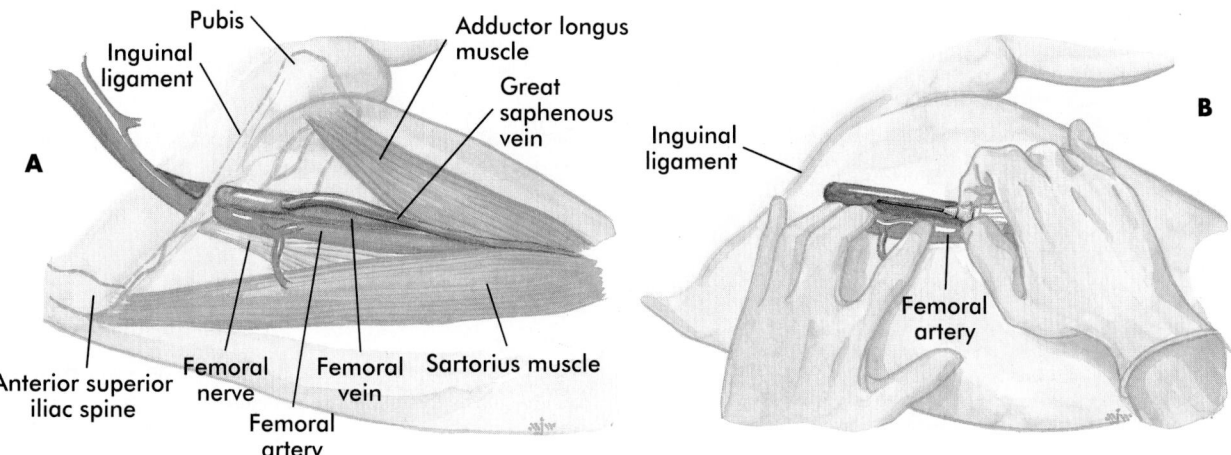

Fig. 13-30 A, Anatomy of the femoral vein. **B,** Femoral venipuncture.

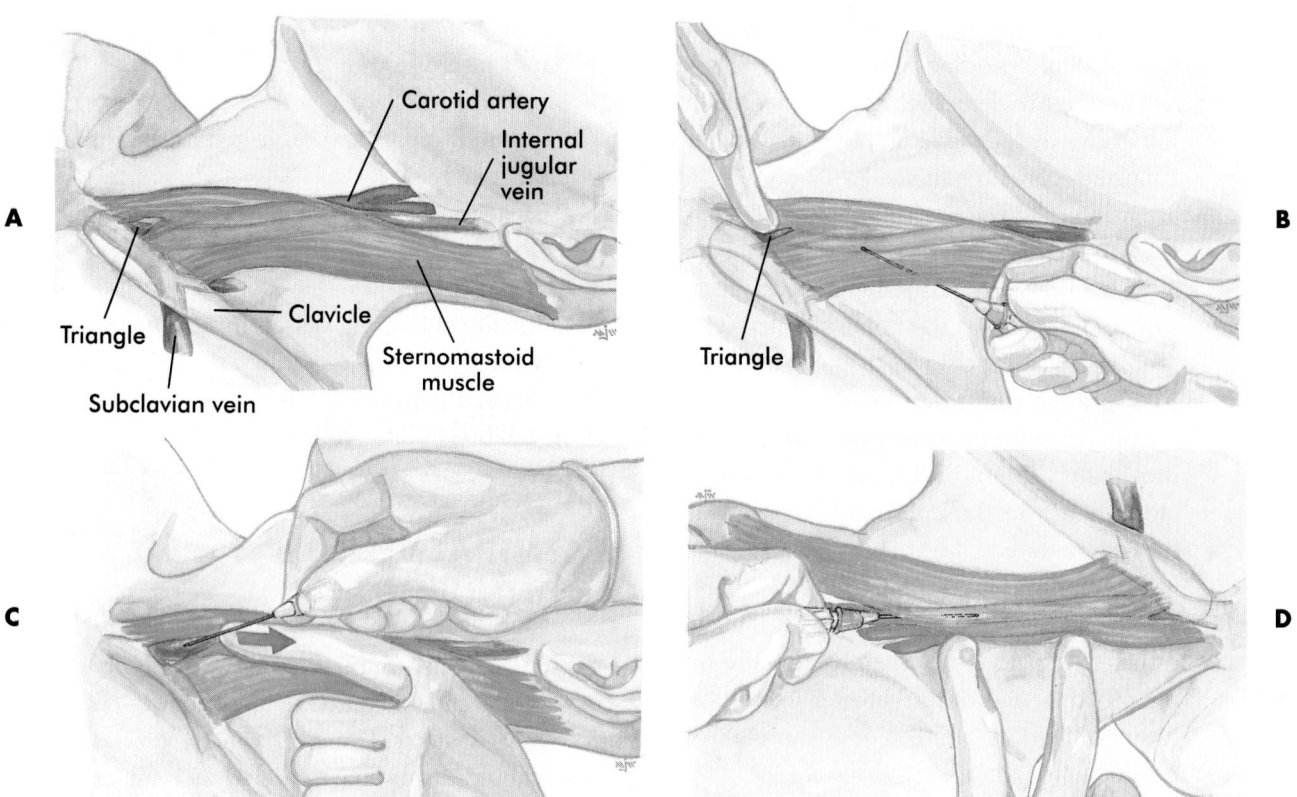

Fig. 13-31 A, Anatomy of the internal jugular vein. **B,** Posterior approach for internal jugular venipuncture. **C,** Central approach for internal jugular venipuncture. **D,** Anterior approach for internal jugular venipuncture.

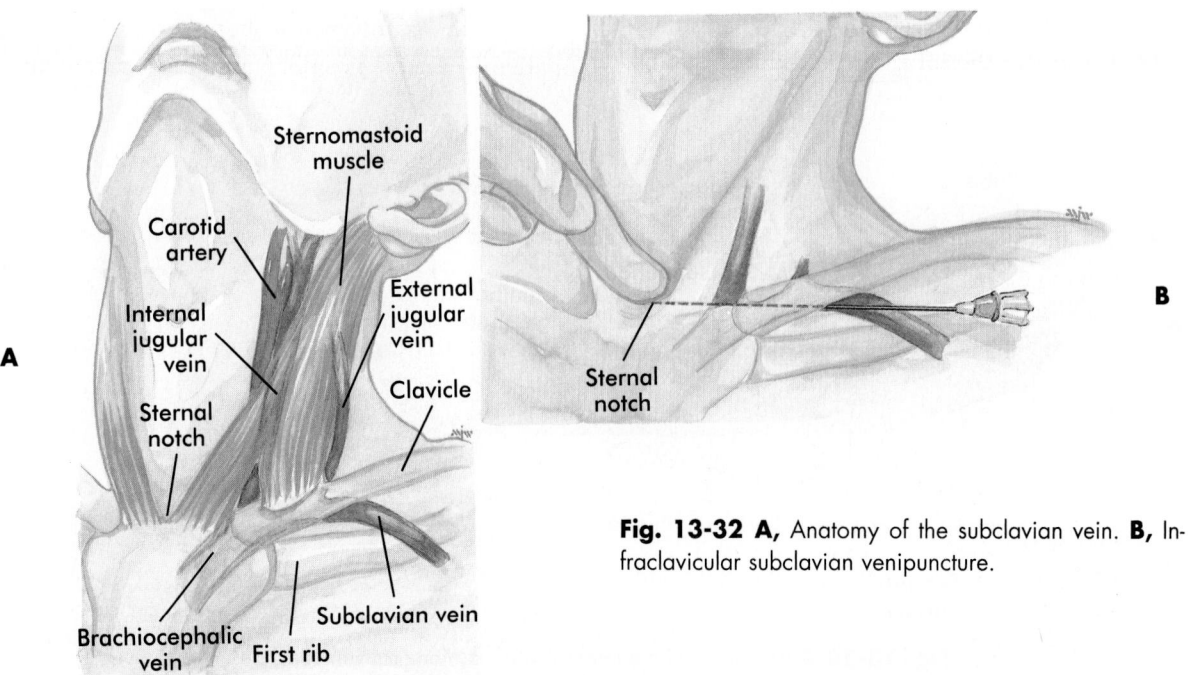

Fig. 13-32 A, Anatomy of the subclavian vein. **B,** Infraclavicular subclavian venipuncture.

knowledge of anatomy and familiarity with the procedure are important in determining the success of this procedure. Central vein cannulation requires special training and authorization from medical control.

Advantages

- Availability when peripheral vessels collapse
- Provision of access to central pressure measurements (in-hospital procedure)
- Safer vasopressor administration

Disadvantages

- Excessive time (5 to 10 minutes) for placement
- Sterile technique (gloves, drape, wipes)
- Special equipment (catheter, large needle, syringe)
- Skill deterioration, which is great (Much practice is required.)
- High complication rate (pneumothorax, arterial injury, abnormal placement)
- Chest x-ray film, which should be obtained immediately after placement to ensure correct position and evaluate for complications
- Inability to initiate procedure while other patient care activities are in progress
- Central placement that is not generally considered to be a useful prehospital technique
- Lower flow rates generally than with peripheral cannulation

● COMPLICATIONS OF ALL INTRAVENOUS TECHNIQUES

Local Complications

- Hematoma formation
- Cellulitis
- Thrombosis
- Phlebitis

Systemic Complications

- Sepsis
- Pulmonary thromboembolism
- Catheter fragment embolism
- Fiber embolism originating from cotton or paper fibers contained in the catheter irrigation solution, leading to foreign body reactions

Infiltration

Infiltration may occur when the needle or catheter has been displaced or when blood or fluid leaks from around the catheter. Signs and symptoms include the following:

- Coolness of skin at the puncture site
- Swelling at the puncture site, with or without pain
- Sluggish or absent flow rate

If infiltration is suspected, the fluid reservoir should be lowered to a dependent position to check for the presence of backflow of blood into the tubing. (The absence of backflow suggests infiltration.) If any of the signs and symptoms are present, the intravenous flow should be discontinued, the needle or catheter immediately removed, and a pressure dressing applied to the site. An alternative puncture site should be chosen and the infusion restarted with new equipment. In addition, the incident should be documented.

Air Embolism

Air embolism is uncommon but can be fatal. Although the volume of air that the human blood stream can tolerate has not been firmly established, fatalities have been reported after 100 ml of air entering the cardiovascular system.[11] A total of 10 ml of air can be fatal in a critically ill patient.

The embolism is caused by air entering the blood stream via the catheter tubing. The risk of air embolism is greatest when a catheter is passed into the central circulation, where negative pressure may actually pull in air. Air can enter the circulation either on insertion of the catheter or when the tubing is disconnected to replace solutions or add new extension tubing. With subsequent pumping, blood foaming occurs in the heart. If enough air enters the heart chamber, it can impede the flow of blood, leading to shock.

Signs and symptoms of air embolism include hypotension; cyanosis; weak, rapid pulse; and loss of consciousness. If air embolism is suspected, the following steps should be taken:

1. Close the tubing.
2. Turn the patient on his or her left side with head down. (If air has entered the heart chambers, this position may keep the air in

the right side of the heart and away from the cardiac valves. The pulmonary artery may absorb small air bubbles.)

3. Check tubing for leaks.
4. Administer high-flow oxygen.
5. Notify medical direction.

The possibility of an air embolism can be minimized by ensuring that all tubing connections are secure and that fluid containers are changed before they are empty.

COMPLICATIONS SPECIFIC TO CENTRAL VENOUS CANNULATION

Cannulation of the central veins presents specific dangers in addition to the complications common to all intravenous techniques. The paramedic must be alert to these dangers because they can be fatal if unrecognized. (Although the femoral vein is not truly a central vein because the catheter is inserted in an area below the diaphragm, it will be included in this section.)

Complications from Femoral Vein Cannulation

- Local complications
  - Hematoma may occur from the vein itself or the adjacent femoral artery.
  - Thrombosis may extend to the deep veins and lead to edema of the leg.
  - Phlebitis may extend to the deep veins.
  - Use of the femoral vein frequently precludes subsequent use of the saphenous vein.
- Systemic complications
  - Thrombosis or phlebitis that may extend proximally to the iliac veins or even the inferior vena cava.

Complications from Internal Jugular and Subclavian Cannulation

- Local complications
  - Hematoma may occur, either from the vein itself or from an adjacent artery.

NOTE:
If a hematoma occurs on one side of the neck, it is hazardous to attempt puncture on the opposite side because of the possibility of bilateral hematomas severely compromising the airway.

  - Damage may occur to an adjacent artery, nerve, or lymphatic duct. Inadvertent puncture of the carotid artery is not uncommon when attempting jugular cannulation.
- Systemic complications.
  - Pneumothorax is common.
  - Hemothorax can occur.
  - Air embolism can occur.
  - Fluid may infiltrate into the mediastinum or the pleural cavity from an extruded catheter.

REGULATING FLUID FLOW RATES

The fluid flow rate should be adjusted as ordered by medical direction. The paramedic must know the volume to be infused, the period of time over which the fluid is to be infused, and the number of drops per milliliter the infusion set delivers. The flow rate is then calculated and adjusted as follows:

$$\text{Drops/min} = \frac{\text{Volume to be infused} \times \text{Drops/ml of infusion set}}{\text{Total time of infusion in minutes}}$$

Example (using a macrodrip infusion set that delivers 10 drops/ml):

Total volume to be infused	120 ml
Infusion set (drops/ml)	10
Time of infusion	60 minutes

$$\text{drops/min} = \frac{120 \text{ ml} \times 10 \text{ drops/ml}}{60 \text{ min}}$$

$$= \frac{120 \times 10}{60} = 20 \text{ drops/min}$$

Example (using a macrodrip infusion set that delivers 10 drops/ml):

Total volume to be infused — 70 ml
Infusion set (drops/ml) — 60
Time of infusion — 60 minutes

$$\text{drops/min} = \frac{70 \text{ ml} \times 60 \text{ drops/ml}}{60 \text{ min}}$$

$$= \frac{4200}{60} = 70 \text{ drops/min}$$

NOTE:
When using microdrip tubing, the number of milliliters per hour equals the number of drops per minute.

REFERENCES

1. Systems of surgery, quoted by Mann FC; *Bull John Hopkins Hospital* 25:205, 1914.

2. Hardaway R, editor: *Shock, the reversible stage of dying,* Littleton, Mass, 1988, PSG Publishing.
3. Giesecke A et al: Fluid therapy and the resuscitation of traumatic shock, *Crit Care Clin* 6(1):61, 1990.
4. Seeley R et al: *Anatomy and physiology,* ed 2, St Louis, 1992, Mosby.
5. McSwain N, Kernstein M: *Evaluation and management of trauma,* Norwalk, Conn, 1987, Appleton-Century-Crofts.
6. Mattox K et al: Prospective MAST study in 911 patients, *J Trauma* 29(8):1104, 1989.
7. McSwain N: Pneumatic anti-shock garment: state of the art 1988, *Ann Emerg Med* 17(5):506, 1988.
8. Chisholm C, Clark D: Effect of the pneumatic anti-shock garment on intramuscular pressure, *Ann Emerg Med* 13:581, 1984.
9. *Some facts about blood,* St Louis, 1984, American Red Cross.
10. Haynes B et al: Catheter introducers for rapid fluid resuscitation, *Ann Emerg Med* 12:606, 1983.
11. *Needle and cannula technique,* Chicago, 1977, Abbott Laboratories.

Summary

Shock is a state of inadequate tissue perfusion that can be caused by a variety of disease states and injuries. If the syndrome is severe or prolonged, it may become irreversible, resulting in multiple organ failure and death. Successful resuscitation of the shock victim depends on recognition of the disease state, airway control, adequate oxygenation and ventilation, fluid replacement, and rapid transport to an appropriate medical facility for definitive care.

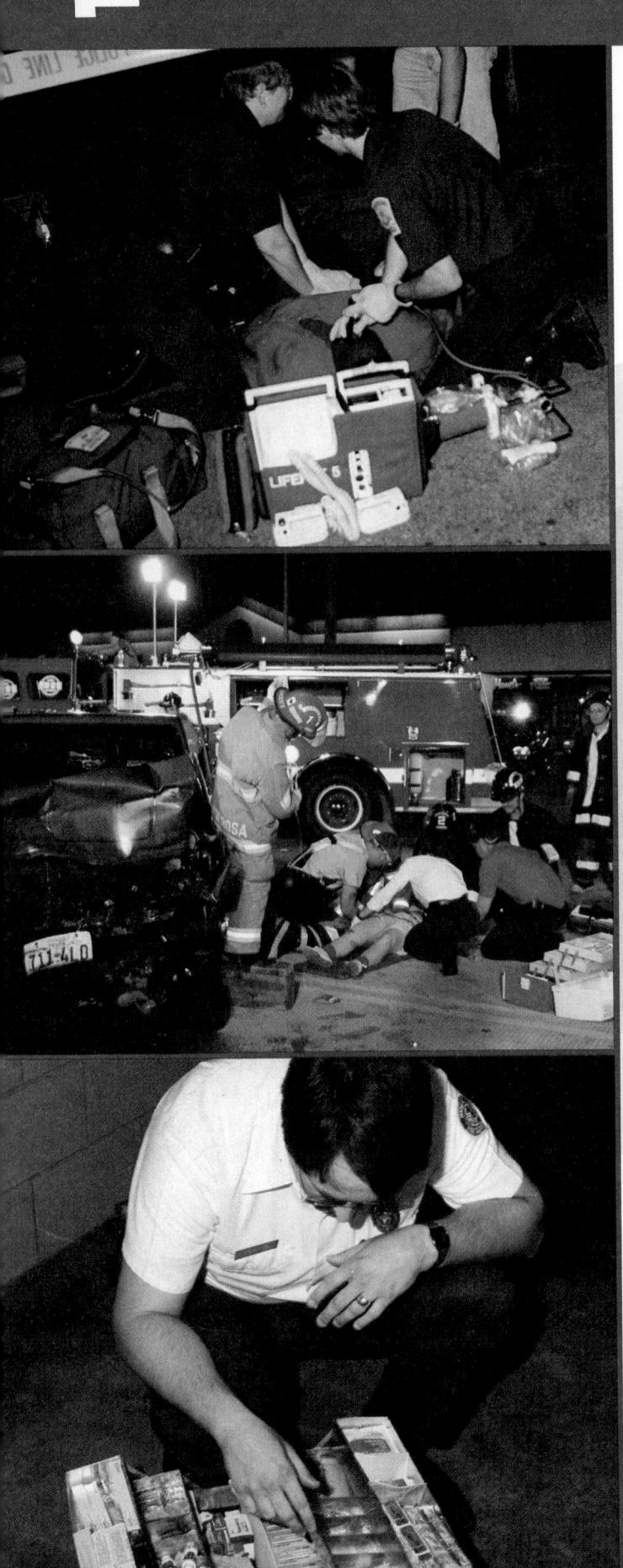

Pharmacological agents have life saving and life-threatening potential. The ability to safely administer prescribed medications and understand the problems that can develop from medication therapy are part of a paramedic's professional patient care responsibilities.

OBJECTIVES

As a paramedic, you should be able to:

1. List five sources of drugs.
2. Identify the four different types of drug names.
3. Outline drug standards and legislation pertinent to the paramedic.
4. Describe the role of drug-control agencies.
5. Distinguish among drug forms.
6. Explain the meaning of drug terms necessary to safely interpret information in drug-reference sources.
7. Discuss factors that influence drug absorption, distribution, and elimination.
8. Describe how drugs react with receptors to produce their desired effects.
9. Outline assessment techniques performed and documented to evaluate the effectiveness of drug therapy.
10. Calculate and correctly measure or infuse the correct volume of drug to be administered for a given situation.
11. Describe steps for ensuring safe administration of drugs.
12. Explain techniques of drug administration by enteral and parenteral routes.
13. Identify special considerations for administering pharmacological agents to pediatric and older patients.
14. List the class, actions, onset, duration, indications, contraindications, adverse reactions, drug interactions, dosage, route of administration, and special considerations for the drugs listed in the Emergency Drug Index.
15. Outline drug actions and considerations for care of the patient who is given drugs that affect the nervous, cardiovascular, respiratory, endocrine, and gastrointestinal systems.

KEY TERMS

absorption: The process involving the movement of drug molecules from the site of entry into the body to the general circulation.

adrenergic: Of or pertaining to the sympathetic nerve fibers of the autonomic nervous system that use epinephrine or epinephrine-like substances as neurotransmitters.

biotransformation: The process whereby a drug is chemically converted to a metabolite.

cholinergic: Of or pertaining to nerve fibers that elaborate acetylcholine at the myoneural junctions.

chronotropic: Pertaining to agents that affect the heart rate; a drug that increases heart rate is said to have a positive chronotropic effect.

contraindication: A medical or physiological factor that makes it harmful to administer a medication that would otherwise have therapeutic value.

distribution: The transport of a drug through the blood stream to various tissues of the body and ultimately to its site of action.

dromotropic: Pertaining to agents that affect conduction velocity through the conducting tissues of the heart; a drug that speeds conduction is said to have a positive dromotropic effect.

drug: Any substance taken by mouth; injected into a muscle, blood vessel, or cavity of the body; or applied topically to treat or prevent a disease or condition.

drug allergy: A systemic reaction to a drug resulting from previous sensitizing exposure and the development of an immunological mechanism. *Continued.*

KEY TERMS—cont'd

drug receptor: Any part of a cell, usually an enzyme or large protein molecule, with which a drug molecule interacts to trigger its desired response or effect.

excretion: The elimination of toxic or inactive metabolites, primarily by the kidney; the intestine, lungs, and mammary, sweat, and salivary glands may also be involved.

parasympatholytic: Anticholinergic producing effects resembling those of interruption or blockade of the parasympathetic nerve supply to effector organs or tissues.

parasympathomimetic: An agent whose effects mimic those resulting from stimulation of parasympathetic nerves, especially the effects produced by acetylcholine.

pharmacodynamics: The study of how a drug acts on a living organism.

pharmacokinetics: The study of the action and effects of drugs within the body, including the routes and mechanisms of absorption and excretion, rate at which a drug's action begins and duration of the effect, and biotransformation.

receptor: A reactive site on the cell surface or within the cell that combines with a drug molecule to produce a biological effect.

side effect: An often unavoidable and undesirable effect of therapeutic doses of a drug; actions or effects other than those for which the drug was originally given.

sympatholytic: Antiadrenergic blocking transmission of impulses from the adrenergic postganglionic fibers to effector organs or tissues.

sympathomimetic: A pharmacological agent that mimics the effects of sympathetic-nervous-system stimulation of organs and structures by acting as an agonist or by increasing the release of the neurotransmitter norepinephrine at postganglionic nerve endings.

NOTE:

This chapter introduces the paramedic to general principles of pharmacology and emergency medications commonly used in the prehospital setting. A more complete description of the emergency drugs included in this chapter can be found in the Emergency Drug Index. Medications described in this section that are included in the Index are denoted by *bold italic* type.

The drug information presented in this section conforms to current medical literature, to manufacturer product monographs, and to the clinical practice of the general medical community at the time of publication. Although every effort has been made to ensure accuracy and completeness, the author, editors, medical advisors, and publisher disclaim liability for any discrepancies, incongruities, undetected errors, omissions in content, or reader misunderstanding. Local protocol regarding drug administration may vary from the information presented in this chapter. The paramedic should follow the guidelines established by medical control.

Section One
Drug Information

● SOURCES OF DRUGS

A **drug** may be defined as "any substance taken by mouth; injected into a muscle, blood vessel, or cavity of the body; or applied topically to treat or prevent a disease or condition."[1] Drugs have been identified or derived from five major sources: plants (for example, digitalis, *morphine sulphate, atropine sulphate*), animals and humans (for example, *epinephrine* [Adrenalin], **insulin,** adrenocorticotropic hormone [ACTH]), minerals or mineral products (for example, iron, iodine, *sodium bicarbonate, calcium chloride*), microorganisms (for example, penicillin, streptomycin), and chemical substances made in the laboratory (for example, *lidocaine* [Xylocaine], *bretylium tosylate* [Bretylol], *diazepam* [Valium]).

● DRUG NAMES

Drugs can be identified by the following four types of names:

1. Chemical name: a precise description of the drug's chemical composition and molecular structure.
2. Generic or nonproprietary name: often a markedly abbreviated form of the chemical name of the drug; more frequently used than the chemical name. Generic medications usually have the same therapeutic efficacy as nongeneric drugs but are generally less expensive.
3. Trade, brand, or proprietary name: a copyrighted name designated by the drug company that sells the medication. Trade names are proper nouns, and thus the first letter is capitalized. This text shows the trade name in parentheses after the generic name of the drug.
4. Official name: The official name of a drug is followed by the initials *USP* or *NF*, denoting its listing in one of the official publications. In most cases, the official name is the same as the generic name.

An example of the four names for a drug follows:

Chemical name: ethyl 1-methyl-4-plenylisonipecotate hydrochloride
Generic name: *meperidine hydrochloride*
Trade name: Demerol Hydrochloride
Official name: meperidine hydrochloride USP

● DRUG STANDARDS AND LEGISLATION

Before 1906, there was little control over the use of medications. Drugs were often sold or distributed by traveling medicine men, drugstores, mail order, and legitimate and self-titled physicians. Listing the ingredients of the medications was not required, and many drug products contained opium, *morphine,* heroin, and alcohol.

In 1906, the Pure Food and Drug Act was enacted by Congress to protect the public from mislabeled or adulterated drugs. This act prohibited the use of false and misleading claims for medications and restricted the sale of drugs with a potential for abuse. The Pure Food and Drug Act also designated the *United States Pharmacopeia (USP)* and the *National Formulary (NF),* as official standards and empowered the federal government to enforce them. Other drug standards and legislation are listed in Box 14-1. Table 14-1 lists characteristics, dispensing restrictions and examples of the five controlled substances.

Drug Regulatory Agencies

In July 1973, the Drug Enforcement Agency (DEA) in the Department of Justice became the nation's sole legal drug-enforcement agency. Additional regulatory bodies or services follow:

- Food and Drug Administration (FDA): The FDA is responsible for enforcing the federal Food, Drug, and Cosmetic Act. The FDA may seize offending goods and criminally prosecute individuals involved.
- Public Health Service: The Public Health Service is an agency within the U.S. Department of Health and Human Services. One duty of this agency is to regulate biological products, which are viruses, therapeutic serums, antitoxins, or analogous products applicable in the prevention or cure of human diseases or injuries. The agency examines and licenses these products and inspects and licenses the establishments that produce them.
- Federal Trade Commission: The Federal Trade Commission is an agency of the federal government directly responsible to the president of the United States. Its principal action with respect to drugs lies in its power to suppress false or misleading advertising to the general public.
- Canadian drug control: In the country of Canada, the Health Protection Branch of the Department of National Health and Welfare is responsible for administering and enforcing the Food and Drugs Act, the Proprietary or Patent Medicine Act, and the Narcotics Control Act.

BOX 14-1

Drug Standards and Legislation

1912: Congress passed the Sherley Amendment prohibiting fraudulent therapeutic claims.

1914: The Harrison Narcotic Act was passed to control the sale of narcotics and to help curb drug addiction or dependence. This was the first narcotic act to be passed by any nation, and it established the word *narcotic* as a legal term.

1938: Prompted by more than 100 deaths in 1937 from ingestion of a diethylene glycol solution of sulfanilamide, the federal Food, Drug, and Cosmetic Act was enacted. This act contained a provision to prevent marketing of a new drug before it was properly tested. In addition, the act required that the label list all ingredients used in preparing the drug and the directions for drug use.

1952: The Durham-Humphrey Amendment changed the 1938 drug act, restricting the dispensing of legend (prescription) drugs. Legend drugs must bear the legend, "Caution: Federal law prohibits dispensing without prescription."

1962: The Kefauver-Harris Amendment required that a new drug's safety and efficacy be proved before it could be approved for use.

1970: The Comprehensive Drug Abuse Prevention and Control Act (also known as the *Controlled Substances Act [CSA]*) superseded the Harrison Narcotic Act of 1914. The CSA classifies a controlled substance by its use and abuse potential. Drugs are classified into numbered schedules from schedule I (drugs with highest abuse potential) to schedule V (drugs with lowest abuse potential). See Table 14-1.

Possession of Controlled Substances

It is illegal for any person to possess a controlled substance unless it has been obtained by a valid prescription or order or unless its possession is pursuant to actions in the course of professional practice. The authority for use of controlled substances and other prescription medications is a function of state agencies operating under federal restrictions provided by the Drug Enforcement Administration (DEA). Paramedics and other allied health professionals who administer medications should be familiar with state laws governing drug administration, storage, and record-keeping requirements. Violations of the CSA are punishable by fine, imprisonment, or both.

- International Drug Control: International control of drugs legally began in 1912 when the first "Opium Conference" was held at The Hague. Various international treaties were adopted, obligating governments to control narcotic substances. These treaties were consolidated in 1961 into one document, known as the *Single Convention on Narcotic Drugs,* which became effective in 1964. Later, the International Narcotics Control Board was established to enforce this law.

Drug References

Several publications provide information on various drugs, their preparation, and recommended administrations. These references include the *American Medical Association (AMA) Drug Evaluation, Hospital Formulary,* medication package inserts, and the *Physician's Desk Reference (PDR)* (Box 14-2). Paramedics should be familiar with these publications and other emergency pharmacology manuals, particularly regarding drugs commonly administered in the prehospital setting.

TABLE 14-1 Controlled Substances

Characteristics	Dispensing Restrictions	Examples (Partial List)
Schedule I Has high abuse potential Has no accepted medical use; for research, analysis, or instruction only May lead to severe dependence	Approved protocol is necessary.	Heroin, marijuana (cannabis), tetrahydrocannabinols, lysergic acid diethylamide (LSD), mescaline, peyote, psilocybin, methaqualone
Schedule II Has high abuse potential Has accepted medical uses May lead to severe physical or psychological dependence, or both	Written prescription is necessary (signed by the practitioner); only emergency dispensing is permitted without written prescription (only required amount may be prescribed for emergency period). No prescription refills are allowed. Container must have warning label.*	Opium, **morphine sulfate,** hydromorphone, **meperidine,** codeine, oxycodone, methadone, secobarbital, pentobarbital, amphetamine, methylphenidate, cocaine, and others
Schedule III Has less abuse potential than drugs in schedules I and II Has accepted medical uses May lead to moderate-to-low physical dependence or high psychological dependence	Written or oral prescription is required. Prescription expires in 6 months. No more than five refills are allowed in a 6-month period. Container must have warning label.*	Preparations containing limited quantities of or combined with one or more active ingredients that are noncontrolled substances (codeine, hydrocodone, **morphine sulfate,** dihydrocodeine, or ethylmorphine) and nonnarcotic drugs such as derivatives of barbituric acid except those that are listed in another schedule, glutethimide, methyprylon, chlorphentermine, paregoric, and others
Schedule IV Has lower abuse potential compared with schedule III drugs Has accepted medical uses May lead to limited physical or psychological dependence	Written or oral prescription is required. Prescription expires in 6 months, with no more than five refills allowed. Container must have warning label.*	Barbital, **phenobarbital,** chloral hydrate, meprobamate, fenfluramine, chlordiazepoxide, **diazepam,** oxazepam, clorazepate, flurazepam, **lorazepam,** dextropropoxyphene, pentazocine, mazindol, alprazolam, and others
Schedule V Has low abuse potential compared with schedule IV drugs Has accepted medical uses May lead to limited physical or psychological dependence	Drug may require written prescription or be sold without prescription (check state law).	Medications, generally for relief of coughs or diarrhea, containing limited quantities of certain opioid controlled substances

*CAUTION: Federal law prohibits the transfer of this drug to any person other than the patient for whom it was prescribed.

BOX 14-2

Drug References

AMA Drug Evaluation: The *AMA Drug Evaluation* provides information on drug groups, dosages, prescribing information, and usage. It also covers valid clinical applications of drug use that differ from those approved by the FDA thus far.

Hospital Formulary: The *Hospital Formulary,* a manual published by the American Society of Hospital Pharmacists, provides an overview in monograph form of nearly every available (approved and unapproved) drug in the United States. It is updated regularly and is available in all hospital pharmacies and in many emergency departments. The *Hospital Formulary* is considered by many to be the most reliable source of information on medications and drugs.

Medication package inserts: Most medications are packaged with written literature describing product use. These inserts provide valuable information as new drugs are introduced and should be consulted to become familiar with the product.

Physician's Desk Reference: The *PDR,* published yearly by the Medical Economics Company, is a concise compilation of drug information, including FDA-approved indications, contraindications, and adverse effects. In addition to providing product information through several cross-referenced indices, it serves as an identification guide by showing actual-size, color pictures of commonly prescribed medications. The *PDR* also lists emergency telephone numbers for poison control centers throughout the United States.

BOX 14-3

Various Forms of Drug Preparations

Preparations for Oral Use
Liquids
   Aqeuous solutions—substances dissolved in water and syrups
   Aqeuous suspensions—solid particles suspended in liquid
   Emulsions—fats or oils suspended in liquid with an emulsifier
   Spirits—alcohol solution
   Elixirs—aromatic, sweetened alcohol and water solution
   Tincture—alcohol extract of plant or vegetable substance
   Fluid extracts—concentrated alcoholic liquid extract of plant or vegetables
   Extracts—syrup or dried form of pharmacologically active drug, usually prepared by evaporating solution

Solids
   Capsules—soluble case (usually gelatin) that contains liquid, dry, or beaded drug particles
   Tablets—compressed, powdered drugs in small disk
   Troches or lozenges—medicated tablets that dissolve slowly in mouth
   Powders or granules—loose or molded drug substance for drug administration, with or without liquids

Preparations for Parenteral Use
   Ampules—sealed glass container for liquid injectable medication
   Vials—glass container with rubber stopper for liquid or powdered medication
   Cartridge or Tubex—single-dose unit of parenteral medication to be used with a specific injecting device

---

● DRUG FORMS AND PREPARATIONS

Drugs and drug preparations are available in many forms, and each has specific indications, advantages, and disadvantages (Box 14-3), which are explained throughout the chapter and in the Emergency Drug Index.

BOX 14-3—cont'd

Intravenous Infusions (Suspended on Hanger at Bedside)

Glass bottles, flexible collapsible plastic bags, and semirigid plastic containers (150 to 1000 ml) used for continuous infusion of fluid replacement with or without medications

Intermittent intravenous infusions—usually a secondary intravenous setup of small plastic or glass bottle (50 to 250 ml) to which medication is added (It runs as a "piggyback," hung separately from the primary intravenous infusion via a secondary administration tubing set usually for 20 to 120 minutes. The primary intravenous solution is run between medication doses.)

Heparin lock—a port site for direct administration of intermittent intravenous medications without the need for primary intravenous solution

Preparations for Topical Use

Liniments—liquid suspensions for lubrication that are applied by rubbing

Lotions—liquid suspensions that can be protective, emollient, cooling, astringent, antipruritic, cleaning

Ointment—semisolid medicine in a base for local protective, soothing, astringent, or transdermal application for systemic effects (such as nitroglycerin, scopolamine, estrogen)

Paste—thick ointment primarily used for skin protection

Plasters—solid preparations that are adhesive, protective, or soothing

Creams—emulsions that contain aqueous and oily bases

Aerosols—fine powders or solutions in volatile liquids that contain a propellant

Preparations for Use on Mucous Membranes

Drops for eyes, ears, or nose—aqueous solutions with or without gelling agent to increase retention time in eye.

Topical instillation of aqueous solution of medications—usually for topical action but occasionally for systemic effects (enema, douche, mouthwash, throat spray, gargle)

Aerosol sprays, nebulizers, and inhalers—aqueous solutions of medication delivered in droplet form to the target membrane, such as bronchial tree (bronchodilators)

Foams—powders or solutions of medication in volatile liquids with propellant (vaginal foams for contraception)

Suppositories—usually medicinal substances mixed in firm but malleable base (cocoa butter) to facilitate insertion into a body cavity (rectum or vagina)

Miscellaneous Drug-Delivery Systems

Intradermal implants—pellets that contain small deposit of medication that are inserted in dermal pocket (They are designed to allow medication to leach slowly into tissue and are usually used to administer hormones such as testosterone or estradiol.)

A micropump system—small, external pump attached by belt or implanted that delivers medication via needle in continuous steady dose (insulin, anticancer chemotherapy, opioids)

Membrane delivery systems—drug-laden membranes instilled in the eye to deliver steady flow of medications (pilocarpine or corticosteroids)

BOX 14-4

Pharmacological Terminology

Antagonism: the opposition of effects between two or more medications occurring when the combined (conjoint) effect of two drugs is less than the sum of the drugs acting separately

Contraindications: medical or physiological factors that make it harmful to administer a medication that would otherwise have therapeutic value

Cumulative action: The tendency for repeated doses of a drug to accumulate in the blood and organs, causing increased and sometimes toxic effects and occurring when several doses are administered or when absorption occurs more quickly than removal by excretion or metabolism

Depressant: a substance that decreases a body function or activity

Drug allergy: a systemic reaction to a drug resulting from previous sensitizing exposure and the development of an immunological mechanism

Drug dependence: a state in which withdrawal of a drug produces intense physical or emotional disturbance; previously termed *habituation*

Drug interaction: beneficial or detrimental modification of the effects of one drug by the prior or concurrent administration of another drug that increases or decreases the pharmacological or physiological action of one or both drugs

Idiosyncrasy: abnormal or peculiar responses to a drug (accounting for 25% to 30% of all drug reactions) thought to result from genetic enzymatic deficiencies or other unique physiological variables leading to abnormal mechanisms of drug metabolism or altered physiological effects of the drug

Potentiation: the enhancement of effect caused by the concurrent administration of two drugs in which one drug increases the effect of the other drug

Side effect: undesirable and often unavoidable effects of using therapeutic doses of a drug; actions or effects other than those for which the drug was originally given

Stimulant: a drug that enhances or increases body function or activity

Summation: the combined effect of two drugs such that the total effect equals the sum of the individual effects of each agent (1 + 1 = 2)

Synergism: the combined action of two drugs such that the total effect exceeds the sum of the individual effects of each agent (1 + 1 = 3 or more)

Therapeutic action: the desired, intended action of a drug

Tolerance: decreased physiological response to the repeated administration of a drug or chemically related substance, possibly necessitating an increase in dosage to maintain a therapeutic effect (tachyphylaxis)

Untoward effect: a side effect that proves harmful to the patient

---

● PHARMACOLOGICAL TERMINOLOGY

Drugs may act in the body in many ways. Some of these actions are desirable (therapeutic effects), and others are undesirable or even harmful (side effects). Drugs may also interact with other drugs to produce uncommon and frequently unpredictable effects. The terminology in Box 14-4 is used to describe various potential reactions to drug therapy.

● ALLERGIC REACTIONS TO DRUGS

Allergic reactions, which account for 6% to 10% of all drug reactions, do not usually occur from the first exposure to a drug. At least one previous exposure is required for the immune system to develop the antibodies that cause the clinical reactions. Because previous exposure is required, patients at risk of developing **drug allergies** can sometimes be identified in interviews. However, patients do not always know the names of drugs they have received, and they may have been unknowingly exposed to a drug through food or milk products (for example, penicillin, which is commonly used in livestock medicine). Another unusual circumstance is cross-reactivity, in which one drug can trigger an allergic reaction in a patient who has never taken that drug but has an allergy to a chemically similar drug. For example, patients with penicillin allergy are also allergic to certain cephalosporins although they have not previously taken a cephalosporin.

Allergic reactions are initiated by the drug in its original form or by a metabolite of the drug formed during its breakdown in the body. Most drugs are not very allergenic, but some drugs elicit strong immune system reactions. Drug allergies can be divided into four classifications based on the mechanism of the body's immune reaction.

Type I, or anaphylactic, reactions occur soon after exposure to a drug. They are caused by a specific type of antibody (immunoglobulin E [IgE]) attached to mast cells. (Classes of immunoglobulins are discussed further in Chapter 22.) When a specific antigen attaches to these IgE antibodies, the chemical substances in the mast cell (including histamine and slow reactive substance of anaphylaxis) are released. These reactions commonly produce urticaria accompanied by severe itching. Type I reactions are not usually serious. However, they can progress to severe reactions involving the cardiovascular and respiratory systems (anaphylaxis). Drugs associated with type I reactions include penicillins, cephalosporins, and iodides. Anaphylaxis is further addressed in Chapter 22.

Type II, or cytotoxic, reactions are delayed reactions that involve certain cytotoxic antibodies of the IgG class. These antibodies are capable of lysing cells and commonly cause hemolytic reactions and destruction of platelets. Examples of type II reactions include drug-induced hemolytic

anemia and conditions resembling systemic lupus erythematosus. Drugs that are associated with type II reactions include quinidine (Duraquin and others), *procainamide* (Pronestyl), and *hydralazine* (Apresoline).

Type III reactions are delayed reactions frequently described as "serum sickness." Like type II reactions, specific antibodies are usually involved. These antibodies (usually IgG) bind the antigen in the blood stream and form complexes. These complexes filter out in various anatomical locations and produce an inflammatory reaction. Symptoms include urticaria, joint pain, swollen lymph nodes, and fever. Drugs associated with type III reactions include penicillins, iodides, sulfonamides, *phenytoin* (Dilantin), and some antitoxins that use horse serum (for example, tetanus antitoxin).

Type IV reactions are those in which contact dermatitis is produced by a topical application of a drug. Type IV reactions are produced by the T lymphocytes, not the hormonal antibodies. They usually require more than 24 hours to become evident. Poison ivy is a prototypical example of a type IV reaction. Drugs associated with type IV reactions include sunscreens, acne preparations, antiinflammatory agents such as topical corticosteroids, and antibiotic powders and ointments.

Section Two
Mechanisms of Drug Action

Drug actions are achieved by a biochemical interaction between the drug and certain tissue components in the body (usually receptors). Note that drugs do not confer any new functions on a tissue or organ in the body; they only modify existing functions. In addition, drugs generally exert multiple actions rather than a single effect. The interactions between a drug and the biological system are divided into two classes: pharmacokinetic interactions (how the body handles the drug) and pharmacodynamic interactions (the drug's effects on the body).

● PHARMACOKINETIC INTERACTIONS

Pharmacokinetics is the study of how the body handles a drug over a period of time, including the processes of absorption, distribution, biotransformation, and excretion. These factors affect a patient's response to drug therapy.

Drug Absorption

Absorption involves the movement of drug molecules from the site of entry to the general circulation. The degree to which drugs attain pharmacological activity depends in part on the rate and extent to which they are absorbed, which in turn depends on the drug's ability to cross the cell membrane. The drug crosses the membrane through the processes of passive diffusion and active transport. Although most drugs enter the cell by passive diffusion, some require a carrier-mediated mechanism to carry them through the membrane.

The cell membrane consists of a lipid bilayer with protein molecules irregularly dispersed throughout. The protein molecules may act as a carrier, enzyme, receptor, or antigenic site (a site capable of binding to and reacting with an antibody). Lipid-soluble drugs can pass through the lipid membrane, but water-soluble drugs cannot. Water-soluble substances such as urea, alcohol, electrolytes, and water must enter the cell through membrane pores.

Absorption begins at the site of administration. The rate and extent of absorption depend on the route of administration, dosage, and dosage form of the drug administered.[2]

Nature of the Absorbing Surface (Cell Membrane) the Drug Must Traverse

If a drug must pass through a single layer of cells (intestinal epithelium), the transport is faster than if it must pass through several layers of cells (skin). In addition, the greater the surface area of the absorbing site, the greater the absorption and the more rapid the drug effect. For example, the small intestine offers a large absorption area, whereas the stomach has a relatively small absorption surface area.

Blood Flow to the Site of Administration

A rich blood supply enhances absorption (sublingual route), and a poor blood supply delays it (subcutaneous route). For example, a patient in shock may not respond to intramuscular administration because diminished circulation decreases absorption. In comparison, intravenous administration of a drug immediately places a drug in the circulatory system, where it is completely absorbed and must be delivered to its target tissue.

Solubility of the Drug

The more soluble the drug, the more rapidly it is absorbed. Parenterally administered nonintravenous drugs prepared in oily solutions are absorbed more slowly than drugs dissolved in water or in isotonic sodium chloride.

pH of the Drug Environment

In solution, many drugs exist in an ionized and unionized form. How and to what extent a drug ionizes depend on whether the drug is an acid or base and on the drug's relative strength. The unionized drug is lipid soluble and readily diffuses across the cell membrane. The ionized drug is lipid insoluble and nondiffusible. An acidic drug (for example, aspirin) is relatively undissociated (unionized) in an acidic environment such as the stomach. The drug then readily diffuses across the membranes into the circulation. A drug that is basic in the same acidic environment tends to ionize and is not easily absorbed through the gastric membrane. The reverse occurs when the drug is in an alkaline medium (Fig. 14-1).

Drug Concentration

Drugs administered in high concentrations tend to be absorbed more rapidly than those administered in low concentrations. In some situations, it is necessary to administer a large dose (loading dose) that temporarily exceeds the body's capacity for excretion of the drug. This rapidly establishes a therapeutic drug level at the receptor site. A smaller dose (maintenance dose) can then be administered to replace the amount of drug excreted. Thus loading doses are based more on the volume of distribution (of which body size is an important component) and less on capacity for excretion

pH effects on drug molecules:

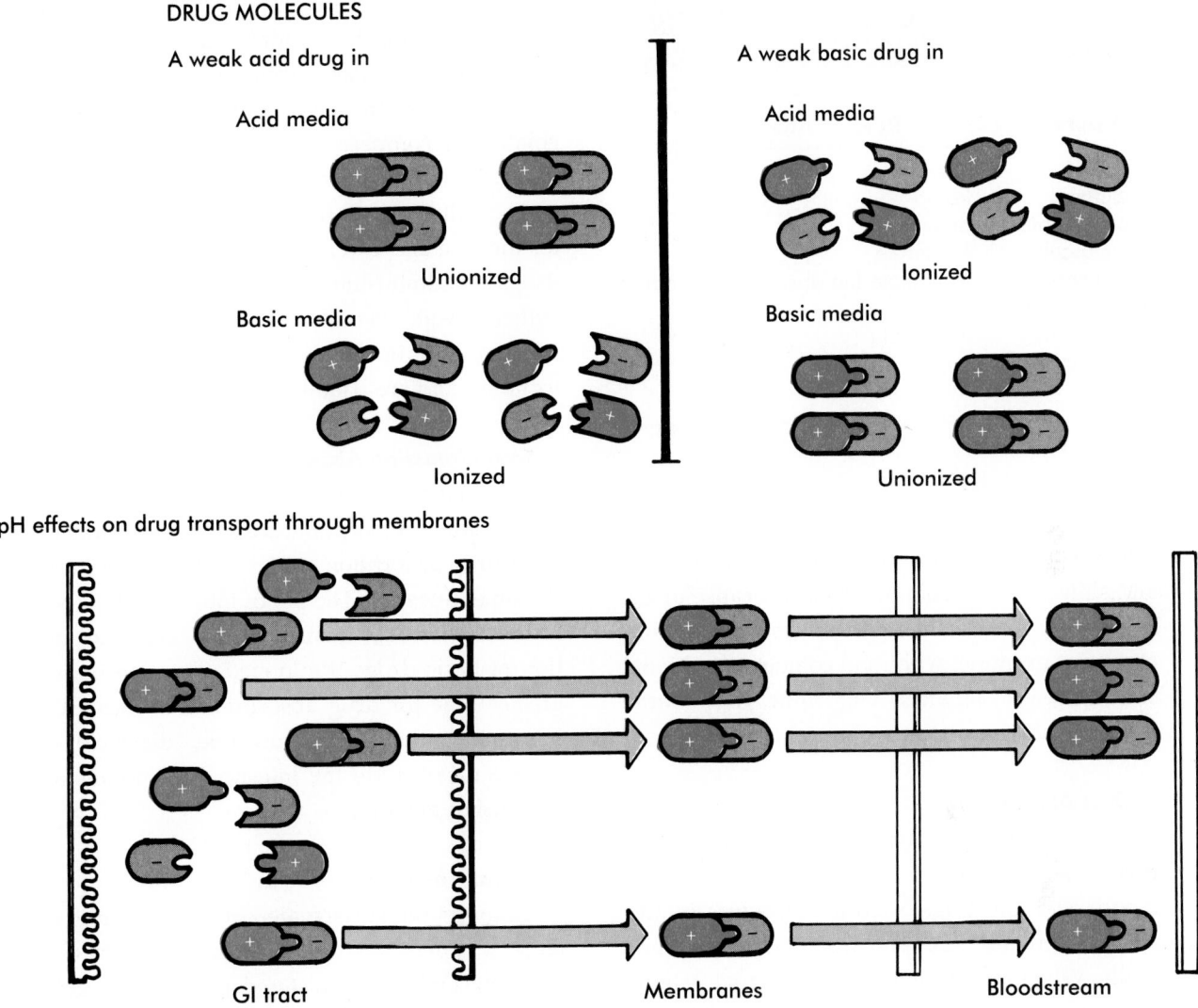

Fig. 14-1 Effect of pH on drug ionization and transport.

(for example, renal failure). Maintenance doses are exactly the opposite.

Drug Dosage Form

Drug absorption can be manipulated by pharmaceutical processing. An example is a combination of an active drug with another substance that is slowly released or a drug that resists digestive action (enteric coatings).

Routes of Drug Administration

As a rule, drugs are administered for local or systemic effects. Some drugs given locally pro-

duce local and systemic effects if they are partly or entirely absorbed. Other drugs are applied for local absorption and yet are targeted solely for systemic effects (for example, *nitroglycerin* and ointment hormones). The route of administration greatly influences drug absorption (Table 14-2). These routes can be classified as enteral, parenteral, pulmonary, and topical.

Enteral Route

Drugs administered along any portion of the gastrointestinal tract are said to use the enteral route. The enteral method of giving drugs is the safest, most convenient, and most economical

TABLE 14-2 Comparison of Drug Absorption Rates by Common Routes of Administration

Route	Rate of Absorption
Enteral	Slow
Sublingual	Rapid
Subcutaneous	Slow
Intramuscular	Moderate
Intravenous	Immediate (no absorption required)
Endotracheal	Rapid
Intraosseous	Immediate
Pulmonary	Rapid
Topical	Moderate

route of administration. It is also the least reliable and slowest of the common routes because of the frequent changes of the gastrointestinal environment (for example, with food contents, emotional state, physical activity). This route allows oral, gastric, small intestinal, and rectal absorption.

Oral Absorption

Although the oral cavity has a rich blood supply, little absorption normally occurs in the mouth. Certain drugs, such as *nitroglycerin* and some hormones, are prepared to be absorbed orally. When administered by sublingual or buccal routes, these drugs rapidly dissolve in the salivary secretions and are absorbed by the oral mucosa. After absorption, the drug enters the systemic circulation, initially bypassing gastrointestinal fluids and the liver.

In sublingual administration, the medication is placed under the tongue and the tablet dissolves in the salivary secretions. The effects from sublingual medication are usually apparent within 2 minutes. In buccal administration, the drug is placed between the teeth and mucous membrane of the cheek. As in sublingual administration, absorption by buccal administration is usually rapid.

Gastric Absorption

The stomach also has a rich blood supply but is not considered an important site for drug absorption. The length of time a medication remains in the stomach varies, depending on the pH of the environment and gastric motility. For example, the pH of the stomach is approximately 1.4. Weakly acidic drugs, such as barbiturates, tend to remain unionized and are readily absorbed into the circulation. In comparison, basic drugs, such as *morphine*, ionize in the stomach and are poorly absorbed. Altering the gastric emptying rate may alter the rate and extent of drug absorption. Many drugs are administered on an empty stomach with sufficient water (8 ounces) to ensure rapid passage into the small intestine. Other drugs cause gastric irritation and are usually given with food.

Small Intestine Absorption

The small intestine has a rich blood supply and thus a larger absorption area than the stomach. Most drug absorption occurs in the upper part of the small intestine. The pH of intestinal fluid is alkaline (7.0 to 8.0), increasing the rate of absorption of basic drugs. Prolonged exposure permits greater time for drug absorption. An increase in intestinal motility (for example, diarrhea) decreases exposure to the intestinal membrane and diminishes absorption.

Rectal Absorption

Although the surface area of the rectum is not large, it is very vascular and capable of drug absorption. Drugs administered rectally are subject to erratic absorption because of rectal contents, local drug irritation, and the uncertainty of drug retention. Rectal medications do not undergo hepatic alteration on first pass through the body, since the blood vessels that perfuse the rectal region bypass the liver.

Parenteral Route

Drugs administered by injection are said to use the parenteral route. Common parenteral routes for administering emergency medications include subcutaneous, intramuscular, intravenous, endotracheal, and intraosseous routes.

Subcutaneous Administration

A subcutaneous injection is given beneath the skin into the connective tissue or fat immediately beneath the dermis. This route is used only for small volumes of drugs (0.5 ml or less) that do not irritate tissue. The rate of absorption is usually slow and can provide a sustained effect.

Intramuscular Administration

An intramuscular injection is given into the skeletal muscle. Absorption generally occurs more rapidly than with subcutaneous injection because of greater tissue blood flow.

Intravenous Administration

An intravenous injection is given directly into the blood stream, bypassing the absorption process. This route produces an almost immediate pharmacological effect. Most intravenous drugs should be administered slowly to help prevent adverse reactions.

Endotracheal Administration

Access to the endotracheal route is generally through an endotracheal tube, permitting drug delivery into the pulmonary alveoli and systemic absorption via the capillaries of the lungs. Because of the large surface area of the alveolar sacs, the rate of absorption by this route is almost as rapid as that of the intravenous route. Endotracheal (ET) tube administration is usually reserved for situations in which an intravenous line cannot be established. Medications that can be administered via the ET tube include *naloxone* (Narcan), *atropine*, *epinephrine* (Adrenalin), and *lidocaine* (Xylocaine). A mnemonic for medications that may be administered via the ET route is L-E-A-N. Several studies suggest that this route is somewhat erratic and less reliable than intravenous or intraosseous delivery and should therefore be used only if these first-line methods are unavailable. It is recommended that 2 to 2½ times the recommended intravenous dose (diluted in 10 ml normal saline) be administered when giving medication by this route.[3]

Intraosseous Administration

Intraosseous (IO) injections are given directly into the bone marrow cavity of pediatric patients through an established, free-flowing IO infusion system. Agents infused by this method are thought to circulate via the medullary cavity of the bone. Through the numerous venous channels of long bones, fluids or drugs rapidly enter the central circulation. Time from injection to entry into the systemic circulation is thought to equal that of the venous route.[4] Emergency medications known to be effective via the IO route include *epinephrine, atropine, sodium bicarbonate, dexamethasone* (Decadron), *dopamine* (Intropin), and *dobutamine* (Dobutrex).

Pulmonary Route

Medication can be administered by inhalation in the form of gas or fine mist (aerosol). The most commonly used inhalation medications are bronchodilators, but the pulmonary circulation can absorb a number of other medications if necessary (for example, drugs for ET administration).

Because of the large surface area and the rich capillary network adjacent to the alveolar membrane, absorption into the blood stream is rapid. Drugs such as bronchodilators, steroids, and antibiotics can be given by various inhalation devices (for example, a nebulizer), propelling the agent into alveolar sacs. This produces primarily local effects but occasionally results in unwanted systemic effects.

Topical Route

In most cases, drugs applied topically to the skin and mucous membranes are rapidly absorbed and are intended to produce a local effect. Only lipid-soluble compounds are absorbed through the skin, which acts as a barrier to most water-soluble compounds. To prevent adverse systemic effects, intact skin surfaces should be used as an administration site. Massaging the skin promotes drug absorption as the capillaries dilate and local blood flow increases.

Drug Distribution

Distribution is the transport of a drug through the blood stream to various tissues of the body and ultimately to its site of action. After a drug has entered the circulatory system, it is rapidly distributed throughout the body. The rate at which this occurs depends on the permeability of capillaries to the drug molecules.

To review, lipid-soluble drugs readily cross capillary membranes to enter most tissues and fluid compartments. Lipid-insoluble drugs require more time to arrive at their point of action. Cardiac output and regional blood flow also affect the rate and extent of distribution into body tissues. Generally, a drug is first distributed to organs that have a rich blood supply (that is, heart, liver, kidney, brain). Then, depending on drug composition, the drug enters tissue with a lesser blood supply, such as muscle and fat.

Drug Reservoirs

Drugs may accumulate at certain locations that function as storage sites, forming reservoirs by binding to specific tissues. As serum levels decline, tissue-bound drug is released from its storage site into the blood stream. The released drug maintains significant serum drug levels and may permit sustained release of the agent, allowing continued pharmacological effect at the receptor site. There are two general types of drug reservoirs: plasma protein binding and tissue binding.

As drugs enter the circulatory system, they may attach to plasma proteins (mainly albumin), forming a drug protein complex. The extent to which this binding occurs affects the intensity and duration of the drug's effect. The albumin molecule is too large to diffuse through the membrane of the blood vessel, so it traps the bound drug in the blood stream. A drug bound to plasma protein is pharmacologically inactive and becomes a circulating drug reservoir. The free drug (unbound drug) exists in equilibrium with the protein-bound fraction and is the only portion of the drug that has biological activity. As the free drug is eliminated from the body, the drug protein complex dissociates, so more drug is released to replace the free portion that was metabolized or excreted. This is summarized in the following equation:

$$\text{Free drug} + \text{Protein} \rightleftarrows \text{Drug protein complex}$$

Although albumin and other plasma proteins provide a number of binding sites, it is possible for two drugs to compete with one another for the same site and displace each other. If certain combinations of drugs are administered simultaneously, this competition can have serious consequences. For example, if a patient taking the anticoagulant medication *warfarin* (Coumadin) is given *quinidine* (Duraquin and others), the quinidine may displace some of the protein-bound warfarin, causing warfarin toxicity, which is usually manifested as severe hemorrhage.

Other factors that influence a drug's binding ability include the concentration of plasma proteins (especially albumin), the number of binding sites on the protein, the affinity of the drug for the protein, and the acid-base balance of the patient. Various disease states, such as hepatic dysfunction (liver disease), alter the body's ability to handle many medications. These alterations result from decreased serum albumin levels (albumin is manufactured by the liver) as well as decreased hepatic metabolism. These and other factors may result in more free drug being available for distribution to tissue sites (increased free drug fraction and enhanced pharmacological response).

A second type of "drug pooling" occurs in fat tissue and bone. Lipid-soluble drugs have a high affinity for adipose tissue, which is where these drugs are stored. Because there is relatively low blood flow in fat tissue, it serves as a stable reservoir for drugs. Some lipid-soluble drugs can remain in body fat for as long as 3 hours after administration. Other drugs (for example, tetracycline) have an unusual affinity for bone. These drugs accumulate in bone after being absorbed onto the bone crystal surface.

Barriers to Drug Distribution

The blood-brain barrier and the placental barrier are protective biological membranes that prevent the passage of certain drugs into these body sites.

The blood-brain barrier consists of a single layer of capillary endothelial cells that line the blood vessels entering the central nervous system. These cells are tightly joined at common borders by continuous intercellular junctions. This special anatomical arrangement permits only lipid-soluble drugs to be distributed into the brain and cerebral spinal fluid (for example, general anesthetics, barbiturates). Drugs that are poorly soluble in fat (for example, many antibiotics) have trouble passing this barrier and cannot enter the brain.

The placental barrier consists of membrane layers that separate the blood vessels of the mother and fetus. Like the blood-brain barrier, the placental barrier is not permeable to many lipid-insoluble drugs, so it provides some protection to the fetus. However, it does allow the passage of certain non-lipid-soluble drugs (that is, steroids, narcotics, anesthetics, some antibiotics). If these drugs are administered to the pregnant mother, they may affect the developing embryo or the neonate.

Biotransformation

After absorption and distribution, the body eliminates most drugs, first by **biotransformation** and then by **excretion.** Biotransformation (metabolism) is a process whereby the drug is chemically converted to a metabolite. The purpose of biotransformation is usually to "detoxify" a drug and render it less active; in some cases, however, this process produces active or even toxic metabolites. (An example is the production of toxic metabolites that results from an acetaminophen overdose.) The liver is the primary site of drug metabolism, but other tissues (plasma, kidneys, lungs, and the intestinal mucosa) can also be involved.

Orally administered drugs absorbed through the gastrointestinal tract normally travel to the liver before entering the general circulation. When this occurs, a significant amount may be metabolized (first-pass metabolism) before the drug reaches the systemic circulation, reducing the amount of drug available for distribution. Medications affected by this initial biotransformation can be given orally in high dosages or administered parenterally to initially bypass the liver.

Individuals metabolize drugs at variable rates. For example, patients with liver and renal disease and cardiovascular dysfunction are expected to have prolonged drug metabolism. Infants with immature metabolic capacity and older adults with degenerative metabolic function experience depressed biotransformation. If drug metabolism is delayed, drug accumulation and cumulative

drug effects may occur. Therefore the paramedic may need to consider dosage reductions (particularly maintenance doses) for patients in these categories (Fig. 14-2).

Excretion

Excretion is elimination of toxic or inactive metabolites. The kidney is the primary organ for excretion; however, the intestine, lungs, and mammary, sweat, and salivary glands may also be involved.

Excretion by the Kidneys

A drug can be excreted in the urine unchanged or as a chemical metabolite of its previous form. Renal excretion consists of three mechanisms: passive glomerular filtration, active tubular secretion, and partial reabsorption (Fig. 14-3).

Passive glomerular filtration is a simple filtration process that can be measured as the glomerular filtration rate (GFR) (see Chapter 10). The GFR is the total quantity of glomerular filtrate (usually expressed in milliliters) formed each minute in all nephrons of both kidneys. The availability of a drug for glomerular filtration depends on its free concentration in plasma. Unbound drugs and water-soluble metabolites are filtered by the glomeruli. Drugs highly bound to protein do not pass through this structure.

After filtration, lipid-soluble compounds are reabsorbed by the renal tubules and thus reenter the systemic circulation. Water-soluble compounds are not reabsorbed and are therefore eliminated from the body. Because of the equilibrium established between free and bound drug, as free drug is filtered from the blood, bound drug is released from its binding sites into the plasma. The rate of excretion depends on the speed of this reaction, thus giving the drug a longer half-life.

Active tubular secretion involves the transport of free drug from the blood across the proximal tubular cell and into the tubular urine by an active process against a concentration gradient. Drugs actively secreted by the renal tubules can be affected by other drugs that compete for the same active transport process. Examples of competitive drug interactions include those between

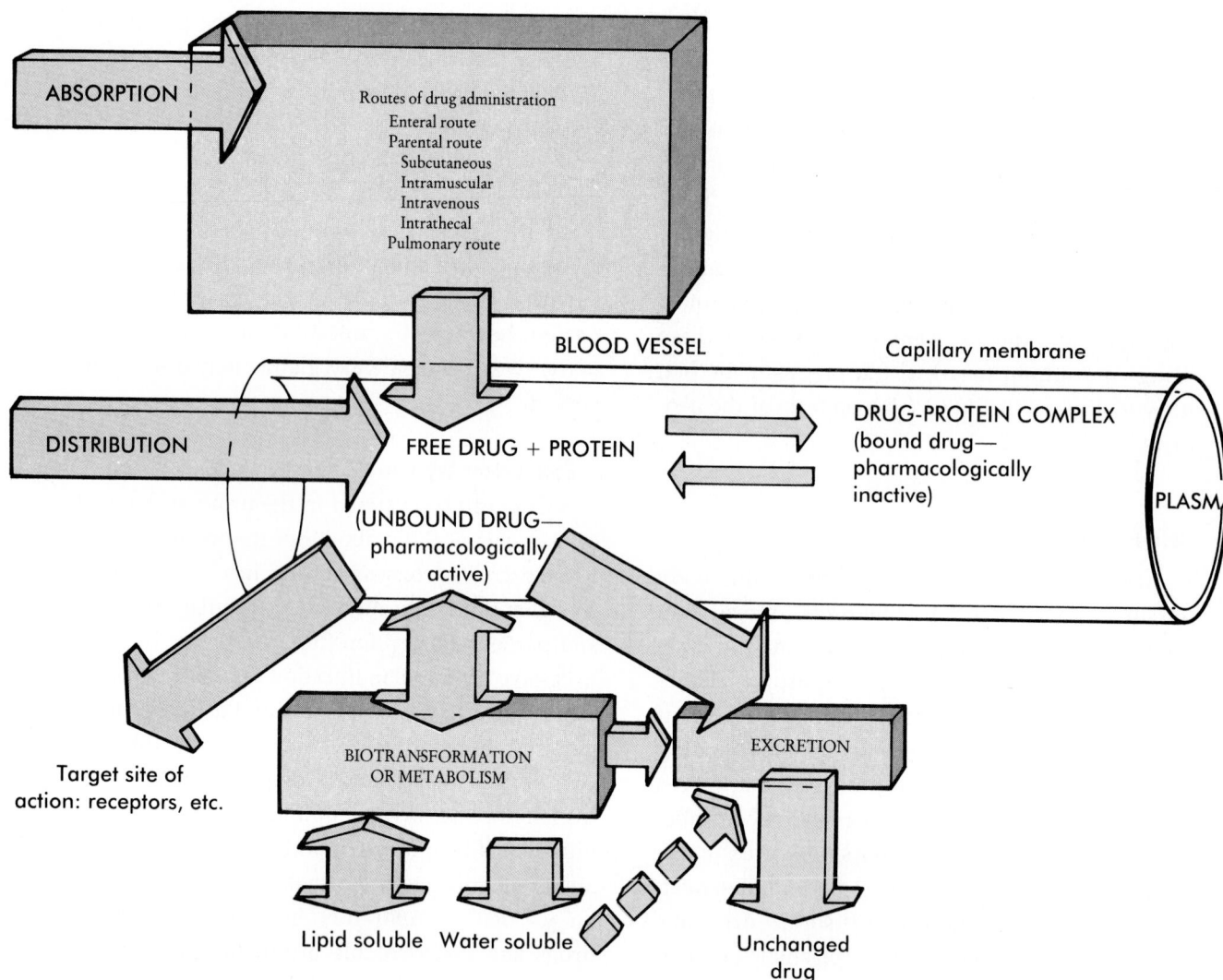

Fig. 14-2 Pharmacokinetic phase of drug action, showing absorption, distribution, biotransformation, and excretion of drugs. Only free drug is capable of movement for absorption, distribution to the target site of action, biotransformation, and excretion; the drug-protein complex represents bound drugs, and because the molecule is large, it is trapped in the blood vessel and serves as a storage site for the drug.

quinidine and *digoxin* and between *verapamil* and *digoxin.* In these examples, the first drug reduces the clearance of the second drug, with a resultant increase in the plasma concentration of the second drug.

Partial reabsorption is reabsorption from the renal tubule by passive diffusion. This reabsorption can be greatly influenced by the pH of the tubular urine, which can vary between 5 and 8. Weak acids are excreted more readily in alkaline urine and more slowly in acidic urine. This is because they are ionized (water soluble) in alkaline urine but nonionized (lipid soluble) in acidic urine. The

reverse is true for weak bases. For example, an increase in urinary pH decreases the reabsorption and increases the clearance of weak acids such as *phenobarbital* and aspirin, whereas a decrease in urinary pH increases the clearance of weak bases such as amphetamine, quinidine, and tricyclic antidepressants.

As a rule, substances that are completely or almost completely excreted by the normal kidney can be removed by an artificial process resembling glomerular filtration. This process, hemodialysis, can be used to remove a wide variety of substances. It is not very effective for drugs that are

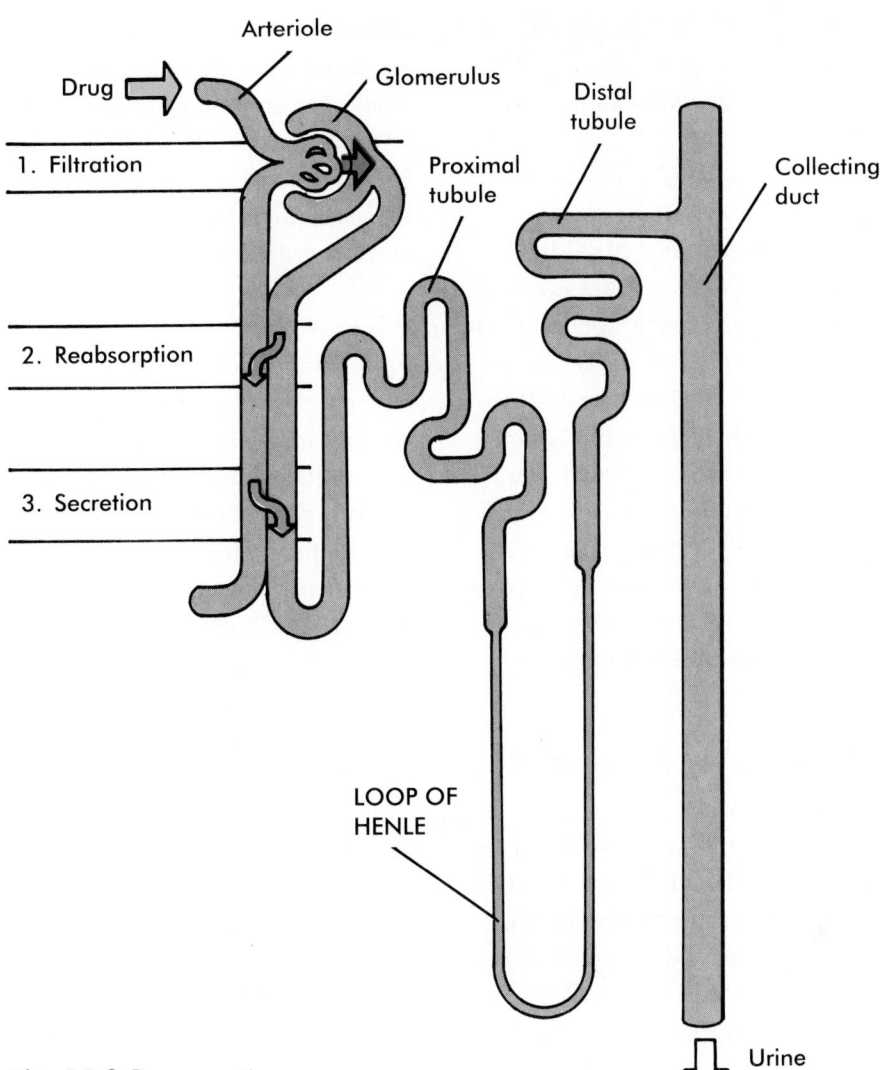

Fig. 14-3 Drug excretion process.

Excretion by the Intestine

Drugs are eliminated through the intestine by biliary excretion. After liver metabolism, the metabolites are carried in bile and passed into the duodenum. The metabolites are then eliminated with the feces. Some drugs are reabsorbed by the blood stream, returned to the liver, and later excreted by the kidneys.

Excretion by the Lungs

Some drugs can be eliminated by the lungs (for example, general anesthetics, volatile alcohols, inhaled bronchodilators). Factors that can alter drug

highly tissue or protein bound and is of limited benefit with rapidly acting toxins.

elimination via the lungs include rate and depth of respiration and cardiac output. Deep breathing and increased cardiac output (which increases pulmonary blood flow) promote excretion. Conversely, the respiratory compromise and decreased cardiac output that may occur during illness or injury can prolong the period required to eliminate drugs through the lungs.

Sweat and Salivary Glands

Sweat is a relatively unimportant means of drug excretion. However, elimination of drugs, their metabolites, or both, via this route can produce some side effects. (Examples include various skin reactions and discoloration of sweat.) Drugs excreted in saliva are usually swallowed and eliminated in the same manner as other orally administered medications. Certain substances given intravenously can be excreted into saliva, causing the individual to describe or complain about the taste of the drug.

Mammary Glands

Many drugs or their metabolites cross the epithelium of the mammary glands and are excreted in breast milk. Breast milk is acidic (pH 6.5), so basic compounds that ionize at this pH (for example, narcotics) achieve high concentrations in this fluid. In contrast, weak acids such as diuretics and barbiturates are less concentrated. Nursing mothers are cautioned not to take any medication except under the supervision of a physician. Mothers are usually advised to take prescribed medications immediately after breast feeding to diminish any risk to the infant.

Factors that Influence the Action of Drugs

Many factors can alter the response to drug therapy, including the age, body mass, gender, pathological state, genetic factors, and psychological factors. The paramedic should recognize these factors and consider individual responses and complications that may result from drug therapy.

Age

It is generally accepted that pediatric and older patients are highly responsive to drugs. This results in part from the immature hepatic and renal systems of the infant and the natural deterioration of these systems in the older adult. These variations in body function can reduce the effectiveness of excretory and metabolic mechanisms. The older patient may also have underlying disease processes that can produce unexpected variations in response to drug therapy. Medication doses for children are usually modified on the basis of body weight or surface area.

Body Mass

Many drugs are given according to body mass (kilograms). There is an indirect relationship between body mass and the final concentration of drug in a particular patient for any given dosage (that is, the larger the patient, the lower the con-

centration for any given dose of drug). The average adult drug dose is calculated on the basis of drug quantity that produces a particular effect in 50% of the population between the ages of 18 and 65 and who weigh approximately 150 pounds (68 kg). The administration of drugs in children is always based on body mass.

Gender

The differences in drug effects on men and women result partially from size differences. Women are usually smaller than men, so they may have higher concentrations of drugs administered without consideration of size. Differences in the relative proportions of fat and water in the bodies of men and women can also produce variations in drug distribution.

Pathological State

Illness or injury and the severity of symptoms can affect the type and amount of drug needed to achieve a desired effect. In addition, underlying disease processes such as circulatory, hepatic, or renal dysfunction can interfere with the physiological processes of drug action and elimination.

Genetic Factors

Genetics can alter the response of some individuals to a number of medications through inherited metabolic (enzymatic) deficiencies or altered receptor-site sensitivities. These pharmacogenetic abnormalities may manifest as idiosyncrasies or be mistaken for drug allergies.

Psychological Factors

A patient's belief in the effects of a drug may strongly influence and potentiate drug effects. For example, a placebo can have the same result as a pharmacological agent if the patient believes the placebo will have the desired effect. In contrast, patient hostility and mistrust can diminish the perceived effects of a drug.

● PHARMACODYNAMIC INTERACTION

One aspect of pharmacodynamics is the study of the mechanism of drug action on living tissue, especially the response of various tissues to specific chemical agents. Drugs do not confer any new function on a tissue or organ of the body. Rather, they modify existing functions. Although there are numerous theories of drug action, most drug actions are thought to result from a chemical interaction between the drug and various receptors throughout the body. The most common form of drug action is the drug receptor interaction.

Drug Receptor Interaction

It is generally believed that most drugs bind to **drug receptors** to produce their desired effect (Box 14-5). According to this theory, a specific portion of the drug molecule (the active site) selectively combines or interacts with some molecular structure (the reactive site on the cell surface or within the cell) to produce a biological effect. These reactive cellular sites are known as **receptors.**

The relationship of a drug to its receptor may be thought of as a key fitting into a lock (Fig. 14-4). The drug represents the key, and the receptor represents the lock. The drug molecule with the best fit to a receptor produces the best response. After absorption, a drug is believed to gain access to a receptor after it leaves the blood stream and is distributed to tissues that contain receptor sites. Drugs that bind to a receptor and cause a physiological response are referred to as *agonists.* Conversely, drugs that bind to a receptor but do not produce any physiological response or whose presence prevents other drugs from binding are referred to as *antagonists.*

Drug Response Relationship

In the prehospital setting, response to drug therapy is usually assessed by observing the pharmacological effect of the drug on easily measured physiological parameters. Examples include monitoring blood pressure after administration of an antihypertensive medication and pain relief after administration of an analgesic. In these situations, the drug response relationship is easily identified and monitored.

Each drug has its own characteristic rate of absorption, distribution, biotransformation, and excretion. Therefore the effectiveness of some drugs cannot be monitored solely by the patient's response. For example, medications such as theophylline, *digoxin* (Lanoxin), and *lidocaine* (Xylocaine) must reach a certain concentration at the target site to achieve the desired effect. Tissue concentrations are often proportional to and can be estimated from serum drug levels. Therapeutic drug levels generally reflect ranges in tissue concentration that relate to a therapeutic response.

Plasma-level profiles (Box 14-6) demonstrate the relationship between the plasma concentration and the level of the therapeutic effectiveness over

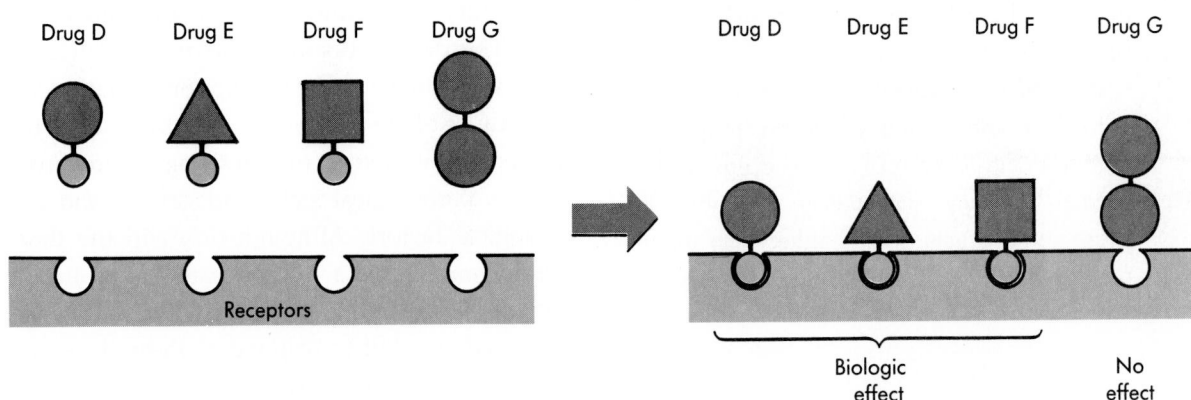

Fig. 14-4 Lock-and-key fit between a drug and the receptors through which it acts. Site on the receptor that interacts with a drug has a definite shape. A drug that conforms to that shape can bind and produce a biological response. In this example, only the shape along the lower surface of the drug molecule is important in determining whether the drug binds to the receptor.

BOX 14-5

Drug Receptor Interaction Terms

Affinity: a drug's propensity to bind or attach itself to a given receptor site

Antagonist: an agent designed to inhibit or counteract effects produced by other drugs; undesired effects caused by cellular components during illness

Efficacy (intrinsic activity): the drug's ability to initiate biological activity as a result of binding to a receptor site

Agonist: a drug possessing affinity and efficacy that combines with receptors and initiates a sequence of biochemical and physiological changes

Antagonist: an agent that inhibits or counteracts effects produced by other drugs or undesired effects caused by normal or hyperactive physiological mechanisms

Competitive antagonist: an agent with an affinity for the same receptor site as an agonist (The competition with the agonist for the site inhibits the action of the agonist; increasing the concentration of the agonist tends to overcome the inhibition. Competitive inhibition responses are usually reversible.)

Noncompetitive antagonist: an agent that combines with different parts of the receptor mechanism and inactivates the receptor so that the agonist cannot be effective regardless of its concentration (Noncompetitive antagonist effects are considered to be irreversible or nearly so.)

Partial antagonist: an agent with affinity and some efficacy but that may antagonize the action of other drugs with greater efficacy (Frequently antagonists share some structural similarities with their agonists.)

BOX 14-6

Plasma-Level Profile Terms

Duration of action: the period from onset of drug action to the time when a drug effect is no longer seen

Loading dose: a bolus of a drug given initially to rapidly attain a therapeutic plasma concentration

Maintenance dose: the amount of drug necessary to maintain a steady therapeutic plasma concentration

Minimum effective concentration: the lowest plasma concentration that produces the desired drug effect

Onset of action or latent period: the interval between the time a drug is administered and the first sign of its effects

Peak plasma level: the highest plasma concentration attained from a dose

Termination of action: the point at which a drug's effect is no longer seen

Therapeutic range: the range of plasma concentrations most likely to produce the desired drug effect with the least likelihood of toxicity (the range between minimum effective concentration and toxic level)

Toxic level: the plasma concentration at which a drug is likely to produce serious adverse effects

---

time (Fig. 14-5). These profiles depend on the rate of absorption, distribution, biotransformation, and excretion after drug administration.

The therapeutic range for most drugs is based on the concentration that provides the highest probability of response with the least risk of toxicity. The dosage (loading and maintenance) required to achieve a therapeutic concentration varies because of the previously described factors that influence the actions of drugs: age, body mass, gender, pathological state, and genetic and psychological factors. Although doses in the therapeutic range have a high probability of efficacy and a low probability of toxicity in most patients, some patients fail to respond to these doses and others may develop toxicity.

Biological Half-Life

The rate of biotransformation and excretion of a drug determines its biological half-life (t½). *Bio-*

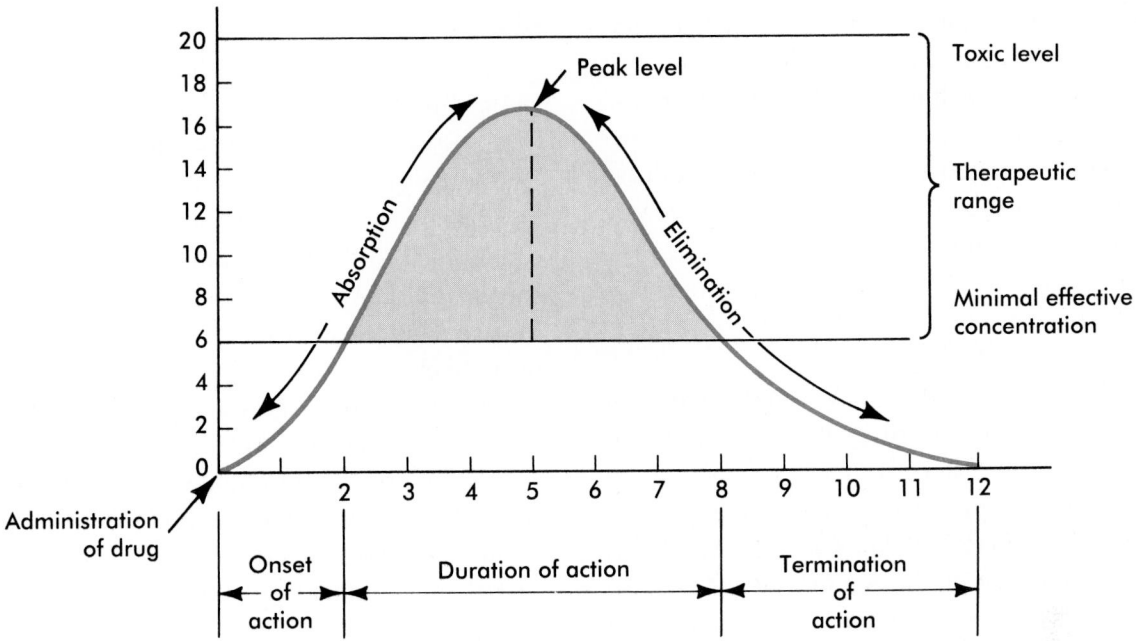

Fig. 14-5 Plasma level profile of a drug.

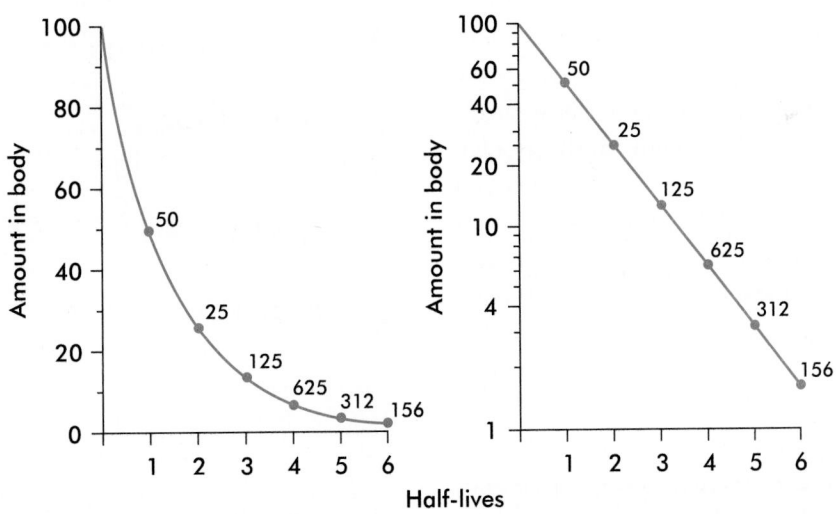

Fig. 14-6 Plots of the amount of drug in the body at each half-life. When the amount is plotted on a cartesian scale *(left)*, an exponential decline is observed. When the amount is plotted on a logarhithmic scale *(right)*, a straight line is observed that is used to determine the half-life.

logical half-life may be defined as the time required to excrete half the amount of drug in the body at the time equilibrium is first established or the time required to excrete half of the total amount of the drug (Fig. 14-6). For example, if a 100-mg injection of *meperidine hydrochloride* (Demerol) is administered and its half-life is 4 hours, 50 mg will be excreted in the first 4 hours, 25 mg (half of the remaining 50 mg) will be excreted in the second 4 hours, and so on. A drug is considered gone from the body after five half-lives have passed.

The half-life of a drug is important when determining the rate of administration. A drug that has a short half-life (for example, 2 to 3 hours) needs to be administered more often to maintain a therapeutic range than a drug with a long half-life, such as 12 hours. The half-life of a drug may be markedly lengthened in persons with hepatic dysfunction or renal disorders. These and other disease processes may require a reduction in drug dosage or an increased interval between doses.

Therapeutic Index

The therapeutic index (TI) is a measurement of the relative safety of a drug. It represents the ratio between two factors: (1) lethal dose 50 (LD 50), the dose of a drug lethal in 50% percent of laboratory animals tested, and (2) effective dose 50 (ED 50), the dose that produces a therapeutic effect in 50% of a similar population. The TI is calculated as follows:

$$TI = \frac{LD\ 50}{ED\ 50}$$

The closer the ratio to 1, the greater the danger in administering the drug to humans. In certain drugs, such as *digoxin* (Lanoxin), the difference between the ED and the LD is small. These drugs are said to have a low TI. In contrast, drugs such as *naloxone* (Narcan) have a wide margin between the ED and LD (a high TI). Paramedics should be familiar with the TIs of emergency medications. Great caution must be taken to avoid toxicity caused by medications administered in the field.

Section Three
Drug Administration

● WEIGHTS AND MEASURES

Three systems for measuring drug dosage are in common use today—the metric system, the apothecary system, and the common household system. Each system deals with units of mass and volume, and any of these three systems may be used by a physician when ordering drugs.

Metric System

The metric system was discussed in Chapter 9, so the following serves as a review (Box 14-7).

The primary unit of mass within the metric system is the gram (g). With prefixes, this unit can be adjusted to express thousands of grams (1 kg equals 1000 g) or thousandths of a gram (1 mg equals 0.001 g). In less common usage are the prefixes *deci* and *centi*, meaning "1/10" and "1/100," respectively.

The primary unit of volume within the metric system is the liter (L). With prefixes, the liter is commonly divided into thousandths (1 L equals 1000 ml) and less commonly into millionths (1 L equals 1,000,000 μl) and hundredths (1 L equals 10 dl). The milliliter (ml) is the metric equivalent of the unit of gas volume, the cubic centimeter (cc).

BOX 14-7

Systems of Equivalents

Metric System
1.0 g = 0.001 kg
1.0 g = 1000 mg
1.0 L = 1000 ml

Apothecary System
1.0 gr = 1/60 dram (dr or l) = 1/480 oz
60 gr = 1 dr
8 dr = 1 oz (or K)
1.0 minim (m) = 1/60 f dr = 1/480 f oz
60 m = 1 f dr (or f l)
8 f dr = 1 f oz (or f K)

Household System
1.0 lb = 16 oz
1.0 pt = ½ quart (qt) = ⅛ gallon (gal)
1.0 pt = 16 f oz = 32 tablespoons (T)
1.0 T = 3 teaspoons (t)
1.0 t = 5 ml
1.0 T = 15 ml
1.0 pt = 480 ml
1.0 qt = 960 ml
1.0 gal = 3.84 L

Apothecary System

The apothecary system is considered less precise and less convenient than the more widely adopted metric system. Only a few medications are now available in units of the apothecary system.

The primary unit of mass in the apothecary system is the grain (gr). The grain was derived from the age-old standard of the weight of a single grain of wheat (approximately 60 mg). Other units of mass used in the apothecary system are the dram, ounce, and pound. A total of 60 gr constitutes 1 dram, and 8 drams equals 1 ounce (see Box 14-7).

The primary unit of volume in the apothecary system is the minim. The minim equals the volume of water that would weigh a grain (approximately 0.005 or 0.006 ml). Other volume measures, which may be considered household measures, are the pint and quart. The equivalent of 60 m is 1 fluid dram (f dr), and 8 f dr equal 1 fluid ounce (f oz).

In written prescriptions, the apothecary system places abbreviations before the numeral. Whole numerical quantities are usually expressed in Roman numerals. (For example, 10 gr would be written as "gr X"). Fractional quantities are usually expressed by Arabic numerals rather than by decimals. (For example, ¼ gr would be written as "gr ¼" rather than "0.25 gr.")

Household System

Household measures include the glass, cup, tablespoon, teaspoon, drop, quart, and pint (see Box 14-7). Standard measures of the household system are not usually available in most homes. For example, the average coffee cup may hold 5 to 9 ounces or more, and the average household teaspoon may hold 4 to 6 ml of liquid. Household measurements are only approximations.

● DRUG CALCULATIONS

While providing emergency care, the paramedic is required to calculate adult and pediatric drug dosages, infusion rates, and the strength of drug solutions and diluted solutions. To perform these tasks, common mathematical skills must be applied in a logical sequence. These skills include a working knowledge of decimals, fractions, and ratios and proportions. This text presents common equations for drug calculations that are accepted within the medical community. Other methods of drug calculations may work as well. The paramedic should choose a method that is precise and reliable. To perform drug calculations:

- Convert all units of measure to the same size and system.
- Assess the computed dosage to determine whether it is reasonable.
- Use one method of dose calculation consistently.

Conversion of All Units of Measure

Units of measure should be converted to the same units as the medication label.

Example: You are to administer 800 μg of **dopamine.** You have 200 mg in 250 ml of intravenous fluid. Convert 800 μg to 0.8 mg so that both measures of weight are in the same units.

When the dose is given per unit of weight, calculate the total dose of drug to be given before performing the drug calculation.

Example: You are to administer 1 mg/kg of lidocaine to a 60-kg patient. Total dose equals 1 mg/kg multiplied by 60 kg, which equals 60 mg.

Assessment of the Computed Dosage

Many emergency drugs are supplied in units that contain enough drug for a normal adult dose. After you have performed your computation, determine whether it is reasonable.

Example: You are to administer 400 mg of **bretylium.** It is supplied in a 10-ml ampule that contains 500 mg of the drug. Therefore a reasonable calculation of volume would be less than 10 ml.

Methods of Calculation

Many drug calculations can be performed almost intuitively, because many drugs are packaged to supply one adult dose. Equations are necessary only when calculations become complicated. There are two methods of calculation in common use:

Method 1:

Method 1 requires that information be substituted in the following formula, which must be memorized for accuracy of computation:

$$\frac{\text{Desired dose to be administered (D)}}{\text{Known dose on hand (H)}} \times$$
$$\text{Unit of measure or volume on hand (Q)} =$$
$$\text{Volume or unit of measure to be administered (X)}$$

$$\frac{D}{H} \times Q = X$$

Example: You are to administer 350 mg of ***aminophylline.*** You have a 10-ml vial that contains 500 mg of the drug. How many milliliters will you give? Using the above formula, calculate the dose.

$$\frac{350 \text{ mg}}{500 \text{ mg}} \times 10 \text{ ml} = X$$
$$\frac{7}{1} \times 1 \text{ ml} = X$$
$$7 \times 1 \text{ ml} = X$$
$$X = 7 \text{ ml}$$

Method 2:

Method 2 uses ratios and proportions to calculate the drug dosage. To use this method, the labeling information should be established initially on one side of the equation. The units of measure must be equivalent throughout the equation:

Desired dose : Desired volume : : Dose on hand :
Volume on hand

Example: You are to administer 40 mg of ***furosemide.*** You have a 10-ml vial that contains 100 mg of the drug. How many milliliters will you give? Using the above formula, calculate the dose.

$$40 \text{ mg} : X : : 100 \text{ mg} : 10 \text{ ml}$$

Multiply inside numbers (means) and outside numbers (extremes).

$$X \times 100 \text{ mg} = 40 \text{ mg} \times 10 \text{ ml}$$

Move all but X to one side of the equation.

$$\frac{X \times 100 \text{ mg}}{100 \text{ mg}} = \frac{40 \text{ mg} \times 10 \text{ ml}}{100 \text{ mg}}$$

Solve for X.

$$X = 4 \text{ ml}$$

Method 2 may also be set up with the ratio expressed as a fraction.

$$\frac{\text{Desired dose}}{X} = \frac{\text{Dose on hand}}{\text{Volume on hand}}$$
$$\frac{40 \text{ mg}}{X} = \frac{100 \text{ mg}}{10 \text{ ml}}$$

Cross multiply.

$$40 \text{ mg} \times 10 \text{ ml} = X \times 100 \text{ mg}$$

Move all but X to one side of the equation.

$$\frac{40 \text{ mg} \times 10 \text{ ml}}{100 \text{ mg}} = \frac{X \times 100 \text{ mg}}{100 \text{ mg}}$$

Solve for X.

$$4 \text{ ml} = X$$

Calculating Infusion Rates

To calculate infusion rates, the paramedic must know the volume to be infused, the period of time over which the fluid is to be infused, and the number of drops per milliliter the infusion set delivers. The infusion rate can then be calculated using the following equation:

$$\text{Drops/min} =$$
$$\frac{\text{Volume to be infused} \times \text{Drops/ml of infusion set}}{\text{Total time of infusion in minutes}}$$

It may be necessary to administer medications via intravenous drip. Calculating the correct drip rate is essential to avoid overdosing or underdosing. To calculate drip rate:

1. Convert all measures to equivalent units.
2. Determine the total volume of drug to be administered (use formula of choice).
3. Calculate the total drops per minute necessary to deliver the prescribed volume over the proper amount of time.

Example: You are to administer a ***lidocaine*** infusion of 2 mg/min. You have a 250-ml bag of fluid that contains 1 g of the drug and microdrip tubing that delivers 60 drops/ml.

Step 1: Convert all units on the drug label (2 mg = 0.002 g).

Step 2: Calculate the correct volume per minute by using an accepted drug formula (for example, ratios, proportions).

$$\frac{D}{H} \times Q = X$$

$$\frac{0.002 \text{ g} \times 250 \text{ ml}}{1 \text{ g}} = X$$

$$X = 0.5 \text{ ml/min}$$

Step 3: Calculate the drip factor using the fluid rate calculation as follows:

$$X = \frac{0.5 \text{ ml} \times 60 \text{ drops/ml}}{1 \text{ min}}$$

Multiply and cancel the appropriate units (ml cancels ml).

$$X = 30 \text{ drops/min}$$

Calculating Pediatric Dosages

The doses of many medications for children are administered in the same proportion to body weight as the doses used for adults. Other medications are given in greatly reduced doses because of differences in the child's ability to metabolize the drug. Pediatric drug doses are often calculated in the prehospital setting using memory aids (for example, charts, dosage books) or with the advice of medical control. Drugs used in the management of pediatric emergencies are further described in the Emergency Drug Index and Chapters 27 and 28.

● DRUG ADMINISTRATION

Safety considerations and procedures should be a high priority during administration of any medication. The paramedic should observe the following guidelines when administering drugs to patients:

- When preparing or giving medicines, concentrate on the procedure and avoid distractions.
- In the prehospital setting, ensure that medication orders received from medical control are clearly understood. Repeat all orders back to medical control for confirmation before administering a drug. If in the emergency department or other patient care areas, make certain that you have a written order for every medication you administer. Verify the patient's name on the armband or identification tag and verify that the patient has no allergy to the medication. Be sure that the *right* patient receives the *right* dose of the *right* drug via the *right* route at the *right* time (the "five patient rights" of drug administration).
- Make a habit of reading the label of the medicine and comparing it to the medication order at least 3 times before administration: when removing the drug from the drug kit or supply area, when preparing the medication for administration, and just before administering it to the patient (before the container is discarded).
- Always verify the route of administration. Some medications can be prepared for administration by several routes (for example, intramuscular or intravenous).
- Make certain that the information on the medication label corresponds exactly to the prescriber's order.
- Never give a medicine from an unlabeled container or from a container on which the label is not legible.
- If you must calculate the dosage of a medication and you are uncertain of your calculation, verify your work on paper and have a co-worker check it.
- Handle multidose vials carefully and with aseptic technique so that medicines are not wasted or contaminated.
- When preparing an injection, always label the syringe immediately. Keep the medication container with the syringe. Do not rely on memory to determine which solution is in which syringe.
- Never administer an unlabeled medication prepared by another person. In doing so, you accept the responsibility for accuracy, dose, and correct medication.
- Never administer a medication that is outdated or that appears discolored, cloudy, or in any other way unusual or tampered with.
- If the patient or your co-workers express doubt or concern about a medication or

dose, recheck to make certain that there is no error before administering the medication. Be aware that the patient has a right to refuse medication.

- Carefully monitor the patient for any adverse effects for at least 5 minutes after administration of any medication. (A longer observation time may be required for intramuscular and oral medications.)
- Document all medications given. This documentation should include the name of the drug, the dosage, and the time and route of administration. When recording parenteral medications, note the site of injection. The patient's response, adverse as well as intended, should be recorded.
- Follow governmental guidelines and local EMS policies regarding the return and disposal of any unused medication.

Medication Errors

Medication errors occur with astonishing frequency. More than 520,000 patients receive the wrong medicine or dose of medicine in U.S. hospitals each year.[5] Common causes of medication errors are:

- A wrong medication dose was ordered by the prescriber.
- Drug calculations were in error.
- Drugs were administered via the wrong route.
- The wrong patient received the drug.

If an incident involving a medication error occurs, the paramedic should:

- Accept professional responsibility for his or her actions.
- Immediately advise medical control or the prescriber.
- Assess and carefully monitor the patient for effects of the drug.
- Document the medication error as required by local and state drug administration policies and those of the medical control institution.
- Modify personal practice to avoid a similar error in the future.

● TECHNIQUES OF DRUG ADMINISTRATION

The various techniques of drug administration used in emergency care include oral, sublingual, parenteral (subcutaneous, intramuscular, and intravenous injections), rectal, ET, skin, and inhalation. Other techniques of drug administration not included in this section are described in pharmacology textbooks.

Oral Route

The oral route is the most frequently used method of drug administration. The patient should be in an upright or sitting position. The pill, tablet, or capsule should be placed in the patient's mouth and swallowed with enough fluid (4 to 8 ounces) to ensure that the drug reaches the stomach.

Many drugs are available in solid and liquid forms. If the medication is in a suspension, the stock bottle or unit dose should be shaken thoroughly before the drug is poured for administration. A drug not packaged as a unit dose should be measured in a medicine cup or by syringe.

Sublingual Route

The most frequently prescribed sublingual drugs are nitrates, which are used to treat angina pectoris. The tablet should be placed under the tongue, where it dissolves. Drinking fluids should be avoided while the drug is being absorbed. If the patient inadvertently swallows the tablet, the effects will be diminished and delayed.

Parenteral Routes

Parenteral administration of drugs includes all forms of drug injection into body tissues or fluids using a syringe and needle or catheter and container. This route of drug administration can be especially hazardous because the drugs given via injection are usually considered irretrievable. In addition, there is a slight chance of infection because the integrity of the skin is broken. Other potential hazards associated with parenteral administration include lipodystrophy, cellulitis or abscess formation, necrosis, skin slough, nerve injury, prolonged pain, and periostitis. Aseptic technique, accurate drug dosage, proper rate of injection, and proper site of injection are essential to avoid harm.

Syringes and Needles

The choice of syringe and needle depends on the route of administration, characteristics of the fluid (for example, aqueous, oil-based), and volume of medication. Syringes in common use today are made of disposable plastic. Sizes range from 1-ml tuberculin and insulin syringes to 60-ml syringes. Tuberculin syringes are marked in 0.01-ml gradients and should be used when the volume to be administered is small. Insulin syringes are available in 0.5- and 1-ml volumes and are marked off in 5-unit increments. When used with the specified strength of insulin, this syringe allows the patient to easily draw up the correct dose without performing calculations. Tuberculin and insulin syringes should not be substituted for each other. Fig. 14-7 illustrates syringes used to accurately measure varying amounts of liquids and liquid medications.

Needles vary in length and gauge from $\frac{3}{8}$ inch to 3 or more inches in length and from 12 gauge (large lumen) to 28 gauge (small lumen). Smaller-lumen (larger gauge) needles are usually used for intradermal injections. Subcutaneous injections are usually given with a $\frac{1}{2}$- or $\frac{5}{8}$-inch, 23- or 25-gauge needle. Intramuscular injections are usually given with a 19- or 21-gauge, $1\frac{1}{2}$- to 2-inch needle; occasionally a 16- or 18-gauge needle is used.

Parenteral Medication Containers

Medications used for injection are usually supplied in single-dose ampules, multidose vials, and prefilled syringes. Single-dose ampules are glass containers that hold one dose of a medication for injection, after which the ampule is discarded. Multidose vials are glass containers equipped with rubber tops that permit several medication doses to be withdrawn for injection.

To prepare a prescribed medication for injection, the paramedic should choose the appropriate needle and syringe. The size of the syringe should be in proportion to the volume of solution to be administered. To withdraw medication from an ampule or vial, the paramedic should follow the following steps (Fig. 14-8):

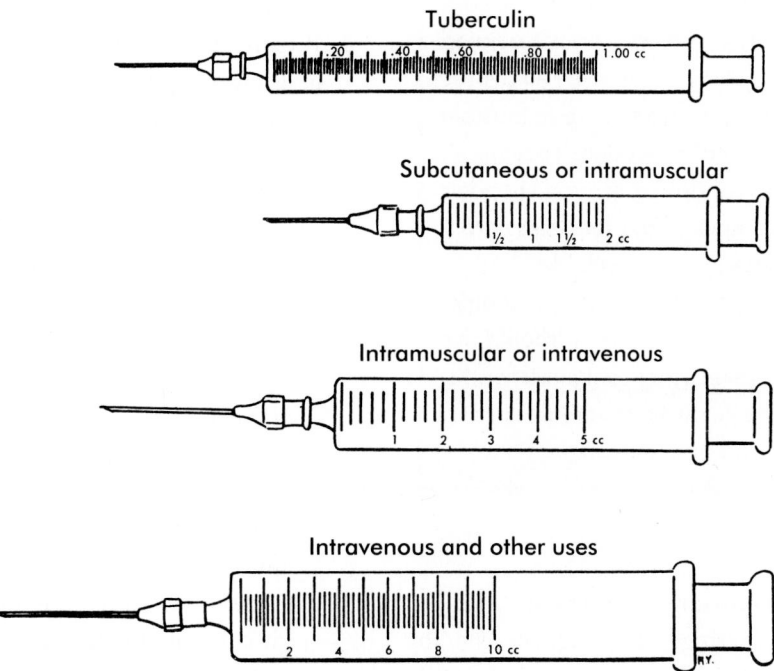

Tuberculin

Subcutaneous or intramuscular

Intramuscular or intravenous

Intravenous and other uses

Fig. 14-7 Syringes used to accurately measure liquids and liquid medication.

Needle Safety

Needle-stick injuries account for a large number of work-related accidents (75 to 150 per 1000 employees each year in teaching hospitals).[6] In addition, the Hepatitis Branch of the Centers for Disease Control has estimated that more than 12,000 health care workers have acquired hepatitis B through needle sticks; 250 to 300 health care workers die each year from the direct or indirect consequences of occupationally acquired hepatitis B. The risk of human immunodeficiency virus (HIV) infection from a single needle-stick exposure to HIV-infected blood is approximately 1 in 200.[7,8] Studies have also reported transmission of at least 20 different pathogens via needle-stick injury, including malaria, syphilis, diphtheria, herpes simplex, herpes zoster, Rocky Mountain spotted fever, and tuberculosis.[9] These findings emphasize the medical consequences of needle-stick injuries. Measures taken to avoid such exposures[9] include:

- Health care personnel should obtain assistance when administering infusion therapy or injections to uncooperative patients.
- Needles should not be recapped, purposely bent or broken by hand, removed from disposable syringes, or otherwise manipulated by hand. If recapping or needle removal is necessary because no alternative is feasible or a specific medical procedure requires it, use of a mechanical device or a one-handed technique is recommended. Needleless products should be used when available.
- Disposable syringes and needles, scalpel blades, and other sharp items should be placed in puncture-resistant containers for disposal and not be allowed to remain among linens or be placed in trash cans.

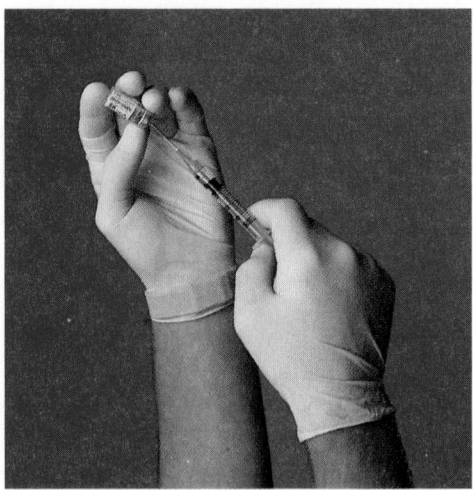

Fig. 14-8 Withdrawing medication from a vial.

1. Assemble the necessary equipment (alcohol swab or gauze, syringe, 18-gauge needle to withdraw medication if using an ampule, and appropriate-gauge needle for injection).
2. Compute the desired volume of medication to be administered.

3. If using a vial:
   a. Clean the rubber stopper with alcohol.
   b. Using the needle chosen for the injection, inject a volume of air into the vial equivalent to the amount of solution to be withdrawn; this prevents a vacuum in the vial, which can make the solution difficult to withdraw. Withdraw the volume required and remove the syringe from the vial.
   c. Gently advance the plunger of the syringe to expel air from the solution.
4. If using an ampule:
   a. Lightly tap or shake the ampule to dislodge any solution from the neck of the container.
   b. Wrap the neck of the glass ampule with an alcohol swab or gauze dressing for protection.
   c. Grasp the ampule, snap off the top, and discard the top in an appropriate medication disposal container. (The ampule is designed to break easily when pressure is exerted at the neck.)
   d. Carefully insert an 18-gauge needle into the solution without allowing it to touch the edges of the ampule and draw the solution into the syringe.
   e. Carefully remove the 18-gauge needle and discard it in the appropriate container. Attach the needle to be used for injection.
   f. Gently advance the plunger of the syringe to expel air.

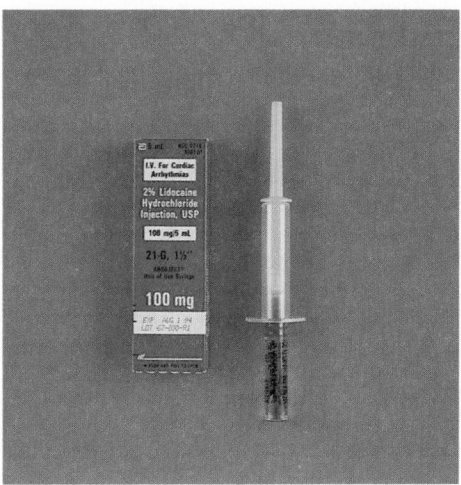

Fig. 14-9 Prefilled syringe for injection of medication.

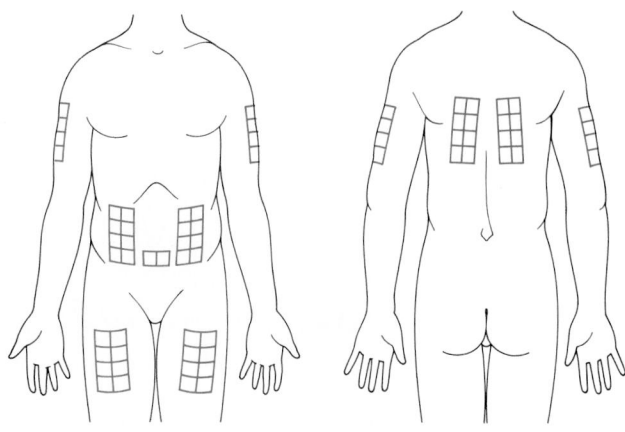

Fig. 14-10 Commonly used subcutaneous injection sites.

> **NOTE:**
> Some hospitals and EMS services require that a filter needle be used as a precaution for glass particles when withdrawing medications from an ampule. An additional precaution is the use of in-line tubing filters for intravenous injections.

There are several manufacturers of prefilled syringes (Fig. 14-9), and the techniques for activating and using the products vary. The paramedic should be familiar with the devices used by particular EMS systems. The technique for activating a common type of prefilled syringe is:

1. Calculate the desired volume of medication to be administered.
2. Pop off the protective caps from the syringe barrel and medication cartridge.
3. Screw the cartridge into the syringe barrel.
4. Gently advance the plunger of the syringe to expel air.

Preparing the Injection Site

The injection site should be prepared in the same manner as for intravenous therapy (see Chapter 13). Cleanse the area with alcohol, iodine swabs, or both, using aseptic technique:

1. Thoroughly scrub the site with alcohol to remove dirt, dead skin, and other surface contaminants.

2. Disinfect the site with overlapping concentric circles, moving outward from the site.
3. Allow the site to dry.

Subcutaneous Injections

Subcutaneous injections are given to place medication below the skin into the subcutaneous layer. The volume of a subcutaneous injection is usually less than 0.5 ml, administered through a ½- or ⅝-inch, 23- or 25-gauge needle. The most common drug administered via this route in the prehospital setting is *epinephrine* (Adrenalin). Common sites for subcutaneous injections are illustrated in Fig. 14-10. The procedure for subcutaneous injections is:

1. Choose the injection site.
2. Hold the skin taut. An alternative method is to elevate the subcutaneous tissue by "pinching" the injection site.
3. With the needle bevel up, insert the needle at a 45-degree angle in one quick motion.
4. Pull back slightly on the plunger (aspirate) to ensure needle placement. If no blood is aspirated, gently but smoothly inject the medication. If blood is present on aspiration, withdraw the needle, discard the medication and equipment, and begin again.
5. After the injection, withdraw the needle at the same angle it was inserted. Use an alcohol swab to massage the site. This helps distribute medication and promote absorption by dilating blood vessels in the area and increasing blood flow.

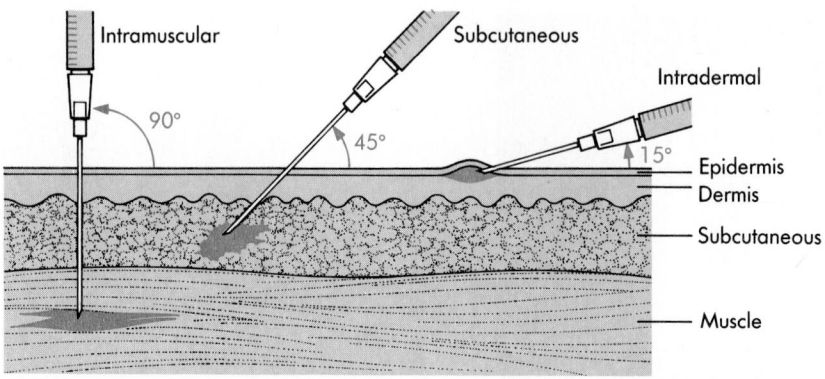

Fig. 14-11 Comparison of angle of injection and location of desposition of medication for intramuscular and subcutaneous injections.

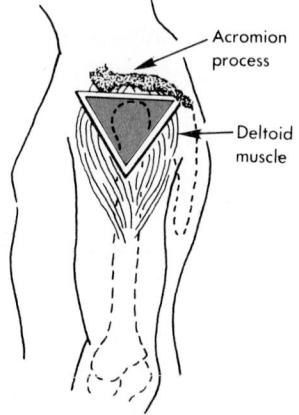

Fig. 14-12 Deltoid muscle injection site roughly forms an inverted triangle, with the acromium process as the base. The muscle may be visible in well-developed patients.

Intramuscular Injections

Deeper injections are made into muscular tissue, passing through the skin and subcutaneous tissue, when a drug is too irritating to be given subcutaneously (although irritation may occur via this route as well) or when a greater volume or faster absorption is desired. A volume up to 5 ml may be given by intramuscular injection.

The type of needle used depends on the site of the injection, condition of the tissue, size of the patient, and nature of the drug to be injected (small lumens for thin solutions and larger lumens for suspensions and oils). Because the muscle layer is below the subcutaneous layer, a longer needle is generally used (usually 1½ inches and 19 or 21

gauge). The procedures for intramuscular injections are the same as those previously described, but the needle is inserted at a 90-degree angle (Fig. 14-11).

Several muscles are commonly used for intramuscular injections, including the deltoid muscle, dorsogluteal site, vastus lateralis muscle, rectus femoris muscle, and ventrogluteal muscle. The deltoid muscle is located in the upper arm. It forms a triangular shape, with the base of the triangle along the acromion process and the peak of the triangle ending approximately a third of the way down the lateral aspect of the upper arm (Fig. 14-12). This muscle is used primarily for vaccinations with small volumes of injection because the muscle is small and can accommodate only small doses of injection (1 ml or less). When injecting in this location, care should be taken to avoid hitting the radial nerve. The patient should be sitting upright or lying flat and should be told to relax the arm muscles.

The dorsogluteal site consists of several gluteal muscles, although the gluteus medius muscle is most commonly used for injection. There are two ways to define this site: (1) Divide the buttocks on one side into imaginary quadrants, and administer the medication into the upper outer quadrant or (2) locate the posterior superior iliac spine and the greater trochanter of the femur, drawing an imaginary line between the two landmarks. The injection is then given up and out from this line (Fig. 14-13). This site should not be used for chil-

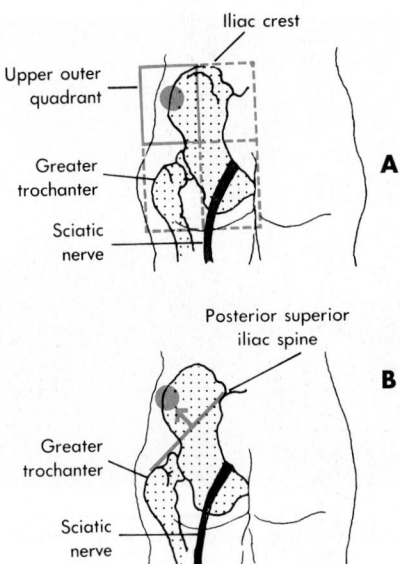

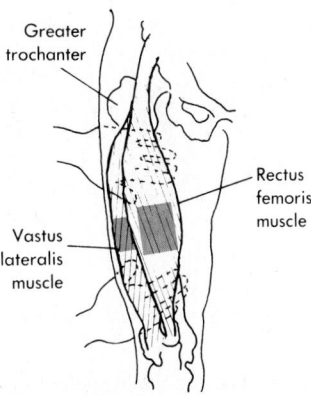

Fig. 14-14 To define the vastus lateralis muscle injection site and the rectus femoral muscle site, place one hand below the patient's greater trochanter and one hand above the knee. The space between the two hands defines the middle third of the underlying muscle. The rectus femoris is on the anterior thigh; the vastus lateralis is on the lateral side.

Fig. 14-13 Two accepted methods for defining the dorsogluteal injection site. **A,** The patient's buttocks can be divided on one side into imaginary quadrants. The center of the upper outer quadrant should be used as the injection site. **B,** The paramedic locates by palpation the posterior superior iliac spine and the greater trochanter and then draws an imaginary line between the two. An injection site up and out from that line should be used.

dren under age 3 because the muscles are not yet well developed and because of the proximity of the sciatic nerve (the largest nerve in the body). Large, well-developed muscles can accommodate an injection up to 5 ml, but anything over 3 ml may be uncomfortable for the patient. When administering an injection via this route, the patient should be lying prone, with the toes pointing inward to promote muscle relaxation. Another complication resulting from gluteal injections is injection into the hip joint, although the risk of this is minimized by attention to anatomical landmarks.

The vastus lateralis and the rectus femoris muscles are located in the thigh and lie side by side. To identify necessary landmarks, the paramedic should place one hand on the patient's upper thigh and one hand on the lower thigh. The area between the paramedic's hands is the middle third of the thigh and the middle third of the underlying muscle (Fig. 14-14). The vastus lateralis lies lateral to the midline and is the preferred injection site for children. It is well developed in all

patients and has few major blood vessels and nerves that can be injured. The rectus femoris is most often used for self-injection because of its accessibility. Acceptable volumes for injection vary with the age of the patient and the size of the muscle. Up to 5 ml may be injected into a well-developed adult. The patient should be sitting upright or lying supine and should be advised to relax his or her muscles.

The ventrogluteal muscle is accessible when the patient lies in a supine or lateral recumbent position. The greater trochanter should be palpated with the palm, with the index finger pointing to the anterior superior iliac spine. The paramedic's remaining three fingers should extend toward the iliac crest. The injection is then made into the center of the V formed between the fingers (Fig. 14-15). This injection site may be used for all patients. It is desirable because the site is free of large nerves and fat tissue. In the adult, this muscle may accommodate up to 5 ml of drug.

Intravenous Injection or Infusion

Medications may be given directly into the vascular system via the intravenous route by injection or infusion. An intravenous injection may be administered through a previously established intravenous infusion line, heparin lock, or implantable

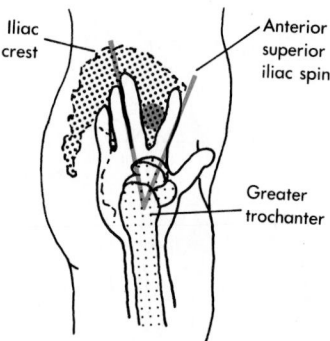

Fig. 14-15 To locate the ventrogluteal muscle injection site, place the palm of one hand on the trochanter of the femur. Make a V with the fingers of that hand, with one side running from the greater trochanter to the anterior-superior iliac spine and the other side running from the greater trochanter to the iliac crest.

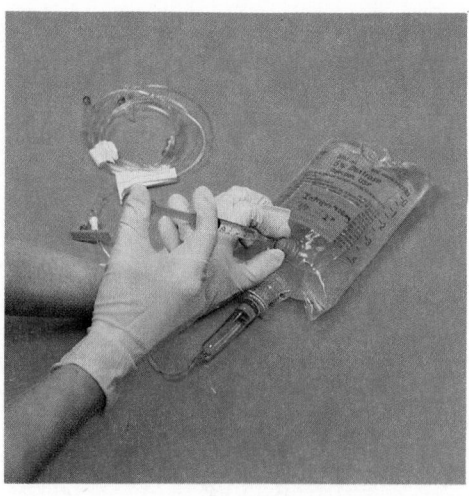

Fig. 14-16 Adding medication to an intravenous reservoir.

port (for example, Port-A-Cath, Hickman catheter). An intravenous infusion is administered by adding a drug to an infusing intravenous solution (for example, normal saline), diluting the drug in a larger volume of fluid and administering the medication through an in-line device (for example, burette, Volutrol, infusion pump), or intermittent infusion ("intravenous piggyback" or "intravenous rider").

Intravenous injections generally consist of a small amount of medication (usually less than 5 ml) and are called *intravenous push* or *intravenous bolus* medications. To administer an intravenous injection, the injection port of the intravenous line should be cleansed with alcohol. The prescribed medication is then injected slowly (usually from 1 to 3 minutes). The rate of injection depends on the type of medication and patient response. Most intravenous tubing is equipped with one-way valves to prevent backflow of medication. If such a value is not present, the tubing above the injection site should be clamped during drug administration. After the injection, the infusion of fluids is continued. Vascular access through implantable ports is described in Chapter 13.

Intravenous infusions can take several forms. To add a medication to the fluid reservoir of an established intravenous line, the paramedic should follow the following steps (Fig. 14-16):

1. Compute the volume of the drug to be added to the fluid reservoir.

2. Draw up the prescribed dose in a syringe. If prefilled syringes are used, note the volume of medication in the syringe and the dose to be used.
3. Cleanse the rubber sleeve of the fluid reservoir with an alcohol swab.
4. Puncture the rubber sleeve and inject the prescribed medication into the fluid reservoir.
5. Withdraw the needle and discard the needle and syringe. Gently mix the medication with the fluid by agitating the reservoir.
6. Label the fluid reservoir with the name of the medication added, amount of the medication added, resultant concentration of the medication in the reservoir, and date, time, and name of the paramedic who prepared the infusion.
7. Calculate the rate of administration in drops per minute as prescribed.

A number of in-line devices allow more accurate delivery of medication diluted in precise amounts of fluids than is possible by simply setting the drip rate. They are often used to administer intravenous medications to children and adults who need precise doses of medication that can readily cause toxicity when administered too rapidly (for example, antidysrhythmics, vasopressors). In-line devices include electronic flow-rate regulators that regulate fluid passage by a magnetically activated metal ball valve and infusion pumps that exert pressure on tubing or fluid by

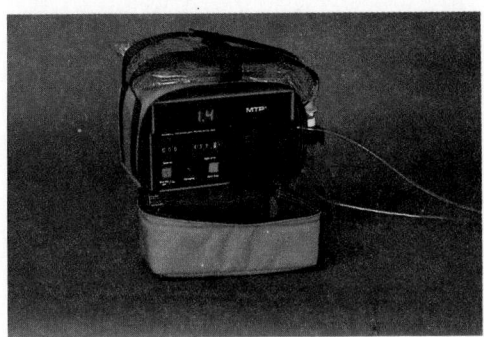

Fig. 14-17 Intravenous infusion pump.

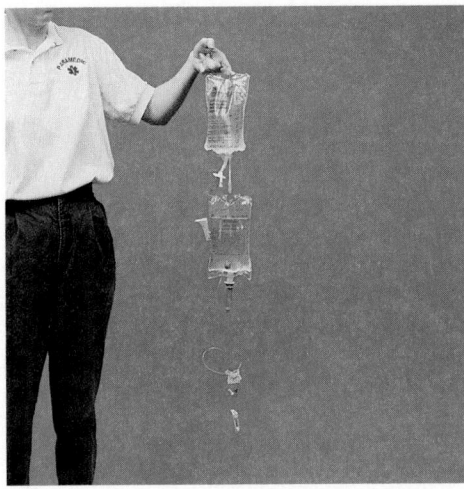

Fig. 14-18 Intravenous piggyback setup.

pumping against pressure gradients. The paramedic should follow the instructions of the equipment manufacturer and become familiar with these devices before using them (Fig. 14-17).

Intermittent infusions are given via a setup that is secondary to the primary intravenous infusion. The piggyback medication is hung in tandem and connected to the primary setup (Fig. 14-18). Most intermittent diluted drug infusions are meant to have a total infusion time of 20 or 30 minutes to 1 hour (depending on the drug and patient response). To prepare an intermittent infusion, the paramedic should follow these steps:

1. Prepare the prescribed medication and add it to the secondary fluid as described above.
2. Bleed the air out of the second administration set and attach a 1-inch, 18-gauge needle.
3. Cleanse the medication port of the primary infusion tubing and insert the needle of the piggyback medication.
4. Tape the needle securely to the medication port.
5. Calculate the flow rate of the secondary infusion in drops per minute.
6. Lower the primary infusion reservoir so that its center of gravity is lower than the secondary infusion reservoir.
7. Open the piggyback line flow clamp, and adjust the flow rate to the desired dose. Clamp the tubing of the primary infusion to allow the piggyback medication to infuse.
8. After administration of the piggyback medication, restart the primary infusion, and discard the piggyback equipment.
9. Always label the bag with the medication.

Another device for intravenous drug administration is a drug "pump." Drug pumps are used by patients who need to slow injection of medication in the home (for example, patients undergoing cancer chemotherapy). These devices usually consist of a syringe with a battery attachment that regulates the injection of medication. Drug pumps are used to administer medication subcutaneously or can be attached to an infusion port such as the Port-A-Cath or Hickman catheter.

Skin Application

In addition to the various emollients and antibiotic ointments, the most commonly used transdermal emergency medication is nitroglycerin. Two types of topical nitroglycerin preparations are available: *nitropaste* (Nitro-Bid Ointment) and transdermal nitroglycerin delivery patches. These medications can be applied to any clean, dry area of the upper arm or hair-free portion of the chest. *Nitropaste* has a lanolin-petrolatum base and is applied in ½-inch increments. Transdermal nitroglycerin patches are adhesive backed and are available in a solid or semisolid form (depending on the manufacturer). The paramedic should always wear gloves when applying or removing these medications to prevent inadvertent self-absorption of the medication. Fig. 14-19 and the Emergency Drug Index offer additional information.

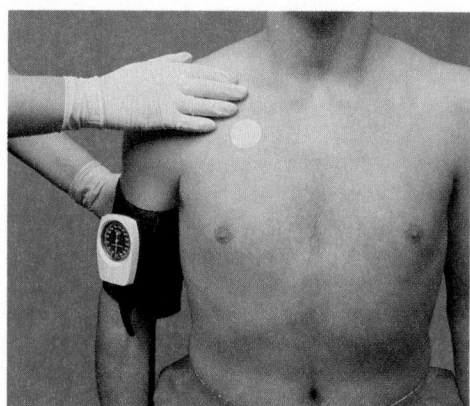

Fig. 14-19 Application of nitroglycerin paste and a nitroglycerin patch.

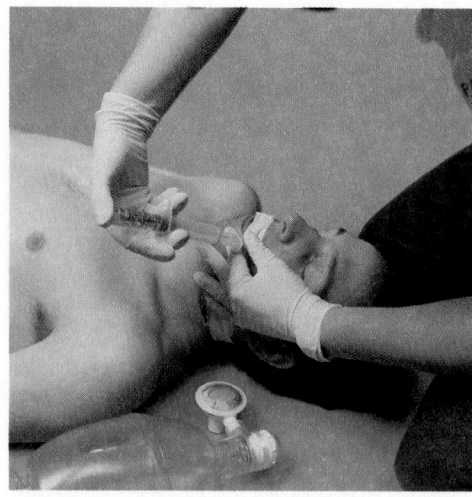

Fig. 14-20 Drug administration via an ET tube.

Drugs such as scopolamine, clonidine, and estrogen are also used in patch form. These drug patches can influence the patient unfavorably during illness. They should be recognized by the paramedic and removed if indicated. Usual sites are postauricular areas and the chest, back, and upper arms.

ET Route

The ET route of drug administration is an alternative that may be used when intravenous access cannot be established. The emergency drugs typically administered via this route include *naloxone* (Narcan), *atropine, epinephrine* (Adrenalin), and *lidocaine* (Xylocaine). When administering medication via this route, the paramedic should follow these steps (Fig. 14-20):

1. Ensure adequate oxygenation and ventilation of the patient's lungs.
2. Prepare the medication (per medical control) so that it is 2 to 2½ times the intravenous dose, and dilute the dose to 10 ml with normal saline.
3. Hyperventilate the patient's lungs.
4. Remove the air source from the ET tube and inject the medication through a catheter deep into the tube.
5. Resume ventilations with several large ventilations to help ensure that the medication

gets as deep into the pulmonary tree as possible (to enhance absorption).
6. Monitor the patient for the desired therapeutic effect and any possible side effects.

Inhalation

In addition to *oxygen* and *nitrous oxide* (Nitronox), several other drugs may be administered via inhalation. These include bronchodilators, corticosteroids, antibiotics, and mucokinetic agents delivered through aerosolization.

Aerosols are liquid or solid particles of a substance dispersed in gas or solution. The effectiveness of aerosolization therapy depends on the number of droplets that can be suspended in the gas or solution, particle size (diameter in microns), output (cc/min), and rate and depth of the patient's breathing. Rapid, shallow breathing decreases the number and retention of droplets reaching the deep bronchioles of the lungs. Delivery of medications by aerosolization offers certain advantages over other routes, including rapid onset and reduced systemic side effects.

Aerosols are produced by devices called *nebulizers*. The most common nebulizers are intermittent positive pressure breathing (IPPB) devices (designed for in-hospital use), metered-dose inhalers (pressure cartridges), and hand-held nebuliz-

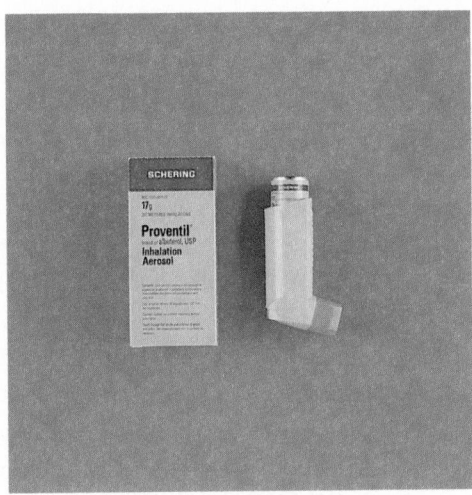

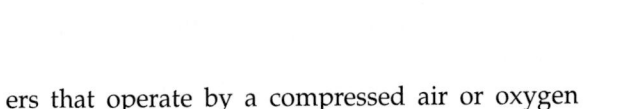

Fig. 14-21 MDI.

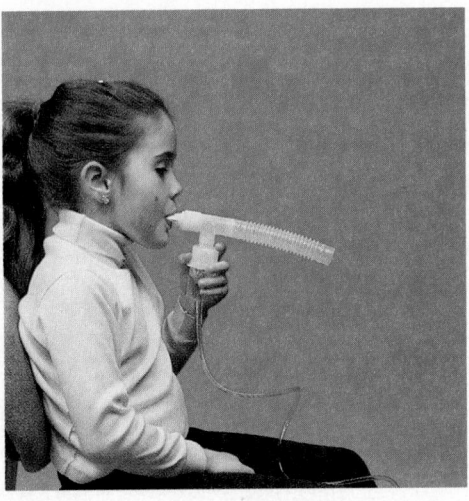

Fig. 14-22 Administration of medication via a hand-held nebulizer.

ers that operate by a compressed air or oxygen source regulated by a flowmeter.

Metered-Dose Inhaler

The metered-dose inhaler (MDI) (Fig. 14-21) has emerged as the most commonly used device in aerosol therapy. It is convenient and delivers a measured dose with each push of the cartridge. MDIs are typically prescribed for self-treatment of asthma, but prehospital use of these devices by paramedics is increasing. Medications prepared in MDIs include *albuterol* (Proventil, Ventolin), *terbutaline* (Brethine), and *isoetharine* (Bronkosol). To prepare a medication for inhalation via this method, the paramedic should follow the following steps:

1. Remove the mouthpiece and protective cap from the bottle.
2. Carefully snap off the cap and turn the mouthpiece sideways.
3. Insert the bottle stem into the hole inside the mouthpiece.
4. Shake the MDI well.
5. Invert the bottle and place the mouthpiece near the patient's mouth. Advise the patient to exhale, pushing as much air from the lungs as possible.
6. Place the mouthpiece in the patient's mouth and instruct the patient to close his or her lips

loosely around it with the tongue underneath the mouthpiece. As the patient inhales deeply over 5 seconds, press the bottle and mouthpiece together quickly and then release it.

7. Instruct the patient to hold his or her breath 5 to 10 seconds before exhaling.
8. Repeat the procedure in 5 to 10 minutes to take advantage of possible deeper penetration by a second round of therapy.

Hand-Held Nebulizers

Hand-held nebulizers are another method of administering some medications via inhalation in the prehospital setting. Disposable nebulizer kits are available from various manufacturers and usually include a mouthpiece, aerosol mask, and reservoir tubing (Fig. 14-22). These devices are attached to a nonhumidified portable or on-board oxygen source and use the Bernoulli principle to create an aerosol mist (sometimes referred to as a *jet* or *pneumatic nebulizer*). Medications appropriate for nebulization therapy include *albuterol* (Proventil, Ventolin), *terbutaline* (Brethine), *metaproterenol* (Alupent), isoetharine (Bronkosol), and *atropine sulfate*.

To administer a medication via a hand-held nebulizer, the paramedic should follow these steps:

NOTE:

The specific procedure may vary slightly depending on the patient's ability to tolerate the treatment by mouthpiece or mask only. A tight seal around the mouthpiece is required, so the patient must be able to cooperate during treatment. (Medication aerosolization may be administered by mouthpiece or mask. Each has an advantage, in that treatment by mouthpiece lessens the amount of medication wasted, but patients with severe dyspnea who are mouth breathers tolerate mask administration much better.)

1. The prescribed drug is mixed (using aseptic technique) with a specified amount of normal saline and instilled in the nebulizer. Some medications are available in a packaged unit dose and contain a fixed amount of diluent (usually 0.9% normal saline).
2. The nebulizer is then attached to a T-piece and mouthpiece and connected to the unit delivering nonhumidified *oxygen* or compressed gas with connecting tubing. (If a patient is unable to use the mouthpiece, a simple face mask may be used in its place.)
3. The oxygen flowmeter should be adjusted to 4 to 6 L/min to produce a steady, visible mist. (A flow rate of 4 to 6 L usually provides a steady production of mist without excessive medication waste. The higher the flow rate, the greater the medication use.) If an aerosol mask is used, the flow rate of *oxygen* should be maintained at 6 to 10 L/min to prevent potential build-up of exhaled carbon dioxide in the mask.
4. When the mist is visible, the patient should begin treatment. Instruct the patient to inhale slowly and deeply by mouth and to hold a breath 3 to 5 seconds before exhaling. This technique causes topical deposition of the aerosol particles deep within the tracheobronchial tree. Inhalation and exhalation should be continued until the aerosol canister is depleted of the medication. Repeat

treatments are usually not given more often than every 15 to 20 minutes (usually to a maximum of three).

Nebulization therapy requires a cooperative patient who can be instructed to breathe deeply so that the drug can be absorbed. If the patient cannot inhale the drug or if the bronchospasm is severe enough to make nebulization therapy ineffective, administration of medication via another route (for example, subcutaneous injection of *epinephrine*) should be considered. If during the course of treatment by aerosolization significant changes in heart rate or dysrhythmias are noted, the treatment should be stopped, and medical control should be contacted for further orders. Paramedics and ambulance crew should avoid the medication vapor stream during nebulization therapy.

● SPECIAL CONSIDERATIONS FOR PEDIATRIC PATIENTS

Pharmacological considerations for pediatric patients have been described throughout this section and are presented during the remainder of this text. The following summary is intended to serve as a review of the pharmacokinetics that influence dosing principles in the neonate and pediatric populations.

Age

The effects of drugs are rather unpredictable among neonates because of the variation in the development and maturation of the different organ systems.

Absorption

Drug absorption in infants and children follows the same general principles as in adults. Factors that influence drug absorption include blood flow at the site of intramuscular or subcutaneous administration as determined by the patient's physiological status and, for orally administered drugs, the underlying gastrointestinal function. Physiological conditions that might reduce blood flow to the muscle and subcutaneous tissue include cardiogenic shock, vasoconstriction caused by sympathomimetic agents, and heart failure. The smaller muscle mass of the infant further complicates drug absorption because of diminished peripheral perfusion to these areas.

Liquids and suspensions disperse quickly in gastrointestinal fluids and are therefore more readily absorbed than tablet or capsule medications. Increases in peristalsis (for example, diarrheal conditions) and lowered gastrointestinal enzyme activities tend to decrease overall absorption of orally or rectally administered medications.

Distribution

Because most drugs are distributed in body water, increases in total body water and extracellular volume can increase the volume of drug distribution. Compared with adults, neonates have proportionately higher volumes of total body water (70% to 75% versus 50% to 60%), and a higher ratio of extracellular to intracellular fluid (40% versus 30%); higher dosages of water-soluble drugs may be needed to achieve effective blood levels in the newborn.

Another major factor determining drug distribution is drug binding to plasma proteins. In general, protein binding of drugs is reduced in the neonate, so the concentration of free drug in plasma is increased. This can result in a greater drug effect or toxicity. Regarding central nervous system effects, the blood-brain barrier in the newborn is much less effective than in adults, allowing drugs greater access to this area.

Biotransformation

Various liver enzyme systems for metabolism generally mature unevenly. Because of the neonate's decreased ability to metabolize drugs, many drugs have slow clearances and prolonged half-lives in the body. This predisposes the neonate toward developing toxicity from drugs metabolized by the liver unless doses are adjusted accordingly.

Elimination

The GFR is much lower in newborns than in older infants, children, and adults. Therefore drugs eliminated through renal function are cleared from the body very slowly in the first few weeks of life. Renal excretory mechanisms progress to maturity after 1 year of age. Before that age, excretion of some substances through the renal system may be delayed because of immaturity, resulting in higher serum levels and a longer duration of action than intended.

Guidelines for Drug Administration

Administering medications to infants and children can be quite difficult, particularly in emergency situations. The following guidelines for drug administration help the paramedic:

- Try to establish a positive relationship and accept the child's fearful or anxious behavior as a natural response.
- Be honest when a medication or procedure will be unpleasant or painful.
- If appropriate, allow the child to help administer the medication (for example, holding the medicine cup or placing a pill in the mouth).
- Use only mild physical restraint if it is required and explain to the child why it is necessary.
- When parenteral medications are required, make certain the injection site is well stabilized and that the injection is given quickly. Two or more persons should be available for children over 4 years of age despite promises that they will "hold still."
- Remember when administering medications that the younger and smaller the child, the narrower the margin for error.

● SPECIAL CONSIDERATIONS FOR OLDER ADULTS

Important changes in drug responses occur with increasing age in most individuals. Factors associated with aging that significantly affect pharmacokinetics include increased incidence of multiple diseases with a concomitant use of medications, nutritional problems, decreasing clearance efficiency, and the possibility of decreased dosing compliance for a variety of reasons. This summary is intended to serve as a review of the pharmacokinetics that influence dosing principles in the older adult.

Age

Declines in the functional capacity of most major organ systems begin in young adulthood and continue throughout life. Thus older adults do not lose specific function at an accelerated rate compared with young and middle-aged adults but rather experience a depleting physiological reserve. It is generally accepted that a linear decrease in physiological function (GFR, cardiac function, maximal breathing capacity) begins no later than age 45. The most important for administration of medications is decreased renal function.

Absorption

Although there is little evidence of major alterations in drug absorption with age, conditions associated with age may alter the rate at which some drugs are absorbed. Examples of these conditions include altered nutritional habits, greater consumption of nonprescription drugs (for example, antacids, laxatives), and changes in gastric emptying. Reduced gastric acid and slowed gastric motility may result in unpredictable rates of dissolution and absorption of weakly acidic drugs.

Distribution

Changes in body composition, such as reduced lean body mass, reduced total body water, and increased fats as a percentage of body mass, have been noted in the older adult. There is also usually a decrease in levels of serum albumin, which binds many drugs, especially weak acids. This affects drug distribution by decreasing the volume in which drugs circulate, which results in increased amounts of free drug in the circulation.

Thus the ratio of bound to free drug in these patients may be significantly altered.

Biotransformation

The capacity of the liver to metabolize drugs does not appear to decline consistently with age for all drugs. However, disorders common with aging, such as congestive heart failure, can impair liver function. In addition, there is a decline of the hepatic recovery from injury such as that caused by alcohol or viral hepatitis.

It is generally believed that certain drugs are metabolized more slowly in the older adult population because of decreased liver blood flow. This decrease may lead to drug accumulation and toxicity. Exercise caution when administering medication metabolized primarily in the liver to a patient with a history of liver disease. Older patients with severe nutritional deficiencies may also have impaired hepatic function.

Elimination

Renal function is the most important factor for clearance of most drugs from the body. The natural reduction in function associated with aging is usually caused by loss of functioning nephrons and decreased blood flow, both of which result in a decreased GFR. A decrease in renal function caused by decreases in renal blood flow may also be secondary to congestive heart failure. The practical result of renal impairment is a marked prolongation of the half-life of many drugs and the possibility of accumulation to toxic levels. Other conditions (for example, dehydration) can cause additional reduction in renal clearance of drugs, which is usually reversible.

Drug Administration Problems

Intentional and unintentional noncompliance with medication therapy may be common in older patients. Although this rarely influences the administration of emergency medications, the paramedic should be familiar with the most common factors that contribute to drug administration problems in older adults, particularly because noncompliance or medication errors may be a precipitating factor in the patient's condition. Some common causes of noncompliance and medication errors are:

- The expense of drugs may lead to noncompliance in patients with fixed incomes. Older patients may not routinely take prescribed medications or may be unwilling to receive medications in emergency situations.
- Noncompliance in taking prescribed medications may result from forgetfulness or confusion, especially if the patient has several prescriptions and different dosing intervals.
- Older patients may forget instructions on the need to complete medication because their symptoms have disappeared. Disappearance of symptoms is often regarded as the best reason to stop the therapy.
- Errors in self-administered medications may result from physical disabilities such as arthritis or visual impairment.
- Noncompliance may be deliberate. A patient may be opposed to taking a drug because of past experiences. A careful drug history is especially important when caring for older adults. The paramedic should remember that the patient usually has the right to refuse medication.

Section Four
Drugs Affecting the Nervous System

● REVIEW OF ANATOMY AND PHYSIOLOGY OF THE NERVOUS SYSTEM

The subdivisions of the nervous system include the central nervous system, the peripheral nervous system, the somatic nervous system, and the autonomic nervous system. The following is a review of the anatomy and physiology of the autonomic division of the peripheral nervous system as it pertains to pharmacology (Box 14-8).

BOX 14-8

Emergency Drugs: Nervous System

atropine sulfate (Atropine)
diazepam (Valium)
dopamine (Dobutrex)
epinephrine (Adrenalin)
isoproterenol (Isuprel)
labetalol (Normodyne)
magnesium sulfate
meperidine (Demerol)
morphine (morphine sulfate)
naloxone hydrochloride (Narcan)
norepinephrine (Levophed)
pancuronium (Pavulon)
phenobarbital (Luminal)
phenytoin (Dilantin)
physostigmine (Antilirium)
propranolol (Inderal)
succinylcholine (Anectine)

Autonomic Division of the Peripheral Nervous System

Anatomical and physiological differences within the autonomic division of the peripheral nervous system are the basis for its further subdivision into sympathetic and parasympathetic components. The cell bodies of the neurons in these two divisions are located in different areas of the central nervous system and leave at different levels, the sympathetic from the thoracic and lumbar regions of the spinal cord and the parasympathetic from the cranial and sacral portions of the spinal cord. Although the two divisions leave at different levels, the heart, many glands, and smooth muscles are innervated by both sympathetic and parasympathetic nerve fibers (Fig. 14-23).

Preganglionic and Postganglionic Neurons

Autonomic intervention by the sympathetic and parasympathetic nervous system may be viewed

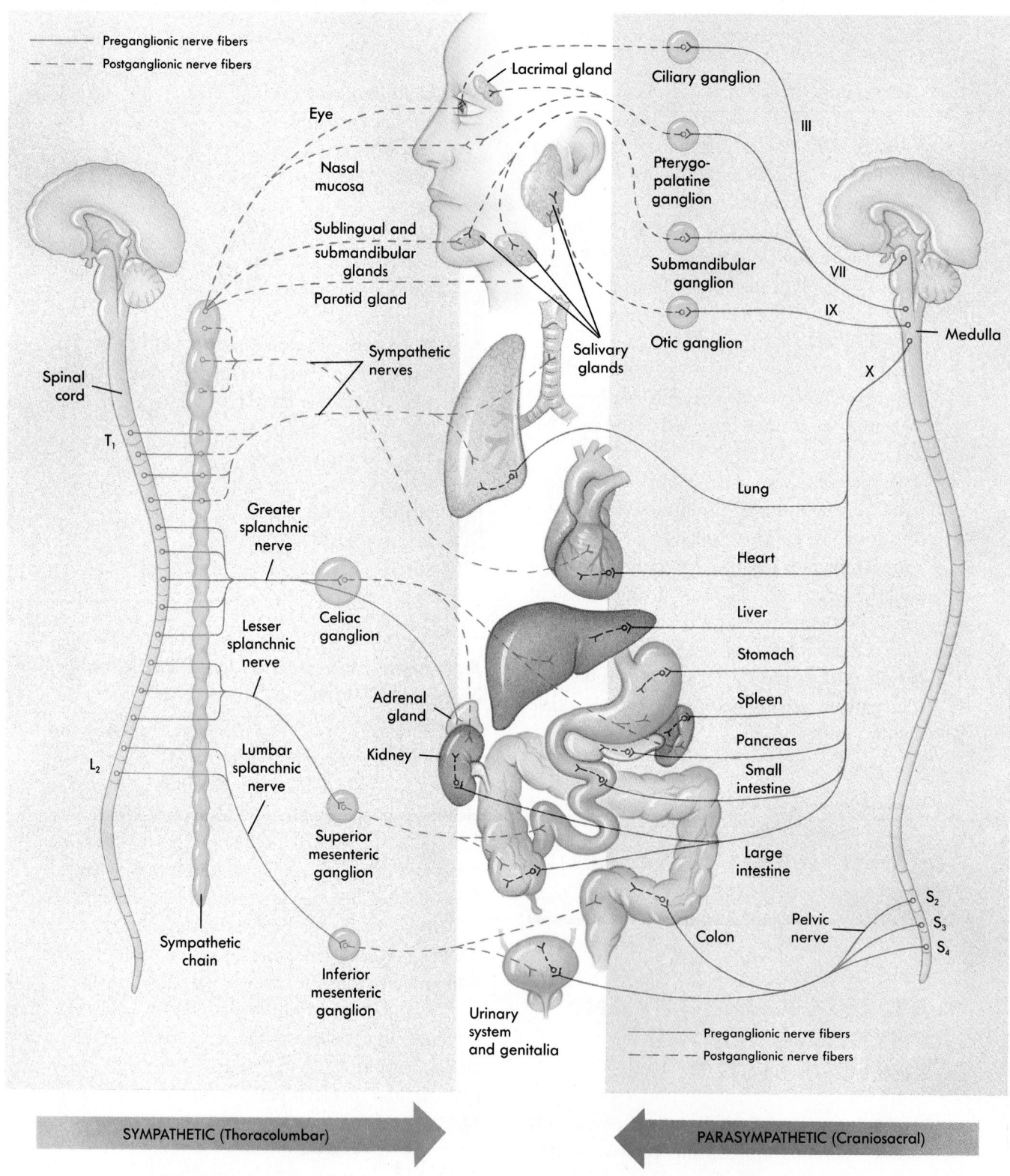

Preganglionic nerve fibers
Postganglionic nerve fibers

Lacrimal gland
Eye
Nasal mucosa
Sublingual and submandibular glands
Parotid gland
Spinal cord
Sympathetic nerves
Salivary glands
Ciliary ganglion
Pterygo-palatine ganglion
Submandibular ganglion
Otic ganglion
Medulla
III
VII
IX
X
T₁
Greater splanchnic nerve
Lesser splanchnic nerve
Celiac ganglion
Adrenal gland
Kidney
Lumbar splanchnic nerve
L₂
Superior mesenteric ganglion
Sympathetic chain
Inferior mesenteric ganglion
Urinary system and genitalia
Lung
Heart
Liver
Stomach
Spleen
Pancreas
Small intestine
Large intestine
Colon
Pelvic nerve
S₂
S₃
S₄
Preganglionic nerve fibers
Postganglionic nerve fibers

SYMPATHETIC (Thoracolumbar)   PARASYMPATHETIC (Craniosacral)

Fig. 14-23 Innervation of major target organs by the autonomic nervous system. Preganglionic fibers are indicated by solid lines, and postganglionic fibers are indicated by broken lines.

as involving a two-neuron chain that exists in a series between the central nervous system and the effector organs. This two-neuron chain comprises a preganglionic neuron located in the central nervous system and a postganglionic neuron located in the periphery. The preganglionic fibers pass between the central nervous system and the ganglia. The postganglionic fibers pass between the ganglia and the effector organ. Many of the sympathetic ganglia lie close to the spinal cord, whereas others lie approximately midway between the spinal cord and the effector organ. The parasympathetic ganglia lie close to or within the walls of the effector organ. The anatomical area that serves as a functional junction between these two neurons is known as a *synapse*.

Cholinergic and Adrenergic Fibers

In sympathetic and parasympathetic divisions, the neurotransmitter for the ganglionic synapse between preganglionic and postganglionic fibers is acetylcholine. The neurotransmitter at the junction between the parasympathetic postganglionic fiber and the effector cell is also acetylcholine. Fibers that release acetylcholine are known as **cholinergic** fibers. All preganglionic neurons of the sympathetic division and all postganglionic neurons of the parasympathetic division are cholinergic.

The neurotransmitter between the sympathetic postganglionic fiber and the effector cell is *norepinephrine,* a member of the catecholamine family. Fibers that release norepinephrine are known as **adrenergic** fibers (a term derived from *noradrenalin,* the British name for norepinephrine). Most postganglionic neurons of the sympathetic division are adrenergic, but a few are cholinergic. The actions of the autonomic nervous system depend on the neurotransmitter released by the ganglionic cells and the effector cells receptor site. For example, stimulation of the sympathetic nerves cause excitatory effects in some organs and inhibitory effects in others. Likewise, parasympathetic stimulation causes excitation in some organs but inhibition in others.

Both systems function continuously, and they occasionally react in a reciprocal fashion. However, most organs are dominantly controlled by one of the two systems. In general, the sympathetic system dominates during stressful events, and the parasympathetic system is most active during periods of emotional and physical calm.

Transmission of Nerve Impulses

The occurrence of neurotransmitters and a number of different receptors provide the basis for the variability in response from stimulation of sympathetic and parasympathetic nerves (excitatory or inhibitory) (Fig. 14-24). For cholinergic synapses, acetylcholine molecules combine with cholinergic receptor molecules. These cholinergic receptors exist in two structurally different forms, nicotinic and muscarinic. Although acetylcholine binds to and activates both types of receptor molecules, nicotine (an alkaloid substance found in tobacco) specifically binds to and activates nicotinic receptors but not muscarinic receptors. Muscarine, an alkaloid extracted from some poisonous mushrooms, specifically binds to and activates muscarinic receptors but not nicotinic receptors. Although nicotine and muscarine are not naturally present in the human body, they demonstrate differences in the two classes of cholinergic receptors.

When acetylcholine binds to nicotinic receptors, there is an excitatory response. When it binds with muscarinic receptors, it results in excitation or inhibition, depending on the target tissue in which the receptors are found. Acetylcholine binding to muscarinic receptors in cardiac muscle causes reduced heart rate; acetylcholine binding to muscarinic receptors in smooth muscle cells of the gastrointestinal tract causes an increased rate and amplitude of contraction. *Atropine* blocks muscarinic but not nicotinic receptor sites (thereby affecting heart rate while not causing paralysis). In contrast, curare is a nicotinic receptor blocker, causing paralysis.

For adrenergic synapses, norepinephrine molecules combine with adrenergic receptor molecules within the membranes of the effector organ. These receptors belong to two structural categories: the alpha adrenergic receptors (alpha receptors), and the beta adrenergic receptors (beta receptors). Norepinephrine binds to and activates

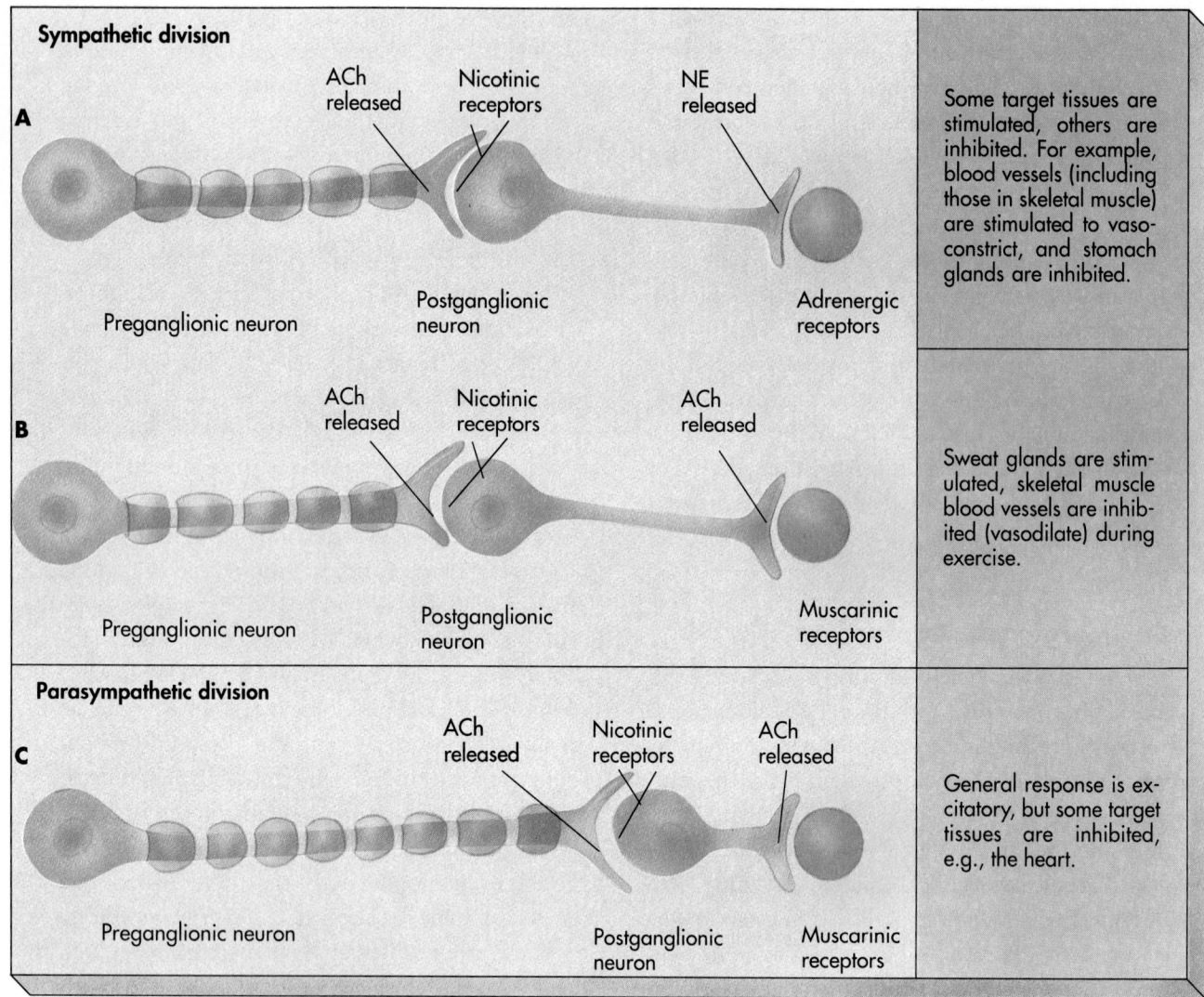

Fig. 14-24 Location of the nicotinic, muscarinic, and adrenergic receptors in the autonomic nervous system. Nicotinic receptors are on the cell bodies of sympathetic and parasympathetic postganglionic cells in the autonomic ganglia. **A,** Adrenergic receptors are in most target tissues innervated by the sympathetic division. **B,** Some sympathetic target tissues have muscarinic receptors. **C,** All parasympathetic target tissues have muscarinic receptors. *NE,* Norepinephrine; *ACh,* acetylcholine.

both types of receptor molecules, although it has more affinity for alpha receptors. *Epinephrine,* a hormone produced by the adrenal medulla, is also classified as an adrenergic substance and has nearly equal affinity for both receptors. In tissues containing alpha and beta receptor cells, one type is more abundant and thus has a dominating effect. Both receptors can be excitatory or inhibitory. For example, beta receptors are stimulatory in cardiac muscle but inhibitory in intestinal smooth muscle (Table 14-3).

● NARCOTIC ANALGESICS AND ANTAGONISTS

Narcotic analgesics relieve pain. Narcotic antagonists reverse the narcotic effects of some analgesics. Pain has two components: the sensation of pain, which involves the nerve pathways and the brain, and the emotional response to pain, which may be a result of anxiety level, previous pain experience, age, gender, and culture. Classifications of pain are listed and defined in Box 14-9.

TABLE 14-3 Autonomic Innervation of Target Tissues

Organ	Effect of Sympathetic Stimulation	Effect of Parasympathetic Stimulation
Heart		
Muscle	Increased rate and force (b)	Slowed rate (c)
Coronary arteries	Dilated (b),* constricted (a)*	Dilation (c)
Systemic blood vessels		
Abdomen	Constricted (a)	None
Skin	Constricted (a)	None
Muscle	Dilated (b, c), constricted (a)	None
Lungs		
Bronchi	Dilated (b)	Constriction (c)
Liver	Release of glucose into blood (b)	None
Skeletal muscles	Breakdown of glycogen to glucose (b)	None
Metabolism	Increase of up to 100% (a, b)	None
Glands		
Adrenal glands	Release of epinephrine and norepinephrine (c)	None
Salivary glands	Constriction of blood vessels and slight production of thick, viscous secretion (a)	Dilation of blood vessels and thin, copious secretion (c)
Gastric glands	Inhibition (a)	Stimulation (c)
Pancreas	Inhibition (a)	Stimulation (c)
Lacrimal glands	None	Secretion (c)
Sweat glands		
Merocrine glands	Copious, watery secretion (c)	None
Apocrine glands	Thick, organic secretion (c)	None
Gut		
Wall	Decreased tone (b)	Increased motility (c)
Sphincter	Increased tone (a)	Decreased tone (c)
Gallbladder and bile ducts	Relaxation (b)	Contraction (c)
Urinary bladder		
Wall	Relaxation (b)	Contraction (c)
Sphincter	Contraction (a)	Relaxation (c)
Eye		
Ciliary muscle	Relaxation for far vision (b)	Contraction for near vision (c)
Pupil	Dilation (a)	Constriction (c)
Arrector pili muscles	Contraction (a)	None
Blood	Increased coagulation (a)	None
Sex organs	Ejaculation (a)	Erection (c)

a, Mediated by alpha receptors; b, mediated by beta receptors; c, mediated by cholinergic receptors.
*Normally there is increased blood flow through coronary arteries as a result of sympathetic stimulation of the heart because of increased demand by cardiac tissue for oxygen. In experiments that isolate the coronary arteries, however, sympathetic nerve stimulation, acting through alpha receptors, causes vasoconstriction. The beta receptors are relatively insensitive to sympathetic nerve stimulation but can be activated by drugs.

Opiates are drugs that contain or are extracted from opium. The term *opioid* designates synthetic drugs that have pharmacological properties similar to those of opium or **morphine,** the chief alkaloid of opium. Opioids work by binding with opioid receptors in the brain and other body organs, altering the patient's pain perception and emotional response to a pain-provoking stimulus. Opioid analgesics include **morphine** (morphine sulfate), codeine (Methylmorphine), hydromorphone (Dilaudid, Dilaudid HP), **meperidine** (Demerol), methadone (Dolophine, Methadose), oxycodone hydrochloride (Percodan, Tylox, Percocet), and propoxyphene (Darvon, Dolene).

Opioid analgesics may produce undesirable effects such as nausea and vomiting, constipation, urinary retention, cough reflex suppression, orthostatic hypotension, and central nervous system depression. Most of these effects can be overcome by careful administration of the analgesic and careful patient monitoring.

Opioid antagonists "block" the effects of opioid analgesics (for example, opioid-induced respiratory depression and sedation) by displacing the analgesics from their effector sites. *Naloxone hydrochloride* (Narcan) and naltrexone (Trexan) are opioid antagonists.

Opioid agonist-antagonist agents have analgesic and antagonist effects. Although the exact mechanism of action is unknown, these medications have pharmacokinetic and adverse effects similar to those of *morphine*. These agents may competitively antagonize some opioid receptor but may have varying degrees of agonist effect at other opioid receptor sites. Examples of these drugs include *butorphanol tartrate* (Stadol), pentazocine (Talwin), and *nalbuphine hydrochloride*

(Nubain). Opioid agonist-antagonist agents generally have a lower dependency potential than opioids, and withdrawal symptoms are not as severe as those of the opioid agonist medications. They may precipitate withdrawal symptoms in addicts.

● NONNARCOTIC ANALGESICS

Nonnarcotic analgesics act by a peripheral mechanism that interferes with local mediators released when tissue is damaged; these mediators stimulate nerve endings and cause pain. When nonnarcotic analgesics are present, the nerve endings in damaged tissues are less frequently stimulated. This mechanism differs from that of narcotic analgesics, which act at the level of the central nervous system. An example of a nonnarcotic analgesic is *ketorolac tromethamine* (Toradol), a nonsteroidal antiinflammatory drug that exhibits analgesic activity.

● ANTIANXIETY AND SEDATIVE-HYPNOTIC AGENTS AND ALCOHOL

Antianxiety and sedative-hypnotic agents and alcohol are presented together because of their similarities in pharmacological action. Antianxiety agents are used to reduce feelings of apprehension, nervousness, worry, or fearfulness.

Sedatives and hypnotics are drugs that depress the central nervous system and that produce a calming effect and help induce sleep. The major difference between a sedative and a hypnotic is the degree of central nervous system depression induced by the agent. For example, a small dose of an agent administered to calm a patient is called a *sedative;* a larger dose of the same agent sufficient to induce sleep would be called a *hypnotic.* Therefore an agent may be a sedative and hypnotic, depending on the dose used.

As previously stated, alcohol has actions characteristic of sedative-hypnotic or antianxiety drugs. The social use of alcohol is mainly as a self-prescribed antianxiety agent; it is considered a major source of drug abuse and dependency.

Scattered throughout the brain stem is a group of nuclei collectively called the *reticular formation.* The reticular formation and its neural pathways constitute a system known as the *reticular activating system,* which is involved with the sleep-wake cycle. Through these pathways, incoming signals from the senses and viscera are collected, processed, and passed to the higher brain centers. The reticular activating system determines the level of awareness to the environment and therefore governs actions and responses to it. Antianxiety and sedative-hypnotic agents and alcohol act by depressing this system.

Classifications

Two prototypical groups of drugs used to treat anxiety or induce sleep are the benzodiazepines and barbiturates, respectively. Benzodiazepines are the drug class most commonly used today to treat anxiety and insomnia. Barbiturates are an older class of drugs with many uses from sedation to anesthesia.

Benzodiazepines

Benzodiazepines were introduced in the 1960s as antianxiety drugs. Today, they are among the most widely prescribed drugs in clinical medicine. This popularity results in part to their very high therapeutic index. Overdoses of 1000 times the therapeutic dose have been reported not to result in death unless taken in conjunction with other central nervous system depressants, such as alcohol.[11] Benzodiazepines are thought to work by binding to specific receptors in the cerebral cortex and limbic system (a major integrating system that governs emotional behavior). These drugs are highly lipid soluble and are widely distributed in the body tissues. They are also highly bound to plasma protein, usually more than 80%. Benzodiazepines have four actions: anxiety reducing, sedative-hypnotic, muscle relaxing, and anticonvulsant. All benzodiazepines are schedule IV drugs because of their potential for abuse. Commonly prescribed benzodiazepines are alprazolam (Xanax), chlordiazepoxide (Librium), clorazepate (Tranxene), *diazepam* (Valium), flurazepam (Dalmane), prazepam (Centrax), *midazolam*

(Versed), *lorazepam* (Ativan), and triazolam (Halcion).

Barbiturates

Barbiturates were once the most commonly prescribed class of medications for sedative-hypnotic effects but have been virtually replaced by benzodiazepines. Barbiturates are divided into four classes according to their duration of action: ultra short acting, short acting, intermediate acting, and long acting. The differences in onset and duration of action depend on their lipid solubility and protein-binding properties. Ultra-short-acting barbiturates are commonly used as intravenous anesthetics. These drugs act rapidly and can produce a state of anesthesia in a few seconds. An example of an ultra-short-acting barbiturate is thiopental sodium (Pentothal).

Short-acting barbiturates produce an effect in a relatively short time (10 to 15 minutes) and peak over a relatively short period (3 to 4 hours). This class of drug is rarely used to treat insomnia; it is more commonly used for preanesthesia sedation and in combination with other drugs for psychosomatic disorders. Examples include pentobarbital (Nembutal) and secobarbital (Seconal).

Intermediate-acting barbiturates have an onset of 45 to 60 minutes and a peak in 6 to 8 hours. Short-acting and intermediate-acting agents have similar patient responses in the clinical setting. Examples of intermediate-acting barbiturates include amobarbital (Amytal) and butabarbital (Butisol).

Long-acting barbiturates require over 60 minutes for onset and peak over a period of 10 to 12 hours. These agents are used to treat epilepsy and other chronic neurological disorders and to sedate patients with severe anxiety. Examples of long-acting barbiturates include mephobarbital (Gemonil) and *phenobarbital* (Luminal).

Miscellaneous Sedative-Hypnotic Drugs

A number of antianxiety and sedative-hypnotic drugs that are occasionally used do not fall into the previously discussed drug classes. These agents are more similar to barbiturates than benzodiazepines in that they are generally shorter acting. Examples of miscellaneous drugs with antianxiety and sedative-hypnotic effects are chloral hydrate (Noctec), ethchlorvynol (Placidyl), and meprobamate (Equanil, Meprospan). In addition to these drugs, antihistamines such as *hydroxyzine hydrochloride* (Vistaril, Atarax) have pronounced sedative effects.

Alcohol Intake And Behavioral Effects

Alcohol is a general central nervous system depressant that can produce sedation, sleep, and anesthesia. In addition, alcohol enhances the sedative-hypnotic effects of other drug classes, including all general central nervous system depressants, antihistamines, phenothiazines, narcotic analgesics, and tricyclic antidepressants. If alcohol is taken with other drugs, this enhancement could result in coma or death. Blood alcohol is measured in milligrams per deciliter. Based on the amount of alcohol consumed and blood alcohol levels, characteristic behavioral effects can be predicted. Behavioral effects associated with alcohol intake are further described in Chapter 23.

● ANTICONVULSANTS

Anticonvulsant drugs are used to treat seizure disorders, most notably epilepsy. Epilepsy is a neurological disorder characterized by a recurrent pattern of abnormal neuronal discharges within the brain. These discharges result in a sudden loss or disturbance of consciousness, sometimes associated with motor activity, sensory phenomena, or inappropriate behavior. It is estimated that epilepsy occurs in approximately 0.5% to 1% of the population. In 50% of these cases, the cause is unknown (primary or idiopathic epilepsy). Secondary epilepsy is epilepsy that can be traced to trauma, infection, a cerebrovascular disorder, or another illness.

The exact mode and site of action of anticonvulsant drugs is not understood. In general, these drugs depress the excitability of neurons that fire to initiate the seizure or suppress generalization of the small focal depolarization that occurs, thus preventing the spread of seizure discharge. Anticonvulsants are presumed to modify the ionic movements of sodium, potassium, or calcium across the nerve membrane, thereby reducing the response to incoming electrical or chemical stimulation. Benzodiazepines also stimulate major inhibitory neurotransmitters in the central nervous system. Many patients require drug therapy throughout their lives to control seizures.

Classifications

Several drugs are available for control of epileptic seizures. The choice of drug depends on the type of seizure disorder (grand mal, petit mal, psychomotor) and the patient's tolerance and response to the prescribed medication. Common anticonvulsants include *phenobarbital* (Luminal), *phenytoin* (Dilantin), *diazepam* (Valium), and *magnesium sulfate.*

● DRUGS AFFECTING THE AUTONOMIC NERVOUS SYSTEM

The nervous and endocrine systems are the major means of controlling and integrating body functions. These two systems share three characteristics: (1) a high-level integration in the brain, (2) the ability to influence processes in distant regions of the body, and (3) the extensive use of negative feedback mechanisms. The major difference between the nervous and endocrine systems is in the mode of transmission of information.

Endocrine system transmission is primarily chemical via blood-borne hormones. The hormones are not targeted for a particular organ but instead diffusely affect many cells and organs concurrently. In contrast, the nervous system primarily relies on rapid electrical transmission of information over nerve fibers, with chemical impulses only carrying signals between nerve cells and their effector cells in a very localized manner, perhaps affecting only a few cells. Drugs affecting the endocrine system are presented later in this section.

Classifications

The autonomic drugs mimic, intensify, or block the effects of the sympathetic and parasympathetic divisions of the autonomic nervous system. These drugs can be classified into four groups:

1. Cholinergic **(parasympathomimetic)** drugs that mimic the actions of the parasympathetic nervous system
2. Cholinergic blocking **(parasympatholytic)** drugs that block the actions of the parasympathetic nervous system
3. Adrenergic **(sympathomimetic)** drugs that mimic the actions of the sympathetic nervous system or the adrenal medulla
4. Adrenergic blocking **(sympatholytic)** drugs that block the actions of the sympathetic nervous system or adrenal medulla

Cholinergic Drugs

Acetylcholine plays an important role in the parasympathetic and sympathetic divisions of the nervous system. It has two major effects in the nervous system: (1) a stimulant effect on the ganglia, adrenal medulla, and skeletal muscle (the "nicotinic effect" of acetylcholine) and (2) stimulant effects at postganglionic nerve endings in cardiac muscle, smooth muscle, and glands (the "muscarinic effect" of acetycholine) (Table 14-4).

Cholinergic drugs act directly by combining with cholinergic receptors in postsynaptic membranes or indirectly by inhibiting the enzyme that normally degrades acetylcholine. This inhibition results in accumulation of acetylcholine, which causes a prolonged and intensified response at various effector sites. Cholinergic drugs have little therapeutic value and are generally not considered emergency medications. The major exception to this is physostigmine (Antilirium), an indirect-acting cholinergic drug that may be used to manage extreme cases of poisoning resulting from atropine-type drugs.

Cholinergic blocking (anticholinergic) agents have many uses in emergency medicine. These drugs work by blocking the muscarinic effects of acetylcholine, thereby decreasing acetylcholine's effect on its effector organ.

The best-known cholinergic blocking drug used in emergency care is *atropine sulfate* (Atropine), a competitive antagonist. It works by occupying muscarinic receptor sites, preventing or reducing the muscarinic response to acetylcholine. Large doses dilate the pupils, inhibit accommodation of the eyes, and increase heart rate by blocking the cholinergic effects of the heart.

Neuromuscular blocking drugs produce complete muscle relaxation and paralysis by binding to the nicotinic receptor for acetylcholine at the

TABLE 14-4 Sites for Muscarinic and Nicotinic Actions of Acetylcholine

Site	Muscarinic Action*	Nicotinic Actions
Cardiovascular		
Blood vessels	Dilation	Constriction } With large doses
Heart rate	Slowed	Increase after atropine
Blood pressure	Decreased	Increase
Gastrointestinal		
Tone	Increased	Increase
Motility	Increased	Increase
Sphincters	Relaxed	—
Glandular secretions	Increased salivary, lacrimal, intestinal, and sweat secretion	Initial stimulation and then inhibition of salivary and bronchial secretions
Skeletal muscle	—	Stimulation
Autonomic ganglia	—	Stimulation
Eye	Pupil constriction	—
	Decreased accomodation	
Blocking agent	Atropine	Tubocurarine
REMARKS	Above effects increase as dosage increases.	Increased dosage inhibits effects and causes receptor blockade.

*Usual sites for therapeutic effects.

neuromuscular junction. Neuromuscular transmission is thus inhibited and remains so for a variable period, depending on the type and amount of neuromuscular blocker used.

These drugs are sometimes used to achieve total paralysis before ET intubation, to relieve muscle spasms of the larynx, to suppress tetany, during electroconvulsive therapy for depression, and to allow for breathing control by a respirator. Because these blocking agents produce complete paralysis, ventilatory support must be provided and the efficacy of ventilation and oxygenation closely monitored. Note that these muscle relaxants do not inhibit pain or seizure activity. Examples of neuromuscular blockers include *pancuronium* (Pavulon), vecuronium (Norcuron), and *succinylcholine* (Anectine).

Adrenergic Drugs

Adrenergic drugs are designed to produce activities like those of neurotransmitters. There are three types: direct acting, indirect acting, and dual acting (direct and indirect) agents.

Direct Acting

Three naturally occurring catecholamines are present in the body: epinephrine, norepinephrine, and dopamine. Epinephrine acts mainly as an emergency hormone released by the adrenal medulla, and norepinephrine acts as an important transmitter of nerve impulses. Dopamine is a precursor of epinephrine and norepinephrine and has a transmitter role of its own in certain portions of the central nervous system. Examples of synthetic catecholamine drugs and the three endogenous catecholamines are *epinephrine* (Adrenalin), *norepinephrine* (Levophed), *isoproterenol* (Isuprel), *dopamine* (Intropin), and *dobutamine* (Dobutrex).

Catecholamines depend on their ability to act directly with alpha and beta receptors. Two subgroups of alpha receptors have been identified: $alpha_1$ and $alpha_2$. $Alpha_1$ are postsynaptic receptors located on the effector organs. The primary role of the $alpha_1$ receptor is to stimulate contraction of smooth muscle. In the vasculature, this results in an increase in blood pressure. $Alpha_2$ receptors are found on the presynaptic nerve endings. When stimulated, these receptors inhibit the further re-

lease of norepinephrine. Like $alpha_1$ receptors, $alpha_2$ receptors mediate vasoconstriction to increase resistance and thus increase blood pressure.

Beta receptors are also subdivided into $beta_1$ and $beta_2$. This classification is based on their response to drugs but also follows anatomical distinctions. $Beta_1$ receptors are located primarily in the heart, whereas $beta_2$ receptors are located predominantly in the bronchiolar and arterial smooth muscle. Beta receptors stimulate the heart; dilate bronchioles; dilate blood vessels in the skeletal muscle, brain, and heart; and aid in glycogenolysis (Table 14-5).

Norepinephrine acts mainly on alpha receptors and causes almost pure vasoconstriction. Epinephrine acts on alpha and beta receptors and produces a mixture of vasodilation and vasoconstriction, depending on the relative number of alpha and beta receptors present in the target tissue. The most important alpha and beta activities in humans are:

- Alpha activities
  - Vasoconstriction of arterioles in the skin and splanchnic area, resulting in a rise in blood pressure and peripheral shunting of blood to the heart and brain resulting from the shifting of blood volume
  - Pupil dilation
  - Relaxation of the gut
- Beta activities
  - Cardiac acceleration and increased contractility
  - Vasodilation of arterioles supplying skeletal muscle
  - Bronchial relaxation
  - Uterine relaxation

Indirect And Dual Acting

Indirect-acting adrenergic drugs act indirectly on receptors by triggering the release of the catecholamines norepinephrine and epinephrine, which then activate the alpha and beta receptors. Dual-acting adrenergic drugs have indirect and direct effects. Drugs in this classification include ephedrine (ephedrine sulfate), phenylephrine (Neo-Synephrine), and metaraminol (Aramine).

Adrenergic blocking agents may be classified into alpha- and beta-blocking drugs. Alpha-

TABLE 14-5 Adrenergic Receptor Stimulation

Effector Organs	Receptor Type	Adrenergic Response
Heart		
Cardiac muscle (atria, ventricles)	Beta$_1$	Increased force of contraction
Sinoatrial node	Beta$_1$	Increased heart rate
Atrioventricular node	Beta$_1$	Increased conduction velocity, shortened refractory period
Conduction tissue	Beta$_1$	
Blood vessels		
Arterioles (smooth muscle)		
Coronary	Alpha, beta$_2$, dopaminergic	Constriction, dilation
Cerebral	Alpha	Constriction
Pulmonary	Alpha, beta$_2$	Constriction, dilation
Mesenteric visceral	Alpha, beta$_2$, dopaminergic	Constriction, dilation
Renal	Alpha, beta$_2$, dopaminergic	Constriction, dilation
Skin, mucosa	Alpha	Constriction
Skeletal muscle	Alpha, beta$_2$	Constriction, dilation
Veins	Alpha$_1$, beta$_2$	Constriction, dilation
Lungs		
Bronchial smooth muscle	Beta$_2$	Bronchodilation (relaxation)
Bronchial glands	Alpha$_2$, beta$_2$	Inhibition
Gastrointestinal tract		
Smooth muscle (motility, tone)	Alpha$_2$, beta$_2$	Decrease
Sphincter	Alpha	Contraction
Secretion	?	Inhibition
Gallbladder and ducts	—	Relaxation
Liver	Beta$_2$	Glycogenolysis, gluconeogenesis
Spleen capsule	Alpha, beta$_2$	Contraction, relaxation
Pancreas: insulin secretion	Alpha	Decrease
Adipose tissue	Beta$_1$	Lipolysis
Urinary bladder		
Detrusor muscle	Beta$_1$	Relaxation
Sphincter	Alpha	Contraction
Kidney ureter	Alpha	Contraction
Kidney secretion (renin)	Beta$_2$	Increase
Uterus		
Pregnant	Alpha	Contraction
Nonpregnant	Beta$_2$	Relaxation
Sex organs, male	Alpha	Ejaculation
Skin		
Pilomotor muscles	Alpha	Contraction
Sweat glands	Cholinergic	Increased secretion
Eye		
Radial muscle, iris (pupil size)	Alpha	Contraction–pupil dilation (mydriasis)
Ciliary muscle	Beta	Relaxation for far vision

blocking drugs block the vasoconstricting effect of catecholamines. They are used in certain cases of hypertension and to help prevent necrosis when *norepinephrine* (Levophed) or *dopamine* (Intropin) has extravasated into the tissues. They have limited clinical application in the prehospital setting.

NOTE: Because of the possibility of extravasation and tissue necrosis, all drugs with alpha effects should be administered through a secure intravenous line well positioned in a large vein.

Beta-blocking agents have greater clinical application and are frequently used in emergency care. These drugs block beta receptors, thereby inhibiting the action at their effector site. Beta-blocking agents are grouped into selective blocking agents, which block beta$_1$ or beta$_2$ receptors, and nonselective blocking agents, which block beta$_1$ and beta$_2$ receptor sites.

Selective beta$_1$-blocking agents are also known as *cardioselective blockers* because they block the beta$_1$ receptors in the heart. An example of an important selective beta$_1$-blocking agent is metoprolol (Lopressor), an antihypertensive. Selectivity is not 100%; even cardioselective drugs may affect the lungs and vice versa.

Nonselective beta-blocking agents inhibit beta$_1$ receptors in the heart and beta$_2$ receptors in the smooth muscle of the bronchioles and blood vessels. Examples include the antianginal antihypertensives nadolol (Corgard) and *propranolol* (Inderal) and the antihypertensive *labetalol* (Normodyne, Trandate). (*Labetalol* also has some alpha-blocking activity.)

Section Five
Drugs Affecting the
Cardiovascular System

● REVIEW OF ANATOMY AND PHYSIOLOGY

The heart is composed of many interconnected branching fibers or cells that form the walls of the two atria and two ventricles. Some of these cells are specialized to conduct electrical impulses. Others have contraction as their primary function. All of these cells are nourished through a profuse network of blood vessels (coronary vasculature). Cardiac drugs are classified by their effects on these tissues. Boxes 14-10 and 14-11 list cardiac drugs and pharmacological terms that describe their actions.

BOX 14-10

Emergency Drugs: Cardiovascular System

adenosine (Adenocard)
amyl nitrite inhalant
anisoylated plasminogen streptokinase activator (Eminase)
bretylium tosylate (Bretylol)
diazoxide (Hyperstat IV)
digoxin (Lanoxin)
diltiazem (Cardizem)
dobutamine (Dobutrex)
epinephrine (Adrenalin)
furosemide (Lasix)
hydralazine hydrochloride (Apresoline)
isoproterenol (Isuprel)
labetalol (Normodyne)
lidocaine (Xylocaine)
nitroglycerin sublingual tablet (Isordil, Sorbitrate)
nitroglycerin paste (Nitro-Bid, Nitrostat, Nitrol)
norepinephrine (Levophed)
phenytoin (Dilantin)
procainamide (Pronestyl)
propranolol (Inderal)
streptokinase (Streptase)
tissue plasminogen activator (t-PA, Alteplase)
verapamil (Isoptin)

● CARDIAC GLYCOSIDES

Cardiac glycosides are naturally occurring plant substances that have characteristic actions on the heart. These compounds contain a carbohydrate molecule (sugar) that, when combined with water, is converted into a sugar plus one or more active substances. Glycosides may work by blocking certain ionic pumps in the cellular membrane, which indirectly increases the calcium concentration to the contractile proteins. An important cardiac glycoside is *digoxin* (Lanoxin), which is used

Pharmacological Terms to Describe Actions of Cardiovascular Drugs

Chronotropic: Chronotropic drugs affect heart rate. If the drug accelerates the heart rate (for example, *isoproterenol*), it is said to have a *positive chronotropic effect*. A drug that decreases the heart rate (for example, *verapamil* [Isoptin]) is said to have a *negative chronotropic effect*.

Dromotropic: Dromotropic drugs affect conduction velocity through the conducting tissues of the heart. If a drug speeds conduction, it is said to have a *positive dromotropic effect*. Examples of drugs with positive dromotropic effects include *isoproterenol* (Isuprel) and *phenytoin* (Dilantin). Drugs with negative dromotropic effects delay conduction (for example, *verapamil* [Isoptin] and *adenosine* [Adenocard]).

Inotropic: Inotropic drugs strengthen or increase the force of cardiac contraction (a positive inotropic effect). Some examples include *digoxin* (Lanoxin), *dobutamine* (Dobutrex), *epinephrine* (Adrenalin), and *isoproterenol* (Isuprel). A drug that weakens or decreases the force of cardiac contraction has a negative inotropic effect. An example of such a drug is *propranolol* (Inderal).

to treat heart failure and to manage certain tachycardias.

Digitalis glycosides can affect the heart in two different ways: (1) They increase the strength of contraction, which is a positive inotropic effect, and (2) they have a dual effect on the electrophysiological properties of the heart. They have a modest negative **chronotropic** effect (causing slight slowing) as well as a more profound negative **dromotropic** effect, decreasing conduction velocity.

Side Effects

Many patients who take cardiac glycosides develop side effects at one time or another because of the small TI. The symptoms may be neurological, visual, gastrointestinal, cardiac, or psychiatric. These symptoms are often vague and can be easily attributed to a viral illness. A high index of suspicion must be maintained. The most common side effects of cardiac glycosides include anorexia, nausea or vomiting, visual disturbances (flashing lights, altered color vision), and cardiac rhythm disturbances (usually slowing with varying degrees of blocked conduction).

The toxic effects of cardiac glycosides are dose related. These effects may be increased by the presence of other drugs, such as diuretics, which may predispose the patient to cardiac rhythm disturbances. Dysrhythmias may include bradycardias, tachycardias, and even ventricular fibrillation. Therefore these patients require close monitoring. Treatment for digitalis toxicity may include correction of electrolyte imbalances, neutralization of the free drug, and use of antidysrhythmics.

● ANTIDYSRHYTHMICS

Antidysrhythmic drugs are used to treat and prevent disorders of cardiac rhythm. The pharmacological agents that suppress dysrhythmias may do so by direct action on the cardiac cell membrane (*lidocaine*), by indirect action that affects the cell (*propranolol*), or both.

Cardiac rhythm disturbances may be caused by ischemia, hypoxia, acidosis or alkalosis, electrolyte abnormalities, excessive catecholamine exposure, autonomic influences, drug toxicity, or scarred and diseased tissue. Dysrhythmias result from disturbances in impulse formation, disturbances in impulse conduction, or both.

Classifications

In recent years, antidysrhythmic drugs have been classified into categories based on their fundamental mode of action on cardiac muscle. Drugs that belong to the same class do not necessarily produce identical actions. However, all antidysrhythmic drugs have some ability to suppress automaticity.

Group I

Group I compounds are subdivided into groups I-A, I-B, and I-C. Group I-A drugs decrease conduction velocity and prolong the electrical potential of cardiac tissue. Examples include quinidine (Quinaglute, Duraquin) and *procainamide* (Pronestyl).

Group I-B drugs increase or have no effect on conduction velocity. Examples include *lidocaine* (Xylocaine) and *phenytoin* (Dilantin).

Group I-C drugs profoundly slow conduction and are indicated only for control of life-threatening ventricular dysrhythmias. Examples include flecainide (Tambocor) and encainide (Enkade).

Group II

Group II drugs are beta-blocking agents that reduce adrenergic stimulation of the heart. An example is *propranolol* (Inderal).

Group III

Group III drugs are antiadrenergic agents that have a positive inotropic action (agonist-antagonist), which increases contractility. Unlike other antidysrhythmic agents, drugs in this group do not suppress automaticity and have no effect on conduction velocity. These drugs are thought to terminate dysrhythmias that result from the reentry of blocked impulses. An example is *bretylium tosylate* (Bretylol).

Group IV

Group IV drugs are also known as *calcium channel blockers*. These drugs are thought to work by blocking the inflow of calcium through the cell membranes of the cardiac and smooth muscle cells. This action depresses the myocardial and smooth muscle contraction, decreases automaticity, and in some cases, decreases conduction velocity. Examples of calcium channel blockers include *verapamil* (Isoptin) and *diltiazem* (Cardizem).

● ANTIHYPERTENSIVES

Hypertension affects approximately 30 million Americans and has been directly related to an increased incidence of stroke, cerebral hemorrhage, heart and renal failure, and coronary heart disease. The exact mechanism of action of many antihypertensive drugs is unknown. The ideal antihypertensive drug should:
- Maintain blood pressure within normal limits for various body positions
- Maintain or improve blood flow without compromising tissue perfusion or blood supply to the brain
- Reduce the work load on the heart
- Have no undesirable side effects
- Permit long-term administration without intolerance

Classifications

Antihypertensive drugs used to reduce blood pressure are classified into four major categories: diuretics, sympathetic blocking agents (sympatholytic drugs), vasodilators, and angiotensin-converting-enzyme (ACE) inhibitors. Calcium channel blockers are also increasingly being used to treat hypertension.

Diuretics

Until recently, diuretics were considered the initial drug of choice in managing mild hypertension. They were also used frequently with other antihypertensives when hypertension could not be controlled by diuretics alone. Use of these medications results in a loss of excess salt and water from the body by renal excretion. The decrease in plasma and extracellular fluid volume (which decreases preload and stroke volume), plus a direct effect on arterioles, results in lowered blood pressure. This response causes an initial decline of cardiac output, followed by a decrease in peripheral resistance and a lowering of the blood pressure.

Thiazides are diuretics that are moderately effective in lowering blood pressure. Many antihypertensive agents cause retention of sodium and water, and thiazides may be given concomitantly to help prevent this side effect. An example of a thiazide diuretic is hydrochlorothiazide (Hydrodiuril).

Loop diuretics are powerful, short-acting agents that inhibit sodium and chloride reabsorption in the loop of Henle. These medications cause excessive loss of potassium and water and an increase in the excretion of sodium. Loop diuretics produce fewer side effects than most other antihypertensives, although hypokalemia and profound dehydration can result from their use. These agents are prescribed to patients who have renal insufficiency or who cannot take other diuretics. An example of a loop diuretic is *furosemide* (Lasix).

Potassium-sparing agents do not result in the potassium loss caused by other diuretics. These medications promote sodium and water loss without an accompanying loss of potassium. Potassium-sparing agents are used to treat hypertensive patients who become hypokalemic with other diuretics or who are apparently resistant to the antihypertensive effects of other diuretics. Potassium-sparing agents can also be used to treat some edematous states such as cirrhosis of the liver with ascites. An example of a potassium-sparing agent is spironolactone (Aldactone).

Combinations of diuretic agents may also be prescribed to lower blood pressure. These combination diuretics usually include hydrochlorothiazide (HCTZ). Examples include Aldactazide, a combination agent with HCTZ and spironolactone, and Dyazide, which contains HCTZ and triamterene. Today, many practitioners are using other agents (such as calcium channel blockers, beta blockers, and ACE inhibitors) for first-line therapy of hypertension. Nonetheless, in patients with hypertension and congestive heart failure, diuretics remain a drug of choice, and they are still a commonly prescribed medication.

Sympathetic Blocking Agents

Sympathetic blocking agents may be classified as beta-blocking agents and adrenergic inhibiting agents. Beta-blocking agents are used to treat cardiovascular disorders, including hypertension. These drugs work by decreasing cardiac output

and inhibiting renin secretion from the kidneys. Both actions result in lower blood pressure. In addition, beta-blocking drugs compete with epinephrine for available beta-receptor sites, inhibiting tissue and organ response to beta stimulation. Examples of beta-blocking agents include:

- Beta$_1$-blocking agents (cardioselective)
  - acebutolol (Sectral)
  - atenolol (Tenormin)
  - metoprolol (Lopressor)
- Beta$_1$- and beta$_2$-blocking agents (nonselective)
  - *labetalol* (Normodyne, Trandate)
  - nadolol (Corgard)
  - *propranolol* (Inderal)

Adrenergic inhibiting agents work by modifying the sympathetic nervous system and are effective antihypertensive drugs. Arterial pressure is influenced through various mechanisms of the heart, blood vessels, and kidneys. Sympathetic stimulation increases heart rate and force of myocardial contraction, constricts arterioles and venules, and causes the release of renin from the kidneys. Blocking this sympathetic stimulation can reduce blood pressure.

Adrenergic inhibiting agents are classified as centrally acting adrenergic inhibitors, peripheral adrenergic inhibitors, and alpha-blocking drugs based on their site of action. The mechanism by which many of these agents work is unknown. It is generally believed that most have multiple sites of action. Examples include the following:

- Centrally acting adrenergic inhibitors
  - clonidine hydrochloride (Catapres)
  - methyldopa (Aldomet)
- Peripheral adrenergic inhibitors
  - guanethidine sulfate (Ismelin)
  - reserpine (Sandril, Serpasil)
- Alpha$_1$- and alpha$_2$-blocking agents (nonselective)
  - prazosin hydrochloride (Minipress)
  - phentolamine (Regitine)
  - phenoxybenzamine (Dibenzyline)

Vasodilator Drugs

Vasodilator drugs act directly on the smooth muscle walls of the arterioles, veins, or both, lowering peripheral resistance and blood pressure. This stimulates the sympathetic nervous system and activates the baroreceptor reflexes, leading to an increase in heart rate, cardiac output, and renin release. Combined therapy is usually prescribed to inhibit the sympathetic response.

In addition to their use as antihypertensives, some vasodilator drugs are effective for treating angina pectoris. For example, nitrates dilate veins and arteries. Their dilating effects on veins lead to venous pooling and a decreased blood return to the heart, thus reducing left ventricular end-diastolic volume and pressure. The subsequent decrease in wall tension helps reduce myocardial oxygen demand and the chest pain associated with myocardial ischemia. Vasodilator drugs are classified as arteriolar dilators and arteriolar and venous dilators. Examples of each are:

- Arteriolar dilator drugs
  - *diazoxide* (Hyperstat IV)
  - *hydralazine hydrochloride* (Apresoline)
  - minoxidil (Loniten)
- Arteriolar and venous dilator drugs
  - *sodium nitroprusside* (Nipride, Nitropress)
  - nitrates and nitrites
    amyl nitrite inhalant
    isosorbide dinitrate (Isordil, Sorbitrate)
    nitroglycerin sublingual tablet (Nitrostat)
    nitroglycerin paste (Nitro-Bid, Nitrostat, Nitrol)
    Intravenous *nitroglycerin*
  - Converting enzyme (ACE) inhibitor

ACE Inhibitor Drugs

The renin-angiotensin-aldosterone system plays an important role in maintaining blood pressure and sodium and fluid balance. A disturbance in this system can result in hypertension. In addition, kidney damage can result in an inability to regulate the release of renin through normal feedback mechanisms, causing elevated blood pressure in some patients.

Angiotensin II is a powerful vasoconstrictor. It raises blood pressure and causes the release of aldosterone, which contributes to sodium and

water retention. By inhibiting conversion of the precursor angiotensin I to the active molecule angiotensin II (which is brought about through ACE), the renin-angiotensin-aldosterone system is suppressed, and blood pressure is lowered. Examples of ACE inhibitors include captopril (Capoten), enalapril (Vasotec), and lisinopril (Prinivil).

Other Antihypertensive Agents

Other antihypertensive drugs include calcium channel blocking drugs and ganglionic blocking agents. Calcium channel blocking agents such as *verapamil* (Isoptin), *nifedipine* (Procardia), and *diltiazem* (Cardizem) reduce peripheral vascular resistance by inhibiting the contractility of vascular smooth muscle. They dilate coronary vessels through the same mechanism. The effects of these drugs are important in treating hypertension, decreasing the oxygen requirements of the heart (through decreased afterload) and increasing oxygen supply (by abolishing coronary artery spasm), thus relieving the causes of angina pectoris. The various drugs in this class differ in degree of selectivity for coronary (and peripheral) vasodilation or decreased cardiac contractility.

Ganglionic blocking agents block sympathetic and parasympathetic ganglia. These drugs decrease peripheral resistance, cardiac output, and stroke volume and are considered less safe than those previously described. They are rarely used today. Their major contribution in the past was to treat hypertension in patients who had dissecting aortic aneurysms. Today, these patients would most likely be treated with a combination beta-blocking agent and *nitroprusside* (Nipride, Nitropress). Examples of these ganglionic blocking agents include trimethaphan (Arfonad), pargyline hydrochloride (Eutonyl), and metyrosine (Demser).

● DRUGS THAT AFFECT THE BLOOD

Bleeding and thrombosis are altered states of hemostasis. Understanding the drugs that affect blood coagulation and the use of thrombolytic agents is a necessary component of prehospital patient management.

Platelets are small cell fragments in blood that provide the initial step in normal repair of blood vessels. Blood coagulation is a process that results in the formation of a stable fibrin clot that entraps platelets, blood cells, and plasma. The end result of this process is called a *blood clot* or *thrombus*. Abnormal thrombus formation (that is, intravascular clotting) is the major cause of myocardial infarction (from coronary thrombosis) and stroke (from cerebral vascular thrombosis).

The coagulation process also occurs in the venous system, although the underlying mechanisms responsible for the thrombosis differ. Arterial thrombi are commonly associated with atherosclerotic plaques, hypertension, and turbulent blood flow that damages the endothelial lining of blood vessels. Damage to the endothelium causes platelets to stick and aggregate in the arterial system. Arterial thrombi are composed mostly of platelets but also involve the chemical substances that contribute to the coagulation process (in particular, fibrinogen and fibrin). Myocardial infarctions and strokes are frequently the result of arterial thrombi.

The three major risk factors for various thromboses are stasis, localized trauma, and hypercoagulable states. Stasis, or reduced blood flow, results from immobilization or venous insufficiency. It is responsible for the increased incidence of deep vein thrombosis (DVT) in most bedridden patients. Localized trauma may initiate the clotting cascade and cause arterial and venous thrombosis. Hypercoagulability is the mechanism behind the increased incidence of DVT in women who take birth control pills and is also responsible for many of the familial thrombotic disorders.

Agents that Affect Blood Coagulation

Drugs that affect blood coagulation may be classified as antiplatelet, anticoagulant, and thrombolytic agents.

Antiplatelet Agents

Drugs that interfere with platelet aggregation are known as *antiplatelet* or *antithrombic drugs.* These drugs are sometimes prescribed prophylactically for patients at risk of developing arterial clots and those who have suffered myocardial infarction or stroke. Antiplatelet agents are also used to treat certain valvular heart diseases, valvular prosthesis, and various intracardiac shunts. Among the most common antiplatelet drugs are aspirin, sulfinpyrazone (Anturane), and dipyridamole (Persantine).

Anticoagulant Agents

Anticoagulant drug therapy is designed to prevent intravascular thrombosis by decreasing blood coagulability. It is commonly used to prevent postoperative thromboembolism; it is also used during hemodialysis. This therapy is primarily prophylactic and has no direct effect on a blood clot that has already formed or on ischemic tissue injured by inadequate blood supply as a result of a thrombus. The major side effect of anticoagulant therapy is hemorrhage, and patients taking anticoagulants are prone to bleeding complications. Examples of anticoagulant agents include warfarin sodium (Coumadin) and *heparin* sodium (Liquaemin).

Thrombolytic Agents

Thrombolytic drugs dissolve clots after their formation by promoting the digestion of fibrin. In recent years, thrombolytic therapy has become the treatment of choice for treating acute myocardial infarction in certain groups of patients. The goal is to re-establish blood flow and prevent myocardial ischemia and tissue death. Thrombolytic therapy has also been used in acute pulmonary embolism, DVT, and peripheral arterial occlusion. The use of thrombolytics in the prehospital setting is being studied in several areas of the United States to determine the safety and efficacy of these agents in this situation. Thrombolytic drugs include *anisoylated plasminogen streptokinase activator* (Eminase), *streptokinase* (Streptase), urokinase (Abbokinase), and *tissue plasminogen activator* (t-PA, Alteplase).

Section Six
Drugs Affecting the Respiratory System

● REVIEW OF ANATOMY AND PHYSIOLOGY

The respiratory system includes all structures involved in the exchange of oxygen and carbon dioxide. Serious narrowing of any portion of the respiratory tract may be an indication for pharmacological therapy (Box 14-12). Emergencies involving the respiratory system are usually caused by reversible conditions such as asthma, emphysema with infection, and foreign body obstruction.

Smooth muscle fibers of the tracheobronchial tree are arranged along the length of the tubular air passage and directly influence the diameter of the airways. The bronchial smooth muscle tone is maintained by impulses from the autonomic nervous system. Parasympathetic fibers from the vagus nerve innervate bronchial smooth muscle through the release of acetylcholine. This neurotransmitter interacts with the muscarinic receptors on the membranes of the cell, producing bronchoconstriction.

BOX 14-12

Emergency Drugs: Respiratory System

albuterol (Proventil, Ventolin)
dexamethasone sodium phosphate (Decadron Phosphate)
diphenhydramine (Benadryl)
epinephrine (Adrenalin)
epinephrine hydrochloride (Adrenalin Chloride) 1:1000
hydroxyzine hydrochloride (Atarax)
promethazine hydrochloride (Phenergan)
racemic epinephrine inhalant (AsthmaNefrin, Micronephrin)
terbutaline sulfate (Brethine, Bricanyl)

Sympathetic fibers primarily affect $beta_2$-receptors through the release of epinephrine from the adrenal medulla and the release of norepinephrine from the peripheral sympathetic nerves. The epinephrine reaches the lungs by way of the circulatory system and interacts with $beta_2$ receptors to produce smooth muscle relaxation and bronchodilation. Thus the $beta_2$ receptor plays the dominant role in bronchial muscle tone. (Although $beta_1$ receptors are also found on bronchial smooth muscle, their ratio to $beta_2$ receptors is 1:3.)

● BRONCHODILATOR DRUGS

Bronchodilator drugs are the primary treatment modality for obstructive pulmonary disease such as asthma, chronic bronchitis, and emphysema. These drugs may be classified as sympathomimetic drugs and xanthine derivatives. Many of these agents are administered by inhalation via a nebulizer or pressure cartridge.

Sympathomimetic Drugs

Sympathomimetic drugs are grouped according to their receptor action: nonselective adrenergic drugs have alpha, $beta_1$ (cardiac), and $beta_2$ (respiratory) activities. Nonselective beta-adrenergic drugs have both $beta_1$ and $beta_2$ effects. Selective $beta_2$-receptor drugs act primarily on $beta_2$ receptors in the lungs (bronchial smooth muscle). Box 14-13 summarizes the alpha, $beta_1$, and $beta_2$ activities of the adrenergic drugs used as bronchodilators.

Nonselective adrenergic drugs stimulate alpha and beta receptors. The alpha activity mediates vasoconstriction to reduce mucosal edema. $Beta_2$ activity produces bronchodilation and vasodilation. Undesirable effects on $beta_1$ receptors include an increase in heart rate and force of contraction. Undesirable $beta_2$ effects include muscle tremors and central nervous system stimulation. Examples of nonselective adrenergic drugs include *epinephrine* inhalation aerosol (Bronkaid Mist, Primatene Mist), *epinephrine* inhalation solution (Adrenalin), and racemic *epinephrine* inhalation solution (AsthmaNefrin, microNephrin, and others).

Because nonselective beta-adrenergic drugs are not selective for beta$_2$ receptors, they have a wide range of effects. These effects have been described previously. Examples of nonselective beta adrenergic drugs include *epinephrine* (Adrenalin, Asmolin, and others), which also has some alpha activity; ephedrine (Ephed II), which also has some alpha activity; ethylnorepinephrine (Bronkephrine), which also has some alpha activity; *isoproterenol* inhalation solution (Aerolone, Vapo-Iso, Isuprel); and *isoproterenol* hydrochloride inhalation aerosol (Isuprel Mistometer, Norisodrine Aerotrol).

The selective action of beta$_2$-selective drugs lessens the incidence of unwanted cardiac effects caused by beta$_1$-adrenergic agents. Patients with hypertension, cardiac disease, or diabetes can better tolerate this group of bronchodilators. Examples of selective beta$_2$ receptor drugs include *albuterol* (Proventil, Ventolin), *terbutaline sulfate* (Brethine, Bricanyl), bitolterol (Tornalate), *epinephrine* suspension (Sus-Phrine) 1:200, *epinephrine hydrochloride* (Adrenalin Chloride) 1:1000, and *isoetharine hydrochloride* (Bronkosol, others).

Xanthine Derivatives

The xanthine group of drugs includes caffeine, theophylline, and theobromine. These drugs relax smooth muscle (particularly bronchial smooth muscle), stimulate cardiac muscle and the central nervous system, increase diaphragmatic contractility, and promote diuresis through increased renal perfusion. The action of various theophylline compounds depends on the content of theophylline, which is the active constituent. Theophylline products vary in their rate of absorption and therapeutic effects. Recently there has been a shift away from the use of theophylline as a first-line drug in the treatment of acute reactive airway disease. There are many theophylline-containing preparations, including aminophylline (Amoline, Somophyllin, Aminophyllin), dyphylline (Dilor, Droxine, Lufyllin), and theophylline (Bronkodyl, Elixophyllin, Somophyllin-T, others).

Other Respiratory Drugs

A variety of other pharmacological agents can be used to treat asthma and other obstructive pul

---

BOX 14-13

Alpha, Beta$_1$, and Beta$_2$ Activities of Adrenergic Drugs Used as Bronchodilators

Alpha Effects (Vasoconstriction)
Systemic Effects
Vasoconstriction
Increased blood pressure

Inhalation
Decreased bronchial congestion
Increased duration of action for coadministered beta$_2$ drugs

Beta$_1$ Effects
Systemic Effects
Cardiac stimulation
  Increased heart rate
  Increased force of contraction
    Possible palpitations and dysrhythmias
Relaxation of gastrointestinal tract

Inhalation
Some bronchodilation and increased heart rate
Fewer effects than with subcutaneous administration

Beta$_2$ Effects
Systemic Effects
Bronchiole dilation
Stimulation of skeletal muscles (tremors)
Vasodilation (mainly in blood vessels supplying muscle)
Glycogenolysis

Central Nervous System Effects
Nervousness
Anxiety
Insomnia
Irritability
Dizziness
Sweating

Inhalation
Lower incidence of systemic effects than with subcutaneous administration

monary diseases. These drugs include prophylactic asthmatic agents such as cromolyn sodium (Intal, Sodium Cromoglycate), aerosol corticosteroid agents such as beclomethasone dipropionate (Vanceril Inhaler, Beclovent), *dexamethasone sodium phosphate* (Decadron Phosphate), and muscarinic antagonists (anticholinergics) such as ipratropium (Atrovent) and glycopyrrolate (Robinul). These medications reduce the allergic or inflammatory response to a variety of stimuli. In the acute care setting, intravenous steroids (Solu-Medrol 125 mg) may be given in an attempt to decrease the inflammatory response and improve airflow.

Antihistamines

Histamine is a chemical mediator found in almost all body tissues. The concentration is highest in the skin, lungs, and gastrointestinal tract. The body releases histamine when exposed to an antigen such as pollen or insect stings. This results in increased localized blood flow, increased capillary permeability, and swelling of the tissues. In addition, histamine produces contractile action on bronchial smooth muscle.

Allergic responses involving histamines and other chemical mediators include local effects such as angioedema, eczema, rhinitis, urticaria, and asthma. Systemic effects from release of histamine as well as certain other mediators may result in anaphylaxis (see Chapter 22).

Antihistamines compete with histamine for receptor sites, thereby preventing the physiological action of histamine. There are two types of histamine receptors: H_1 receptors (acting primarily on the blood vessels and the bronchioles) and H_2 receptors (acting mainly on the gastrointestinal tract). Older antihistamines are specific antagonists for the H_1 receptors.

In addition to blocking some actions of histamine, antihistamines also have anticholinergic or atropine-like action. This may result in the inhibition of secretions, tachycardia, constipation, drowsiness, and sedation. In addition, most antihistamines have a local anesthetic effect that may sooth the skin irritation caused by an allergic reaction. The primary clinical use of antihistamines is for allergic reactions, but they are also sometimes prescribed to control motion sickness or as a sedative or antiemetic. Examples of antihistamines are dimenhydrinate (Dramamine), *diphenhydramine* (Benadryl Hydrochloride), *hydroxyzine hydrochloride* (Atarax), *hydroxyzine pamoate* (Vistaril), meclizine hydrochloride (Antivert), and *promethazine hydrochloride* (Phenergan, others).

Section Seven
Drugs Affecting the Endocrine System

● REVIEW OF ANATOMY AND PHYSIOLOGY

The endocrine system is a major means of controlling and integrating body functions (Box 14-14). Information from various regions in the body to distant sites is transmitted via blood-borne hormones.

Hormones are natural chemical substances that act after secretion into the blood stream from endocrine glands (ductless glands that secrete internally). These glands include the anterior and posterior pituitary, thyroid, parathyroid, and adrenal glands and the thymus, pancreas, testes, and ova-

BOX 14-14

Emergency Drugs: Endocrine System
dexamethasone (Decadron)
dextrose 50%
glucagon
insulin
methylprednisolone sodium succinate (Solu-Medrol)
oxytocin (Pitocin, Syntocinon)

ries. Although this discussion is limited to pancreatic hormones, hormones from the various endocrine glands work together to regulate vital processes, including:

- Secretory and motor activities of the digestive tract
- Energy production
- Composition and volume of extracellular fluid
- Adaptation, such as acclimatization and immunity
- Growth and development
- Reproduction and lactation

● PANCREAS

The pancreas lies beneath the peritoneum, between the greater curvature of the stomach and the duodenum. The pancreas is an exocrine gland (providing digestive juices to the small intestine) and an endocrine gland. The endocrine portion of the pancreas consists of pancreatic islets (islets of Langerhans), which produce the hormones that enter the circulatory system.

Hormones of the Pancreas

The pancreatic hormones play an important role in regulating the concentration of certain nutrients in the circulatory system. The two major hormones secreted by the pancreas are *insulin* and *glucagon.*

Insulin is the primary hormone that regulates glucose metabolism. In general, it increases the ability of the liver, adipose tissue, and muscle to take up and use glucose. Glucose not immediately needed as an energy source is stored in the skeletal muscle, liver, and other tissues as glycogen.

Glucagon primarily influences the liver, although it has some effect on skeletal muscle and adipose tissue. In general, *glucagon* stimulates the liver to break down glycogen so that glucose is released into the blood. *Glucagon* also inhibits the uptake of glucose by muscle and fat cells. The balancing action of these two hormones protects the body from hyperglycemia and hypoglycemia.

This balance of hormonal actions is important when considering the metabolic derangements that can occur in diabetes mellitus. The relationship of *glucagon* and *insulin* to other hormones and substances such as *dextrose 50%* (D_{50}) and *thiamine* (vitamin B_1) is addressed in Chapter 19.

Section Eight
Drugs Affecting the
Gastrointestinal Tract

Conditions of the stomach or gastrointestinal tract that may require emergency drug therapy are usually limited to nausea and vomiting. Emergency drugs (Box 14-15) used to treat these disorders are classified as emetics and antiemetics.

● EMETICS AND ANTIEMETICS

Vomiting is an involuntary action coordinated by the emetic center of the medulla. It may be initiated through the central nervous system as a secondary reaction to emotion, pain, or disequilibrium (motion sickness); through irritation of the mucosa of the gastrointestinal tract or bowel; and through stimulation from the chemoreceptor trigger zone of the medulla by circulating drugs and toxins (for example, opiates and digitalis).

BOX 14-15

Emergency Drugs: Gastrointestinal System
activated charcoal
diphenhydramine hydrochloride (Benadryl)
hydroxyzine pamoate (Vistaril)
promethazine hydrochloride (Phenergan)
syrup of ipecac

Emetics

Drugs used to induce vomiting are administered as part of the treatment for certain drug overdoses and poisonings. These drugs include apomorphine and *syrup of ipecac.* The treatment of drug overdoses and poisonings is further addressed in Chapter 23.

Antiemetics

Drugs used to treat nausea and vomiting include antagonists of histamine, acetylcholine, and dopamine, as well as other drugs whose actions are not clearly understood. These drugs are most effective when administered before rather than after nausea and vomiting have begun. For example, drugs used to treat motion sickness or vertigo should be taken 30 minutes before traveling. Listed are common antiemetics:

- Anticholinergic agents
  - scopolamine (Transderm-Scop)
- Antihistaminic agents
  - dimenhydrinate (Dramamine)
  - *diphenhydramine hydrochloride* (Benadryl)
  - *hydroxyzine pamoate* (Vistaril)
  - meclizine hydrochloride (Antivert)
  - *promethazine hydrochloride* (Phenergan)
- Antidopaminergic agents
  - chlorpromazine hydrochloride (Thorazine)
  - fluphenazine hydrochloride (Prolixin)
  - *haloperidol* (Haldol)
  - prochlorperazine (Compazine)
- Miscellaneous agents
  - dronabinol (Marinol)
  - nabilone (Casamet)
  - benzquinamide hydrochloride (Emete-Con)

REFERENCES

1. Glanze W, editor: *Mosby's medical, nursing, and allied health dictionary,* ed 3, St Louis, 1990, Mosby.
2. McKenry L, Salerno E: *Mosby's pharmacology in nursing,* ed 18, St Louis, 1992, Mosby.
3. American Heart Association: Guidelines for cardiopulmonary resuscitation and emergency cardiac care, *JAMA* 268(16):2172, 1992.
4. Pratt J: Intraosseous infusion, *Int Pediatr* 4(1):19, 1989.
5. *St. Louis Post Dispatch,* St Louis, Mo, July 7, 1988, p. 1D.
6. Fedson D: *Immunizations for health care workers and patients in hospitals. Prevention and control of nosocomial infections,* Baltimore, 1987, Williams & Wilkins.
7. Protection against occupational exposure to hepatitis B virus (HBV) and human immunodeficiency virus (HIV), *Federal Register,* Washington, DC, 1987, Department of Labor, Department of Health and Human Services.
8. National Institute for Occupational Safety and Health, Centers for Disease Control: *Guidelines for prevention of transmission of human immunodeficiency virus and hepatitis B virus to health-care and public-safety workers,* Atlanta, 1989, The Centers.
9. Collier C: *Recommendations for needle-stick, puncture wounds, and muco-cutaneous blood and body fluid exposure in health care workers,* Jefferson City, Mo, 1992, Missouri Department of Health Bureau of Communicable Disease Control.
10. Clark J et al: *Pharmacologic basis of nursing practice,* ed 4, St Louis, 1993, Mosby.
11. Syverud S et al: Prehospital use of neuromuscular blocking agents in a helicopter ambulance program, *Ann Emerg Med* 17(3):237, 1988.

Summary

Pharmacological agents have lifesaving and life-threatening potential. Whether a paramedic is administering medication or obtaining a patient history, an understanding of the pharmacological properties of drugs is an important part of emergency care.

Throughout the years, I've seen many paramedics become overwhelmed by the severity of a trauma call. Remember, most trauma patients who show signs and symptoms of shock will require blood replacement and surgery. It is important to expedite transport for definitive care, using good basic skills first.

Ray McDowell
Paramedic Field Supervisor
Crowley, Louisiana

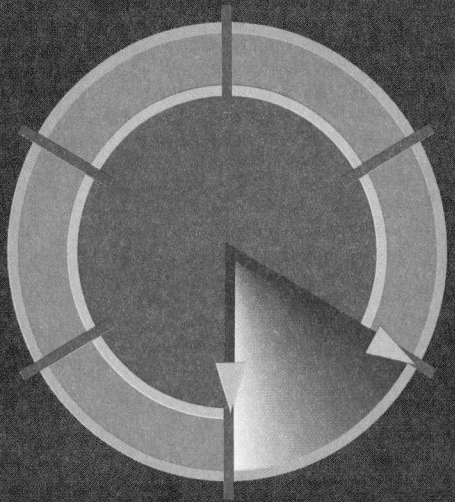

15 TRAUMA

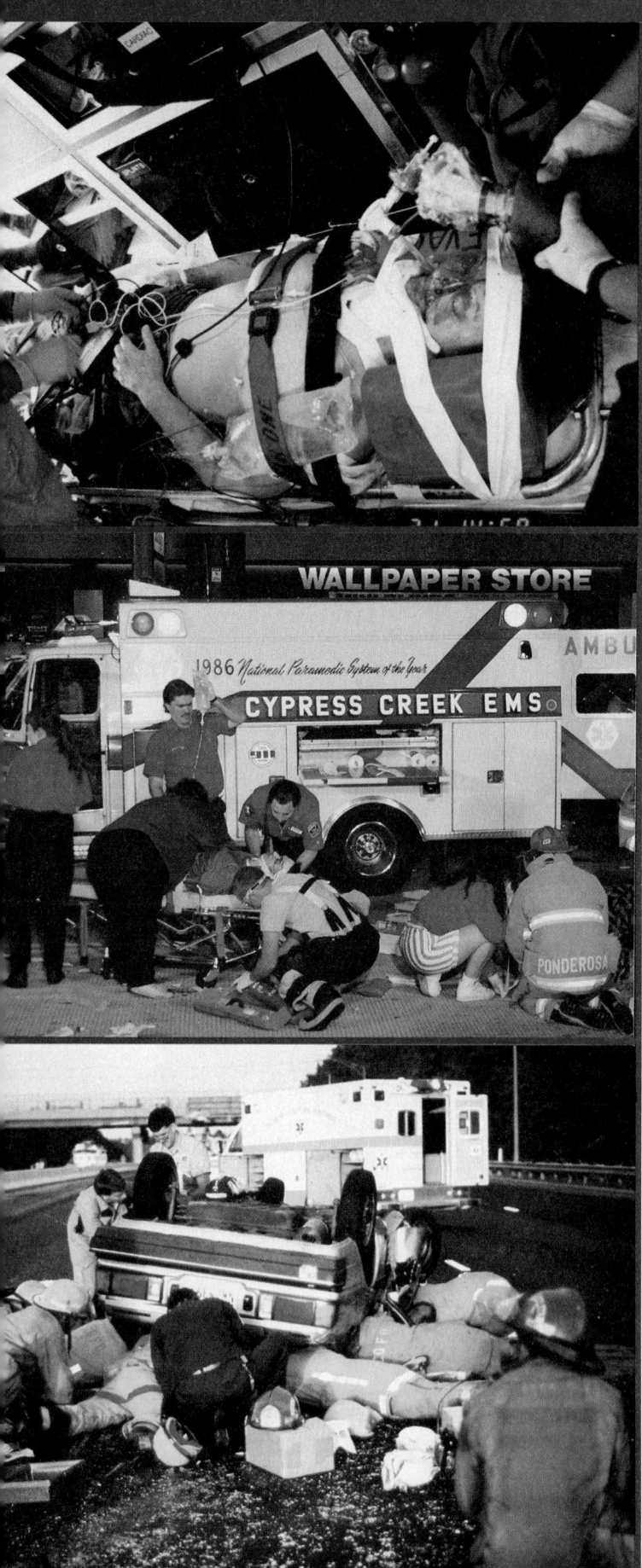

Victims of trauma may require lifesaving surgery to repair an injury. The paramedic must be able to recognize this category of patient, stabilize the patient's injury when possible, and provide rapid transportation to an appropriate medical facility for definitive care.

● INCIDENCE OF TRAUMA

Trauma is a devastating medical and social problem. It is the leading cause of death and disability among Americans between the ages of 1 and 37 years and the fourth leading cause of death among all Americans.[1] In 1990, there were approximately 93,500 accidental deaths in the United States; the National Safety Council estimates that the total number of injures in the United States approaches 60 million annually.[2] Of these injuries, 9 million are disabling, 350,000 result in permanent

KEY TERMS

blunt trauma: An injury produced by the wounding forces of compression and change of speed, both of which may disrupt tissue.

cavitation: A temporary or permanent opening produced by a force that pushes body tissues laterally away from the track of a projectile.

Glasgow coma scale: A standardized system for assessing the degree of conscious impairment in the critically ill and for predicting the duration and ultimate outcome of coma.

kinematics: The process of predicting injury patterns that may result from the forces and motions of energy.

pediatric trauma score: An injury severity index that grades six components commonly seen in pediatric trauma patients: size (weight), airway, central nervous system, systolic blood pressure, open wound, and skeletal injury.

revised trauma score: An injury severity index that uses the Glasgow coma scale with measurements for systolic blood pressure and respiratory rate.

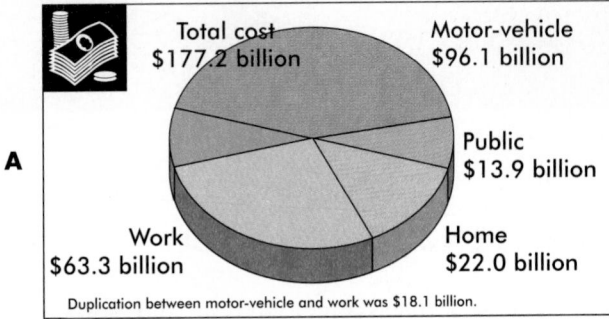

A

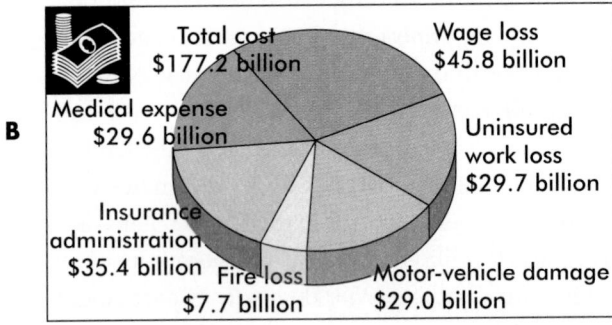

B

Fig. 15-1 A, Costs of accidents by class, 1991. **B,** Costs of accidents by component, 1991.

BOX 15-1

The Golden Hour

The first hour after severe injury is known as the *golden hour*. It is a critical period in which surgical intervention for the trauma patient can enhance survival and reduce complications. The paramedic must recognize patients in this category and ensure that prehospital care activities do not unnecessarily delay patient transport. These patients are best served by rapid assessment, stabilization of life-threatening injuries, and rapid transportation to an appropriate medical facility for definitive care.

---

impairment, and 8,400,000 result in temporary disabilities. In 1991, the cost of trauma to society in terms of lost productivity exceeded 177 billion dollars. The breakdown of trauma-related accident costs in the United States for 1991 is illustrated in Fig. 15-1.

Prevention of Trauma Deaths

Deaths from trauma can be categorized as occurring in three periods: immediate, early, and late. Each period presents its own unique problems.[3]

Immediate

The first peak of the distribution is immediate death, which occurs within seconds or minutes of the injury. Lacerations of the brain, brain stem, upper spinal cord, heart, aorta, or other large vessels usually cause these deaths. Few if any patients in this category can be saved. The number of these deaths can be reduced only through effective injury-prevention programs.

Early

The second death peak occurs within the first 2 to 3 hours after injury (Box 15-1). These deaths are usually caused by subdural or epidural hematoma, hemopneumothorax, ruptured spleen, lacerated liver, pelvic fracture, or multiple injuries associated with significant blood loss. Most of these injuries are treatable with available techniques, but the time lapse between injury and definitive care is critical.

Late

The third peak of the distribution is death that occurs days or weeks after the injury. These deaths most often result from sepsis, infection, or multiple organ failure. Prehospital emergency care focused on early recognition and treatment of life-threatening injury can play an important role in preventing these late deaths from trauma.

**Section One
Kinetics of Trauma**

● WOUNDING FORCES OF TRAUMA

Trauma injuries are those caused by a transfer of energy from some external source to the human body. The extent of injury is determined by the type of energy applied, how quickly it is applied, and to what part of the body. To understand the transfer of energy, four basic laws of physics must be considered:

1. Newton's first law of motion: An object, whether at rest or in linear motion, remains in that state unless force is applied.
2. Conservation of energy law: Energy cannot be created or destroyed; it can only change form. The forms energy can take are mechanical, thermal, electrical, and chemical.
3. Newton's second law of motion: Force equals mass multiplied by acceleration or deceleration.
4. Kinetic energy (KE) equals half the mass (M) multiplied by the velocity squared (V^2).

As the formula indicates, velocity is much more important than mass in determining total kinetic energy.

Example: An automobile and its unrestrained 150-pound driver are traveling 60 miles per hour. According to Newton's first law of motion, the auto remains in motion until acted on by an outside force. If the driver gradually applies the brakes, the mechanical energy of the auto is slowly converted to thermal injury (conservation of energy law) by the friction of the brakes; the energy transfer occurs gradually through the slow deceleration.

If the auto strikes a tree, however, and is instantaneously stopped, the mechanical energy is absorbed by the tree, the auto, and the driver. When the front of the car has stopped, the rear of the car continues forward until all of the energy of its motion is absorbed. The driver is traveling in the same direction and at the same speed as the auto before impact, so like the rear of the car, the driver continues forward. The driver suffers injuries in anatomical areas that strike the vehicle.

In this sequence, then, the motion of the front of the car is stopped by the tree; the steering column continues forward and stops against the dashboard; the driver's sternum stops against the steering column; and the driver's chest cavity and its contents hit the sternum and are crushed from behind by the posterior thorax, deforming the entire chest.

The kinetic energy would be calculated as follows:

$$KE = \frac{1}{2}(MV^2)$$

$$KE = \frac{150}{2} \times 60^2$$

$$KE = 270,000 \text{ units of energy}$$

As shown in this calculation, the 150-pound driver traveling 60 miles per hour must change 270,000 units of kinetic energy (known as *foot*

pounds, calculated as pounds multiplied by miles per hour) into another form of energy when he or she stops. In addition, since force equals mass multiplied by acceleration (Newton's second law of motion), the 150-pound driver is moving forward in the vehicle with approximately 9000 foot-pounds of force when stopped by the steering column. The energy of the body's motion causes tissue destruction as this energy is absorbed into the body cells when the body stops. This example illustrates the principle, but the actual total force would also be determined by the true rate of deceleration or "g" force and a variety of other factors.)

Kinematics

The process of predicting injury patterns that may result from the forces and motions of energy is known as **kinematics.** Certain types and patterns of injuries are associated with certain mechanisms of trauma. In addition to individual factors such as age and protective factors (for example, restraint systems, helmets, air bags), the paramedic should consider the following when evaluating the trauma patient:

- Mechanism of injury
- Force of energy applied
- Anatomy
- Energy (for example, mass; velocity; distance; thermal, electrical, chemical forms)

Section Two
Blunt Trauma

● BLUNT TRAUMA

Blunt trauma is an injury produced by the wounding forces of compression and change of speed, which may disrupt tissue.

Direct compression or pressure on a structure is the most common type of force applied in blunt trauma. The amount of injury depends on the length of time of compression, the force of compression, and the area compressed. For example, compression of the thorax may lead to fractured ribs or pneumothorax. Other compression injuries include contusions and lacerations of solid organs and rupture of hollow (air-filled) organs.

Acceleration is an increase and a decrease in the velocity of a moving object; both may produce significant injury. For example, when a vehicle stops abruptly, the occupant's body continues its constant velocity after the impact and decelerates as it strikes the steering wheel, restraint system, or dashboard. The body is forcibly stopped, but the contents of the cranial, thoracic, and peritoneal body cavities remain in motion because of inertia. Tissues may be stretched, crushed, ruptured, lacerated, or sheared from their points of attachment as a result. Examples of change-of-speed injuries include concussion, bony fracture, organ laceration, and aortic tear.

● MOTOR VEHICLE COLLISION

The various injuries produced by blunt trauma can be best illustrated by examining motor vehicle collisions, although forces that cause blunt trauma can result from a variety of impacts. As described in the example, a motor vehicle collision involves three separate impacts as the energy is transferred: (1) the vehicle strikes an object, (2) the occupant collides with the inside of the car, and (3) the internal organs collide inside the body. The injuries that result from automobile crashes depend on the type of collision, the position of the occupant inside the vehicle, and the use or nonuse of personal restraints.

Motor vehicle collision may be classified by type of impact. These include head on, lateral, rear end, rotational, and roll over. The forces of compression and change of speed produce predictable injury patterns in each type of collision.

Head-On (Frontal) Impact

Head-on collisions result when forward motion stops abruptly (for example, when one automobile collides with another traveling in the opposite direction). The first collision occurs when the auto hits the second vehicle, resulting in damage to the front of the car. As the vehicle abruptly stops, the occupant continues to move at the speed of the auto before impact. The front seat occupant continues forward into the steering column or dashboard, resulting in the second collision. The occupant usually travels in one of two pathways in relationship to the dashboard: down and under or up and over. The precise course of this pathway determines how the organs collide inside the body and the extent of tissues damaged.

In the down-and-under pathway, the occupant travels downward into the vehicle seat and forward into the dashboard or steering column (Fig. 15-2). The knees become the leading part of the body, striking the dashboard; the upper legs absorb most of the impact. Predictable injuries include dislocated knees, patellar fractures, fractured femurs, posterior fractures or dislocation of the acetabulum, vascular injury, and hemorrhage. After the initial impact of the knees into the dashboard, the body rotates forward. As the chest wall hits the steering column or dashboard, the head and torso absorb energy as indicated in the description of the up-and-over pathway.

In the up-and-over pathway, as the body in forward motion strikes the steering wheel, the momentum of the thorax is absorbed by the ribs and underlying structures (Fig. 15-3). Predictable injuries from this transfer of energy include fractured

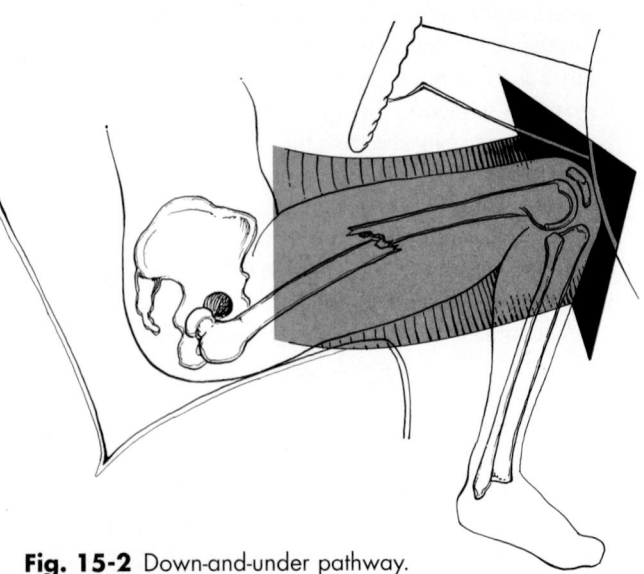

Fig. 15-2 Down-and-under pathway.

ribs, ruptured diaphragm, hemopneumothorax, pulmonary contusion, cardiac contusion, myocardial rupture, and vascular disruption (most notably, aortic rupture).

If the abdomen is the point of impact, compression injuries can occur to the hollow abdominal organs, the solid organs, and the lumbar vertebrae. The kidneys, liver, and pancreas are subject to vascular tears from supporting tissue, including the disruption of renal vessels from their points of attachment to the inferior vena cava and descending aorta. Predictable injuries include lacerated liver, ruptured spleen, internal hemorrhage, and abdominal organ incursion into the thorax (ruptured diaphragm).

If the occupant's head is the leading point of impact, the continued momentum of the body is absorbed by the cervical vertebrae. Cervical flexion or hyperextension may produce severe angulation of the neck, resulting in fracture or dislocation of the cervical vertebrae. In addition, angulation and direct in-line compression of the cervical vertebrae may damage the soft tissues of the neck and cause spinal cord injury and spinal instability. Other predictable injuries include trauma to the brain (for example, concussion, contusion, edema) and vascular disruption resulting in subdural or epidural hematoma.

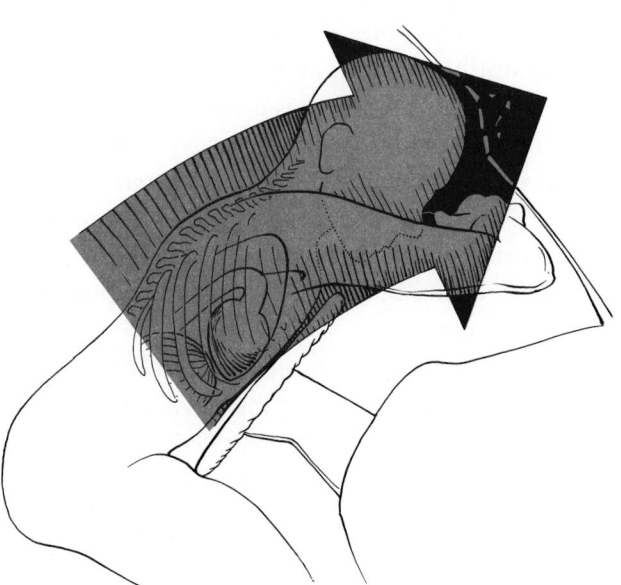

Fig. 15-3 Up-and-over pathway.

Lateral Impact

Lateral impact occurs when a vehicle is struck from the side. Injury patterns depend on whether the damaged automobile remains in place or moves away from the point of impact. The external shell of an auto that remains in place after impact usually intrudes into the passenger compartment, directing force at the lateral aspect of the occupant's body. Predictable injuries result from compression to the torso, pelvis, and extremities. Examples of these injuries include fractured ribs, pulmonary contusion, ruptured liver or spleen (depending on the side involved), fractured clavicle, fractured pelvis, and head and scalp injury.

If the damaged vehicle moves away from the point of impact, the occupant is also pulled away from the point of impact, moving laterally with the car. The effects of inertia on the head, neck, and thorax produce lateral flexion and rotation of the cervical spine. This movement can result in neurological injury and tears or strains of the lateral ligaments and supporting structures of the neck. Injuries can also occur on the side of the passenger opposite the impact as the occupant is propelled toward the other side of the car. If other occupants are in the auto, secondary collision with other passengers is likely.

Rear-End Impact

A vehicle struck from behind rapidly accelerates, causing the auto to move forward under the occupant. The greater the difference in the forward speed of the two vehicles, the greater the force and damaging energy of the initial impact. For example, if a stationary vehicle is struck from behind by a vehicle traveling 50 mph, the damaging energy is greater than when a vehicle traveling 30 mph is struck by a vehicle traveling 50 mph. Thus in forward collisions, the *sum* of both vehicles' speeds is the velocity that produces damage. In rear-end collisions, the *difference* between the two speeds is the damaging velocity.

Predictable injuries in rear-end collisions include back injuries; fractures of the femur, tibia, fibula, and ankles; and cervical strain or fracture caused by hyperextension. If the auto undergoes a second collision by striking an object in front of it, injuries associated with frontal impact should also be suspected.

Rotational Impact

Rotational impacts occur when an off-center portion of the automobile (usually the front quarter) strikes an immoveable object or one that is moving slower or in the opposite direction. The part of the vehicle striking the object stops during impact. The remainder of the vehicle continues in forward motion until the energy is completely transformed. The occupant moves inside the vehicle with the forward motion and is usually struck by the side of the car as the vehicle rotates around the point of impact. A rotational impact results in injuries common to both head-on and lateral collisions.

Roll-Over Accidents

In roll-over accidents, the occupant tumbles inside the auto and is injured wherever the body strikes the vehicle. The various impacts occur at many different angles, providing the potential for multiple-system injuries. Predictable injuries sustained in roll-over collisions are difficult to categorize. These accidents may produce any of the injury patterns associated with other types of collisions.

● RESTRAINTS

Public awareness programs in personal safety and various state laws regarding lap belt protection have increased auto occupant use of personal restraints to an estimated 82% in 1990.[4] The National Highway Traffic Safety Administration (NHTSA) reports that, from 1983 through 1990, an estimated 24,886 lives were saved by safety belts and that another 5765 lives would have been saved if all 50 states had belt use laws in effect. According to the NHTSA, of all passenger fatalities, restrained passengers comprise 26.9%, and unrestrained passengers comprise 51.2%.

A significant hazard to unrestrained occupants is ejection from the vehicle after impact. Accord-

ing to 1990 data supplied by the NHTSA, 17.9% of unrestrained occupants were totally ejected, and 74% of these occupants were fatally injured. Ejection from vehicles accounts for 27% of trauma deaths that occur each year. A total of 1 of every 13 ejection victims suffers a spinal fracture, and ejected victims are killed 6 times as often as those who are not ejected.[5] The high mortality rate among ejected victims results in part from the occupant being subjected to a second impact as the body strikes the ground or another object outside the vehicle.

The three restraining systems available in the United States are lap belts, diagonal shoulder straps, and air bags, all of which significantly reduce injuries. If they are inappropriately worn, however, these protective devices can also produce injuries.

Lap Belts

The lap belt (alone or in combination with a diagonal shoulder strap) is the most commonly used restraint system. When properly applied, the lap belt should be directed at a 45-degree angle to the floor and be positioned between the anterior-superior iliac spine and the femur. A lap belt worn tightly enough to remain in this position absorbs energy forces and protects the abdominal cavity by transferring energy to the strong, bony pelvis.

If the lap belt is incorrectly worn above the anterior-iliac spine, the forward motion of the body during impact is absorbed by vertebrae T12, L1, and L2. As the thorax is propelled forward, the abdominal organs are compressed between the vertebral column and the lap belt, causing potential injury to the liver, spleen, duodenum, and pancreas. An indicator of these abdominal injuries is the presence of abrasions or a lap belt imprint over the abdomen.

Significant injury may result even when a lap belt is used correctly. These injuries occur from angulation of the lumbar spine, pelvis, thorax, and head around the restraint system and from failure of the restraint system to sufficiently decrease the impact forces. Injuries that may occur with high-speed impacts include sternal fractures, chest wall injuries, lumbar vertebral fractures, head injuries, and maxillofacial trauma.

Diagonal Shoulder Straps

Use of a diagonal shoulder strap helps absorb the forward motion of the thorax after impact. When worn in conjunction with the lap belt, the shoulder strap prevents the thorax, face, and head from striking the dashboard, windshield, or steering column. Clavicular fractures may result from the position of the shoulder strap. Organ collision inside the body, cervical fracture, and spinal cord injury may still injure internal organs during high-speed impacts, even when personal restraint systems are used.

Air Bags

Air bags inflate from the center of the steering wheel and dashboard during frontal impact. They are most effective in cushioning the forward motion of the occupant when used with a lap belt. Air bags deflate immediately and are effective only with an initial frontal collision. They are ineffective in lateral or roll-over impacts. These systems do not prevent movement in the down-and-under pathway. Thus the occupants' knees may still be the point of impact, resulting in leg, pelvis, and abdominal injuries. Any special considerations regarding air bags are addressed in Chapter 5.

Child Safety Seats

The leading cause of death in children under age 4 is injuries sustained in motor vehicle crashes; for each of these deaths, the U.S. Department of Health, Education, and Welfare estimates that thousands more suffer debilitating injury. The NHTSA reports that approximately 1546 children under the age of 5 were saved from 1982 through 1990 as a result of child restraint use; in 1990, 295 unrestrained children under the age of 5 died in passenger cars.[4]

Child safety seats are now required in all 50 states for selelct age groups of children. The seats are available in several shapes and sizes to accommodate the different stages of physical development, including infant carriers, booster seats, and toddler seats. Child safety seats use a combination of lap belts, shoulder belts, full body harnesses, and harness-and-shield apparatus to protect the child during vehicle collision. Predictable injuries likely to occur even with the appropriate use of child safety seats include blunt abdominal trauma, change-of-speed injuries from deceleration forces, and spinal injury.

● ORGAN COLLISION INJURIES

Organ motions and their injuries are a result of deceleration and compression forces. Recognition of these injuries requires a high degree of suspicion using the principles of kinematics.[6]

Deceleration Injuries

When body organs are put into motion after an impact, they continue to move in opposition to the structures that attach them to the body. Therefore there is a risk of separation of body organs from their attachments. Injury to the vascular pedicle or mesenteric attachment may lead to brisk or exsanguinating hemorrhage.

Head Injuries

When the head strikes a stationary object, the cranium comes to an abrupt stop, but brain tissue inside the cranium continues to move until it is compressed against the skull (Fig. 15-4). During this movement, brain tissue may be bruised or crushed, and blood vessels attached to the brain and skull may be torn, producing intracranial hemorrhage. Other injuries associated with deceleration of the head include central nervous sys-

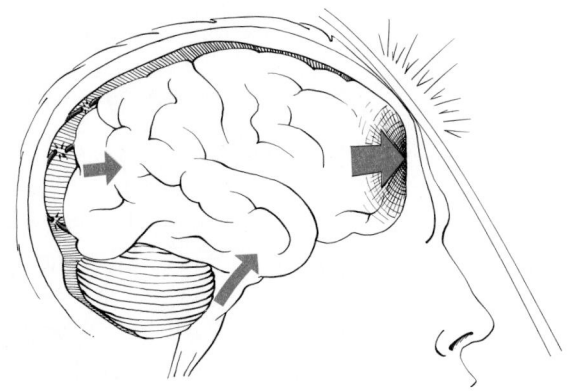

Fig. 15-4 After cessation of forward motion of the skull, the brain continues its motion, resulting in possible contusion and intracerebral hemorrhage.

tem injury from stretching of the spinal cord and its attachments and cervical fracture.

Thoracic Injuries

The aorta is frequently injured by severe deceleration forces. It is affixed at several points, most proximally by the aortic valve, below the arch by the ligamentum arteriosum, and along the descending aorta by its attachment to the thoracic spine. As the thorax strikes a stationary object, the heart and aorta continue in motion in opposition to their attachment at the lower end of the aortic arch. The aorta is usually sheared at the level of its ligamentum arteriosum attachment (Fig. 15-5). Frank rupture of the aorta leads to rapid exsanguination, but transection and dissection can tamponade, allowing patients to arrive at an emergency department and survive the injury.

Abdominal Injuries

When deceleration forces are applied to the abdomen, intraabdominal organs and retroperitoneal structures (most commonly the kidneys) are affected. The forward motion of the kidneys may shear them away from their vascular pedicle (Fig. 15-6); the forward motion of the small and large intestine may result in mesenteric tears. The downward and forward motion of the liver may cause separation at its midpoint from its vascular and hepatic duct pedicle, and the forward motion of the spleen, which is restrained by the diaphragm and abdominal wall attachments, may result in tear of the splenic capsule.

Compression Injuries

Compressive forces can injure any portion of the body. This discussion is limited to injuries of the head, thorax, and abdomen.

Head Injuries

Compression injuries to the head may result in open fractures, closed fractures, and bone fragment penetration. Associated injuries include brain contusion and lacerations of brain tissue. Compression forces to the skull can also produce hemorrhage from fractured bone, meningeal vessels, or the brain itself. If facial structures are involved in the injury, soft tissue trauma and facial bone fractures may occur. Central nervous system injury and cervical fracture should also be considered when evaluating injuries to the head.

Thoracic Injuries

The lungs and heart are frequently involved in compression injury to the thorax. Associated inju-

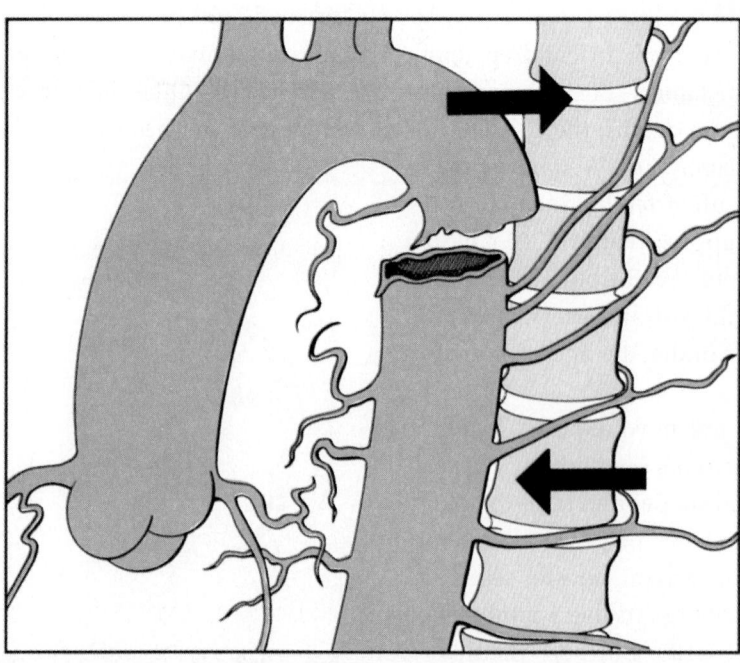

Fig. 15-5 Shearing forces along the descending aorta move in opposition to the attachments at the lower end of the aortic arch.

ries to external structures include fractured ribs and sternum, which may lead to an unstable chest wall, open pneumothorax, or both.

A serious lung injury that can occur from compression forces results from a "paper-bag effect." This injury occurs when increased intrathoracic pressure causes rupture of the lungs. For example, when an automobile driver is threatened by an approaching vehicle, he or she notes the potential collision and instinctively takes a deep breath and holds it. This protective inhalation fills the lungs (paper bag) with air against the closed glottis and creates a closed container (Fig. 15-7). As the thorax strikes the steering column, the inward motion of the chest wall causes an increase in lung pressure, resulting in alveolar rupture (as when a hand strikes the paper bag). This phenomenon is thought to be responsible for the majority of pneumothoraces after automobile trauma.[6] Penetration of a fractured rib through the pleura or laceration of the lung also contributes to pneumothorax after blunt trauma to the chest.

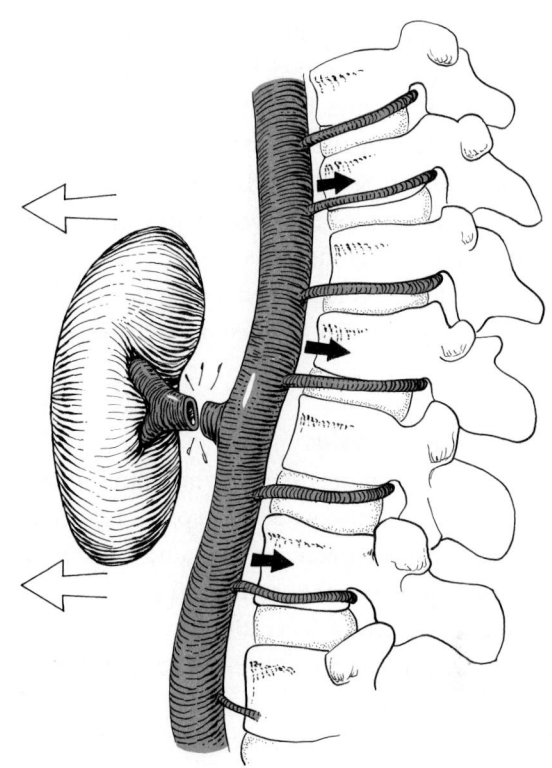

Fig. 15-6 Forward motion of the kidney may cause separation at its midpoint from its vascular pedicle.

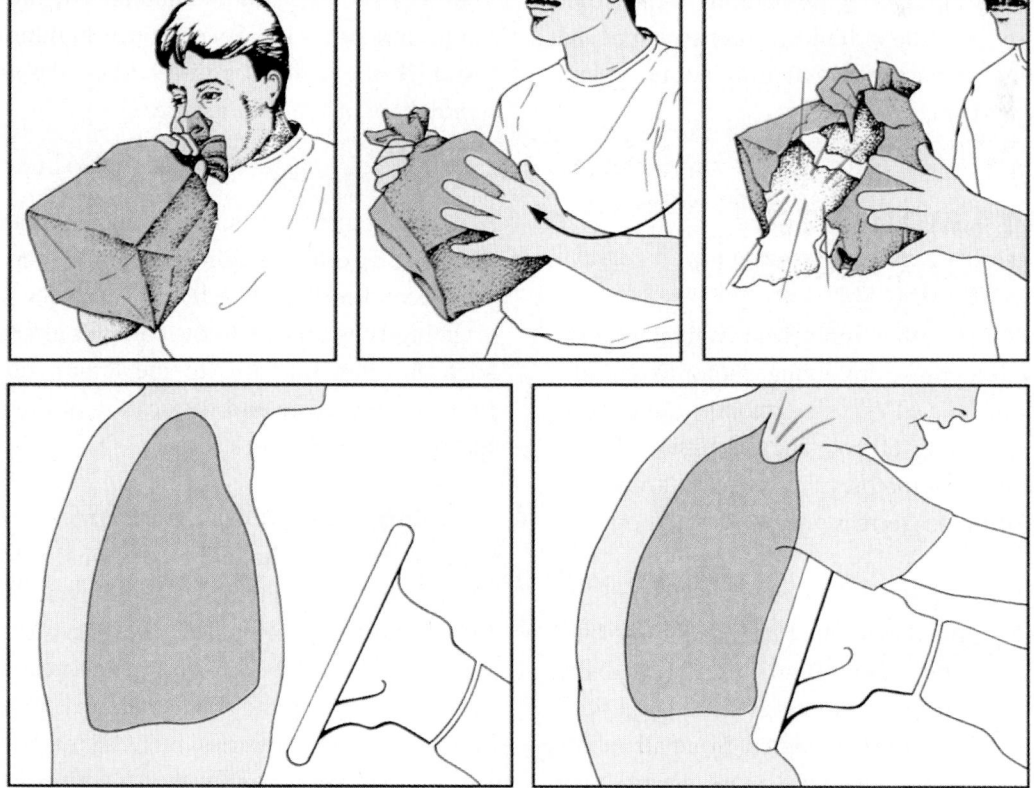

Fig. 15-7 In an accident, the lungs are similar to a paper bag held tightly at the neck and compressed with the other hand. Thoracic compression against the closed glottis causes the lungs to pop, just like the paper bag.

During compression injury to the thorax, the heart may become trapped between the sternum and the thoracic spine. Depending on the force of energy applied, increased intraabdominal compression and retrograde hydrostatic pressure on the aorta can rupture the aortic valve. Compression of the patient's heart between the sternum and the vertebral column can cause cardiac dysrhythmias, myocardial contusion, or rupture of the ventricle.

Abdominal Injuries

Compression injuries to the abdominal cavity can have serious effects such as solid organ rupture, vascular organ hemorrhage, and hollow organ perforation into the peritoneal cavity. Common injuries include lacerations to the spleen, liver, and kidney and rupture of the bladder, especially if it is full.

Just as the paper-bag effect produces a pneumothorax in thoracic injury, compression of the abdominal cavity can cause increases in intraabdominal pressure that exceed the tensile strength of the abdominal compartment. Predictable injuries include rupture or herniation of the diaphragm and rupture of hollow organs such as the gallbladder, urinary bladder, duodenum, colon, stomach, and small bowel.

● OTHER MOTORIZED VEHICULAR ACCIDENTS

Injuries from other motorized vehicular accidents include those involving motorcycles, all-terrain vehicles (ATVs), snowmobiles, and farm machinery, among others. The discussion in this text is limited to motorcycles and ATVs because of their common recreational use and popularity.

Small motorized vehicles are considered by many to be more dangerous than other motor vehicles because they offer minimal protection to the rider from the transfer of energy associated with collisions. The injuries sustained in small motor vehicle accidents are usually more severe than those received from automobile crashes. As with other types of motor vehicle collision, predictable injuries depend on the type of collision that occurs.

Motorcycle Collision

Common motorcycle collisions result from head-on impact and angular impact and from laying the motorcycle down.

Head-On Impact

A motorcycle's center of gravity is above the front axle, forward of the rider's seat. When the motorcycle strikes an object that stops its forward motion, the rest of the bike and the rider continue forward until acted on by an outside force. Typically, the motorcycle tips forward and the rider is propelled over the handlebars. The forward motion of the rider is stopped by secondary impacts with the handlebars or other objects. Predictable injuries caused by these secondary impacts include head and neck trauma and compression injuries to the chest and abdomen. If the feet remain on the foot rests during impact, the rider's forward motion is absorbed by the midshaft of the femur. This may result in bilateral fractures to the femur and lower leg. Severe perineal injuries may result if the rider's groin strikes the tank or handlebars of the motorcycle.

Angular Impact

When a motorcycle strikes an object at an angle, the rider is often caught between the cycle and the second object. Predictable injuries include crushing-type injuries to the patient's affected side such as open fractures to the femur, tibia, and fibula and fracture and dislocation of the malleolus.

Laying The Motorcycle Down

Professional racers and recreational riders may use the strategy of laying the motorcycle down before striking an object. This protective maneuver separates the rider from the motorcycle and the object by allowing the rider to slide away from the bike. Predictable injuries include massive abrasions ("road rash") and minor fractures to the affected side as the rider slides on the ground or pavement. Although these injuries may be severe, they are usually less serious than those that might occur from other types of impacts.

ATVs

Injuries from accidents involving ATVs are quite different from those seen in motorcycle collisions. ATVs have a higher center of gravity than motorcycles and a large, flat front tire that makes them somewhat difficult to steer. These factors require a specific balance much different than that required for motorcycles or bicycles to keep the ATV from overturning.

The natural tendency of the rider to put a foot down to support the ATV when stopping may lead to the rear tire running over the rider's foot, catching the leg, and throwing the rider forward off the vehicle and onto his or her shoulder. Predictable injuries from ATV accidents include extremity injury and fracture, clavicular fracture, and serious head and neck injuries.

Personal Protective Equipment

Protective equipment for riders of small motor vehicles includes boots, leather clothing, eye protection, and helmets. Helmets are structured to absorb the energy of an impact, thereby reducing injuries to the face, skull, and brain. According to the NHTSA, there were 3270 fatalities in 1990 from motorized cycle crashes; in that year, three of every five riders in fatal crashes did not wear helmets.[4] (Nonuse of helmets increases head injuries by more than 300%.[5])

● PEDESTRIAN ACCIDENTS

In 1988, 70,000 people were injured in auto-pedestrian collisions in the United States. Of those injuries, 8500 were fatal.[7] All auto-pedestrian collisions have great potential to produce serious injuries and require a high degree of suspicion for multiple-system trauma.

There are three primary mechanisms of injury (multiple impacts) in auto-pedestrian collisions. The first impact occurs when the bumper of the vehicle strikes the body, the second occurs as the pedestrian strikes the hood of the vehicle, and the third occurs when the pedestrian strikes the ground or another object.

Predictable injuries depend on whether the pedestrian is an adult or a child. Variations in the height of the pedestrian in relation to the bumper and hood of the car affect the injury pattern. The velocity of the vehicle is also a major factor. However, even low speeds can result in serious trauma because of the mass of the vehicle and the transfer of energy. Another consideration in evaluating a pedestrian accident is the possibility of the patient suffering a second pedestrian-auto collision from another vehicle.

Adult Pedestrian

Most adult pedestrians threatened by an approaching vehicle attempt to protect themselves by turning away from the oncoming auto. Therefore injuries are often a result of lateral or posterior impacts. During the initial impact, the adult is usually struck by the vehicle bumper in the lower legs, producing lower extremity fractures.

The second impact occurs as the pedestrian falls toward the hood of the vehicle. This impact may result in fractures to the femur, pelvis, thorax, and spine and produce intraabdominal or intrathoracic injury. The head and spine may also be injured if the victim strikes the hood or windshield.

The third impact occurs as the victim strikes the ground or is thrown against another object. This may result in significant damage to the hip and shoulder of the affected side as the body makes contact with the landing surface. Fractures, internal hemorrhage, and head and spinal injury may be caused by the sudden deceleration and compression forces associated with this impact.

Child Pedestrian

Unlike adults, who try to protect themselves from auto-pedestrian injury, children tend to face the oncoming vehicle. Therefore their injuries are often the result of a frontal impact. Because children are smaller than most adults, the initial impact of the auto occurs higher on the body, usually above the knees or pelvis. Predictable injuries from the initial impact include fractures to the femur and pelvic girdle as well as internal hemorrhage.

The second impact occurs as the front of the vehicle's hood continues forward, making contact with the victim's thorax. The victim is immediately thrown backward, forcing the head and neck to flex forward. Depending on the position of the patient in relation to the auto, the child's head and neck may contact the vehicle's hood. Predictable injuries include abdominal-pelvic and thoracic trauma, facial trauma, and head and neck injury.

The third impact occurs as the child is thrown downward to a landing surface. Because of the child's smaller size and weight, he or she may fall under the vehicle and be dragged for some distance or fall to the side of the vehicle and be run over by the front or rear wheels. Predictable injuries consist of all of those previously described and may include traumatic amputation.

● OTHER CAUSES OF BLUNT TRAUMA

Sports Injuries

Sports are practiced by participants of all ages. Common sports associated with frequent injuries include contact sports such as football, basketball, hockey, and wrestling; high-velocity activity sports such as downhill skiing, water skiing, bicycling, and skate boarding; racquet sports; and swimming and diving.

Although sporting activities provide a variety of health benefits, they can also produce severe injury. For example, sports-related injuries are the third most common cause of cervical spine injury, preceded only by motor vehicle crashes and falls.[8]

Sport-related injuries are caused by forces of acceleration and deceleration, compression, twisting, hyperextension, and hyperflexion. Using the general principles of kinematics, potential injuries can be predicted by ascertaining the following:

- What energy forces were transferred to the patient?
- To what part of the patient's body was the energy transferred?
- What associated injuries should be considered as a result of the energy transfer?

- How sudden was the acceleration or deceleration?
- Was compression, twisting, hyperextension, or hyperflexion involved in the injury?

If the patient used protective equipment, it should be evaluated to help determine the mechanism of injury. For example, the condition and structural stability of a helmet may provide clues as to the amount of energy transferred to the patient during the accident. Other examples include broken skis, broken hockey sticks, and structural deformities of bicycles.

Blast Injuries

Blast injury is a general term used to describe damage to a patient exposed to a pressure field produced by an explosion of volatile substances. Explosions of this nature have primarily been a wartime concern. In recent years, however, the number of blast injuries from homemade bombs used in social protests and terrorist activities has increased. Other causes include exploding automobile batteries, industrial use of volatile substances, accidents in clandestine drug laboratories, explosions in mining, and transportation accidents involving hazardous materials.

Blasts release large amounts of energy in the form of pressure and heat. If this release of energy is confined in a casing (for example, a bomb), the pressure ruptures the casing and ejects fragments of the housing at high velocity. The remaining energy is transmitted to the surrounding environment and may severely injure bystanders. Blast injuries may be classified as primary, secondary, tertiary, and miscellaneous injuries.

Primary blast injuries result from sudden changes in environmental pressure. These injuries usually occur in gas-containing organs and cause the most severe damage when poorly supported tissue is displaced beyond its elastic limit. The organs and tissues most vulnerable to primary blast injury are the ears, lungs, central nervous system, and gastrointestinal tract. Predictable damage to these areas includes hearing loss, pulmonary hemorrhage, cerebral air embolism, abdominal hemorrhage, or bowel perforation.

Thermal burns may also result from the release of energy in the form of heat. These injuries are likely to occur on unprotected areas (for example, face, hands) that are close to the source of explosion (see Chapter 16).

Secondary blast injuries usually result when bystanders are struck by flying debris (for example, glass, metal, falling mortar). In addition to the obvious injuries such as lacerations and fractures, flying debris may cause high-velocity missile-type injuries if nails, screws, or casing fragments are part of the debris.

Tertiary blast injuries occur when victims are propelled through space by an explosion and strike a stationary object. These injuries are similar to those sustained in vertical falls and ejections from automobiles or small motor vehicles. In most cases, the sudden deceleration from the impact causes more damage than the acceleration through space because the deceleration is much more sudden. Injuries from these forces include damage to the abdominal viscera, central nervous system, and musculoskeletal system.

Miscellaneous blast injuries result from radiation exposure and inhalation of dust and toxic gases. Predictable injuries include those to the eyes, lungs, and soft tissues.

Vertical Falls

According to the National Safety Council, falls accounted for 12,200 deaths in 1991; they were the second leading cause of accidental death in the United States.[1] In predicting injuries associated with falls, the paramedic should evaluate the distance fallen, the body position of the patient on impact, and the type of landing surface struck. Injuries associated with vertical falls are a result of deceleration and compression.

Falls from distances greater than 3 times the height of an individual (15 to 20 feet) may be associated with severe injuries. As a point of reference for these distances, the roof of a one-story house is approximately 15 feet and a two-story house approximately 30 feet from the ground.

Adults who have fallen more than 15 feet usually land on their feet. A predictable injury from this vertical fall is bilateral calcaneus fractures. As the energy dissipates from the initial impact, the head, torso, and pelvis push downward, and the body is forced into flexion. When this occurs, hip dislocations and compression fractures of the spinal column in the thoracic and lumbar areas are seen. If the patient leans forward or attempts to break the fall with outstretched hands, bilateral Colles' fractures (clinically evident by the so-called silver fork deformity) to the wrists are likely.

If the distance fallen is less than 15 feet, most adults land in the position in which they fell. For example, an adult who falls head first will strike the landing surface with the head, arms, or both. Predictable injuries depend on the body part that strikes the landing surface and the route of transfer of energy through the body. Internal injuries should be suspected if the trunk of the body is the initial impact area.

Children tend to fall head first, regardless of distance fallen or body position during the fall because their heads are proportionally larger. For this reason, children are usually victims of head injury.

The ability of the landing surface to absorb energy influences the severity of injury. For example, less damage would be expected from a fall on a soft, grassy surface than a fall on asphalt or concrete.

Section Three
Penetrating Trauma

● PENETRATING TRAUMA

All penetrating objects, regardless of velocity, cause some form of tissue disruption. This damage occurs as a result of two types of forces: crushing and stretching. The character of the penetrating object, its speed of penetration, and the type of body tissue it passes through or into determine which of the two mechanisms of injury predominates.

Cavitation is a temporary or permanent opening produced by a force that pushes body tissues laterally away from the tract of a projectile. The amount of cavitation produced by the transfer of energy is directly related to the density of tissue in a given body area and the ability of the body tissue to return to its original shape and position. For example, a patient who has received a high-velocity blow to the abdomen experiences abdominal cavitation at the moment of impact. Because of the density of the abdominal musculature, however, the cavitation is temporary even in the presence of severe intraabdominal injury.

Permanent cavities are produced by penetrating injuries in which the transfer of energy exceeds the tensile strength of the tissue. Certain injuries (for example, a stab wound to the abdomen) may produce temporary and permanent cavitations as tissues are displaced in frontal and lateral directions.

● BALLISTICS

The effect of a projectile on the body is determined primarily by the energy created and dissipated by the object into surrounding tissues. In dealing with injuries from penetrating trauma, the principles of kinematics should be considered. To review, kinetic energy equals half the mass of an object multiplied by the square of its velocity.

With reference to ballistic trauma, doubling the mass doubles the energy, but doubling the velocity quadruples the energy. Therefore a small-caliber bullet traveling at high speed can produce more serious injury than a large-caliber bullet traveling at a lower speed, provided that it does not strike a major vessel or organ.

Damage And Energy Levels of Projectiles

Injuries caused by penetrating trauma may be classified as those resulting from three energy levels: low, medium, and high. For the purpose of this text, nonbullet weapons are considered low-energy projectiles, and bullets are considered medium- and high-energy projectiles.

Low-energy projectiles such as knives, needles, and ice picks cause tissue damage by their sharp, cutting edges (Fig. 15-8). The amount of tissue crushed in these injuries is usually minimal be-

cause the amount of force applied in the wounding process is small. The more blunt the penetrating object, the more force that must be applied to cause penetration. The more force needed to cause penetration, the more tissue crushed. The damage of tissue from low-energy injuries is usually limited to the pathway of the projectile.

When evaluating a patient with a stab wound, the paramedic should attempt to identify the type of wounding object. In addition, the possibility of multiple wounds, embedded penetrating objects, extensive internal damage to organs of the thorax and abdomen, and penetration of multiple body cavities should be considered. A high degree of suspicion is also indicated for stab wounds to areas of the back and flank, since these may be associated with penetrating hollow visceral injuries and potential injuries to retroperitoneal organs. Penetrating injuries of the thorax may involve the abdomen, just as abdominal injuries may involve the thorax.

Medium-energy injuries are usually caused by firearms that have a muzzle velocity of less than 1500 feet per second. All handguns and some rifles are considered medium-energy weapons. The injury track produced by medium-energy weapons is usually 2 to 3 times the diameter of the projectile.

High-energy injuries are usually caused by firearms with a muzzle velocity of more than 1500 feet per second. Examples of high-energy weap-

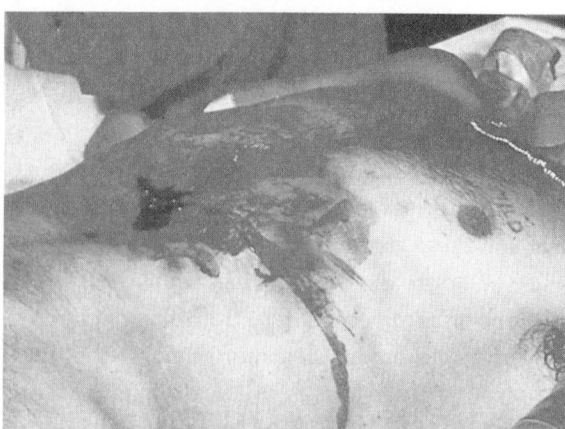

Fig. 15-8 Stab wound in which a knife had pierced the liver and pancreas and entered the splenic vein.

ons include military rifles, M-15s, M-16s, and some deer rifles. As with medium-energy injuries, the injury track produced by high-energy weapons is usually 2 to 3 times the diameter of the projectile.

Wounding Forces of Medium- and High-Energy Projectiles

A firearm cartridge is composed of a bullet made of metal, gunpowder to propel the bullet, a primer to explode and ignite the gunpowder, and a cartridge case that surrounds these components. When the trigger is pulled, the metal hammer strikes the firing pin, which ignites the primer. The gunpowder ignites and forces the bullet to exit the cartridge case.

The mechanism of injury from firearms is related to the energy created and dissipated by the bullet into the surrounding tissues. When a firearm is discharged, several events affect this dissipation of energy and ultimately the wounding forces of the missile:

1. As the missile travels through air, it experiences wind resistance, or drag. The greater the drag, the greater the slowing effect on the missile. Therefore a firearm discharged at close range usually produces a more severe injury than the same firearm discharged at a greater distance.

2. As the missile travels through air, a sonic pressure wave spreads out behind the missile during its flight through the air. Because the speed of sound in tissue is approximately 4 times the speed of sound in air, the sonic pressure wave jumps ahead and precedes the missile through the tissue. This pressure wave displaces tissue and sometimes stretches it dramatically.

3. Tissue disruption is caused by the localized crush of tissue in the missile's path and the momentary stretch of the surrounding tissue.

When a projectile strikes a body, tissue stretches at the point of impact to allow entry of the penetrating object (temporary cavitation). Because the projectile's energy exceeds the tensile strength of the tissue, tissue crush occurs, impelling surrounding tissues outward from the path of the projectile (permanent cavitation). The differences in wounds caused by projectiles vary with the amount and location of crushed and stretched tissue (Fig. 15-9).

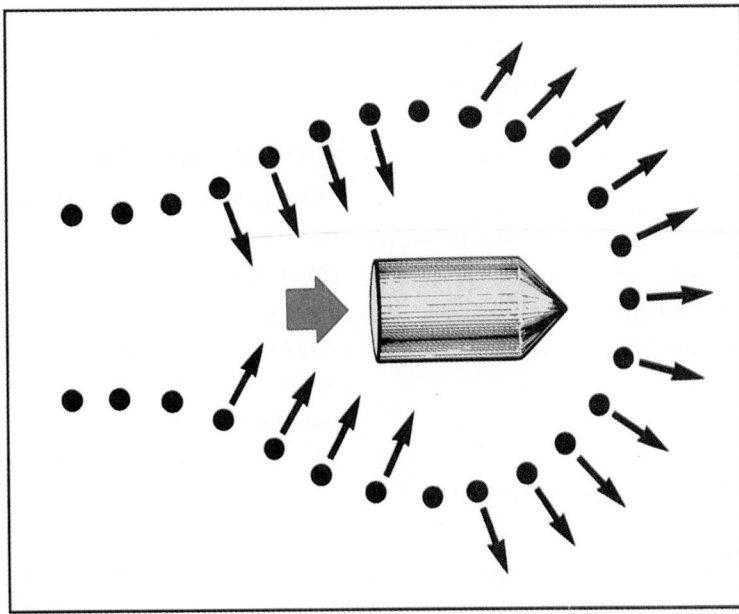

Fig. 15-9 Bullet passing through tissue. The temporary cavity is created by outward stretching of the permanent cavity as the tissue particles move away from the penetrating missile.

The wounding forces of a missile depend on the projectile mass, deformation, fragmentation, type of tissue struck, striking velocity, and range.[6]

Projectile Mass

Tissue crush is limited by the physical size or profile of the projectile. If the missile strikes point first, the crushed area will be no larger than the diameter of the bullet. If the missile is tilted as it strikes the body, the amount of crushed tissue will be no larger than the length and longitudinal cross section of the bullet.

Deformation

Some firearm missiles deform when striking tissue (for example, expanding hollow- or soft-point hunting bullets). The points of these projectiles typically flatten on impact. The diameter of the bullet is thus expanded, creating a larger area of crushed tissue. Military use of these bullets in war has been forbidden.

Fragmentation

Each piece of missile crushes its own path through tissue, causing extensive tissue damage. These fragments produce a larger frontal area than a single, solid bullet and disperse energy into the surrounding tissues very rapidly. Tissues weaken from the multiple fragment tracks and increase the subsequent stretch of the temporary cavity. The higher the velocity, the more likely the bullet is to fragment. If a bullet fragments, there may be no exit wound.

Type of Tissue Struck

Tissue disruption varies greatly with tissue type. For example, elastic tissues such as the bowel wall, lung, and muscle tolerate stretch much better than nonelastic organs such as the liver.

Striking Velocity

The velocity of a missile determines the extent of cavitation and tissue deformation. Low-velocity missiles localize injury to a small radius from the center of the injury tract and have little disruptive effect, pushing the tissue aside. High-velocity missiles produce more serious injuries because they lose more energy to the tissues and produce more cavitation.

Bullet yaw or tumble in tissue also contributes to cavitation and tissue damage. A wedge-shaped bullet's center of gravity is nearer to the base than the nose. As the missile strikes body tissue, it slows rapidly. Momentum carries the base of the bullet forward and the center of gravity becomes the leading part of the missile. This forward rotation around the center of mass causes an end-over-end motion, producing more energy exchange and more tissue damage.

Range

The distance of the weapon from the target is a significant factor in the severity of ballistic trauma. Air resistance (drag) slows the missile significantly; therefore increasing the distance of the projectile from the target decreases the velocity at the time of impact.

If the firearm is discharged at close range (within 3 feet), cavitation may occur from the combustion of powder and the forceful expansion of gases. The gas and powder may enter the body cavity and cause internal explosion of tissue. (This is common with shotgun wounds but less common with handguns because the latter produce a small amount of gas and create a small entrance wound.) The expansion of only gas can cause extensive tissue destruction, especially in an enclosed area (for example, the skull).

Shotgun Wounds

Shotguns are short-range, low-velocity weapons. These firearms fire multiple lead pellets, which are encased in a larger shell. Each pellet (there may be 9 to 400 or more, depending on pellet size and gauge of gun) is considered a missile capable of producing tissue damage. Each shell contains pellets, gunpowder, and a plastic or paper wad that separates the pellets from the gunpowder. This wad of unsterile material increases the potential for infection in shotgun wounds.

The energy transferred to body tissue and the resultant tissue damage depends on the gauge of the gun, size of the pellets, powder charge, and distance from the victim. For example, a 12-gauge, full-choke shotgun with number 6 shot (275 pellets) concentrates 95% of the pellets into a 7-inch circle at 10 yards. At close range, a shotgun injury has the potential for creating extensive tissue damage similar to that from a high-velocity missile weapon.

Entrance and Exit Wounds

The appearance of entrance and exit wounds is affected by a variety of factors, including range, barrel length, caliber, powder, and weapon (Fig. 15-10). In general, an entrance wound over soft tissue is round or oval and may be surrounded by an abrasion rim or collar. If the firearm was discharged at intermediate or close range, powder burns (tattooing) may also be present.

Exit wounds, if present, are generally larger than entrance wounds because of the cavitational wave that occurred as the bullet passed through the tissues. As the bullet exits the body, the skin may "explode," resulting in ragged and torn tis-

Forensic Considerations in Managing Gunshot Wounds

Lifesaving procedures always take precedence over forensic considerations. However, the paramedic should not touch or move weapons or other environmental clues unless it is absolutely necessary for patient care procedures. Other forensic considerations follow:

- Document the exact condition of the patient and wound appearance on arrival at the scene, including environment of the patient, body position in relation to objects, doorways.
- Disturb the scene as little as possible.
- If possible, cut or tear clothing along a seam to avoid altering tears made by a penetrating object.
- Avoid cutting through a bullet hole in the clothing.
- Do not shake clothing.
- Keep all clothing in a paper bag rather than a plastic bag that may alter evidence and do not give it to the victim's family members.
- Save any avulsed tissue for forensic pathology.
- If the bullet is retrieved, place it in a padded container to prevent marring and secure the evidence until it is delivered to the authorities (obtain a receipt).

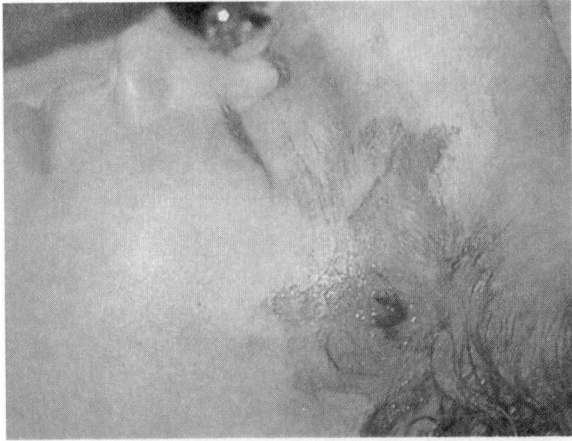

A

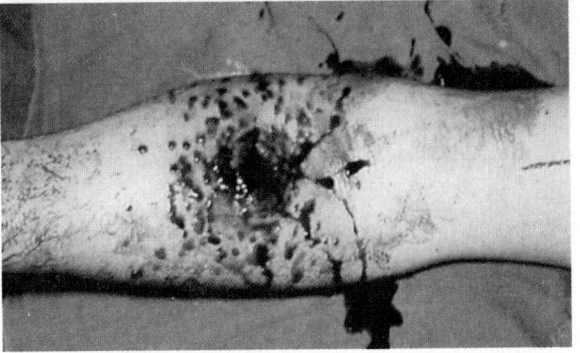

B

Fig. 15-10 A, The powder marks show that this 0.22-caliber bullet wound was inflicted at close range. **B,** A short-range shotgun wound to the forearm. **C,** Exit wound caused by a powerful shotgun fired at close range.

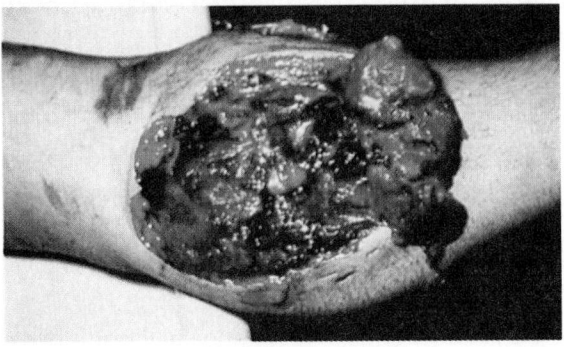

C

sue. This splitting and tearing often produces a star-burst or stellate wound.

If the muzzle is in direct contact with the skin at the time of firearm discharge, expanding gases may enter the tissue and produce crepitus on examination. These burning gases may also produce thermal injury at the entrance site and along the injury track.

Special Considerations for Specific Injuries

Identification of ballistic injuries requires a thorough examination and a high degree of suspicion. This is because penetrating trauma from high- and medium-velocity missiles is unpredictable.

Head Injuries

Gunshot wounds to the head are typically devastating because of direct destruction of brain tissue and subsequent swelling. In addition, patients with head wounds frequently sustain severe face and neck injuries, resulting in significant blood loss, difficulty in maintaining airway control, and spinal instability.

As a medium-energy projectile penetrates the skull, the energy is absorbed within the closed space of the cranium. The resulting force of the injury compresses brain tissue against the cranial cavity, often fracturing orbital plates and separating the dura from the bone. Depending on the characteristics of the missile, the bullet may not have sufficient force to exit the skull after penetration, as occurs with 0.22- and 0.25-caliber handguns. In these injuries, the bullet follows the curvature of the skull's interior, producing significant damage.

High-velocity wounds to the skull produce massive destruction as pieces of skull and brain are typically blown away. At close range, this results in part from the large quantities of gas produced by combustion of the propellant. If the weapon is held in contact with the head, the gas follows the bullet into the cranial cavity, producing an explosive effect.

Thoracic Injuries

Gunshot wounds to the thorax may result in severe injury to the pulmonary and vascular sys-

tems. If the lungs are penetrated by a missile, the pleura and pulmonary parenchyma are likely to be disrupted, producing a pneumothorax. On occasion, the pulmonary defect allows air to continue to flow into the thoracic cavity that cannot be expelled. The subsequent increase in pressure may eventually cause collapse of the lung and a shift in the mediastinum to the unaffected side (tension pneumothorax).

Vascular trauma from penetrating injuries may result in massive internal and external hemorrhage. For example, if the pulmonary artery or vein, vena cava, or aorta is destroyed, exsanguination may occur within minutes. Other vascular injuries from penetrating trauma to the thorax include hemothorax and, if the heart is involved, myocardial rupture or pericardial tamponade.

Penetrating injury can cause thoracic trauma in the absence of visible chest wounds. For example, a bullet may enter the abdomen and travel upward through the diaphragm and into the thorax. All victims of gunshot wounds to the abdomen should accordingly be evaluated for thoracic injury, and victims of thoracic gunshot wounds should be evaluated for abdominal injury.

Abdominal Injuries

Gunshot wounds to the abdomen usually require surgical assessment to determine the extent of injury. Penetrating trauma may affect multiple organ systems, causing damage to air-filled and solid organs, vascular injury, trauma to the vertebral column, and spinal cord injury. A high degree of suspicion should be maintained when treating victims of penetrating abdominal trauma, even if they appear to be stable.

Extremity Injuries

Gunshot wounds to the extremities are occasionally life threatening and may result in lifelong disability. Special considerations with these injuries include vascular injury with bleeding into soft tissues and damage to nerves, muscles, and bones. Any extremity that has sustained penetrating trauma should be evaluated for bone injury, motor and sensory integrity, and the presence of adequate blood flow.

Vessels may be injured by being struck by the bullet or by temporary cavitation. Either mechanism can damage the lining of the blood vessel, producing hemorrhage or thrombosis. Penetrating trauma can damage muscle tissue by stretching it as the muscle expands away from the path of the missile. Stretching exceeding the tensile strength of the muscle produces hemorrhage.

Bone struck by a penetrating object may be deformed and fragmented. If this occurs, the transfer of energy causes pieces of bone to act as secondary missiles, crushing their way through surrounding tissue. This may result in extensive damage and additional tissue disruption.

Section Four
Assessment and Management of the Trauma Patient

● ASSESSMENT PROTOCOLS

Several assessment protocols or injury rating systems (also known as *indices* or *scales*) are used to triage, guide patient care, predict patient outcome, identify changes in patient status, and evaluate trauma care in epidemiological studies and quality-assurance reviews. These indices are especially important to prehospital personnel in determining patient care needs with reference to hospital resources. Local protocols should be followed, and medical control should always be consulted before transport of any patient.

The assessment protocols addressed there are Glasgow coma scale, trauma score, revised trauma score, and pediatric trauma score. Many local and state EMS agencies use the data generated by these indices to monitor hospital trauma care and to help determine the allocation of hospital resources.[2] These indices become more reliable as indicators of patient outcome when combined with other measures of physiological status.

Glasgow Coma Scale

The **Glasgow coma scale** (GCS) evaluates eye opening, verbal response, motor responses, and

brain stem reflex function. The scale is considered one of the best indicators of eventual clinical outcome[2] and should be part of any neurological examination for patients with head injury (Table 15-1).

Trauma Score

The trauma score (TS) was developed in 1980 to predict outcome for patients with blunt or penetrating injuries (Table 15-2). It was based on the trauma index, an earlier measurement introduced in 1971, that used a numerical injury rating system based on a patient's injured body region, type of injury, and cardiovascular, central nervous system, and respiratory status. The TS modified the trauma index to include systolic blood pressure, respiratory rate, and the GCS. The TS has limited use in the prehospital setting.

Revised Trauma Score

The **revised trauma score** (RTS) uses the GCS with measurements for systolic blood pressure and respiratory rate that are divided into five intervals (Table 15-3). A range of values for these physiological measurements is assigned a number

TABLE 15-1 Glasgow Coma Score			
Eye Opening			Total GCS Points
Spontaneous	4		14-15 = 5
To voice	3		11-13 = 4
To pain	2		8-10 = 3
None	1		5-7 = 2
			3-4 = 1
Verbal Response			
Oriented	5		
Confused	4		
Inappropriate words	3		
Incomprehensible words	2		
None	1		
Motor Response			
Obeys command	6		
Localizes pain	5		
Withdrawn (pain)	4		
Flexion (pain)	3		
Extension (pain)	2		
None	1		
Total trauma score			1-16

TABLE 15-2 Calculation of Trauma Score Using the Glasgow Coma Scale

Glasgow Coma Scale		
Eye-opening response	Spontaneous	4
	To voice	3
	To pain	2
	None	1
Best verbal response	Oriented	5
	Confused	4
	Inappropriate words	3
	Incomprehensible sounds	2
	None	1
Best motor response	Obeys command	6
	Localizes pain	5
	Withdraws (pain)	4
	Flexion (pain)	3
	Extension (pain)	2
	None	1
TOTAL	Apply this score to GCS portion of TS below:	3-15
Trauma Score		
GCS (total points from above)	14-15	5
	11-13	4
	8-10	3
	5-7	2
	3-4	1
Respiratory rate	10-24/min	4
	25-35/min	3
	36/min or greater	2
	1-9/min	1
	None	0
Respiratory expansion	Normal	1
	Retractive/none	0
Systolic blood pressure	90 mm Hg or greater	4
	70-89 mm Hg	
	50-69 mm Hg	
	0-49 mm Hg	1
	No pulse	0
Capillary refill	Normal	2
	Delayed	1
	None	0
TOTAL TRAUMA SCORE		1-16

Trauma score	16	15	14	13	12	11	10	9	8	7	6	5	4	3	2	1
Percentage survival	99	98	96	93	87	76	60	42	26	15	8	4	2	1	0	0

TABLE 15-3 Revised Trauma Score

GCS	SPB	RR	Coded Values
13-15	>89	10-29	4
9-12	76-89	>29	3
6-8	50-75	6-9	2
4-5	1-49	1-5	1
3	0	0	0

SPB, Systolic blood pressure, *RR*, respiratory rate.

between 0 and 4. These numbers are then added to give a total between 0 and 12. The American College of Surgeons recommends that patients who have a revised trauma score of 11 or less be transferred to level I trauma centers.[2]

Pediatric Trauma Score

The **pediatric trauma score** (PTS) grades six characteristics commonly seen in pediatric trauma

TABLE 15-4 Components of the Pediatric Trauma Score

Component	Values		
	+2	**+1**	**−1**
Size	≥20 kg	10-20 kg	≤10 kg
Airway	Normal	Maintainable	Unmaintainable
CNS	Awake	Obtunded	Coma
SBP	≥90 mm Hg	50-90 mm Hg	≤50 mm Hg
Open wound	None	Minor	Major
Skeletal injuries	None	Closed fracture	Open or multiple fractures

CNS, Central nervous system; *SPB,* systolic blood pressure.

BOX 15-2

CUPS System of Patient Categorization

CPR: The patient is in respiratory or cardiac arrest.

Unstable: The patient is in shock, with or without accompanying respiratory distress.

Potentially unstable: The patient has marginal vital signs and requires close monitoring. The victim's survivability may well be affected by transport or treatment delay.

Stable: The patient is in no distress. Vital signs are within normal limits, and there are no respiratory problems.

---

patients: size (weight), airway, central nervous system, systolic blood pressure, open wound, and skeletal injury (Table 15-4). The American College of Surgeons recommends that any pediatric trauma patient with a PTS of less than 8 be transported to a level I trauma center. Although specifically designed for pediatric patients, the PTS has demonstrated no advantages over the RTS. Pediatric trauma is further addressed in Chapter 27.

In addition to these assessment protocols, the paramedic may use other methods to categorize patients and to determine the need for immediate transport. One method of patient status coding is the CUPS system, which assigns patients to one of four categories (Box 15-2). Regardless of the method chosen, the paramedic must remember that assessment is a dynamic process in which patients' conditions frequently change. Constant monitoring of the patient is crucial, and changes in patient status may alter the course of a treatment plan.

● MANAGEMENT OF THE TRAUMA PATIENT

As discussed in Chapter 11, the prehospital management of a trauma patient may be limited to airway control, spinal immobilization, major fracture stabilization, fluid replacement, and rapid transportation to an appropriate medical facility. Prehospital management of specific traumatic injury is presented thorughout this chapter by body system.

● HEAD TRAUMA

Head injuries affect nearly 2 million people each year in the United States and account for approximately 50% to 55% of all prehospital deaths.[9] The categories of head trauma discussed in this section include maxillofacial trauma; ear, eye, and dental trauma; and trauma to the skull and brain.

Maxillofacial Trauma

In descending order of frequency, major causes of maxillofacial trauma are motor vehicle crashes, home accidents, athletic injuries, animal bites, intentional violent acts, and industrial injuries.[9] Maxillofacial trauma may be classified as soft tissue injuries and facial fractures.

Soft Tissue Injuries

The face receives its blood supply from the branches of the internal and external carotid arteries. Because of this rich vascular supply, soft tissue injuries to the face often appear to be quite serious (Fig. 15-11). With the exception of compromised upper airway and the potential for significant bleeding, however, damage to the tissues of the maxillofacial area is seldom life threatening. Depending on the mechanism of injury, facial

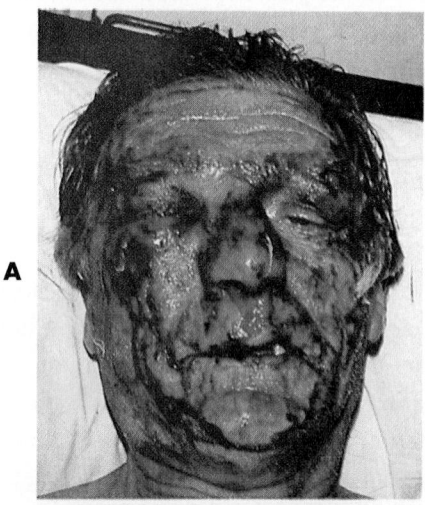

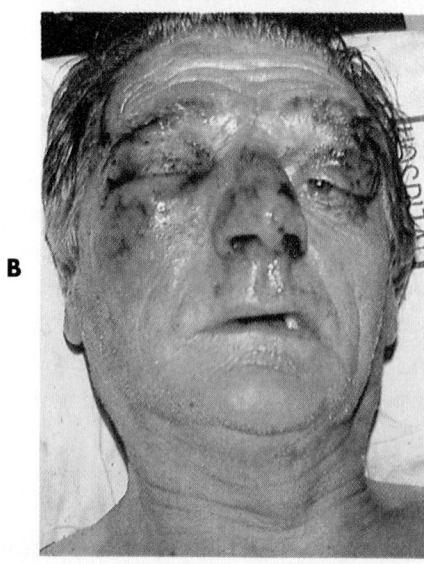

Fig. 15-11 A, Appearance of a patient after being attacked. **B,** Appearance of same man after cleansing.

trauma may range from minor cuts and abrasions to more serious injuries involving extensive soft tissue lacerations and avulsions.

Management

1. Use spinal precautions.
2. Assess the airway for obstruction caused by blood, vomitus, bone fragments, broken teeth, dentures, and damage to the anterior neck.
3. Apply suction as needed.
4. Secure and maintain the airway through oral or nasal adjuncts, tracheal intubation, or cricothyrotomy as indicated.
5. Ensure adequate ventilation and oxygenation.
6. Control bleeding through direct pressure and pressure bandages.

Facial Fractures

Although facial bones can withstand tremendous forces from energy impact, facial fractures are common after blunt trauma. The anatomical structure of the facial bones allows stepwise fracture to absorb the impact of blunt trauma. Blunt trauma injuries may be classified as fractures to the mandible, midface, zygoma, orbit, and nose. Signs and symptoms of facial fractures include:

- Pain
- Swelling
- Ecchymosis
- Lacerations
- Dental malocclusion
- Limitation of mandibular excursion
- Visual disturbances
- Limited ocular movements
- Asymmetry of cheekbone prominences
- Discontinuity of the orbital rim
- Crepitus
- Displacement of the nasal septum

Fractures of the Mandible

The mandible is the single facial bone in the lower third of the face. Because of its prominence, fractures to this bone rank second in frequency after nasal fractures. The mandible is a hemicircle of bone and may break in multiple locations, often distant from the point of impact. Signs and symptoms specific to mandibular fractures include malocclusion (patients may complain that their teeth do not "feel right" when their mouths are closed), numbness in the chin, and patients' inability to open their mouths. The patient may also have difficulty swallowing and excessive salivation. Most patients with mandibular fractures require hospitalization.

Anterior dislocation of the mandible in the absence of fracture may also occur as a result of blunt trauma to the face (rare), an abnormally wide yawn, and dental treatment requiring that the jaws be open for long periods. In these movements, the condylar head advances forward beyond the articular eminence of the temporal bone. The jaw-closing muscles spasm, and the mouth becomes locked in a wide-open position. The patient usually experiences severe pain from the muscle spasm and anxiety and discomfort that perpetuate the spasm. Mandibular dislocations are manually reduced in the emergency department with the aid of a muscle relaxant, sedative, or general anesthetic.

Fractures of the Midface

The middle third of the face includes the maxilla, zygoma, floor of the orbit, and nose. Fractures to this region result from direct or transmitted force (for example, blunt trauma to the mandible transmitted to produce fractures to the maxilla). They are often associated with central nervous system injury and spinal trauma (Fig. 15-12).

In 1901, a cadaver study done by LeFort described three patterns of injuries that can be produced in the midface region. These fractures bear his name (Fig. 15-13). A LeFort I fracture involves the maxilla up to the level of the nasal fossa. The LeFort II involves the nasal bones and medial orbits and is generally shaped like a pyramid. The LeFort III entails craniofacial dislocation involving all the bones of the face. Depending on the severity of injury, different combinations of LeFort fractures may be present.

Signs and symptoms specific to midface fractures include midfacial edema, unstable maxilla, lengthening of the face ("donkey face"), epistaxis, numb upper teeth, nasal flattening, and cerebrospinal fluid rhinorrhea (cerebrospinal fluid leakage caused by ethmoid cribriform plate fracture). Patients with midface fractures are usually hospi-

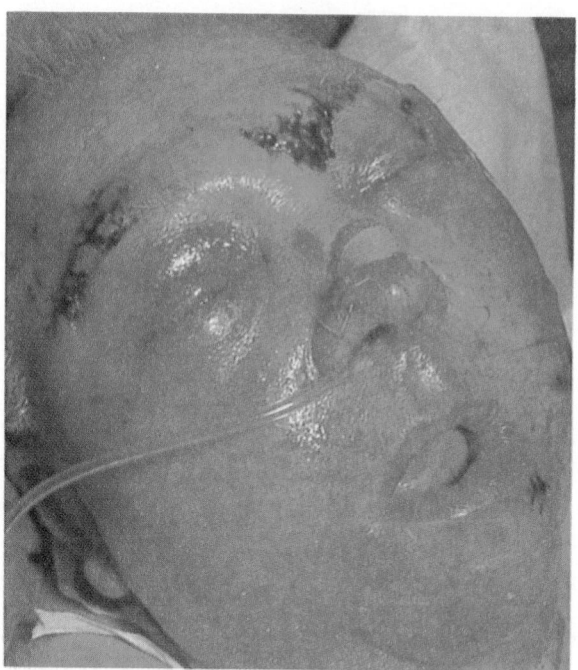

Fig. 15-12 Fracture of the middle third of the face.

talized. These patients are at risk (particularly those with LeFort II and III fractures) of having a seriously compromised airway and of having nasogastric or even nasotracheal tubes placed intracranially.

Fractures of the Zygoma

The zygoma (malar eminence) articulates with the frontal, maxillary, and temporal bones. It is commonly called the *cheekbone* and is seldom fractured because of its sturdy construction. When fractures occur, they are usually a result of physical assaults and motor vehicle crashes. Zygomatic fractures are frequently associated with orbital fractures and manifest similar clinical signs (Fig. 15-14). They are differentiated with radiological imaging. Signs and symptoms specific to zygomatic fractures include flatness of a usually rounded cheek area; numbness of the cheek, nose, and upper lip (particularly if an orbital fracture is involved); epistaxis; and altered vision.

Fractures of the Orbit

The orbital contents are protected by a bony ring that resembles a pyramid, with the apex pointed toward the back of the head. The bones of the walls, floor, and roof of the orbit are quite

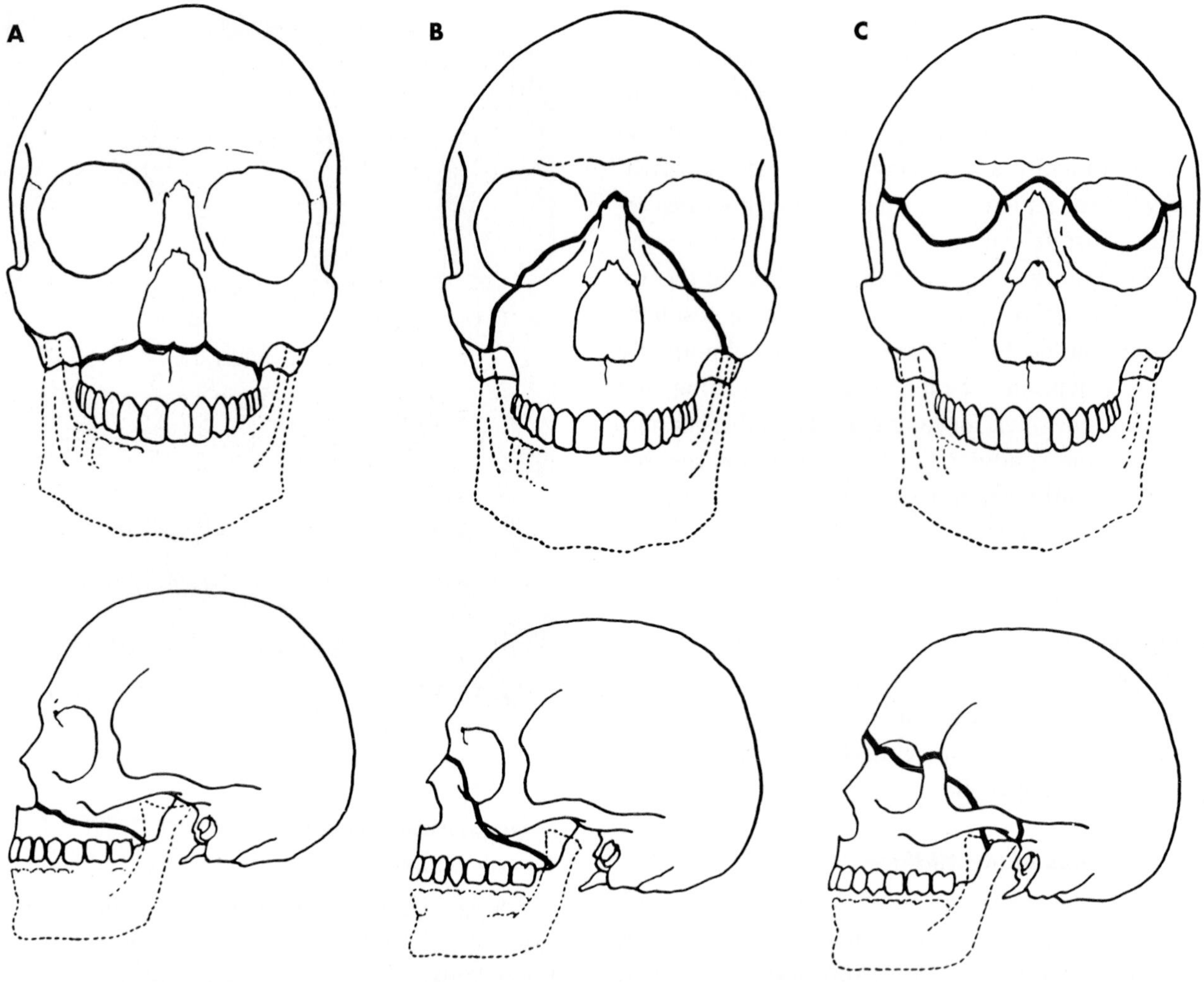

A   B   C

Fig. 15-13 A, LeFort I facial fractures (lateral and frontal views). **B,** LeFort II fractures (lateral and frontal views). **C,** LeFort III fractures (lateral and frontal views).

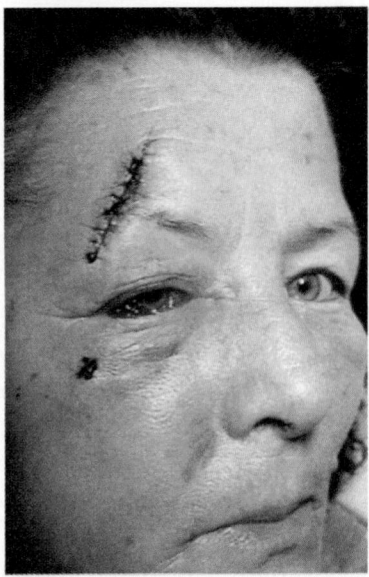

Fig. 15-14 Fracture of the zygomatic bone.

thin and are easily fractured by direct blows and transmitted forces (Fig. 15-15). In addition, many orbital fractures are associated with other facial injuries such as LeFort II and III fractures.

Blowout fractures to the orbit occur when an object of greater diameter than that of the bony orbital rim strikes the globe of the eye and surrounding soft tissue. This impact pushes the globe into the orbit, compressing the orbital contents. The sudden increase in intraocular pressure is transmitted to the orbital floor, the weakest part of the orbital structure. If the orbital floor fractures, the orbital contents may herniate into the maxillary sinus, where soft tissue and extraocular muscles may be entrapped in the defect. Signs and symptoms of blowout fractures include periorbital edema, subconjunctival ecchymosis, diplopia, en-

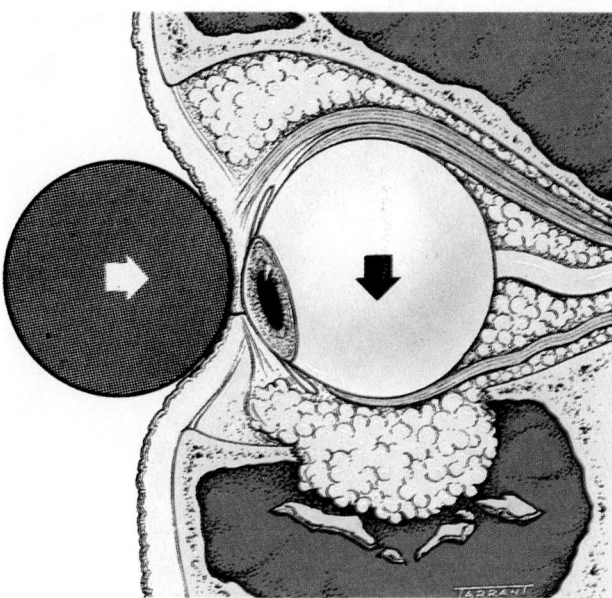

Fig. 15-15 Artist's impression of a blowout fracture caused by the impact of a ball.

ophthalmos (recessed globe), epistaxis, anesthesia in the region of the infraorbital nerve (anterior cheek), and impaired extraocular movements.

Orbital fractures are often associated with other fractures, such as Lefort II and III injuries, and those of the zygomatic complex. In addition, injury to the orbital contents is common and should be suspected with any facial fracture.

Fractures of the Nose

Of all the facial bones, the nasal bones have the least structural strength and are fractured most frequently. The external portion of the nose, formed mostly of hyaline cartilage, is supported mainly by the nasal bones and the frontal processes of the maxillary bones. Injuries to the nose may depress the dorsum of the nose, displace it to one side, or result only in epistaxis and swelling without apparent skeletal deformity. Fractures to the orbit may also be present. In children, minimal displacement of nasal bones can result in growth changes and ultimate deformity.

Management

1. Assume that the spine has been injured and use spinal precautions (facial fractures are as-

sociated with a high percentage of concomitant cervical spine fractures).
2. Assess the airway for obstruction caused by blood, vomitus, bone fragments, broken teeth, dentures, and damage to the anterior neck.
3. Apply suction as needed.
4. Secure and maintain the airway through oral or nasal adjuncts, tracheal intubation, or cricothyrotomy as indicated.

> **NOTE:**
> **Beware of nasal intubations in suspected midface and cribriform plate fractures.**

5. Ensure adequate ventilation and oxygenation.
6. Control bleeding through direct pressure and pressure bandages.
7. Control epistaxis by external direct pressure (compression of the anterior nares).

Ear, Eye, and Dental Trauma

The ears, eyes, or teeth may be injured separately or in association with other forms of head trauma. Injury to these regions may be minor or may result in permanent sensory function loss and disfigurement. Regardless of the severity, ear, eye, and dental trauma should be evaluated and treated only after life-threatening problems (for example, airway control with spinal precautions, breathing, circulation) have been addressed.

Ear Trauma

Trauma to the ear may include lacerations and contusions, thermal injuries, chemical injuries, traumatic perforations, and barotitis.

Lacerations and Contusions

Lacerations and contusions usually result from blunt trauma and are particularly common in victims of domestic violence (Fig. 15-16). These injuries are treated by direct pressure to control bleeding and the application of ice to decrease soft tissue swelling. If a portion of the ear has been avulsed, the avulsed tissue should be retrieved if

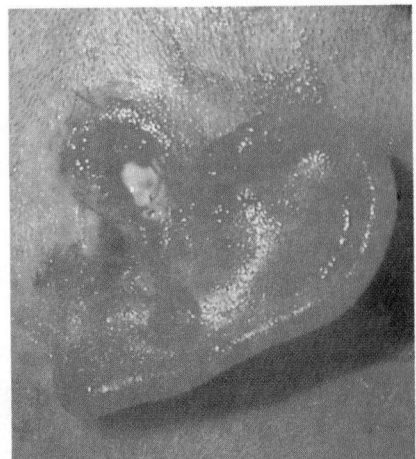
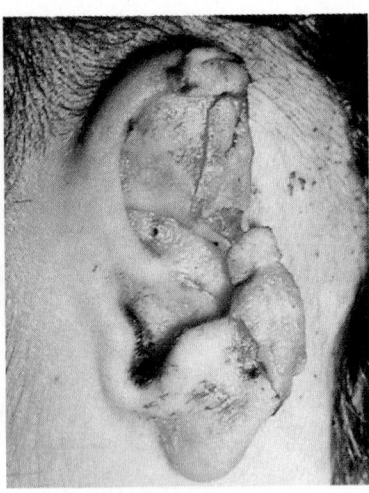

Fig. 15-16 A, Partially detached pinna. **B,** Loss of rim.

possible, wrapped in moist gauze, sealed in plastic, placed on ice, and transported with the patient for surgical repair (see Chapter 16).

Thermal Injuries

Thermal injuries may occur from prolonged exposure to extreme cold or exposure of lesser duration to extreme heat. Contact with hot liquids or electrical currents can also lead to thermal injury. Prehospital management is usually limited to soft tissue dressings to prevent contamination and patient transportation. Thermal injuries are further discussed in Chapters 16 and 25.

Chemical Injuries

Strong acids or alkali produce burns on contact. Emergency care consists of copious irrigation. After irrigation, the ear and ear canal should be bathed with saline or sterile water, allowing the irrigation liquid to remain in the ear canal for 2 to 3 minutes. This procedure should be repeated 3 to 4 times, after which the ear should be dried and covered to prevent contamination. The patient should be transported for physician evaluation.

Traumatic Perforations

The tympanic membrane can be perforated by penetrating objects such as a cotton-tipped applicator or from great pressure differentials resulting from explosions or scuba diving (barotrauma). These injuries usually heal spontaneously without treatment, but evaluation by a physician is recommended.

If the injury is caused by a penetrating object, it should be stabilized in place and the ear should be covered to prevent further contamination. If the ear canal has been contaminated (for example, by swimming water or a foreign object), antibiotic therapy is usually prescribed. Serious complications that may result from perforations include facial nerve palsy frequently accompanied by temporal bone fractures, hearing loss, and vertigo.

Barotitis

Barotitis occurs when an individual is exposed to changes in barometric pressure great enough to produce inflammation and injury to the middle ear. Barotitis can result, for example, from flying at high altitudes (including patient transport by air ambulance) and from scuba diving.

Gas pressure in the air-filled spaces of the middle ear is normally in equilibrium with the environment. Boyle's law states that at constant temperature, the volume of gas is inversely proportional to the pressure. On ascent, gas expands, and on descent, it contracts. Therefore when gases become trapped or partially trapped, they expand in direct proportion to the decrease in pressure. When trapped gas cannot equilibrate with ambient pressure, pain and the sensation of a blocked ear may develop. To equalize the pressure in the middle ear, the patient can be directed to bear down (Valsalva maneuver), yawn, swallow, and move the lower jaw. These methods may cause the eustachian tube to open, equalizing pressure in the middle ear cavity.

Eye Trauma

It is estimated that over 2000 eye and orbital injuries occur each day in the United States.[9] Common causes of eye injury are blunt and penetrating trauma from motor vehicle crashes, sport and recreational activities, and violent altercations; chemical exposure from household and industrial accidents; foreign bodies; and animal bites and scratches.

Evaluation

Acute eye injuries may be difficult to identify because a patient with normal vision may have a serious underlying injury. Symptoms requiring a high degree of suspicion includes obvious trauma with eye injury; visual loss or blurred vision that does not improve with blinking, indicating possible damage to the globe, ocular contents, or optic nerve; and loss of a portion of the visual field, indicating possible detachment of the retina, hemorrhage into the eye, or optic nerve injury. Evaluation of eye injury should include a thorough history and measurement of visual acuity, pupillary reaction, and extraocular movements.

History

A thorough history should include the following information:
- Exact mode of injury
- Previous ocular, medical, and drug history, including cataracts, glaucoma, and presence of hepatitis or the human immunodeficiency virus (HIV)
- Use of eye medications
- Use of corrective glasses or contact lenses
- Presence of ocular prosthesis
- Duration of symptoms and treatment interventions that may have been attempted before EMS arrival

Visual Acuity

Measurement of visual acuity is usually the first step in any examination of the patient's eyes. (The exception is a chemical burn to the eye; in this case, irrigation should precede visual acuity measurement.) To measure visual acuity, the paramedic should use a hand-held visual acuity chart or any printed material with small, medium, and large point sizes (for example, an intravenous fluid bag). The distance that the printed matter was held from the patient's face should be recorded.

The vision of each eye should be measured separately while covering the untested eye with material that will occlude vision without applying pressure. The injured eye should be tested first for acuity comparison to the uninjured eye. If corrective lenses are worn, acuity should be measured with lenses first and then without lenses. Illiteracy or foreign language limitations may require alternative methods of evaluation, such as finger-counting, hand motion, and presence or absence of light perception. Abnormal responses to any of these methods indicate significant loss of vision.

Pupillary Reaction

Pupils should be black, round, and equal in size and should react to light in concert; both eyes should constrict in response to light and dilate in response to dark. Abnormal pupillary responses after blunt trauma to the eye are common. They may be caused by tearing but are more commonly caused by direct trauma to the pupillary sphincter. They may also suggest a more serious injury involving the optic nerve or globe. Causes of pupil abnormalities in the absence of recent injury include drug use, cataracts, previous surgical procedures, ocular prosthesis, anisocoria (normal or congenital unequal pupil size), central nervous system disease, strokes, and previous injury. All of the patient's pupil abnormalities should be documented.

Extraocular Movements

Extraocular muscles are responsible for movements of the globe. Voluntary muscles, which are innervated by cranial nerves III, IV, and VI, are attached to the outside of the eyeball and bones of the orbit and move the globe in any desired direction. Involuntary eye muscles, which are innervated by sympathetic nerves, are located within the eye. Examples of involuntary eye muscles are the iris and the ciliary muscle, which dilate constrict the pupil and change the shape of the lens, respectively.

To evaluate the eyes' extraocular movement, instruct the patient to visually track the movement of an object (for example, finger, pencil, penlight) up, down, to the right, and to the left. Abnormalities in movement may indicate orbital content edema, cranial nerve injury, contusions or lacerations of extraocular muscles, or muscle entrapment in a fracture. Patients with limited or abnormal extraocular movements frequently complain of double vision in one or more directions of gaze. All findings should be documented.

Evaluation and Management of Specific Eye Injuries

Although few eye injuries are truly urgent, all victims of ocular trauma should be evaluated by a physician. Some patients require specialized care by an ophthalmologist. If a serious injury that may require specialized care is suspected, medical control should be advised as soon as possible so that services will be available when the patient arrives in the emergency department (Fig. 15-17).

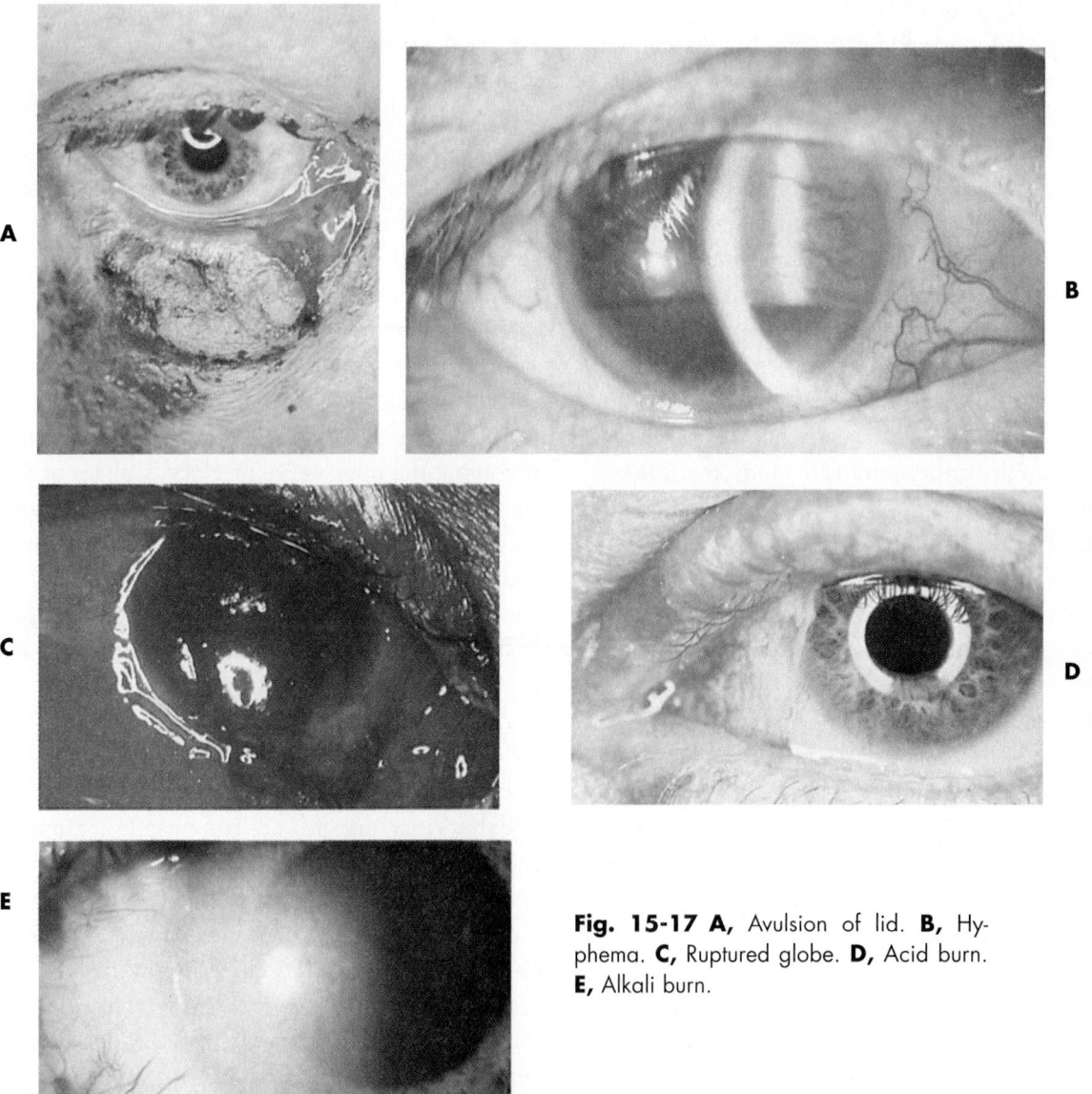

Fig. 15-17 A, Avulsion of lid. **B,** Hyphema. **C,** Ruptured globe. **D,** Acid burn. **E,** Alkali burn.

Foreign bodies in the cornea, conjunctiva, or eyelid are usually evidenced by a patient complaint of foreign body sensation (especially on opening and closing the eyelids) and by profuse tearing. If a foreign body is suspected, the inner surface of the upper and lower lid and conjunctiva should be inspected and the foreign body removed by gentle, copious irrigation with clear fluid (for example, tap water, normal saline, or sterile water).

Corneal abrasion occurs when the outer layers of the cornea are rubbed off. The injury often results from a foreign body scratching the cornea, and it is also common in those who wear contact lens. Patients with a corneal abrasion usually complain of pain and foreign body sensation under the upper eyelid, photophobia (abnormal light sensitivity), excessive tearing, and sometimes a decrease in visual acuity. Often, these signs and symptoms are delayed. Prehospital management of corneal abrasion is gentle irrigation with clear fluid and the application of a double patch to both of the patients eyes to prevent consensual eye movement and resultant aggravation (Fig. 15-18). Corneal abrasions generally heal within 24 to 48 hours.

Blunt trauma to the eye or its adjacent structures may result in a contusion injury, traumatic hyphema (bleeding into the anterior chamber), or globe or scleral rupture. Signs and symptoms of these injuries are:

- Contusion injury
  - Traumatic dilation or constriction of the pupil
  - Pain
  - Photophobia
  - Blurred vision
  - Tears of the iris (tear-shaped pupil)
- Traumatic hyphema
  - Traumatic dilation or, less commonly, constriction of the pupil
  - Decrease in visual acuity
  - Blood in the anterior chamber (may be visible with penlight)
- Globe or scleral rupture
  - Decrease in visual acuity to hand movements or light perception
  - Lowered intraocular pressure (soft eye)
  - Pupil irregularity
  - Hyphema

Blunt injury to the eye may be associated with other serious injuries, such as orbital fracture, vitreous hemorrhage, and dislocation of the lens. Prehospital care should be limited to control of any bleeding with gentle, direct pressure; protection of the affected eye with a metal shield or cardboard cup; and rapid transportation for physician evaluation. If traumatic hyphema or globe or scleral rupture is suspected, immobilize the patient's head and spine, elevate the head of spine board 40 degrees to decrease intraocular pressure, and instruct the patient to avoid any ac-

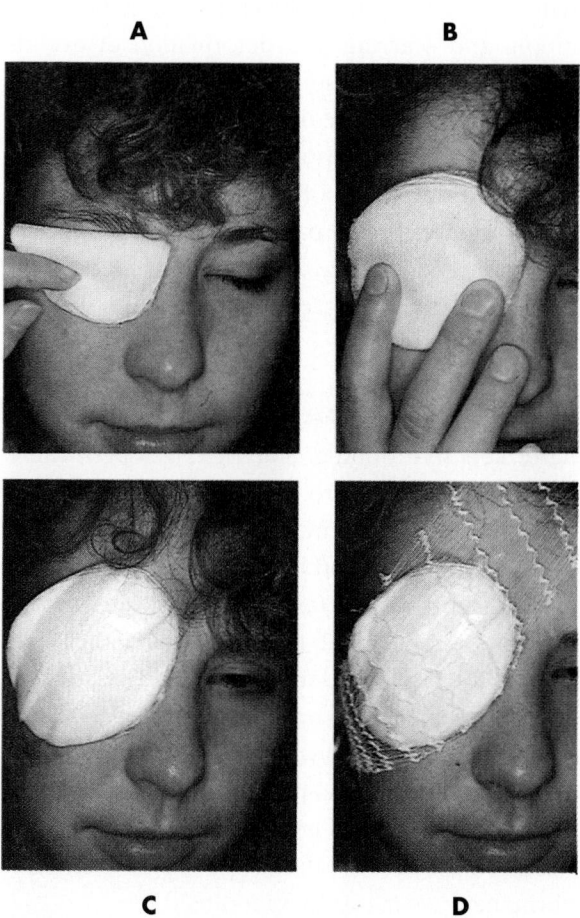

A   B

C   D

Fig. 15-18 A, A folded pad is placed over the closed eye. **B,** A second unfolded pad is placed over the top of the first pad. **C,** Tape is applied along the length of the pad. **D,** The pads are secured firmly in place.

Removal of Contact Lenses

Removal of Hard and Rigid Gas-Permeable Lenses

1. With gloved hands, separate the eyelids so that the margins of the lids are beyond the top and bottom edges of the lens.
2. Gently press the eyelids down and forward to the edges of the lens.
3. Move the eyelids toward each other, forcing the lens to slide out between them.
4. Store the lens in a container with water or saline and label the container with the patient's name. If a contact lens container is not available, store each lens in a separate container and label as left or right.
5. If lens removal is difficult, the lens should be gently moved downward from the cornea to the conjunctiva overlying the sclera until arrival in the emergency department.

NOTE: Special suction cups are also available for the removal of hard and rigid contact lenses. This device should be moistened with saline or sterile water before contacting the lens.

Removal of Soft Lenses

1. With gloved hands, pull down the lower eyelid.
2. Gently slide the soft lens down onto the conjunctiva.
3. Using a pinching motion, compress the lens between the thumb and index finger.
4. Remove the lens from the eye.
5. Store the lens in a container (marked right or left) with water or saline and label the container with the patient's name.

tivity that might increase intraocular pressure (for example, straining, coughing).

Penetrating injury to the eye may be associated with embedded foreign bodies, lid avulsions, and lacerations to the lids, sclera, or cornea. Penetrating globe injuries can damage retinal structures and cause a loss of vitreous humor and subse-

quent blindness. Any bleeding should be controlled by gentle, direct pressure, and the globe should be protected from dehydration or contamination from foreign bodies by covering the orbital area with plastic or damp dressings and an eye shield.

Protruding intraocular foreign bodies should be stabilized and covered with a cardboard cup secured with tape, and the unaffected eye should be covered to prevent consensual movement. No attempt should be made to remove the object. If necessary, the penetrating object may be shortened judiciously to facilitate transport (consult with medical control). Oxygen and intravenous fluids may also be recommended in these patient situations.

Chemical injury to the eye may be associated with loss of corneal epithelial tissue, globe perforation, and scarring and deformation of eyelids and conjunctiva. These injuries are true emergencies and require immediate intervention. A chemical exposure generally mandates extensive, continuous irrigation of both eyes with a neutral fluid for 20 minutes before patient transport if effective irrigation is being performed and while en route to the emergency department.

Contact Lenses

There are three general types of contact lenses: hard, soft hydrophilic, and rigid gas-permeable. Hard lenses are microlenses that are sometimes prescribed for astigmatism. (These lenses are rarely used today.) Soft hydrophilic lenses are usually large in diameter (extending onto the conjunctiva) and retain 25% to 85% hydration. Soft lenses may be designed for daily or extended wear. Rigid gas-permeable lenses are similar in size to microlenses and have a low water content and high oxygen permeability. Gas-permeable lenses are generally removed at the end of each day but may be designed for intermediate wear (up to 7 days) or permanent wear (up to 3 months).

As a rule, EMS personnel should not attempt to remove contact lenses in patients with eye injuries. To do so may cause additional damage and aggravate the injury. If management of an eye injury is complicated by the presence of contact lenses (for example, chemical burns to the eyes), medical control may recommend that the lenses be removed. If the patient is unable to remove the lenses, the paramedic may be instructed to do so.

Dental Trauma

There are 32 teeth in the normal adult mouth. Each tooth consists of two sections: the crown, which projects above the gingiva (the portion of the oral mucosa surrounding the tooth), and the root, which fits into the bony socket (alveolus) of the maxilla or mandible. Three layers make up the hard tissues of the teeth: the enamel, the dentin (ivory), and the cementum. The soft tissues of the teeth include the pulp and the periodontal membrane (Fig. 15-19).

The teeth and associated alveolar process may be injured alone or in combination with fractures of the jaw or facial bones. The two most common types of dental trauma involve fractures and avulsions of the anterior teeth. If a tooth is fractured, the oral cavity should be carefully searched for tooth fragments. Removal of fragments reduces the risk of aspiration and obstruction of the airway.

More than 2 million teeth are avulsed each year, and 90% can be saved with proper emergency treatment. Permanent teeth that have been avulsed have a good survival rate if replanted and stabilized within 1 hour. (Deciduous teeth or "milk teeth" are not generally replanted because they may become fused to the bone, delaying formation and eruption of the permanent tooth.) If the avulsed tooth has been extraoral for less than 15 minutes, medical control may recommend re-

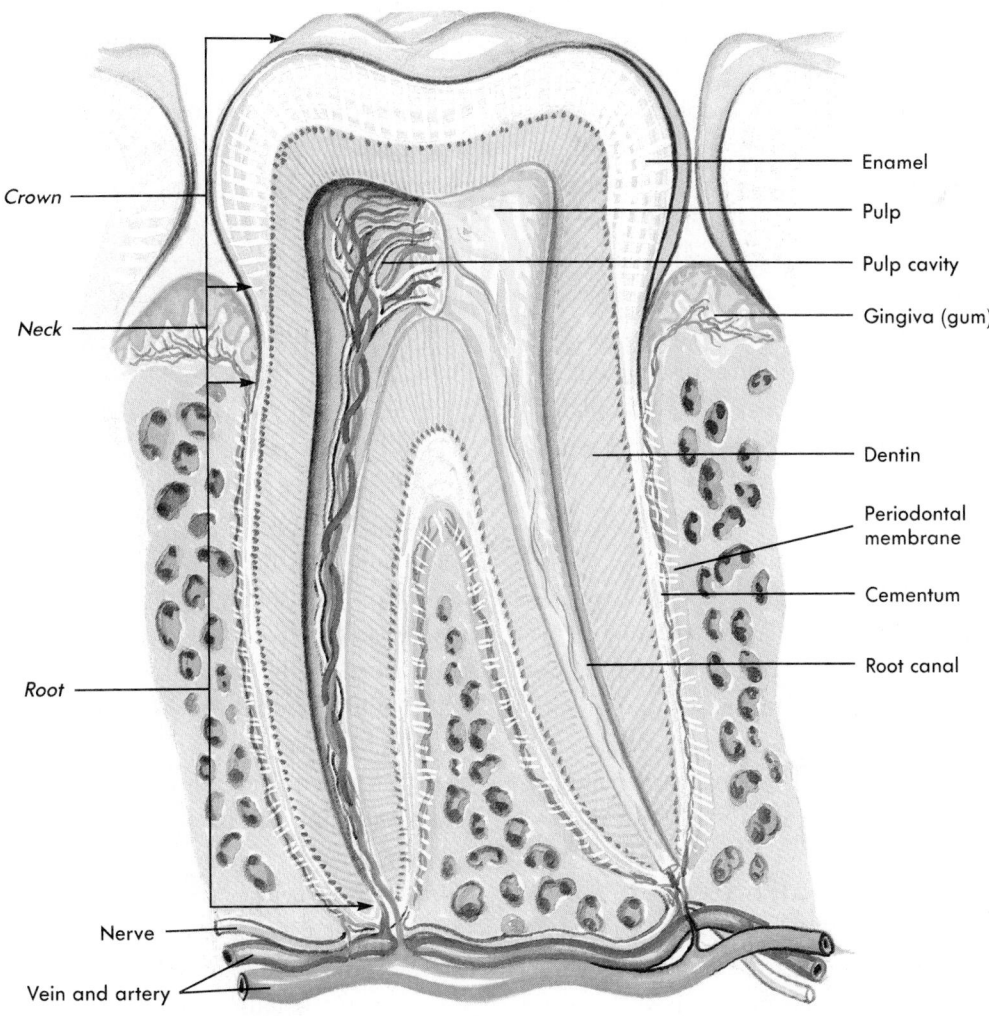

Fig. 15-19 Longitudinal section of a tooth.

planting the tooth into the original socket. Take care not to replant the tooth backwards, and be alert for possible aspiration. If replantation is impossible, follow the five guidelines of the American Dental Association and the American Association of Endodontists[10]:

1. Never place an avulsed tooth in anything that can dry or crush the outside of the tooth.
2. Do not handle the tooth roughly. Do not rinse it off or rub, scrape, or disinfect the outside of the tooth in any way. (Any adherent membrane or fibrous tissue should be left in place to avoid stripping off the periodontal membrane and ligament, which are critical to the survival of a replanted tooth.)
3. Place the tooth in a nurturing break-resistant storage device with a tightly fitted top and soft inner walls. An example of such a device is the commercially prepared *Emergency Tooth Preserving System.*
4. Store the tooth in a pH-balanced, isotonic, glucose-, calcium-, and magnesium-enriched cell-preserving fluid (for example, Hank's solution). Use refrigerated fresh whole milk as the best alternative storage medium (powdered milk is not suitable). For very short periods (1 hour or less), use sterile saline. Do not use tap water because it damages the periodontal ligament.
5. Advise medical control of avulsed teeth so that appropriate services will be available when the patient arrives in the emergency department.

Trauma to the Skull and Brain

The anatomical components of the skull are the scalp, followed by the cranial vault, under which are the dural membrane, the arachnoid membrane, the pia, and the brain substance. Injuries to the skull may be classified as soft tissue injuries to the scalp and skull fractures.

Soft-Tissue Injuries to the Scalp

The most common scalp injury is an irregular linear laceration. Like the face, the scalp is very vascular. Therefore scalp lacerations may give rise to profuse bleeding and resultant hypovolemia, particularly in infants and children. Other, less-

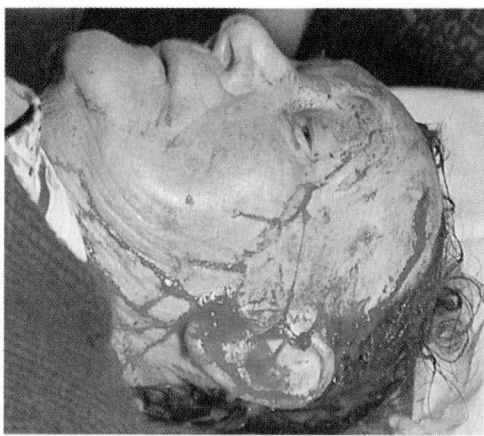

Fig. 15-20 Even small wounds from the scalp can bleed profusely.

frequent scalp injuries include stellate wounds, avulsions, and subgaleal hematomas (Fig. 15-20).

Management of soft tissue injuries to the scalp includes efforts to prevent contamination of open wounds, use of direct pressure or pressure dressings to decrease blood loss, and fluid replacement if needed. The paramedic should also consider the potential for underlying skull fracture and brain and spinal trauma as indicated by the mechanism of injury. Aside from the possibility of excessive blood loss, scalp lacerations that occur as a single entity rarely produce life-threatening complications.

Skull Fractures

Skull fractures may be classified as linear fractures, basilar fractures, depressed fractures, and open vault fractures (Fig. 15-21). Complications associated with these injuries are cranial nerve injury, vascular involvement (for example, meningeal artery, dural sinuses), infection, underlying brain injury, and dural defects caused by depressed bone fragments. With all injuries to the head, the paramedic should consider the potential for spinal injury and take appropriate precautions.

Linear Fractures

Linear fractures (seen as straight lines on x-ray film) account for 70% of all fractures to the skull. They are not usually depressed and often occur without an overlying scalp laceration. As an isolated injury, these fractures generally have a low rate of complication. However, if the fracture is associated with scalp laceration, infection is possible. In addition, linear fractures that cross the meningeal groove in the temporal-parietal area, midline, or occipital area may lead to epidural bleeding from vascular involvement.

Basilar Skull Fractures

Basilar skull fractures are usually associated with major impact trauma. These injuries may occur when the mandibular condyles perforate into the base of the skull but more commonly result from an extension of a linear fracture into the floor

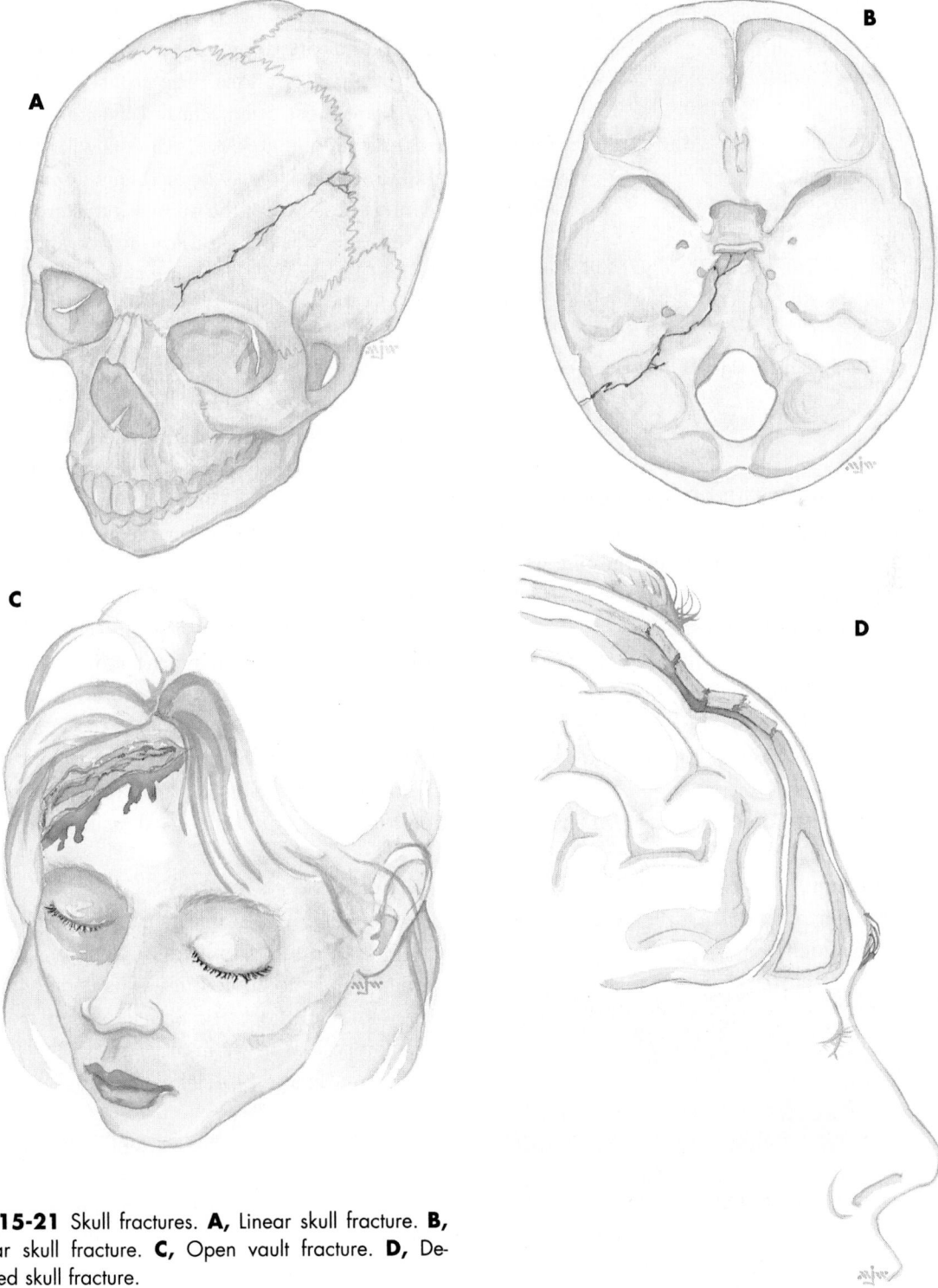

Fig. 15-21 Skull fractures. **A,** Linear skull fracture. **B,** Basilar skull fracture. **C,** Open vault fracture. **D,** Depressed skull fracture.

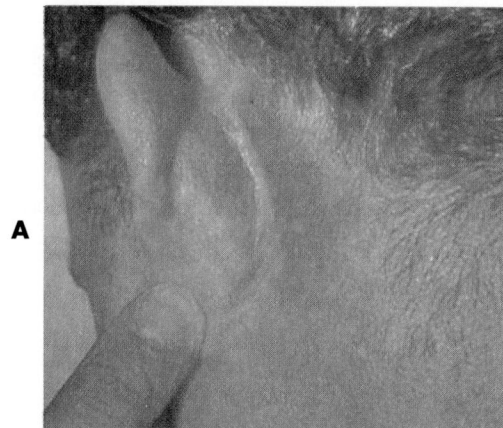

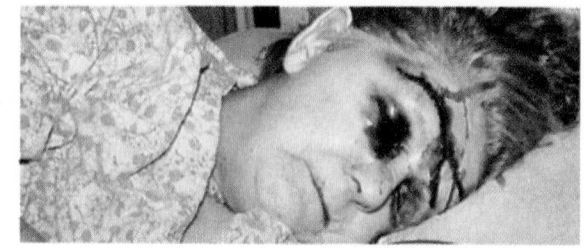

Fig. 15-22 A, Battle's sign. **B,** Raccoon's eyes.

of the anterior and middle fossae. Basilar skull fractures can be difficult to see on x-ray films and are usually diagnosed clinically by the following signs and symptoms:

- Ecchymosis over the mastoid process resulting from fracture to the temporal bone (Battle's sign) (Fig. 15-22, *A*)
- Ecchymosis of one or both orbits caused by fracture of the base of the sphenoid sinus (raccoon's eyes) (Fig. 15-22, *B*)
- Blood behind the tympanic membrane caused by fractures of the temporal bone (hemotympanum)
- Cerebral spinal fluid leakage, which can result in bacterial meningitis

NOTE:

Battle's sign and raccoon's eyes do not usually occur until some time after the injury. If they are present on EMS arrival, the ecchymosis probably results from a previous injury.

Other complications associated with basilar skull fractures include cranial nerve injuries and massive hemorrhage from vascular involvement of the carotid artery. Treatment for basilar skull fractures includes bed rest, in-hospital observation, and antibiotic prophylaxis (controversial).

Depressed Skull Fractures

Depressed skull fractures usually result from a relatively small object striking the head at high speed and are therefore commonly associated with scalp lacerations. The frontal and parietal bones are most often affected by these fractures. It is estimated that 30% of patients with depressed skull fractures have associated hematomas and cerebral contusions. If the depression is greater than the thickness of the skull, dural laceration is also likely. Patients with depressed skull fractures frequently require surgical removal of the bone fragments (craniectomy).

Open-Vault Fractures

Open-vault fractures result when there is direct communication between a scalp laceration and cerebral substance (Fig. 15-23). Because of the nature of these injuries and the force required to produce them, they are often associated with multiple-system trauma and a high mortality rate. Communication between the intracranial contents and the external environment may lead to infection (meningitis). Open-vault fractures require surgical repair. Prehospital management is usually limited to spinal immobilization, ventilatory support, efforts to prevent contamination, and rapid transportation to an appropriate medical facility.

Cranial Nerve Injuries

Twelve pairs of cranial nerves leave the brain and pass through openings in the skull called foramina. Injury to cranial nerves is usually associated with skull fractures. Signs and symptoms of common cranial nerve injuries are:

- Cranial nerve I (olfactory nerve)
  - Loss of smell
  - Impairment of taste (dependent on food aroma)
  - Hallmark of basilar skull fracture

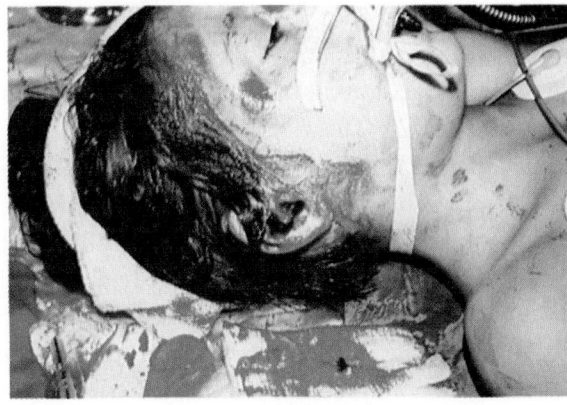

Fig. 15-23 Severe fracture of the base of the skull.

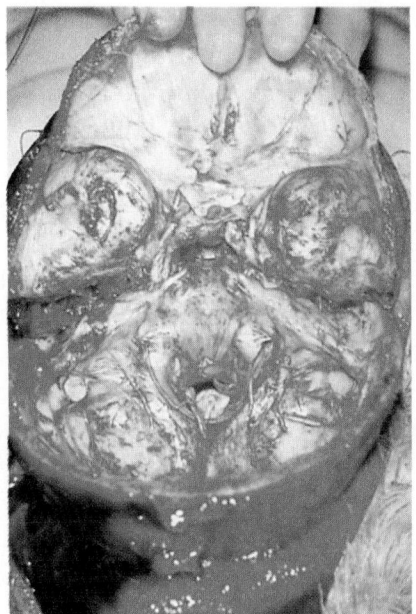

- Cranial nerve II (optic nerve)
  - Blindness in one or both eyes
  - Visual field defects
- Cranial nerve III (oculomotor nerve)
  - Ipsilateral, dilated, fixed pupil
  - Especially compression by the temporal lobe
  - Mimicking of direct ocular trauma
- Cranial nerve VII (facial nerve)
  - Immediate or delayed facial paralysis
  - Basilar skull fracture
- Cranial nerve VIII (auditory nerve)
  - Deafness
  - Basilar skull fracture

Trauma to the Brain

Damage to the brain and associated intracranial hemorrhage may occur with or without scalp lacerations or skull fractures. These injuries result from mechanical forces to the skull (blunt and penetrating trauma) and brain movement within the skull (a result of acceleration or deceleration forces). Brain injury may result from contusion, hemorrhage (for example, subdural, epidural, or cerebral hematoma), edema with associated increased intracranial pressure, and ischemia. Temporary dysfunction may occur with concussive injuries.

Anatomy of the Skull and Brain

The brain is divided into four areas: the brain stem (consisting of the medulla, pons, and midbrain), the diencephalon (including the thalamus and hypothalamus), the cerebrum, and the cerebellum. The intracranial contents consist of brain water (58%), brain solids (25%), cerebrospinal fluid (7%), and intracranial blood (10%).

Concussion

Concussion is a fully reversible brain injury that does not result in structural damage to the brain. It is caused by mild-to-moderate impact to the skull, movement within the cranial vault, or both. It occurs when the function of the brain stem (particularly the reticular activating system) or both cerebral cortices is temporarily disturbed, resulting in a brief altered level of consciousness, usually less than 5 minutes.

> **NOTE:**
> If the patient has been unconscious for more than 5 minutes, the paramedic should suspect a more serious injury caused by contusion or hemorrhage.

The loss of consciousness is usually followed by periods of drowsiness, restlessness, and confusion, with a fairly rapid return to normal behavior. The patient may have no recall of the events before the injury (retrograde amnesia) or immediately after recovery of consciousness (antegrade amnesia). This short-term memory loss may produce anxiety, and the patient frequently asks repetitive questions (for example, "Where am I? What happened?"). Other signs and symptoms of concussion are vomiting, combativeness, transient visual disturbances (for example, light flashes, wavy lines), defects in equilibrium and coordination, and changes in blood pressure, pulse rate, and respiration (rare). After physician evaluation, treatment generally consists of in-hospital or home observation by a reliable observer for 24 to 48 hours.

A concussion injury affects the patient most severely at the time of impact and is followed by improvement. It is the most common and least serious type of brain injury. *Any patient whose condition worsens over time or whose level of consciousness deteriorates rather than improves must be suspected of having a more serious injury.* Therefore it is important to document baseline measurements of level of consciousness, memory status, and neurological function in any victim of head injury.

Cerebral Contusion

A cerebral contusion is bruising of the brain in the area of the cortex or deeper within the frontal, temporal, or occipital lobes. This bruising produces a structural change in the brain tissue and results in greater neurological deficits and abnormalities than are seen with concussions. These abnormalities may include seizures, hemiparesis, aphasia, and personality changes. If the brain stem is also contused, the patient may lose consciousness. In some cases, the comatose state may be prolonged, lasting hours to days or longer. Of the patients who die from head injury, 75% have cerebral contusions at autopsy.

If applied force is sufficient to cause the brain to be displaced against the irregular surfaces of the skull, tiny blood vessels in the pia matter may rupture. The brain substance may be damaged locally at the site of impact (coup) or on the contralateral side (contrecoup) opposite the site of impact. Contrecoup injuries are commonly caused by deceleration of the head, as in a fall or motor vehicle crash.

As a rule, cerebral contusions usually heal without intervention. Like patients with concussion, these patients usually improve, although the time to heal and level of improvement differ in these two conditions. The most important complication associated with cerebral contusion is increased intracranial pressure manifested by headache, nausea, vomiting, seizures, and a declining level of consciousness. These signs are usually delayed responses that are not seen in the prehospital emergency setting.

Edema

Significant injuries to the brain often result in swelling of the brain tissue with or without associated hemorrhage. The swelling, which results from humoral and metabolic responses to injury, leads to marked increases in intracranial pressure. This can in turn lead to decreased cerebral perfusion or herniation.

Ischemia

Ischemia can result from vascular injuries, secondary vascular spasm, or increased intracranial pressure. In any case, focal or more global infarcts can result.

Hemorrhage

The same forces that result in concussion and contusion may also cause serious vascular damage with resultant hemorrhage into or around brain tissue. These injuries may cause epidural or subdural hematomas that compress the underlying brain tissue or intraparenchymal hemorrhage (bleeding directly into the brain tissue). Hemorrhage is often associated with cerebral contusions and skull fractures.

Cerebral Blood Flow

Although the brain accounts for only 2% of adult weight, 20% of total body oxygen use and 25% of total body glucose use are devoted to brain metabolism. Oxygen and glucose delivery are controlled by cerebral blood flow.

Cerebral blood flow is a function of cerebral perfusion pressure (CPP) and resistance of the cerebral vascular bed. CPP is determined by the mean arterial pressure (MAP) (the diastolic pressure plus one-third pulse pressure minus intracranial pressure). Therefore when intracranial pressure increases, CPP decreases.

Vascular tone in the normal brain is regulated by carbon dioxide pressure (P_{CO_2}), oxygen pressure (P_{O_2}), and autonomic and neurohumoral control; P_{CO_2} has the greatest effect on intracerebral vascular diameter and subsequent resistance. For example, if P_{CO_2} is increased from 40 to 80 torr, cerebral blood flow is doubled, resulting in increased brain blood volume and intracranial pressure. If P_{CO_2} is decreased to 30 torr, cerebral blood flow is reduced (thus the rationale for hyperventilating the lungs of a patient with head injury).

Intracranial Pressure

The normal range of intracranial pressure is 0 to 15 torr. When intracranial pressure rises above this level because of an expanding mass or diffuse swelling, the body's ability to maintain CPP is compromised, and cerebral blood flow is diminished. As the cranial vault continues to fill (because of brain edema or expanding hematoma, the body attempts to compensate for the decline in CPP by a rise in MAP (Cushing reflex). However, this increase in cerebral blood flow further elevates the intracranial pressure. As it continues to rise, cerebrospinal fluid is displaced to compensate for the expansion. If unresolved, the brain substance may herniate over the edge of the tentorium or through the foramen magnum (Fig. 15-24).

Early signs and symptoms of increased intracranial pressure include headache, nausea and vomiting, and altered level of consciousness. These are eventually followed by increased systolic pressure, widened pulse pressure, and a decrease in the pulse and respiratory rate (Cushing's triad). As the volume continues to expand in the cranial vault, herniation of the temporal lobe through the tentorium causes compression of cranial nerve III, producing a dilated pupil and loss of the light reflex on the side of compression. The patient rapidly becomes unresponsive to verbal and painful stimuli and may exhibit the ominous signs of decorticate posturing (characterized by extension of the legs and flexion of the arms at the elbows) or decerebrate posturing (characterized by extension of all four extremities) (Fig. 15-25).

Respiratory Patterns

As intracranial pressure continues to rise, abnormal respiratory patterns (see Chapter 11) may develop. Respiratory abnormalities associated with increased intracranial pressure and significant brain-stem injury include hypoventilation, Cheyne-Stokes breathing (which may accompany decorticate posturing), central neurogenic hyperventilation (a very fast, shallow panting that may accompany decerebrate posturing), and ataxic breathing. The clinical significance of decorticate and decerebrate posturing and respiratory patterns are not of major clinical importance other than to identify the need for intervention and treatment (intubation, hyperventilation, and consideration for surgery).

Types of Brain Hemorrhage

Traditionally, brain hemorrhages are classified according to their location as epidural, subdural, or cerebral (intraparenchymal) (Fig. 15-26).

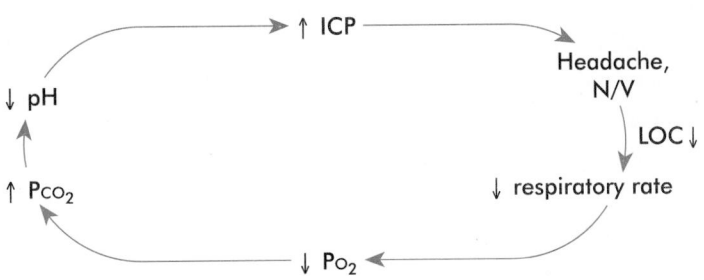

Fig. 15-24 Effects of increased intracranial pressure.

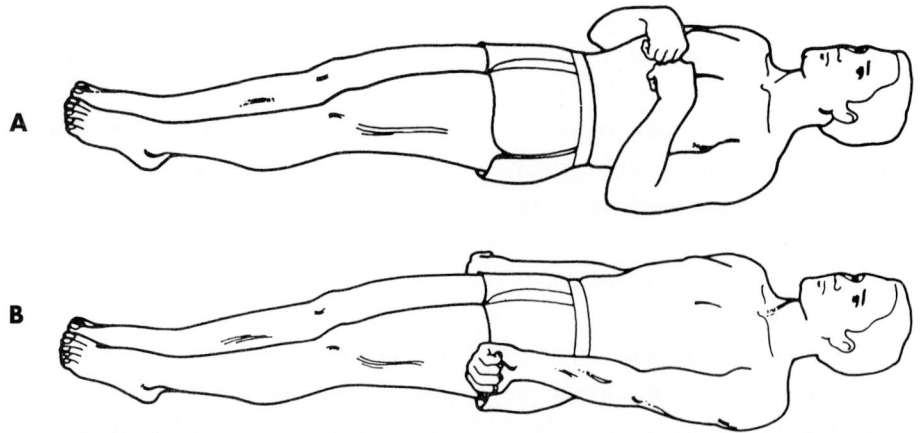

Fig. 15-25 A, Abnormal flexion (decorticate posturing). **B,** Abnormal extension (decerebrate posturing).

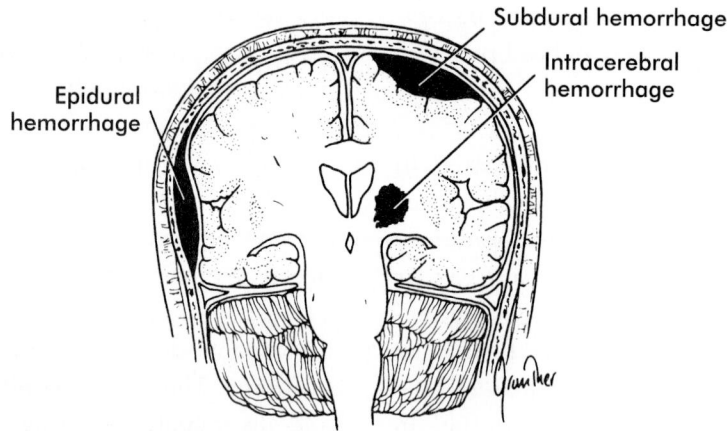

Fig. 15-26 Varieties of intracranial hemorrhage.

Epidural Hematoma

An epidural hematoma is a collection of blood between the cranium and the dura in the epidural space. It is usually a rapidly developing lesion associated with a laceration or tear of the middle meningeal artery. This hemorrhage frequently occurs as a result of a linear or depressed skull fracture in the temporal bone, although bleeding from other sites can also produce epidural hemorrhage. If the source of hemorrhage is predominantly venous, deterioration is not usually as rapid because low-pressure vessels bleed more slowly.

A total of 50% of patients with epidural hematoma have a transient loss of consciousness, followed by a lucid interval in which neurological status returns to normal. (The remaining 50% of patients with acute epidural hematoma never recover consciousness.) The lucid interval usually lasts between 6 and 18 hours, during which time the hematoma enlarges. As intracranial pressure rises, the patient develops a headache with lethargy, decreasing level of consciousness, and contralateral hemiparesis. In the early stages of an epidural hematoma, the patient's only complaints may be a headache and drowsiness. Immediate recognition and rapid transportation to an appropriate medical facility for surgical intervention are the cornerstones of definitive therapy.

Common causes of epidural hematoma include low-velocity blows to the head, violent altercations, and deceleration injuries. Approximately 15% to 20% of these patients die.

Subdural Hematoma

A subdural hematoma is a collection of blood between the dura and the surface of the brain in the subdural space. This injury usually results from bleeding of the veins that bridge the subdural space. Associated contusion or laceration of the brain is frequently present. It is often the result of blunt head trauma and is commonly associated with skull fracture. Subdural hematomas are classified as acute (50% to 80% mortality rate), subacute (25% mortality rate), and chronic (20% mortality rate), depending on the time lapse between the injury and development of symptoms. As a general rule, if symptoms occur within 24 hours, the hematoma is considered acute; between 2 and 10 days, subacute; and after 2 weeks, chronic.

Signs and symptoms of subdural hematoma are similar to those of epidural hematoma and include headache, nausea and vomiting, decreasing level of consciousness, coma, abnormal posturing, paralysis, and in infants, bulging fontanelles. These findings may be quite subtle because of the slow evolution of the hematoma in the subacute and chronic phases. Definitive care consists of surgical evacuation of the hematoma. Individuals at increased risk of developing subdural hematoma include older adults and patients with clotting deficiencies (for example, alcoholics, hemophiliacs, persons who take anticoagulants) and patients with cortical atrophy (older adults, alcoholics).

Cerebral Hematoma

An *intracerebral hematoma* may be defined as a collection of more than 5 ml of blood somewhere within the substance of the brain, most commonly in the frontal or temporal lobe. This injury usually results from multiple lacerations produced by penetrating head trauma or a high-velocity deceleration injury in which vessels are torn as the brain moves across rough surfaces of the skull. It may also occur as the brain is compressed and distorted from increased intracranial pressure.

Cerebral hematoma is often associated with subdural hemorrhage and skull fracture. Signs and symptoms may be immediate or delayed, depending on the size and location of the hemorrhage. Once symptomatology presents, the patient usually deteriorates rapidly. The mortality rate after surgical evacuation of the hematoma is more than 40%.

Penetrating Injury

Penetrating injuries to the brain are usually caused by missiles fired from handguns and stab wounds caused by sharp instruments such as knives, scissors, or screwdrivers. Less frequently, penetrating trauma may result from falls and high-velocity motor vehicle crashes. Associated injuries include skull fracture; damage to cerebral arteries, veins, or venous sinuses; and intracranial hemorrhage. Complications include infection and posttraumatic epilepsy. Definitive care for these injuries requires neurosurgical intervention.

Assessment and Neurological Evaluation

Prehospital management of the head-injured patient is determined by a number of factors, including the mechanism and severity of injury and the patient's level of consciousness; associated injuries affect priorities of emergency care.

Airway and Ventilation

Initial steps in treating all patients with head trauma are to ensure an open airway with spinal precautions and provide adequate ventilatory support with high-concentration oxygen. Airway management may include oral or nasal adjuncts, esophageal obturator airway, esophageal gastric tube airway, or nasal or tracheal intubation to maintain and protect the airway. Tracheal intubation and ventilatory support are usually recommended in all head-injured patients who have GCS scores of 8 or less.

Head-injured patients are likely to vomit. If the patient has a decreased level of consciousness, a nasogastric tube should be inserted to decompress the stomach. In the presence of facial fractures, rhinorrhea, or otorrhea, an orogastric tube rather than a nasogastric tube should be inserted to avoid possible intubation of the cranial cavity through the fracture site. In addition, the patient's condition should be well stabilized on a long spine board for safe repositioning, and suction equipment with large-bore suction catheters should be available.

Ventilatory support should be focused on maintaining adequate oxygenation and optimizing cerebral perfusion while decreasing abnormally high intracranial pressure. The P_{CO_2} can increase cerebral blood flow and lead to an increase in intracranial pressure. By decreasing the P_{CO_2} to a range of 25 to 30 torr through hyperventilation (respiratory rate of 24 to 30 breaths per minute), intracranial pressure can be lowered. An elevated P_{O_2} and, in particular, a lowered P_{CO_2} help buy time against the ill effects of intracranial hemorrhage and elevated intracranial pressure.

Circulation

After the airway has been secured while maintaining spinal protection, maintaining the patient's cardiovascular function becomes the next priority. Major external bleeding should be controlled, and the patient's vital signs should be assessed to establish a baseline for future evaluations. A cardiac monitor will detect changes in rhythm (particularly bradycardias and tachycardias) that can occur with increasing intracranial pressure and brain-stem injury.

Persistent hypotension that results from an isolated head injury is a rare and terminal event with the exception of head injury in infants and small children. *Head injury does not produce hypovolemic shock.* Therefore a head-injured patient who is also hypotensive should be evaluated for other sources of hemorrhage and the possibility of neurogenic shock from spinal cord trauma.

The blood pressure of every patient should be maintained at normal levels with fluid replacement or pneumatic antishock garment (PASG) per protocol. Choice of intravenous fluids is somewhat controversial. Isotonic fluids should be used for hemorrhagic shock but probably should be used cautiously in patients with evidence of hypotension secondary to neurogenic shock. In the latter patient group, vasopressors may also be quite helpful. Neurogenic shock can often be distinguished from hemorrhagic shock by the following:

- A relatively bradycardic response (for example, a pulse of 80 with a blood pressure of 80)
- Skin that is often warm and dry (not cool and clammy)
- No evidence of significant blood loss or hypovolemia
- Paralysis and loss of spinal reflexes

Neurological Examination

The conscious patient should be interviewed to determine his or her memory status before and after the injury and to learn of significant medical history (for example, heart disease, hypertension, diabetes, epilepsy, medication use, alcohol or drug use, allergies). The history should also include the mechanism of injury and the events leading up to the injury (for example, loss of consciousness before or after the accident).

The conscious patient's motor skills should be evaluated to determine his or her ability to follow commands and to note any paralysis. (Hemiparesis or hemiplegia, especially with a sensory deficit on the same side, indicates brain damage rather than spinal trauma.) If the patient is unconscious on EMS arrival, bystanders should be interviewed about the history of the event and the length of time the patient has been unconscious. The most important indicator of increasing intracranial pressure is deterioration in the patient's sensorium. Therefore level of consciousness should be evaluated by use of AVPU Scale or by the GCS and revaluated several times during the encounter with the patient.

The patient's pupils should be assessed for position, size, and reactivity to light. Abnormal pupillary responses may indicate an increase in intracranial pressure and cranial nerve involvement. However, alcohol and some drugs can cause abnormal pupillary reactions, but they are commonly bilateral (except for certain eye drops, if placed in one eye). If the patient is conscious, extraocular movement should also be evaluated.

Fluid Therapy

Fluid therapy should normally be restricted in a patient with head injury to minimize cerebral edema. If the patient is hemodynamically stable, an intravenous line of crystalloid fluid should be established to keep the vein open. If significant hypovolemia is present from another injury, the patient should be managed with aggressive fluid therapy, use of PASG per protocol, and rapid transportation to an appropriate medical facility. In this circumstance, the injury causing hypovolemia usually is more immediately life threatening than the head injury.

Drug Therapy

Drug therapy in the prehospital setting for head injury is controversial. Pharmacological agents that may be prescribed by medical control to decrease cerebral edema or circulating blood volume include *mannitol* (Osmotrol), *furosemide* (Lasix), and other diuretics. If used, medical-control agencies may require the insertion of an indwelling urinary catheter to carefully monitor urine output before administration of these agents. Hypotension leading to hypoperfusion may occur as a complication of diuretic use in patients with head injuries.

Dexamethasone (Decadron) is a commonly used steroid that works as an antiinflammatory agent. Although steroid use in the treatment of head-injured patients is controversial, some medical-control agencies occasionally recommend them to reduce the inflammation that leads to postinjury cerebral edema and pulmonary congestion. Although steroids are not currently popular in the management of acute head injury, there has been a resurgence in the use of high-dose steroids in patients with blunt spinal cord injury. The doses are so large, however, that the medication is usually administered in emergency departments.

Anticonvulsant agents such as *phenytoin* (Dilantin), *diazepam* (Valium), and *phenobarbital* are generally reserved for head-injured patients who develop seizure activity. As a rule, these drugs are not used in the initial management of head injuries because of their sedating effects. Some medical control agencies may prescribe anticonvulsant agents as a prophylactic measure to prevent a rise in intracranial pressure that often accompanies sudden seizure activity. Intravenous *lidocaine* (Xylocaine) has been shown to blunt increases in intracranial pressure that normally occur during endotracheal intubation.

● ANTERIOR NECK AND SPINE TRAUMA

Trauma to the anterior neck and spine may result in critical injuries that can seriously endanger the patient's life. Emergency care procedures for these patients may include aggressive management to correct life-threatening airway compromise, hemorrhage control from venous or arterial bleeding, and spinal immobilization to prevent irreversible spinal cord injury and paralysis.

Anterior Neck Trauma

Anterior neck injuries are caused by blunt and penetrating trauma (Fig. 15-27). These injuries may result in damage to the skeletal structures, vascular structures, nerves, muscles, and glands of the neck. (With both blunt and penetrating neck injuries, cervical spine injury must be assumed until ruled out by cervical radiography.) Common mechanisms of injury to the anterior neck are:
- Motor vehicle crashes
  - Neck striking dashboard or steering column
  - Hyperextension and hyperflexion injuries

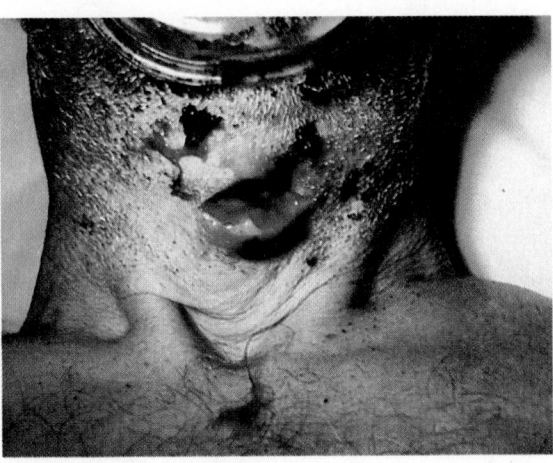

Fig. 15-27 A self-inflicted stab wound that had entered the pharynx.

- Sport and recreational activities
  - Contact sports (boxing, karate, basketball, football, hockey)
  - Small motor vehicles ("clothesline" injuries to the neck from running into wires, ropes, fences)
  - Water sports (jet skiing, water skiing)
  - Snow skiing
  - Horseback riding
- Industrial accidents
  - "Strangulation" injuries from clothing, jewelry, or personal equipment getting caught in machinery
- Violent altercations
  - Stab wounds (knives, screwdrivers, ice picks)
  - Missile injury from firearms
  - Blows to the neck
- Hangings

Evaluation

For purposes of evaluating the trauma patient, the neck can be divided into three zones defined by horizontal planes (Fig. 15-28).[2] Zone I represents the base of the neck, extending from the sternal notch to the top of the clavicles or the cricoid cartilage. Injuries to this zone carry the highest mortality rate because of the risk of injury to major vascular and thoracic structures (subclavian vessels and jugular veins, lungs, esophagus, trachea, cervical spine, cervical nerve roots).

Zone II extends from the clavicles or cricoid cartilage cephalad to the angle of the mandible. The carotid artery, jugular vein, trachea, larynx, esophagus, and cervical spine are the vital structures in this zone. Because of its relative size, zone II injuries are the most common but have a lower mortality rate than zone I injuries.

Zone III is the part of the neck above the angle of the mandible. The risk of injury to the distal carotid artery, salivary glands, and pharynx is greatest in this zone.

Soft Tissue Injuries

Soft tissue injuries to the neck from blunt trauma often produce hematomas and associated edema or direct laryngeal or tracheal injury, both of which can result in airway compromise. Penetrating trauma may produce lacerations and puncture wounds with resultant vascular, laryngeal-tracheal, or esophageal injury. Uncommonly, blunt trauma may also cause vascular injuries. As with all other scenarios of trauma, initial evaluation and resuscitation must begin with rapid assessment, control of the airway, and consideration for spinal injury.

Hematomas and Edema

Edema of the pharynx, larynx, trachea, epiglottis, and vocal cords may produce enough pressure in the neck tissues to completely obstruct the airway. If the airway is compromised (evidenced by dyspnea, inspiratory stridor, cyanosis, or changes in voice quality), oral or nasal intubation with spinal precautions should be considered. Intubation stabilizes damaged areas of the neck, protects the airway, and provides a means for ventilatory support. (A smaller endotracheal tube may be needed to ensure passage through the airway.)

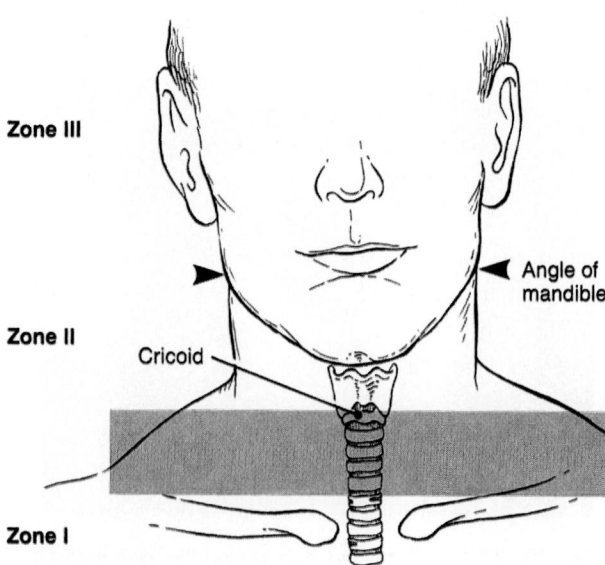

Fig. 15-28 Zones of the neck. The junction of zone 1 and zone 2 is variously described as the cricoid cartilage or top of the clavicles.

> **NOTE:**
> Fractured or transected airways may be totally obstructed or occluded by attempts at oral or nasal intubation. In these cases (if the patient is moving air), rapid transportation with high-concentration oxygen is perhaps the most prudent course.

If blood or vomitus that cannot be cleared with suction obstructs the airway or if progressive edema makes direct intubation impossible, cricothyrotomy or transtracheal jet insufflation may be indicated. Other measures that may prove helpful in treating edematous airways include the administration of cool, humidified oxygen and slight elevation of the patient's head (if not contraindicated by the injury).

Lacerations and puncture wounds

Lacerations and puncture wounds may be superficial or deep. Superficial injuries can usually be managed by covering the wound to prevent further contamination. Deep, penetrating wounds are associated with more serious injuries to underlying structures. These injuries may require aggressive airway therapy and ventilatory support, suction, hemorrhage control by direct pressure, and fluid replacement. Signs and symptoms of significant penetrating neck trauma include:

- Shock
- Active bleeding
- Large or expanding hematoma
- Pulse deficit
- Neurological deficit (cerebrovascular accident, brachial plexus injury, spinal cord injury)
- Dyspnea
- Hoarseness
- Stridor
- Subcutaneous emphysema
- Hemoptysis
- Dysphagia
- Hematemesis

Vascular Injury

Blood vessels are the most commonly injured structures in the neck; they may be injured by blunt or penetrating trauma. Vessels at risk of injury include the carotid, vertebral, subclavian, innominate, and internal mammary arteries and the jugular and subclavian veins. Laceration of these major vessels can result in rapid exsanguination if bleeding is not controlled.

After securing the airway with spinal precautions and providing adequate ventilatory support, prehospital management of vascular injury to the anterior neck should be directed at controlling hemorrhage by constant, direct pressure. The paramedic should apply pressure only to the affected vessels, so blood flow to the brain is not obstructed. If bleeding cannot be controlled in this manner, medical control may advise tamponading the vessels with direct, gloved finger pressure.

> **NOTE:**
> Under no circumstances should cervical vessels be clamped with hemostats in the prehospital setting. Doing so may traumatize critical vascular structures and produce permanent nerve injury.

If a venous injury is suspected, the patient should be kept supine or in a slight Trendelenburg position to prevent air embolism (a rare but lethal complication). If an air embolism is suspected, the immobilized patient should be turned on the left side, head lower than feet, to attempt to trap the air embolus in the right ventricle.

Fluid replacement for hypovolemia should be aggressive, using large-bore catheters and isotonic crystalloid. The use of PASG in this setting is controversial and may actually be detrimental. If penetrating injury to the base of the neck (zone I) has occurred, placement of at least one intravenous line in a lower extremity should be considered in the event that upper-extremity venous drainage has been compromised by the laceration. The second intravenous line should be placed in the upper extremity on the side opposite the injury.

Laryngeal or Tracheal Injury

Injury secondary to blunt or penetrating trauma to the anterior neck may cause fracture or dislocation of the laryngeal and tracheal cartilages, hemorrhage, or swelling of the air passages, all of which can significantly compromise the airway and cause respiratory distress. According to the American College of Surgeons, airway injury is the second most common cause of death in head and neck trauma patients.[2] Therefore rapid and judicious control of the airway and prevention of aspiration can save the lives of many patients with this injury. In addition, a high degree of suspicion for associated vascular disruption and esophageal, chest, and intraabdominal injury are important aspects of preventing death. Injuries that may be associated with laryngeal and tracheal trauma include:

- Fracture of the hyoid bone resulting in laceration and distortion of the epiglottis
- Separation of the hyoid and thyroid cartilages resulting in epiglottis dislocation, aspiration, and subcutaneous emphysema
- Fractures of the thyroid cartilage resulting in epiglottis and vocal cord avulsion, arytenoid dislocation, and aspiration of blood and bone fragments
- Dislocation or fracture of the cricothyroid resulting in long-term laryngeal stenosis, laryngeal nerve paralysis, and laryngotracheal avulsion
- Fracture to the trachea resulting in tracheal avulsion, complete airway obstruction, and subcutaneous emphysema

Emergency airway management of laryngeal and tracheal trauma is controversial. Some medical control agencies recommend oral or nasal intubation; others may feel that intubation attempts may contribute to the potential for anoxic injury and further damage the airway structures. Alternative methods of airway management include use of bag-valve-mask ventilation, cricothyrotomy, and transtracheal jet insufflation.

> **NOTE:**
> Airway procedures involving entry through the neck are generally avoided in the field because of associated risks. In general, these patients should be well ventilated with a bag-value-mask device and rapidly transported to the receiving facility for surgical tracheostomy. Transtracheal jet insufflation is hazardous in the presence of a complete airway obstruction, since the technique, if not modified carefully, does not provide adequate expiratory volume and may result in carbon dioxide retention as well as significant barotrauma.

If penetrating trauma causes complete disruption of the laryngotracheal complex, medical control may recommend dissection through the wound so that the exposed distal trachea can be directly cannulated with a cuffed endotracheal tube. Regardless of the method chosen, emergency care is directed at securing the airway with spinal precautions, providing adequate ventilatory support, controlling hemorrhage, treating for shock, and providing rapid transport to an appropriate medical facility for definitive surgical care.

Esophageal Injury

Esophageal injuries should be suspected in patients with trauma to the neck or chest. Specific injuries that require a high degree of suspicion for associated esophageal injury include tracheal fractures, penetrating trauma from stab or gunshot wounds, and ingestion of caustic substances.

Esophageal injury is difficult to diagnose and may be overlooked as the paramedic focuses on more obvious life-threatening injuries. Signs and symptoms include subcutaneous emphysema, neck hematoma, and oropharyngeal or nasogastric blood (indicating esophageal perforation).

> **NOTE:**
> Esophageal perforation is associated with a high mortality rate from mediastinitis, caused by the release of gastric contents into the thoracic cavity. If not contraindicated by mechanism of injury, the patient with a suspected esophageal tear should be placed in a semi-Fowler's position to prevent reflux of gastric contents.

Spinal Trauma

According to the National Spinal Cord Injury Register, more than 10,000 new spinal cord injuries occur each year in the United States. Of these patients, an estimated 4200 die before admission to a hospital.[8] Most of these injuries result from motor vehicle crashes (41%), falls (13%), firearms (9%), and recreational activities (5%).

Spinal Anatomy and Physiology

The spinal column is composed of 33 bones (vertebrae) divided into five sections: 7 cervical, 12 thoracic, 5 lumbar, 5 sacrum (fused), and 4 coccyx (fused). The anterior elements of the spine include vertebral bodies, intervertebral disks, and anterior and posterior longitudinal ligaments that connect the vertebral bodies anteriorly and inside the canal.

Each vertebra consists of a solid body (bearing most of the weight of the vertebral column), a posterior and anterior arch, a posterior spinous process, and in some vertebrae, a transverse process. Ligaments between the spinous processes provide support for the movements of flexion and extension, whereas those between the lamina provide support during lateral flexion. The spinal cord lies in the spinal canal, with the spinal nerve roots passing out through the vertebral foramen.

Mechanism of Injury

Spinal trauma most commonly results from the spine being forced beyond its physiological limits of motion (Fig. 15-29). The adult skull, which weighs approximately 16 to 22 pounds, sits on top of the first cervical vertebrae (C1), or the atlas. The second cervical vertebrae (C2), or the axis and its odontoid process, allow the head to move with approximately an 180-degree range of motion. Because of the weight and position of the head in relation to the thin neck and cervical vertebrae, the cervical spine is particularly susceptible to injury (27% to 33% of all cervical spine injuries occur in the C1 to C2 region). Other spinal components that

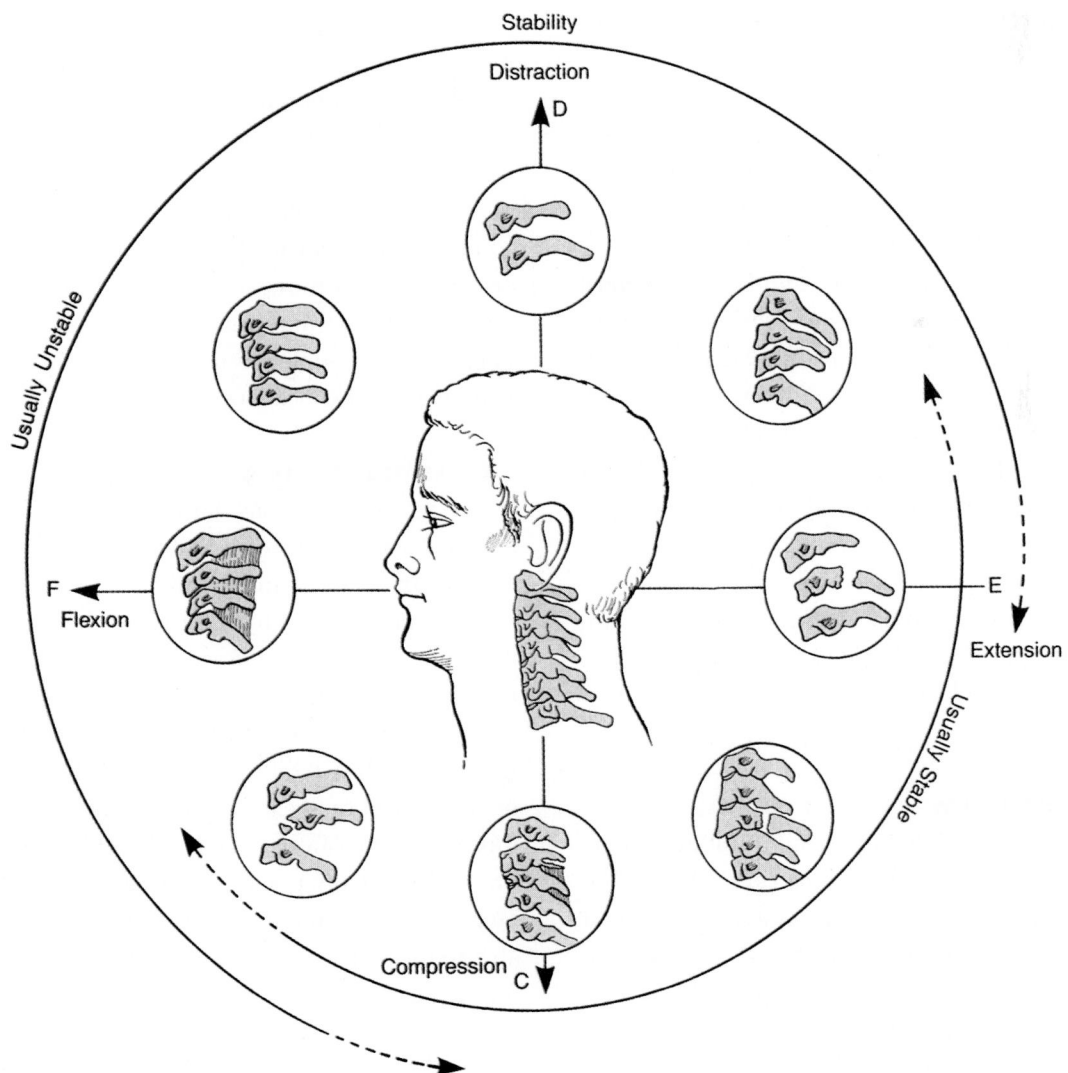

Fig. 15-29 Mechanisms of cervical spine injury and fracture or dislocation. The mechanism of cervical injury (flexion versus extension) determines the type of cervical spine fracture or dislocation.

affect physiological limits of motion are the posterior neck muscles, which permit up to 60 degrees of flexion and 70 degrees of extension without stretching of the spinal cord, and the sacrum, which is joined to the pelvis by immoveable joints.

The specific mechanisms of injury that frequently cause spinal trauma are axial loading; extremes of flexion, hyperextension, or hyperrotation; excessive lateral bending; and distraction. These energy forces may result in stable and unstable injuries, based on the extent of disruption to spinal structures and the relative strength of the structures remaining intact.

Axial Loading

Axial loading (compression) of the spine results when direct forces are transmitted along the length of the spinal column. Examples include striking the head against a windshield of an automobile, shallow diving accidents, vertical falls, and being struck on the head or a helmet with a heavy object.

Flexion, Hyperextension, and Hyperrotation

Extremes in flexion, hyperextension, or hyperrotation may result in fracture, ligamentous injury, or muscle injury. Spinal cord injury is caused by impingement into the spinal canal by subluxation of one or more cervical vertebrae. Examples of these motion extremes include rapid acceleration or deceleration forces from motor vehicle crashes, hangings, and midfacial skeletal or soft tissue trauma. Serious injuries often result from a combination of loading *and* rotational forces, producing displacement or fracture of one or more vertebrae.

Lateral Bending

Excessive lateral bending may result in dislocations and bony fractures to the cervical and thoracic spine. The injury occurs as a sudden lateral impact moves the torso sideways. Initially, the head tends to remain in place until pulled along by the cervical attachments. Examples of lateral bending include side or angular collisions from motor vehicle crashes and injuries from contact sports. The mechanism of this lateral force requires less movement before injury than flexion or extension caused by frontal or rear impacts.

Distraction

Distraction may occur if the cervical spine is suddenly stopped while the weight and momentum of the body pull away from it. This force or stretching may result in tearing and laceration of the spinal cord. Examples of distraction include intentional or accidental hangings (suicide, schoolyard or playground accidents).

Other less common mechanisms of spinal injury include blunt and penetrating trauma and electrical injury. The spinal cord, like the brain, may become concussed, contused, and lacerated and may develop hematomas and edema in response to blunt trauma. Examples include spinal injuries that result from direct blows, as from falling tree limbs or other heavy objects.

Penetrating trauma to the spine may be caused by missile-type injuries or stab wounds to the neck, chest, or abdomen. These forces may result in laceration of the spinal cord or nerve roots over a wide area and may occasionally produce a complete transection. In addition, areas of edema or contusion adjacent to the laceration may disrupt or cavitate cord tissue.

Spinal trauma may occur from direct electrical injury or by the violent muscle spasms that accompany electrical shock (see Chapter 16).

Classifications of Cervical Injury

Cervical injuries may be classified as sprains and strains, fractures and dislocations, cord lesions (transections), and sacral and coccygeal fractures. Many cervical injuries can result in irreversible spinal cord injury. Regardless of the specific injury, all patients with suspected spinal trauma should be immobilized, and unnecessary movement should be avoided until injury to the spine or spinal cord can be excluded by radiography. An unstable spine can only be ruled out by radiography or lack of any potential mechanism for the injury. As a guideline, the presence of spine injury and an unstable spine should be assumed with the following:

- Significant trauma and use of intoxicating substances
- Seizure activity
- Complaints of pain in the neck or arms (or paresthesia in the arms)
- Neck tenderness on examination

- Unconsciousness as a result of head injury
- Injury above the clavicle
- A fall more than 3 times the patient's height
- A fall and fracture of both heels (associated with lumbar fractures)
- Injury from a high-speed motor vehicle crash

The damage produced by the injury forces can be further complicated by the patient's age (calcification from the aging process), preexisting bone diseases (osteoporosis, spondylosis, rheumatoid arthritis, Paget's disease), and congenital spinal cord anomalies (for example, fusion, narrow spinal canal). Spinal cord neurons do not regenerate to any great extent. Therefore any injury to the central nervous system that produces cellular death often results in irreparable damage and permanent loss of function. The role of the paramedic in protecting this critical area cannot be overemphasized.

Sprains and Strains

Sprains and strains usually result from hyperflexion and hyperextension forces. A hyperflexion sprain occurs when the posterior ligamentous complex tears at least partially. This sprain can also result in tears of the joint capsules and may allow partial dislocation (subluxation) of the intervertebral joints. Hyperextension strains are common in low-velocity, rear-end automobile collisions and are commonly known as *whiplash*. Injury occurs as the occiput is thrown backward against the posterior thorax during impact, damaging anterior soft tissues of the neck.

With both sprains and strains, local pain may be produced by spasms of the neck muscles and injury to the vertebrae, intervertebral disks, and ligamentous structures. The pain is usually described as a nonradiating, aching soreness of the neck or back muscles. Discomfort usually varies in intensity with changes in posture.

On examination, a deformity of the spine may be palpable if subluxation has occurred, and the patient may complain of associated point tenderness and swelling. Until the diagnosis is excluded by radiography, these patients should be treated as if they have an unstable cervical spine injury with a potential for spinal cord damage. Treatment of cervical sprain or strain is usually symptomatic and may occasionally include a cervical

collar to decrease neck movement, heat application, and analgesics.

Fractures and Dislocations

The most frequently injured spinal regions in descending order are C5 to C7, C1 to C2, and T12 to L2. Of these injuries, the most common are wedge-shaped compression fractures and "teardrop" fractures or dislocations. Neurological deficits associated with these fractures and dislocations vary with the location and extent of injury. Although the spine and spinal cord are anatomically closely related, the spine can be fractured without spinal cord injury and vice versa. In addition, multiple-level spinal injuries are common.

Wedge-shaped fractures are hyperflexion injuries that usually result from compressive force applied to the anterior portion of the vertebral body with stretching of the posterior ligament complex (commonly seen in industrial accidents and falls). These fractures usually occur in the mid or lower cervical segments or at T12 and L1. They are generally considered stable because the posterior ligamentous complex is rarely totally disrupted.

Teardrop fractures and dislocations are extremely unstable injuries that result from a combination of severe hyperflexion and compression forces commonly seen in motor vehicle crashes. During impact, the vertebral body is fractured, the anterior-inferior corner of the vertebral body being displaced anteriorly. Unlike simple wedge fractures, these fractures may be associated with neurological abnormalities. These are among the most unstable injuries of the cervical spine. A number of other spinal injuries are associated with the mechanisms of flexion, extension, rotation, and axial loading. Most of these are unstable and require careful immobilization.

Cord Lesions

Lesions to the spinal cord are classified as complete or incomplete. Complete lesions are usually associated with spinal fracture or dislocation. Patients have total absence of pain, pressure, and joint sensation and complete motor paralysis below the level of injury. Autonomic dysfunction may be associated with complete cord lesions, depending on the level of cord involvement. Manifestations of autonomic dysfunction include:

- Bradycardia caused by loss of sympathetic autonomic activity
- Hypotension caused by loss of vasomotor control and peripheral vascular resistance
- Priapism
- Loss of sweating and shivering
- Poikilothermy (body temperature varying with ambient temperature)
- Loss of bowel and bladder control

The paramedic should be familiar with several incomplete spinal cord syndromes. Knowledge of these syndromes helps the EMS provider understand the mechanism of injury and the potential for further injury. The three syndromes indicating incomplete lesions of the spinal cord are:

1. Central cord syndrome: Central cord syndrome, commonly seen with hyperextension or flexion cervical injuries, is characterized by greater motor impairment of the upper than lower extremities. Signs and symptoms of central cord syndrome are:
   a. Paralysis of the arms
   b. Sacral sparing (the preservation of sensory or voluntary motor function of the perineum, buttocks, scrotum, or anus)
2. Anterior cord syndrome: Anterior cord syndrome, usually seen in flexion injuries, is caused by pressure on the anterior aspect of the spinal cord by a ruptured intervertebral disk or fragments of the vertebral body extruded posteriorly into the spinal canal. Signs and symptoms include:
   a. Decreased sensation of pain and temperature below the level of the lesion (including lesions of the sacral region)
   b. Intact light touch and position sensation
   c. Paralysis
3. Brown-Séquard syndrome: Brown-Séquard syndrome is a hemitransection of the spinal cord. It may result from a ruptured intervertebral disk or encroachment on the spinal cord by a fragment of vertebral body, often after knife or missile injuries. Pressure on half of the spinal cord results in weakness of the upper and lower extremities on the ipsilateral side and loss of pain and temperature on the contralateral side.

Sacral and Coccygeal Fractures

The majority of serious spinal injuries occur in the cervical, thoracic, and lumbar regions. This is partly because of the location of the spinal cord and its termination in the adult spine at approximately L2 and because of the protection provided by the ring structure of the pelvis and the musculature of the buttocks and lower back. However, fractures through the foramina of S1 and S2 are fairly common and may compromise several sacral nerve elements. They may result in loss of perianal sensory motor function and in bladder and sphincter disturbances.

The sacrococcygeal joint may also be injured as a result of direct blows and falls. Patients frequently complain that they have "broken their tailbone" and experience moderate pain from the mobile coccyx. Diagnosis is usually confirmed by a physician through a rectal examination.

Evaluation

Spinal cord trauma should only be evaluated after all life-threatening injuries have been assessed and treated. As with any scenario of serious illness or injury, the paramedic's first priority must be scene survey and assessment of the patient's airway, breathing, and circulation. The second priority is to preserve spinal cord function and avoid secondary injury to the spinal cord.

The primary injury to the spine occurs at impact. Therefore the critical role of EMS providers is to prevent secondary injury that could result from unnecessary movement of an unstable spinal column, hypoxemia, edema, or shock (which may reduce perfusion of the injured cord). These goals are best met by maintaining a high degree of suspicion for the presence of spinal trauma (based on scene survey, kinematics, and history of the event), by providing early spinal immobilization, and by rapidly correcting any volume deficit through fluid replacement, PASG application (per protocol), and oxygen administration.

After any life-threatening problems encountered in the primary or secondary surveys are treated, a neurological examination should be performed. This examination may be done in the field or en route to the receiving hospital if the patient's condition requires rapid transportation. Thorough documentation of the paramedic's findings provides an important baseline for further assessment and evaluation after the patient is delivered to the emergency department.

The components of the neurological examination include evaluation of motor and sensory findings and reflex responses.

> **NOTE:**
> Any movement of the patient for performing a general or neurological examination must be accompanied by continuous, manual protection and stabilization of the spine.

Motor Findings

Conscious patients should be questioned about pain in the neck or back, any feelings of numbness or tingling in the body, and ability to move arms and legs. If possible, the strength and motion of all four extremities should be tested by asking the patient to flex the elbows (biceps, C6), grasp and squeeze the examiner's fingers (finger flexors, C8), and extend the elbows (triceps, C7). In unconscious patients, painful stimuli in the hands and lower extremities may initiate an involuntary muscle reflex unless the patient is in profound coma.

Sensory Findings

In conscious patients, sensory examination should be performed with light touch on each hand and each foot to evaluate the ability to feel this type of stimuli. If the patient cannot feel light touch or is unconscious, sensation may be evaluated by gently pricking the hands and soles of the feet with a sharp object. The examination should proceed from head to toe; the level at which sensation stops or the unconscious patient ceases to respond to a painful stimulus should be recorded by marking that location on the patient's skin with ink or a marker. (These marks make it possible to accurately compare sensory level after repeated examinations.) Lack of response to pinprick in the upper extremities indicates cord damage in the cervical region; failure of only the lower extremities to respond indicates cord injury in the thoracic region, lumbar regions, or both.

Dermatomes (see Chapter 10) correspond to spinal nerves, so the following four landmarks may be useful for sensory evaluation:

1. C2 to C4 dermatomes provide a collar of sensation around the neck and over the anterior chest to below the clavicles.
2. T4 dermatome provides sensation to the nipple line.
3. T10 dermatome provides sensation to the umbilicus.
4. S1 dermatome provides sensation to the soles of the feet.

Reflex Responses

Reflex responses are seldom evaluated in the prehospital setting. Some abnormal responses are easily observed, however, and may indicate autonomic injury. These responses include loss of temperature control, hypotension, bradycardia, and priapism. Another pathological reflex includes the presence of Babinski's sign (the plantar reflex), which is a reflex movement in which the great toe bends upward when the outer edge of the sole of the foot is scratched (Fig. 15-30). (Babinski's sign is a normal and expected response in children under 2 years of age.)

Other Methods of Evaluation

Visual inspection may also indicate the presence of injury and its level. For example, transection of the cord above C3 often results in respiratory arrest. Lesions that occur at C4 may result in paralysis of the diaphragm, whereas transections that occur at C5 to C6 usually spare the diaphragm, permitting diaphragmatic breathing. This is because the intercostal muscles are sequentially innervated between C4 to C5 and T12. Accordingly, intercostal muscle groups may be paralyzed with cervical or thoracic lesions below the level where diaphragmatic innervation takes place. (The higher the lesion, the greater the loss of intercostal muscle function.)

The patient's body position may also provide clues about neurological injury. For example, a pa-

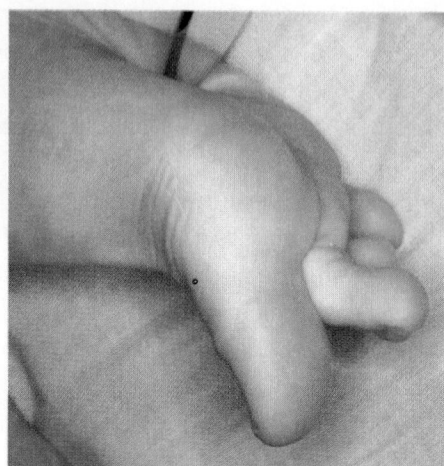

Fig. 15-30 Babinski's sign: dorsiflexion of the great toe with or without fanning of the toes.

tient with a spinal cord injury at C6 may lie with the arms flexed at the elbows and wrists ("hold-up" position).

Management of Spinal Injuries

The absence of neurological deficits does not rule out significant spinal injury. More than 50% of patients with cervical spinal injuries have normal responses to motor, sensory, and reflex examinations.[2] Therefore if the paramedic suspects a spinal injury for any reason, the patient's spine must be protected. In addition, the patient's ability to walk should not be a factor in determining the need for spinal precautions. As previously stated, an unstable spine can only be ruled out by radiography and the lack of any potential mechanism for spinal injury.

Spinal Immobilization Techniques

Immediately on recognizing a possible or potential spine injury, the patient's head and neck should be manually protected. The basic principle to follow is that the head and neck must be maintained in line with the long axis of the body. If other injuries require treatment, the patient's head and neck position must be maintained without interruption.

There are a number of commercial immobilization devices designed for prehospital use. When properly applied to patients who are sitting,

standing, or lying, these devices can provide adequate spinal protection. However, no mechanical device should be considered for application until the head and neck have been stabilized with manual in-line immobilization.

> **NOTE:**
> All spinal immobilization techniques presented in this text follow the guidelines recommended by the Prehospital Trauma Life Support Committee of the National Association of Emergency Medical Technicians in cooperation with the Committee on Trauma of the American College of Surgeons.[5]

Manual In-Line Immobilization

Manual in-line immobilization should be applied without traction, applying only enough traction to relieve the weight of the head from the cervical spine. After manual immobilization has been initiated, it must be continued without interruption until the head and spine are immobilized to an appropriate mechanical device (short spine board or vest, long spine board). Contraindications for moving the patient's head to an in-line position are listed. If any of these contraindications occur, all manual movement of the patient's head should stop, and the head and neck should be stabilized in the position found:

- Resistance to movement
- Neck muscle spasm
- Increased pain
- The presence or increase in neurological deficits during movement (for example, numbness, tingling, loss of motor function)
- Compromise of the airway or ventilation
- Severe misalignment of the head away from the midline of the shoulders and body axis (rare)

Manual in-line immobilization can be accomplished from almost any patient position.

Manual Immobilization from the Sitting or Standing Patient's Side

1. Stand alongside the patient, holding the back of the head with one hand. Place the thumb and first finger of the other hand on each

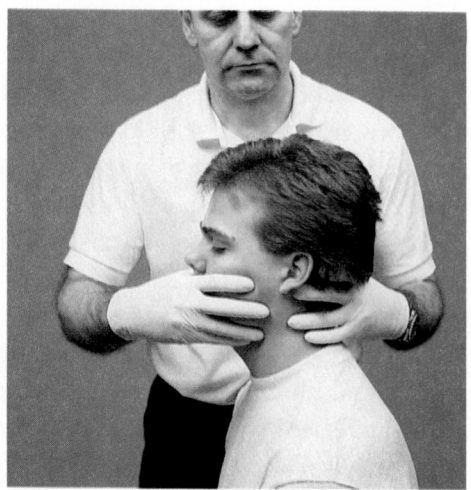

Fig. 15-31 Manual in-line immobilization from the side.

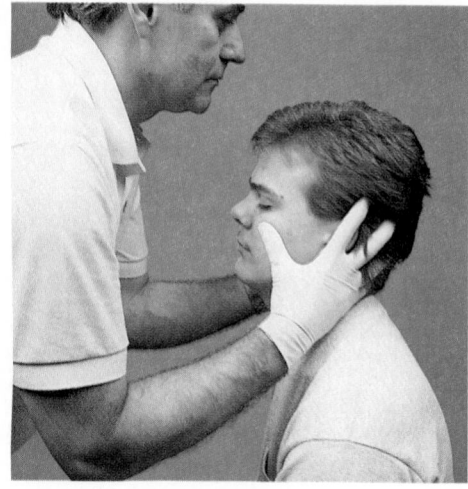

Fig. 15-32 Manual in-line immobilization from the front.

cheek, just below the zygomatic arch (Fig. 15-31).

2. Tighten the position of both hands without moving the head or neck.

3. Move the head to an in-line position if needed. Maintain this position by bracing the elbows against your torso for support.

Manual In-Line Immobilization from the Front of the Sitting or Standing Patient

1. Stand in front of the patient and place the thumb of each hand on the patient's cheeks, just below the zygomatic arch.

2. Place the little fingers of each hand on the posterior aspect of the patient's skull.

3. Spread the remaining fingers of each hand on the lateral planes of the head and increase the strength of the grip (Fig. 15-32).

4. Move the head to an in-line position if needed. Maintain this position by bracing the elbows against your torso for support.

Manual In-Line Immobilization with a Supine Patient

1. Kneel or lie at the patient's head and place the thumbs of each hand just below the zygomatic arch of each cheek (Fig. 15-33).

2. Place the little fingers of each hand on the posterior aspect of the patient's skull.

3. Spread the remaining fingers of each hand on the lateral planes of the head and increase the strength of the grip.

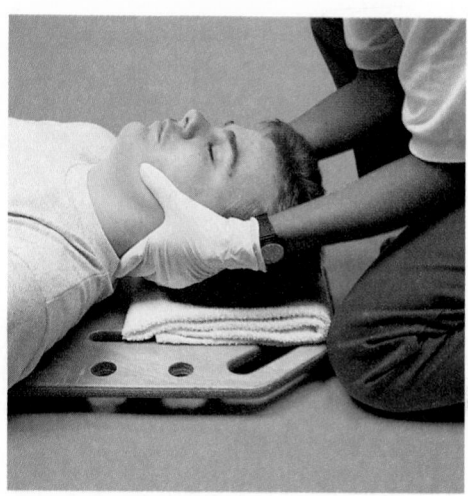

Fig. 15-33 Manual in-line immobilization with a supine patient.

4. Move the head to an in-line position if needed. Maintain this position by bracing the elbows against your torso or ground surface for support.

Log-Roll with Spinal Precautions

Log-rolling methods are used when it is necessary to move patients with possible spinal injury. Examples include moving patients onto a mechanical immobilization device and turning patients from a prone to a supine position. Log-rolling maneuvers require a minimum of four rescuers to provide adequate spinal protection.

NOTE:

The position of the patient's arms during log-rolling maneuvers may affect thoracolumbar motion and further compromise spinal instability. Recent studies have demonstrated that lateral motion can be minimized by positioning patients with arms extended at the side, palms on lateral thighs.[11] This method uses the patient's arms to splint the body, maintains neutral alignment of the pelvis and legs, and minimizes movement.

Log-roll of the supine patient

1. Rescuer 1 should be positioned at the patient's head, providing in-line manual stabilization (Fig. 15-34). A rigid cervical collar should be applied and a long spine board placed at the patient's side. (If there is an obvious spinal injury with paralysis or if shock is suspected, the PASG should be prepared on the spine board per protocol.)
2. Rescuers 2 and 3 should be positioned at the patient's midthorax and knees. The patient's arms should be extended at the sides, palms

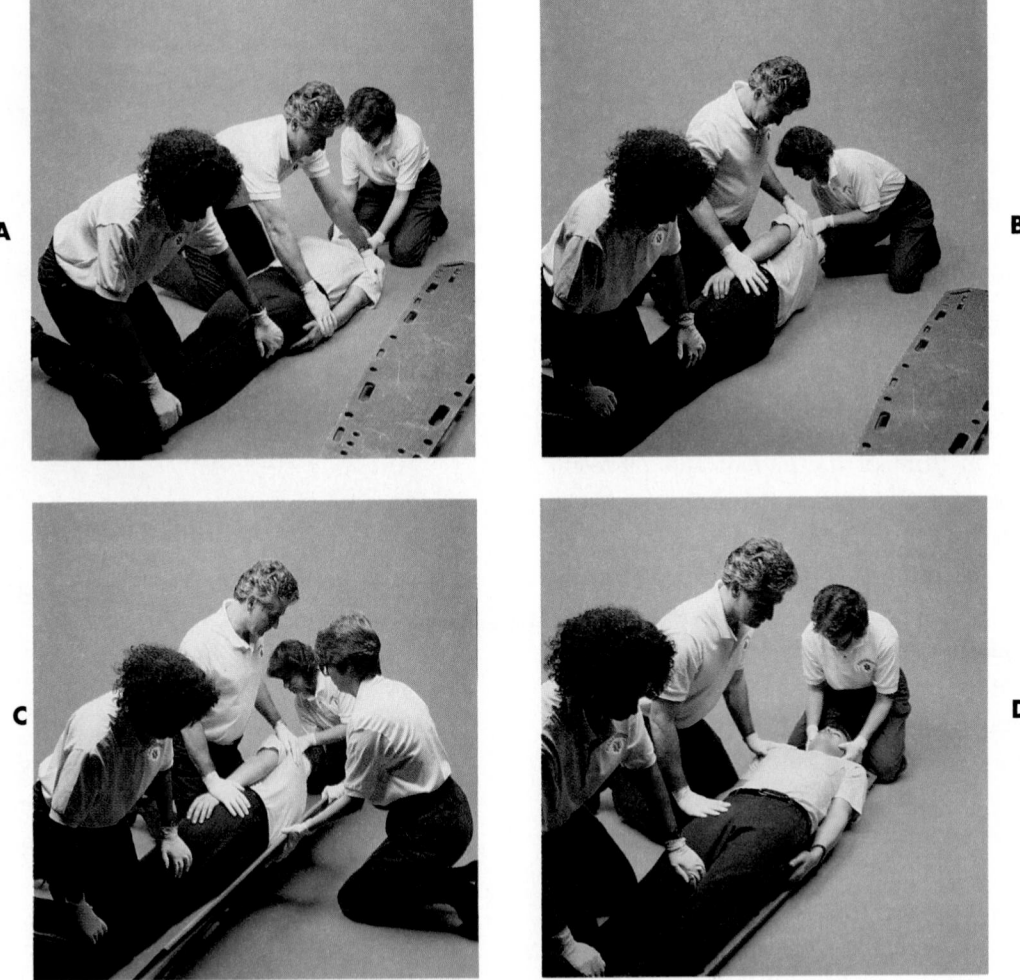

Fig. 15-34 A, To log-roll a supine patient, rescuer 1 is positioned at the patient's head, providing in-line manual stabilization. Rescuers 2 and 3 are positioned at the patient's midthorax and knees. **B,** While maintaining immobilization, the rescuers slowly log-roll the patient onto his or side perpendicular to the ground in one organized move. **C,** Rescuer 4 positions the long spine board by placing the device flat on the ground or at a 30- to 40-degree angle against the patient's back. **D,** In one organized move, the rescuers slowly log-roll and center the patient onto the long spine board.

on lateral thighs. The legs should be brought together for neutral alignment.

3. Rescuer 2 grasps the far side of the patient at the shoulder and wrist. Rescuer 3 grasps the hips (just distal of the wrists) and both lower extremities at the ankles.

4. In one organized move, the rescuers slowly log-roll the patient onto his or her side, perpendicular to the ground. In-line support of the patient's head must be maintained by rotating it exactly with the torso to avoid flexion or hyperextension. In addition, the ankles must be slightly elevated to maintain lateral and anterior-posterior alignment.

5. Rescuer 4 positions the long spine board by placing the device flat on the ground or at a 30- to 40-degree angle against the patient's back.

6. In one organized move, the rescuers slowly log-roll and center the patient on the long spine board.

Log-roll of the prone patient. The general principles used in log-rolling supine patients can be applied to a patient who is in a prone or semiprone position. The procedure incorporates the same initial alignment of the patient's arms and legs and the same rescuer responsibilities for maintaining alignment. The two major differences in this log-roll maneuver are rescuer 1's hand position during the log-roll and the application of the rigid cervical collar, which can only be applied after the patient is in a supine position (Fig. 15-35).

1. Rescuer 1 places his or her hands in a position that provides in-line stabilization and

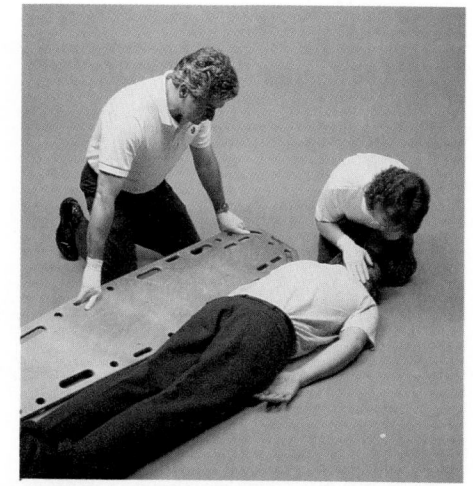

A

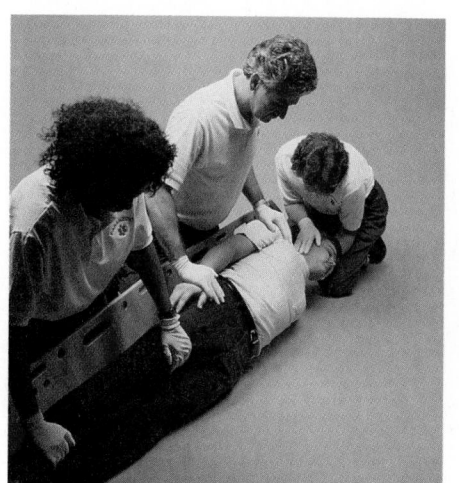

B

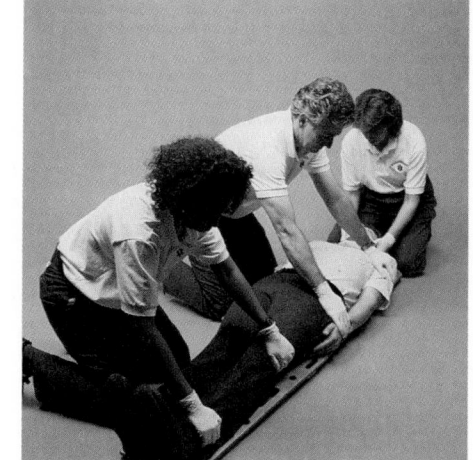

C

Fig. 15-35 A, Rescuer 1 places his or her hands in a position that provides in-line stabilization and that accommodates the rotation of the patient with the torso. Rescuer 2 positions the long spine board. **B,** In one organized move, the patient is rotated away from the direction of his or her initial prone position. **C,** In one organized move, the rescuers slowly log-roll and center the patient onto the long spine board. A rigid cervical collar is then applied.

that accommodates rotation of the patient with the torso.

2. In one organized move, the patient is rotated away from the direction of the initial prone position.
3. The long spine board is placed on a flat surface or positioned between the patient's back and the rescuers at the patient's side.
4. In one organized move, the rescuers slowly log-roll and center the patient on the long spine board.
5. A rigid cervical collar is applied.

Mechanical Devices

Spinal immobilization equipment covered includes rigid cervical collars, short spine boards, and long spine boards. For this text, only *general* principles of spinal immobilization by mechanical devices are presented. The specific methods of ap-

plication vary by device. Paramedics should familiarize themselves with the equipment used in their locale and follow the application guidelines of the equipment manufacturer.

Rigid Cervical Collars

Rigid cervical collars are designed to protect the cervical spine from compression. Although these devices may reduce movement and some range of motion of the head, they do not by themselves provide adequate immobilization of the spine. These mechanical devices must always be used in conjunction with manual in-line stabilization or mechanical immobilization by a suitable device (for example, vest, short spine board, long spine board). To apply a rigid cervical collar, the paramedic should follow these general steps, which demonstrate the application of the Stifneck Collar (Fig. 15-36):

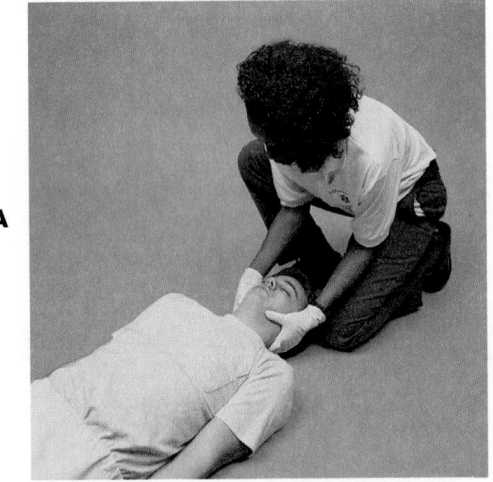

A

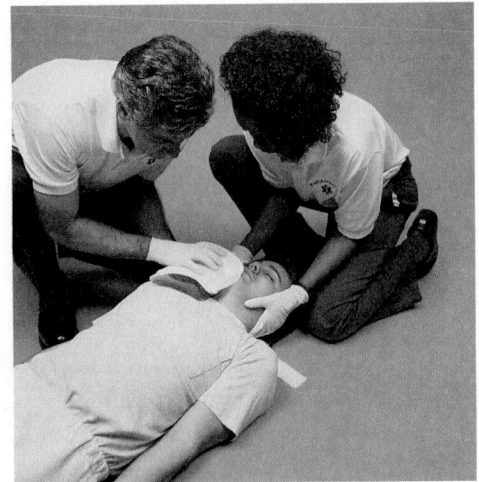

B

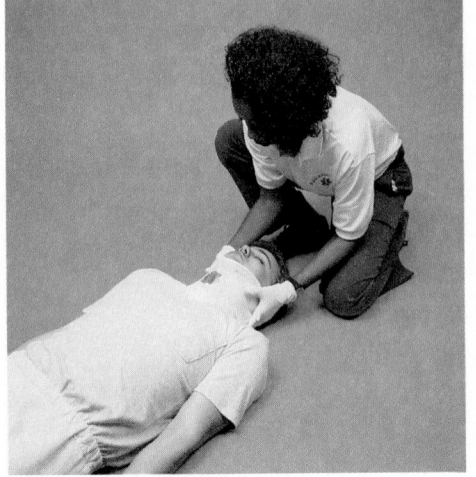

C

Fig. 15-36 A, Rescuer 1 applies manual, in-line immobilization and maintains this position throughout the procedure. **B,** Rescuer 2 positions the collar and secures it with Velcro straps. **C,** Rescuer 1 spreads fingers and maintains support until the patient is secured to a short or long spine board.

1. Rescuer 1 applies manual in-line immobilization from behind the patient and maintains this position throughout the procedure.
2. Rescuer 2 properly angles the collar for placement.
3. Rescuer 2 positions the collar bottom.
4. Rescuer 2 sets the collar in place around the patient's neck.
5. Rescuer 2 secures the collar with the Velcro straps.
6. Rescuer 1 spreads his or her fingers and maintains support until the patient is secured to a short or long spine board.

Rigid cervical collars are available in a number of sizes to accommodate the various physical characteristics of patients (Fig. 15-37). Choosing the appropriate size reduces flexion or hyperextension that may occur during patient extrication and packaging and as a result of acceleration and deceleration forces that normally occur during patient transportation in emergency vehicles. The following guidelines apply to the use of rigid cervical collars:

- Rigid cervical collars must not inhibit the patient's ability to open his or her mouth or to clear his or her airway in case vomiting occurs.
- Rigid cervical collars must not obstruct airway passages or ventilations.
- Rigid cervical collars should only be applied after the head has been brought into a neutral in-line position.

Short Spine Boards

Short spine boards or other short spine extrication devices are used to splint the cervical and thoracic spine. These mechanical devices vary in design and are available from a number of equipment manufacturers (Fig. 15-38). Short spine boards are generally used to provide spinal immobilization in situations in which the patient is in a sitting position or a confined space. After short spine board immobilization, the patient is transferred to a long spine board device for complete spinal immobilization. Examples of short spine boards include the wooden half backboard, the Kendrick's Extrication Device (KED), the Oregon Spine Splint II, and the Hare Extrication Device. General principles of short spine board application, demonstrated with the KED, are (Fig. 15-39):

1. After manual in-line immobilization and the application of a rigid cervical collar, the short

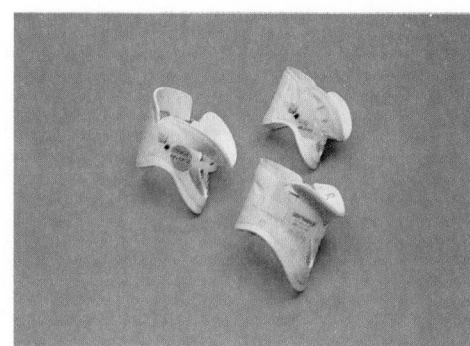

Fig. 15-37 Cervical collars.

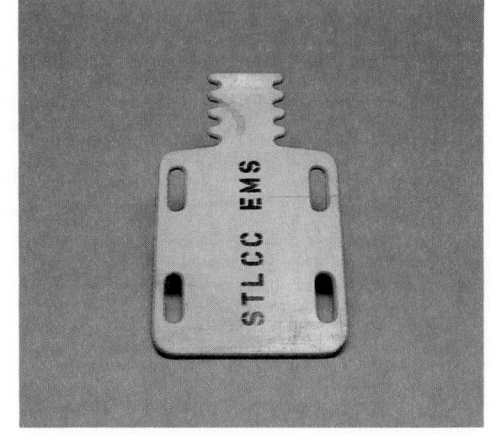

A

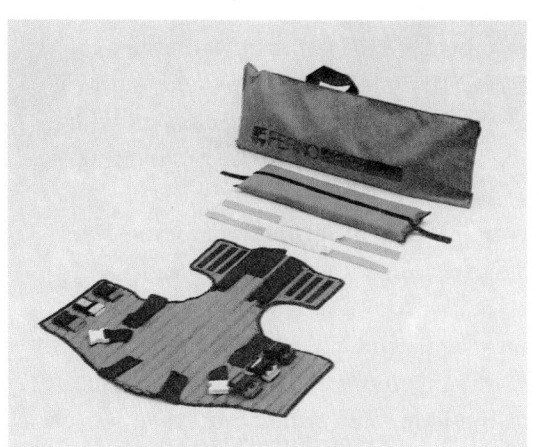

B

Fig. 15-38 A, Wooden short spine board. **B,** KED.

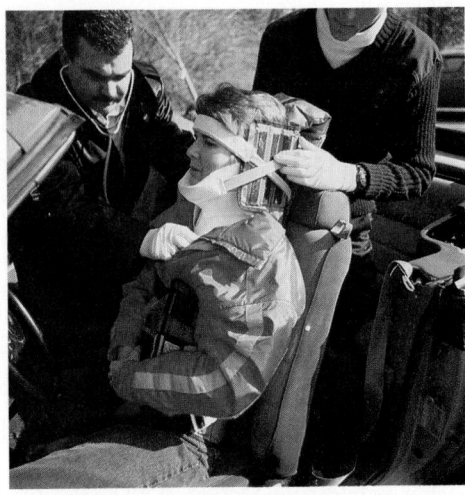

Fig. 15-39 KED application.

NOTE:
Short spine board application should only be considered if the patient's condition allows. If the patient is unstable because of a life-threatening injury or if the time required to apply the device would jeopardize the patient's life (for example, a burning vehicle), the patient's head and neck should be stabilized with manual in-line support, and the patient should be moved as a unit to a long spine board.

spine board device is placed behind the patient. It should be positioned snugly beneath the patient's axillae to prevent it from moving up the torso.

2. Immobilize the upper and middle torso by fastening the upper, middle, and lower chest straps. The upper strap can be relatively tight without impairing chest excursion. The middle and lower straps should be snug so that fingers cannot be slipped beneath the straps. Readjust as needed.

3. Position and fasten each groin strap separately, forming a loop. These straps prevent the KED from moving up and the lower end from moving laterally.

4. Pad and secure the head to the short spine board.

5. Carefully move the patient as a unit to a long spine board by rotating the patient and KED onto the board. The legs are held proximal to the knees and are lifted during the transition.

6. Center the patient on the long spine board and slowly lower the patient's legs to an in-line position.

7. Secure the patient and KED to the long spine board, maintaining a neutral in-line position with the long axis of the body. Then loosen the KED chest straps.

The steps required for this rapid extrication are (Fig. 15-40):

1. Rescuer 1 supports the patient's head and neck and uses manual in-line stabilization from behind the patient or from the patient's side. This stabilization is maintained by rescuer 1 throughout the extrication procedure.

2. After a rapid primary assessment, a rigid cervical collar is applied, and a long spine board is positioned near the vehicle.

3. Rescuer 2 helps support the patient's midthorax as rescuer 3 frees the patient's lower extremities for extrication.

4. On rescuer 2's command, the patient is rotated so that his or her back faces the open doorway. The patient's feet are positioned on the passenger seat by rescuer 3. Each movement during the rotation of the patient should be coordinated, stopping so that the rescuers and the patient can be repositioned as needed to limit unwanted patient movement.

5. The long spine board should be inserted on the car seat at the patient's buttocks, and the patient should be carefully lowered onto the backboard.

6. The patient is centered on the long spine board and secured as described below.

Long Spine Board with Supine Patient

Like short spine boards, long spine boards are available in a variety of configurations. These include wooden spine boards, metal alloy spine boards, vacuum mattress splints, and split litters

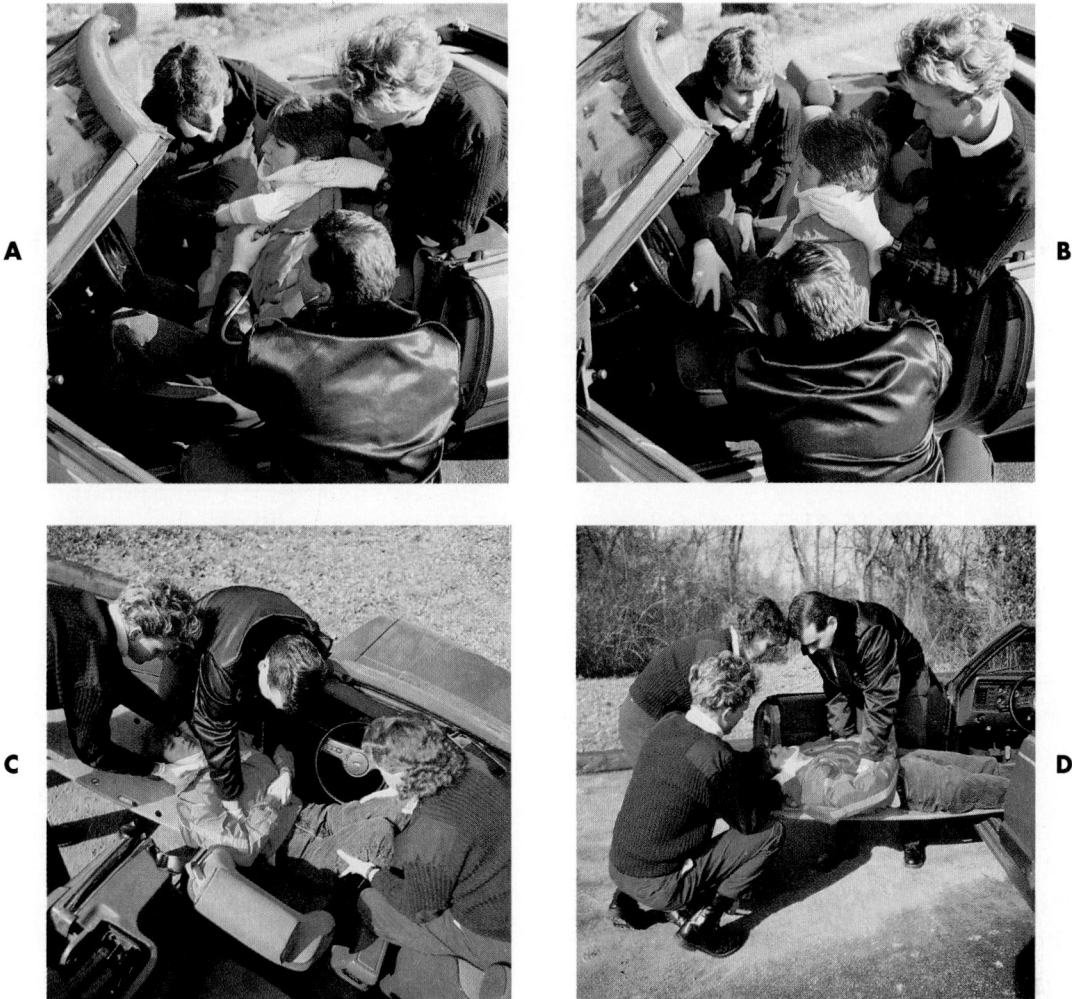

Fig. 15-40 A, Rescuer 1 supports the patient's head and neck and uses manual in-line stabilization throughout the procedure. **B,** After a rapid primary assessment, rescuer 2 helps support the patient's midthorax as rescuer 3 frees the patient's lower extremities for extrication. **C,** The patient is carefully lowered onto the long spine board. **D,** The patient is centered and secured on the long spine board.

(scoop stretchers) that must be used in conjunction with a long spine board. The following description of securing patients on a long spine board may be applied to any long spinal immobilization device.

Immobilizing the torso to a long spine board must always precede immobilization of the head to prevent angulation of the cervical spine. The torso must not be allowed to move up, down, or to either side. Straps should be placed at the shoulders or chest to avoid compression and lateral movement of the thorax, around the mid-torso, and across the iliac crest to prevent movement of the lower torso. Care should be taken not to tighten the straps to the point that chest excursion is inhibited.

After immobilization of the torso, the head and neck should be immobilized in a neutral, in-line position. When most adults are placed on a long or short spinal device, a significant space is produced between the back of the head and the spine board. Therefore noncompressible padding (for example, commercial padding, folded towels) should be added before securing the head (Fig. 15-

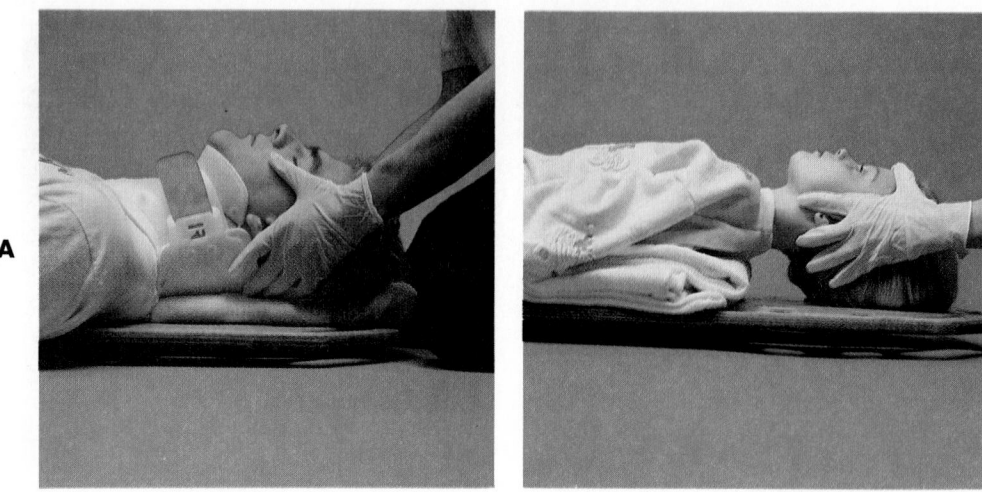

Fig. 15-41 Padding requirements for adult **(A)** and pediatric **(B)** patients.

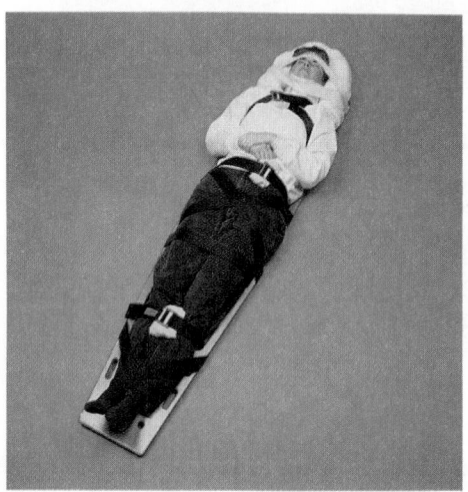

Fig. 15-42 Long spine board immobilization (supine patient).

41, *A*). The amount of padding required for in-line immobilization varies by patient and must be evaluated on an individual basis. Too little padding may cause hyperextension of the head, and too much padding may cause flexion; both may increase spinal cord damage. Children have proportionally larger heads than adults and may require padding under the torso to allow the head to lie in a neutral position on the board (Fig. 15-41, *B*). The padding (if needed) should be firm and extend the full length and width of the torso from the buttocks to the top of the shoulders to prevent movement and misalignment of the spine.

The head is secured to the spinal device by placing commercial pads or rolled blankets on both sides of the head and securing them with 2- to 3-inch tape strips or a self-adhering firm wrap such as Colban, Medi-Rip, or Elastoplast. (Elastic or gauze bandages do not provide adequate fixation.) The upper forehead should be secured across the supraorbital ridge. The lower portion of the head should be secured across the anterior portion of the rigid cervical collar. Chin straps, sandbags, and intravenous bags are considered less optimal in immobilizing the head to a spinal device.

The patient's legs should be secured to the long spine board, with two or more straps applied above and below the knees. Towels, blankets, or suitable padding may be placed on both sides of the patient's lower legs to minimize movement and help maintain the patient's central position on the spinal device. The ankles and feet should be tied together with a cravat (Fig. 15-42).

Before moving the patient, the patient's arms should be secured to the spinal device for safety. This is best accomplished by placing the patient's arms at his or her side (palms in) and securing them with a separate strap placed across the forearms and torso.

Long Spine Board with Standing Patient
Patients who are standing may also be secured to a long spine board using the following technique (Fig. 15-43):

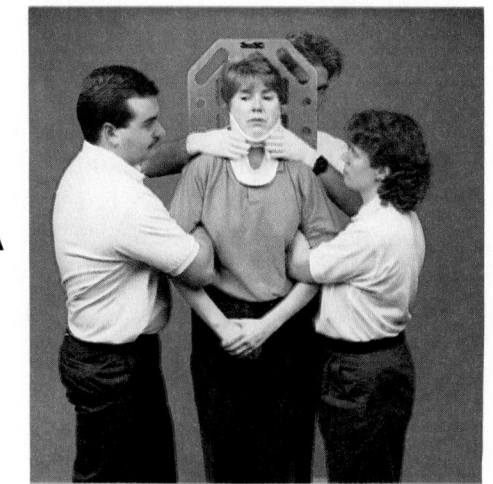 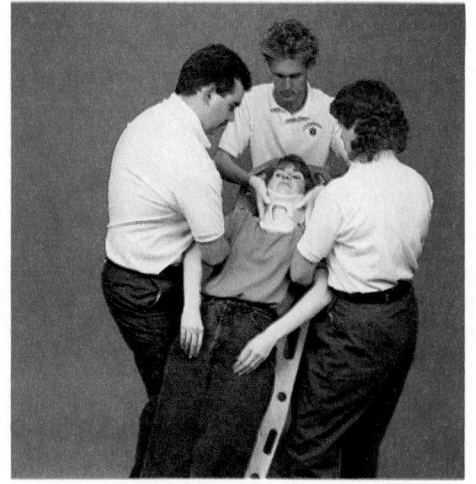

Fig. 15-43 A, While rescuer 1 maintains manual in-line stabilization, the patient is supported by rescuers 2 and 3. **B,** In one organized move, the patient is lowered to the ground on the long spine board for further immobilization.

1. Rescuer 1 applies manual, in-line immobilization from behind the patient and maintains this position throughout the procedure. A rigid cervical collar is applied.
2. Rescuer 2 slides the long spine board behind the patient from the side, and the patient's upper and lower torso are secured to the spine board.
3. Padding (if needed) is placed behind the patient's head, and the head is secured to the spine board.
4. After immobilization of the patient's torso, neck, and head, the patient is lowered halfway to the ground by rescuers 1 and 2. Rescuer 3 stabilizes the foot end of the spinal device. As the spine board is lowered approximately halfway, movement of the board stops to reposition hand-holds on the board.
5. The patient is lowered to the ground and secured to the board as described.

> **NOTE:**
> If the patient becomes unstable during the backboarding procedure, manual in-line stabilization should be maintained, and the patient should be supported by rescuers 2 and 3 as he or she is lowered to the ground on the long spine board for further immobilization.

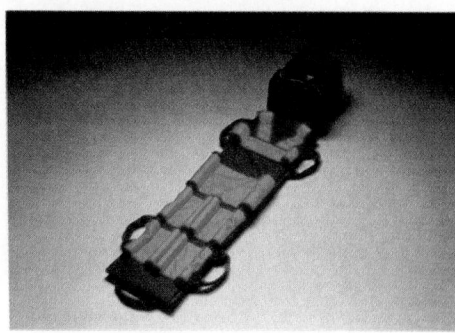

Fig. 15-44 Infant and pediatric immobilization board.

Immobilizing Pediatric Patients

As with adult patients, prehospital care of a pediatric patient with suspected spine trauma should be managed with manual in-line immobilization, a rigid cervical collar, and a long spinal immobilization device. A variety of pediatric immobilization devices are available from various equipment manufacturers (Fig. 15-44). If special pediatric immobilization devices are not available, children may be secured on an adult long spine board.

Helmet Removal

As a rule, full-face helmets should be removed in the prehospital setting to allow access to the patient's airway and to provide in-line immobilization of the head and neck. Consult medical control if the patient complains of increased pain during removal or if the helmet is difficult to remove. The following steps in helmet removal are recommended by the American College of Surgeons Committee on Trauma (Fig. 15-45):

1. Rescuer 1 immobilizes the helmet and head in an in-line position. This is accomplished by the rescuer pressing his or her palms on each side of the helmet with the fingertips curled over its lower margin.

2. Rescuer 2 removes the face shield and chin strap, assessing the patient airway and ventilatory status.

3. Rescuer 2 grasps the patient's mandible by placing the thumb at the angle of the mandible on one side and two fingers at the angle on the other side. Rescuer 2's other hand is placed under the neck at the base of the skull, taking over in-line immobilization of the patient's head.

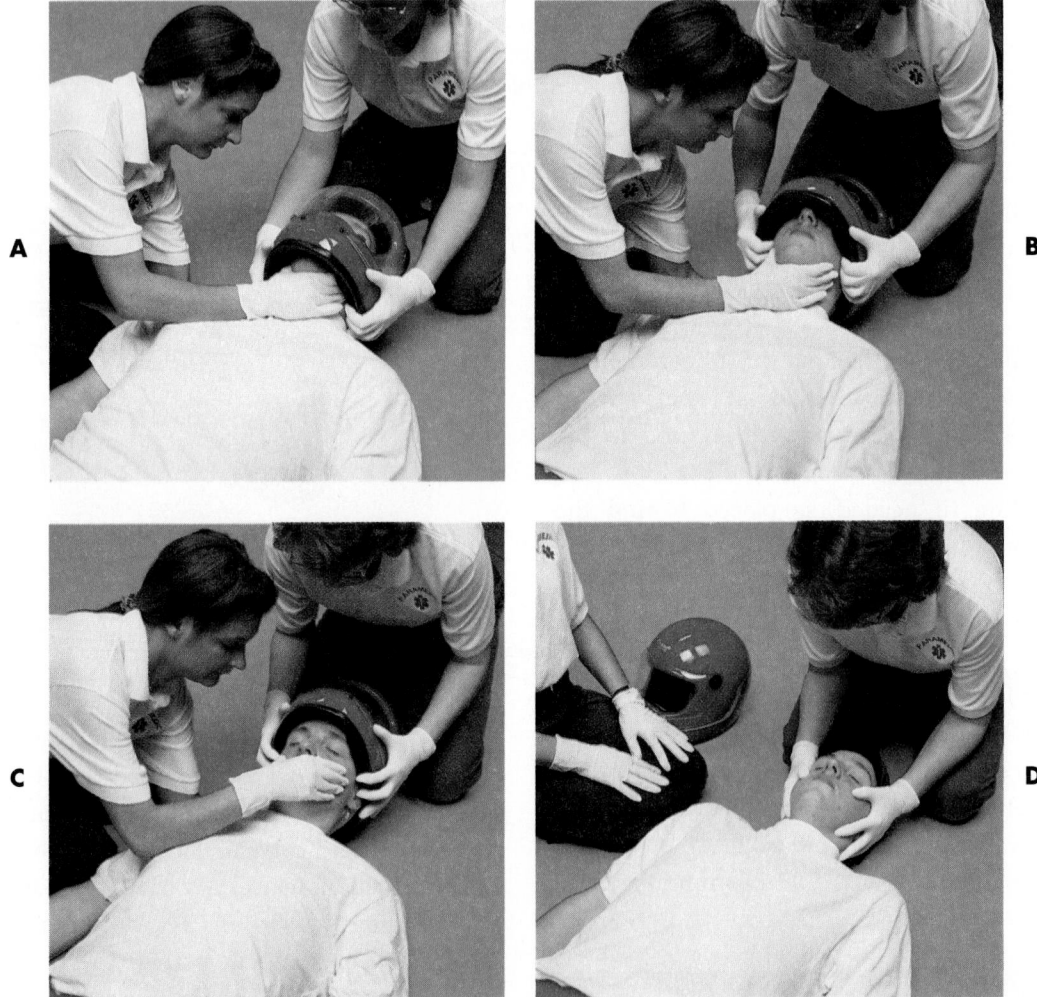

Fig. 15-45 A, Rescuer 1 immobilizes the helmet and head in an in-line position. Rescuer 2 grasps the patient's mandible by placing the thumb at the angle of the mandible on one side and two fingers at the angle on the other side. Rescuer 2's other hand is placed under the neck at the base of the skull, producing in-line immobilization of the patient's head. **B,** Rescuer 1 carefully spreads the sides of the helmet away from the patient's head and ears. **C,** The helmet is then rotated toward the rescuer to clear the nose and removed from the patient's head in a straight line. **D,** After removal of the helmet, rescuer 1 applies in-line immobilization. A rigid cervical collar is applied.

4. Rescuer 1 carefully spreads the sides of the helmet away from the patient's head and ears. The helmet is then rotated toward the rescuer to clear the patient's nose and removed from the patient's head in a straight line. Just before removing the helmet from under the patient's head, rescuer 1 assumes in-line immobilization by squeezing the sides of the helmet against the patient's head.

5. Rescuer 2 repositions his or her hands to support the head and to prevent it from dropping as the helmet is completely removed. This is accomplished by the rescuer placing a hand further up on the occipital area of the head and by grasping the maxilla with the thumb and first fingers of the other hand on each side of the nose. After this position is secured, rescuer 2 takes over in-line immobilization.

6. Rescuer 1 rotates the helmet approximately 30 degrees, following the curvature of the patient's head. The helmet is completely removed by carefully pulling it in a straight line.

7. After removal of the helmet, rescuer 1 applies in-line immobilization, and a rigid cervical collar is applied.

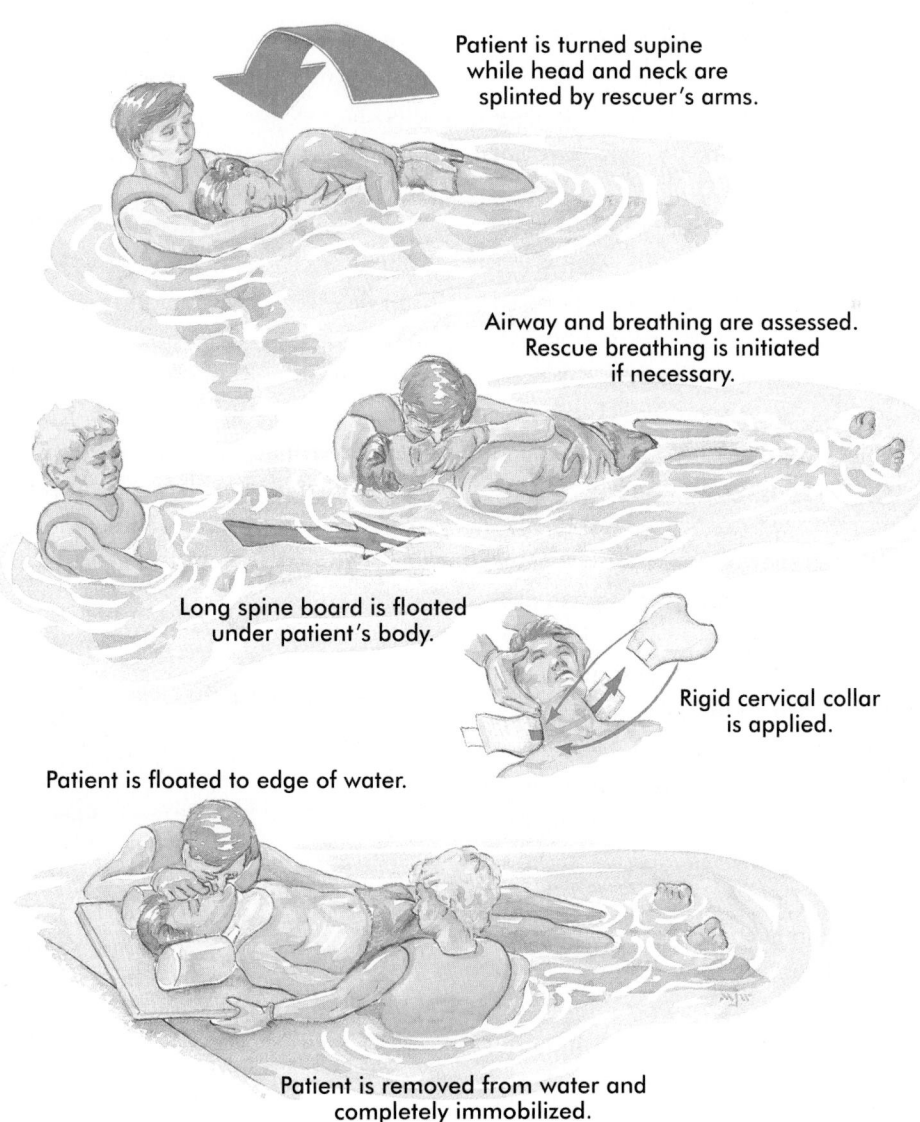

Patient is turned supine while head and neck are splinted by rescuer's arms.

Airway and breathing are assessed. Rescue breathing is initiated if necessary.

Long spine board is floated under patient's body.

Rigid cervical collar is applied.

Patient is floated to edge of water.

Patient is removed from water and completely immobilized.

Fig. 15-46 Extrication of a diving accident victim.

NOTE:

A key point to remember during helmet removal is that in-line immobilization must be maintained throughout the procedure. Therefore the rescuers should never move their hands at the same time. In addition, the helmet must be rotated in one direction to clear the nose and in the opposite direction to clear the back of the patient's head.

Spinal Immobilization In Diving Accidents

Most diving accidents involve injury to the patient's head, neck, and spine. If the patient is still in the water when EMS arrives, the patient should be managed as follows (Fig. 15-46):

1. Only rescuers trained in water rescue should enter the water.
2. A supine patient should be floated to a shallow area without unnecessary movement of the spine.
3. A prone patient should be approached from the top of the head. One arm of the rescuer should be positioned under the patient so that the head, neck, and torso are supported. The rescuer's other arm should be placed across the patient's head and back, splinting the head and neck between the rescuer's arms. The patient should be carefully turned to a supine position, and airway and breathing should be quickly assessed by the paramedic. (Rescue breathing may be initiated in the water.)
4. A second rescuer slides a long spine board or other rigid device under the patient's body while the first rescuer continues to support the patient's head and neck. A rigid cervical collar should be applied. Manual in-line immobilization must be maintained throughout the rescue.
5. The spinal immobilization device should be floated to the edge of the water and lifted out.
6. The patient should be completely immobilized on the long spine board as previously described.

● THORACIC TRAUMA

Chest injuries are directly responsible for more than 25% of the 50,000 to 60,000 deaths that result from motor vehicle crashes each year and contribute significantly to another 25% to 50%.[8] Chest injuries are caused by blunt trauma, penetrating trauma, or both, and frequently result from motor vehicle crashes, falls from heights, blast injuries, blows to the chest, chest compression, gunshot wounds, and stab wounds. Thoracic trauma may be classified as skeletal injury, pulmonary injury, heart and great vessel injury, and diaphragmatic injury.

Skeletal Injury

Skeletal injuries can be caused by blunt and penetrating trauma. Specific injuries discussed in this chapter are clavicular fractures, rib fractures, flail chest, and sternal fractures.

Clavicular Fractures

Fractured clavicles usually result from direct trauma and are seldom by themselves significant injuries (Fig. 15-47). They are common in children who fall on their shoulders or outstretched arms and in athletes involved in contact sports. Treatment is usually accomplished with a sling and swathe that immobilizes the affected shoulder and arm or a clavicle strap. These injuries usually heal well within 4 to 6 weeks.

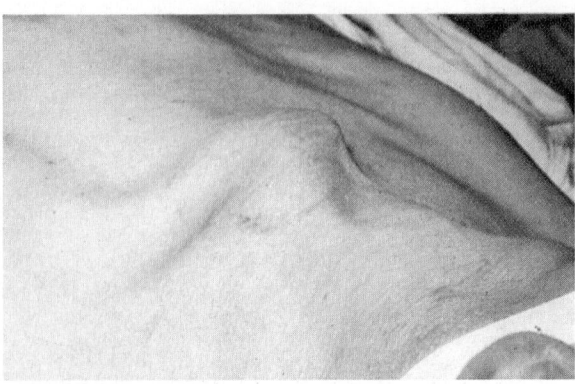

Fig. 15-47 Fracture of the left clavicle seen from above the left shoulder.

Signs and symptoms of clavicular fractures include pain, point tenderness, and evident deformity. A complication that may be associated with clavicular fracture is injury to the subclavian vein or artery from bony fragment penetration, producing a hematoma or venous thrombosis.

Rib Fractures

Rib fractures most commonly occur on the lateral aspect of ribs 3 through 8 where they are least protected by musculature (Fig. 15-48). Fractures are more likely in adults than in children because younger patients have more resilient cartilage.

Simple rib fractures are usually very painful but rarely life threatening. Most patients can localize the fracture by pointing to the area (confirmed by palpation). Occasionally movement or crepitation can be felt. Treatment is aimed at relieving pain

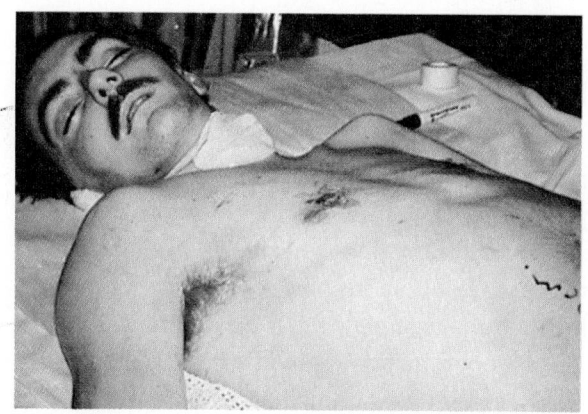

Fig. 15-48 Chest wall asymmetry caused by rib fractures.

that may interfere with ventilation. This may be accomplished by splinting the patient's arm against the chest wall with a sling and swathe. Based on the mechanism of injury, the paramedic should consider the possibility of more serious trauma such as closed pneumothorax and internal bleeding. (Fractures to the lower ribs, 8 through 12, may be associated with spleen, kidney, or liver injuries.)

Great force is required to fracture the first and second ribs because of their shape and the protected location provided by the scapulae, clavicles, and upper chest musculature. Fractures to these ribs are often associated with myocardial contusion, bronchial tears, and vascular injury.

Flail Chest

A flail chest may occur when two or more adjacent ribs are fractured in two or more places (Fig. 15-49). This injury is not usually detected in the prehospital setting because of the muscle spasm that accompanies the injury. However, within 2 hours after the injury, the muscle spasm subsides and the injured segment of the chest wall may begin to move in a paradoxical fashion with inspiration and expiration.

During inspiration the diaphragm descends, lowering the intrapleural pressure. The unstable chest wall is pushed inward by the outside atmospheric pressure as the rest of the chest wall expands. During expiration, the diaphragm rises and the intrapleural pressure exceeds atmospheric pressure, causing the unstable chest wall to move

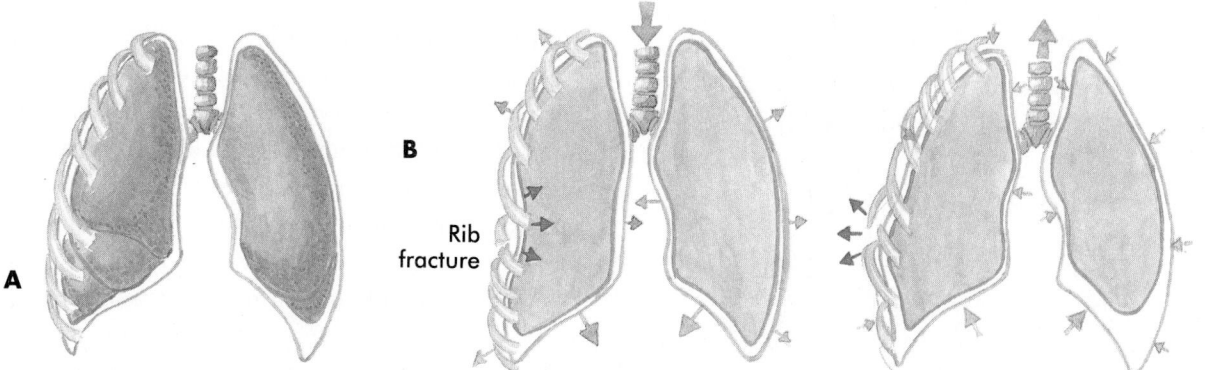

Fig. 15-49 Flail chest. **A,** Normal lungs. **B,** Flail chest during inspiration. **C,** Flail chest during expiration.

outward. Patients with flail chest often develop hypoxia because of the underlying pulmonary contusion usually associated with this injury. The contusion, which results from interstitial and alveolar hemorrhage, is associated with decreased vital capacity and vascular shunting of deoxygenated blood. Signs and symptoms of flail chest include tenderness and bony crepitus on palpation and paradoxical motion (a late sign).

Prehospital management of patients with flail chest includes assisting ventilation with positive pressure via a bag-valve-mask, high-concentration supplemental oxygen, and fluid replacement as needed. Field stabilization of the flail segment is somewhat controversial. In one method, the paramedic attempts to splint the flail segment in the inward position with simple hand pressure or bulky dressings or towels taped to the chest wall. Although this splinting can reduce vital capacity, it may increase the efficiency of ventilation. Most authorities, however, recommend intubation and positive-pressure ventilation in patients with respiratory distress and a flail chest. Medical control may also recommend intubation, particularly if the chest injury is associated with shock, other severe injuries, head injury, or pulmonary disease

or if it occurs in patients over age 65. A large percentage of patients with significant chest injury progress to respiratory failure, requiring long-term ventilatory support and hospitalization.

Sternal Fractures

Sternal fractures are uncommon but serious. They usually result from a direct blow to the chest, as when it strikes a steering column, or from a massive crush injury (Fig. 15-50). Sternal fractures are usually very painful and may be associated with an unstable chest wall, myocardial injury, or cardiac tamponade. Signs and symptoms include a history of significant anterior chest trauma, tenderness, and abnormal motion or crepitation over the sternum. Prehospital management includes maintaining a high degree of suspicion for associated injuries, airway maintenance, ventilatory support, and rapid transportation to an appropriate medical facility.

Pulmonary Injury

Pulmonary injuries may be classified as closed pneumothorax, tension pneumothorax, open pneumothorax, hemothorax, pulmonary contusion, and traumatic asphyxia. Any of these injuries can result in respiratory insufficiency. Prehospital management must be directed at ensuring an open airway, providing ventilatory support, correcting immediately life-threatening ventilatory problems (for example, tension pneumothorax), and rapid transportation for definitive care.

Closed Pneumothorax

A closed pneumothorax is caused by the presence of air in the pleural space and a partially or totally collapsed lung (Fig. 15-51). A common cause of pneumothorax is a fractured rib pushed inward after blunt thoracic trauma. Pneumothoraces may also occur in the absence of rib fractures from excessive pressure on the chest wall against a closed glottis (paper-bag effect).

Signs and symptoms of a closed pneumothorax include chest pain, dyspnea, and tachypnea. Auscultation may disclose decreased or absent breath sounds on the affected side. Prehospital manage-

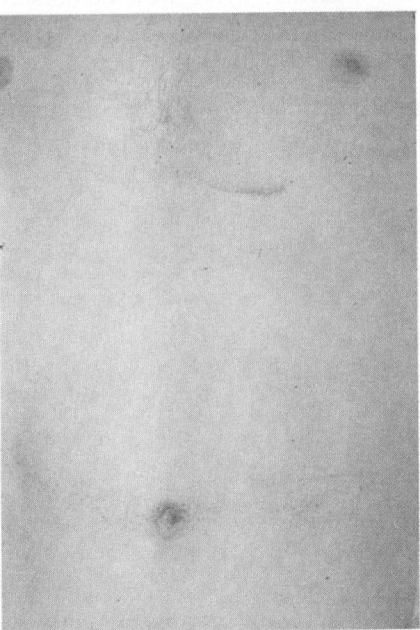

Fig. 15-50 A well-marked band of spotty bruising caused by a steering wheel impact.

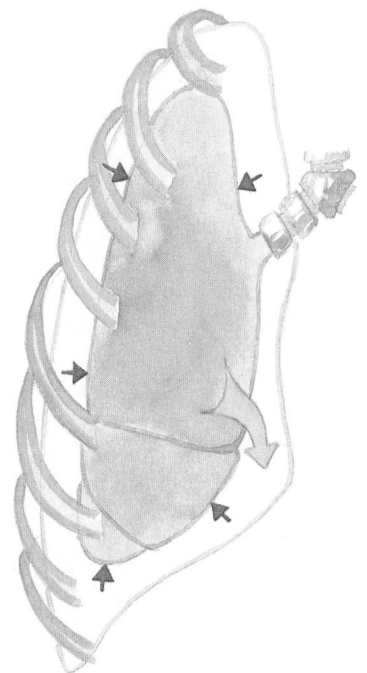

Fig. 15-51 Simple pneumothorax.

ment is directed at ventilatory support with high-concentration oxygen and careful monitoring for signs of a tension pneumothorax. The patient should be transported in a semisitting position of comfort unless this is contraindicated by the mechanism of injury. If the patient's respirations are fewer than 12 or more than 28 per minute, ventilatory assistance with a bag-valve-mask may be indicated.

Most healthy patients have large circulatory and ventilatory reserve capacities. Therefore closed pneumothoraces are not usually life threatening. Life-threatening consequences may develop, however, if the pneumothorax is a tension pneumothorax, if it occupies more than 40% of the hemithorax, or if it occurs in a patient with shock or pre-existing pulmonary or cardiovascular diseases.

Open Pneumothorax

An open pneumothorax develops when penetrating injury to the chest allows the pleural space to be exposed to atmospheric pressure, as occurs with gunshot wounds, stab wounds, and impaled objects (Fig. 15-52). The severity of the injury is directly proportional to the size of the wound.

When a chest wound is larger than the normal pathway for air through the nose and mouth, atmospheric pressure forces the air through the open wound and into the thoracic cavity during inspiration. As the air accumulates in the pleural space, the lung on the injured side collapses and begins to shift toward the uninjured side. Very little air enters the tracheobronchial tree to be exchanged with intrapulmonary air on the affected side, which results in decreased alveolar ventilation and decreased perfusion. The normal side is also adversely affected because expired air may enter the lung on the collapsed side, only to be rebreathed into the functioning lung with the next ventilation. This may result in severe ventilatory dysfunction, hypoxemia, and death unless rapidly recognized and corrected.

Signs and symptoms of open pneumothorax include shortness of breath, pain, and a sucking or gurgling sound as air moves in and out of the pleura space through the open chest wound (giving rise to the name *sucking chest wound*). Prehospital management of an open pneumothorax entails:

1. Closing the chest wound. This may be accomplished through applying an occlusive petroleum gauze dressing (covered with sterile dressings) and securing it with tape. Medical control may advise that only three sides of the dressing be taped to provide for a "venting" mechanism (or one-way valve) that allows spontaneous decompression of a developing tension pneumothorax.
2. Providing ventilatory support with high-concentration oxygen. Airway management may include assisted ventilations with a bag-valve-device and intubation.
3. Treating for shock through the administration of crystalloid. (Use of a PASG is controversial and is generally contraindicated in chest trauma.)
4. Rapidly transporting the patient to an appropriate medical facility.

Tension Pneumothorax

When air within the thoracic cavity cannot exit the pleural space, a tension pneumothorax may develop (Fig. 15-53). This is a true emergency that

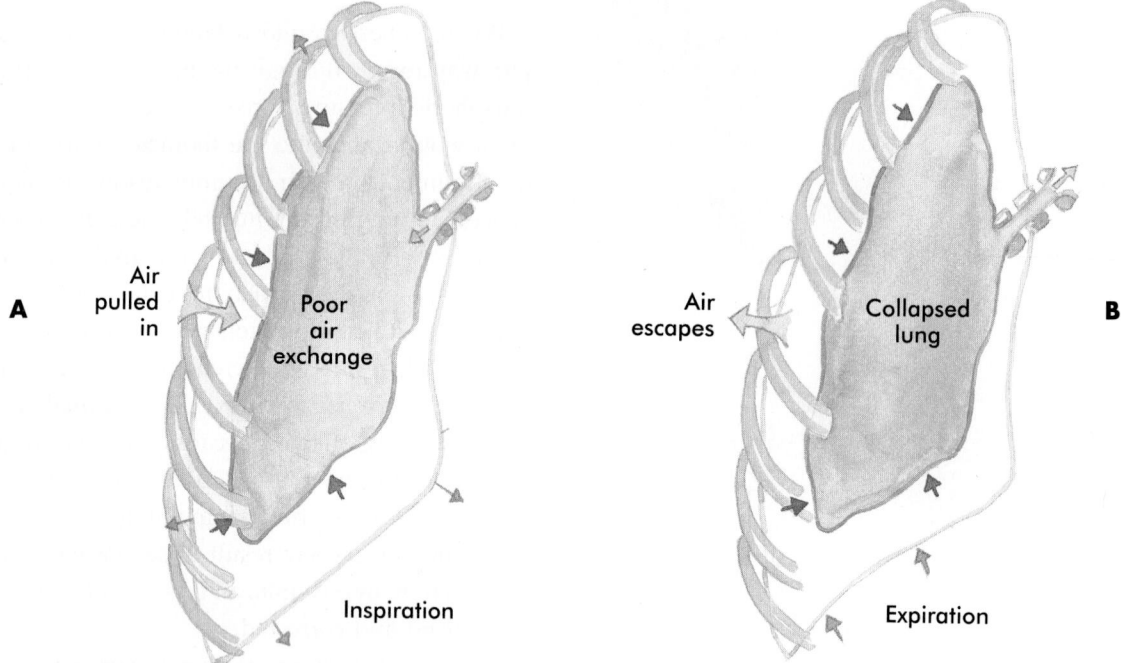

Fig. 15-52 Open pneumothorax. **A,** Air enters pleural cavity during inspiration. **B,** Air exits pleural cavity during expiration.

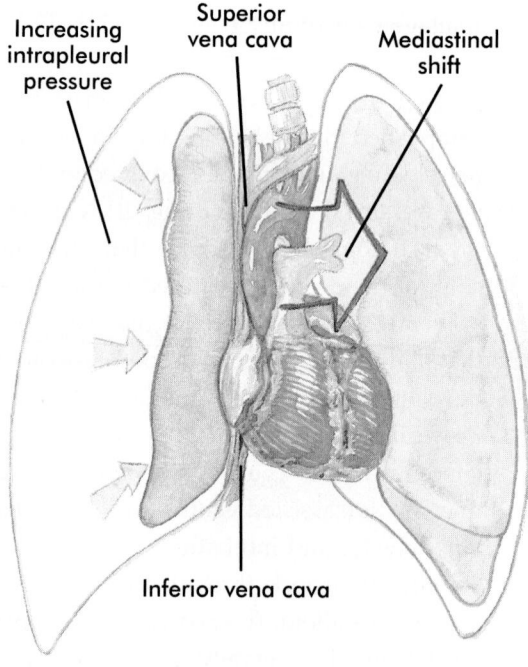

Fig. 15-53 Tension pneumothorax.

results in death if not immediately recognized and treated.

When air is allowed to leak into the pleural space during inspiration and becomes trapped during expiration, an increase in pleural pressure results. The increase in pressure produces a shift in the mediastinum and further compresses the lung on the uninjured side. In addition, venous return to the heart is decreased by compression of the vena cava, resulting in decreased cardiac output. Signs and symptoms of a tension pneumothorax are listed below:

- Anxiety
- Cyanosis
- Increasing dyspnea
- Tracheal deviation (a late sign)
- Tachycardia
- Hypotension
- Diminished or absent breath sounds on the injured side
- Distended neck veins (unless hypovolemic)
- Unequal expansion of the chest (tension does not fall with respiration)
- Subcutaneous emphysema

Tension pneumothoraces may be confirmed by radiography in the hospital setting, although waiting for x-ray confirmation is considered less-than-optimal management. In the prehospital setting, a suspected tension pneumothorax evidenced by increasing dyspnea, compromised ventilation, tachycardia, tachypnea, and unilateral decreased or absent breath sounds should be treated aggressively. Emergency care is directed at reducing the pressure in the pleural space (returning the intrapleural pressure to atmospheric or subatmospheric levels).

Tension Pneumothorax Associated with Penetrating Trauma

An open pneumothorax that has been sealed with an occlusive dressing may result in a tension pneumothorax. In such cases, increased pleural pressure can be relieved by momentarily removing the dressing. When the dressing has been lifted from the wound, there should be an audible release of air from the thoracic cavity. If this does not occur and the patient's condition remains unchanged, the paramedic should gently spread the chest wound open to allow the trapped air to escape. After the pressure has been released, the wound should again be sealed.

> **NOTE:**
> This maneuver of removing the dressing to relieve pleural pressure may need to be done periodically during patient transport. If the tension is not relieved with this procedure, thoracic decompression should be attempted.

Tension Pneumothorax Associated with Closed Trauma

A tension pneumothorax that develops in a patient with closed chest trauma must be relieved through thoracic decompression with either a large-bore needle or commercially available thoracic decompression kit. The paramedic should consult with medical control before initiating this procedure.

Needle decompression is accomplished by inserting a 2-inch 14- or 16-gauge hollow needle or catheter into the affected pleural space, usually in the second intercostal space in the midclavicular line (Fig. 15-54). The needle should be inserted just above the third rib to avoid the nerve, artery, and vein that lie just beneath each rib. After insertion of the needle, there should be an audible rush of air as pressure escapes from the pleural space (confirming the tension pneumothorax). The needle or catheter should be secured in place with tape.

If time and circumstances allow, the hub of the needle can be occluded during inspiration by a one-way valve to prevent reentry of air into the pleural space. This can be accomplished by cutting a finger from a sterile glove (rinsed with sterile water) and creating a small hole at the finger tip. The finger is slipped over the hub of the needle and secured with a rubber band. An alternative method is to attach special tubing and a flutter valve to the hub of the needle instead of a finger from a sterile glove. Both methods permit air to escape from but not enter the pleural space.

Hemothorax

A hemothorax is the accumulation of blood in the pleural space caused by bleeding from the lung parenchyma or damaged vessels (Fig. 15-55). Blood loss may be massive in these patients; each side of the thorax can hold 30% to 40% of the patient's blood volume. Therefore patients with a hemothorax frequently have hypovolemia and hypoxemia.

> **NOTE:**
> If the injury was produced by penetrating trauma, there may be an associated pneumothorax. This condition is referred to as a *pneumohemothorax* or *hemopneumothorax*.

As blood continues to fill the pleural space, the lung on the affected side may collapse, and rarely, the mediastinum may even shift away from the hemothorax, compressing the unaffected lung. The resultant respiratory and circulatory compromise are responsible for the following signs and symptoms:

- Tachypnea
- Dyspnea
- Cyanosis (often not evident in hemorrhagic shock)
- Diminished or decreased breath sounds
- Hypovolemia
- Tracheal deviation to the unaffected side (rare)

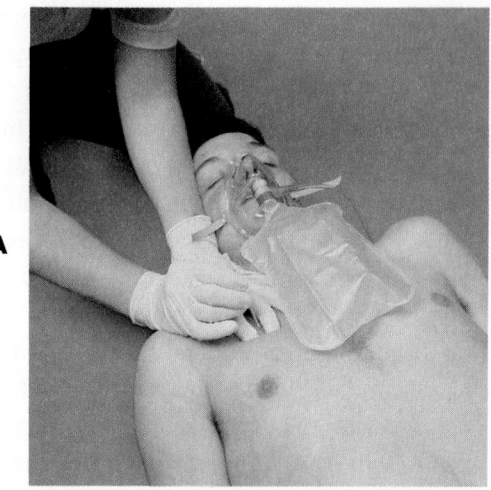
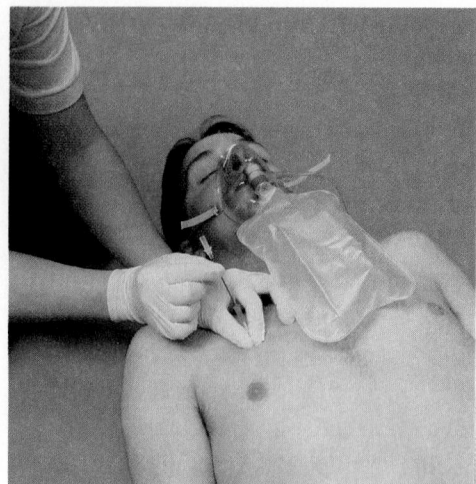
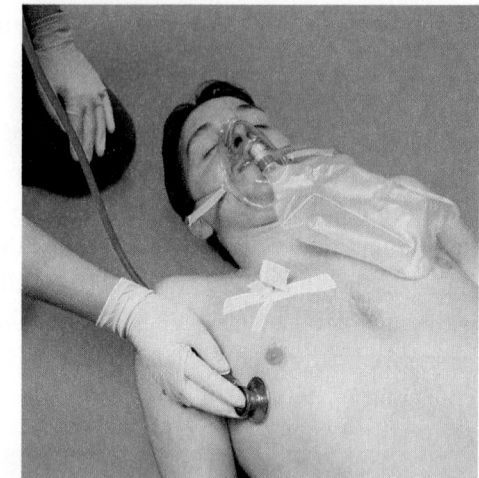

Fig. 15-54 A, Insert a 2-inch, 14- or 16-gauge hollow needle or catheter into the affected pleural space, usually in the second intercostal space in the midclavicular line. **B,** After needle insertion, there should be an audible rush of air as pressure escapes from the pleural space. **C,** Secure the catheter in place with tape, and prevent the reentry of air into the pleural space. Carefully monitor the patient's respiratory status.

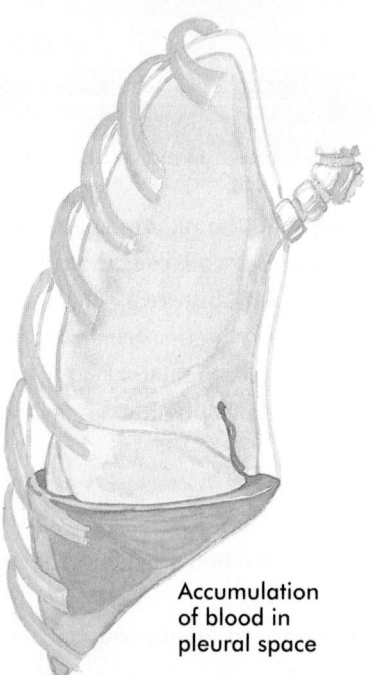

Accumulation
of blood in
pleural space

Fig. 15-55 Hemothorax.

Prehospital care for patients with a hemothorax is directed at correcting ventilatory and circulatory compromise. This entails administering high-concentration oxygen; ventilatory support with bag-valve-mask, intubation, or both; administration of volume-expanding fluids to correct the hypovolemia; and rapid transportation to an appropriate medical facility.

Pulmonary Contusion

Pulmonary contusion is most commonly caused by rapid deceleration forces that cause the lung to contact the chest wall (for example, motor vehicle crashes, injuries producing a flail chest). These forces result in rupture of the alveoli with hemorrhage and interstitial edema. Because the contused area of the lung is not able to function properly after injury, profound hypoxemia may develop. The degree of respiratory complication is directly

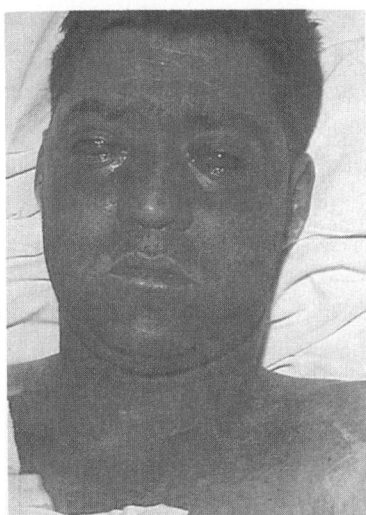

Fig. 15-56 The discoloration of traumatic asphyxia, which results from forcible compression of the chest.

related to the size of the contused area. Signs and symptoms of pulmonary contusion are initially subtle and should be suspected based on the kinematics of the event and the presence of associated injuries.

Emergency care for pulmonary contusion includes ventilatory support and high-concentration oxygen administration. Patients with associated injuries or preexisting pulmonary or cardiovascular disease should be closely monitored for the need to assist ventilations with a bag-valve-device, intubation, or both. Although pulmonary contusions can be associated with major thoracic injury, they generally heal spontaneously over several weeks.

Traumatic Asphyxia

Traumatic asphyxia is a term used to describe a severe crushing injury to the chest and abdomen (Fig. 15-56). It results from an increase in intrathoracic pressure that forces blood from the right side of the heart into the veins of the upper thorax, neck, and face. Although the forces involved in this phenomenon may produce lethal injury, traumatic asphyxia alone is not life threatening (although brain hemorrhages, seizures, coma, and death have been documented as occasional sequela).[2]

Signs and symptoms of traumatic asphyxia include reddish-purple discoloration of the face and neck, jugular vein distention, and swelling or hemorrhage of the conjunctiva (subconjunctival petechiae may appear). Emergency care for the patient is directed at ensuring an open airway, providing adequate ventilation, and caring for associated injuries.

Heart and Great Vessel Injury

Trauma to the heart and great vessels may result from blunt or penetrating injury and associated forces. The injuries discussed in this section are myocardial contusion, pericardial tamponade, and traumatic aortic rupture.

Myocardial Contusion

Myocardial contusion, the most common cardiac injury after blunt trauma to the chest, is due to the anatomical arrangement in which the heart is located between the sternum anteriorly and the spine posteriorly. The clinical findings in myocardial contusion are often subtle and frequently overlooked for the following reasons: (1) multiple injuries direct attention elsewhere, (2) there is often little evidence of thoracic injury, and (3) signs of cardiac injury may not be present on initial examination.

Contusions to the myocardium usually result from motor vehicle collision as the chest wall strikes the dashboard or steering column. Therefore a deformed dashboard or steering column should alert the paramedic to the possibility of a cardiac injury. The extent of injury may vary from a localized bruise to a full-thickness injury to the wall of the heart, resulting in a traumatic myocardial infarction.

Patients with a myocardial contusion may have no symptoms or may complain of chest pain similar to that of a myocardial infarction. Other signs and symptoms include electrocardiogram (ECG) abnormalities, tachycardia, and palpitations. Emergency care for these patients is similar to that used for myocardial infarction: oxygen administration, ECG monitoring, and pharmacological therapy for dysrhythmias. Any intervention that increases myocardial oxygen consumption should be avoided. Myocardial contusion has been reported in approximately 20% of patients with severe blunt chest trauma, but it is rarely fatal.

Pericardial Tamponade

Blunt or penetrating trauma may cause tears in the heart chamber walls, allowing blood to leak from the heart. If the pericardium has been torn sufficiently, this blood leaks into the thoracic cavity and the patient rapidly exsanguinates. However, the pericardium often remains intact, in which case the blood enters the pericardial space, causing increased pericardial pressure. If 150 to 200 ml of blood enters the pericardial space acutely, pericardial tamponade develops. (Smaller volumes can also produce significant clinical changes.) The fluid in the pericardial space markedly increases pericardial pressure and does not allow the heart to expand and refill with blood, resulting in a decrease in stroke volume and cardiac output. (Penetrating injuries such as those from some knife and gunshot wounds may result in exsanguination rather than tamponade because the pericardium has too large a wound to maintain the blood in the pericardial space.)

Most patients with pericardial tamponade initially demonstrate peripheral vasoconstriction (which tends to raise the diastolic blood pressure more than the systolic blood pressure, causing a decrease in pulse pressure) and an increase in heart rate to compensate for the decrease in cardiac output. Up to this point, pericardial tamponade and hemorrhagic shock have similar manifestations. However, one very important clinical finding often allows differentiation of the two forms of shock. This clinical finding was first described by Beck in 1935 and, with two other clinical clues, makes up what is known as *Beck's triad.*

Beck's triad consists of elevated central venous pressure evidenced by jugular vein distention, muffled heart sounds, and narrowing pulse pressure. A pulsus paradoxus may also occur in pericardial tamponade. This is evidenced by a systolic blood pressure that drops more than 10 to 15 mm Hg during inspiration compared with expiration. The first element of Beck's triad, elevated venous pressure, has come to be seen as the single best way to distinguish hemorrhagic shock from pericardial tamponade. It is important to stress, however, that certain other entities can present with hypotension and elevated central venous pressure. These are most notably tension pneumotho-

rax in the trauma victim and cardiogenic shock. It is also true that patients with tamponade and hemorrhage may not initially demonstrate elevated venous pressure.

Pericardial tamponade is a true emergency. These patients must have pericardial blood removed and the source of the bleeding stopped to survive the injury. Prehospital management includes careful monitoring, oxygen administration, fluid replacement, and rapid transport to an appropriate medical facility. Some medical control agencies may authorize the prehospital use of needle pericardiocentesis to aspirate blood from the pericardial sac in the prehospital setting. Although this procedure is usually limited to the emergency department, it is described here for reference.

> **NOTE:**
> Needle pericardiocentesis requires special training and authorization from medical control. Complications of this procedure include laceration of a coronary artery, laceration of the lung, laceration of the ventricle, cardiac dysrhythmias, increased tamponade, and laceration of the liver.

Pericardiocentesis

1. Using aseptic technique, insert a 3-inch, 16- or 18-gauge needle (attached to a 50-cc syringe) at the angle of the xiphoid cartilage and the seventh rib.
2. Advance the needle at a 45-degree angle to the skin toward the right or left midclavicular line while aspirating the syringe with negative pressure. If the needle is advanced too far, a pulsation will be felt through the needle and syringe.
3. Aspirate as much fluid as possible. Fluid is usually encountered at a depth of 3 to 4 cm. (Removal of as little as 20 to 25 ml of blood from a distended pericardium may produce a dramatic blood pressure response.)
4. After withdrawing blood from the pericardial sac, attach a surgical clamp to the needle at the level of the skin to avoid accidental advancement of the needle.

5. If tamponade recurs, aspirate blood again if necessary.

Traumatic Aortic Rupture

Traumatic aortic rupture is thought to be the result of shearing forces that develop between tissues that decelerate at different rates (Fig. 15-57). Common mechanisms of injury include rapid deceleration in high-speed motor vehicle crashes, falls from great heights, and crushing injuries. It has been estimated that one out of every six people who die in motor vehicle crashes sustains a rupture of the aorta.[12] Of these patients, 80% to 90% die at the scene as a result of massive hemorrhage. Approximately 10% to 20% of patients survive the first hour because the bleeding is tamponaded by the surrounding adventitia of the aorta and intact visceral pleura. Of these, however, 30% have ruptures within 6 hours—thus the need for a rapid and pertinent evaluation and transportation to an appropriate medical facility.

The usual site of damage to the aorta is in the distal arch just beyond the take-off of the left subclavian artery and proximal to the ligamentum arteriosum. The ligamentum arteriosum and descending thoracic arch are relatively fixed, whereas the transverse portion of the arch is relatively mobile. If shearing forces exceed the tensile strength of the arch, the junction of the mobile and fixed points of attachment may be partially torn. If the outer layer of tissue surrounding the aorta remains intact, the patient may survive long enough for surgical repair.

Because aortic rupture is a severe injury (with an 80% to 90% fatality rate within the first hour), the paramedic should always consider the possibility of this injury in any trauma patient who has unexplained shock and an appropriate mechanism of injury (rapid deceleration). Upper-extremity hypertension can occur in patients with aortic rupture. This is thought to result from compression of the aorta by the expanding hematoma. Other patients have generalized hypertension secondary to increased sympathetic discharge. Approximately 25% of these patients have a harsh systolic murmur over the pericardium. Rarely, paraplegia is seen with a normal cervical and thoracic spine. This is secondary to decreased blood flow through the anterior spinal artery, which is in the thoracic region composed of branches from the posterior intercostal arteries, which in turn are branches from the thoracic aorta.

Prehospital management of these patients includes advising medical control of the suspected rupture, high-concentration oxygen administration, ventilatory support with spinal precautions, fluid replacement, and rapid transportation for surgical intervention.

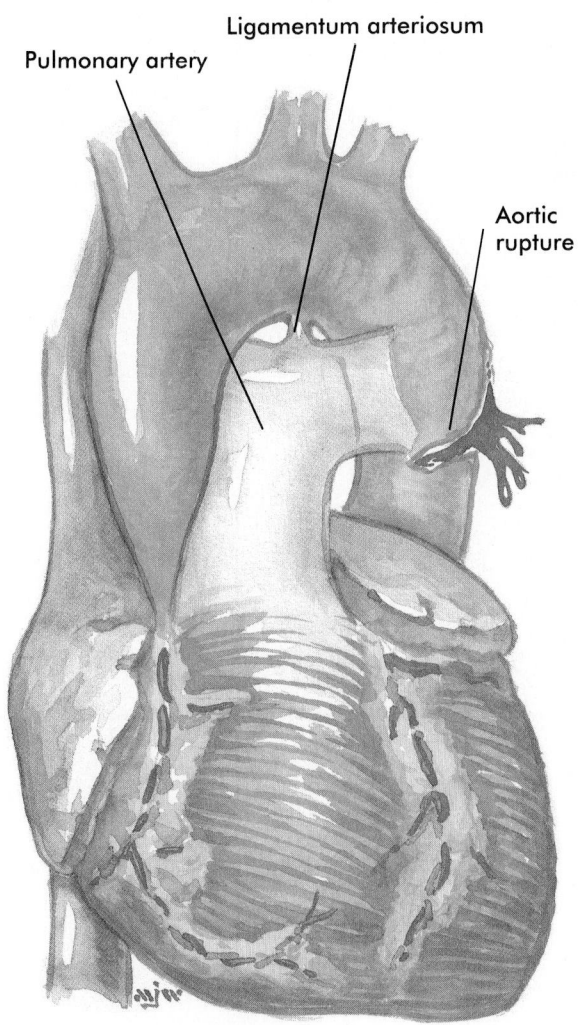

Pulmonary artery

Ligamentum arteriosum

Aortic rupture

Fig. 15-57 Aortic rupture.

> **NOTE:**
> Patients who are normotensive should have limited replacement fluids to prevent an increase in pressure in the remaining aortic wall tissue.

Diaphragmatic Rupture

The diaphragm is a sheet of voluntary muscle that separates the abdominal cavity from the thoracic cavity. When rapid compression of the abdomen results in a sharp increase in intraabdominal pressure (for example, blunt trauma to the trunk), the pressure differences may cause abdominal contents to rupture through the thin diaphragmatic wall and enter the chest cavity (Fig. 15-58). Diaphragmatic ruptures more commonly occur on the left side than on the right because of the location of the liver, which somewhat protects the right hemidiaphragm. Ruptures on either side can allow intraabdominal organs to enter the thoracic cavity, where they may cause compression of the lung with a reduction in ventilation, a decrease in venous return, a decrease in cardiac output, and shock. Multiple injuries are often present in patients with diaphragmatic rupture because of the mechanical forces involved.

Signs and symptoms of a ruptured diaphragm include abdominal pain, shortness of breath, and decreased breath sounds. If a majority of the abdominal contents are displaced into the chest, the abdomen may have a hollow or empty appearance. Prehospital management includes oxygen administration, ventilatory support as needed, volume-expanding fluids, and rapid transport to an appropriate medical facility for surgical repair. Some medical control agencies may also recommend that a nasogastric tube be placed to decompress the stomach.

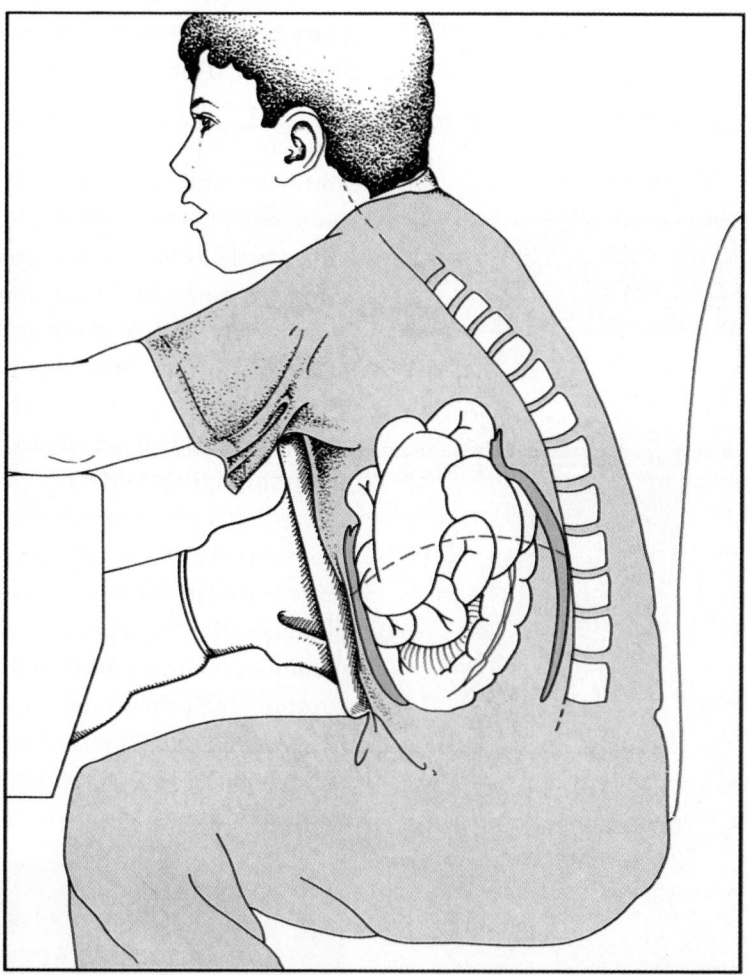

Fig. 15-58 Diaphragmatic rupture. A rapid compression of the abdomen may increase intraabdominal pressure, causing the abdominal contents to rupture through the thin diaphragmatic wall and enter the chest cavity.

● ABDOMINAL TRAUMA

Abdominal trauma may be difficult to evaluate in the prehospital setting. This is due to the wide spectrum of potential injuries to multiple organs, physical findings that are sometimes lacking or exaggerated, and altered levels of pain perception that occur as a result of preexisting conditions, shock, alcohol or drug use, head injury, and other factors. Therefore a high degree of suspicion must be exercised based on the mechanism of injury and kinematics.

Mechanisms of Abdominal Injury

Abdominal injury may result from blunt or penetrating trauma. Regardless of the organ injury, prehospital management is usually limited to securing the airway with spinal precautions, providing ventilatory support, providing wound management, treating shock with fluid replacement and PASG (per protocol), and rapidly transporting the patient for definitive care.

Blunt trauma to abdominal organs usually results from compression or shearing forces. Compression forces may cause the abdominal viscera to be crushed between solid objects, for example, the steering column and spinal vertebrae. Shearing forces may produce a tear or rupture of the solid organs or blood vessels as they become stretched at their points of attachment (stabilizing ligaments or blood vessels). The degree of injury is usually related to the quantity and duration of force applied and the type of abdominal structure injured (fluid filled, gas filled, solid, hollow).

Penetrating injury may result from stab wounds, gunshot wounds, or impaled objects. Major complications of penetrating trauma are hemorrhage from a major vessel or solid organ and perforation of a segment of bowel. As a rule, injuries from penetrating trauma do not have as high a mortality rate as those that result from blunt trauma.

Specific Abdominal Injuries

Abdominal injury may be classified as solid organ, hollow organ, retroperitoneal organ, pelvic organ, or vascular injury.

Solid Organ Injury

Injury to solid organs usually results in significant blood loss. The two solid organs most commonly injured are the liver and spleen; both are primary sources of exsanguination.

The liver is the largest organ in the abdominal cavity. Because of its location, it is commonly injured from trauma to the eighth through twelfth ribs on the right side of the body and from trauma to the upper central part of the abdomen. Injury to the liver should be suspected in any patient with a steering wheel injury or a history of epigastric trauma. After injury, blood and bile escape into the peritoneal cavity, producing signs and symptoms of peritoneal irritation and shock.

The spleen lies in the upper left quadrant of the abdomen and is slightly protected by the organs surrounding it medially and anteriorly and by the lower portion of the rib cage. Injury to this organ is commonly associated with other intraabdominal injuries. Splenic injury should be suspected in motor vehicle crashes and in falls or sport injuries in which there was an impact to the lower left chest, flank, or upper left abdomen. A common complaint associated with splenic injury is pain in the left shoulder (Kehr's sign), thought to be caused by referred pain secondary to irritation of the adjacent diaphragm from splenic hematoma or hemoperitoneum.

Hollow Organ Injury

Injuries to the hollow abdominal organs can result in sepsis, wound infection, and abscess formation, particularly if trauma to the intestine remains undiagnosed for an extended period. In contrast to solid organ injury, in which hemorrhage is the major cause of symptoms, injury to the hollow organs results in symptoms from spillage of their contents (resulting in peritonitis).

The stomach is not commonly injured after blunt trauma because of its protected location in the abdomen. Penetrating trauma, however, may cause gastric transection or laceration. Patients with this condition may exhibit signs of peritonitis rather rapidly from leakage of acidic gastric contents. Diagnosis of injury to the stomach is usually confirmed during surgery unless nasogastric drainage returns blood.

The colon and small intestine are similar to the stomach and duodenum in that injury to these organs is probably a result of penetrating trauma (for example, a gunshot wound to abdomen or buttocks) rather than blunt trauma. However, the large and small bowel may also be injured by compression forces in high-speed motor vehicle crashes and in deceleration injuries associated with wearing personal restraints. Because of the amount of force required to injure the colon and small intestine, other injuries are usually present. As previously stated, a common problem associated with these injuries is peritoneal contamination with bacteria.

Retroperitoneal Organ Injury

Retroperitoneal organ injury may occur as a result of blunt or penetrating trauma to the anterior abdomen, posterior abdomen (particularly the flank area), or thoracic spine. Hemorrhage within the retroperitoneal area may be massive, as much as 20 units of blood.

The kidneys are solid organs that lie in the retroperitoneal space but that may be injured with abdominal trauma as well. Injuries may involve contusion fracture and laceration (resulting in hemorrhage, urine extravasation, or both). Contusions are usually self-limiting and heal with bed rest and forced fluids. Fractures and lacerations are more severe and may require surgical repair, depending on which part of the kidney is damaged.

The ureters are hollow organs rarely injured by blunt trauma because of their flexible structure. When injury occurs, it usually results from penetrating abdominal or flank wounds (for example, stab wounds, firearm injuries).

The pancreas is a solid organ that lies within the retroperitoneal space. Injury, though rare, is usually caused by compressive or penetrating forces applied to the upper left quadrant, as in steering wheel and bicycle handlebar impalement. The pancreas is more commonly injured in penetrating trauma (particularly firearms) than in blunt trauma.

The duodenum lies across the lumbar spine and is seldom injured because of its location in the retroperitoneal area, near the pancreas. When great force from blunt trauma or penetrating injury occurs, the duodenum may be crushed or lacerated. Injury to this organ is usually associated with concurrent pancreatic trauma; it is confirmed through surgery.

Pelvic Organ Injury

Injury to pelvic organs usually results from motor vehicle crashes that produce pelvic fractures. Other less frequent causes of pelvic organ injury are penetrating trauma, straddle-type injuries from falls, pedestrian accidents, and some sexual acts. Because the pelvis provides support and protection for multiple organ systems, there is great potential for associated injury. The most common associated injuries are those to the urinary bladder and urethra.

The urinary bladder is a hollow organ that may be ruptured by blunt trauma, penetrating trauma, or pelvic fracture. Rupture is more likely if the bladder is distended at the time of injury. With rupture, the integrity of the peritoneum may be broken, and urine may extravasate into the peritoneal cavity. Bladder injury should be suspected in inebriated patients subjected to lower abdominal trauma. Gross hematuria may be present, or the patient may complain that he or she is unable to void.

Urethral disruption occurs more frequently in men and is usually secondary to blunt trauma associated with pelvic fracture. The patient usually complains of an inability to urinate and abdominal pain. Blood at the meatus indicates urethral injury.

> **NOTE:**
> Passage of an indwelling urinary catheter is contraindicated in these patients.

Vascular Structure Injury

Intraabdominal arterial and venous injuries may be life threatening because of their potential for massive hemorrhage. These injuries usually occur from penetrating trauma but may also arise from compression or deceleration forces applied to the abdomen. As in solid organ injury, vascular injury usually presents as hypovolemia and is occasionally associated with a palpable abdominal mass. The major vessels most frequently injured are the aorta, inferior vena cava, and the renal, mesenteric, and iliac arteries and veins.

Assessment

The most significant indicator of severe abdominal trauma is the presence of unexplained shock. In addition to mechanism of injury and classic presentation of hypovolemia, other signs and symptoms that should alert the paramedic to the possibility of severe abdominal trauma are:

- Bruising and discoloration to the abdomen
- Abrasions
- Obvious bleeding
- Pain, abdominal tenderness or guarding
- Abdominal rigidity, distention
- Evisceration
- Rib fractures
- Pelvic fractures

Management

Emergency care of patients with abdominal trauma is usually limited to stabilizing the patient and rapid transportation to an appropriate medical facility for surgical intervention. The most important components of on-scene care are:

- Rapid evaluation of the patient and mechanism of injury
- Airway maintenance with spinal precautions
- Oxygen administration
- Ventilatory support as needed
- Reduction of continued hemorrhage by pressure
- Fluid replacement with volume expanders and PASG (per protocol)
- Cardiac monitoring

● EXTREMITY TRAUMA

Extremity or musculoskeletal trauma may occur as an isolated injury or with other injuries. Although these injuries are seldom life threatening, their early recognition and treatment may prevent long-term, debilitating complications. Extremity trauma usually results from motor vehicle crashes, falls, and contact sports.

Classifications

The musculoskeletal system and associated neurovascular structures comprise bones, nerves, vessels, muscles, tendons, ligaments, and joints. Injuries that can result from application of traumatic forces to these tissues include fractures, sprains, strains, and joint dislocations. The paramedic should not attempt to differentiate these injuries in the prehospital setting. Patients with suspected extremity trauma should be treated as though a fracture exists.

Fractures

A fracture is any break in the continuity of bone or cartilage (Fig. 15-59). It may be complete or in-

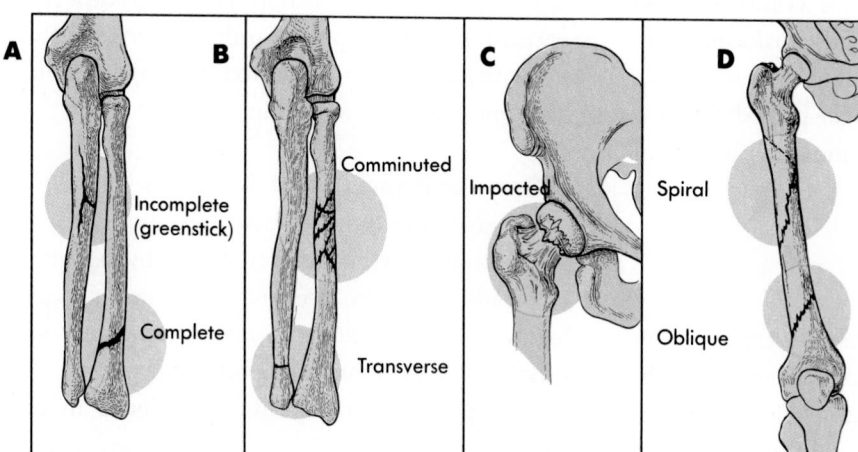

Fig. 15-59 Bone fractures. **A,** Complete and incomplete. **B,** Comminuted and transverse. **C,** Impacted. **D,** Oblique and spiral.

complete, depending on the line of fracture through the bone. Fractures are also classified as open or closed, depending on the integrity of the skin near the fracture site. Fractures of long bones may result in moderate-to-severe hemorrhage, releasing as much as 2 units of blood in the lower leg and 4 units in the thigh (third-space bleeding).

Sprains

A sprain is partial tearing of a ligament caused by a sudden twisting or stretching of a joint beyond its normal range of motion. Two common areas for sprains are the knee and ankle.

Sprains are graded by severity. A first-degree sprain has no joint instability because only a few ligamentous fibers are torn. Swelling and hemorrhage are minimal. A second-degree sprain causes more disruption than first-degree injuries. The joint is usually still intact, but there is increased swelling and ecchymosis. In third-degree sprains, the ligaments are totally disrupted. If third-degree sprains are accompanied by a dislocation, nerve or vascular compromise to the extremity is possible.

Strains

A strain is an injury to the muscle or its tendon from overexertion or overextension. They commonly occur in the back and arms and may be accompanied by a significant loss of function. Severe strains may cause an avulsion of bone from the attachment site.

Joint Dislocations

A joint dislocation occurs when the normal articulating ends of two or more bones are displaced. Joints that are frequently dislocated are shoulders, elbows, fingers, hips, knees, and ankles. The injury should be suspected when a joint is deformed or does not move with normal range of motion.

Signs and Symptoms

Signs and symptoms of extremity trauma may range from subtle complaints of discomfort to obvious deformity or open fracture. Field evaluation should be rapid, assuming significant injury.

Common signs and symptoms of extremity trauma include:

- Pain on palpation or movement
- Swelling, deformity
- Crepitus
- Decreased range of motion
- False movement
- Decreased or absent sensory perception or circulation distal to the injury (evidenced by alterations in skin color and temperature, distal pulses, capillary refill)

> **NOTE:**
> This text presents immobilization strategies for fractures and dislocations as they pertain to isolated extremity injuries. Again, extremity trauma is seldom life threatening, so patients with multiple-systems traumatic injury should first be treated for conditions that compromise airway, breathing, circulation (including internal and external hemorrhage in the extremities), and spinal stability. If rapid transportation is indicated by the patient's condition or mechanism of injury, injured extremities can be stabilized by fully immobilizing the patient on a long spine board.

Management

Evaluation of an injured extremity should always include an assessment for the "five Ps": pain, pallor, pulselessness, paresthesias, and paralysis. The assessment should also include a comparison with the opposite, uninjured extremity. If extremity trauma is suspected, the injury should be immobilized by splinting.

General Principles of Splinting

The goal of splinting is immobilization of the injured body part. Immobilization by splinting helps alleviate pain; decrease tissue injury, bleeding, and contamination in an open wound; and simplify and facilitate transport of the patient. The general principles of splinting are listed in Box 15-3.

Types of Splints

A wide variety of splints and splinting materials are available through a number of equipment manufacturers. These splints can be broadly categorized as rigid, soft or formable, and traction splints.

BOX 15-3

General Principles of Splinting

• Expose and examine the injured extremity. Look for a wound, tenting of the skin, or obvious discoloration that may indicate the presence or potential of an open fracture.

• Support the body part.

• Remove jewelry or constrictive items of clothing.

• Assess and document sensory and circulatory status before immobilization. If there is no palpable, distal pulse, medical control may recommend applying gentle traction along the long axis of the extremity (distal to the injury) until the distal pulse is palpable.

• Immobilize the extremity so that the splint includes the joints above and below the fracture or the bones above and below the dislocation. Avoid excessive movement of the body part. (Movement may increase bleeding into the tissue space, increase the risk of fat embolus, or convert a closed fracture to an open fracture.)

NOTE: Immobilization requires a minimum of two rescuers.

• When applying splints applied to the hand or foot, leave the fingers or toes exposed to provide for inspection and evaluation of neurovascular status.

• Reevaluate and document sensory and circulatory status after immobilization. If a nerve or pulse deficit develops after splinting, remove the splint and place the extremity in its original position.

Rigid splints cannot be changed in shape and require that the body part be positioned to fit the splint's design. Examples of rigid splints include board splints, contoured metal and plastic splints, and some cardboard splints (Fig. 15-60). Rigid splints should be padded before use to accommodate for anatomical shape and patient comfort.

Soft or formable splints can be molded into various shapes and configurations to accommodate the injured body part. Examples of soft or formable splints include pillows, blankets, slings and swathes, vacuum splints, some cardboard splints, and wire ladder splints (Fig. 15-61). Inflatable air splints are also considered to be soft or formable

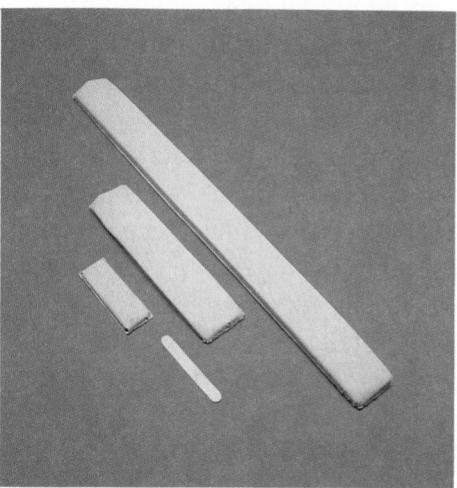

Fig. 15-60 Rigid splints.

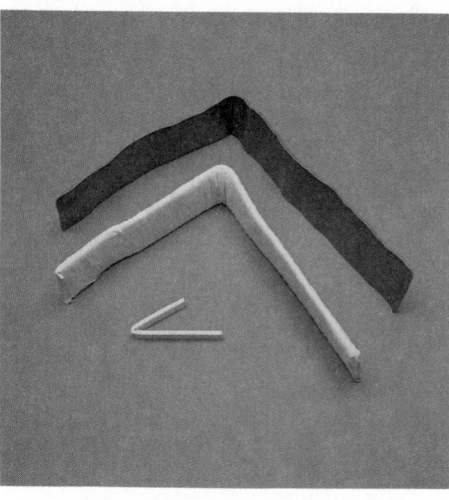

Fig. 15-61 Formable splints.

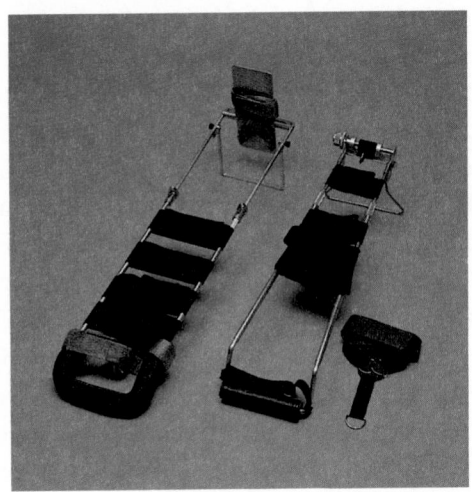

Fig. 15-62 Traction splints.

splints, but they are not designed to be used for injuries proximal to the knee or elbow.

Traction splints are specifically designed for midshaft femur fractures. These splints do not apply or maintain sufficient traction to reduce a femoral fracture but provide enough traction to stabilize and align it. Examples include Thomas Half Ring, Hare Traction, and Sager Traction (Fig. 15-62).

Upper-Extremity Injuries

Upper-extremity injuries can be classified as fractures or dislocations to the shoulder, humerus, elbow, radius and ulna, wrist, hand, and finger (Fig. 15-63). Clavicular injury was discussed in the section on thoracic trauma. Most upper-extremity injuries can be adequately immobilized by application of a sling and swathe.

Shoulder Injury

Shoulder injuries are common in the older adult because of weaker bone structure and frequently result from a fall on an outstretched arm. Management includes:

1. Assessment of neurovascular status
2. Application of sling and swathe (Fig. 15-64)
3. Application of a cold pack

Humerus Injury

Upper-arm fractures are common in older adults and children. Radial nerve damage may be present if a fracture occurs in the middle or distal portion of the humeral shaft, and a fracture of the humeral neck may cause axillary nerve damage. Internal hemorrhage may also be a complication. Management includes:

1. Assessment of neurovascular status
2. Traction if there is vascular compromise
3. Application of a rigid splint and sling and swathe (Fig. 15-65)
4. Application of a cold pack

Elbow Injury

Elbow injuries are common in children and athletes. The mechanism of injury usually involves falling on an outstretched arm or flexed elbow. Associated complications include laceration of the brachial artery and radial nerve damage. Management includes:

1. Assessment of neurovascular status
2. Splinting in the position found with a pillow, blanket, rigid splint, or sling and swathe (Fig. 15-66)
3. Application of a cold pack

Radius, Ulnar, or Wrist Injury

Like most other upper-extremity injuries, injuries to the radius, ulna, and wrist are usually a result of a fall on an outstretched arm. Wrist injuries may involve the distal radius, ulna, or any of the eight carpal bones. The most common wrist injury involves a fracture of the distal radius with dorsal angulation (Colles' fracture). Forearm injury is common in both children and adults. Management includes:

1. Assessment of neurovascular status
2. Splinting in the position found with rigid or formable splints or sling and swathe (Fig. 15-67)
3. Application of a cold pack and elevation

Hand (Metacarpal) Injury

Injury to the hand frequently results from contact sports, violence (fighting), and crushing in industrial contexts. A common metacarpal injury is boxer's fracture, which results from direct trauma to a closed fist fracturing the fifth metacarpal bone. These injuries may also be associated with hematomas and open wounds. Although the boxer's fracture is the most common metacarpal

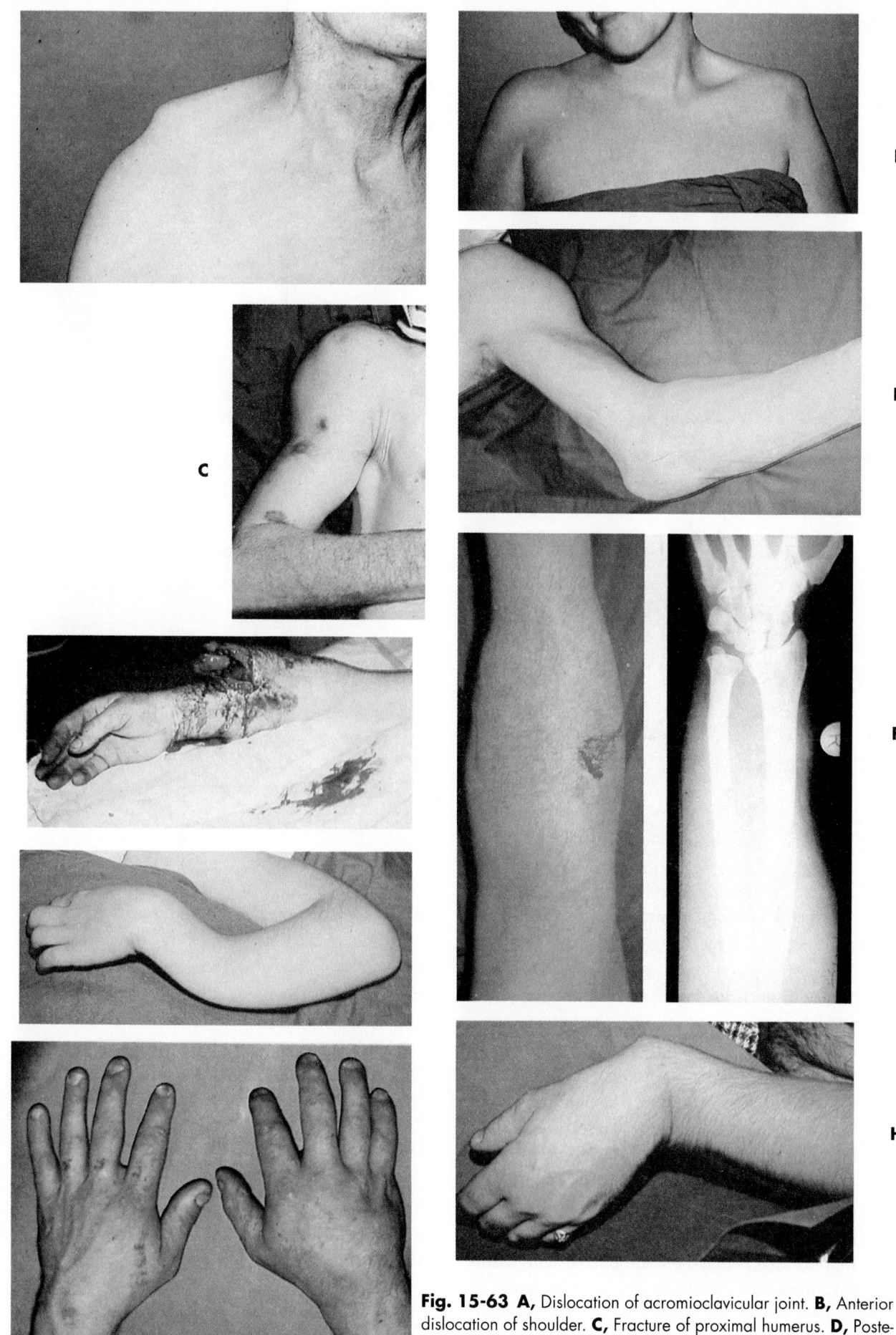

Fig. 15-63 A, Dislocation of acromioclavicular joint. **B,** Anterior dislocation of shoulder. **C,** Fracture of proximal humerus. **D,** Posterior dislocation of elbow joint with marked deformity. **E,** Severe open fracture of forearm. **F,** Penetration of forearm caused by nail gun. **G,** Greenstick fracture with marked deformity. **H,** Fracture of distal radius. **I,** Hand injury from motorcycle crash.

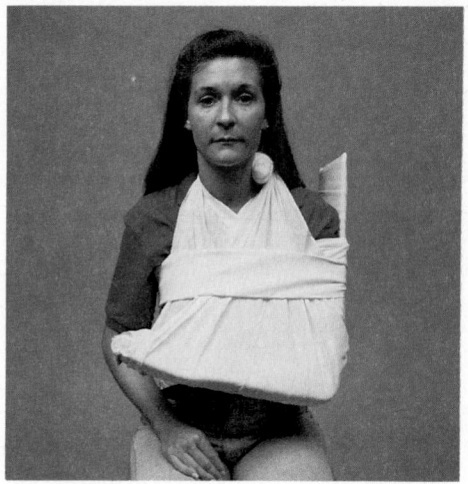

Fig. 15-64 Immobilization of the shoulder.

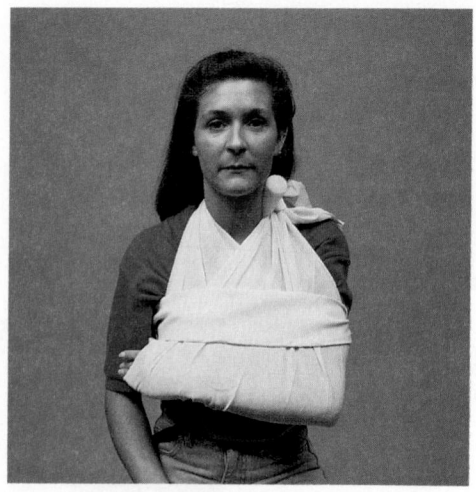

Fig. 15-65 Immobilization of the humerus.

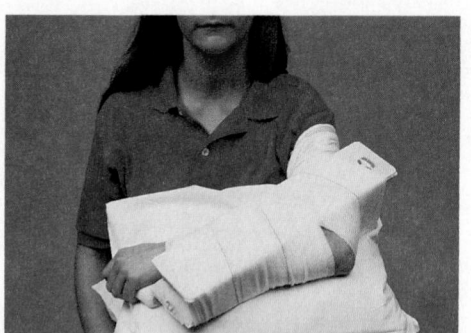

Fig. 15-66 Immobilization of the elbow.

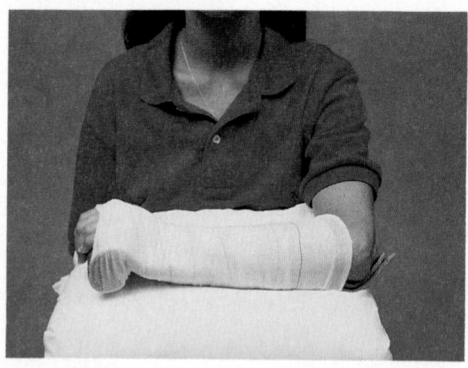

Fig. 15-67 Immobilization of the forearm.

fracture, any of the metacarpals can be fractured, depending on the mechanism of injury. Hand injuries should be splinted in the position found with rigid or formable splints (previously described for a radius, ulnar, or wrist injury). Management includes:

1. Assessment of neurovascular status
2. Splinting with a rigid or formable splint (pillow, blanket) in a position of function (as with a hand grasping a football)
3. Application of a cold pack and elevation

Finger (Phalangeal) Injury

Injured fingers may be immobilized with foam-filled aluminum splints or tongue depressors or by simply taping the injured finger to an adjacent one ("buddy splinting"). Although finger injuries are common, they should not be considered trivial. Serious injuries include thumb metacarpal fractures and any open or markedly comminuted metacarpal or proximal phalanx fracture (see Fig. 15-82). Management includes:

1. Assessment of neurovascular status
2. Splinting as previously described (Fig. 15-68)
3. Application of a cold pack and elevation

Lower-Extremity Injuries

Lower-extremity injuries include fractures or dislocations to the hip, femur, knee and patella, tibia and fibula, ankle and foot, and phalanx (Fig. 15-69). Pelvic fractures have been discussed.

Hip Injury

Hip injuries commonly occur in older adults as a result of a fall and in younger patients as a re-

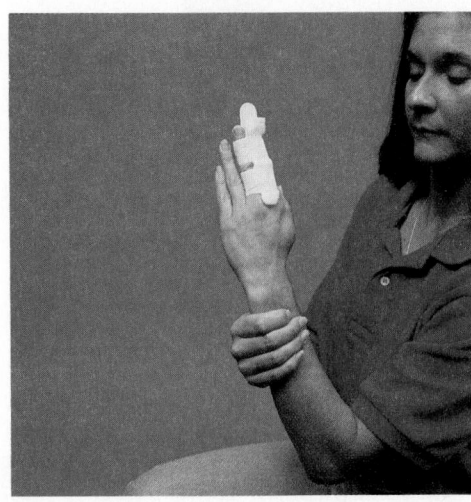

Fig. 15-68 Immobilization of the finger.

sult of major trauma. If the hip is fractured at the femoral head and neck, the affected leg is usually shortened and externally rotated. By comparison, dislocations of the hip are usually evidenced by a shortened and internally rotated leg. Management includes:

1. Assessment of neurovascular status
2. Splinting with a long spine board and generously padding patient for comfort during transport. (Slight flexion of knee or padding beneath knee may improve comfort [Fig. 15-70].)
3. Frequent monitoring of vital signs

Femur Injury

Injury to the femur usually results from major trauma, as in motor vehicle and pedestrian accidents. It is also a fairly common result of child abuse.

Fractures to the femur are usually evident from the powerful thigh muscles producing overriding of the bone fragments. The patient generally has a shortened leg that is externally rotated and midthigh swelling from hemorrhage (which can be life threatening). These fractures should be immobilized in the field with a traction splint. Management includes:

1. Oxygen administration
2. Treatment for shock
3. Assessment of neurovascular status
4. Application of a traction splint (Fig. 15-71)
5. Careful monitoring of vital signs

NOTE:
Traction splints are only to be used to immobilize midshaft femur fractures. They are contraindicated for fractures to the lower third of the leg, pelvic fractures, hip injury, knee injury, and avulsion or amputation of the ankle and foot. It is recommended that the patient be positioned on a long spine board before traction splint application.

If concurrent injuries are contributing to the development of shock and if local protocol advocates the use of PASG in conjunction with a traction splint, the traction splint should be applied *over* the PASG only after it has been inflated. Any traction device placed under the PASG may promote continued hemorrhage, tissue damage, and compromised circulation to the injured extremity.

Knee and Patella Injury

Fractures to the knee (supracondylar fracture of the femur, intraarticular fracture of the femur or tibia) and fractures and dislocations of the patella commonly result from motor vehicle crashes, pedestrian accidents, contact sports, and falls on a flexed knee. The relationship of the popliteal artery to the knee joint is important and may give rise to vascular injury (particularly with posterior dislocations). Management includes:

1. Assessment of neurovascular status
2. Splinting in the position found with rigid or formable splint (Fig. 15-72)
3. Application of a cold pack and elevation, if possible

Tibia and Fibula Injury

Injuries to the tibia and fibula may result from direct or indirect trauma or twisting injury. If associated with the knee, popliteal vascular injury should be suspected. Management includes:

1. Assessment of neurovascular status
2. Splinting with a rigid or formable splint (Fig. 15-73)
3. Application of a cold pack and elevation

Foot and Ankle Injury

Fractures and dislocations of the foot and ankle may result from a crush injury, a fall from a height,

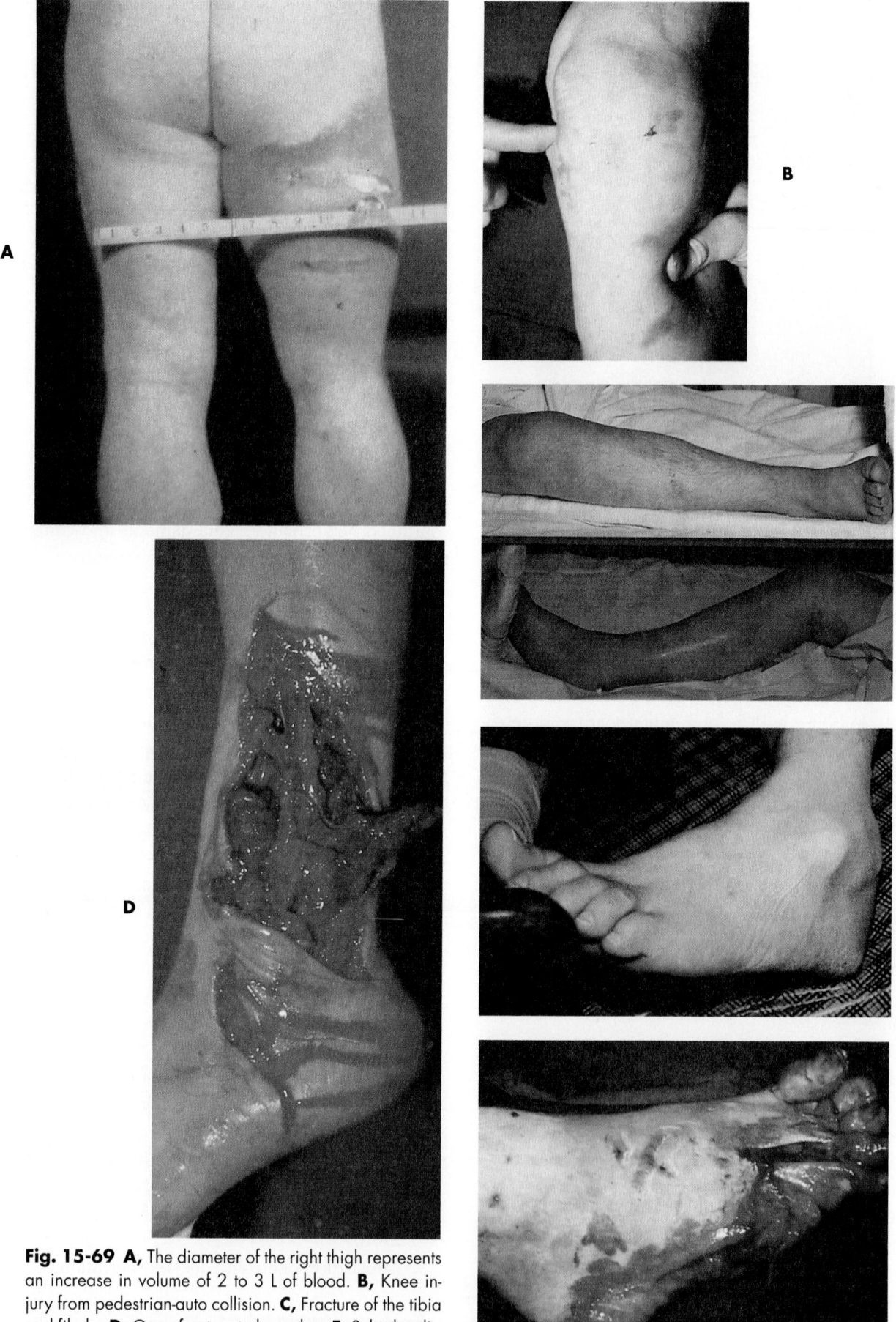

Fig. 15-69 A, The diameter of the right thigh represents an increase in volume of 2 to 3 L of blood. **B,** Knee injury from pedestrian-auto collision. **C,** Fracture of the tibia and fibula. **D,** Open fracture to lower leg. **E,** Subtalar dislocation. **F,** A foot that had been run over by the wheel of a railway coach.

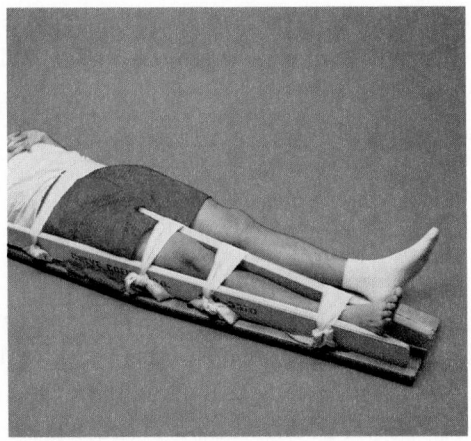

Fig. 15-70 Immobilization of the hip.

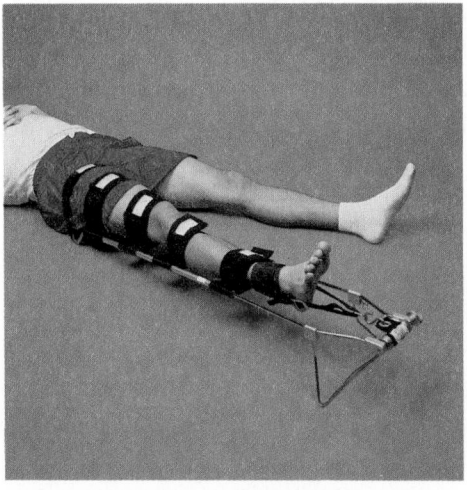

Fig. 15-71 Application of traction splint.

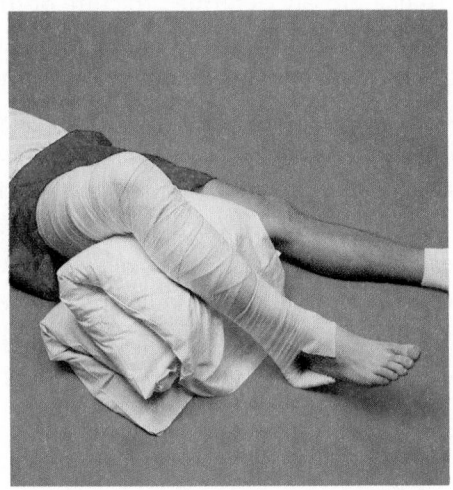

Fig. 15-72 Immobilization of the knee.

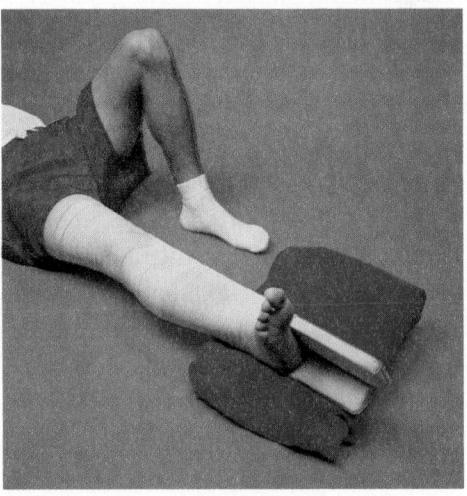

Fig. 15-73 Immobilization of the lower leg.

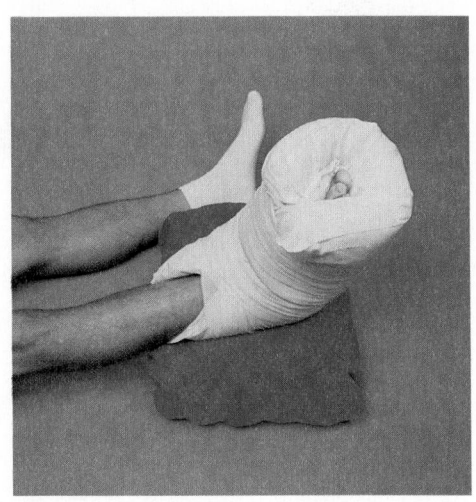

Fig. 15-74 Immobilization of the foot and ankle.

or a violent rotary force. The patient usually complains of point tenderness and is hesitant to bear weight on the extremity. Management includes:

1. Assessment of neurovascular status
2. Application of a formable splint, such as a pillow, blanket, or air splint (Fig. 15-74)
3. Application of a cold pack
4. Elevation

Phalanx Injury

Toe injuries are often caused by "stubbing" the toe on an immoveable object. These injuries are usually managed by buddy taping the toe to an adjacent toe for support and immobilization. Management includes:

1. Assessment of neurovascular status
2. Buddy splinting
3. Application of a cold pack
4. Elevation

Open Fractures

Patients with open fractures require special care and evaluation by the paramedic. Fractures may be open in two ways: from within, as when a bone fragment pierces the skin, or from without, after a gunshot wound, for example. An open fracture may have also made contact with the skin some distance from the fracture site. Although most open fractures are obvious because of associated hemorrhage, a small puncture wound may not be immediately apparent, and bleeding may be minimal. Therefore the paramedic must consider any soft tissue wound in the area of a suspected fracture to be evidence of an open fracture.

Open fractures are considered a true surgical emergency because of the potential for infection. Most authorities agree that open wounds associated with fractures should be covered with sterile, dry dressings. They should not be irrigated in the field or soaked with any type of antiseptic solution. Hemorrhage should be controlled with direct pressure and pressure dressings.

If a bone end or bone fragment is visible, it should be covered with a dry, sterile dressing and splinted. Bone ends that slip back into the wound during immobilization should be noted and reported to the receiving hospital so that surgical debridement can take place.

Straightening Angular Fractures and Dislocations

Angular fractures and dislocations may pose significant problems regarding splinting and, in some situations, patient extrication and transportation. If the paramedic feels it is necessary to attempt manipulation of a fracture or dislocation to facilitate transport or to improve the vascular integrity of the injured extremity, medical control should be consulted.

As a rule, a grossly deformed fracture or dislocation can often be aligned if necessary without causing additional damage or extreme discomfort to the patient. (Analgesics may be used if not contraindicated by other injuries.) The injury should be handled carefully, and gentle, firm traction should be applied in the direction of the long axis of the extremity. If there is obvious resistance to alignment, the extremity should be splinted without repositioning. *Dislocations with obvious deformity around a joint should never be realigned in the prehospital setting.*

REFERENCES

1. National Safety Council: *Accident facts*, Chicago, 1992, The Council.
2. Moore E et al: *Early care of the injured patient*, ed 4, Philadelphia, 1990, BC Decker.
3. Baker C et al: Epidemiology of trauma deaths, *Am J Surg* 140:144, 1980.
4. US Department of Transportation, National Highway Traffic Safety Administration: *1990 traffic fatality facts*, Washington, DC, 1991, The Department.
5. McSwain N et al, editors: *Prehospital trauma life support*, ed 2, Akron, Oh, 1990, Emergency Training.
6. McSwain N, Kerstein M: *Evaluation and management of trauma*, Norwalk, Conn, 1987, Appleton-Century-Crofts.
7. National Safety Council: *Accident facts*, Chicago, 1989, The Council.
8. Tintinall J et al, editors: *Emergency medicine: a comprehensive study guide*, ed 2, New York, 1988, McGraw-Hill.
9. Trunkey D, Lewis F: *Current therapy of trauma*, ed 3, Philadelphia, 1991, BC Decker.
10. Krasner P: Management of avulsed teeth, *JEMS* 18(6):31, 1989.
11. Suter R, Tighe T: Thoraco-lumbar spinal instability during variations of the log-roll maneuver, *Prehosp Disast Med* 5(3):306, 1990.
12. Baxt W: *Trauma: The first hour,* Norwalk, Conn, 1985, Appleton-Century-Crofts.

Summary

Although the vast majority of all injuries are not life threatening or permanently disabling, trauma is the leading cause of death among all ages in this country. Priorities of emergency care include rapid assessment of life-threatening injury, airway management with spinal precautions, ventilatory support, fluid resuscitation, and rapid patient transport to an appropriate medical facility for surgical intervention. If these elements of emergency care can be provided within the golden hour after critical injury, the likelihood of minimizing mortality and maintaining a functional human being is greatly enhanced.

16 SOFT TISSUE INJURIES AND BURNS

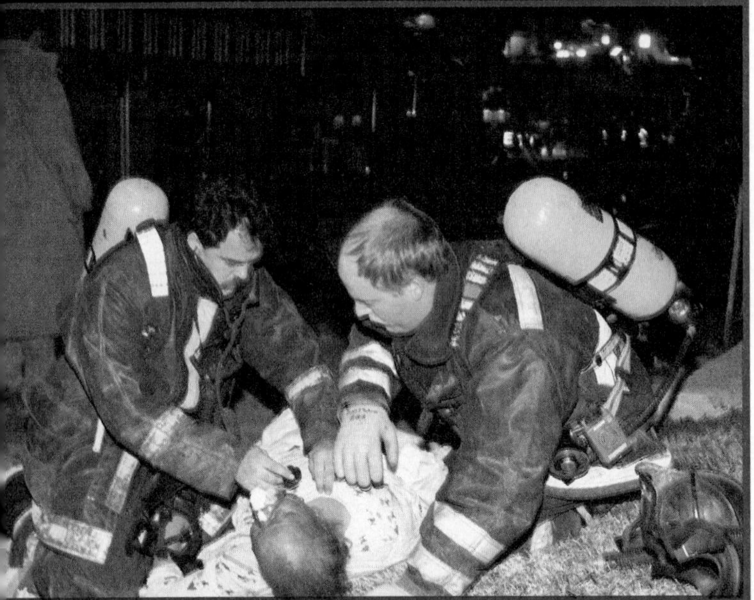

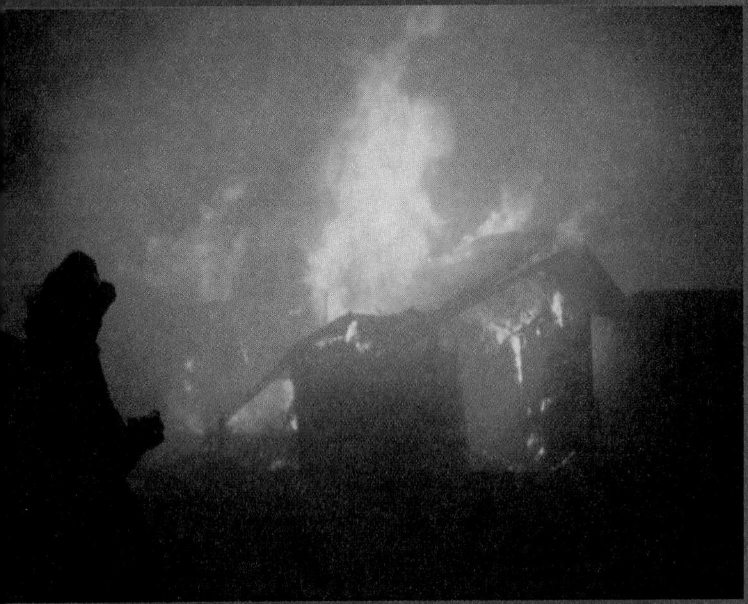

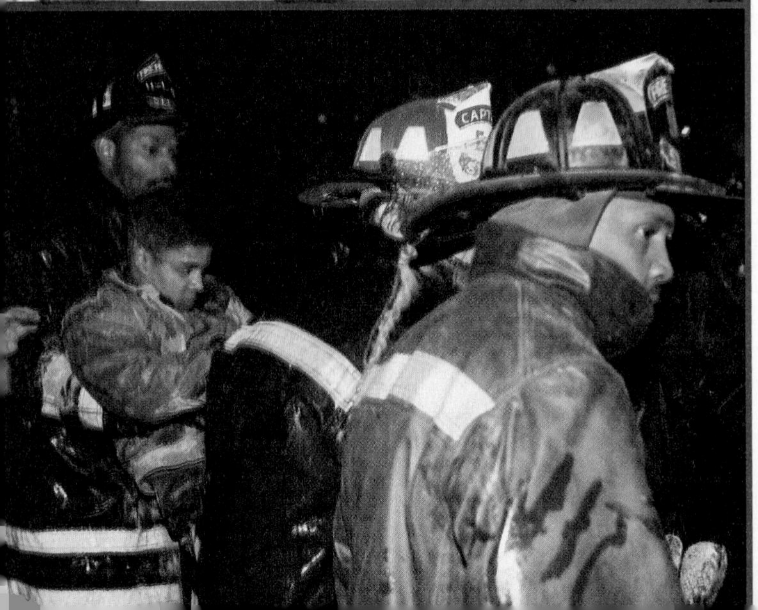

The skin and its accessory organs are the primary cosmetic structures of the body and perform many functions that are critical to survival. Therefore soft tissue injuries or burns may be life threatening and emotionally devastating. The paramedic must thoroughly understand soft tissue trauma to quickly assess life-threatening injury and to intervene to promote normal healing and function.

As a paramedic, you should be able to:

1. Describe the normal structure and function of the integumentary system.
2. Describe the pathophysiology of soft tissue injury.
3. Describe in the correct sequence patient-management techniques for control of hemorrhage.
4. Discuss pathophysiology as a basis for key signs and symptoms and describe the mechanism of injury, assessment, and management of specific soft tissue injuries.
5. Identify sources of burn injury.
6. Describe the pathophysiology of burn injury in local and systemic responses.
7. Classify burn injury according to depth, extent, and severity based on established standards.
8. Describe the assessment of the burn-injured patient.
9. Outline the prehospital management of the burn-injured patient.
10. Discuss pathophysiology as a basis for key signs, symptoms, and management of the patient with an inhalation injury.
11. Outline the general assessment and management of the patient who has a chemical injury.
12. Describe specific complications and management techniques for selected chemical injuries.
13. Describe the physiological effects of electrical injury as they relate to each body system based on an understanding of key principles of electricity.
14. Outline assessment and management of the patient with electrical injury.
15. Describe the distinguishing features of radiation injury.

Section One
Soft Tissue Injuries

● ANATOMY AND PHYSIOLOGY

The skin is a tough, supple membrane that covers the entire body surface. It constitutes the larg-

KEY TERMS

compartment syndrome: A crush injury that usually results from compressive forces or blunt trauma to muscle groups confined in tight fibrous sheaths with minimal ability to stretch.

crush injury: Injury from a compressive force sufficient to interfere with the normal structure and metabolic function of the involved cells and tissues.

crush syndrome: A life-threatening and sometimes preventable complication of prolonged immobilization or compression; a pathological process that destroys or alters muscle tissue.

zone of coagulation: In a burn, the central area that has sustained the most intense contact with the thermal source and in which coagulation necrosis of the cells has occurred and the tissue is nonviable.

zone of hyperemia: An area lying at the periphery of the zone of stasis in which blood flow is increased as a result of the normal inflammatory response to injury.

zone of stasis: The area of burn tissue that surrounds the critically injured area and that consists of potentially viable tissue despite the serious thermal injury.

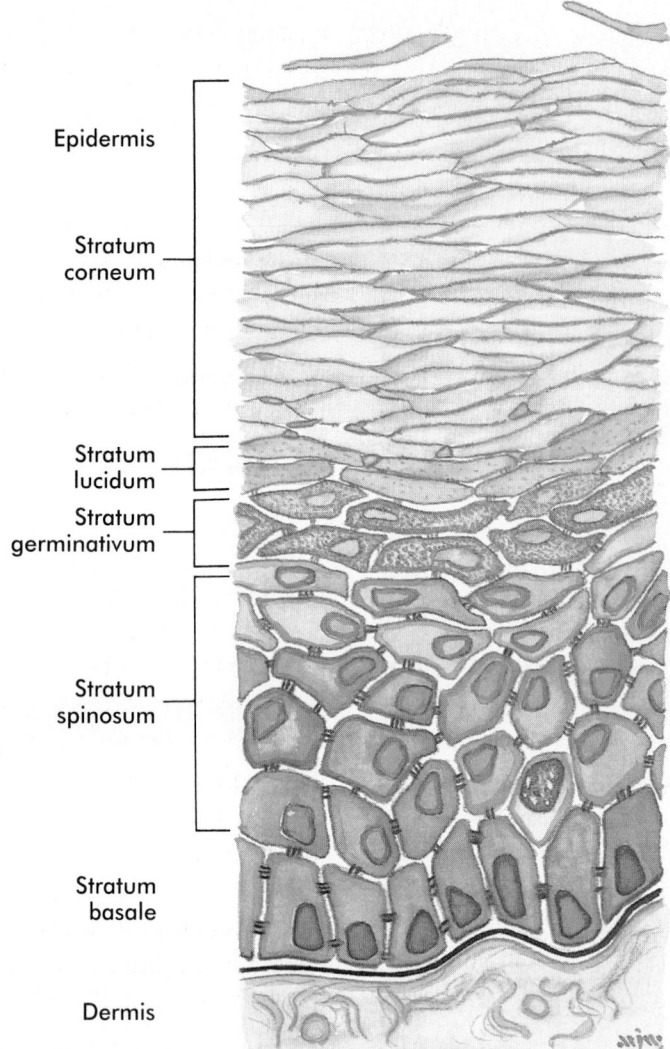

Fig. 16-1 Five layers of the epidermis.

est and most dynamic organ of the body, covering more than 20 square feet and composing 16% of total body weight. The skin is composed of two distinct layers of tissue: the outer layer, or epidermis, and the inner layer, or dermis.

Epidermis

The epidermis is a thin, avascular epithelial tissue that derives its nourishment from the capillaries of the dermis. Although it is only as thick as the page of this text, the epidermis is composed of five layers: the stratum basale, the innermost layer; the stratum spinosum; the stratum granulosum; the stratum lucidum; and the stratum cor-

neum, the most superficial layer of the epidermis, composing approximately 20 layers of dead skin cells that are filled with the waterproofing protein keratin. (Fig. 16-1).

Dermis

The dermis lies beneath the epidermis and contains connective tissue, elastic fibers, blood vessels, lymph vessels, and motor and sensory fibers. The dermis also houses other structures of the integumentary system, including hair, nails, and sebaceous and sweat glands. These specialized structures are formed from cells of the stratum basale layer.

Connective tissue and elastic fibers in the dermis give skin its strength and elasticity. Blood vessels in the dermis nourish all skin cells. The blood vessels also aid in body temperature regulation whereby body heat is conserved or released to the surrounding environment through vasoconstriction or vasodilation. Nerves in the dermis generate impulses to dermal muscles and glands and carry impulses away from sensory receptors in the skin. In addition, the dermis has a reservoir of defensive and regenerative elements that combat infection and repair deep wounds by specialized white blood cells, lymphatics, and other cellular components.

The subcutaneous tissues that underlie the dermis are composed of adipose and connective tissue. Their functions include insulation, cushioning, caloric reserve, and body substance and shape. To summarize, the skin is a primary sense organ whose key functions include:

- Shielding underlying tissues from fluid loss
- Protecting internal structures from mechanical injury
- Preventing the entrance of infectious organisms

● PATHOPHYSIOLOGY

Surface trauma may interfere with the normal preservation of body fluids and electrolytes and with the maintenance of body temperature. The two physiological responses to surface trauma are vascular and inflammatory reactions that may lead to healing, scar formation, or both. The extent and success of these responses are influenced by the amount of tissue disruption caused.

Hemostasis

Hemostasis is the initial physiological response to wounding. This vascular reaction involves vasoconstriction, formation of a platelet plug, coagulation, and the growth of fibrous tissue into the blood clot that permanently closes and seals the injured vessel.

Vasoconstriction secondary to injury is rapid but temporary. In response to injury, severed blood vessels constrict and retract with the aid of the surrounding subcutaneous tissues. This vessel spasm slows blood loss immediately and may completely close the ends of the injured vessels. The vasoconstriction response is typically sustained for as long as 30 minutes, during which time blood coagulation mechanisms are activated to produce a blood clot.

Platelets adhere to injured blood vessels and to collagen in the connective tissue that surrounds the injured vessel. As platelets contact collagen, they swell, become sticky, and secrete chemicals that activate other surrounding platelets. This process causes the platelets to adhere to one another and creates a "platelet plug" in the injured vessel. If the opening in the vessel wall is small, the plug may be sufficient to stop blood loss completely. For larger wounds, however, a blood clot is necessary to arrest the flow of blood (Fig. 16-2).

Blood coagulation occurs as a result of a chemical process that begins within seconds of a severe vessel injury and within 1 to 2 minutes of a minor wound. Coagulation progresses rapidly; within 3 to 6 minutes after the rupture of a vessel, the entire end of the vessel is filled with a clot. Within 30 minutes, the clot retracts and the vessel is further sealed. The blood-clotting mechanism is a complex biological process that includes the following three mechanisms:

1. Prothrombin activator is formed in response to rupture or damage of the blood vessel.
2. Prothrombin activator stimulates the conversion of prothrombin to thrombin.
3. Thrombin acts as an enzyme to convert fibrinogen into fibrin threads that entrap platelets, blood cells, and plasma to form the clot.

The process of hemostasis is a normal protective mechanism necessary for survival. However, in certain circumstances the mechanism, once triggered, results in responses that threaten life and function. These situations include blood clots that form because of accumulation of plaque in vessels afflicted by atherosclerosis. When this occurs in the coronary arteries, it may result in myocardial infarction; in the cerebral vasculature, it may produce stroke.

Hemostasis can also be impaired by certain diseases or genetic factors that interrupt the clotting

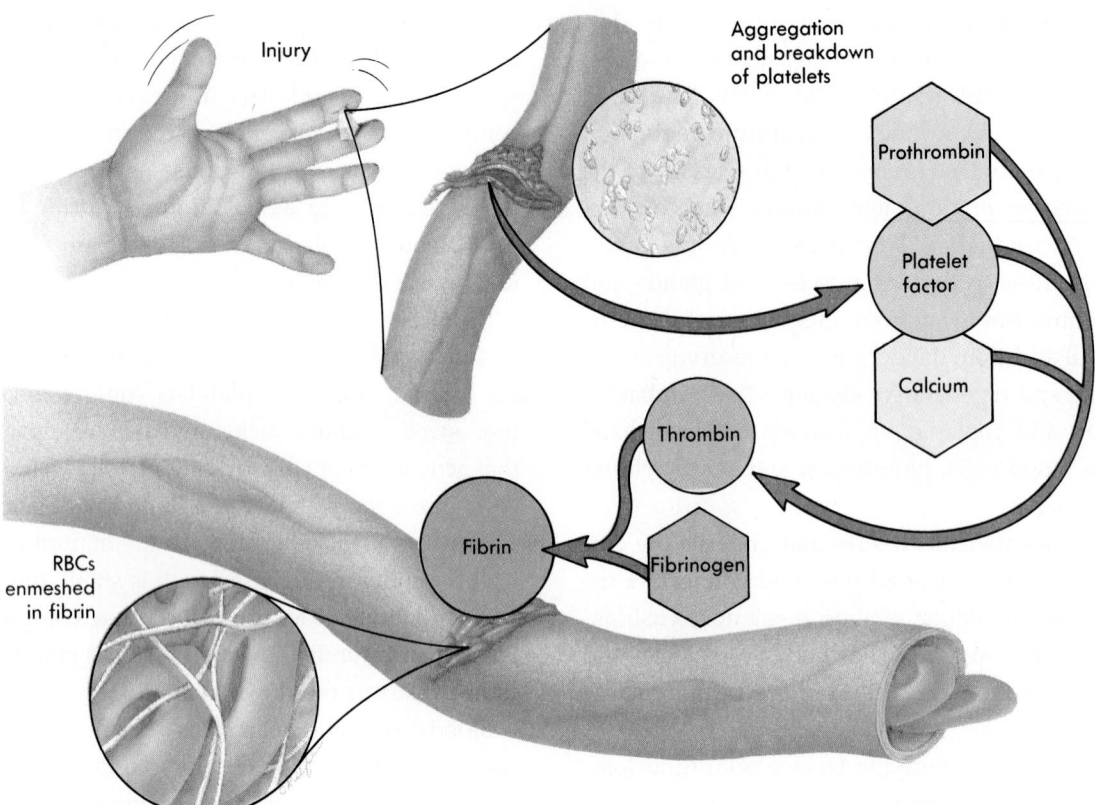

Fig. 16-2 The complex clotting mechanism can be distilled into three basic steps: release of platelet factors at the injury site, formation of thrombin, and trapping of red blood cells in fibrin to form a clot.

cascade, thereby retarding the process of clot formation. Examples include hemophilia, thrombocytopenia (a platelet deficiency), and liver disease, which affects the production of clotting factors. Various medications can also impair coagulation. Aspirin decreases platelet activity, and warfarin sodium (Coumadin) suppresses the liver's ability to make certain clotting factors. In any patient with impaired hemostasis, even minor trauma can result in uncontrollable and life-threatening hemorrhage.

Inflammatory Response

The release of chemicals from the injured vessel and various blood components (platelets, white blood cells) causes localized vasodilation of arterioles, precapillary sphincters, and venules, increasing the permeability of the affected capillaries and vessels. Plasma, plasma proteins, electrolytes, and chemical substances from the leaking venules accumulate in the extracellular space for approximately 72 hours after the injury. Blood flow increases to the area of injury to supply the metabolic demands of the tissues during healing and results in the redness, swelling, and pain associated with inflammation.

The transport of specialized white blood cells to the injured area also increases local blood flow. The white cells prepare the wound for eventual healing by clearing foreign bodies and dead tissue. Within hours of the injury, new epithelial cells are regenerated and begin the process of healing. It can take as long as 12 weeks for the injured tissue to regain its full strength and function.

● HEMORRHAGE AND CONTROL OF BLEEDING

Blood loss is frequently associated with soft tissue injury and may be the result of damage to ar-

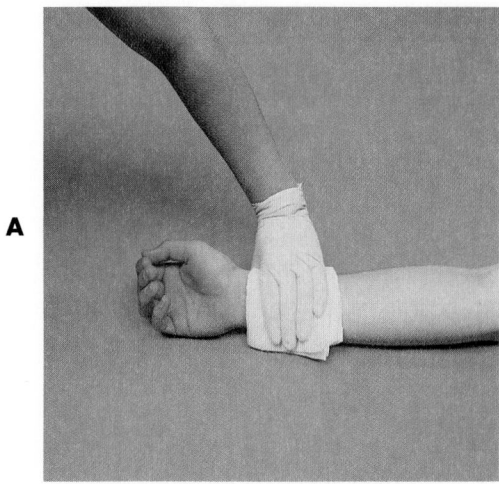

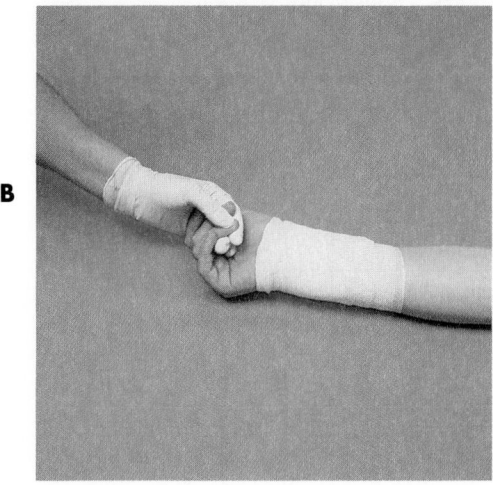

Fig. 16-3 A, Application of direct pressure to control hemorrhage. **B,** Pressure dressing.

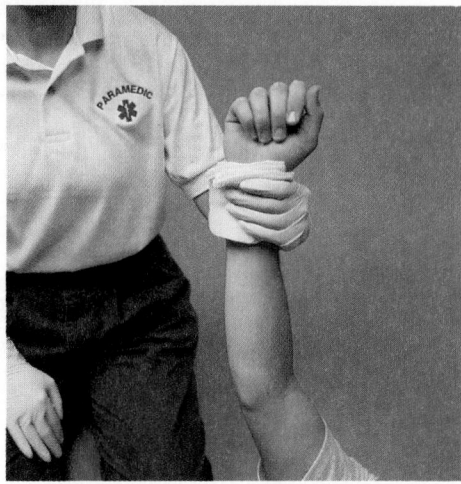

Fig. 16-4 Elevation to control hemorrhage.

teries, veins, capillaries, or a combination thereof. Generally, arterial bleeding is characterized as bright red and spurting, venous bleeding as dark reddish-blue and oozing, and capillary bleeding as bright red and flowing. However, it is often difficult to differentiate the types of vessel hemorrhage. In the prehospital setting, the primary concern in hemorrhage, regardless of origin, is to control the bleeding process.

Methods of hemorrhage control include direct pressure, elevation, pressure point, immobilization by splinting, pneumatic pressure devices (air splints, pneumatic antishock garment [PASG]), and use of tourniquets. A brief description of each method follows. As in any patient encounter where contact with body fluids is likely, personal protective measures should be taken.

Direct Pressure

External hemorrhage is best controlled by applying direct pressure over the injury site (Fig. 16-3, *A*). Direct pressure, applied with the rescuer's gloved hand or a hand-held dressing, controls most types of hemorrhage within 4 to 6 minutes. To maintain control, a pressure dressing may be applied over the site and held in place with a self-adherent roller bandage wrapped tightly over the dressing but not so tightly that it acts as a tourniquet (Fig. 16-3, *B*). After a dressing is applied, it should not be removed because removal may disrupt the fresh blood clot. If bleeding resumes and the dressing becomes soaked with blood, another dressing should be placed atop the initial dressing and held in place with direct pressure until the bleeding is again controlled.

Elevation

Venous bleeding that occurs in an extremity may be controlled or reduced by elevating the extremity above the level of the heart (Fig. 16-4). Elevation by itself does not usually control hemorrhage and should be considered a supplement to direct pressure.

Pressure Point

Pressure-point control should be attempted in cases in which direct pressure and elevation have

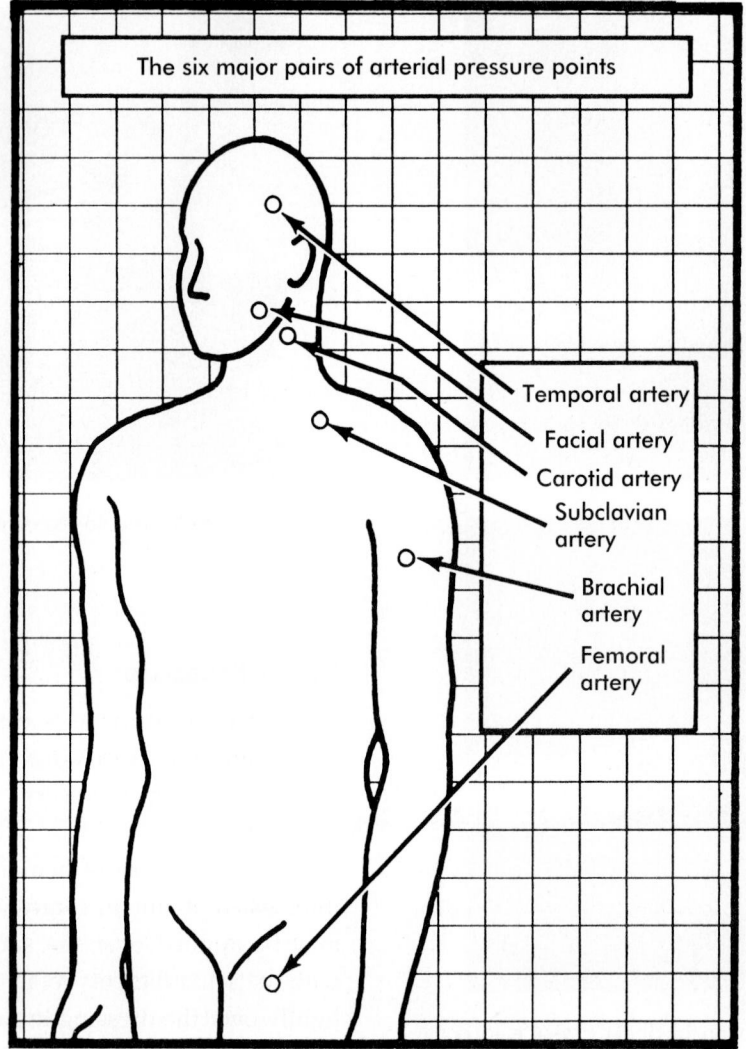

Fig. 16-5 Arterial pressure points.

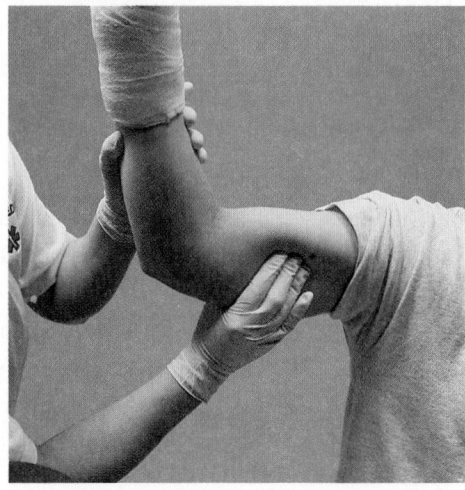

Fig. 16-6 Pressure-point control.

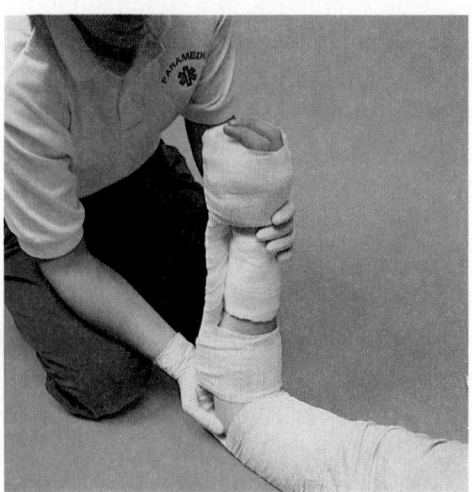

Fig. 16-7 Immobilization by splinting to control hemorrhage.

not controlled hemorrhage. The chosen artery must be proximal to the injury site and must over-lie a bony structure against which it can be compressed. Examples of pressure-point sites include the temporal artery to control bleeding from the scalp, the brachial artery to control bleeding from the forearm, and the femoral artery to control bleeding from the leg (Fig. 16-5). Pressure-point control (Fig. 16-6) should be maintained for at least 10 minutes and may require continued compression during patient transport. Combinations of direct pressure, elevation, and proximal pressure-point compression may be required to control vigorous hemorrhage.

To apply pressure and free the paramedic's hands for other tasks, applying a blood pressure cuff over the pressure point (brachial artery) may be useful. This effectively acts as a tourniquet, so time of application should be noted on the cuff itself.

Immobilization by Splinting

Patient movement promotes blood flow and may disrupt the clot or increase vascular injury. Therefore the patient should be well immobilized whenever possible (Fig. 16-7). Extremity injuries may be immobilized with appropriate splinting devices, or the patient may be fully immobilized with a long spine board. Immobilization is not effective by itself as a method to control bleeding and should be used as an adjunct.

Pneumatic Pressure Devices

Pneumatic pressure devices, such as inflatable air splints applied to an extremity or PASG, may help provide uniform direct pressure to an injury site as well as immobilization. If used, these devices should be applied over a dressed wound and only after the bleeding has been controlled by other methods (Fig. 16-8).

Tourniquet

There is little or no indication for tourniquet use in the emergency management of hemorrhage. Use of a tourniquet may be associated with dam-

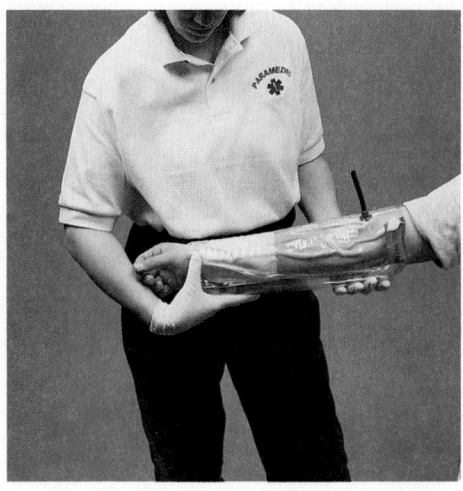

Fig. 16-8 Application of pneumatic pressure device to control hemorrhage.

age to nerves and blood vessels and eventual loss of the extremity. Another hazard is that an inadequately applied tourniquet may only produce venous occlusion, restricting the outflow but not the inflow of blood and producing an *increase* in blood loss. Therefore a tourniquet should only be considered as a last resort when all other methods have failed and when its use is essential to save the patient's life. An example of such an extreme circumstance is a partial or complete traumatic amputation of a limb. Even in these cases, other methods of hemorrhage control are often effective. Guidelines for applying a tourniquet are listed below (Fig. 16-9):

1. Consult with medical control.
2. Select a site for the tourniquet. The site should be approximately 2 inches proximal to the wound and over the supplying brachial or femoral artery.
3. Place the tourniquet (commercially prepared or wide, flat material) over the artery to be compressed. Never use thin material such as rope or twine because it may damage underlying tissue. (If a blood pressure cuff is used as a tourniquet, inflate the cuff until the cuff pressure exceeds the arterial pressure or to the point at which the hemorrhage stops.)
4. Place the pad (a roll of gauze or thick folded dressings) over the artery to be compressed.

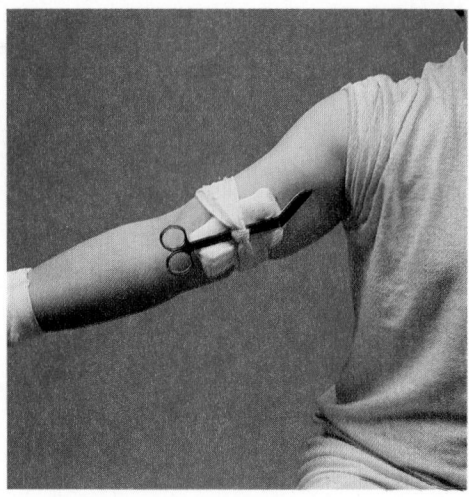

Fig. 16-9 Application of a tourniquet to control hemorrhage.

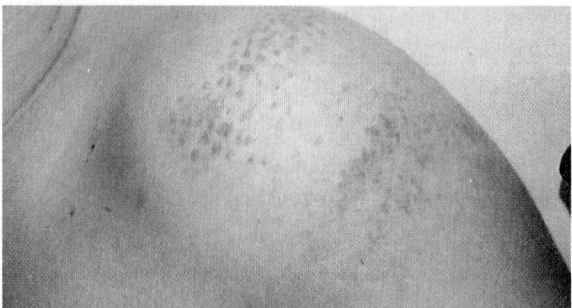

Fig. 16-10 Spotty bruising on a well-padded part of the shoulder.

5. Encircle the tourniquet twice around the extremity and pad, then tie it in a half knot over the pad.
6. Place a windlass (stick, pen, or similar object) on the half knot and secure it in place with a square knot.
7. Tighten the windlass by twisting *only* until hemorrhage stops. Secure the windlass in that position. Once it is tightened, never loosen the tourniquet.
8. Note the time of tourniquet application and secure it to the patient, or clearly mark *TK* on the patient's forehead. Document the tourniquet procedure on the patient's trip ticket.

> **NOTE:**
> A tourniquet should never be covered or obstructed from view. When the patient is delivered at the receiving hospital, immediately advise emergency department personnel that a tourniquet has been applied.

● SPECIFIC SOFT TISSUE INJURIES

Soft tissue injuries may be classified as closed or open as determined by the absence or presence of a break in the continuity of the epidermis. Although soft tissue wounds are often the most evident injury, they are generally considered low-priority injuries unless life-threatening hemorrhage or associated airway compromise is present.

Closed Wounds

Closed soft tissue injuries are usually associated with minimal blood loss, although as described in Chapter 15, some closed injuries may cause significant blood loss in the cavities of the thorax, abdomen, pelvis, or soft tissues of the legs. For the purpose of this text, closed wounds are classified as contusion, hematoma, and crushing injuries, including crush injury, compartment syndrome, and crush syndrome.

Contusions and Hematomas

Contusions and hematomas are caused by blunt trauma and are characterized by blood vessel disruption beneath the epidermis, resulting in ecchymosis; leakage of blood in the deeper tissues, resulting in a hematoma; or both (Fig. 16-10). These wounds are usually superficial but may also be associated with underlying fractures and vascular involvement. Four general principles of treatment for contusion and hematoma are:

1. Apply ice or cold packs to the injured area to stimulate vasoconstriction and reduce hemorrhage.
2. Apply compression to decrease bleeding with manual pressure, a compression bandage, or an air splint.

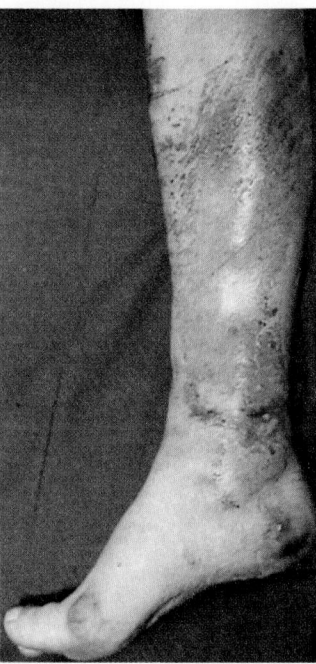

Fig. 16-11 Appearance of a women's leg after it had been run over by the wheel of a milk van.

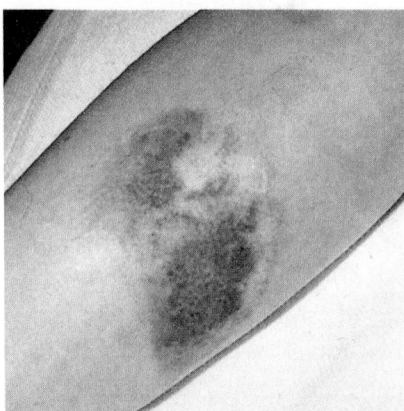

Fig. 16-12 Appearance that can follow prolonged crushing, as occurs when an unconscious person lies on the body part for several hours.

3. Elevate the injured body part so that it rests above the level of the heart.
4. Immobilize the injury with splinting devices to prevent body motion.

Crush Injury

Crush injury is one of the three injuries that may occur when tissue is exposed to a compressive force sufficient to interfere with the normal structure and metabolic function of the involved cells and tissues (Fig. 16-11). The degree of injury produced by the crushing force depends on the amount of pressure applied to the body, the amount of time the pressure remains in contact with the body, and the specific body region in which the injury occurs.

Crush injury usually involves the upper or lower extremities, the torso, or the pelvis. It may result from entrapment under a heavy object, as in a foundation collapse, or from some other massive compressive force. A massive crush injury to vital organs may cause immediate death. The signs and symptoms of major crush injury to an extremity are those of vascular insufficiency (the "five Ps"):

1. Pain
2. Paresis (a late finding)
3. Paresthesia
4. Pallor (variable)
5. Pulselessness (late finding)

Prehospital management of patients with major crush injury includes airway and ventilatory support, oxygen administration, fluid replacement as needed, immobilization, and rapid transport to an appropriate medical facility.

Compartment Syndrome

Compartment syndrome is a continuation in the disease spectrum of crush injury and is a surgical emergency (Fig. 16-12). It usually results from compressive forces or blunt trauma to muscle groups confined in tight fibrous sheaths with minimal ability to stretch (below the knee, above the elbow). Other less-common causes of compartment syndrome include:

- Extreme exertional exercise
- Low-level repetitive injury
- Electrical shock
- Hemorrhage into a compartment (for example, coagulopathy among hemophiliacs)
- Circumferential deep burns and electrical burns
- Vascular occlusion
- Immobilization with pressure necrosis (for example, among alcoholics, drug addicts, victims of cerebrovascular accident)

Compartment syndrome develops as associated hemorrhage and edema increase pressure in the closed fascial space (compartment). This results in ischemia to the muscle, which causes further muscle cell swelling. As the intracompartmental pressure continues to rise, circulation is compromised, and irreversible ischemic damage to tissue develops within several hours to several days after injury. In addition to muscular damage, any nerves that travel through the compartment may also undergo necrosis if the condition remains untreated. Signs and symptoms of compartment syndrome include:

- Pain seemingly out of proportion to injury
- Swelling (tautness of the compartment)
- Tenderness to palpation
- Weakness of the involved muscle groups
- Pain on passive stretch (earliest finding)
- Ischemic changes at the site of compression (the five Ps of vascular insufficiency)

Prehospital care for compartment syndrome includes airway and ventilatory support, oxygen administration, immobilization, fluid replacement as needed, and rapid transport to an appropriate medical facility. Definitive care is directed at restoring compromised circulation and correcting metabolic derangements (metabolic acidosis, hyperkalemia). If the patient proves to have elevated intracompartmental pressure, a rapid fasciotomy is performed to decompress the compartment and restore circulation.

Recognition of compartment syndrome requires a high degree of suspicion based on patient history and mechanism of injury. Though most frequently associated with tibial fracture of the lower leg, compartment syndrome may also occur with crush injury or fracture of the femur, forearm, or upper arm. Delayed treatment can result in nerve death, muscle necrosis, and crush syndrome.

Crush Syndrome

Crush syndrome is a life-threatening and sometimes preventable complication of prolonged immobilization or compression. It is a pathological process that causes destruction or alteration of muscle tissue. Crush syndrome is relatively rare and is most likely in catastrophic events in which patient rescue and extrication are delayed beyond 4 to 6 hours (for example, earthquake, building collapse). Prehospital management of crush syndrome often determines patient outcome.

The exact mechanism of crush syndrome is unknown. It is believed that the compressive forces of entrapment produce a pathological process that disrupts vascular integrity and causes loss of cellular architecture and structure of the membrane system. Patients with crush syndrome may appear stable for hours or days, as long as the compressive forces remain in place. When the patient is released from the entrapment, however, three detrimental processes occur simultaneously that may ultimately lead to death:

1. Oxygen-rich blood returns to the ischemic extremity, producing a pooling of intravascular volume into crushed tissue. This reduces circulating volume, often leading to the onset of clinical shock.
2. With the return of oxygen-rich blood, various toxic substances and waste products of anaerobic metabolism are released into the systemic circulation, causing metabolic acidosis. High levels of intracellular solutes and water are released from damaged cells, resulting in hyperkalemia, hyperuricemia, hypocalcemia, and hyperphosphatemia.
3. Myoglobin is released from the damaged cells of the injured extremity and filtered through the kidneys, resulting in acute renal failure.

Crush syndrome is a complex entity that is difficult to diagnose and treat because of the many variables involved, such as the extent of tissue damage, duration and force of compression, patient's general health, and associated injuries. Management of crush syndrome is controversial, and prehospital care must be supervised through a medical control physician familiar with this pathological process.

EMS personnel should consider the potential for crush syndrome when prolonged immobilization or compression occurs. Emergency care must be coordinated with rescue efforts so that the timing of the release from entrapment follows medical treatment to prevent the development of hypovolemic shock and crush syndrome. Patient care measures include:

1. Airway and ventilatory support
2. High-concentration oxygen administration
3. Maintenance of body temperature
4. Aggressive hydration to maintain urine output
5. Pharmacological agents (controversial)
   a. *Sodium bicarbonate*
   b. *Mannitol*
   c. *Furosemide*
   d. *Calcium chloride*
   e. Inhalation of beta agonists
6. Arterial tourniquets (controversial)
7. Surgical amputation (by physician) when extrication is impossible

Open Wounds

Open soft tissue injuries may be classified as abrasion, laceration, puncture, avulsion, amputation, and bites.

Abrasion

An abrasion is a partial-thickness injury caused by the scraping or rubbing away of a layer or layers of skin (Fig. 16-13). The wound usually results from friction with a hard object or surface (as occurs, for example, in sporting accidents and motorcycle crashes).

The wound should be assessed for size, depth, location, and contamination. Abrasions involving a large body surface area may cause significant loss of body fluids and the development of shock (rare). Prehospital care is usually limited to cleaning the injured surface of gross contaminants and lightly covering the wound with a sterile dress-

ing. Extensive debridement should not be attempted in the prehospital setting.

Laceration

A laceration results from a tear, a split, or an incision of the skin (Fig. 16-14). These injuries may be caused by blunt forces, which typically produce a jagged injury, or by a knife or other sharp object, resulting in a linear wound, or incision. The sizes and depths of lacerations can vary greatly, depending on the injury sites and wounding mechanism, and may be sources of significant bleeding. Initial prehospital care is usually directed at hemorrhage control through direct pressure. If internal bleeding is suspected, the patient should be closely monitored for signs of hypovolemic shock.

Puncture

A puncture wound (Fig. 16-15) commonly results from contact with a sharp, pointed object such as a wooden splinter, needle, staple, glass, or nail. Although the entrance wound is generally small, these injuries may be associated with deep penetration and injury to underlying tissues. All punctures should be evaluated for depth, contamination, evidence of retained foreign bodies, and associated injury. Punctures may be difficult to assess in the prehospital setting—an injury that appears to be minor can conceal a considerable amount of internal damage.

In some penetrating injuries, the wounding object may remain embedded or impaled in the

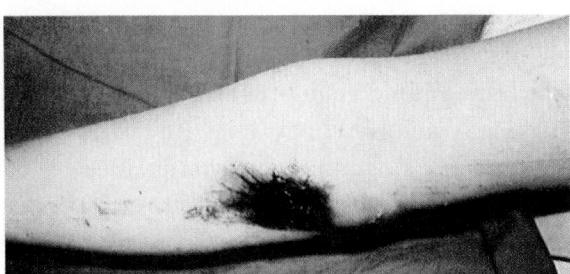

Fig. 16-13 Deep abrasion caused by a fall from a bicycle.

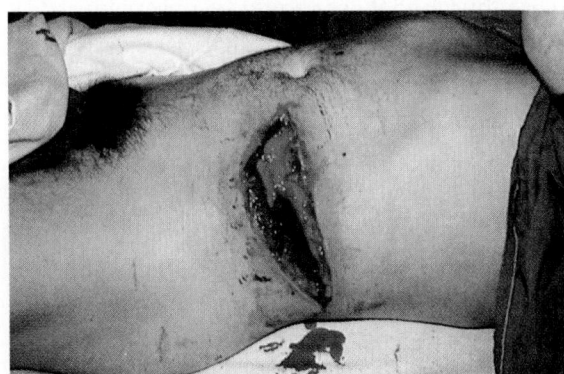

Fig. 16-14 Large wound caused by a broken power saw.

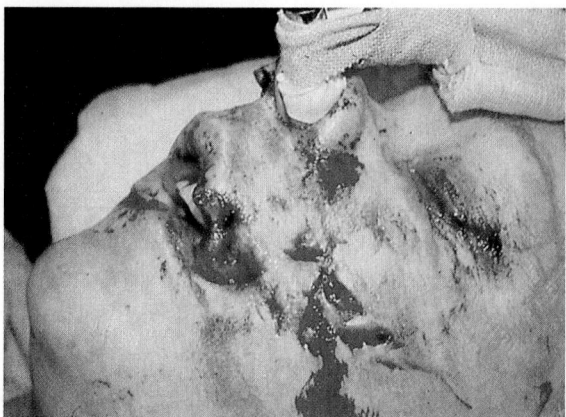

Fig. 16-15 Puncture wounds caused by broken glass from a shattered windshield.

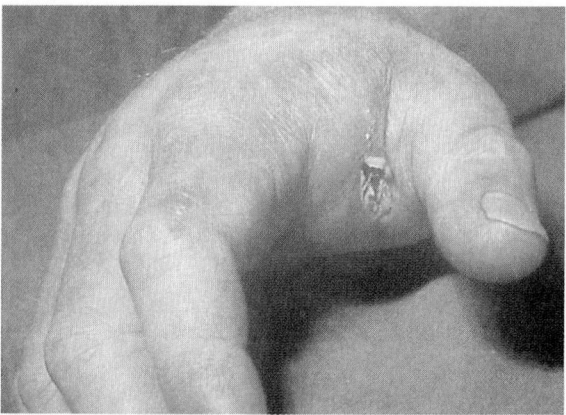

Fig. 16-17 Injection of paraffin into the hand resulted in amputation of the index finger.

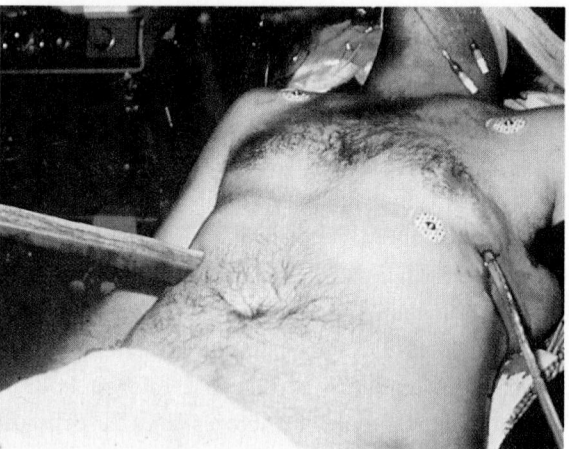

Fig. 16-16 Piece of wood impaled in the right chest, piercing the diaphragm and lacerating the spleen, stomach, and liver.

wound (Fig. 16-16). If an impaled object is present, these four guidelines should be observed:

1. Do not remove the impaled object—severe hemorrhage or damage to underlying structures may occur.

> ### NOTE:
> Medical control may recommend that an impaled object in the facial area that interferes with airway control or ventilation be removed at the scene. If removal is necessary, severe hemorrhage should be anticipated and direct pressure applied.

2. Do not manipulate the impaled object unless it is necessary to shorten the object for extrication or for patient transport.
3. Control bleeding with direct pressure applied around the impaled object.
4. Stabilize the object in place with bulky dressings and immobilize the patient to prevent movement.

Another type of puncture wound may result from injection of a substance into the body under high pressure, (for example, grease, paint, turpentine, dry-cleaning fluids, molten plastics [Fig. 16-17]). These injuries often have life- or limb-threatening potential. Rapid surgical decompression and debriding are indicated. These injuries are usually associated with minimal bleeding and numbness and blanching of the involved area and may not appear to be serious. However, definitive care generally requires hospitalization and surgical intervention to prevent infection. Amputation may be necessary if treatment is delayed.

Avulsion

An avulsion is a full-thickness skin loss in which the wound edges cannot be approximated. Frequently involved body areas are the ear lobes, nose tip, and fingertips. Avulsion injuries are often caused by industrial equipment, such as meat slicers or sawing devices, and domestic violence such as human bites (Fig. 16-18). Prehospital management of avulsed tissue varies by protocol, but these two guidelines generally apply:

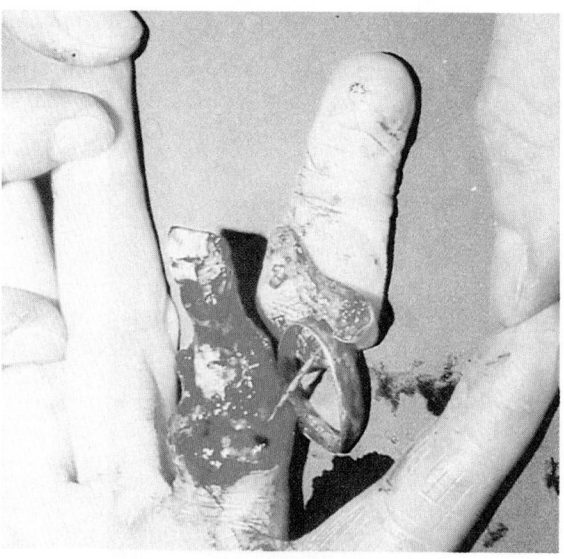

Fig. 16-18 Ring avulsion injury.

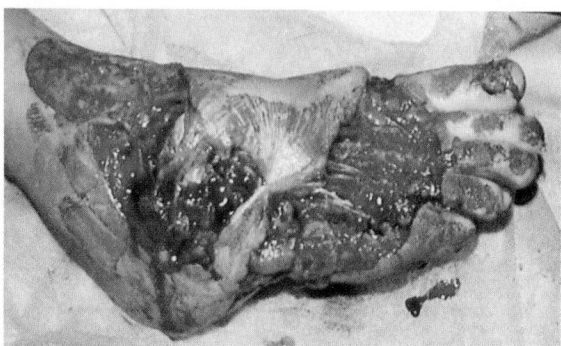

Fig. 16-19 Degloving injury of the foot.

> **NOTE:**
> To prevent additional tissue damage, it is generally recommended that the tissue not be placed directly on ice.

1. If the tissue is still attached to the body:
   a. Clean the wound surface of gross contaminants with sterile saline.
   b. Gently fold the skin back to its normal position.
   c. Control bleeding and dress the wound with bulky pressure dressings.
2. If the tissue is completely separated from the body:
   a. Control the bleeding with application of direct pressure.
   b. Retrieve the avulsed tissue if possible.

> **NOTE:**
> Patient transport should not be delayed in an effort to find avulsed tissue or amputated body parts if they are not readily available. Law enforcement officers or other health care providers at the scene should be notified of the ambulance destination so that the avulsed tissue or amputated body part can be transported at a later time, if found.

   c. Wrap the tissue in gauze, either dry or moistened with lactated Ringer's or saline solution (per protocol).
   d. Seal the tissue in a plastic bag.
   e. Place the sealed bag on crushed ice.

A degloving injury is a type of avulsion in which shearing forces separate the skin from the underlying tissues (Fig. 16-19). Common causes of degloving injury are industrial machinery that entangles an extremity, producing circumferential tearing; finger jewelry caught on a stationary object, producing a shearing of the soft tissue and possibly of the bone of the digit; and machinery that entraps hair, resulting in scalp avulsion.

Degloving injuries may be associated with underlying skeletal damage and massive loss of tissue in the affected area. Bleeding may be significant. Emergency care of these injuries is the same as for other types of soft tissue trauma. Special attention should be paid to control of bleeding, and affected extremities should be splinted. The patient must be transported to an appropriate medical facility to manage the complicated neurovascular problems frequently associated with these injuries.

Amputation

Traumatic amputation involves a complete or partial loss of a limb secondary to mechanical force (Fig. 16-20). The digits, lower leg, hand and forearm, and the distal portion of the foot are most frequently injured in this fashion. Bleeding is a potentially fatal complication of amputation injury. In situations in which a complete amputation has

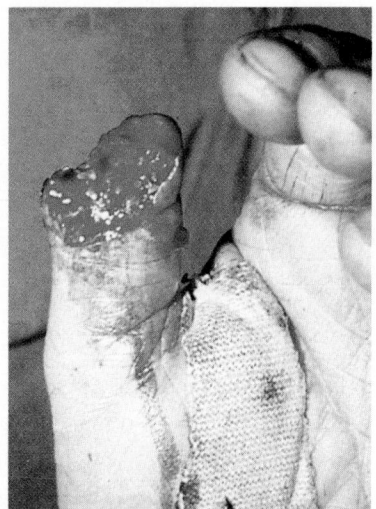

Fig. 16-20 Amputation of the fingertip.

occurred, however, injured arteries often retract, and hemorrhage may be less severe than in partial amputation injuries.

As with other open wounds, initial attempts at hemorrhage control should begin with direct pressure and elevation. Although a tourniquet may be required, it should be avoided if possible as the resultant damage might interfere with replantation attempts. The amputated limb should be retrieved and managed in the same manner as avulsed tissue.

Bites

An animal or human bite wound is frequently a combination of puncture, laceration, avulsion, and crush injury (Fig. 16-21). The great pressure of the injuring jaw, which may be as great as 400 psi in some dog bites, can involve deep structures such as tendons, muscles, and bones. Complications from bite wounds (particularly human bites) include abscesses, lymphangitis, cellulitis, osteomyelitis, tenosynovitis, tuberculosis, hepatitis B, and tetanus. Other less common complications of mammalian bites include the transmission of diseases such as actinomycosis, syphilis, and rarely, rabies. Although it is theoretically possible for the human immunodeficiency virus (HIV) to be contracted from a human bite, the Centers for Disease Control suggest that the potential for salivary transmission of the virus is remote.[1] All patients should be advised to seek physician evaluation.

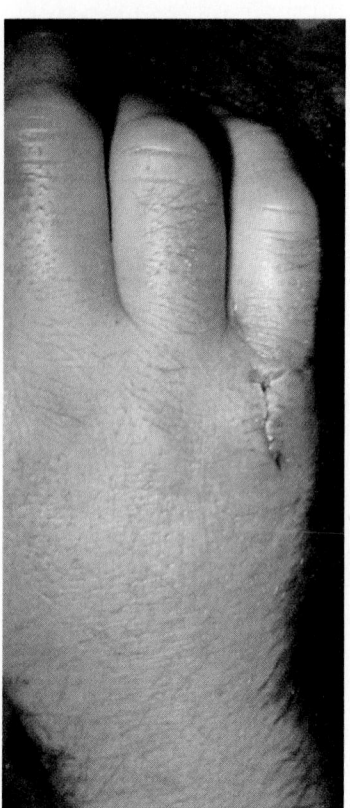

Fig. 16-21 Human bite to the hand.

In addition to the general principles of the care of soft tissue injury, a thorough history of the wounding force should be obtained from the patient so that potential complications can be evaluated. If the wound resulted from a human bite and the perpetrator is available and cooperative, a medical history from the perpetrator should be obtained to determine if he or she is known to have or be a carrier of any infectious diseases. In the case of an animal wound, law-enforcement or animal-control agencies should be contacted per protocol. Scene safety should be a prime concern when a response is made to a reported animal bite to avoid injury to the paramedic crew.

● GENERAL WOUND ASSESSMENT

Assessment of life-threatening injuries and resuscitation necessarily precede evaluation and intervention of non-life-threatening soft tissue injuries. Wounds that do not pose a threat to life are evaluated in the secondary survey. General wound assessment should include a history of the wounding event and careful examination of the injury.

Wound History

A wound history should include the following:
- Time of injury
- Environment where the injury occurred (risk of infection is greater in unclean environments)
- Mechanism of injury and likelihood of concurrent or associated injuries
- Volume of blood loss
- Severity of pain
- Previous medical history, including use of medications that may impair hemostasis
- Tetanus immunization

Physical Examination

A physical examination of a wound should include the following:
- Inspection of the wound for bleeding, size, depth, presence of foreign bodies, amount of tissue lost, edema, and deformity
- Inspection of the area surrounding the wound for damage to underlying structures, arteries, nerves, tendons, or muscle
- Assessment of sensory or motor function of the extremity
- Evaluation of the perfusion status of the wound and tissue distal to the wound
- Palpation of the injury and associated structures to evaluate capillary refill, distal pulses, tenderness, temperature, edema, and crepitus (if underlying bony injury is suspected)

Section Two
Burn Injuries

● INCIDENCE AND PATTERNS OF BURN INJURY

Burns are a devastating form of trauma associated with high mortality rates, lengthy rehabilita-

tion, cosmetic disfigurement, and permanent physical disabilities. Each year, more than 2.5 million Americans seek medical attention for burns. Of these, 100,000 are hospitalized and 12,000 die as a result of thermal injury.[2]

Morbidity and mortality rates from burn injury follow significant patterns with regard to gender, age, and socioeconomic status. For example, two thirds of all fire fatalities are males, the death rate from thermal injury is highest among children and older adults, and three fourths of all fire deaths occur in the home, with the highest incidence in lower-income households.[3] A key component of the professional role of the paramedic is community education to stress prevention as the most effective management of these injuries.

Major Sources

A burn injury is caused by an interaction between energy (thermal, chemical, electrical, or radiation) and biological matter. The majority of burns are thermal and commonly result from flames, scalds, or contact with hot substances. Frostbite, also considered a thermal injury, is addressed in Chapter 25.

Chemical burns are caused by substances capable of producing chemical changes in the skin, with or without heat production. Although heat may be generated during the burning process, the chemical changes in the skin, not the heat, produce the greatest injury. Chemical burns differ from thermal burns in that the topical agent generally adheres to the skin for prolonged periods, producing continuous tissue destruction. The severity of the chemical injury is related to the type of agent, its concentration and volume, and the duration of contact. Chemical agents that frequently cause burn injury include acids and alkalis, which are found in many household cleaning products.

Electrical injuries entail direct contact with an electric current or arcing of electricity between two contact points near the skin. In direct contact injury, the current itself is not considered to have any thermal properties, but the potential energy of the current is transformed into thermal energy when it meets the electrical resistance of biological tissue interposed between the entrance and exit sites. Arc injuries are localized at the termination of current flow and are caused by the intense heat or flash that occurs. Flame burn may also occur as a result of arcing if the heat generated ignites clothing.

Radiation injury is caused by ionizing and nonionizing radiation (see Chapter 7). Burns may result from a high level of radiation exposure to a specific body area, but radiation injuries make up a very small percentage of burn injuries.

● PATHOPHYSIOLOGY

Studies have shown that surface temperatures of 44° C (111° F) do not produce burns unless exposure time exceeds 6 hours.[3] At temperatures between 44° and 51° C (111° and 124° F), the rate of epidermal necrosis approximately doubles with each degree of temperature rise. At 70° C (185° F) or greater, the exposure time required to cause transepidermal necrosis is less than 1 second. The degree of tissue destruction depends on the temperature and duration of exposure. Factors that influence the body's ability to resist burn injury include the water content of the skin tissue; thickness and pigmentation of the skin; presence or absence of insulating substances such as skin oils or hair; and peripheral circulation of the skin, which affects dissipation of heat.

Local Response to Burn Injury

Burn injury immediately destroys cells or so completely disrupts their metabolic functions that cellular death ensues. Cellular damage is distributed over a spectrum of injury. Some cells are destroyed instantly, others are irreversibly injured, and some injured cells may survive if rapid and appropriate intervention is provided in the prehospital setting.

Major burns have three distinct zones of injury, which usually appear in a "bull's eye" pattern (Fig. 16-22). The central area of the burn wound, which has sustained the most intense contact with the thermal source, is the **zone of coagulation.** In this area, coagulation necrosis of the cells has occurred and the tissue is nonviable. The **zone of stasis** surrounds the critically injured area and consists of potentially viable tissue despite the serious thermal injury. In this zone, cells are ischemic because of clotting and vasoconstriction. The cells die within 24 to 48 hours after injury if no supportive measures are undertaken. At the periphery of the zone of stasis is the **zone of hyperemia.** This zone has increased blood flow as a result of the normal inflammatory response. The tissues in this area recover in 7 to 10 days if infection or profound shock does not develop.

Tissue damage from burns depends on the degree of heat and duration of exposure to the thermal source. As a rule, the burn wound swells rap-

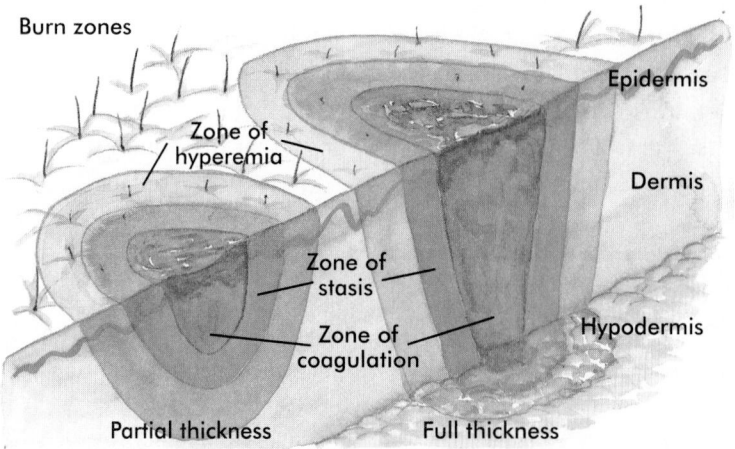

Fig. 16-22 Three zones of intensity: (1) zone of hyperemia (peripheral), (2) zone of stasis (intermediate), and (3) zone of coagulation (central).

idly because of the release of chemical mediators, which cause an increase in capillary permeability and a fluid shift from the intravascular space into the injured tissues. The increased permeability is accentuated by injury to the sodium pump in the cell walls. As sodium moves into the injured cells, it causes an increase in osmotic pressure that increases the inflow of vascular fluid into the wound. Finally, the normal process of evaporative loss of water to the environment is dramatically accelerated (5 to 15 times that of normal skin) through the burned tissue. In a small wound, these physiological alterations produce a classic local inflammatory response (pain, redness, swelling) without major systemic effects. If the wound covers a large body surface area, however, these local tissue responses can produce major systemic effects and life-threatening hypovolemia.

Systemic Response to Burn Injury

As local events occur at the injury site, other organ systems become involved in a general response to the stress caused by the burn, which may compromise patient outcome. One of the earliest manifestations of the systemic effects of a large thermal injury is hypovolemic shock with a decrease in venous return, decreased cardiac output, and increased vascular resistance (except in the hyperemic zone). This hypovolemic state, when added to hemolysis (destruction of red blood cells) and rhabdomyolysis (muscle necrosis) with subsequent hemoglobinuria and myoglobinuria, often leads to renal failure. Other systemic responses to major burn injury include:

- Pulmonary response
  - Hyperventilation to meet increased metabolic needs
- Gastrointestinal response
  - Decrease in splanchnic perfusion that may lead to mucosal hemorrhage and transient adynamic ileus
  - Vomiting and aspiration
  - Stress ulcers
- Musculoskeletal response
  - Decreased range of motion from immobility and edema

  - Possible osteoporosis and demineralization (late)
- Neuroendocrine response
  - Increased amounts of circulating epinephrine and norepinephrine and transient elevation of aldosterone levels
- Metabolic response
  - Elevated metabolic rate, particularly with infection or surgical stress
- Immune response
  - Altered immunity, resulting in increased susceptibility to infection
  - Depressed inflammatory response
- Emotional response
  - Physical pain
  - Isolation from loved ones and familiar surroundings
  - Fear of disfigurement, deformities, and disability
  - Altered self-image
  - Depression

● CLASSIFICATIONS

Burns (body surface area involvement and depth) must be assessed and classified as accurately as possible in the field to ensure appropriate treatment and to monitor progression of tissue damage. However, this not typically possible in the prehospital setting because of the progressive nature of the injury. With a burn, the amount of tissue damage may not be evident for hours or sometimes days after the injury.

Depth of Burn Injury

Burns are classified in terms of depth as first, second, and third degree. First- and second-degree burns are partial-thickness burns that usually heal without surgery. Third-degree burns are full-thickness burns that usually require skin grafts.

First-Degree Burns

First-degree burns are characteristically painful, red, and dry, and they blanch with pressure (Fig.

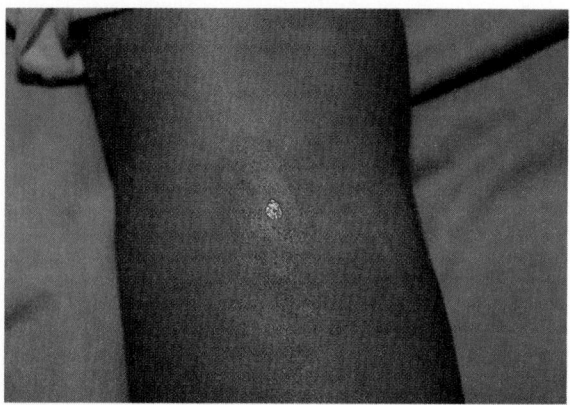

Fig. 16-23 First-degree burn.

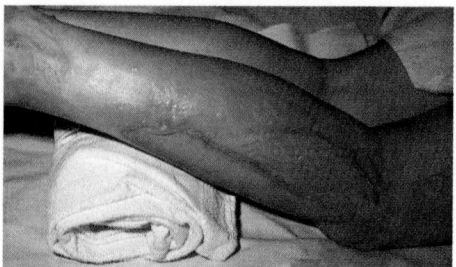

Fig. 16-25 Deep partial-thickness burn.

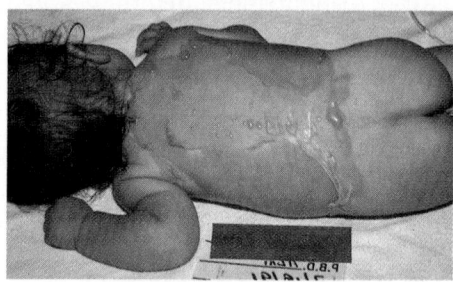

Fig. 16-24 Superficial partial-thickness second-degree burn.

16-23). They typically occur secondary to prolonged exposure to low-intensity heat or a short-duration flash exposure to a heat source. In first-degree burns, only a superficial layer of epidermal cells is destroyed, and they slough (peel away from healthy tissue underneath the wound) without residual scarring. These injuries usually heal within 2 to 3 days. An example of a first-degree burn is sunburn.

Second-Degree Burns

Second-degree burns may be divided into two groups: superficial partial-thickness and deep partial-thickness wounds. The superficial partial-thickness injury is characterized by blisters and is commonly caused by skin contact with hot but not boiling water or other hot liquids, explosions producing flashburns, hot grease, and flame.

In superficial partial-thickness second-degree burns (Fig. 16-24), injury extends through the epidermis to the dermis, but the basal layers of the skin are not destroyed, and the skin regenerates within a few days to a week. Edema fluid infiltrates the dermal-epidermal junction, creating the blisters characteristic of this depth of wound. Intact blisters provide a seal that protects the wound from infection and excessive fluid loss. For this reason, blisters should never be broken in the prehospital setting. The injured area is usually red, wet, and painful and may blanch when the tissue around the injury is compressed. In the absence of infection, these wounds heal without scarring, usually within 14 days.

If the depth of the second-degree burn involves the basal layer of the dermis, it is considered a deep partial-thickness burn (Fig. 16-25). As in superficial partial-thickness burns, edema forms at the epidermal-dermal junction. Sensation in and around the wound may be diminished because of the destruction of basal-layer nerve endings. The injury may appear red and wet or white and dry, depending on the degree of vascular injury. Wound infection and subsequent sepsis and fluid loss are major complications of these injuries. If uncomplicated, deep partial-thickness burns generally heal within 3 to 4 weeks. Skin grafting may be necessary to promote timely healing and to minimize thick scar tissue formation, which may severely restrict joint movements and cause persistent pain and disfigurement.

Third-Degree Burns

In third-degree burns, the entire thickness of the epidermis and dermis is destroyed; thus skin

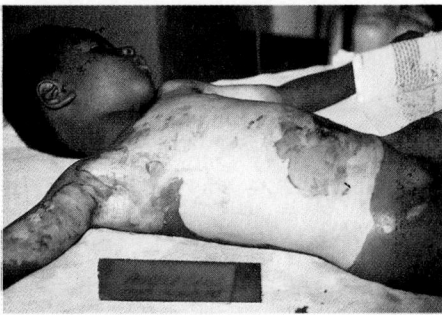

Fig. 16-26 Third-degree burn.

grafts are necessary for timely and proper healing (Fig. 16-26). The wound is characterized by coagulation necrosis of the cells and appears pearly white, charred, or leathery. A definitive sign of third-degree burn is a translucent surface in the depths of which thrombosed veins are visible. Eschar, a tough, nonelastic coagulated collagen of the dermis, is present in these injuries.

Sensation and capillary refill are absent in third-degree burns because small blood vessels and nerve endings are destroyed. This often results in large plasma volume loss, infection, and sepsis. Natural wound healing may produce contracture deformity and severe scarring. Therefore surgical intervention with skin grafting is necessary to close full-thickness wounds, to minimize complications, and to allow restoration of maximal function.

Some burn classifications also include a fourth-degree burn to describe a full-thickness injury that penetrates the subcutaneous tissue, muscle, fascia, periosteum, or bone. These burns usually result from incineration-type exposure and electrical burns in which heat is sufficient to destroy tissues below the skin.

Extent and Severity of Burn Injury

There are several methods to evaluate the extent of burn injury. Two common methods include the "rule of nines" and the Lund and Browder chart. In addition, the American Burn Association has devised a categorization of burns to determine severity. Use of any of these methods to evaluate a burn injury should never delay patient care or transport.

Rule of Nines

The rule of nines is commonly used in the pre-hospital setting. The measurement divides the total body surface area (TBSA) into segments that are multiples of 9%. This method provides a rough estimate of burn injury size and is most accurate for adults and for children older than 10. Fig. 16-27 explains the rule of nines.

If the burn is irregularly shaped or has a scattered distribution throughout the body, the rule of nines is difficult to apply. In these situations, burn size can be estimated by visualizing the patient's palm as an indicator of percentage. The surface of the patient's palm equals approximately 1% of the total body surface area.

Lund and Browder Chart

The Lund and Browder chart (Fig. 16-28) is a more accurate method of determining the area of burn injury because it assigns specific numbers to each body part. It is used to measure burns in infants and young children because it allows for developmental changes in percentages of body surface area. For example, the adult head is 9% of TBSA, but the newborn head is 18% TBSA.

American Burn Association Categorization

Using the criteria established by the American Burn Association, burn injuries are categorized as major, moderate, and minor (Box 16-1).

In determining severity, factors such as the patient's age, the presence of concurrent medical or surgical problems, and the complications that accompany certain types of burns such as those of the face and neck, hands and feet, and genitalia must also be considered. For example, burns of the face and neck may cause respiratory compromise or interfere with the ability to eat or drink. Burns of the hands and feet may interfere with ambulation and activities of daily living. Perineal burns present a high risk of infection because of the contaminants in this region and may disrupt the normal patterns of elimination.

Burn Center Referral Criteria

Many EMS services use the categorizations previously described or other criteria as bases for de-

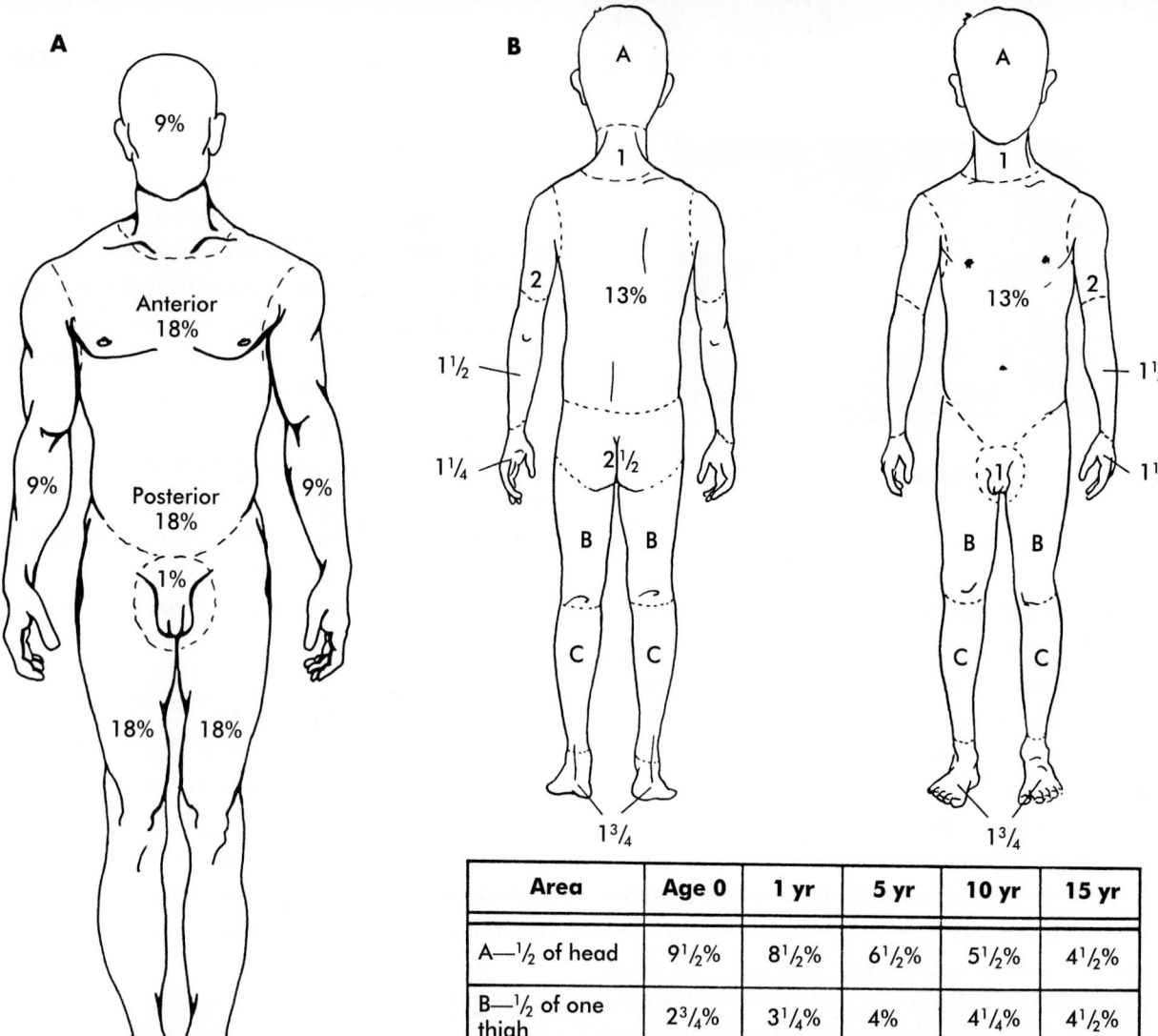

Area	Age 0	1 yr	5 yr	10 yr	15 yr
A—$\frac{1}{2}$ of head	$9\frac{1}{2}$%	$8\frac{1}{2}$%	$6\frac{1}{2}$%	$5\frac{1}{2}$%	$4\frac{1}{2}$%
B—$\frac{1}{2}$ of one thigh	$2\frac{3}{4}$%	$3\frac{1}{4}$%	4%	$4\frac{1}{4}$%	$4\frac{1}{2}$%
C—$\frac{1}{2}$ of one leg	$2\frac{1}{2}$%	$2\frac{1}{2}$%	$2\frac{3}{4}$%	3%	$3\frac{1}{4}$%

Fig. 16-27 A, Rapid estimation of burn extent can be determined by the rule of nines. Only partial-thickness (second-degree) and full-thickness (third-degree) burns are considered for percentage area determination. **B,** Estimation of burn size in children. Note that the relative area sizes change significantly with age.

BOX 16-1

American Burn Association Categorization

Major Burn

25% of the body surface or greater

Functionally significant involvement of hands, face, feet, or perineum

Electrical or inhalation injury

Concomitant injury

Severe preexisting medical problems

Moderate Burn

15% to 25% body surface area

No complications or involvement of hands, face, feet, or perineum

No electrical injury, inhalation injury, concomitant injury, or severe preexisting medical problem

Minor Burn

15% or less body surface area

No involvement of face, hands, feet, or perineum

No electrical burns, inhalation injury, severe preexisting medical problems, or complications

Age	0-1	1-4	5-9	1-14	15
A—$\frac{1}{2}$ of head	$9\frac{1}{2}$%	$8\frac{1}{2}$%	$6\frac{1}{2}$%	$5\frac{1}{2}$%	$4\frac{1}{2}$%
B—$\frac{1}{2}$ of one thigh	$2\frac{3}{4}$%	$3\frac{1}{4}$%	4%	$4\frac{1}{4}$%	$4\frac{1}{2}$%
C—$\frac{1}{2}$ of one leg	$2\frac{1}{2}$%	$2\frac{1}{2}$%	$2\frac{3}{4}$%	3%	$3\frac{1}{4}$%

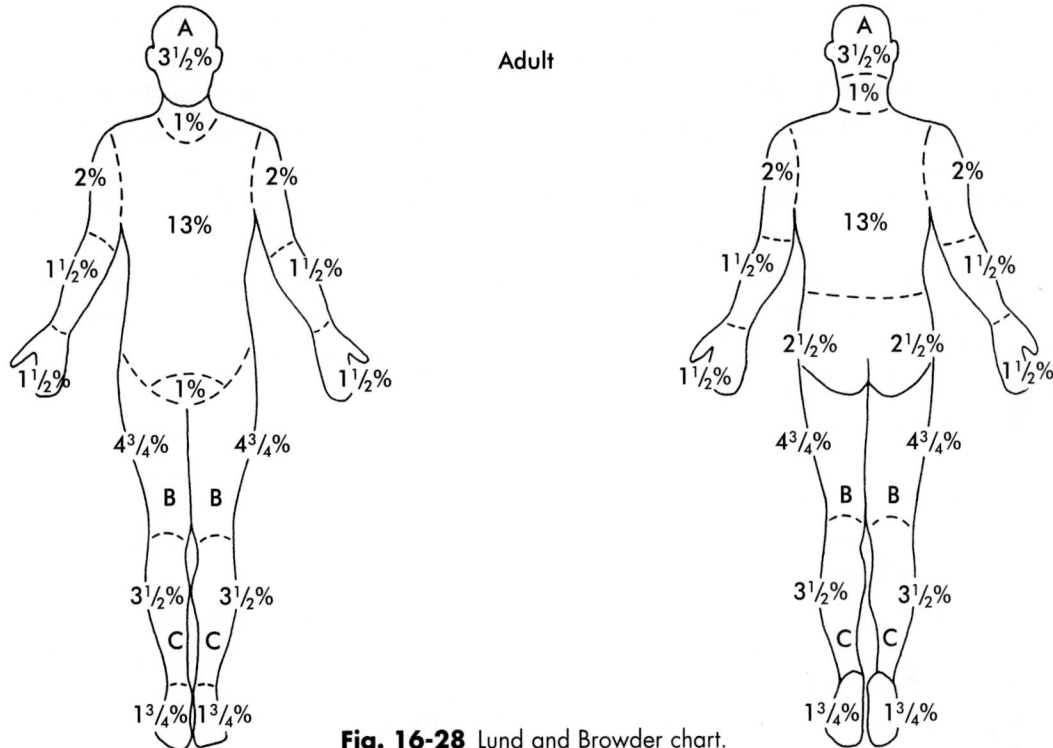

Fig. 16-28 Lund and Browder chart.

termining which patients need transport to specialized burn centers. According to the Committee on Trauma of the American College of Surgeons and the American Burn Association, burn injuries usually requiring referral to a burn center include[4] the following eleven guidelines:

1. Second- and third-degree burns that in combination cover more than 10% of the body surface area in patients under 10 or over 50 years of age
2. Second- and third-degree burns that in combination cover more than 20% of the body surface area of patients in the other age groups
3. Second- and third-degree burns that involve the face, hands, feet, genitalia, or perineum or those that involve skin overlying major joints
4. Third-degree burns over more than 5% body surface area in any age group

5. Significant electrical burns, including lightning injury
6. Significant chemical burns
7. Inhalation injury
8. Burn injury in patients with preexisting illnesses that could complicate management, prolong recovery, or affect mortality
9. Burns in any patient in whom concomitant trauma poses an increased risk of morbidity or mortality and who may be initially treated in a trauma center until stable before transfer to a burn center
10. Burns in children seen in hospitals without qualified personnel or equipment for their care (should be transferred to a burn center with these capabilities)
11. Burn injuries in patients who require special social and emotional or long-term rehabilitative support, including cases involving suspected child abuse and neglect

● PATHOPHYSIOLOGY OF BURN SHOCK

Shock after thermal injury results from edema and accumulation of vascular fluid in the tissues in the area of injury. Locally, there is a brief initial decrease in blood flow to the area followed by a marked increase in arteriolar vasodilation. A concurrent release of vasoactive substances from the burned tissue causes increased capillary permeability, producing intravascular fluid loss and wound edema. The fluid loss into the injured tissues and the marked increase in evaporative fluid loss secondary to the break in the epithelial barrier contribute to produce hypovolemia.

The greatest loss of intravascular fluid occurs in the first 8 to 12 hours, followed by a continued, moderate loss over the next 12 to 16 hours. At some point within 24 hours, the extravasation of fluid greatly diminishes and equilibrium between the intravascular space and the interstitial space is reached. Shock and organ failure (most commonly acute renal failure) can occur as a consequence of hypovolemia. Fluid volume replacement for burned patients in the prehospital setting may be indicated in cases of prolonged extrication, when discovery of the patient is delayed several hours, and during interhospital transfer to a burn center.

> **NOTE:**
> Hypovolemia secondary to burn trauma is usually not seen in the prehospital setting because burn edema develops over the first several hours after the burn. Therefore a patient with burns who is hypovolemic should be evaluated for other injuries that may be responsible for the volume loss.

Fluid Replacement

The increase in capillary permeability associated with burns prevents the creation of an osmotic gradient between the intravascular and extravascular space, allowing colloid solutions to quickly equilibrate across the capillary barrier and into the interstitium. In addition, sodium is the ion lost from the circulation in disproportionate amounts. Consequently, salt-containing crystalloid solution is usually considered the fluid of choice in the initial resuscitation of burn patients in the first 24 hours. In the second 24-hour period, capillary permeability returns toward normal, with restoration of functional capillary integrity. Therefore colloid solutions may be given in the second day to minimize intravenous fluid loading.

Several fluid resuscitation formulas that take body size and extent of burned body surface area into account have proved clinically useful in replacing fluids. The two most common formulas for estimating fluid replacement are the Parkland formula and the modified Brooke formula. These have been combined into the consensus formula. All three formulas call for half of the total calculated amount of fluid to be infused over the first 8 hours from the time of the injury and the second half to be infused over the following 16 hours.

Fluid resuscitation in burn patients remains controversial. Paramedics should consult with medical control and follow local protocol. Regardless of therapy, fluid resuscitation must be guided by regular monitoring of measures of hemodynamic function (for example, vital signs, respiratory rate, lung sounds, capillary refill, urinary output). *When determining the percentage of burn for fluid resuscitation, calculate only second- and third-degree burns.*

Consensus Formula

1. The first 24 hours: 2 to 4 ml lactated Ringer's multiplied by kg multiplied by percent TBSA burn
   a. 50% of the calculated amount infused in the first 8 hours
   b. 25% of the calculated amount infused in the second 8 hours
   c. 25% of the calculated amount infused in the third 8 hours

Example: A 100-kg patient has 30% TBSA. Total fluid to be infused in the first 24 hours at 2 ml/kg is calculated as follows: 2 ml × 30 × 100 = 6000 ml. Of the 6000 ml, 3000 ml should be infused in the first 8 hours, a rate of 375 ml/hr. The volume of fluid actually infused may be adjusted according to individual patient needs as prescribed by medical control.

2. The second 24 hours:
   a. The amount and composition of fluids required after the first 24 hours are vastly

different from those administered during the first 24 hours. Fluid replacement is dictated by the patient's response to the burn and the treatment regimen.

● ASSESSMENT OF THE BURN PATIENT

Emergency care for a burn patient, like any other trauma patient, begins with the primary survey to recognize and treat life-threatening injuries. In burn patients, however, the dramatic appearance of burns and the characteristic odor of burnt flesh may easily distract the paramedic from life-threatening problems. It is important that the EMS provider be confident in the assessment and direct efforts away from the burn wound and toward the patient as a whole.

Primary Survey

Evaluation of the patient's airway is a major concern in the primary survey, particularly for the patient with an inhalation injury. The paramedic should observe for stridor (an ominous sign that indicates the patient's upper airway is at least 80% narrowed), facial burns, soot in the nose or mouth, singed facial or nasal hair, edema of lips and the oral cavity, coughing, inability to swallow secretions in the pharynx, hoarse voice, and circumferential neck burns. Airway management should be aggressive with these patients.

Breathing should be evaluated for rate, depth, and the presence of wheezes, crackles, or rhonchi. The patient's circulatory status should be evaluated by assessing the presence, rate, character, and rhythm of pulses; capillary refill; skin color and temperature; and obvious arterial bleeding.

The patient's neurological status should be determined by using the AVPU scale or a similar method. Deviations from the norm should be carefully evaluated for underlying cause. Abnormalities include hypoxia, decreased cerebral perfusion from hypovolemia, and cerebral injury resulting from head trauma. After completing the primary survey, a history of the event should be obtained while a secondary survey is performed.

An accurate history from the patient or bystanders can help the paramedic determine the potential for inhalation injury, concomitant trauma, or preexisting conditions that may influence the physical examination or patient outcome. When obtaining the patient history, the following information should be ascertained:

- What is the patient's chief complaint?
- What were the circumstances of the injury?
  - Did it occur in an enclosed space?
  - Were explosive forces involved?
  - Were hazardous chemicals involved?
  - Is there related trauma?
- What was the source of the burning agent (for example, flame, metal, liquid, chemical)?
- Does the patient have any significant medical history?
- What medications does the patient take (including recent ingestion of illegal drugs or alcohol)?
- Did the patient lose consciousness at any time? (Suspect inhalation injury.)
- What is the status of tetanus immunization?

Secondary Survey

At the beginning of the secondary survey, a complete set of vital signs should be assessed. The blood pressure should be obtained in an unburned extremity, if available. If all extremities are burned, sterile gauze may be placed under the blood pressure cuff and an attempt made to auscultate a blood pressure. Patients with severe burns or preexisting cardiac or medical illness should be monitored by electrocardiogram (ECG). Lead placement may need to be modified to avoid placing electrodes over burned areas. Field care and hospital destination are determined by the depth, size, and extent of burned tissue and the presence of associated illness or injury.

● GENERAL PRINCIPLES IN BURN MANAGEMENT

Goals for prehospital management of the severely burned patient include preventing further tissue injury, maintaining airways, administering oxygen and ventilatory support, providing fluid resuscitation, providing rapid transport to an appropriate medical facility, and using aseptic technique to minimize the patient's exposure to infectious agents. Patients with burns should also be evaluated for other types of life-threatening trauma; some will have additional injuries associated with the burn event. Examples include blunt or penetrating trauma sustained in automobile crashes, blast injury, and skeletal or spinal injury from attempts to escape the thermal source.

Stopping the Burning Process

The first step in managing any burn is to stop the burning process. This step must be accomplished with the safety of the emergency crew in mind because it often occurs in close proximity to the source that caused the burn. With minor first-degree burns, the burning process can be terminated by cooling the local area with cold water. Ice, snow, or ointments should never be applied to the burn because they may increase the depth and severity of thermal injury. In addition, ointments may impair or delay assessment of the injury when the patient arrives in the emergency department.

In cases of severe burns, the patient should be rapidly and safely moved from the burning source to an area of safety if possible. If the person's clothing is in flames or is smoldering, he or she should be placed on the floor or ground and rolled in a blanket to smother the flames or doused with large quantities of the cleanest available water. Contaminated water sources, such as a lake or river, should be avoided. These patients should never be allowed to run or remain standing. Running may fan the flame, and an upright position may increase the likelihood of the patient's hair being ignited. (Stop! Drop! Roll!)

The patient's clothing should be completely removed while cooling the burn so that heat is not trapped under the smoldering cloth. If pieces of smoldering cloth have adhered to the skin, they should be cut (not pulled) away. Melted synthetic fabrics that cannot be removed should be soaked in cold water to stop the burning process. After the burn is cooled, the patient with a large body surface area injury should be covered with a clean, preferably sterile sheet, over which blankets are placed when ambient temperatures are low.

Airway, Oxygen, and Ventilation

The adequacy of airway and ventilatory efforts should be evaluated in all burn patients. High-concentration humidified oxygen should be administered to any patient with severe burns, and ventilation should be assisted as needed. If inhalation injury is suspected, the patient should be closely observed for signs of impending airway obstruction. Life-threatening laryngeal edema may be progressive and may make tracheal intubation difficult if not impossible. The decision to intubate these patients should not be delayed.

Circulation

The need for fluid resuscitation is based on the severity of the injury, the patient's vital signs, and transport time to the receiving hospital. In the critically burned patient, prompt initiation of intravenous therapy is essential to prevent long-term complications such as burn shock and renal failure.

If possible, intravenous therapy should be initiated with a large-bore catheter in an unburned upper extremity. If an unburned site is not available, the catheter may be inserted through burned tissue (although the risk of subsequent infection is greater). Care should be taken to secure the catheter with a dressing; tape may not adhere to the injured areas as it begins to leak fluid.

If transport of the burn patient is delayed or a lengthy interfacility transport is anticipated, other patient care procedures may be required. These include administration of analgesics, placement of a nasogastric tube to prevent gastric distention or vomiting, and placement of an indwelling urinary catheter to measure urine output and to maintain patency of the urethra in patients with burns to the genitalia. Procedures for nasogastric tube insertion are presented in Chapter 21.

Special Considerations

Although all burn injuries warrant good patient assessment and care, burns of specific body regions require special consideration. These include burns to the face and extremities and circumferential burns.

Burns of the face swell rapidly and may be associated with airway compromise. The head of the ambulance stretcher should be elevated at least 30 degrees (if not contraindicated by spinal trauma) to minimize the edema. If the patient's ears are burned, the use of a pillow should be avoided to minimize additional injury to the area.

If burns involve the extremities, all rings, watches, and other jewelry should be removed to prevent vascular compromise with increased wound edema. Peripheral pulses should be reassessed frequently, and the burned limb should be elevated above the patient's heart if possible.

Burn injuries that encircle a body region can pose a threat to the patient's life. Circumferential burns that occur to an extremity may produce a tourniquet-like effect that may quickly compromise circulation and cause irreversible damage to the limb. Circumferential burns of the chest can severely restrict movement of the thorax and may significantly impair chest wall compliance. If this occurs, the depth of respirations is reduced, tidal volume is decreased, and the patient's lungs may become difficult to ventilate, even by mechanical means. Definitive treatment for circumferential burns involves an in-hospital surgical procedure known as *escharotomy*, whereby incisions are made through deep burns to reduce compartment pressure and allow adequate blood flow to occur to and from the affected limb or thorax.

● INHALATION INJURY

Smoke inhalation injury is present in approximately 20% to 30% of all patients admitted to burn centers; more than 50% of the 12,000 fire deaths each year are directly related to smoke inhalation or inhalation injury.[2] Prehospital considerations in caring for patients with inhalation injury include recognition of the dangers inherent in the fire environment, pathophysiology of inhalation injury, and early detection and treatment of impending airway or respiratory problems.

Smoke inhalation most commonly occurs in a closed environment such as a building, automobile, or airplane and is caused by the accumulation of toxic byproducts of combustion. However, inhalation injury can also occur in an open space, and all burn victims should be evaluated for this injury. Dangers that contribute to inhalation injury in a fire environment are:

- Consumption of oxygen by the fire
- Production of carbon monoxide
- Production of other toxic gases

Pathophysiology

Smoke inhalation and inhalation injury compose a broad group of consequences secondary to combustion. For this text, these consequences are classified as carbon monoxide poisoning, inhalation injury above the glottis, and inhalation injury below the glottis.

Carbon Monoxide Poisoning

Carbon monoxide is a colorless, odorless, tasteless gas produced by incomplete combustion of carbon-containing fuels. Carbon monoxide does not physically harm lung tissue, but it causes a reversible displacement of oxygen on the hemoglobin molecule, forming carboxyhemoglobin (COHb). The result is low circulating volumes of oxygen despite normal partial pressures. In addition, the presence of COHb causes a shift in the hemoglobin dissociation curve to the left, requiring that tissues be very hypoxic before oxygen is released from the hemoglobin to fuel the cells.

Carbon monoxide has approximately 250 times the affinity for hemoglobin that oxygen has. Therefore small concentrations of carbon monoxide in inspired air can result in severe physiological impairments, including tissue hypoxia, inadequate cellular oxygenation, inadequate cellular and organ function, and eventually death. The physical effects of carbon monoxide poisoning are related to the level of COHb in the blood. Levels less than 10% do not usually cause symptoms; they are common in smokers, traffic police, truck drivers, and others who are chronically exposed to carbon monoxide. At levels of 20%, a healthy patient may complain of headache, nausea, vomiting, and loss of manual dexterity. At 30% the patient may become confused and lethargic, and ECG abnormalities may be present. At levels between 40% and 60%, coma may develop. Levels above 60% are often fatal. Tachypnea and cyanosis are not usually present in these patients because arterial oxygen tension is normal. Patients with high COHb levels may have a skin appearance that is bright red, but more commonly the patient has normal or pale skin and lip coloration.

Treatment of the patient with carbon monoxide poisoning includes ensuring a patent airway, providing adequate ventilation, and administering high-concentration oxygen. (As discussed in Chapter 12, pulse oximeter use is unreliable in determining effective patient oxygenation in carbon monoxide poisoning.) The half-life of carbon monoxide at room air is approximately 4 hours. This can be reduced to 30 to 40 minutes if 100% oxygen and adequate ventilation are provided. The use of hyperbaric oxygen therapy (see Chapter 25) in treating carbon monoxide poisoning is controversial, and the paramedic should follow local protocol.

Inhalation Injury Above the Glottis

The structure and function of the airway superior to the glottis make it particularly susceptible to injury if exposed to high temperatures. The upper airway is very vascular and has a large surface area, which allows it to normalize temperatures of inspired air. Because of this design, actual thermal injury to the lower airway is rare because the upper airway sustains the impact of injury when environmental air is superheated.

Thermal injury to the airway can result in immediate edema of the pharynx and larynx (above the level of the true vocal cords), which can rapidly progress to complete airway obstruction. Signs and symptoms of upper airway inhalation injury include (Fig. 16-29):

- Facial burns
- Singed nasal or facial hairs
- Carbonaceous sputum
- Edema of the face, oropharyngeal cavity, or both
- Signs of hypoxemia
- Hoarse voice
- Stridor
- Brassy cough
- Grunting respirations

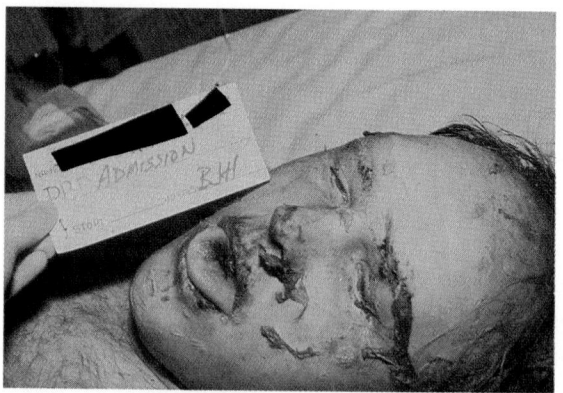

Fig. 16-29 Inhalation injury.

Prompt recognition and protection of the airway are critical in these patients. If impending airway obstruction is suspected, early nasotracheal or orotracheal intubation may be warranted because progressive edema can make emergency intubation extremely hazardous if not impossible.

Inhalation Injury Below the Glottis

The two primary mechanisms of direct injury to the lung parenchyma are heat and toxic material inhalation. Thermal injury to the lower airway is rare; causes include inhalation of superheated steam, which has 4000 times the heat-carrying capacity of dry air; aspiration of scalding liquids; and explosions, which occur as the patient is breathing high concentrations of oxygen under pressure.

Most fire-related lower-airway injuries result from the inhalation of toxic chemicals such as the gaseous byproducts of burning materials. Signs and symptoms of lower-airway injury may be immediate but are more frequently delayed, beginning several hours after the exposure. These include:

- Wheezes
- Crackles or rhonchi
- Productive cough
- Signs of hypoxemia
- Spasm of bronchi and bronchioles

Prehospital care should be directed at ensuring a patent airway and providing high-concentration oxygen and ventilatory support. Specific airway and ventilatory management, which may include nasal or oral tracheal intubation and pharmacological therapy with bronchodilators, should be coordinated with on-line medical control.

● CHEMICAL INJURY

More than 60,000 people seek medical attention for chemical injuries each year; of these, more than 3000 die.[5] Exposure to chemical irritants is common because as caustic chemicals are frequently present in the home and workplace.

Three types of caustic agents are frequently associated with burn injuries: alkalis, acids, and organic compounds. Alkalis, strong bases with a high pH, occur in hydroxides and carbonates of sodium, potassium, ammonium, lithium, barium, and calcium. These compounds are commonly found in oven cleaners, household drain cleaners, fertilizers, heavy industrial cleaners, and the structural bonds of cement and concrete. Strong acids are in many household cleaners, such as rust removers, bathroom cleaners, and swimming pool acidifiers.

Organic compounds are chemicals that contain carbon. Most organic compounds are harmless chemicals such as wood and coal. However, several organic compounds produce caustic injury to human tissue. These include phenols and creosote and petroleum products such as gasoline. In addition to their role in producing chemical burns, organic compounds may be absorbed by the skin, causing serious systemic effects. As previously stated, the severity of chemical injury is related to the chemical agent, the concentration and volume of the chemical, and the duration of contact.

Assessment

These exposure factors can often be assessed during the patient history. When dealing with a chemical exposure, the paramedic should ascertain the following:

- Type of chemical substance (If the container is available and can be safely transported, it should be taken to the medical facility.)
- Concentration of chemical substance
- Volume of chemical substance
- Mechanism of injury (local immersion of a body part, injection, splash)
- Time of contamination
- First aid administered before EMS arrival
- Pain

Management

As with all burn injuries, the safety of the rescuers must be the first consideration in managing the victim of chemical injury. The paramedic must consider the use of protective gear before approaching the scene. Depending on the chemical agent involved, personal protection may include gloves, eye shields, protective garments, and appropriate breathing apparatus.

The treatment of chemical injuries varies little from that of thermal burns during the primary survey. After the primary survey, treatment is directed at stopping the burning process. This can best be accomplished by the following:

1. Remove all clothing, including shoes, which can trap concentrated chemicals.
2. Brush off powdered chemicals.
3. Irrigate the affected area with copious amounts of water.
   a. In otherwise stable patients, irrigation takes priority over transportation unless irrigation can be continued en route to the emergency department.
   b. If a large body surface area is involved, a shower should be used for irrigation, if readily available.
4. If chemical exposure involves the eyes, irrigate copiously with lactated Ringer's or a saline solution and continue it until arrival at the medical center.
   a. Consider the use of eye irrigation devices such as the Morgan lens (see Chapter 7).

Use of Antidotes or Neutralizing Agents

According to the American Burn Association, no agent has been found to be superior to water for treating most chemical burns.[2] Consequently, the use of antidotes or neutralizing agents should be avoided in initial prehospital management of most burn injuries. Many neutralizing agents produce heat and may increase injury when applied to the wound.

In special circumstances, such as when an industrial complex within a response area is known to use a chemical agent with a specific antidote, medical control may elect to have the ambulance stock the neutralizer. In this situation, paramedics should receive special training on the indications, use, and side effects of these agents.

Specific Chemical Injuries

Although the primary treatment for most chemical burns is copious irrigation with water, several specific chemical injuries warrant further discussion. These include petroleum, hydrofluoric acid, phenols, ammonia, and alkali metals.

Petroleum

In the absence of flame, products such as gasoline and diesel fuel can cause significant chemical burns if prolonged contact occurs. Initially the injury appears to be only a first- or second-degree burn when in fact it may be a full-thickness injury. Systemic effects such as central nervous system depression, organ failure, and death may result from the absorption of various hydrocarbons. In addition, lead toxicity can occur if the exposure was from gasoline containing tetraethyl lead.

Hydrofluoric Acid

Hydrofluoric acid, one of the most corrosive materials known, is used in industry for cleaning fabrics and metals, for glass etching, and in the manufacture of silicone chips for electronic equipment. Both the hydrogen ion and the fluoride ion are damaging to tissue. Fluoride inhibits several chemical reactions essential to cell survival, and it continues to penetrate and kill cells when it is neutralized by binding to calcium or magnesium. Thus endogenous or exogenous hydrofluoric acid has the potential to produce very deep and severe injuries. If large body surface areas are involved, the patient may experience severe hypocalcemia and even death. Even the most minor-appearing wounds that involve hydrofluoric acid should be evaluated at an appropriate medical facility.

Irrigation of the exposed area with copious amounts of water should be initiated in the prehospital setting. On arrival in the emergency department, patient treatment may include subcutaneous administration of a 10% calcium gluconate solution directly into the burn site.

Phenol

Phenol (carbolic acid) is an aromatic hydrocarbon derived from coal tar. It is widely used in industry as a disinfectant in cleaning agents and in the manufacture of plastics, dyes, fertilizers, and explosives. Skin contact with phenol can result in local tissue coagulation and systemic toxicity if the agent is absorbed. A soft tissue injury from phenol exposure may be painless because of the agent's anesthetic properties. Minor exposures may cause central nervous system depression and dysrhythmias. Patients with significant exposures (10% to 15% TBSA) may require systemic support and should be carefully observed for signs of respiratory failure.

Wounds should be copiously irrigated with large volumes of water. After irrigation, medical control may recommend that the wound be swabbed with a suitable solvent such as glycerol, vegetable oil, or soap and water to bind phenol and prevent its systemic absorption.

Ammonia

Ammonia is a noxious, irritating gas and strong alkali that is very soluble in water. It is an extremely hazardous solution if introduced into the eye and may result in tissue necrosis and blindness. The patient with an ammonia "burn" to the eye will probably have swelling or spasm of the eyelids. These patient injuries must be irrigated with water or a balanced salt solution for up to 24 hours.

Respiratory injury from ammonia vapors depends on the concentration and duration of exposure. For example, short-term, high-concentration exposure usually results in upper-airway edema, whereas long-term low-concentration exposure may damage the lower respiratory tract. Initial care for patients with respiratory injury includes high-concentration oxygen administration, ventilatory support as needed, and rapid transport to an appropriate medical facility.

Alkali Metals

Sodium and potassium are highly reactive metals that can ignite spontaneously. Water is generally contraindicated when these metals are imbedded in the skin, since they react with water and produce large amounts of heat. Physically removing the metal or covering it with oil minimizes the thermal injury.

● ELECTRICAL INJURY

Electrical injuries account for 3% to 5% of admissions to burn centers and are responsible for more than 1000 deaths each year.[6] An understanding of the principles of current and the path of destruction it may produce in the body is essential for good patient care and personal safety at the scene of an electrocution.

Principles of Electricity

Tissue damage produced by electric current is a function of six factors: amperage, voltage, resistance, type of current, current pathway, and duration of current flow.

Amperage is a measure of the current flow (intensity) per unit time. One ampere (amp) is a passage of 1 coulomb of charge per second past any point in the circuit. Thus a 10-amp flow means that 10 coulombs of electricity are passing a point per second.

Voltage is a continuous force (tension) applied to any electric circuit that produces a flow of electricity. Volts are the potential driving force for electrical current. One volt is the force needed to drive 1 amp of current in a circuit with 1 ohm of resistance. High-voltage electrical injuries result from contact with a source of 1000 volts or greater. High-tension accidents commonly range from 7200 to 19,000 volts but may involve current with as high as 100,000 to 1 million volts.

An ohm is a measure of the resistance of an electrical conductor. Electrical resistance is composed of four factors: (1) resistivity, the capacity of a material to resist current flow; (2) the size of the object pathway; (3) the length of the object pathway; and (4) temperature. Resistance to the flow of electricity varies greatly within the body because various tissues have different resistance to current flow. Tissue resistance to electrical flow in the body is highest in bone, decreasing progressively through the fat, skin, muscle, blood, and nerve tissue.

Two basic forms of electric current are in common usage: direct current (DC) and alternating current (AC). The type of current can influence patterns and severity of injury. DC flows in one direction only. It is frequently used in industry and is the type of current produced by batteries. DC is commonly used in electrosurgical devices and defibrillators and is characterized by high amperage and low voltage.

AC reverses the direction of flow at regular intervals (60-cycle current has 60 reversals per second). These alterations in current direction can cause tetanic muscle contractions, which may "freeze" the victim to the source until the current is terminated. Household current in the United States is generally AC and either 120 or 220 volts. AC is a more common cause of electrical injury.

Electricity normally flows along a continuous pathway known as an *electric circuit*. Although the current pathway can be somewhat unpredictable, as a rule, low-voltage current (less than 1000 volts) follows the path of least resistance and high-voltage current follows the shortest path. In either case, the greater the current flow, the greater the heat generated.

The pathway of the current through the body is important because it gives a clue as to what anatomical structures are damaged. For example, if the current travels from one hand to the other, it may flow across the heart and provoke ventricular fibrillation or other dysrhythmias.

Tissue injury results from the conversion of electrical energy into heat. The amount of heat produced is directly proportional to the square of the current strength multiplied by the resistance of the tissue multiplied by the duration of the current flow (Joule's law). Therefore injury is directly proportional to the duration of contact with the electrical source.

Types of Electrical Injury

Three basic types of injury may occur as a result of contact with electric current: direct contact burns, arc injuries, and flash burns. Direct contact burns occur when electric current directly penetrates the resistance of the skin and underlying tissues. The hand and wrist are common entrance sites, and the foot is a common exit site (Fig. 16-30.) Although the skin may initially resist the flow of current, continued contact with the source lessens resistance and permits increased current flow. The greatest tissue damage occurs directly under and adjacent to the contact points and may include fat, fascia, muscle, and bone. Although tissue destruction may be massive at the entrance and exit sites, it is the area between these wounds that poses the greatest threat to the patient's life.

Arc injuries occur when a person is close enough to a high-voltage source that the current between two contact points near the skin overcomes the resistance in the air, passing the current flow through the air to the bystander. Temperatures generated by these sources can be as high as 2000° to 4000° C (3632° to 7232° F), and the arc may jump as far as 10 feet.

Flash burns are produced when the heat of electric current ignites a nearby combustible source.

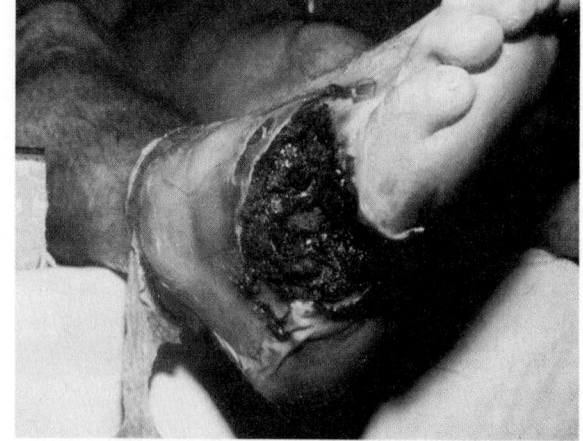

Fig. 16-30 Direct contact burn. **A,** Entry wound (hand). **B,** Exit wound (foot).

Common injury sites include the face and eyes. Flash burns may also ignite a person's clothing or cause fire in the surrounding environment. No electrical current passes through the body in this type of burn.

Effects of Electrical Injury

Electrical injuries are often unpredictable and vary according to the parameters described. However, certain physiological effects should be anticipated by the paramedic crew.

The skin is almost always the first point of contact with electrical current. Direct contact and passage of current through tissue may produce extensive areas of coagulation necrosis. The entrance site is often a characteristic bull's-eye wound and may appear dry, leathery, charred, or depressed. The exit wound may be ulcerated and may have an "exploded" appearance where areas of tissue are missing.

Oral burns are frequently seen in children under the age of 2. These wounds are typically caused by a child chewing or sucking on a low-tension electrical cord. Oral burns may be associated with injury to the tongue, palate, and face.

Electrical current may cause significant dysrhythmias and damage to the myocardium as it passes through the body. Immediate cardiac arrest is the most common cause of death after electrical injury, and ventricular fibrillation is often the presenting rhythm. Experts believe that DC, such as a lightning strike, is likely to produce asystole, whereas 60-amp AC is more likely to produce ventricular fibrillation. It does not take a large amount of current to produce dysrhythmias (100 milliamperes can cause ventricular fibrillation). If early rescue and resuscitation can be initiated by the paramedic, success rates are high. Hypertension associated with a large release of catecholamines is also a common finding in electrical injury.

Nerve tissue is an excellent conductor of electrical current and may therefore be commonly affected in electrical injuries. Central nervous system damage may result in seizures or coma with or without focal neurological findings; peripheral nerve injury may lead to motor or sensory deficits, which may be permanent. If the current passes through the brain stem, respiratory arrest or depression or cerebral edema or hemorrhage may rapidly lead to death.

Electrical injury can cause extensive necrosis of blood vessels. These injuries, although they may not be evident on EMS arrival, can cause immediate or delayed internal hemorrhage or arterial or venous thrombosis and embolism with subsequent complications.

Damage within the extremities after an electrical burn is similar to crush injury in that severe muscle necrosis releases myoglobin, and hemolysis releases hemoglobin, which can precipitate in the renal tubules, producing acute renal failure.

Acute renal failure is a serious complication that affects approximately 10% of significant direct-contact electrical injuries. It may result from a combination of myoglobin or hemoglobin sludging in the renal tubules, disseminated intravascular coagulation secondary to tissue damage, hypovolemic shock, and DC damage. Although acute renal failure is not of immediate consequence in the prehospital environment, prompt fluid resuscitation and management of shock may have a positive impact on a significant number of these patients.

Ventilation may be impaired when electrical burns produce central nervous system injury or chest wall dysfunction. If the respiratory center is disrupted, hypoventilation can lead to immediate patient death. Contact with any AC sources has also been documented to produce respiratory arrest and death from tetany of the muscles of respiration.

In the electrocuted patient, severe muscle spasms can produce bony fractures and dislocations, even of major joints. In addition, a patient may fall after the electrical shock and sustain significant skeletal trauma, including damage to the cervical spine.

Conjunctival and corneal burns and ruptured tympanic membranes are common in some electrical injuries. Cataracts and hearing loss may also appear as late as 1 year after the event.

Numerous other internal structures may be damaged secondary to electrical injury, including the abdominal organs and urinary bladder. Submucosal hemorrhage may occur in the bowel, and various forms of ulceration are possible. Each patient requires a thorough physical assessment and a high degree of suspicion for associated trauma.

Assessment and Management

Patient assessment should begin by ensuring that no hazards exist for the rescuers or bystanders. If the patient is still in contact with the electrical source, the electric company, fire department, or other specially trained personnel should be summoned before approaching the patient. Once the scene is safe, patient intervention may begin.

Primary Survey

The primary survey should proceed as for all other trauma patients, with particular care being taken to immobilizing the cervical spine. If the patient is not breathing, artificial ventilation should proceed immediately. Intubation should be performed as soon as possible because apnea may persist for lengthy periods. A patient who is breathing should have a patent airway maintained and respirations supported with supplemental high-concentration oxygen. If the patient is in cardiac arrest, resuscitation efforts should be implemented according to protocol. If possible, a history should be obtained, including the following:

- Patient's chief complaint
- Source and voltage of the electrical injury
- Duration of contact
- Level of consciousness before and after the injury
- Past significant medical history

Secondary Survey

The secondary survey should be particularly thorough to search for entrance and exit wounds or any associated trauma caused by tetany or a fall. The paramedic should remember that there may have been multiple pathways of current and therefore multiple wounds. All of the patient's clothing and jewelry should be removed and the areas between the patient's fingers and toes examined for sites of entry or exit. Distal pulses, motor function, and sensation should be carefully assessed in all extremities and well documented to monitor for possible development of compartment syndrome. Entrance and exit wounds should be covered with sterile dressings, and any associated trauma should be managed with appropriate treatment modalities.

Internal damage from electrical current may be much more significant than external wounds, and frequent reassessment is necessary because of the progressive nature of electrical injury. In addition, ECG monitoring is implemented at the scene and continued during patient transport. As previously discussed, electrical injury may cause a variety of dysrhythmias, some of which can be lethal.

Management

Early fluid resuscitation is critical in managing patients with severe electrical injury to prevent hypovolemia and subsequent renal failure. If possible, two large-bore intravenous lines should be established in an extremity without entry or exit wounds. The fluid of choice is generally lactated Ringer's solution, which should be infused with an initial fluid challenge of 20 to 40 ml/kg.

In the emergency department or during interhospital transfer, the patient's intravenous fluid rates will be regulated to maintain a urine output of 75 to 100 ml/hr, which decreases the potential for renal damage caused by myoglobin. In addition, emergency-department management may include administration of *sodium bicarbonate* to maintain an alkaline urine, which increases the solubility of hemoglobin and myoglobin and thus minimizes the incidence of renal failure. *Mannitol* may also be used to increase urinary output and excretion of the hemoglobin and myoglobin proteins.

Lightning Injury

Lightning strikes the earth approximately 7.4 million times each year[7] and accounts for 200 to 300 deaths annually in the United States.[8] It comprises DC of up to 200,000 amps at a potential of 100 million or more volts, with temperatures that vary between 16,000° and 60,000° F. Lightning injuries can occur from a direct strike or by a side flash (splash) between a victim and a nearby object that has been struck by lightning. A total of 30% of those struck by lightning die.

Lightning strikes produce tissue injuries that differ from other types of electrical injury (Fig. 16-

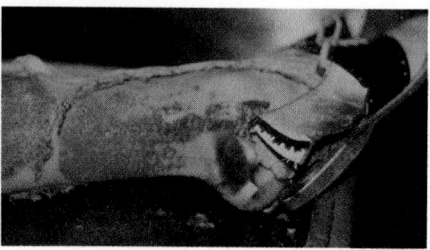

Fig. 16-31 Lightning injury.

31). Because the duration of the lightning is short (1/100 to 1/1000 second), skin burns are less severe than those seen with other high-voltage current, and third-degree burns are rare. Common lightning burns are linear, feathery, and punctate (pinpoint) in appearance. In addition, depending on the severity of the strike, the patient may suffer cardiac and respiratory arrest, which are the most common causes of death in lightning injuries.

Lightning injuries may be classified as minor, moderate, or severe. Patients with minor lightning injuries are usually conscious and are frequently confused and amnestic. Burns or other signs of injury are rare, and vital signs are usually stable.

Patients with moderate injury may be combative or comatose and may have associated injuries from the impact of the lightning strike. First- and second-degree burns are common, as is tympanic membrane rupture. These patients may have serious internal organ damage and should be carefully observed for signs and symptoms of cardiorespiratory dysfunction.

Severe lightning injuries include those that cause immediate brain damage, seizures, respiratory paralysis, and cardiac arrest. Prehospital care is directed at basic and advanced life support measures and rapid transport to an appropriate medical facility.

Assessment and Management

As in any emergency response, scene safety is the first priority. If the electrical storm is still in progress, all patient care activities should take place in a sheltered area. To prevent injury from subsequent lightning strikes, the paramedic crew should stay away from objects that project from the ground, including trees, fences, and high buildings, and avoid areas of open water. If rescue attempts in an open area are necessary, the paramedic should stay low to the ground.

Prehospital management of lightning injuries is the same as for other severe electrical injuries. Initial patient care is directed at airway and ventilatory support, basic and advanced life support, patient immobilization, fluid resuscitation to prevent hypovolemia and renal failure, pharmacological therapy to promote excretion of myoglobin and to treat dysrhythmias, wound care, and rapid transport to an appropriate medical facility. Cardiopulmonary resuscitation should be initiated immediately for patients who appear "dead" because resuscitation is possible after lightning injury.

Radiation Injury

Burns from radiation exposure are rare and are treated like all other kinds of burns. The wounds should be covered with a sterile dressing. Associated injuries are assessed and treated, and the patient is transported for physician evaluation. Special considerations in radiation accidents and personal precautions are described in Chapter 7.

REFERENCES

1. Centers for Disease Control: US Department of Health and Human Services, Public Health Service: *Guidelines for prevention of transmission of human immunodeficiency virus and hepatitis B virus to health-care and public safety workers*, Atlanta, 1989, The Department.
2. Nebraska Burn Institute: *Advanced burn life support course provider's manual*, Lincoln, 1990, The Institute.
3. Achauer B: *Management of the burned patient*, Norwalk, Conn, 1987, Appleton & Lange.
4. Committee on Trauma American College of Surgeons: *Resources for optimal care of the injured patient*, Chicago, 1990, The Committee.
5. McLaughlin E: *Critical care of the burned patient*, Rockville, Md, 1990, Aspen.
6. Martyn J: *Acute management of the burned patient*, Philadelphia, 1990, WB Saunders.
7. Linn A: Avoiding bolts from the blue, *St. Louis Post Dispatch*, August 23, 1988, p. 1D.
8. Fontanarosa P: Boom: lightning and related injuries, *JEMS* 13(7):36, 1988.

Summary

Management of soft tissue injuries and burns often presents a challenge for the emergency care provider. Understanding the consequences of these injuries and appropriate prehospital management can reduce morbidity and mortality in this complex patient group.

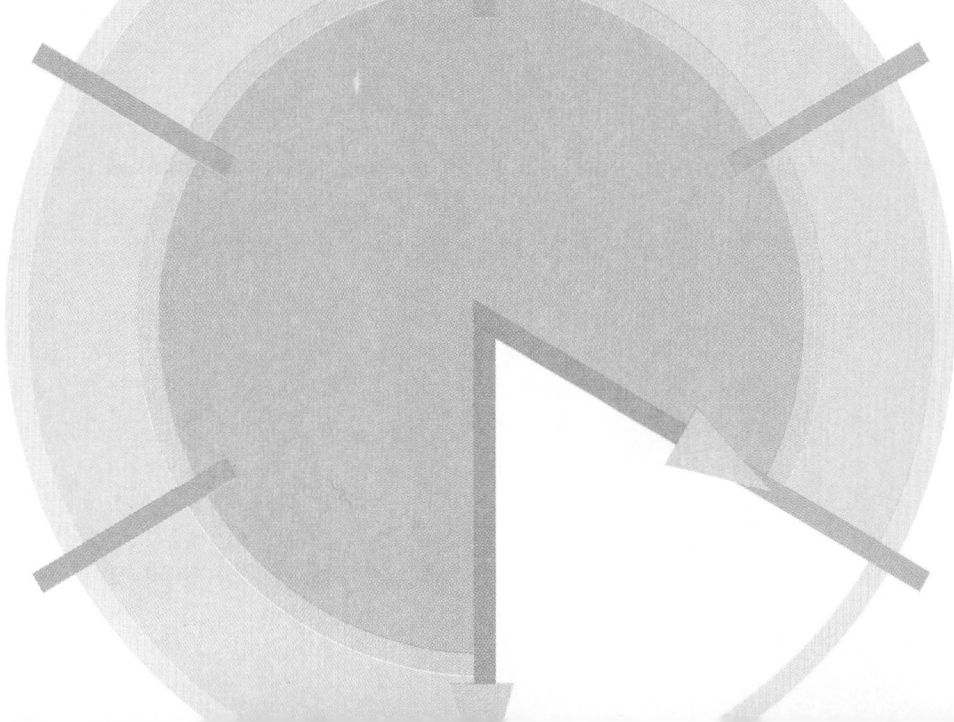

MEDICAL

DIVISION FOUR

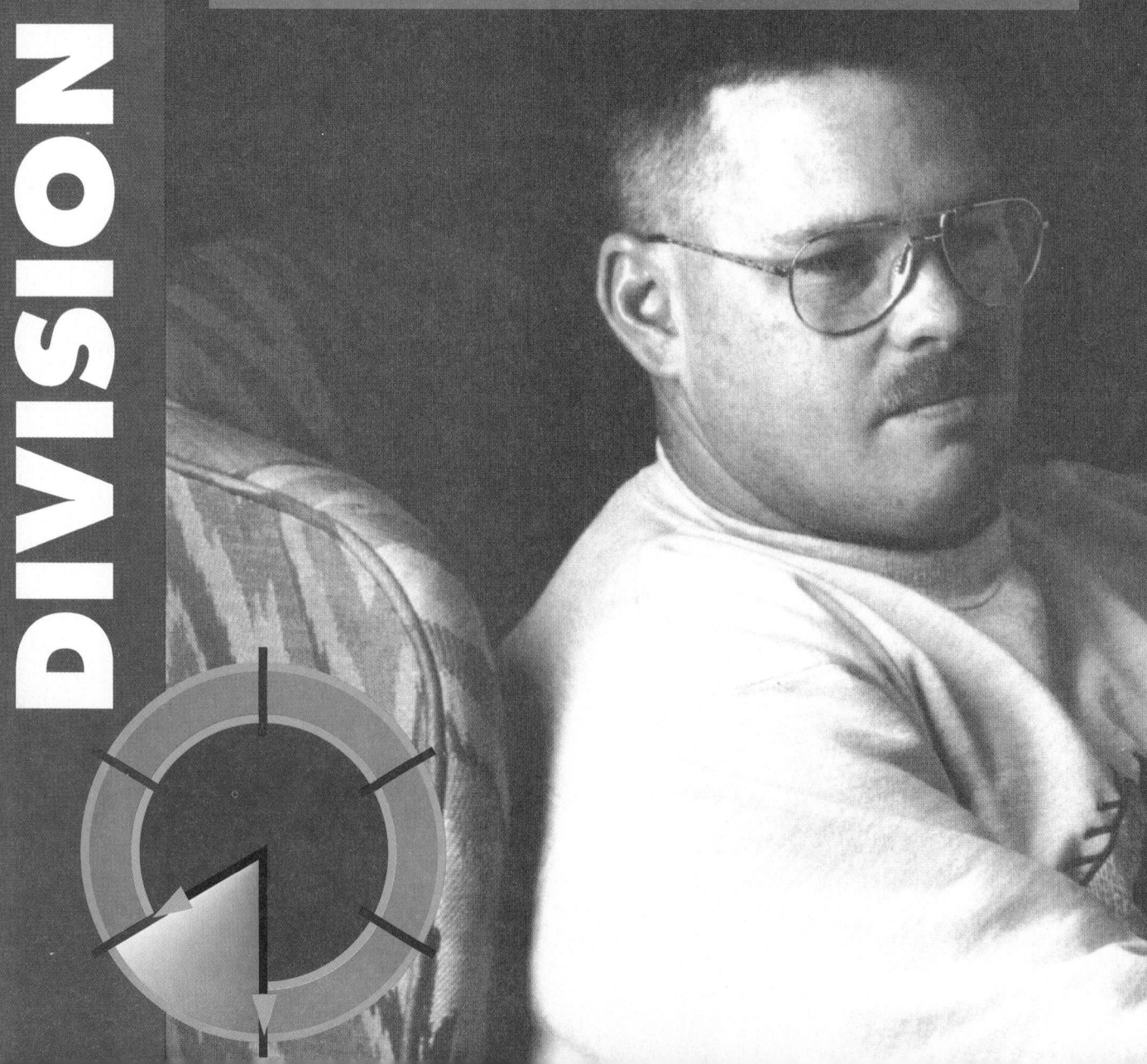

My first experience with a cardiac arrest patient will always be a memorable one. Upon arrival, the rescue squad was performing CPR. The patient was in V-fib, and in two shocks, he regained a sinus rhythm with a perfusing pulse. I intubated him, started an IV, and administered cardiac drugs. En route, the patient regained consciousness and was able to answer questions. Unfortunately, not all cardiac arrest calls are success stories, as I learned in my career!

Rick Gower, TSgt, USAF, NREMT-P
Andrews Air Force Base, Maryland

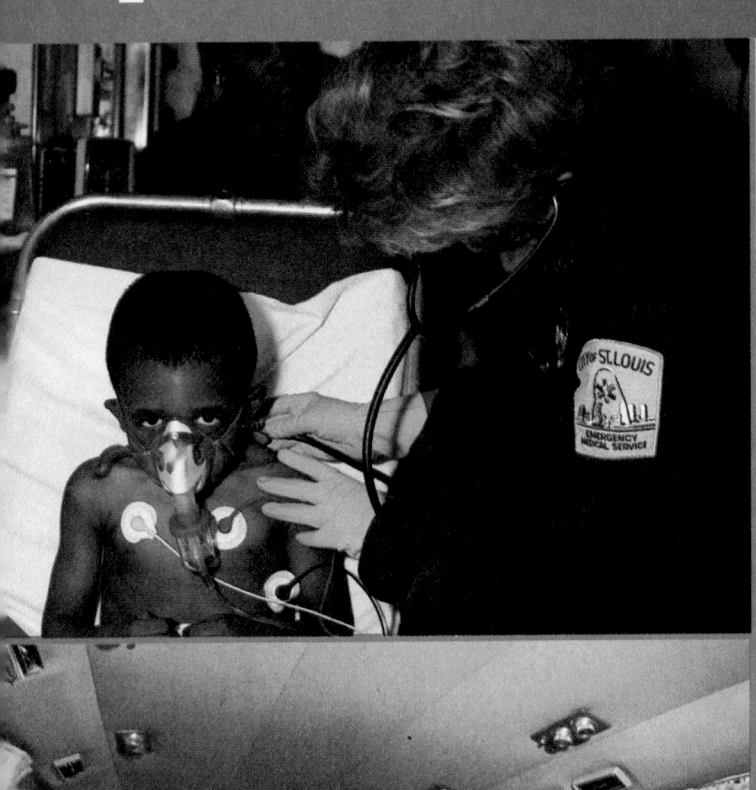

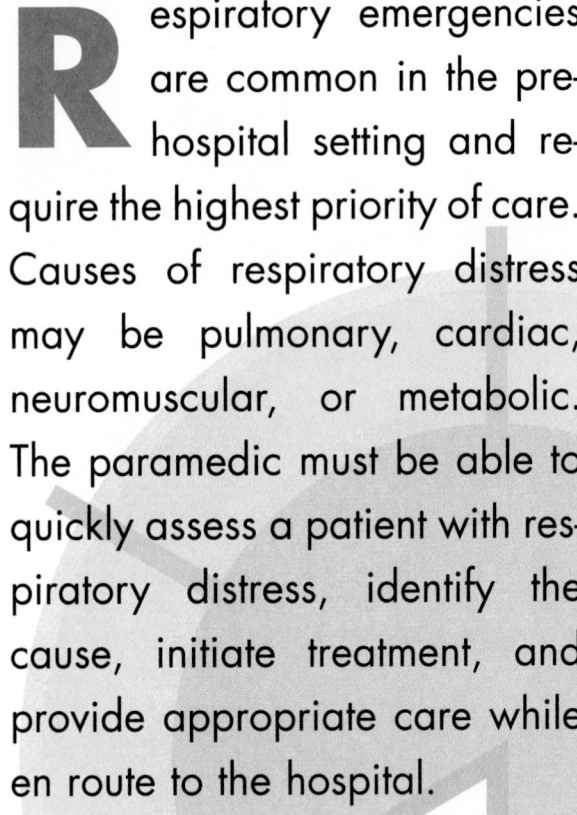

Respiratory emergencies are common in the prehospital setting and require the highest priority of care. Causes of respiratory distress may be pulmonary, cardiac, neuromuscular, or metabolic. The paramedic must be able to quickly assess a patient with respiratory distress, identify the cause, initiate treatment, and provide appropriate care while en route to the hospital.

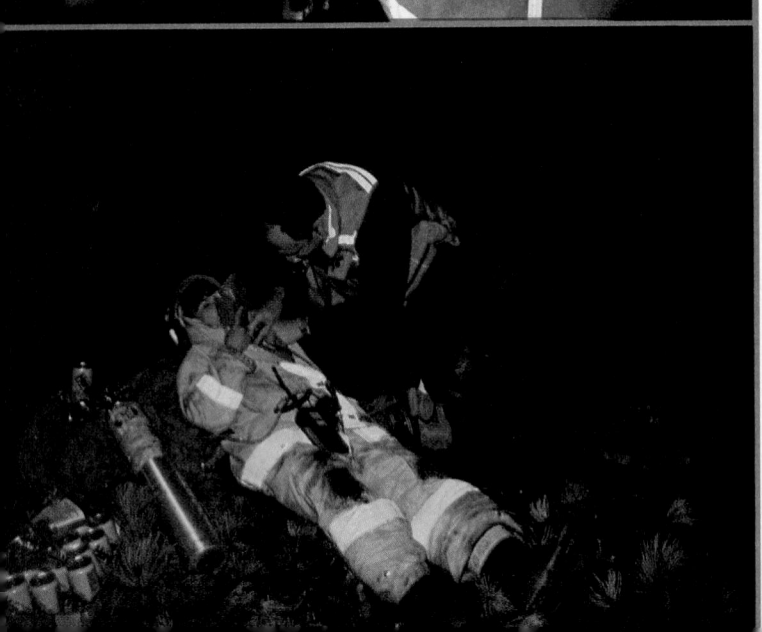

OBJECTIVES

As a paramedic, you should be able to:

1. Describe pathophysiology, assessment, and management of the following non-infectious respiratory disorders:
   a. Adult respiratory distress syndrome
   b. Obstructive airway disease
   c. Chronic obstructive pulmonary disease
   d. Asthma
   e. Cystic fibrosis
   f. Pulmonary embolism
   g. Pickwickian syndrome
   h. Central nervous system dysfunction
2. Describe pathophysiology as a basis for key signs and symptoms, patient assessment, and management of the following infectious respiratory disorders:
   a. Pleurisy
   b. Influenza
   c. Pneumonia
   d. Legionnaire's disease
   e. Tuberculosis

● NONINFECTIOUS RESPIRATORY DISORDERS

Noninfectious respiratory disorders result from serious injury or illness such as chronic obstructive pulmonary disease, asthma, cystic fibrosis, pulmonary embolism, Pickwickian syndrome, and central nervous system dysfunction.

Adult Respiratory Distress Syndrome

Adult respiratory distress syndrome (ARDS) (also known as *noncardiogenic pulmonary edema*) is a term used to describe a complex ventilation disorder caused by increased capillary permeability. The syndrome develops as a complication of in-jury or illness such as trauma, inhaled toxins, gastric aspiration, hematological disorders, infections, drug overdose, or toxic metabolic disorders. Regardless of the specific cause, increased capillary permeability results in a clinical condition in which the lungs are wet and heavy, congested, hemorrhagic, and stiff, with decreased perfusion capacity across alveolar membranes. As a result, there is a decrease in pulmonary compliance, requiring higher airway pressure for each breath.

ARDS leads to severe hypoxemia, intrapulmonary shunting, reduced lung compliance, and in some cases, irreversible parenchymal lung damage. Unique to this syndrome is that most patients who develop ARDS have healthy lungs before the event that caused the disease. ARDS is more common in men than women and has a mortality rate of over 50%. Complications include respiratory failure, cardiac dysrhythmias, disseminated intra-

KEY TERMS

asthma: A respiratory disorder characterized by recurring episodes of paroxysmal dyspnea, wheezing on expiration caused by constriction of the bronchi, coughing, and viscous mucoid bronchial secretions.

chronic obstructive pulmonary disease: A progressive and irreversible condition characterized by diminished inspiratory and expiratory capacity of the lungs.

pulmonary embolism: The blockage of a pulmonary artery by foreign matter such as fat, air, tumor tissue, or a thrombus, which usually arises from a peripheral vein.

pulmonary hypertension: A condition of abnormally high pressure within the pulmonary circulation.

tubercle: A characteristic lesion that results from infection by tubercle bacilli.

vascular coagulation, barotrauma, congestive heart failure, and renal failure.

Management

Patients with ARDS usually have tachypnea, labored breathing, and impaired gas exchange 12 to 72 hours after the initial injury or medical crisis. Because the syndrome is often a complication of another illness or injury, the paramedic should consider the pathophysiology of the underlying problem and provide supplemental oxygen and ventilatory support to improve arterial oxygenation.

Most patients with moderate-to-severe respiratory distress require mechanical ventilatory support with positive end expiratory pressure (PEEP). PEEP maintains a degree of positive pressure at the end of exhalation to keep alveoli open and to push fluid from the alveoli back into the interstitium or capillaries. Ventilatory support with PEEP can be accomplished in the prehospital setting through intubation and the use of a Boehringer valve, a cylinder in which a metal ball is suspended (Fig. 17-1). The Boehringer valve is connected to the expiratory port of a bag-valve device and creates PEEP by forcing the patient to exhale against the weight of the metal ball (available in 5-, 10-, and 15-cm water pressures).

> **NOTE:**
> This type of ventilatory support requires special training and authorization from medical control. PEEP may cause adverse circulatory effects (including decreased venous return, decreased cardiac output, and decreased oxygen delivery) and pulmonary barotrauma (pneumothorax and pneumomediastinum).

Depending on the underlying cause of ARDS, prehospital management may also include fluid replacement to maintain cardiac output and peripheral perfusion, drug therapy to support mechanical ventilation, and the use of pharmacological agents such as corticosteroids and diuretics (all of which are controversial in treating ARDS).

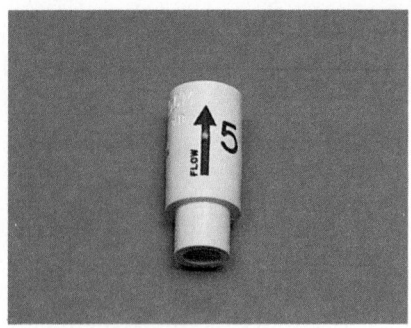

Fig. 17-1 Boehringer valve.

Obstructive Airway Disease

Obstructive airway disease is a major health problem in the United States, affecting some 17 million Americans. According to the National Health Institute, pulmonary disease is responsible for one of every eight deaths and is a significant factor in one of every four deaths.[1] Predisposing factors that contribute to obstructive pulmonary disease include smoking, environmental pollution, industrial exposures, and various pulmonary infectious processes during childhood.

Obstructive airway disease is a triad of distinct diseases that often coexist: chronic bronchitis and emphysema (together referred to as **chronic obstructive pulmonary disease** [COPD]) and asthma, which may progress to COPD. Although these diseases are presented separately in this chapter, the paramedic should remember that different degrees of each are frequently present in the same patient.

Chronic Bronchitis

Chronic bronchitis is a clinical description that refers to excessive mucous secretions and inflammatory changes in the bronchial tree (Fig. 17-2). It results from prolonged exposure to irritants (most commonly, cigarette smoke) and is clinically diagnosed by the presence of cough with sputum occurring on most days for at least 3 months in the year and for at least 2 consecutive years. The alveoli are not seriously affected, and diffusion remains relatively normal.

Patients with severe chronic bronchitis (sometimes called *blue bloaters* when they appear cyanotic) have a low oxygen pressure (Po_2) because

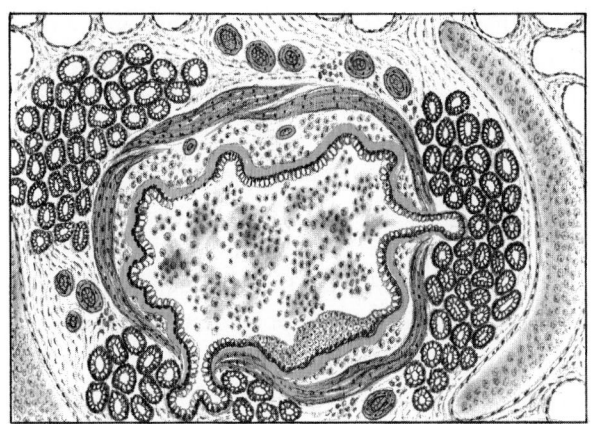

Fig. 17-2 Chronic bronchitis. Bronchi are filled with excess mucus.

of altered ventilation-perfusion relationships in the lung and hypoventilation. The hypoventilation leads to hypercapnia, hypoxemia, and increases in arterial carbon dioxide pressure (P_{CO_2}). The increase in P_{CO_2} constricts the pulmonary circulation, leading to pulmonary hypertension and eventually cor pulmonale.

Patients with chronic bronchitis have frequent respiratory infections that eventually result in scarring of lung tissue. In time, irreversible changes occur in the lung, with resultant emphysema or bronchiectasis (an abnormal dilation of the bronchi caused by a pus-producing infection of the bronchial wall).

Pulmonary Hypertension

Pulmonary hypertension in an elevation of mean pulmonary artery pressure and systolic pulmonary artery pressure under resting conditions. The syndrome usually results from progressive disease of pulmonary vessels or lung parenchyma, but often the exact cause remains unknown. This discussion is limited to pulmonary hypertension resulting from chronic lung disease.

In obstructive lung disease, several factors contribute to chronic vasoconstriction, including parenchymal lung damage, hypoxemia, erythrocytosis, and the possible release of chemical mediators. The vasoconstriction of the pulmonary vessels increases the force required by the right ventricle to pump blood through the lungs. Over time, the right ventricle hypertrophies and further increases

its systolic pressure. Eventually, right-sided heart failure occurs.

In early stages, right-sided heart failure from pulmonary disease occurs only during periods of increased stress on the heart. In later stages, these stresses are consistently present, evidenced by jugular vein distention, hepatomegaly, and peripheral edema. A complication of pulmonary hypertension is cor pulmonale.

Cor Pulmonale

Cor pulmonale is a secondary condition of pathological hypertrophy and dilation of the right ventricle of the heart. It results from disease processes that affect the function or structure of the lung or its vasculature. Cor pulmonale may occur with or without congestive heart failure. The most common causes of cor pulmonale are obstructive lung disease, restrictive lung disease, and vascular diseases. COPD is responsible for approximately 75% of cases of cor pulmonale in the United States.

Emphysema

Emphysema is an anatomical description of pathological changes in the lung; it is the end stage of a process that progresses slowly for many years. The disease is characterized by permanent abnormal enlargement of the air spaces beyond the terminal bronchioles, destruction of the alveoli, and failure of the supporting structures to maintain alveolar integrity (Fig. 17-3). Besides reducing the alveolar functional surface area, it reduces elasticity, leading to trapping of air. Thus residual volume increases while vital capacity remains relatively normal.

The associated reduction in arterial P_{O_2} leads to increased red blood cell production and polycythemia (an elevated hematocrit). This elevation in hematocrit is much more common in the "blue bloater" (chronic bronchitis) than the "pink puffer" (predominantly emphysema) because the former is more often chronically hypoxemic. Decreases in alveolar membrane surface area and in the number of pulmonary capillaries in the lung decrease the area for gas exchange and increase resistance to pulmonary blood flow, ultimately causing pulmonary hypertension.

Patients with emphysema have some resistance to airflow in and out of the lungs, but most of the hyperexpansion results from air trapping secondary to the loss of elastic recoil (Fig. 17-4). Chronic bronchitics have increased airway resistance in inspiration and expiration, whereas emphysema patients have increased airway resistance only on expiration. Normally an involuntary act, expiration becomes a muscular act in patients with COPD. Over time, the chest becomes rigid (barrel shaped), and the patient must use accessory muscles of the neck to breathe. Full deflation of the lungs become increasingly difficult and finally impossible. Often, the patient with emphysema is thin because of poor dietary intake and the increased caloric consumption required for the work of breathing. The patient with chronic bronchitis, by comparison, does not usually appear thin because of edema secondary to right ventricular failure.

Pulmonary hypertension may ultimately lead to cor pulmonale and death in emphysemic or bronchitic patients, but it is a late finding in patients with predominantly emphysema. These categories are not pure and exclusive. Most patients have pathological changes consistent with emphysema *and* bronchitis, but frequently one or the other dominates the clinical findings.

Assessment

Patients with COPD are generally aware of and have adapted to their illness. A request for emer-

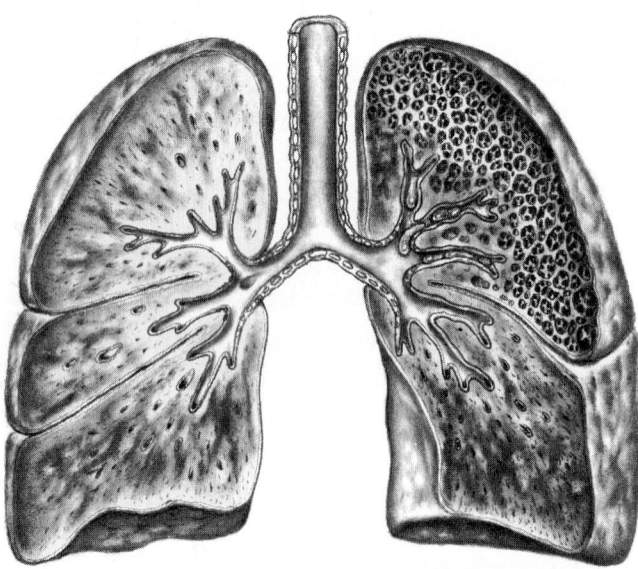

Fig. 17-3 Cystic changes of lobar emphysema resulting from destruction of alveoli.

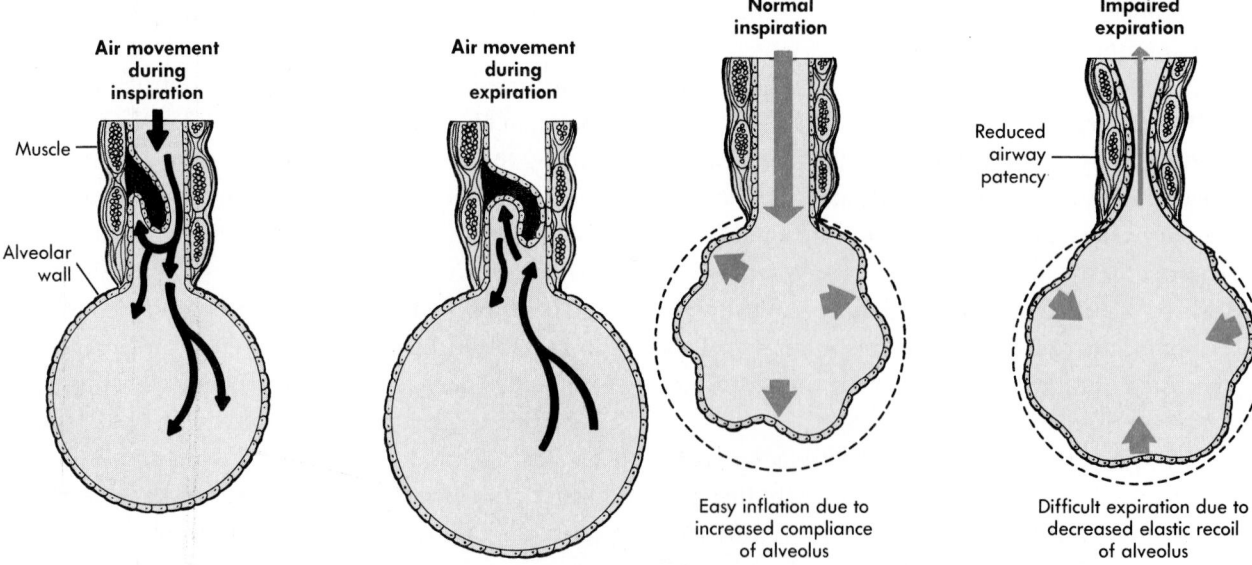

Fig. 17-4 Mechanism of air trapping in COPD: Mucous plugs and narrowed airways cause air trapping and hyperinflation on expiration. During inspiration, the airways enlarge, allowing gas to flow past the obstruction. This mechanism of air trapping occurs in asthma and chronic bronchitis. Mechanism of air trapping in emphysema: Damaged or destroyed alveolar walls no longer support and hold open the airways, and alveoli lose their property of elastic recoil. Both of these factors contribute to collapse during expiration.

gency care indicates that a significant change has occurred in the patient's condition. The patient with COPD usually presents with an acute episode of worsening dyspnea that is manifested even at rest, an increase or change in sputum production, or an increase in the malaise that accompanies the disease. Other common complaints include inability to sleep and recurrent headache.

On EMS arrival, the patient with COPD is likely to be in respiratory distress. Often, the patient is sitting upright and leaning forward to facilitate breathing; such patients frequently use pursed-lip breathing with a long expiratory effort to expel trapped air. In addition, use of accessory muscles needed for trying to ventilate against an obstructive lesion in the airway can result in respiratory fatigue. Increases in hypoxemia and hypercarbia may be evidenced by tachypnea, diaphoresis, cyanosis, confusion, irritability, and drowsiness.

Other physical findings include wheezes, rhonchi, and crackles, which occur mainly on inspiration. Breath sounds and heart sounds may also be diminished because of reduced air exchange and the increased diameter of the thoracic cavity. In late stages of decompensation, the patient may have peripheral cyanosis, clubbing of the fingers, and signs of right-sided heart failure. The electrocardiogram (ECG) may reveal cardiac dysrhythmias or signs of atrial enlargement.

Management

The primary goal of prehospital care for these patients is correction of hypoxemia through improved airflow. This can be accomplished through oxygen administration and pharmacological therapy. Either therapy can produce serious side effects and complications, particularly if the patient has used medication before EMS arrival. Therefore it is important for the paramedic to obtain a thorough medical history regarding medication use, home oxygen use, and drug allergies.

All patients should have an intravenous line established and kept open and a cardiac monitor applied. If the patient has a productive cough, coughing should be encouraged. Any sputum should be collected and delivered with the patient for laboratory analysis.

Patients with COPD rely on a hypoxic drive for their ventilatory effort, so most authorities recommend that supplemental oxygen be administered judiciously by nasal cannula at initial flow rates of 2 L/min or less. If the hypoxia does not improve or if respiratory distress continues, the concentration of delivered oxygen should be increased in increments (steps of 2 L/min for several minutes at each step), with constant monitoring and reassessment. *The paramedic should never withhold oxygen because of fear of decreasing hypoxic drive.* Pulse oximetry to measure oxygen saturation should be considered and ventilations assisted as needed.

Medications useful in treating the reversible components of COPD in the prehospital setting include beta agonists (*terbutaline, albuterol*) and occasionally xanthine bronchodilators such as *aminophylline.* (Refer to Chapter 14 and the Emergency Drug Index for specific drug therapy.)

Asthma

Asthma, or reactive airway disease, is a common disorder that affects nearly 10 million Americans and is responsible for 4000 to 5000 deaths each year.[2] Asthma is most common in children and young adults but can occur in any decade of life. The disease may be divided into two types: extrinsic and intrinsic. Extrinsic asthma commonly has onset in childhood, whereas intrinsic asthma more commonly has adult onset. Childhood asthma often improves or resolves with age, but adult asthma is usually persistent. A total of 50% of all asthma develops in patients before the age of 10 and another 33% before age 30. There may be a familial tendency toward the disease of asthma.

There are differences in the factors that precipitate intrinsic and extrinsic asthma attacks. Intrinsic asthma results from hypersensitivity to allergens such as dust, lint, insecticides, food, and pollen and to drugs such as aspirin (which accounts for 10% of attacks). Cold temperature, respiratory infections, vigorous exercise, and emotional stress, on the other hand, can trigger both attacks. Regardless of the cause, the pathophysiological sequence is similar (Fig. 17-5).

Pathophysiology of an Asthma Attack

Asthma generally occurs in acute attacks of variable duration, between which the patient is

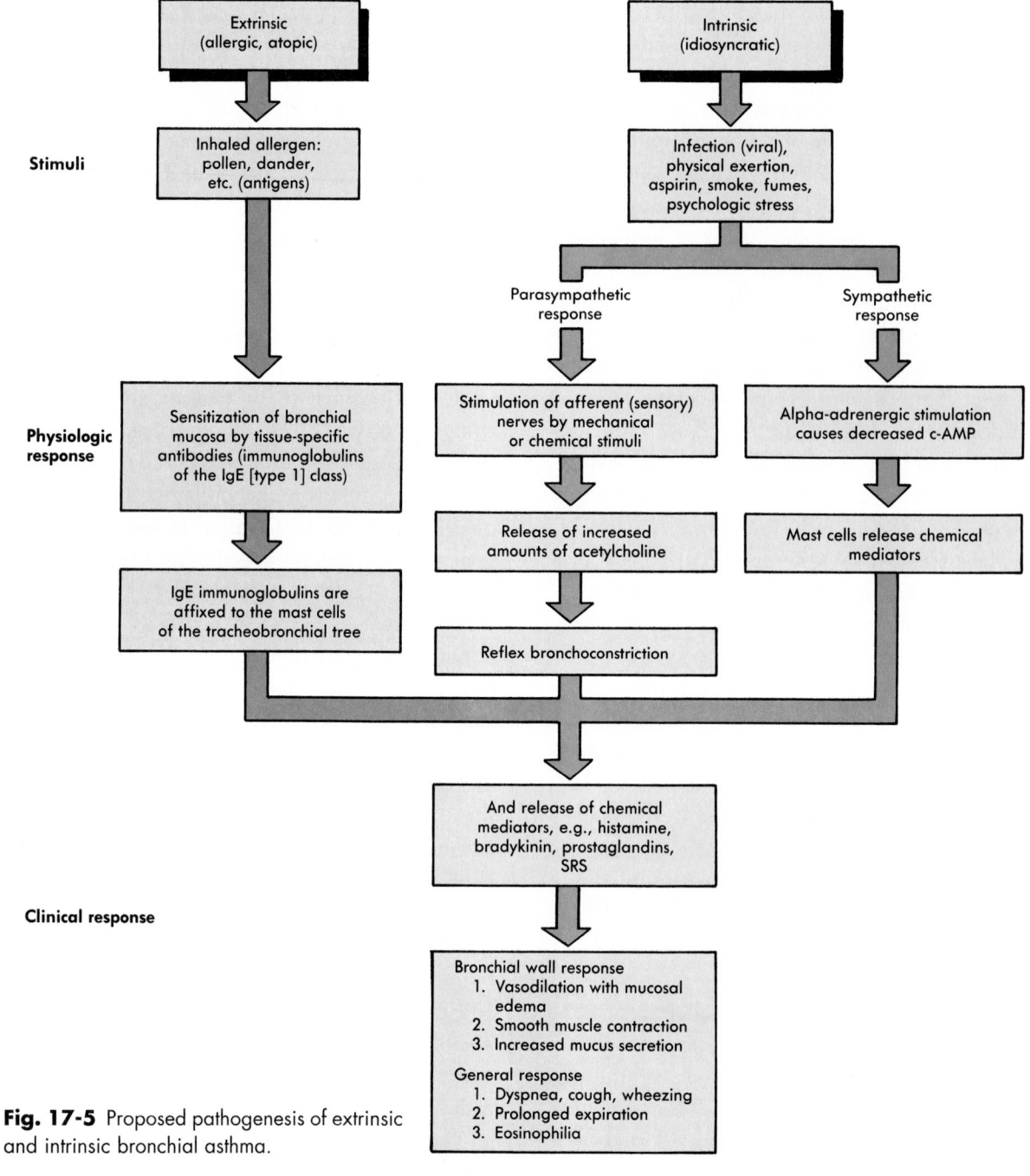

Fig. 17-5 Proposed pathogenesis of extrinsic and intrinsic bronchial asthma.

relatively symptom free. The attack is characterized by reversible airflow obstruction caused by bronchial smooth muscle contraction, hypersecretion of mucus resulting in bronchial plugging, and inflammatory changes in the bronchial walls (Fig. 17-6). With increased resistance to airflow, there is alveolar hypoventilation and marked ventilation-perfusion mismatching (leading to hypoxemia) and carbon dioxide retention (stimulating hyper-

ventilation). The increased airway resistance also leads to air trapping.

During an acute attack, the combination of increased airway resistance, increased respiratory drive, and air trapping creates excessive demand on the muscles of respiration. This leads to greater accessory muscle use and increases the potential for respiratory fatigue. If labored breathing continues, excessive negative intrathoracic pressure

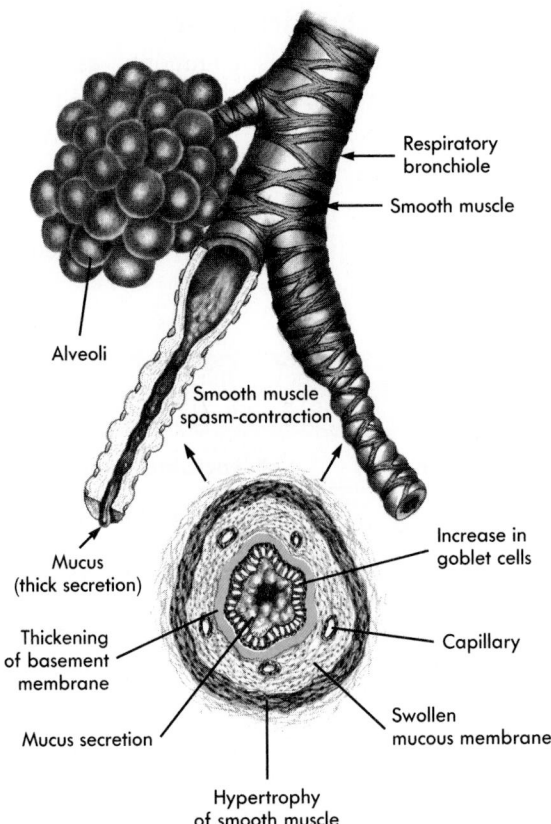

Fig. 17-6 With bronchial asthma, the bronchiole is obstructed on expiration, particularly by muscle spasm, edema of the mucosa, and thick secretions.

may decrease left ventricular preload. The result is a transient reduction in cardiac output and systolic blood pressure, with the subsequent physical findings of a pulsus paradoxus (a decrease in systolic pressure of more than 10 mm Hg during inspiration when compared with that during expiration). If the attack remains unabated, hypoxemia and perhaps the hemodynamic alterations may lead to death.

Assessment

On EMS arrival, the patient is usually sitting upright, leaning forward with hands on knees (tripod position), and using accessory muscles to facilitate breathing. The typical asthmatic is in obvious respiratory distress, with rapid and loud respirations. Audible wheezing may be present. The patient's mental status should be noted and monitored carefully. Lethargy, exhaustion, agitation, and confusion are ominous signs of impending respiratory failure. An initial history must be quickly obtained. Questions regarding onset, relative severity, medication use, and precipitating cause of the attack should be specific and to the point. If the asthmatic attack is so severe that the patient cannot speak, P_{O_2} is probably less than 40 torr.

On auscultation, there may be a prolonged expiratory phase, usually with wheezing from the movement of air through the narrowed airways. Inspiratory wheezing (unlike inspiratory stridor) does not indicate upper airway occlusion but suggests that the large and midsize muscular airways are obstructed to a greater degree than if only expiratory wheezes are heard. Inspiratory wheezes (also known as *rhonchi*) may also suggest large airway secretions. A silent chest indicates such severe obstruction that flow rates are too low to generate breath sounds. Other signs of severe asthma include:

- Diaphoresis and pallor
- Retractions
- Inability to speak
- Pulse rate greater than 130 beats per minute
- Respirations greater than 30 breaths per minute
- Pulsus paradoxus above 20 mm Hg
- Altered mental status

> **NOTE:**
> Asthma patients are true medical emergencies. Treatment should be aggressive, and observation for deterioration, which can be unexpected, rapid, and fatal, must be vigilant. Initial patient management should be directed at ensuring an adequate airway, providing humidified supplemental oxygen, and reversing the bronchospasm.

Management

Pharmacological therapy is based on the patient's age and medication use before EMS arrival. The initial medications prescribed by medical control will probably be those with a short onset of action (for example, *epinephrine, albuterol,* or *terbutaline).* Medical control can also prescribe rehydration through the administration of intravenous fluids. All patients with acute asthma should be transported in a position of comfort to maximize use of respiratory muscles and monitored for cardiac rhythm disturbances.

Status Asthmaticus

Status asthmaticus refers to a severe, prolonged asthma attack that cannot be broken with repeated doses of bronchodilators. It may be of sudden onset (resulting from spasm of the airways), or it may be more insidious. Frequently it is precipitated by a viral respiratory infection. Status asthmaticus is a true emergency that requires early recognition and immediate transport. These patients are in imminent danger of respiratory failure.

Patient management guidelines for status asthmaticus are the same as those for acute asthma attacks, but the urgency of rapid transport is more important. In addition, these patients are usually dehydrated and require intravenous fluid administration. The patient's respiratory status should be closely monitored, and the paramedic should anticipate the need for intubation and aggressive ventilatory support.

Differential Considerations

Although wheezing is commonly associated with asthma, it may also be present with other diseases that cause dyspnea (Table 17-1). For example, tachypnea, wheezing, and respiratory distress may indicate heart failure, pneumonia, pulmonary edema, pulmonary embolism, pneumo-

TABLE 17-1 Diseases and Symptoms Associated with Wheezing

Disease	Associated Symptoms
Asthma	Productive cough, tightness in chest
Bacterial pneumonia	Productive cough, pleuritic pain
Chronic bronchitis	Chronic, productive cough
Emphysema	Cough
Foreign body aspiration	Cough
Heart failure	Cough, orthopnea, nocturnal dyspnea
Pneumothorax	Sudden, sharp pleuritic pain
Pulmonary congestion	Tachypnea, cough
Pulmonary embolism	Sudden, sharp pleuritic pain
Toxic inhalation	Cough, pain

Fig. 17-7 CF is a disorder of the exocrine glands that causes those glands to produce abnormally thick secretions of mucus. The glands most affected are the respiratory, pancreatic, and sweat glands.

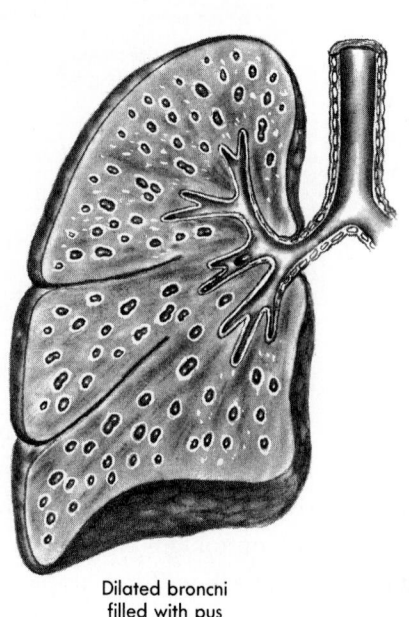

Dilated broncni filled with pus

Increased goblet cells in airway epithelium
Increased submucosal size glands

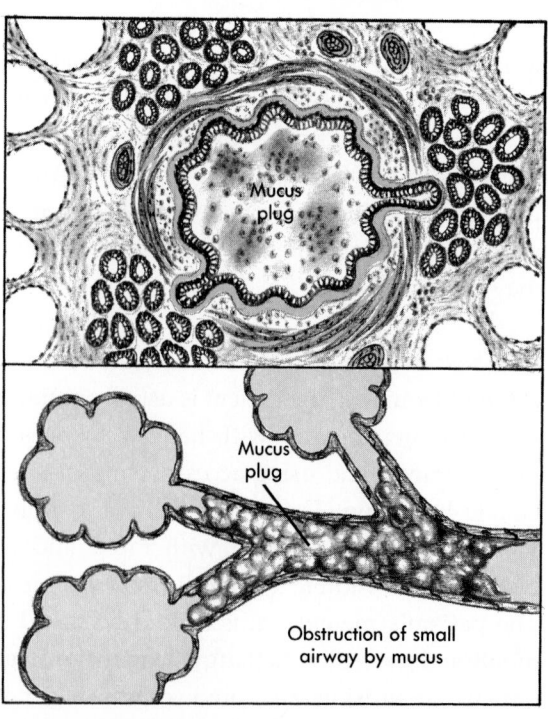

Mucus plug

Mucus plug

Obstruction of small airway by mucus

thorax, toxic inhalation, foreign body aspiration, and various other pathological states. Only through gathering a complete history and performing a thorough patient assessment can appropriate emergency care decisions be made.

Cystic Fibrosis

Cystic fibrosis (CF) is an inherited disorder of the exocrine glands that causes abnormal secretion of thick mucus, which plugs the bronchi (Fig. 17-7). It is the most common cause of life-threatening pulmonary disease of European Americans during childhood and adolescence. The disease is less prevalent among African Americans, Native Americans, and Asian Americans. CF is a fatal illness, the median age of death being approximately 22 years for women and 28 years for men. Death is usually a result of respiratory insufficiency and secondary pulmonary hypertension and cor pulmonale.

Patients with CF have associated chronic bronchitis, chronic sinusitis, emphysema, and respiratory failure, which usually develop at an early age (2 to 20 years). Thick mucous plugs cause bronchial obstruction leading to areas of atelectasis and hyperinflation. As the disease progresses, hypoxia, hypercapnia, acidosis, pulmonary hypertension, and cor pulmonale ensue. In addition, these patients usually suffer from pancreatic insufficiency and increased sweat-chloride levels.

Signs and Symptoms

Patients with CF may have severe dyspnea and respiratory distress similar to those of patients with other forms of obstructive pulmonary disease. Most of these patients have wheezing on auscultation (if tidal volumes are sufficient to produce audible wheezing). Other signs and symptoms include cough, tachypnea, tachycardia, cyanosis, chest hyperexpansion, and diminished breath sounds. Use of accessory muscles during ventilation is common. Most patients are aware of their disease.

Management

Emergency care for patients with CF includes airway management, supplemental oxygen ad-

ministration, and in severe cases of respiratory distress, the use of bronchodilators (beta-adrenergic sympathomimetics). Definitive care usually includes in-hospital therapy to minimize bronchial plugging and inhibit bacterial colonization.

Pulmonary Embolism

Pulmonary embolism (PE) refers to blockage of a pulmonary artery by a clot or other foreign material that has traveled there from another place of origin, usually the lower extremities (Fig. 17-8). It is a relatively common disorder that affects approximately 650,000 individuals each year in the United States. Of this number, approximately 38% of the patients die from the emboli, 10% within the first hour after blockage.[3]

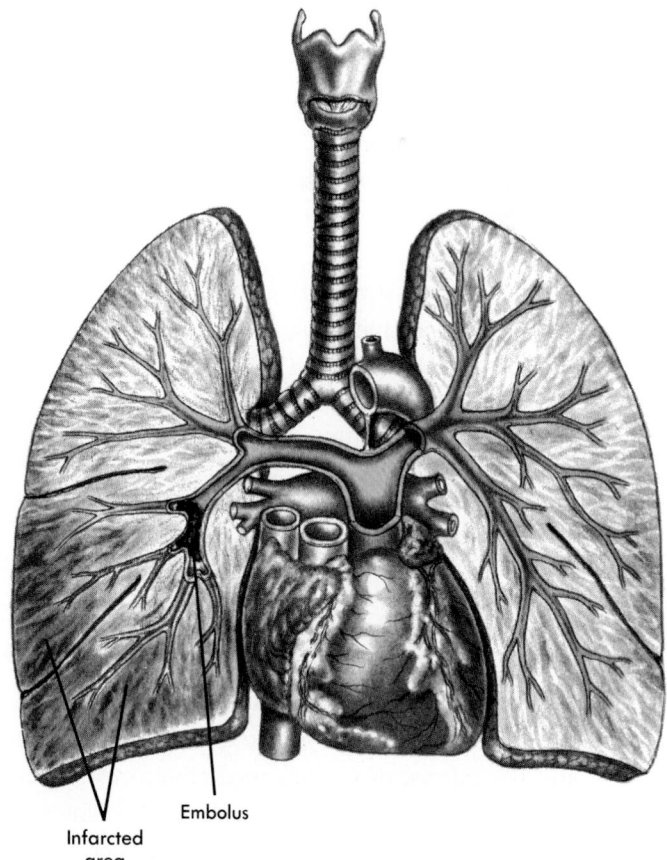

Embolus

Infarcted area

Fig. 17-8 PE is the blockage of a pulmonary artery by foreign matter, such as a thrombus, that usually arises from a peripheral vein, fat, air, or tumor tissue. The blockage obstructs blood supply to the lung tissue.

PE usually begins as venous disease. It is most often caused by migration of a thrombus from the large veins of the lower extremities, but it can also occur as a result of fat, air, or tumor tissue. The clot or embolus dislodges and travels through the venous system to the right side of the heart. From there it migrates to the pulmonary arteries, obstructing blood supply to the lung. The most common sites for thrombus formation are the deep veins of the legs and pelvis. Six factors that contribute to the development of venous thrombosis are:

1. Venostasis
   a. Extended travel
   b. Prolonged bed rest
   c. Obesity
   d. Advanced age
   e. Burns
   f. Varicose veins
2. Venous injury
   a. Surgery of the thorax, abdomen, pelvis, or legs
   b. Fractures of the pelvis or legs
3. Increased blood coagulability
   a. Malignancy
   b. Oral contraceptives
4. Pregnancy
5. Disease
   a. Chronic lung disease
   b. Congestive heart failure
   c. Atrial fibrillation
   d. Myocardial infarction
   e. Previous pulmonary embolism
   f. Previous deep vein thrombosis
   g. Infection
   h. Diabetes mellitus
6. Multiple trauma

When one or more pulmonary arteries occlude, the embolism produces an area of lung that is ventilated but hypoperfused. In response, a reflex bronchoconstriction results from hypocarbia and the release of various mediators (most notably, histamine and serotonin) from the clot formation, causing blood vessels to constrict. If the patient's vascular obstruction is severe (60% or greater pulmonary occlusion), hypoxemia, acute pulmonary hypertension, systemic hypotension, and shock may rapidly occur, with subsequent death.

Signs and Symptoms

The cross-sectional area of pulmonary vasculature obstructed may be small, moderate, or massive; therefore pulmonary embolus may present very differently. Signs and symptoms depend on the location and size of the clot and may include dyspnea, cough, hemoptysis, pain, anxiety, syncope, hypotension, diaphoresis, tachypnea, tachycardia, fever, and distended neck veins. In addition, chest splinting, pleuritic pain, pleural friction rub, crackles, and localized wheezing may be present. The paramedic should consider a PE in any patient who has cardiorespiratory problems that cannot be otherwise explained, particularly when the risk factors are present.

Management

Prehospital care is primarily supportive. Supplemental oxygen should be administered, a cardiac monitor applied, and an intravenous line of normal saline or lactated Ringer's solution established. The patient should be transported in a position of comfort. Definitive care requires hospitalization and anticoagulant therapy.

Pickwickian Syndrome

Pickwickian syndrome (from the description of a character in Dickens's *Pickwick Papers*) is a term used to describe a condition of extreme obesity, somnolence, and apneic episodes. The syndrome is thought to be a form of sleep apnea sometimes accompanied by cardiac rhythm disturbances.

Patients with pickwickian syndrome usually complain of headache and episodes of inappropriate dozing. Cyanosis from hypoventilation, muscle twitching, and signs of right-sided heart failure may be present. Prehospital management is primarily supportive: ventilation assistance as needed, oxygen administration, cardiac monitoring, and transportation for physician evaluation. Definitive treatment is directed toward weight reduction, although surgery and tracheostomy may be required.

Central Nervous System Dysfunction

Central nervous system injury, cerebral vascular accident, and the use of some drugs, including narcotics and barbiturates, can depress or alter respiratory muscles or the nerves that supply them. In addition, diseases of the respiratory muscles or nerves may affect an individual's ability to respond to the respiratory drive. These diseases include myasthenia gravis and Guillain-Barré syndrome.

Myasthenia Gravis

Myasthenia gravis is a relatively uncommon disease characterized by pronounced muscular weakness. Although it probably has multiple etiologies, the condition is usually associated with circulating antiacetylcholine-receptor antibodies that affect postsynaptic acetylcholine-receptor sites. Therefore the nerve impulses that cause muscle contraction do not easily reach the muscles.

The onset of myasthenia gravis is gradual, and the course of the disease varies greatly from one person to another. In myasthenia crisis, there may be a sudden onset of respiratory paralysis. When this occurs, the prognosis is usually poor. Signs and symptoms of the disease include:

- Increasing fatigue
- Poor inspiratory effort
- Delayed recovery of muscle strength
- Weak eye, facial, and jaw muscles
- Diplopia
- Dysphagia
- Inability to handle secretions (potential for aspiration)

Prehospital care of these patients is usually limited to supportive airway therapy and transportation for physician evaluation. Definitive care includes administration of drugs (cholinergics, steroids, or immunosuppressants), surgery (thymectomy), or both.

Guillain-Barré Syndrome

Guillain-Barré syndrome is a symptom complex thought to follow infectious diseases, exposure to toxins, and collagen vascular diseases. The illness is also thought to develop after certain vaccinations or immunizations; a disproportionately large number of cases were reported after massive immunization against the "swine flu" in 1976.[4] In approximately 50% of cases, the syndrome follows an acute febrile episode associated with a mild upper respiratory or gastrointestinal infection.

The syndrome usually presents first with weakness and paralysis of the lower extremities, which are more severely affected than the upper extremities. Progression may be rapid or take several days. If the medulla is involved, respiratory arrest or cardiovascular collapse can occur. Prehospital management consists of general supportive care and transportation for physician evaluation. Signs and symptoms of Guillain-Barré syndrome are:

- Tingling sensation in the extremities (for hours to days)
- Severely depressed deep tendon reflexes
- Symmetrical paralysis, usually beginning in the lower extremities and gradually ascending to the respiratory muscles
- Much more prominent motor involvement than sensory involvement (helps to differentiate from cord lesion)

● INFECTIOUS RESPIRATORY DISORDERS

The respiratory tract is the most common site of infection, and respiratory infections are the most common category of disease in the industrialized world. Contributing to susceptibility to respiratory infections are exposure to infectious persons, chronic lung disease, immune deficiency disorders, malnourishment, and extremes in age (older adults and children). The infectious respiratory disorders discussed in this chapter are pleurisy, influenza, pneumonia, Legionnaires' disease, and tuberculosis. (Epiglottitis, bronchiolitis, and croup, which are common respiratory disorders in children, are addressed in Chapter 27.) Health care providers are susceptible to these and other infectious diseases, so personal protective measures, including the use of masks for the patient and paramedic, should always be taken when providing patient care.

Pleurisy

Pleurisy is the result of inflammation of the pleura. It is a common manifestation of a number of respiratory diseases, including bacterial or viral respiratory infection, tuberculosis, lung tumor (particularly pleural based), pulmonary embolism, rib fractures or contusions, and intercostal muscle involvement. In addition, pleurisy can result from direct pulmonary trauma.

Pleurisy may be classified as pleurisy with effusion, in which large amounts of fluid collect in the pleural cavity, and dry pleurisy, in which very little exudate is produced. The pain of pleurisy results when the pleural surfaces rub together during respiration, often producing an audible pleural friction rub. The patient usually complains of a sharp, sudden pain in the chest wall or back that increases with inspiration. If the pleuritic area affects the border of the diaphragm, the pain may also be referred to the shoulder. Pleurisy with effusion may be associated with dyspnea, elevated body temperature, and a recent history of dry pleurisy.

Management

Emergency care for these patients includes calming measures, oxygen administration, cardiac monitoring, and transportation for physician evaluation. General patient management usually consists of bed rest, antiinflammatory agents, analgesics, antipyretics, and treatment of the underlying disease or infection. This condition cannot be diagnosed in the prehospital setting. Therefore more serious etiologies of chest pain should always be considered.

Influenza

Influenza is a generalized, acute, febrile disease associated with upper and lower respiratory tract viral infection. It is usually characterized by the abrupt onset of a severe and protracted cough, fever, headache, myalgia, and mild sore throat. Of all the viruses, influenza and parainfluenza viruses are the most common causes of serious respiratory infections and have significant morbidity and mortality rates.

Influenza viruses A, B, and C (and their many mutagenic strains) are known for their potential to cause respiratory infections rapidly after exposure (usually within 24 to 48 hours). The viruses are inhaled in aerosolized mucous droplets from infected persons and are deposited on and penetrate the surface of upper respiratory tract mucosal cells (Fig. 17-9). The virus-containing exudate eventually spreads to the lower respiratory tract, causing interstitial inflammation and destruction of the ciliated epithelium. The impaired mucociliary clearance often leads to a secondary bacterial infection, which may result in pneumonia or acute respiratory failure, particularly in patients with chronic lung disease.

Influenza is particularly significant because of the potential for widespread epidemics of the disease in high-risk populations (for example, adults and children with chronic cardiorespiratory or metabolic disorders, residents of nursing homes and other institutions, health care workers). Current vaccines with minimal side effects are effective against some strains of the virus. If uncomplicated, influenza is self-limiting. Acute symptoms last 2 to 7 days and are followed by a convalescent period of approximately 1 week. Complications of influenza are pneumonia and Reye syndrome (see Chapter 27).

Management

Prehospital care for patients with influenza is generally supportive. Depending on the patient's condition, supplemental oxygen and intravenous fluid administration may be indicated. After physician evaluation, these patients may be managed with specific antiinfective agents to counteract bacterial complications and are given antipyretics and antitussives for symptomatic relief. Amantadine has been shown to be effective in treating influenza A infection if given early enough.

Pneumonia

Pneumonia is an acute inflammatory process of the respiratory bronchioles and the alveoli. It is caused by bacterial, viral, or fungal infection (Fig. 17-10). It is the most common cause of death from infectious disease in North America, accounting for 27.7 of every 100,000 deaths.[1] These diseases may be spread by droplets or contact with infected persons (mycoplasma, viruses) or through aspiration of bacteria from one's own nasooropharynx

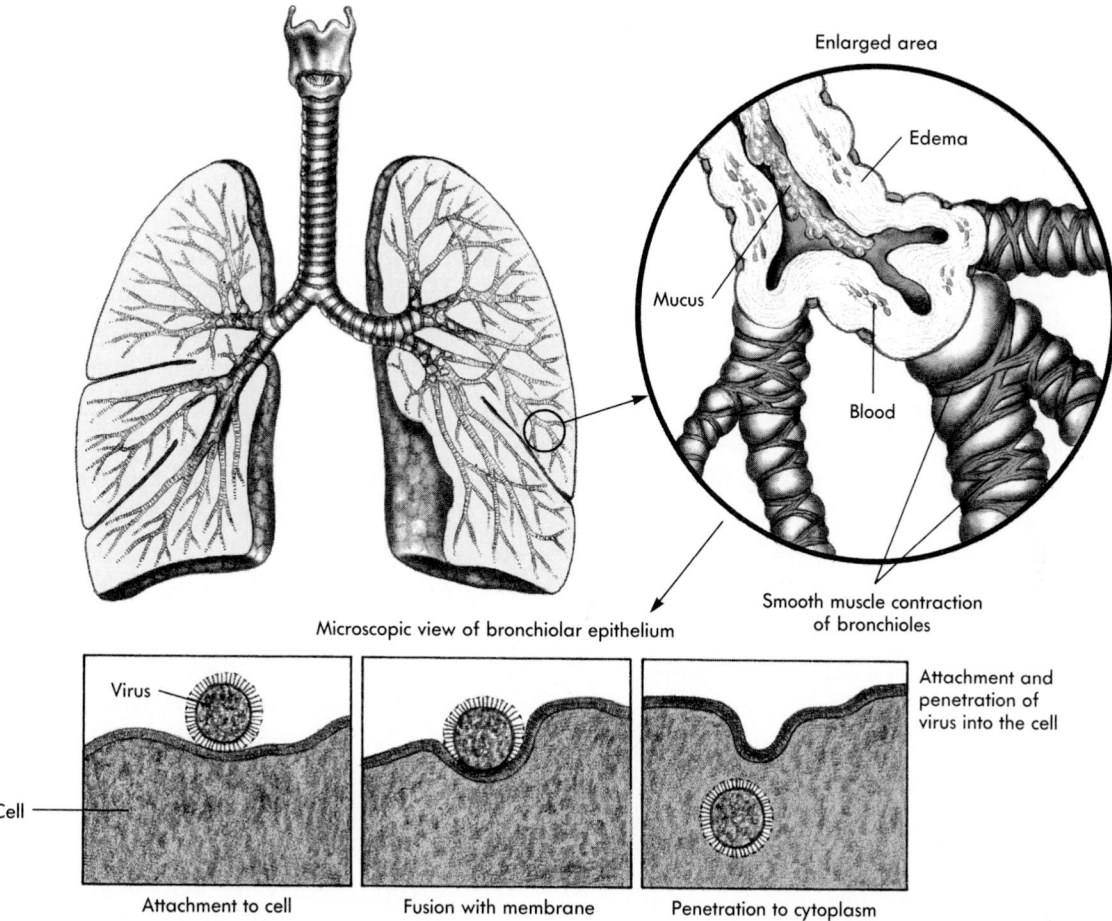

Fig. 17-9 Influenza is a generalized, acute, febrile disease associated with upper and lower respiratory tract viral infection.

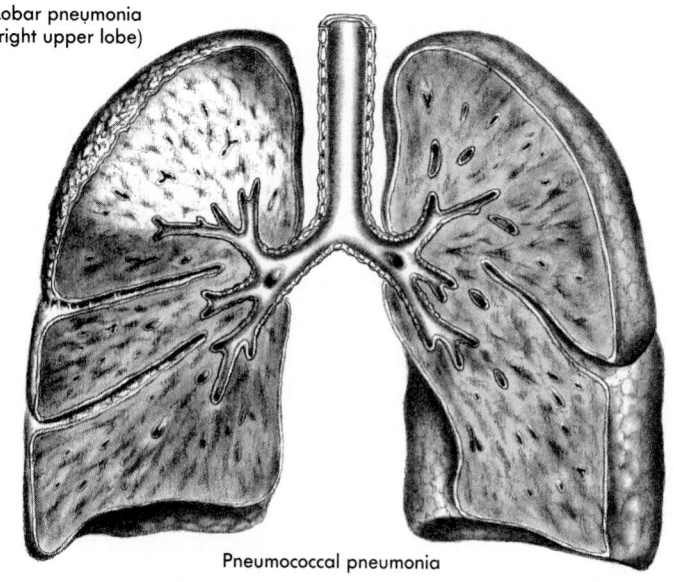

Lobar pneumonia (right upper lobe)

Pneumococcal pneumonia

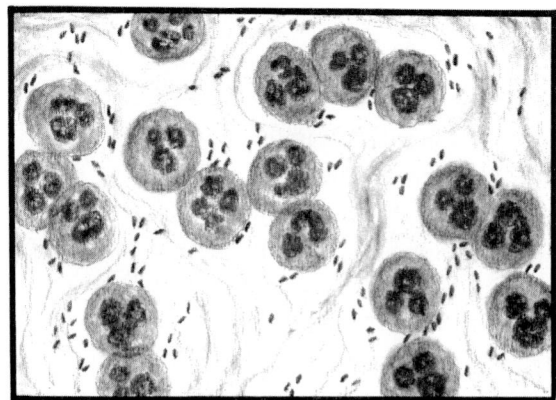

Purulent sputum with pneumococci and polymorphonuclear leukocytes

Fig. 17-10 Pneumonia is an inflammatory process of the respiratory bronchioles and alveoli that is caused by infection.

(pneumococcus). Pneumonia may be classified as viral, bacterial, mycoplasma, or aspiration pneumonia.

Viral Pneumonia

Influenza A is the most common type of viral pneumonia. It often occurs as epidemics in populations of small groups such as school children or army recruits. The interstitial infection caused by the virus predisposes the patient to secondary bacterial pneumonia.

Bacterial Pneumonia

The pneumococcus bacillus (*Bacillus pneumoniae*) accounts for 90% of all bacterial pneumonias. It affects 1 in 500 persons annually, with a peak incidence in winter and early spring. A vaccine now available is 80% to 90% effective against this type of pneumonia in adults. Most bacterial pneumonia results from aspiration of oropharyngeal contents. Thus patients in coma or with seizures, suppressed cough reflex, and increased secretions are predisposed to develop it. Other contributing factors to bacterial pneumonia include:

- Infection
  - Upper respiratory infection (influenza)
  - Postoperative infection
- Foreign body aspiration
- Alcohol or other drug addiction
- Cardiac failure
- Stroke
- Syncope
- PE
- Chronic illness
  - Chronic respiratory disease
  - Diabetes mellitus
  - Congestive heart failure
- Prolonged immobilization of patients
- Compromised immune status

Mycoplasmal Pneumonia

Mycoplasmal pneumonia is caused by infection with *Mycoplasma pneumoniae*. Exposure to the organism causes mild upper respiratory infection in school-age children and young adults. Transmission is believed to be through infected respiratory secretions, so the condition spreads quickly among family members. This form of pneumonia may be treated effectively with erythromycin or tetracycline.

Aspiration Pneumonia

Aspiration pneumonia is an inflammation of the lung parenchyma resulting from introduction of foreign material into the tracheobronchial tree. The syndrome is common in patients who have an altered level of consciousness (for example, from seizure activity, use of alcohol or other drugs, anesthesia, infection, shock), in intubated patients, and in those who have aspirated foreign bodies. Factors common to patients of aspiration include depression of the cough or gag reflex, inability of the patient to handle secretions or gastric contents, and alterations in physiological mechanisms to protect the airway.

Aspiration pneumonia may be nonbacterial (for example, after aspiration of stomach contents, toxic materials, inert substances) or bacterial (as a secondary complication). Bacterial aspiration pneumonia has a poor prognosis, even with antibiotic therapy.

Management

The pathophysiology of pneumonia depends on the etiological agent. In viral and mycoplasma pneumonias, the inflammatory response in the bronchi damages the ciliated epithelium, causing congestion and in some cases hemorrhage. Signs and symptoms include chest pain, cough, fever, and dyspnea. Patients usually complain of general malaise and upper respiratory and gastrointestinal symptoms. Auscultation of the chest may reveal wheezing and fine crackles. If uncomplicated, symptoms usually abate in 7 to 10 days.

Bacterial pneumonia begins with infection in the alveoli progressively filling the alveoli with fluid and purulent sputum. As the infection spreads from alveolus to alveolus, large areas of the lung, sometimes entire lobes, can become consolidated (filled with fluid and cellular debris). Consolidation reduces the available surface area of respiratory membrane and decreases the ventilation-perfusion ratio, both of which may lead to hypoxemia. Patients with bacterial pneumonia usually have acute shaking chills, tachypnea, tachycardia, cough, and sputum production.

The sputum may be rust colored (classic for pneumococcus) but is more commonly yellow, green, or gray. Additional symptoms include malaise, anorexia, flank or back pain, and vomiting. If the disease is uncomplicated and treated with antibiotics, the patient begins to recover within 3 to 5 days, although antibiotics are usually continued for a total of 7 to 10 days.

The physiological effects of aspiration pneumonia are based on the volume and pH of the aspirated substances. If the pH is below 2.5, as may occur in aspiration of stomach contents, atelectasis, pulmonary edema, hemorrhage, and cell necrosis may occur. In addition, the alveolar-capillary membrane may be damaged, leading to exudation and, in severe cases, ARDS. Patient presentation varies with the scenario and the severity of the insult (for example, near-drowning, foreign body aspiration, aspiration of gastric contents). Clinical features may include dyspnea, cough, bronchospasm, wheezes, rhonchi, crackles, cyanosis, and pulmonary and cardiac insufficiency. Of these patients, 25% to 45% develop pulmonary infection.

Prehospital care for patients with pneumonia includes airway support, oxygen administration, ventilatory assistance as needed, intravenous administration, cardiac monitoring, and transportation for physician evaluation. In cases of aspiration, suctioning of the airway may be required. General patient management usually includes bed rest, analgesics, decongestants, expectorants, and antibiotic therapy. In severe cases, bronchoscopy and mechanical ventilation may be part of definitive patient care.

Legionnaires' Disease

Legionnaires' disease (legionellosis) is an acute bacterial infection that results from *Legionella pneumophila*, a bacterium found in natural and synthetic water systems and cultured from dry soil and mud. The disease was named (before identifying the etiological agent) because of a 1976 outbreak of an unknown illness in 200 people at the American Legion Convention in Philadelphia. More than 700 cases of Legionnaires' disease are reported each year, and the infectious agent is thought to be responsible for 4% to 22.5% of all bacterial pneumonias.

Legionnaires' disease progresses rapidly during the first 4 to 6 days of clinical illness. Signs and symptoms are similar to those of bacterial pneumonia and include fever, anorexia, weakness, malaise, shaking chills, diarrhea, nausea, and vomiting. Some patients also complain of dyspnea, pleuritic chest pain, and a nonproductive cough. Coma occurs in 15% to 20% of these patients. Complications include renal failure, septicemia, and respiratory failure resulting in death (15%).

Management

As in other forms of infectious respiratory disease, emergency care includes airway support, oxygen administration, ventilatory assistance as needed, intravenous fluids, cardiac monitoring, and transportation for physician evaluation. After stabilization, patients are generally treated with antibiotic agents. In severe cases, renal dialysis and aggressive ventilatory support are needed.

Tuberculosis

Tuberculosis (TB) is an airborne disease transmitted primarily by inhalation of a minute, dried-droplet nuclei coughed or sneezed into the air by a patient whose sputum contains the virulent bacilli *Mycobacterium tuberculosis* (the most common etiological agent in human TB). In the early 1900s, at least 80% of the U.S. population was infected with TB before reaching the age of 20.[2] After a period of decline beginning in the early 1950s, the incidence of outbreaks is now increasing among the homeless, migrants, people who are immune compromised, and those in correctional facilities. TB is characterized by stages of early infection, latency, and potential reactivation of the disease.

> **NOTE:**
> **Paramedics must recognize the risk of exposure to TB, use respiratory isolation (mask for the patient and paramedic), and maintain an updated record of personal TB skin testing regularly.**

Early Infection

After the TB bacilli enter the body, they multiply slowly, forming a primary focus of infection. Within 3 weeks, the bacilli pass into the lymphatic vascular system, infecting the entire body. The most common site for primary TB infection is the lung. Less common sites include the spine and other bony areas, the meninges, the kidney, the liver, and the spleen. Previously unexposed persons have no defense against multiplication of the organism for approximately 2 to 10 weeks. During this stage of the disease, the primary infection is generally asymptomatic, but a cellular and humoral immune response can be detected by a skin test.

Latency

Eventually the immune response results in a "walling-off" of the lesion by fibrous tissue to form a **tubercle** (a characteristic lesion that results from infection by TB bacilli). A total of 85% to 95% of these patients enter the latent stage of the disease and remain disease free for variable periods. During this stage, reinfection with subsequent exposure is possible.

In approximately 5% to 15% of all infected persons with pulmonary TB, the walling-off process fails. The bacilli spread throughout the lungs, causing many areas of fibrosis. The disease reduces the total amount of functional lung tissue, vital capacity, and total respiratory-membrane surface area and produces an abnormal ventilation-perfusion ratio.

Reactivation

The pulmonary focus is reactivated within the first year in 4% to 5% of patients and then occurs at a rate of approximately 1% per year thereafter, accounting for most of the active TB diagnosed today. In the remainder of cases, the infection is contained, and the patients remain immune from primary infection for life.

Reactivation is most common in older persons and in those with chronic and debilitating disease. The classic symptoms of pulmonary TB are fever, night sweats, malaise, weight loss, and cough with sputum production (generally green to yellow). In advanced stages of the disease, dyspnea, hemoptysis, and other signs of respiratory failure may be present.

Management

Prehospital care for patients with TB includes airway support, oxygen administration, ventilatory assistance as needed, intravenous fluids, cardiac monitoring, and transportation for physician evaluation. Patients who are sputum positive are generally hospitalized with isolation procedures to prevent the spread of the disease. After initial stabilization, the patient is usually managed with a selection of antiinfective agents, with periodic reculturing of sputum.

REFERENCES

1. Wilson S, Thompson J: *Respiratory disorders*, St Louis, 1990, Mosby.
2. Hale D: Asthma deaths on rise in U.S., *New York Times*, Aug 2, 1990, p. 24.
3. Callaham M: *Current practice of emergency medicine*, ed 2, Philadelphia, 1991, BC Decker.
4. O'Doherty D, Fermaglich J: *Handbook of neurologic emergencies*, Flushing, NY, 1977, Medical Examination Publishing.

Summary

Evaluation and management of respiratory distress is of utmost importance in any patient care encounter. Compromise of the respiratory system greatly reduces the patient's chance for survival and may negate all other steps taken to manage significant illness or injury to other body systems. From the time the paramedic crew arrives at the scene until the patient is delivered to the receiving hospital, attention must be focused on this basic principle of emergency care.

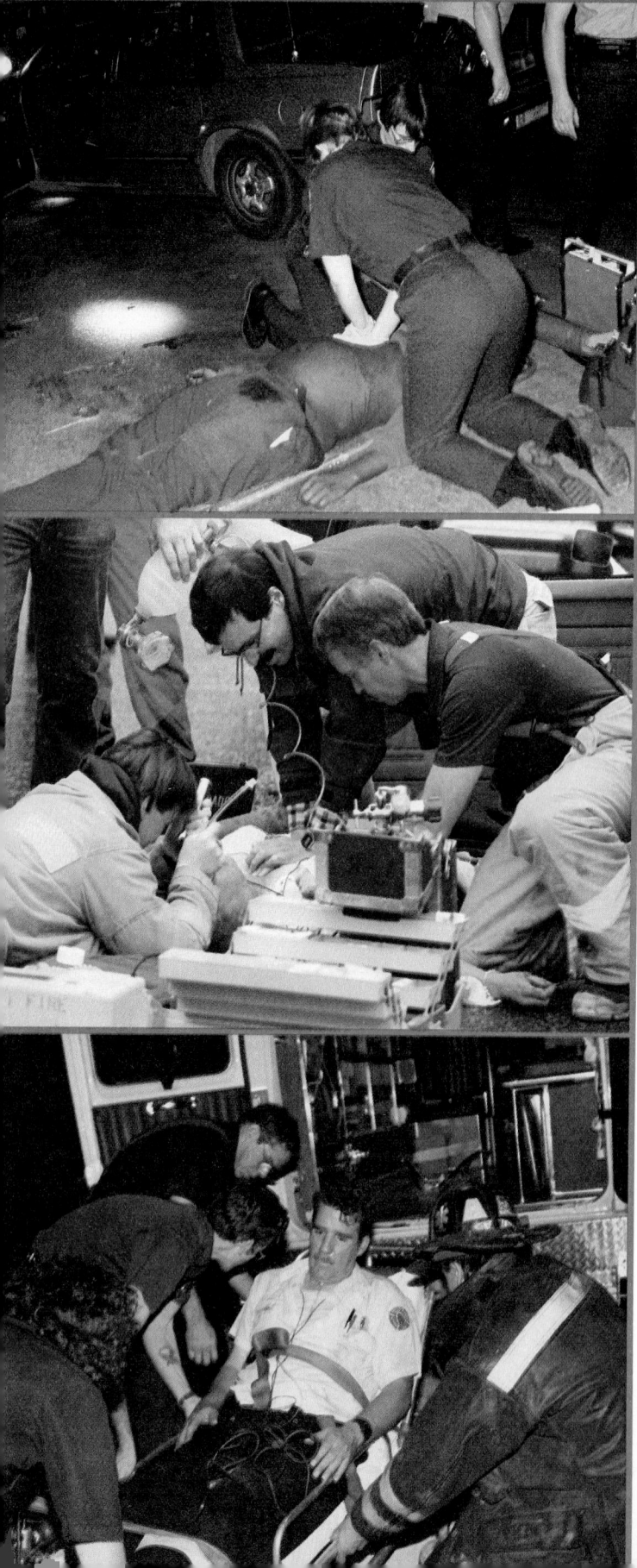

Diseases of the heart are primarily related to obstruction of the coronary arteries due to spasm or formation of plaque. Cardiovascular disease is responsible for approximately 1 million deaths in the United States each year; more than half of these result from myocardial infarction.[1] It has been estimated that 100,000 to 200,000 of these victims could survive if given prompt cardiopulmonary resuscitation (CPR) and early initiation of advanced cardiac life support.[2]

OBJECTIVES

As a paramedic, you should be able to:

1. Describe the normal physiology of the heart and vascular system.
2. Discuss electrophysiology as it relates to the normal electrical events in the cardiac cycle.
3. Describe the mechanical activity of the cardiac cells.
4. Detail in the correct sequence the electrical conduction system in the heart.
5. Describe basic monitoring techniques that permit clear electrocardiogram interpretation.
6. Explain the relationship of the electrocardiogram tracing to the heart's electrical activity.
7. Describe in sequence the steps in electrocardiogram interpretation.
8. Identify the characteristics of normal sinus rhythm in lead II.
9. Interpret electrocardiogram tracings.
10. Given a dysrhythmia, identify the site of origin, discuss its possible causes, recognize its critical features in monitoring lead II, interpret a selected rhythm tracing, describe prehospital management, and describe treatment.
11. Assess a patient who may be suffering from a cardiovascular disorder.
12. Describe patient assessment and management of selected cardiovascular diseases based on knowledge of the pathophysiology of the illness.
13. List indications, contraindications, and mechanism of action for pharmacological agents for cardiovascular disease.
14. Identify critical patient care measures for a person in cardiac arrest.
15. Given a scenario, state correct interventions according to the American Heart Association.

KEY TERMS

action potential: A change in membrane potential in an excitable tissue that acts as an electrical signal and is propagated in an all-or-none fashion.

coarse ventricular fibrillation: Fibrillatory waves greater than 3 mm in amplitude.

depolarization: A change in electrical charge difference across the cell membrane that causes the difference to be smaller or closer to 0 millivolts. A phase of the action potential in which the membrane potential moves toward 0 or becomes positive.

ectopic focus: Cardiac dysrhythmia caused by irritation of an excitation impulse at a site other than the sinus node.

excitability: The property of a cell that enables it to react to irritation or stimulation.

fine ventricular fibrillation: Fibrillatory waves less than 3 mm in amplitude.

P wave: The first complex of the electrocardiogram, representing depolarization of the atria.

pacemaker cells: Certain myocardial cells capable of initiating an electrical impulse.

paroxysmal supraventricular tachycardia: An ectopic rhythm in excess of 100 beats per minute and usually faster than 170 beats per minute that begins abruptly with a premature atrial or junctional beat and is supported by an antrioventricular nodal reentry mechanism or by an atrioventricular reentry mechanism involving an accessory pathway.

PR interval: The time elapsing between the beginning of the P wave and the beginning of the QRS complex in the electrocardiogram.

Continued.

539

KEY TERMS—cont'd

premature atrial contraction: A cardiac dysrhythmia characterized by an atrial beat occurring before the expected excitation and indicated on the electrocardiogram as an early P wave.

premature junctional contraction: A single contraction that occurs during sinus rhythm earlier than the next expected sinus beat and caused by premature discharge of an ectopic focus in the atrioventricular junctional tissue.

premature ventricular contraction: A cardiac dysrhythmia characterized by a ventricular beat preceding the expected electrical impulse and indicated on the electrocardiogram as an early, wide QRS complex without a preceding related P wave.

QRS complex: The principal deflection in the electrocardiogram, representing ventricular depolarization.

QT interval: The time elapsing from the beginning of the QRS complex to the end of the T wave, representing the total duration of electrical activity of the ventricles.

refractory period: The period after effective stimulation during which excitable tissue fails to respond to a stimulus of threshold intensity.

resting membrane potential: The electrical charge difference inside a cell membrane measured relative to just outside the cell membrane.

ST segment: The early part of repolarization in the electrocardiogram of the right and left ventricles.

Starling's law of the heart: A rule that the force of the heartbeat is determined by the length of the fibers comprising the myocardial walls.

T wave: Deflection in the electrocardiogram after the QRS complex, representing ventricular repolarization.

KEY TERMS—cont'd

U wave: Gradual deviation from the T wave in the electrocardiogram thought to represent the final stage of repolarization of the ventricles.

ventricular tachycardia: A tachycardia that usually originates in the Purkinje fibers.

Section One
Anatomy and Physiology
of the Heart

● ANATOMY

The anatomy of the heart is described and illustrated in Chapter 10. Readers are encouraged to refer to that chapter for a review.

Blood enters the right side of the heart through the inferior and superior vena cavae. The four pulmonary veins bring oxygenated blood to the left side of the heart. The cells of the myocardium, however, do not exchange nutrients and metabolic end products with the blood within the heart chambers. Like perfusion of all other organs, cardiac tissue perfusion is supplied by arteries that branch from the aorta: the right and left coronary arteries (Fig. 18-1).

The coronary arteries are the exclusive suppliers of arterial blood to the heart muscle, delivering 200 to 250 ml of blood to the myocardium each minute during rest. The left coronary artery carries approximately 85% of the blood supply to the myocardium, and the right coronary artery carries the remainder. The coronary arteries originate just above the aortic valve and divide into smaller vessels that encircle the heart.

The left main coronary artery subdivides into the left anterior descending and circumflex arteries. The former supplies the anterior wall of the

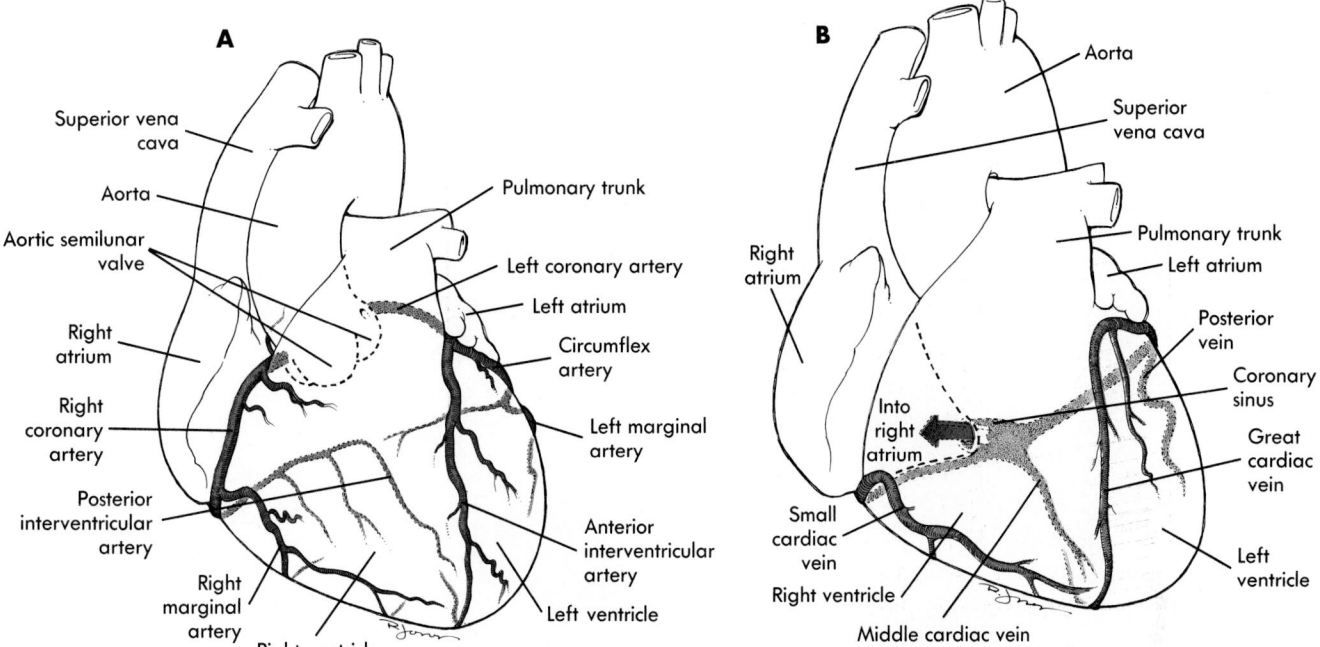

Fig. 18-1 Blood vessels providing circulation of the heart. **A,** Arteries. **B,** Veins. The anterior surface of the heart is represented. The vessels of the anterior surface are seen directly and have a darker color, whereas the vessels of the posterior surface are seen through the heart and have a lighter color.

more muscular left ventricle and the interventricular septum. The latter feeds the lateral and posterior portions of the left ventricle as well as part of the right ventricle. The right coronary artery and the left anterior descending artery, depending on which is more dominant in a particular heart, supply most of the right atrium and ventricle and the inferior aspect of the left ventricle. In addition to the blood supply provided by these arteries, many anastomoses exist between arterioles of coronary arteries that allow the development of collateral circulation. These anastomoses play an important role in providing alternative routes of blood flow in the event of blockage in one or more of the coronary vessels.

Coronary capillaries permit the exchange of nutrients and metabolic wastes. The capillaries merge to form coronary veins. These veins deliver most of the blood to the coronary sinus, which empties directly into the right atrium. The coronary sinus is the major vein draining the myocardium of the left ventricle.

● PHYSIOLOGY

The heart can be thought of as two pumps in one: a low-pressure pump (right atrium and right ventricle) supplying the pulmonary vasculature and a high-pressure pump (left atrium and left ventricle) supplying the systemic vasculature. The right atrium receives venous blood from the systemic circulation via the superior and inferior vena cavae and from the heart itself by way of the coronary sinus. This deoxygenated blood flows across the tricuspid valve into the right ventricle. From there, it is pumped through the pulmonic valve and into the lungs via the pulmonary artery. From the pulmonary artery, the blood enters the pulmonary capillary bed, where gas exchange takes place.

From the lungs, the blood travels through four pulmonary veins back to the left atrium. The mitral valve opens, and blood flows to the left ventricle. As the ventricle contracts, blood is propelled through the aortic valve into the aorta. From the

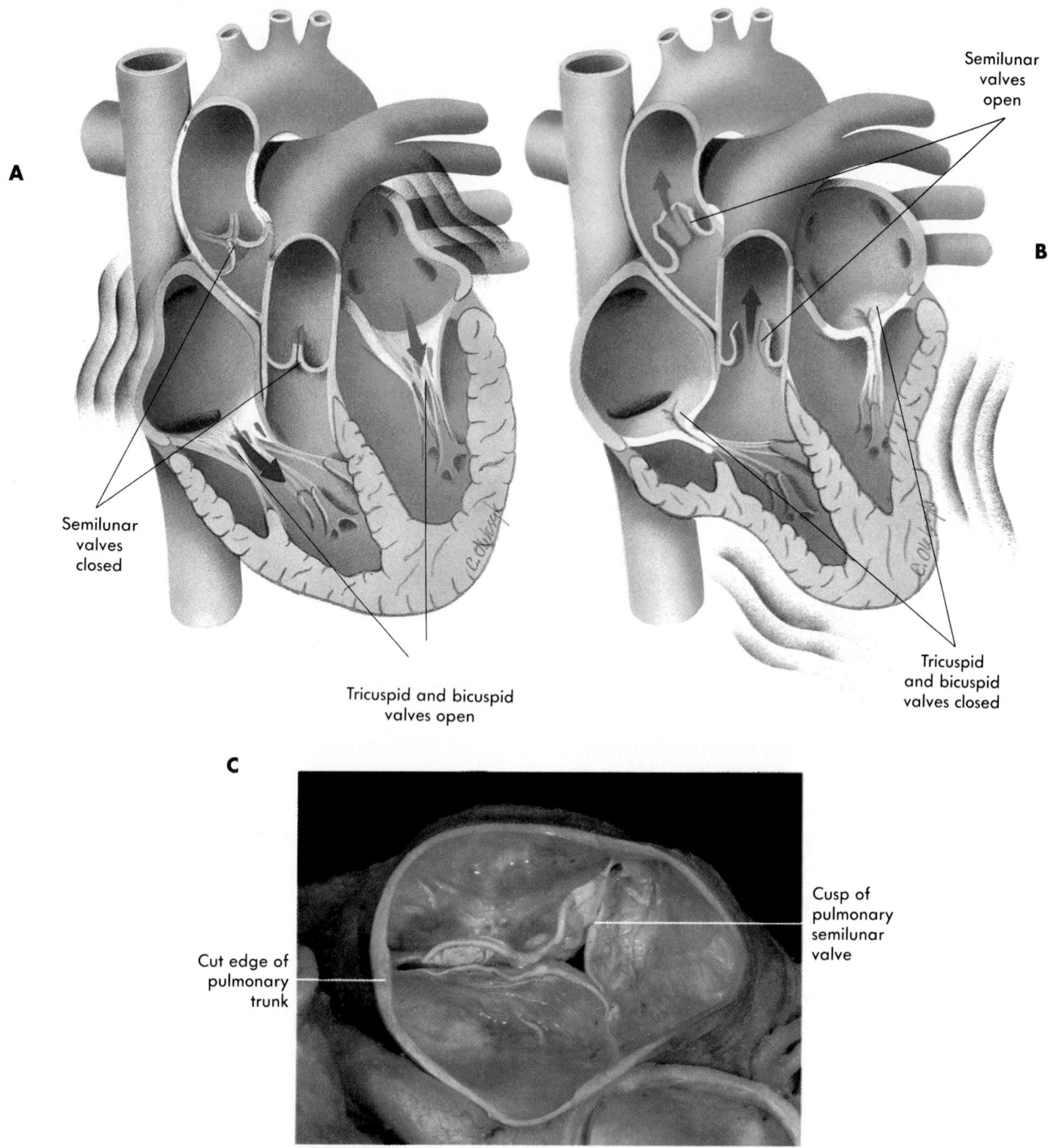

Fig. 18-2 Heart action. **A,** During atrial systole (contraction), cardiac muscle in the atrial wall contracts, forcing blood through the atrioventricular valves and into the ventricles. **B,** During the ventricular systole that follows, the atrioventricular valves close, and blood is forced out of the ventricles through the semilunar valves into the arteries. **C,** The pulmonary semilunar valves as seen from above (superior).

aorta, blood is distributed throughout the systemic arterial circulation.

Cardiac Cycle

The pumping action of the heart is a product of rhythmic, alternate contraction (systole) and relaxation (diastole) of the atria and ventricles. (When *systole* and *diastole* are used without reference to specific chambers, they mean *ventricular systole or diastole*.) These heartbeats occur approximately 70 times per minute in resting adults. One complete heartbeat (systole and diastole) lasts approximately 800 milliseconds (ms) or 0.8 second (1 ms = 0.001 second). Pressure changes produced within the heart chambers by contraction are responsible for blood movement as blood moves from areas of high pressure to areas of low pressure (Fig. 18-2).

Atrial Systole and Diastole

The right and left atria serve as reservoirs and "booster pumps" to increase blood volume into the ventricles, which fill primarily by passive pressure differences. At the beginning of ventricular diastole, pressure in the ventricles falls below the pressure within the atria. The tricuspid and mitral valves open, and blood rushes into the ventricles from the atria. Nearly 70% of the blood that enters the ventricles does so while the atria and ventricles are in diastole. When blood moves from atrium to ventricle, the valves lie open against the ventricular wall.

Toward the end of ventricular diastole (less than 0.2 second before ventricular contraction), both atria contract almost simultaneously, squeezing approximately 20% more blood into the ventricle's chambers. This "atrial kick" contributes significantly to stroke volume. Atrial diastole lasts approximately 700 ms, and atrial systole lasts 100 ms.

As previously stated, the atria function primarily as reservoirs. Under most conditions, the ventricles can pump sufficient blood to maintain homeostasis even if the atria do not contract at all. However, under conditions of stress, when the heart may pump 300% to 400% more blood than during rest, atrial systole becomes important in maintaining pumping efficiency.

Ventricular Systole and Diastole

As the ventricular myocardium begins to contract during ventricular systole, ventricular pressure exceeds atrial pressure and the atrioventricular (AV) valves close. As the contraction proceeds, ventricular pressure continues to rise until it exceeds that in the pulmonary artery on the right side or in the aorta on the left side of the heart. At that time, the pulmonary and aortic valves open, and blood flows from the ventricles into those arteries (ejection). During ejection, ventricular volume decreases, and blood is no longer forced from the ventricles, even though contraction continues. Ventricular systole lasts for approximately 300 ms and is nearly simultaneous in both ventricles.

After ventricular contraction, ventricular relaxation begins, and ventricular pressure falls rapidly. When the pressure falls below the pressure in the aorta or the pulmonary trunk, blood is forced back toward the ventricles, closing the pulmonary and aortic valves. As ventricular pressure drops below atrial pressure, the tricuspid and mitral valves open, and blood flows from the atria into the ventricles. Ventricular diastole lasts for approximately 500 ms, 100 of which overlap the entire period of atrial systole.

Stroke Volume

The stroke volume (SV) is the amount of blood ejected from each ventricle with one contraction. SV depends on preload (end-diastolic volume), afterload, and myocardial contractility.

Preload

During diastole, blood flows from the atria into the ventricles, and the volume of each ventricle (end-diastolic volume) normally reaches 120 to 130 ml. As the ventricles empty during systole, their volume decreases to 50 to 60 ml (end-systolic volume). Therefore the amount of blood ejected during each cardiac cycle (SV) is approximately 70 ml (SV equals end-diastolic volume minus end-systolic volume).

Increased preload usually leads to increased SV. In a patient with a healthy heart, the capacity to increase SV is great. For example, during exercise when the heart contracts strongly, the end-systolic volume can fall to as little as 10 to 30 ml. If large amounts of blood flow into the ventricles during diastole, their end-diastolic volume can become as great as 200 to 250 ml in the normal heart. As a result, the SV may be nearly 200 ml. Therefore by increasing the end-diastolic volume and decreasing the end-systolic volume, the SV can be increased to more than double that of normal. The heart's ability to pump more strongly when it has a larger preload is explained by a concept known as **Starling's law of the heart.**

Starling's Law of the Heart

According to Starling's law, myocardial fibers contract more forcefully when stretched. (This ability of stretched muscle to contract with increased force is characteristic of all striated muscle, not just cardiac muscle.) The primary mechanism by which Starling's law affects SV and ultimately cardiac output is as follows: When the ventricles are filled with larger-than-normal volumes of blood (increased preload), they contract with greater-than-normal force to deliver their entire contents to the systemic circulation.

The most important feature of the heart's ability to adapt itself to changing volumes in venous return is that, within reasonable limits, changes in arterial pressure have minimal effect on cardiac output. In other words, the heart can pump either a small amount of blood or a large amount, depending on the amount of venous return. Because of Starling's law, the heart automatically adapts as long as the total quantity of blood does not exceed the physiological limit the heart can pump. Therefore regardless of arterial pressure, venous return is still the most important factor in SV.

The theory of Starling's law and its effect on SV can only be applied up to a certain limit of muscle fiber stretching (atrial pressure of up to 170 mm Hg). Beyond that limit, muscle fiber stretch actually diminishes the strength of contraction, and the heart begins to fail.

Afterload

Afterload is a result of peripheral vascular resistance, the total resistance against which blood must be pumped. An increase in peripheral vascular resistance decreases SV because of the in-

creased pressure in the aorta that the ventricular muscle must overcome to open the aortic valve and push blood through. Conversely, a decrease in peripheral vascular resistance increases SV if there is sufficient volume of fluid in the system. Preload is a more important factor than afterload in determining cardiac output.

Myocardial Contractility

The intrinsic state of the myocardium, along with the activity of the autonomic nervous system, plays a major role in the function of the heart. Ischemia or various medications can decrease myocardial contractility by decreasing the number of functional myocardial cells (as occurs in myocardial infarction) or by decreasing the ability of the individual myocardial cells to contract (for example, as a result of hypoxia or the administration of beta blockers). The state of the myocardium may be the overriding factor in the heart's ability to pump effectively. If the myocardium is normal, preload (with Starling's mechanism), afterload, and the state of autonomic activity are all factors in cardiac function.

Cardiac Output

Cardiac output, the amount of blood pumped by each ventricle per minute, is closely related to SV. Cardiac output can increase by increasing the heart rate, SV, or both, and is calculated as follows:

$$\text{Cardiac output} = \text{SV} \times \text{Heart rate}$$

Peripheral vascular resistance modifies cardiac output through its effect on SV. Vasodilation of the arteries, for example, decreases peripheral vascular resistance and arterial pressure (afterload), thereby producing an increase in cardiac output. In contrast, vasoconstriction of arteries and the smaller arterioles increases peripheral vascular resistance and tends to decrease cardiac output. However, constriction of the venous circulation by increasing the filling of the heart through Starling's mechanism causes the heart to contract more forcefully and thereby maintains cardiac output. Since blood pressure is a function of cardiac output and peripheral vascular resistance, the systolic pressure rises.

Nervous System Control of the Heart

In addition to the body's intrinsic control in regulating the heart, extrinsic control by the parasympathetic and sympathetic nerves of the autonomic nervous system is a major factor influencing heart rate, conductivity, and contractility. Control is achieved by a group of nerves, the cardiac plexus, that innervates the atria and ventricles. The atria are well supplied with large numbers of sympathetic and parasympathetic nerve fibers, but the ventricles are supplied mainly by sympathetic nerves.

The parasympathetic nervous system is concerned primarily with vegetative functions, whereas the sympathetic nervous system helps prepare the body to respond to stress. These sympathetic and parasympathetic control systems directly oppose one another and are generally balanced to maintain a normal state of cardiac function.

Parasympathetic Control

Parasympathetic nerve fibers are carried to the heart through the vagus nerve. Innervation by these fibers has a continuous inhibitory influence on the heart, primarily by decreasing heart rate and to a lesser extent contractility. The vagus nerve may be stimulated in several ways. Examples include the Valsalva maneuver, carotid sinus pressure, nausea or vomiting, pain, and distention of the urinary bladder. Acetylcholine is the chemical mediator that transmits parasympathetic nerve impulses.

Although strong parasympathetic stimulation can decrease the heart rate to 20 or 30 beats per minute, it generally has little effect on SV. In fact, SV may increase with a decreased heart rate because the longer time interval between heart beats allows the heart to fill to a greater capacity (Starling's law).

Sympathetic Control

Sympathetic nerve fibers originate in the thoracic region of the spinal cord and form the thoracic and cervical sympathetic ganglia. Their postganglionic fibers release the chemical mediator norepinephrine, which stimulates the heart rate (positive chronotropic effect) and the force of

muscle contraction (positive inotropic effect). Sympathetic stimulation of the heart causes dilation of coronary blood vessels, probably by indirect effects. Along with the constriction of peripheral vessels, this tends to ensure that increased oxygen demands on the heart are met by an increased oxygen supply. The cardiac effects of norepinephrine result from stimulation of cell surface alpha- and beta-adrenergic receptors. Other beta-receptor responses include bronchodilation and peripheral vasodilation. Peripheral alpha-receptor stimulation results primarily in peripheral vasoconstriction.

Strong sympathetic stimulation of the heart may increase the heart rate significantly; the exact number of beats depends on the patient's age and whether the heart stays in a normal rhythm or develops an abnormal rhythm. When rates are markedly accelerated (greater than 150 beats per minute), the time available for diastolic filling decreases, and the heart may have a smaller end-diastolic volume. If the heart rate becomes too great, diastole is so short that ventricular filling is markedly reduced. This produces a decrease in SV. This process occurs at slower rates in sedentary people than it does in well-trained athletes. Cardiac output may be maintained by the increased heart rate (since cardiac output equals SV multiplied by heart rate), but under extreme conditions, cardiac output also decreases.

Hormonal Regulation of the Heart

Sympathetic impulses are transmitted to the adrenal medulla at the same time they are transmitted to all blood vessels. These impulses cause the adrenal medulla to secrete the hormones epinephrine and norepinephrine into the circulating blood. These hormones are secreted in response to increased physical activity, emotional excitement, or stress.

Epinephrine has essentially the same effect on cardiac muscles as norepinephrine and therefore increases the rate and force of contraction. In addition, epinephrine causes blood vessels to constrict in the skin, kidneys, gastrointestinal tract, and other viscera and causes dilation of blood vessels in skeletal muscles and cardiac muscle. Epinephrine takes longer to act on the beta-adrenergic receptors of the heart than direct sympathetic innervation does, but the effect lasts longer because the hormonal release is slower in onset and slower in decline. Norepinephrine causes constriction of peripheral blood vessels in most areas of the body and stimulates cardiac muscle.

Role of Electrolytes

Myocardial cells, like all other cells of the human body, are bathed in an electrolyte solution. The major electrolytes that influence cardiac function are calcium, potassium, and sodium. Magnesium, a major intracellular cation, appears to be important as well.

Section Two
Electrophysiology of the Heart

Much coronary care is based on the electrical and mechanical properties of cardiac function. The paramedic must thoroughly understand the biochemistry and physiology of cardiac cells to provide appropriate emergency care. The two basic groups of cells within the myocardium important for cardiac function are the specialized cells of the electrical conduction system responsible for the formation and propagation of electric current and the working myocardial cells that possess the property of contractility.

● ELECTRICAL ACTIVITY OF CARDIAC CELLS

Most biochemical reactions produce metabolites whose sum of positive and negative charges is neutral. However, the dielectric field of the physiological medium, determined by acid-base balance and ionized particles, profoundly affect metabolism and electrophysiology. Nearly all biochemical reactions involve charged intermediate groups, and most involve reactions with water split into a proton and hydroxyl ions or other charged substrates.

● MEMBRANE POTENTIALS

Ions are charged particles that are electrically positive or negative, depending on their ability to accept or donate electrons. In solutions containing electrolytes, the electrostatic attraction of particles with unlike charges and the repulsion between particles with like charges result in a tendency to produce ion pairs, which maintain electrical neutrality throughout the solution.

Electrically charged particles may be thought of as small magnets. They require energy to push them apart if they have opposite charges and to push them together if they have like electrical charges. Thus separated particles with opposite charges have an electrical magnetic-like force of attraction that gives them *potential* energy. The effect of this is to establish a membrane potential between the inside and the outside of the cell. The electrical charge (potential difference) between the inside and outside of cells can be measured by a voltmeter or oscilloscope and is expressed in millivolts (mV) (1 mV = 0.001 volt). This potential energy is released when the cell membrane separating the positively charged ions inside the cell and the negatively charged ions outside the cell becomes permeable to them.

The total concentration of positive ions roughly equals the intracellular and extracellular compartments. What leads to an overall negative charge intracellularly is the presence of large negatively charged proteins that cannot diffuse out of the cell.

Resting Membrane Potential

When the cell is in an unstimulated or "resting" state, the electrical charge difference is referred to as a **resting membrane potential** (RMP). The term *potential* is used in the electrical sense, as a synonym for *voltage*, since opposite charges have the ability to do work when separated. Because the inside of the cell is negative compared with the outside of the cell membrane, RMP is reported as a negative number (approximately −90 mV).

The RMP is the result of an equilibrium between two opposing forces: the concentration gradient of permeable ions (primarily potassium) across the cell membrane and the electrical forces across the cell membrane produced by the separation of positively charged ions from their negative ion pair. The RMP is primarily established by the difference between the intracellular potassium ion concentration and the extracellular potassium ion level. The ratio of 148 to 5 produces a large chemical gradient for potassium ions to leave the cell, but the negative intracellular membrane charge relative to the extracellular membrane charge tends to keep potassium ions in the cell (Fig. 18-3).

Changes in potassium ion concentration on either side of the cell membrane or in cell membrane permeability to potassium ions quickly establish a new equilibrium across the cell membrane. If this equilibrium results in a decreased charge difference across the cell membrane, the RMP becomes *less* negative **(depolarization)**. In comparison, an increased charge difference across the cell membrane causes the RMP to become *more* negative (hyperpolarization).

The sodium ion, on the other hand, has a chemical and electrical gradient, which would tend to cause it to move intracellularly. Because the membrane is permeable only to sodium ions at specific times in the depolarization cycle, it plays a dominant role only at that time, such as during the rapid phase of depolarization (phase 0) (Fig. 18-4).

The contribution of unpaired ions to the RMP depends on two factors: (1) the active transport of ions through the membrane by way of the sodium-potassium exchange pump, which creates an imbalance of negative and positive charges on the two sides of the membrane, and (2) diffusion of ions through the membrane by way of the ion channels, which also creates an imbalance of charges.

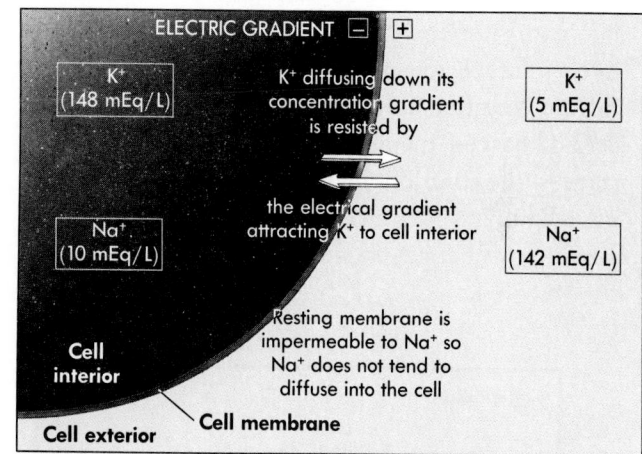

Fig. 18-3 At equilibrium (resting conditions), the tendency for potassium ions to diffuse out of the cell is opposed by the potential difference (electrical gradient) across the cell membrane. Because the resting membrane is not permeable to sodium ions, sodium ions do not tend to diffuse into the cell.

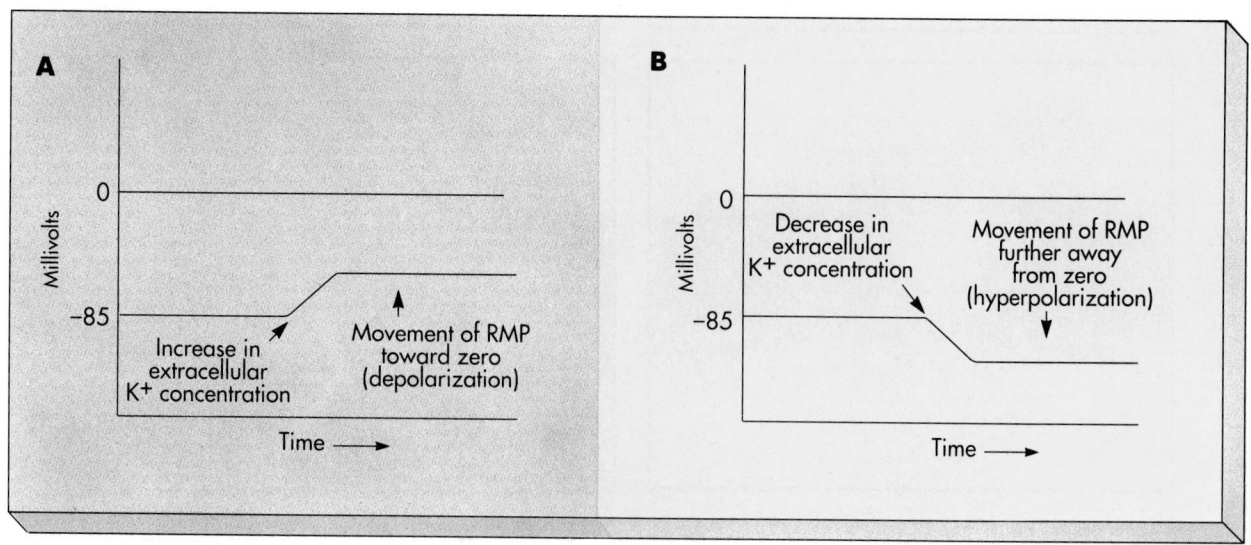

Fig. 18-4 Changes in the RMP caused by changes in extracellular potassium ion concentration. **A,** Elevated extracellular potassium ion concentration causes depolarization. **B,** Decreased extracellular potassium ion concentration causes hyperpolarization.

Sodium-Potassium Exchange Pump

The specialized sodium-potassium exchange pump actively pumps sodium ions out of the cell and potassium ions in, thus separating the ions across the membrane against their concentration gradients. Potassium ions are transported into the cell, increasing their concentration in the cell; sodium ions are transported out of the cell, increasing their concentration outside (Fig. 18-5).

The sodium-potassium exchange pump normally transports three sodium ions out for every two potassium ions taken in. Therefore more positively charged ions are transferred outward than inward, creating unequal concentrations of ions across the cell membrane. Under these circumstances, the contribution of this pump to the resting membrane potential in most cells is small compared with that generated by diffusion.

Diffusion Through Ion Channels

The cell membrane is selectively permeable, allowing some but not all substances to pass through the membrane. It is relatively permeable to potassium, somewhat less permeable to calcium chloride, and minimally permeable to sodium. The cell membrane appears to have individual protein-lined channels that allow passage of a specific ion or group of ions. Movement in these channels may be regulated by voltage-dependent changes in permeability. These permeability characteristics are influenced by their electrical charge, their size, and the proteins that open and close the channels (gating proteins).

The potassium ion channels are smaller than the sodium ion channels and thus prevent sodium from passing. Potassium ions are small enough to pass through sodium ion channels, but the con-

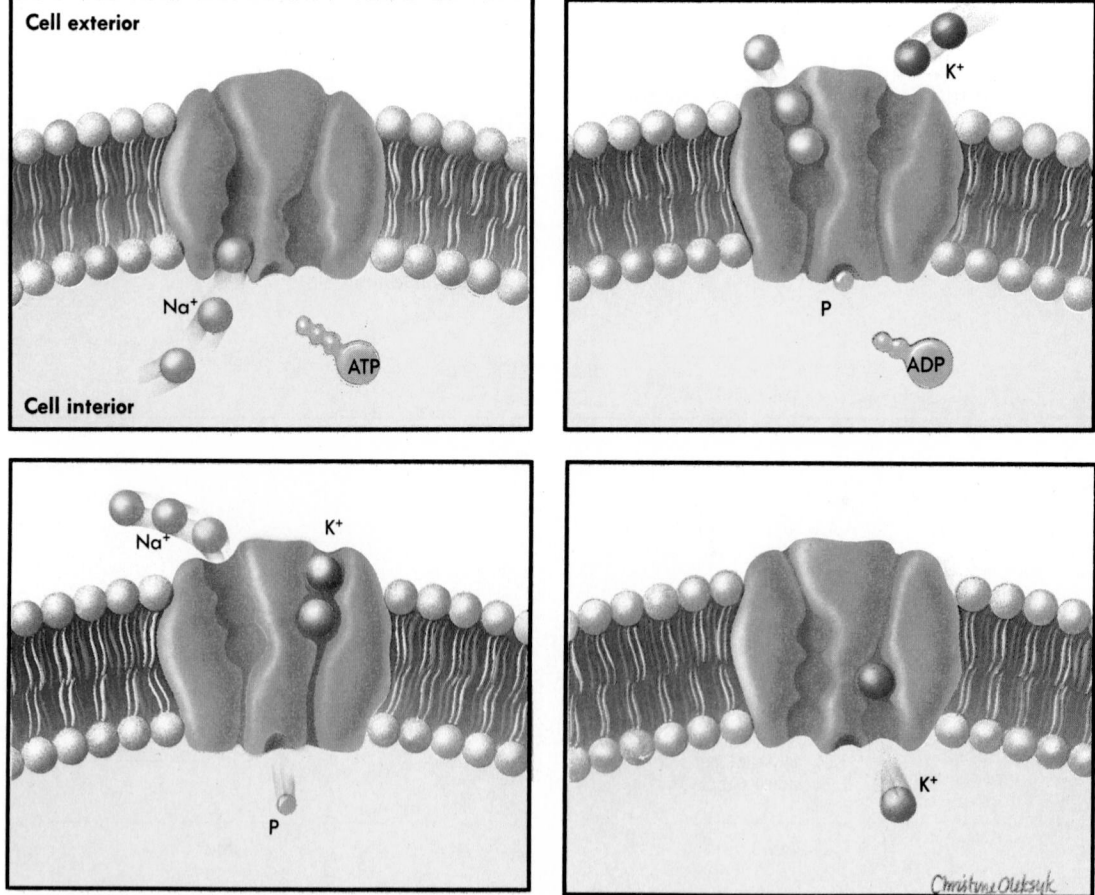

Fig. 18-5 The sodium-potassium exchange pump actively transports sodium ions out of the cell across the cell membrane and potassium ions into the cell across the cell membrane. Adenosine triphosphate is used as the energy source, and the pump can transport up to three sodium ions for every two potassium ions transported.

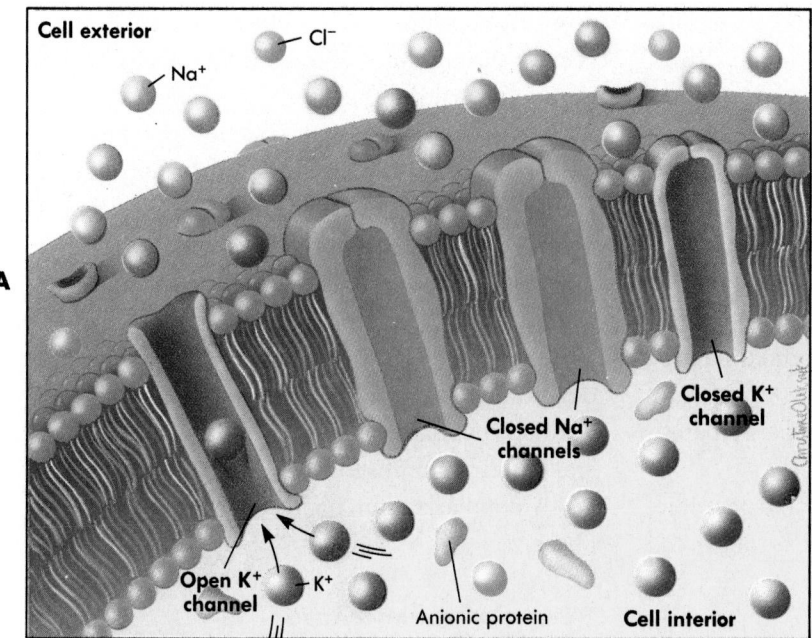

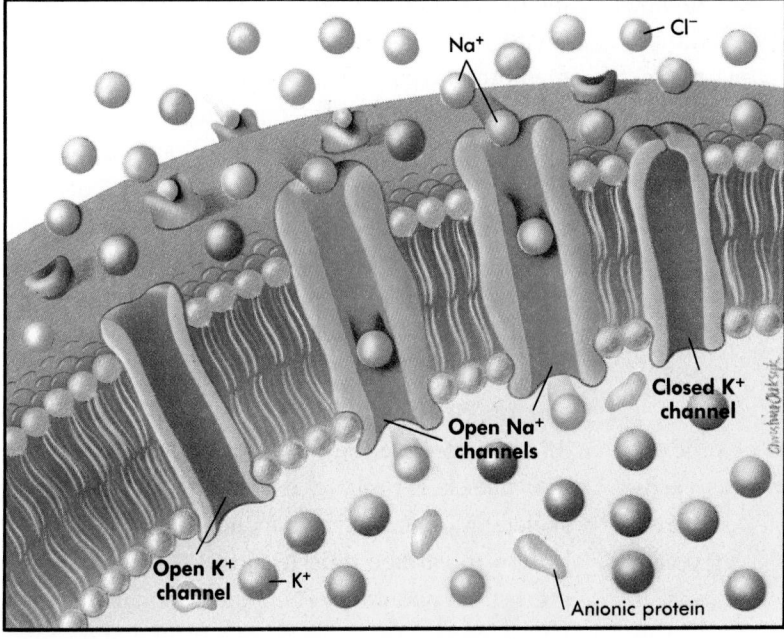

Fig. 18-6 Effect of a stimulus that causes a voltage change across the cell membrane on the permeability of the cell membrane. **A,** Sodium channels remain closed in a resting or unstimulated cell membrane. **B,** Depolarization of the cell membrane causes sodium channels to open. Sodium ions then diffuse down their concentration gradient into the cell, causing depolarization of the cell membrane.

centration gradient and strong electrical gradient for sodium ions from the outside to the inside of the cell favor the intracellular passage of sodium ions through the sodium ion channels over the egress of potassium ions during phase 0 depolarization. Gating proteins open and close the sodium ion channels, and their activity is influenced by the RMP as well as by the extracellular concentration of various ions.

Gating proteins allow depolarization (the inward passage of sodium ions when the membrane potential of the cell changes). Rapid depolarization creates a local area of current known as the **action potential**. After one patch of membrane is depolarized, the electrical charge spreads along the cell surface, opening more channels (Fig. 18-6).

Pharmacological Actions

In cardiac muscle, sodium and calcium ions can enter the cell through two separate channel systems in the cell membrane: fast channels and slow channels. Fast channels are sensitive to small changes in membrane potential. As the cell drifts toward threshold level (perhaps because of a slow leak of potassium), a point is reached where the fast channels open (approximately −75 mV), resulting in a rush of sodium ions intracellularly and in very rapid depolarization (phase 0). The slow channel has selective permeability to calcium and to a lesser extent to sodium. This channel opens at membrane potentials of approximately −50 mV. It normally is responsible for the plateau phase of depolarization (phase 2) and participates in muscular contraction.

Delineation of the concept of slow and fast ion channels has led to the development of pharmacological blocking agents that selectively affect either channel. Of particular importance to prehospital pharmacology are the calcium channel blockers (which selectively block the slow channel), *verapamil* and *nifedipine.* These slow channel-blocking agents specifically prevent the movement of calcium ions into the cell without altering its voltage dependence. In contrast, *procainamide* (a type I antidysrhythmic) owes much of its antidysrhythmic effects to its ability to block the fast inward sodium channel.

● CELL EXCITABILITY

Nerve and muscle cells are capable of producing action potentials, a property known as **excitability.** When these cells are stimulated, a series of changes in the RMP normally causes depolarization of a small region of the cell membrane. If the stimulus is strong enough to depolarize a cell membrane to a level called the *threshold potential,* an explosive series of permeability changes takes place to produce an action potential that spreads over the entire cell membrane.

Propagation of Action Potential

An action potential at any point on the cell membrane acts as a stimulus to adjacent regions of the cell membrane. Therefore the excitation process, once started, is propagated (or spread) down the length of the cell and conducted across synapses from cell to cell. This local flow of electrical current through the cell membrane opens sodium channels sensitive to changes in voltage, which results in an action potential. Action potentials occur in response to a stimulus or do not occur at all, depending on whether the threshold potential is reached (the all-or-none principle).

The characteristics of action potentials vary somewhat from one cell type to another. Skeletal muscle fibers and peripheral nerves have brief action potentials, which generally last less than 5 ms. Cardiac cells have action potentials that last several hundred milliseconds. The action potential has a depolarization phase and a repolarization phase.

Depolarization Phase

The depolarization phase occurs when the membrane potential is less negative than the RMP (that is, closer to zero). In the resting state, the cell membrane is 50 to 75 times more permeable to potassium than to sodium ions. During an action potential, the permeability of the membrane to sodium and potassium ions changes markedly, and sodium ions rush into the cell. The resting potential moves from a negative value toward zero and then becomes positive on the inside and negative on the outside of the membrane.

In many respects, the action potential in skeletal muscle is similar to the action potential in cardiac muscle, but the depolarization phase of cardiac muscle is prolonged in comparison to that of skeletal muscle. The prolonged period of depolarization in cardiac muscle is the plateau phase of the action potential. The plateau phase lasts as long as two to three tenths of a second and causes contraction of the heart muscle during this period.

Repolarization Phase

The cell repolarizes slightly before the plateau phase because of the closing of sodium channels, but the bulk of repolarization occurs after the plateau phase and is caused by potassium leakage out of the cell and the return of the cell membrane to its resting permeability state. In some instances, more positive ions leave the cell than are needed to reach the normal resting membrane potential. When this occurs, the membrane is said to be *hy-*

perpolarized, resulting in a brief period in which the cell's interior is more negative than it was in its resting state.

Refractory Period of Cardiac Muscle

Cardiac muscle, like all excitable tissue, has a **refractory period** associated with the action potential. During the absolute refractory period, the cardiac muscle cell is completely insensitive to further stimulation. Because the depolarization phase of cardiac muscle is prolonged, the refractory period is also prolonged.

The refractory period ensures that the cardiac muscle is completely relaxed before another action potential can be initiated. The refractory period of the ventricles is 0.25 to 0.3 second, approximately the duration of the action potential. The refractory period of the atrial muscle is much shorter than that of the ventricles, approximately 0.15 second. Therefore the rate of atrial contraction can be much faster than that of the ventricles. There is also a relative refractory period (approximately 0.05 second), during which the muscle cell is more difficult than normal to excite, but nonetheless can be stimulated.

Phases of Cardiac Action Potential

The cardiac action potential (representing the changes in membrane potential) can be divided into five phases, phases 0 through 4 (Fig. 18-7).

Phase 0 (the rapid depolarization phase) represents the very rapid upstroke of the action potential, which occurs when the cell membrane reaches the threshold potential (approximately −70 mV). During this phase, the fast sodium channels open momentarily, permitting rapid entry of sodium into the cell. As the positively charged ions flow into the cell, the interior of the cell becomes electrically positive (+20 to +30 mV with respect to its exterior). During the upstroke the cell depolarizes, initiating a cascade of events that leads to muscular contraction. Phase 0 is immediately followed by repolarization, which is divided into three phases.

Phase 1 (the early rapid repolarization phase) represents the phase in which the fast sodium channels close, the flow of sodium ions into the cell terminates, and the loss of potassium from the cell continues. The result is a decrease in the number of positive electrical charges within the cell and a drop in the membrane potential to approximately 0 mV.

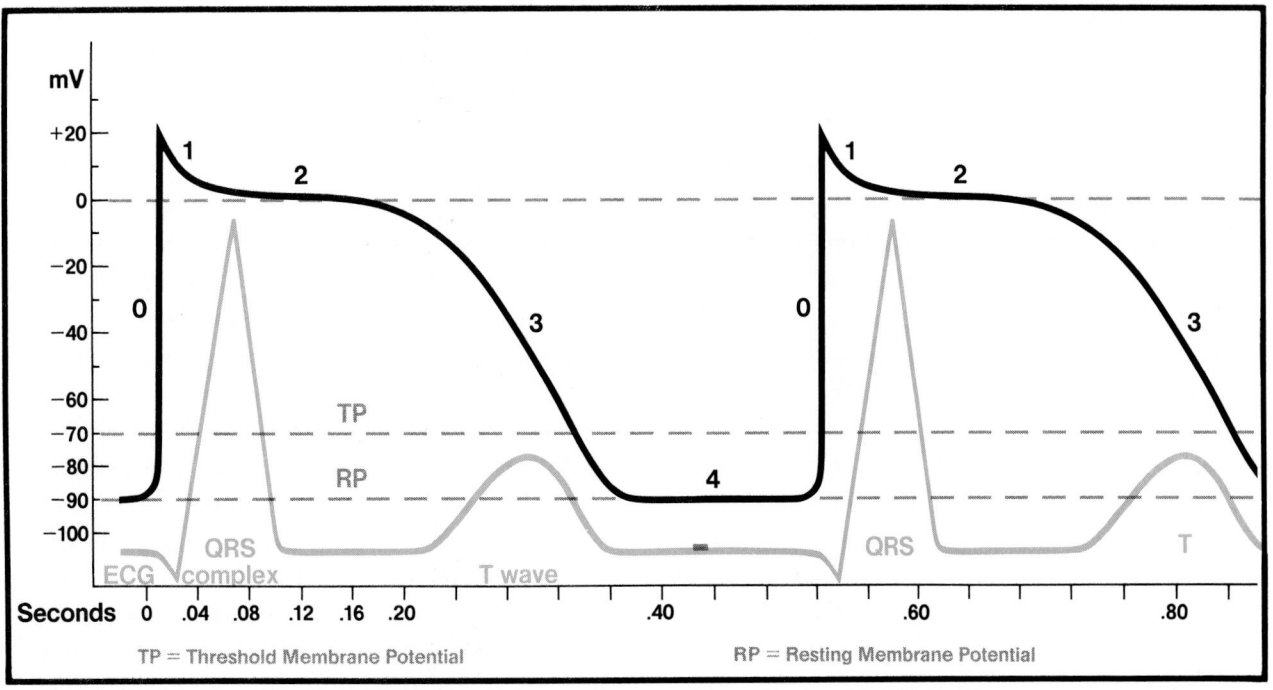

Fig. 18-7 Cardiac action potential of myocardial cells.

Phase 2 (the plateau phase) is the prolonged phase of slow repolarization of the action potential. During this phase, calcium enters the myocardial cells, triggering a larger secondary release of calcium from intracellular storage sites (the sarcoplasmic reticulum) and initiating contraction. Membrane potentials remain at approximately 0 mV during the plateau phase because of the slow rate of repolarization. Calcium slowly enters the cell through the slow calcium channels as potassium continues to leave the cell. The inward calcium current has the following three main functions:

1. Prolongation of the refractory period. It maintains the cell in a prolonged depolarized state, allowing time for completion of one muscle contraction before another depolarization begins.
2. Delivery of calcium.
3. Stimulation of the sarcoplasmic reticulum. This stimulation causes the release of the intracellular stores of calcium that also take part in the contraction process.

Phase 3 (the terminal phase of rapid repolarization) results in the inside of the cell becoming markedly negative and the membrane potential returning to approximately -90 mV (its resting level). Phase 3 is initiated by the closing of the slow calcium channels and by an increase in permeability, with outflow of potassium down its concentration gradient. Repolarization is completed by the end of this phase.

Phase 4 represents the period between action potentials, when the membrane has returned to its RMP. During phase 4, the inside of the cell is negative (-90 mV) with respect to the outside, but there is still an excess of sodium in the cell and potassium outside the cell. This activates the sodium-potassium exchange pump, and the excess sodium is transported out of the cell and the potassium back in. During phase 4, certain myocardial cells (**pacemaker cells**) have a slow depolarization from their most negative membrane potential to a level at which the threshold is reached and phase 0 begins all over again. Other cells that are not normally pacemaker cells tend to maintain a stable RMP until depolarized by a propagating current.

● MECHANICAL ACTIVITY OF CARDIAC CELLS

Cardiac muscle cells or fibers are elongated, branching cylindrical cells that contain one or occasionally two centrally located nuclei and a large number of mitochondria. These striated cells are bound end to end and laterally to adjacent cells by specialized cell-to-cell contacts (intercalated disks). Intercalated disks contain gap junctions that function as areas of low electrical resistance between the cells, allowing action potentials to pass from one cell to adjacent cells. Each cardiac muscle cell is surrounded by a semipermeable cell membrane called the *sarcolemma*. The sarcolemma allows certain charged particles, such as sodium, potassium, and calcium ions, to flow in and out of cardiac cells during the various phases of the pumping action of the heart.

Cardiac muscle cells are so tightly bound together and their membranes so permeable to electrical impulse that they act as a mass of merged cells (a single cell) known as a *syncytium*. Within the heart are two separate syncytiums, the atrial syncytium and the ventricular syncytium. These are separated from one another by the fibrous structure that supports the valves and physically separates the atria from the ventricles.

Structure and Arrangement of Cardiac Muscle Cells

Cardiac muscle cells contain the contractile proteins actin and myosin arranged as myofilaments. The actin and myosin myofilaments are organized in highly ordered units called *sarcomeres,* which are joined end to end to form myofibrils.

Cardiac cells also contain a number of perpendicular invaginations known as *transverse tubes (T tubules)* and a plentiful supply of mitochondria, the combination of which is known as a *diad* (Fig. 18-8). T tubules appear to provide a direct pathway for material from the extracellular space (for example, calcium ions) to reach the myofibrils. Mitochondria play an important role in the aerobic energy production of the cell. In addition, the mitochondria are thought to serve as an intracellular storehouse for calcium ions. The fundamental

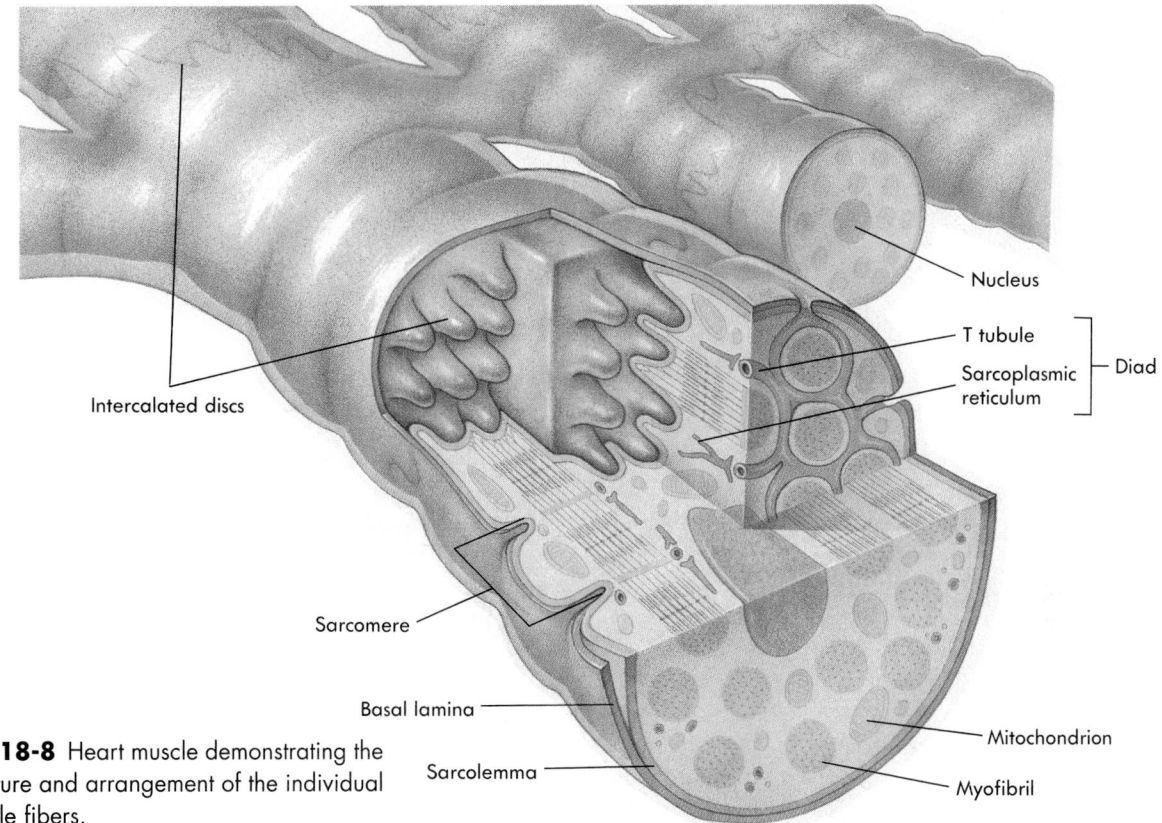

Fig. 18-8 Heart muscle demonstrating the structure and arrangement of the individual muscle fibers.

(Labels: Intercalated discs, Nucleus, T tubule, Sarcoplasmic reticulum, Diad, Sarcomere, Basal lamina, Sarcolemma, Mitochondrion, Myofibril)

contraction process for cardiac and skeletal muscle is believed to be activated by calcium ions, resulting in a binding between myosin and actin myofilaments.

● ELECTRICAL CONDUCTION SYSTEM OF THE HEART

The conduction system of the heart is composed of two nodes and a conducting bundle (Fig. 18-9). The two nodes are contained within the walls of the right atrium and are named according to their location. The sinoatrial (SA) node is medial to the opening of the superior vena cava, and the AV node is medial to the right AV valve. The AV node and the bundle of His form the AV junction. This bundle passes through a small opening in the fibrous skeleton to reach the interventricular septum, where it divides into right and left bundle branches. The left bundle branch then subdivides into the anterior and posterior fascicles, which provide pathways for impulse conduction. (Recently a third fascicle of the left bundle branch that innervates the interventricular septum and the base of the heart has been identified.)

The right and left bundle branches extend beneath the endocardium on either side of the septum to the apical portions of the right and left ventricles, respectively. The bundle branches subdivide into smaller branches and become Purkinje fibers (large-diameter cardiac muscle fibers). The terminal Purkinje fibers contact unspecialized myocardial fibers through which electrical impulses spread from cell to cell in the remaining myocardium. The rapid conduction along these fibers causes depolarization of all right and left ventricular cells more or less simultaneously, ensuring a single coordinated contraction.

Pacemaker Activity

In skeletal and most smooth muscle, the individual cells contract only in response to impulses

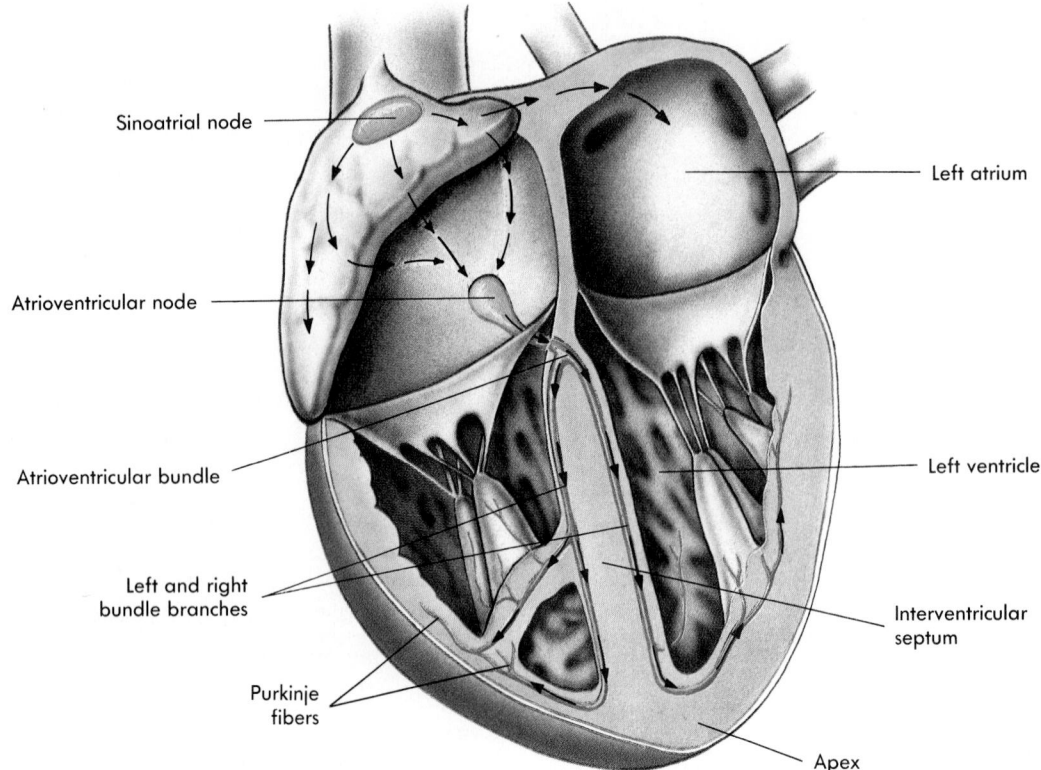

Fig. 18-9 Conduction system of the heart. Impulses *(arrows)* travel across the wall of the right atrium from the sinoatrial node to the AV node. The AV bundle extends from the AV node through the fibrous skeleton and into the interventricular septum, where it divides into right and left bundle branches. The bundle branches descend to the apex of the ventricle and then branch repeatedly for distribution throughout the ventricular walls.

arising from hormonal stimulation or neurotransmitters from the efferent branch of the central nervous system. However, unlike most other muscle cells, cardiac fibers have specialized cells capable of generating electrical impulses spontaneously (a property known as *automaticity*). Such cells are called *pacemaker cells*. Pacemaker cells depolarize in a repetitive manner. This rhythmic activity occurs because these tissues do not have a stable RMP. Instead, the RMP gradually decreases with time from its maximum repolarization potential until it reaches a critical threshold, at which time depolarization results. If the normal pacemaker cells of the heart fail to generate an electrical impulse, other pacemaker cells take over. These pacemaker cells are also capable of depolarization and subsequent propagation of an action potential, although it occurs usually at a slower intrinsic rate.

Sequence of Excitation in Cardiac Muscle

Under normal circumstances, the dominant pacemaker function of the heart is supplied by the SA node. This is because the SA node reaches its threshold for depolarization at a faster rate than other specialized tissues. The rapid rate of the SA node normally prevents the discharge of slower pacemakers from becoming dominant. If impulses from the SA node do not develop normally, however, the next specialized tissue to reach its threshold level would assume the pacemaker duties.

Cardiac cells with their characteristic automaticity serve as a "fail-safe" mechanism for initiating electrical impulses. The "back-up" (intrinsic pacemakers) are arranged in cascade fashion; the farther from the SA node, the slower the intrinsic firing rate. In order, the location of cells with pacemaker capabilities and rates of spontaneous discharge are the SA node (60 to 100/min), AV junctional tissue (40 to 60/min), and the ventricles, including the bundle branches and Purkinje fibers (20 to 40/min).

From the SA node, the excitation spreads throughout the right atrium, passing cell to cell by way of the gap junctions. Through internodal tracts, impulses travel directly to the left atrium and to the base of the right atrium, resulting in virtually simultaneous contraction of both atria. Approximately 0.04 second is required for the impulse of the SA node to spread to the AV node. From there, propagation of the action potentials within the AV node is slow compared with the rate in the remainder of the conducting system. As a result, there is a delay of 0.11 second from the time the action potentials reach the AV node until they pass to the AV bundle. The total delay of 0.15 second allows atrial contraction to be completed before ventricular contraction begins.

After leaving the AV node, the impulse travels through the bundle of His and the left and right bundle branches. As the action potential passes through the individual Purkinje fibers, the velocity of conduction increases, ending in near-simultaneous contraction of the left and right ventricles. Ventricular contraction begins at the apex. Once stimulated, the special arrangement of muscle layers in the wall of the heart produce a wringing action that proceeds toward the base of the heart. Total time for ventricular contraction is 0.08 to 0.09 second.

Autonomic Nervous System Effects on Pacemaker Cells

The effects of autonomic nervous system stimulation on the heart rate are mediated through the chemical neurotransmitters acetylcholine and norepinephrine. Acetylcholine causes the cell membrane of the SA node to become more permeable to potassium ions, resulting in hyperpolarization and a decrease in the slope of phase 4 depolarization. This a delays the pacemaker reaching threshold and therefore decreases the heart rate. Parasympathetic effects may also result from stimulation of the cardiac branch of the vagus nerve to

the heart, as occurs in vigorous carotid sinus massage, which may abolish the threshold potential altogether.

Norepinephrine increases the heart rate by increasing the rate of phase 4 depolarization. The result is an increase in pacemaker discharge rate in the SA node and Purkinje fibers. Norepinephrine also increases the flow of potassium and calcium ions into the cell during depolarization and the plateau phase of the action potential. As a result, sympathetic stimulation leads to an increase in heart rate and the force of cardiac contraction.

Mechanisms of Ectopic Electrical Impulse Formation

An ectopic beat results when the pacemaker function is assumed for one beat by cells other than those in the SA node. These isolated events are sometimes referred to as *premature beats* because they occur early in diastole before the SA node is normally scheduled to discharge. The new pacemaker is called an **ectopic focus.** Depending on the location of the ectopic focus, the premature beats may be of atrial origin, **premature atrial contractions** (PACs); junctional origin, **premature junctional contractions** (PJCs); or ventricular origin, **premature ventricular contractions** (PVCs). The ectopic focus may be intermittent or sustained and may assume the pacemaker duties of the heart.

The two basic mechanisms by which ectopic electrical impulses can be generated in the heart are enhanced automaticity and reentry. Abnormal impulse formation, with abnormal impulse conduction, is the basis of cardiac dysrhythmias.

Enhanced Automaticity

Enhanced automaticity is caused by an acceleration of phase 4 depolarization that commonly results from an abnormally high leakage of sodium ions into the cells, causing the cells to reach threshold prematurely. As a result, the rate of electrical impulse formation in potential pacemakers increases beyond their inherent rate (Fig. 18-10).

Enhanced automaticity is responsible for dysrhythmias in Purkinje fibers and other myocardial

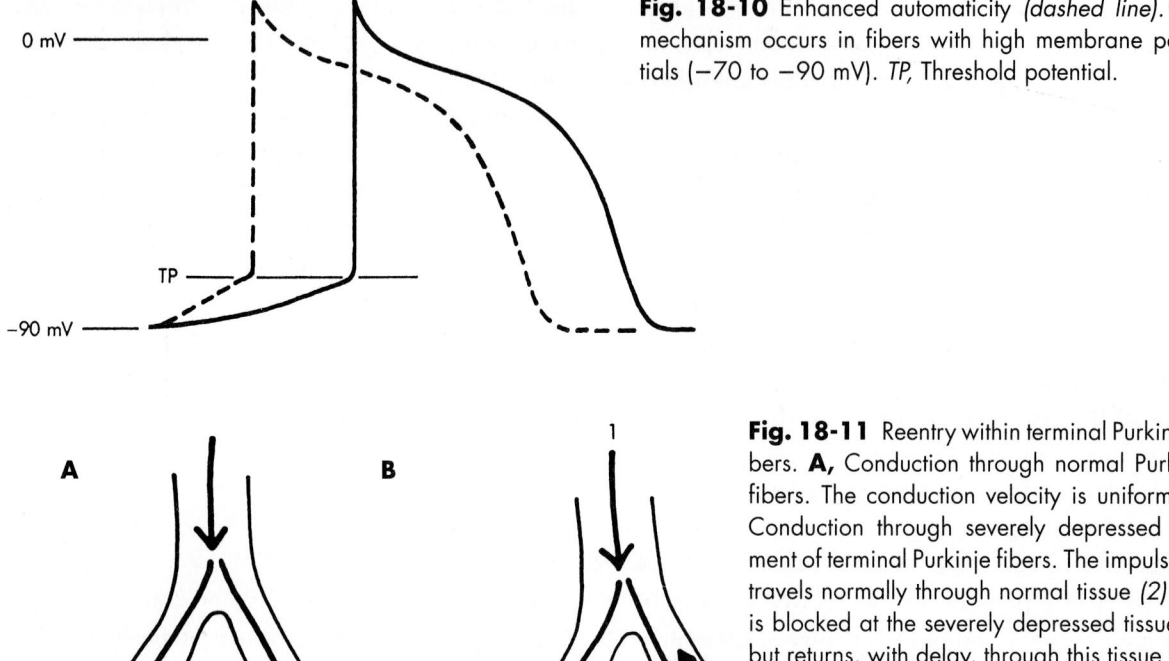

Fig. 18-10 Enhanced automaticity *(dashed line).* This mechanism occurs in fibers with high membrane potentials (−70 to −90 mV). *TP,* Threshold potential.

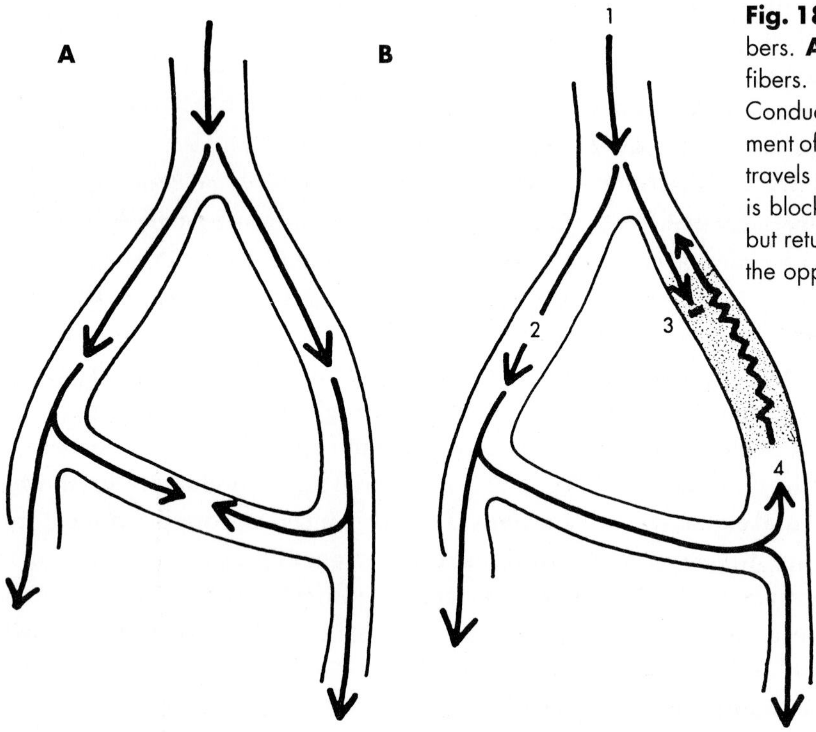

Fig. 18-11 Reentry within terminal Purkinje fibers. **A,** Conduction through normal Purkinje fibers. The conduction velocity is uniform. **B,** Conduction through severely depressed segment of terminal Purkinje fibers. The impulse *(1)* travels normally through normal tissue *(2)* and is blocked at the severely depressed tissue *(3)* but returns, with delay, through this tissue from the opposite direction.

cells with a high resting membrane potential. Enhanced automaticity may be secondary to excess catecholamines, digitalis toxicity, hypoxia, hypercapnia, myocardial ischemia or infarction, increased venous return (stretching of the heart), hypokalemia, hypocalcemia, heating or cooling of the heart, or *atropine* administration.

Reentry

Reentry is the reactivation of tissue by a returning impulse (Fig. 18-11). It occurs when the progression of an electrical impulse is delayed, blocked, or both, in one or more segments of the heart's electrical conduction system, whereas the electrical impulse is conducted normally through the rest of the heart. A delayed or blocked impulse that enters cardiac cells that have just become repolarized may produce single or repetitive ectopic beats. Reentry dysrhythmias can occur in the SA node, atria, AV junction, bundle branches, or Purkinje fibers. Reentry is the sustaining mechanism in some cases of ventricular bigeminy or trigeminy, **ventricular tachycardia,** and **paroxysmal supraventricular tachycardia** (PSVT).

The reentry mechanism requires that, at some point, conduction through the heart takes parallel pathways, each having a different conduction speed and refractory characteristics. A premature impulse, for example, may find one branch of a conducting pathway still refractory from the passage of the last normal impulse. If the impulse passes (somewhat slowly) along a parallel conducting pathway, by the time the impulse reaches the previously blocked pathway, it may have had time to recover its ability to conduct. If the two parallel paths connect at an area of excitable myocardial tissue, the depolarization process from the slower path may enter the faster conducting pathway and travel in a retrograde manner back to the origin of the impulse. If the delay in the conduction of the impulse is constant for each beat, the abnormal beat usually follows the normal beat at exactly the same interval of time (the constant coupling interval).

Because one factor favoring reentry is delayed conduction, rhythms that depend on reentry for their development are disorders of conduction rather than of impulse formation. Common causes of delayed or blocked electrical impulses are myocardial ischemia, certain medications, and hyperkalemia. These can decrease the rate of rise of phase 0 of the action potential and increase times for action potential duration as well as repolarization.

Section Three
Introduction to ECG Monitoring

The electrocardiograph (ECG) is a graphic representation of the heart's electrical activity generated by depolarization and repolarization of the atria and ventricles. It is a valuable diagnostic tool for identifying a number of cardiac abnormalities, including abnormal heart rates and rhythms, abnormal conduction pathways, hypertrophy or atrophy of portions of the heart, and the approximate location of ischemic or infarcted cardiac muscle.

Evaluation of the ECG requires a systematic approach that includes descriptive analysis (assessing the ECG tracing) and clinical impression (applying ECG analysis in assessing the patient). The ECG tracing is only a reflection of the heart's electrical activity. It does not provide information on mechanical events; neither force of contraction nor blood pressure can be measured from the ECG.

● BASIC CONCEPTS OF ECG MONITORING

The summation of all the action potentials transmitted through the myocardium during the cardiac cycle can be measured on the surface of the body. This measurement is obtained by applying electrodes on the body's surface that are connected to an appropriate recording device. The voltage changes are fed to an ECG machine, amplified, and displayed visually on the oscilloscope, graphically on ECG paper, or both. Voltage may be positive (seen as an upward deflection on the ECG tracing), negative (seen as a downward deflection on the ECG tracing), or isoelectric, when no electrical current is detected (seen as a straight baseline on the ECG tracing). The continuous curve of waves or deflections comprises the ECG.

The ECG was historically monitored by using three locations for electrode sensors—the patient's right arm, left arm, and left leg—forming an equilateral triangle called *Einthoven's triangle* (Fig. 18-12). It is assumed that the heart lies in the center of the electrical field defined by the axes of the three electrodes. Although this is not precisely true, as a practical matter this concept still provides the basis for ECG today.

ECG Leads

ECG machines can provide many views of the heart's electrical activity by monitoring voltage changes between any number of electrodes applied in various places on the body. Each pair of electrodes is referred to as a *lead*. A standard ECG performed in the hospital is recorded by viewing the heart's electrical activity from 12 leads. Although some EMS services have equipment that provides 12-lead recording, equipment providing 3- and 4-lead recording is more common in the prehospital setting.

An ECG lead consists of two surface electrodes of opposite polarity (one positive and the other negative) or one positive surface electrode and one reference point. A lead composed of two electrodes of opposite polarity is called a *bipolar lead*. A lead composed of a single positive electrode and a reference point is a *unipolar lead*. Bipolar leads

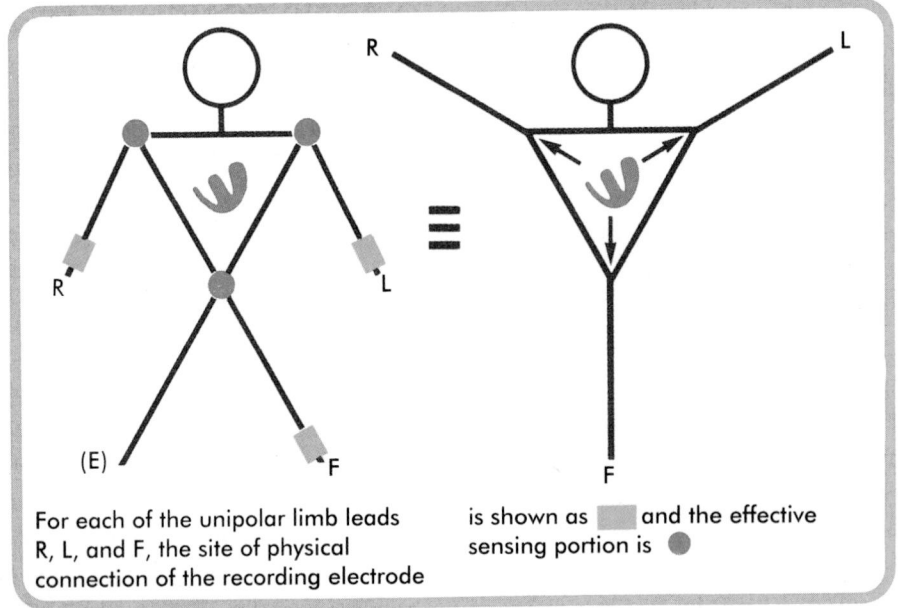

For each of the unipolar limb leads R, L, and F, the site of physical connection of the recording electrode is shown as ▨ and the effective sensing portion is ●

Fig. 18-12 Einthoven's triangle. Electrodes are placed on the right and left arms and the left leg, forming a triangle.

constitute the standard limb leads (I through III). Unipolar leads make up the augmented limb leads (aV$_R$, aV$_L$, and aV$_F$) and the precordial leads (V$_1$ through V$_6$).

The ECG machine makes it possible to make any electrode positive or negative, depending on which lead the machine is monitoring. Each lead assesses the electrical activity of the heart from a slightly different angle. The various leads produce different ECG tracings. The wave of depolarization is a progressive wave of positive charges. If the depolarization moves toward a positive electrode or away from a negative electrode, the ECG tracing for that particular lead shows an upward deflection. If the wave moves away from a positive electrode, a negative deflection shows on the ECG tracing.[3]

Standard Limb Leads

Standard limb leads record the difference in electrical potential between the left arm, the right arm, and the left leg electrodes, which represent the axes of the standard limb leads. If these axes are moved so that they cross a common midpoint without changing their orientation, they form a triaxial reference system (three intersecting lines

of reference). Lead I is a lateral (leftward) lead that assesses the heart's electrical activity from a vantage point defined as 0 degrees on a circle divided into an upper negative 180 degrees and a lower positive 180 degrees. Leads II and III are inferior leads that assess the heart's electrical activity from vantage points of +60 degrees and +120 degrees, respectively (Fig. 18-13). The electrodes of the three bipolar leads are placed on the following areas of the body:

Lead	Positive Electrode	Negative Electrode
I	Left arm	Right arm
II	Left leg	Right arm
III	Left leg	Left arm

Augmented Limb Leads

Augmented limb leads record the difference in electrical potential between the respective extremity lead sites and a reference point with zero electrical potential at the center of the electrical field of the heart. As a result, the axis of each lead is formed by the line from the electrode site (on the right arm, left arm, or left leg) to the center of the heart. The aV$_R$, aV$_L$, and aV$_F$ leads intersect at different angles than the standard limb leads and

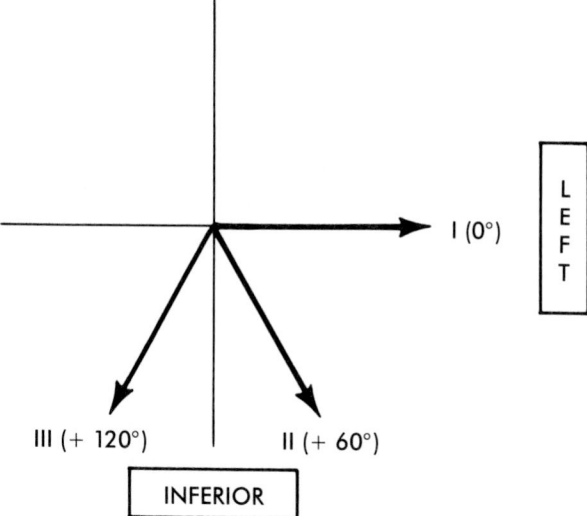

Fig. 18-13 Electrical vantage points of the three standard limb leads.

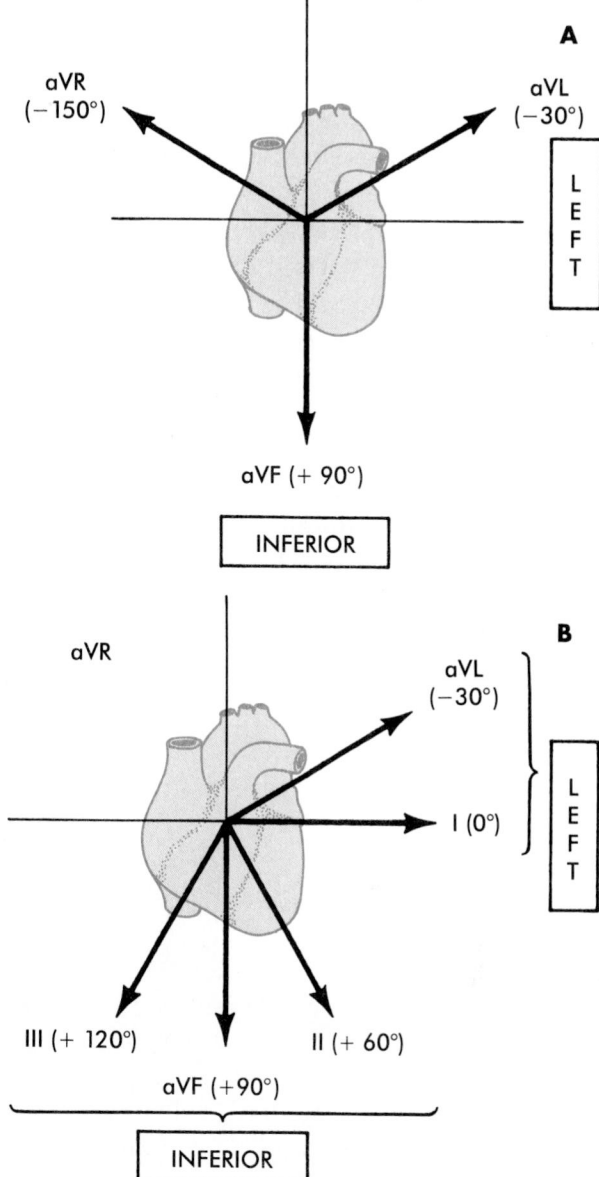

Fig. 18-14 A, Electrical vantage points of the three augmented limb leads. **B,** Combined electrical vantage points. Leads II, III, and aV$_F$ are considered inferior leads; I and aV$_L$ are considered lateral leads.

produce three other intersecting lines of reference, which together with the standard limb leads make up the hexaxial reference system. Augmented limb leads use the same set of electrodes as the standard limb leads. They measure an axis between the two bipolar leads by electronically combining the negative electrodes. By proper switching of the ECG machine, augmented limb leads can be obtained.

Lead aV$_L$ acts as a lateral (leftward) lead that records the heart's electrical activity from a vantage point that looks down from the left shoulder (-30 degrees). Lead aV$_F$ acts as an inferior lead, recording the heart's electrical activity from a vantage point that looks up from the left lower extremity ($+90$ degrees). Lead aV$_R$ is a distant recording electrode that looks down at the heart from the right shoulder. (Lead aV$_R$ is seldom used in ECG analysis.) Based on these lead descriptions, the lateral or left-sided leads are I and aV$_L$, and the inferior leads are II, III, and aV$_F$ (Fig. 18-14).

Precordial Leads

The six precordial leads are projected through the anterior chest wall toward the patient's back (the negative end of each chest lead). These positive leads are placed on the chest in reference to

the thoracic landmarks and record the heart's electrical activity in the transverse or horizontal plane.

Accurate placement of precordial leads is crucial to avoid incorrect readings of morphology or amplitude. Correct placement of electrodes requires identifying the angle of Louis (or sternal angle) on the patient's sternum. This landmark can be located by palpating the horizontal ridge where the manubrium joins the body of the sternum. The second rib attaches to the sternum at this point, so the second intercostal space lies just below this point. Dropping down two additional intercostal spaces and moving just to the right of the sternum indicates the reference position for lead V_1. The anatomical landmarks for properly placing V_2 through V_6 are shown in Fig. 18-15. In women, electrodes should be placed under the left breast to avoid any errors in the ECG tracing that may occur from a potentially large interposing mass.

Leads V_1 and V_2 are septal leads; V_2 through V_4 are anterior leads; and V_4 through V_6 are lateral precordial leads. The wall of the right ventricle (denoted by X in Fig. 18-15) and the posterior wall of the left ventricle (denoted by Y) are areas of the heart that are not well visualized by the six precordial leads.

Modified Lead Recording

Placement of the electrodes for the precordial leads is sometimes changed slightly to better evaluate conduction of a specific area of the heart. These leads are then referred to as *modified chest leads* (a modification of the original CL [chest left], CR [chest right], and CF [chest foot] leads) and become MCL_1, MCL_2, MCL_3, etc. Modified chest leads useful for monitoring cardiac activity in the prehospital setting are MCL_1 and MCL_6. These leads may help distinguish between supraventricular tachycardia with aberration and ventricular tachycardia and can help diagnose conduction blocks in the bundle branches.

When MCL_1 is viewed, the positive electrode is placed in the V_1 position and the negative electrode is placed anteriorly, just below the lateral end of the left clavicle. The ground electrode is placed in a similar position below the right

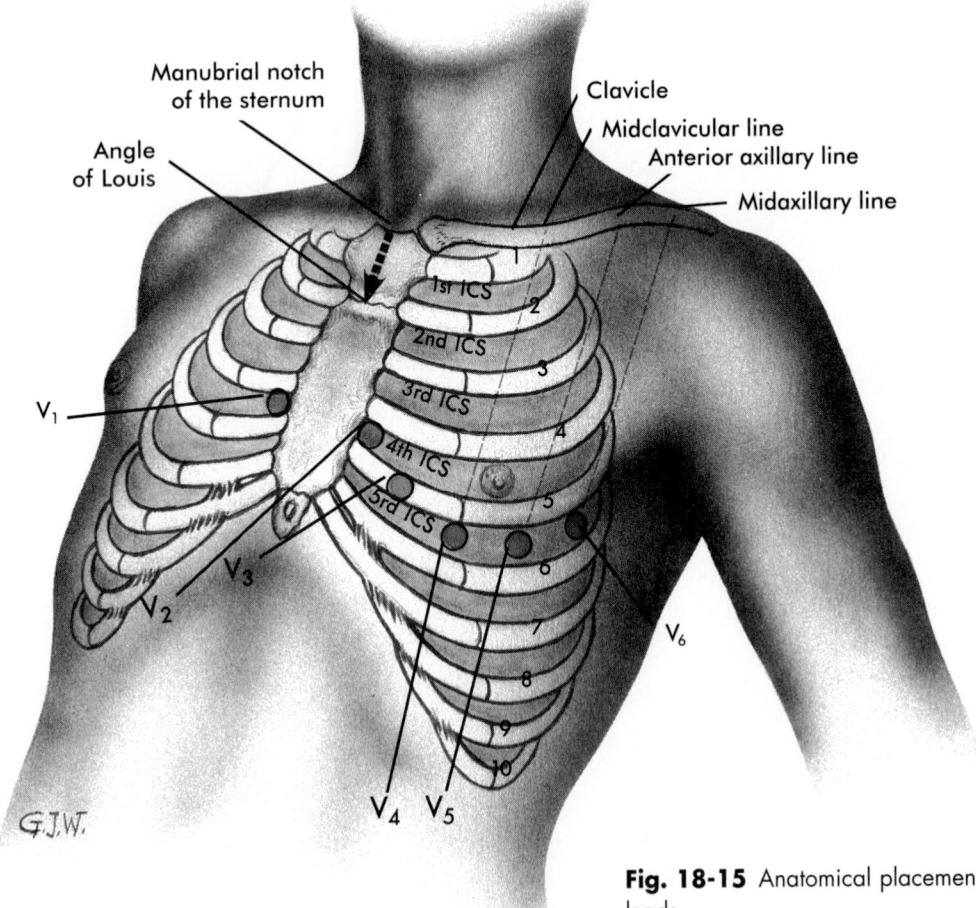

Fig. 18-15 Anatomical placement of the six precordial leads.

clavicle. Electrical activity in MCL_6 is observed by placing the positive electrode on the left midaxillary line at the level of the fifth intercostal space (as for lead V_6). The negative electrode is placed anteriorly, just below the right shoulder. The ground electrode is placed anteriorly, just below the left shoulder (Fig. 18-16).

Routine ECG Monitoring

Routine monitoring of cardiac rhythm in the prehospital setting, emergency department, or coronary care unit is usually obtained in lead II or MCL_1, which are the best leads to monitor for dysrhythmias because of their ability to visualize P waves. Considerable information can be gathered from a single monitoring lead, and in most situations, cardiac monitoring by a single lead is sufficient. For example, a paramedic can determine how fast the heart is beating, how regular the heartbeat is, and how long conduction is taking in different parts of the heart. Single-lead monitoring has limitations, however; it may fail to reveal various abnormalities (particularly ischemic ST-segment changes) in the ECG tracing. The sequence for field evaluation of a patient's ECG should include a sequential assessment of leads I, II, III, and MCL_1 or MCL_6 to ensure that treatment decisions are based on the best possible informa-

tion, particularly with suspected myocardial infarction.

Application of Monitoring Electrodes

The most commonly used electrodes for continuous ECG monitoring are pregelled, stick-on disks that can be easily applied to the chest wall. The following guidelines should be observed to minimize artifacts in the signal and to make effective contact between the electrode and the skin:

1. Choose an appropriate area of skin, avoiding large muscle masses and large quantities of hair that may prevent the electrode from lying flat against the skin.
2. Cleanse the area with alcohol to remove dirt and body oil. When attaching electrodes to the extremities, use the inner surfaces of the arms and legs. If necessary, excess body hair should be shaved before placing the electrodes. If the patient is extremely diaphoretic, use tincture of benzoin to aid in securing application.
3. Attach the electrodes to the prepared site.
4. Attach the ECG cables to electrodes. Most ECG cables are marked for right arm, left arm, and left leg application.
5. Turn on the ECG monitor and obtain a baseline tracing.

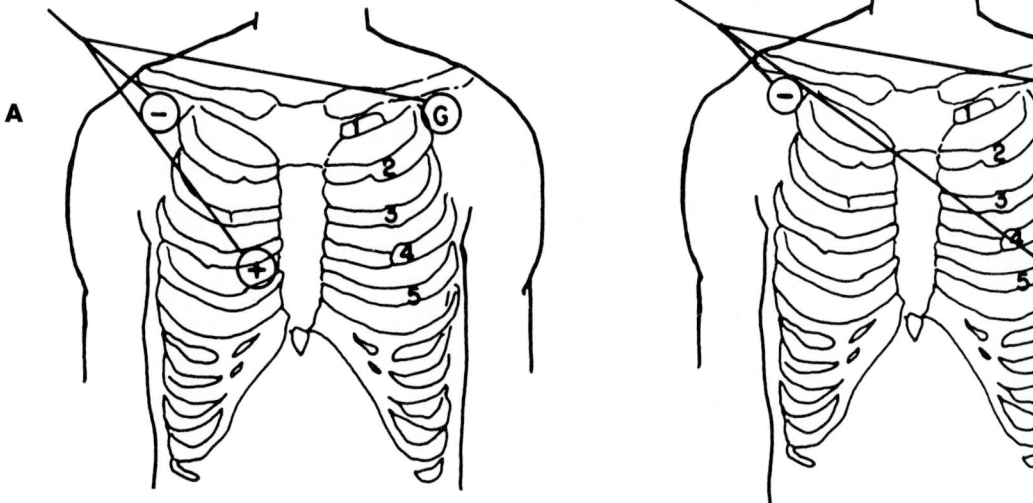

Fig. 18-16 Monitor lead placement for MCL_1 **(A)** and MCL_6 **(B).**

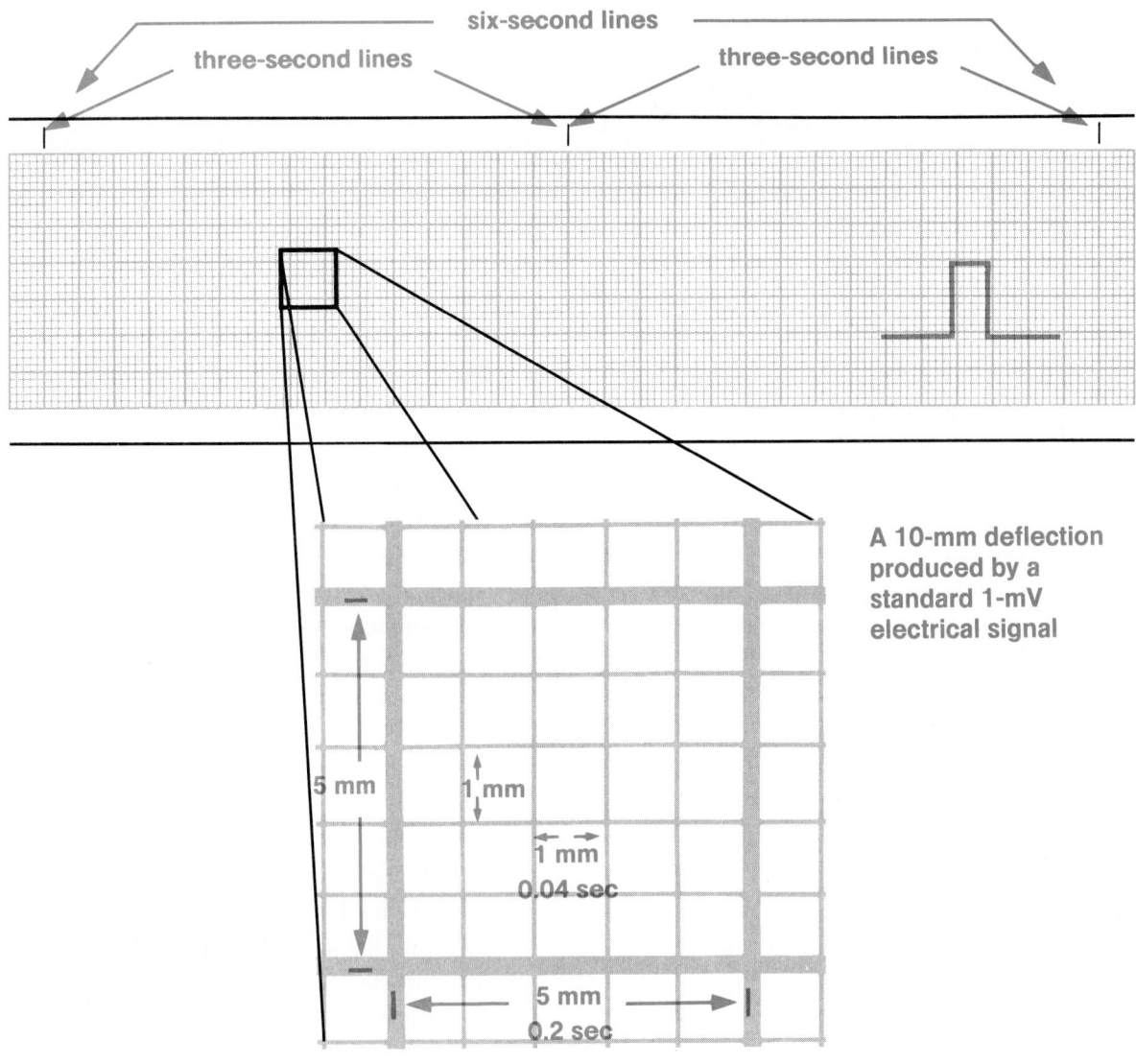

Fig. 18-17 ECG graph paper.

If the signal is poor, the paramedic should recheck the cable connections and the effectiveness of the patient's skin contact to the electrodes. Other common causes of a poor signal include excessive body hair, dried conductive gel, poor electrode placement, and diaphoresis.

ECG Graph Paper

The paper used in recording ECGs is standardized to allow comparative analysis of an ECG wave. The graph paper is divided into squares 1 mm in height and width. The paper is further divided by darker lines every fifth square, both vertically and horizontally. Each large square is 5 mm high and 5 mm wide (Fig. 18-17).

As the graph paper moves past the stylus of the ECG machine, it measures time and amplitude. Time is measured on the horizontal plane (side to side). When the ECG is recorded at the standard paper speed of 25 mm/sec, each small square equals 0.04 second (1 mm) and each large square (the dark vertical lines) equals 0.20 second (5 mm). These squares measure the length of time it takes an electrical impulse to pass through a specific part of the heart.

Amplitude is measured on the vertical axis (top to bottom) of the graph paper. Each small square

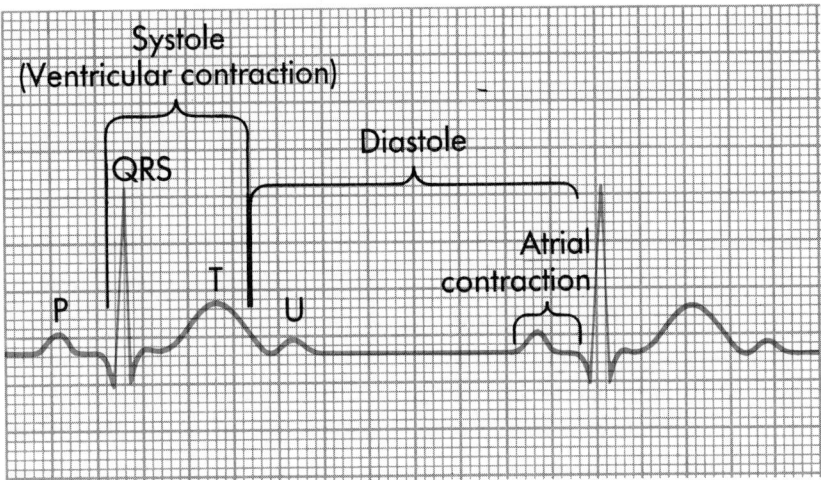

Fig. 18-18 Summary of the electrical basis of the ECG.

of the graph paper equals 1 mV, and each large square (five small squares) equals 5 mV. The sensitivity of the ECG machine is standardized. When properly calibrated, a 10-mV electrical signal produces a 10-mm deflection (two large squares) on the ECG tracing. ECG machines equipped with calibration buttons should have a calibration curve placed at the beginning of the first ECG tracing.

Time interval markings are denoted by short vertical lines and are usually located on the top of the ECG graph paper. When the ECG is recorded at the standard paper speed, the distance between each short vertical line is 75 mm (3 seconds). Each 3-second interval contains 15 large squares (0.2 second multiplied by 15 squares equals 3 seconds). These markings are used to calculate heart rate.

● RELATIONSHIP OF ECG TO ELECTRICAL ACTIVITY

Each wave form seen on the oscilloscope or recorded on the ECG graph paper represents the conduction of an electrical impulse through a specific part of the heart. All wave forms begin and end at the isoelectric line, which represents the absence of electrical activity in cardiac tissue. In lead II, a deflection above the baseline is positive and

indicates an electrical flow toward the positive electrode. A deflection below the baseline is negative and indicates an electrical flow away from the positive electrode.

The normal ECG consists of a **P wave, QRS complex,** and **T wave.** Occasionally, a **U wave** can also be seen after the T wave. If present, it is usually a positive deflection and may be associated with electrolyte abnormalities. Other key components of the ECG that should be evaluated include the **PR interval, ST segment,** and **QT interval.** The combination of these waves represents a single heartbeat or one complete cardiac cycle (Fig. 18-18). The electrical events of the cardiac cycle are followed by their mechanical counterparts. The descriptions of ECG wave form components refer to those that would be seen in lead II monitoring.

P Wave

The P wave is the first positive (upward) deflection on the ECG, representing atrial depolarization. It is usually rounded and precedes the QRS complex. The P wave begins with the first positive deflection from the baseline and ends at the point where the wave returns to the baseline. The duration of the P wave is normally 0.10 second or less, and its amplitude is 0.5 to 2.5 mm. The P wave is usually followed by a QRS complex. However, if conduction disturbances are present, a QRS complex does not always follow each P wave.

PR Interval

The PR interval is the time it takes for an electrical impulse to be conducted through the atria and the AV node up to the instant of ventricular depolarization. The PR interval is measured from the beginning of the P wave to the beginning of the next deflection on the baseline (the onset of the QRS complex). The normal PR interval is 0.12 to 0.20 second (three to five small squares on the graph paper) and depends on the heart rate and the conduction characteristics of the AV node. When the heart rate is fast, the PR interval is normally of shorter duration than when the heart rate is slow. A normal PR interval indicates that the electrical impulse has been conducted through the atria, AV node, and bundle of His normally and without delay.

QRS Complex

The QRS complex is generally composed of three individual waves: the Q, R, and S waves. The QRS complex begins at the point where the first wave of the complex deviates from the baseline and ends where the last wave of the complex begins to flatten at, above, or below the baseline. The direction of the QRS complex may be predominantly positive (upright), predominantly negative (inverted), or biphasic (partly positive, partly negative). The shape of the normal QRS complex is narrow and sharply pointed. Its duration is generally 0.08 to 0.12 second (one to three small

squares on the graph paper) or less, and its amplitude normally varies from less than 5 mm to more than 15 mm.

The Q wave is the first negative (downward) deflection on the ECG, although it may not be present in all leads, and represents depolarization of the interventricular septum. The R wave is the first positive deflection after the P wave. Subsequent positive deflections in the QRS complex that extend above the baseline and that are taller than the first R wave are called *R prime* (R'), *R double prime* (R''), and so on. The S wave is the negative deflection that follows the R wave. Subsequent negative deflections are called *S prime* (S'), *S double prime* (S''), and so on. Although there may be only one Q wave, there can be more than one R wave and one S wave in the QRS complex. The R and S waves represent the sum of electrical forces resulting from simultaneous depolarization of the right and left ventricles (Fig. 18-19).

The QRS complex follows the P wave and marks the approximate beginning of mechanical systole, which continues through the T wave. The QRS complex represents ventricular depolarization, or the conduction of an electrical impulse from the AV node through the bundle of His, Purkinje fibers, and the right and left bundle branches that results in ventricular depolarization.

ST Segment

The ST segment represents the early part of repolarization of the right and left ventricles. It immediately follows the QRS complex and ends with the onset of the T wave. The point at which it "takes off" from the QRS complex is called the J

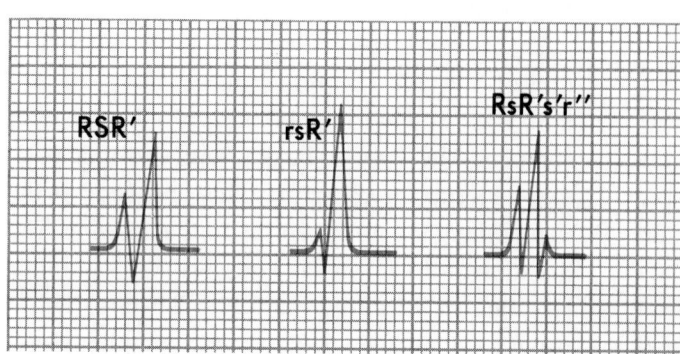

Fig. 18-19 QRS complexes with more than one positive or negative deflection.

point. In a normal ECG, the ST segment begins at baseline and has a very slight upward slope. The duration of the ST segment is approximately 0.20 second, depending on the heart rate.

The position of the ST segment is commonly judged as normal or abnormal using the baseline of the PR interval as a reference. Deviations above this baseline are referred to as *ST-segment elevation,* and those below it are referred to as *ST-segment depression* (Fig. 18-20). Certain conditions occasionally cause depression or elevation of the PR interval, thus affecting the reference for ST-segment abnormalities. Usually the baseline from the end of the T wave or U wave to the beginning of the P wave maintains its isoelectric position. Abnormal ST segments may be seen in infarction, ischemia, and pericarditis; after digitalis administration; and in other disease states.

T Wave

The T wave represents repolarization of the ventricular myocardial cells and occurs during the last part of ventricular systole. The T wave is identified as the first deviation from the ST segment and ends where the wave returns to the baseline. This wave may be above or below the isoelectric line and is usually slightly rounded and slightly asymmetrical. Depressed T waves may indicate previous or current cardiac ischemia. The duration of the T wave is 0.10 to 0.25 second, and the amplitude is usually less than 5 mm. A T wave elevated more than half the height of the QRS complex (peaked T wave) may indicate new ischemia of the myocardium or hyperkalemia.

QT Interval

The QT interval is the period from the beginning of ventricular depolarization (onset of the QRS complex) until the end of ventricular repolarization, or the end of the T wave (Fig. 18-21). During the initial portion of this interval, the heart is completely refractory to all premature stimuli (the absolute refractory period). During the latter portion of this interval, the conduction system is in a relative refractory period in which premature impulses may occur while the heart is vulnerable. Commonly prescribed medications that prolong the QT interval include quinidine, *procainamide,*

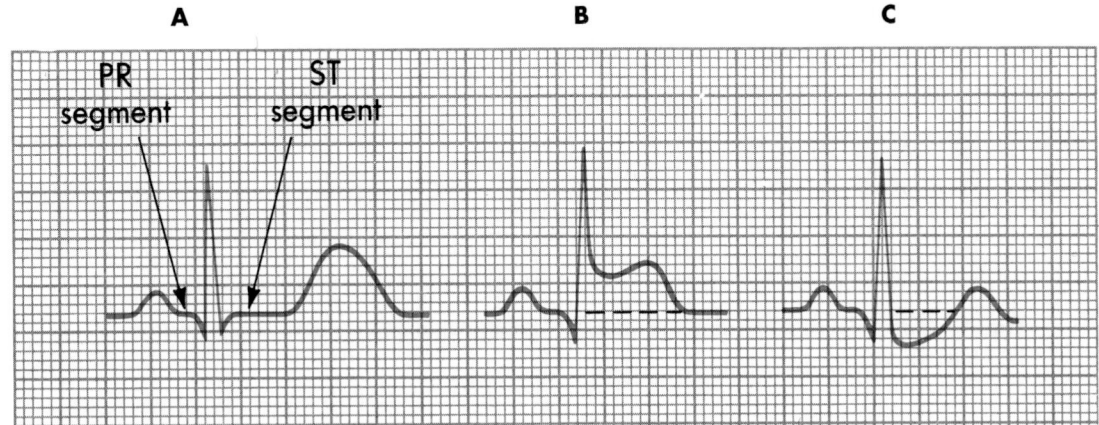

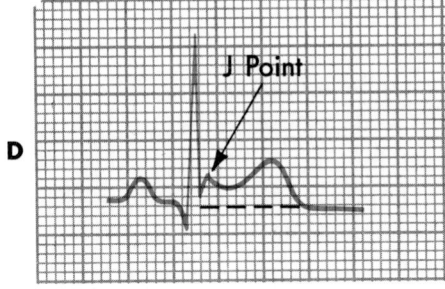

Fig. 18-20 ST-segment deviations. **A,** Use of the PR segment as a baseline. **B,** The ST segment is elevated with respect to the PR-segment baseline. **C,** The ST segment is depressed with respect to the PR-segment baseline. **D,** J point (ST-segment elevation). A prominent notch marks the takeoff of the ST segment.

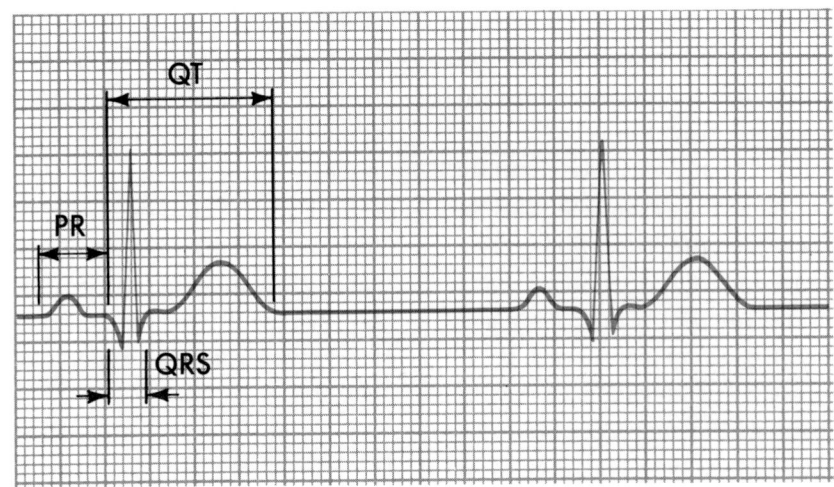

Fig. 18-21 PR, QT, and QRS intervals.

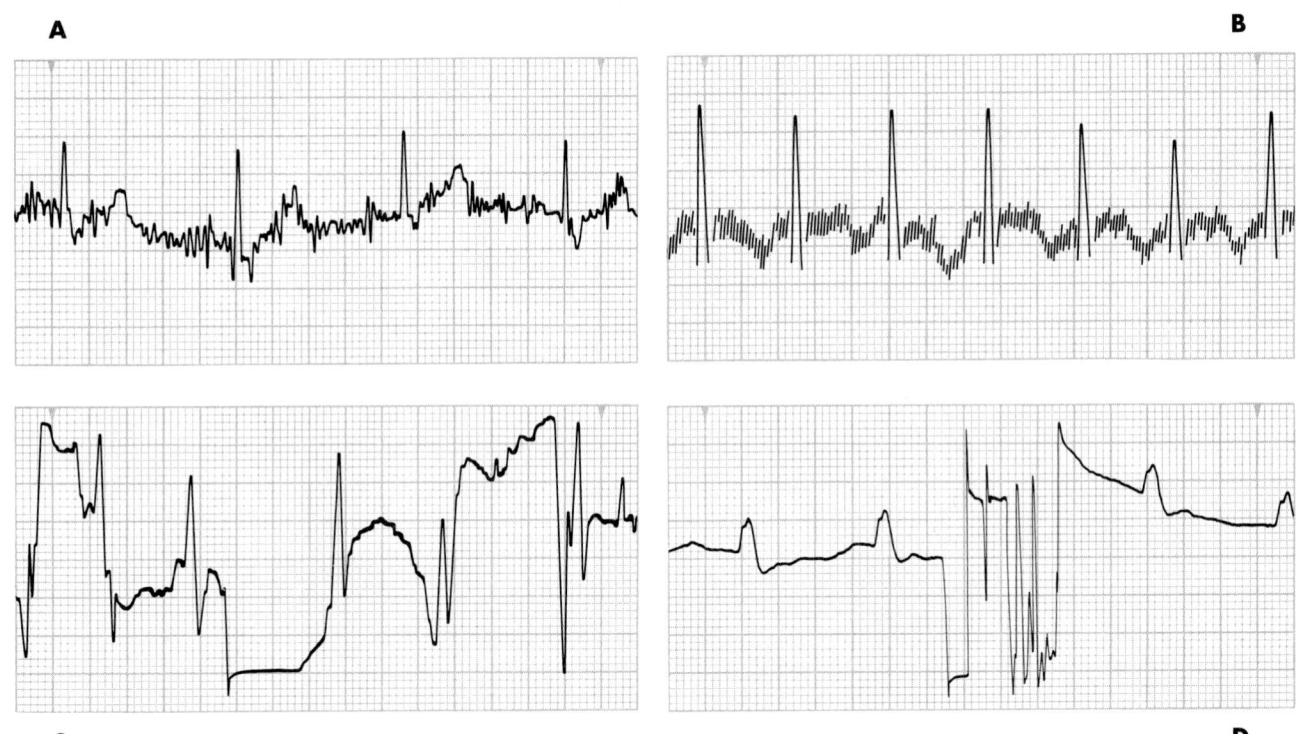

Fig. 18-22 Artifacts. **A,** Muscle tremor. **B,** AC (60-cycle) interference. **C,** Loose electrodes. **D,** Biotelemetry.

and disopyramide (type IA antidysrhythmics). These antidysrhythmics, by virtue of their effect on the QT interval, may lead to potentially lethal dysrhythmias, including ventricular tachycardia, ventricular fibrillation, and an unusual bidirectional ventricular dysrhythmia called *torsades de pointes*.

Artifacts

Artifacts are deflections on the ECG display or tracing produced by factors other than the heart's electrical activity (Fig. 18-22). Common causes of artifacts are improper grounding of the ECG machine, patient movement, loss of electrode contact with the patient's skin, patient shivering, and external chest compression. Two types of artifact that deserve special mention are alternating current interference (60-cycle interference) and biotelemetry-related interference.

Alternating-current (AC) interference may occur in a poorly grounded AC-operated ECG machine or when an ECG is obtained near high-tension wires or transformers. This results in a thick baseline composed of 60-cycle waves. The P waves may not be discernable because of the interference, but the QRS complex is usually visible. AC interference may also be caused by the patient or the lead cable touching a metal object such as a bed rail. Placing a blanket between the metal object and the patient may correct the interference.

Biotelemetry-related interference may occur when biotelemetry ECG signals are poorly received. This may result from weak batteries or from ECG transmission in areas with poor signaling conditions or at great distances from a base station receiver. Biotelemetry-related interference may produce sharp spikes and waves that have a jagged appearance.

Section Four
ECG Interpretation

● STEPS IN RHYTHM ANALYSIS

Evaluation of an ECG requires a systematic approach to analyzing a given rhythm. Paramedics are encouraged to memorize the "rules" for each dysrhythmia presented in this chapter and to use a consistent format to analyze rate, rhythm, QRS complex, P waves, and PR interval.

Step 1: Analyze the Rate

Analyzing the heart rate is usually the first step in interpreting an ECG. This may be done in a number of ways. The methods for calculating the heart rate presented in this text are heart rate calculator rulers, the triplicate method, the R-R method, and the 6-second count method.

In most cases, the heart rate is determined by analyzing the ventricular rate (the QRS complex). However, if the atrial and ventricular rates are different, as may occur in certain dysrhythmias, they must be calculated separately. The paramedic should remember that the normal heart rate is between 60 and 100 beats per minute. If the rate is below 60, it is considered a bradycardia; if the rate is above 100, it is considered a tachycardia.

Heart Rate Calculator Rulers

Heart rate calculator rulers (Fig. 18-23) are available from a number of manufacturers, and the directions for use supplied with them should be followed. Heart rate calculator rulers are reasonably accurate if the rhythm is regular. However, the paramedic should not rely solely on a mechanical device or tool to determine heart rate because they may not be readily available.

Triplicate Method

The triplicate method of determining heart rate (Fig. 18-24) is accurate only if the rhythm is regular and greater than 50 beats per minute. The

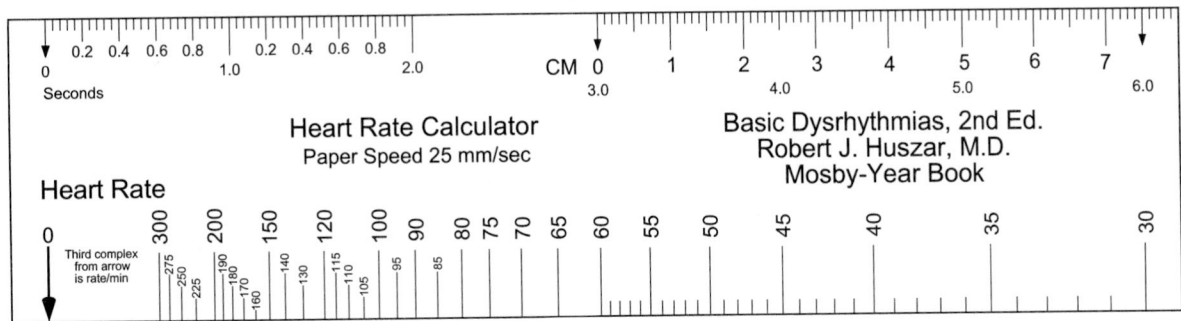

Fig. 18-23 Heart rate calculator ruler.

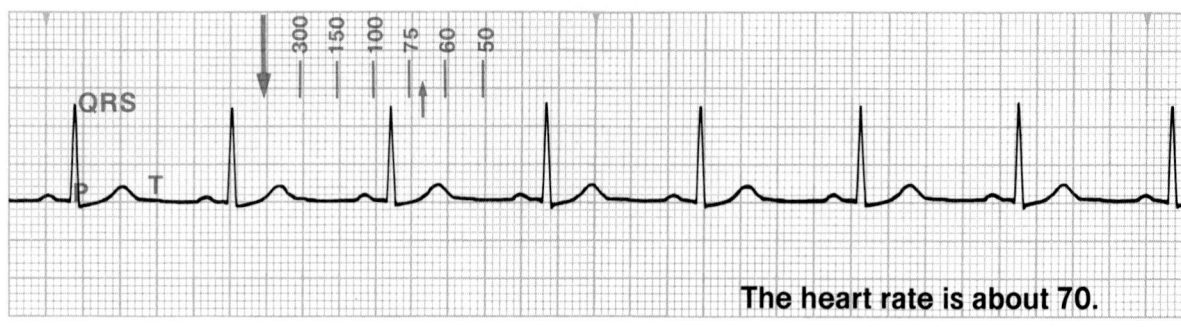

Fig. 18-24 Triplicate method.

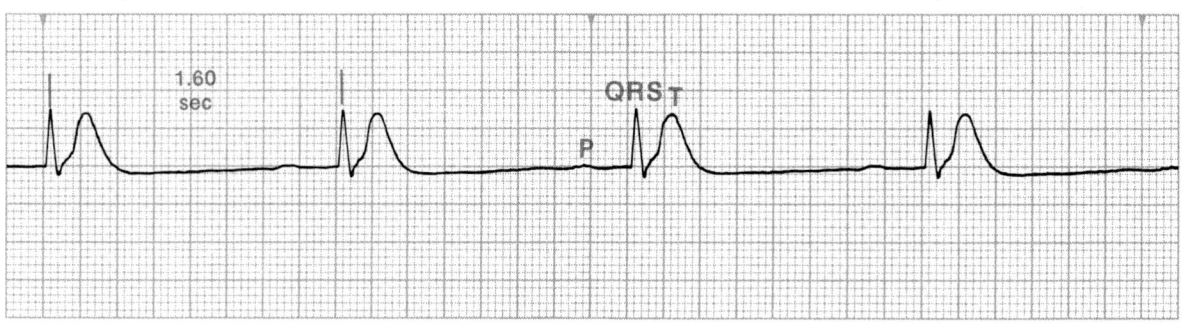

The heart rate = $\dfrac{60}{1.60\ \text{sec}}$ = 37.5 or, rounded off, 38.

Fig. 18-25 R-R interval method 1.

method requires memorizing two sets of numbers: 300-150-100 and 75-60-50. These numbers are derived from the distance between the heavy black lines (each representing 1/300 minute). Therefore two 1/300-min units equals 2/300 min equals 1/150 min or a heart rate of 150/min; three 1/300-min units equals 3/300 min equals 1/100 min or a heart rate of 100/min. Using these triplicates, the heart rate can be calculated as follows:

1. Select an R wave that lines up with a dark vertical line.
2. Number the next six dark vertical lines consecutively from left to right as 300-150-100 and then 75-60-50.
3. Identify where the next R wave falls with reference to the six dark vertical lines. If the R wave falls on 75, the heart rate is 75 beats per minute. If the R wave falls halfway between 100 and 150, the heart rate is approximately 125 beats per minute.

R-R Method

The R-R method may be used several different ways to calculate the heart rate. Like the triplicate method, the rhythm must be regular to obtain an accurate reading. However, the R-R method works equally well for slow rates.

Method 1.
Measure the distance in seconds between the peaks of two consecutive R waves and then divide this number into 60 to obtain the heart rate (Fig. 18-25).

Method 2.
Count the large squares between the peaks of two consecutive R waves and divide this number into 300 to obtain the heart rate (Fig. 18-26).

Method 3.
Count the small squares between the peaks of two consecutive R waves and divide this number into 1500 to obtain the heart rate (Fig. 18-27).

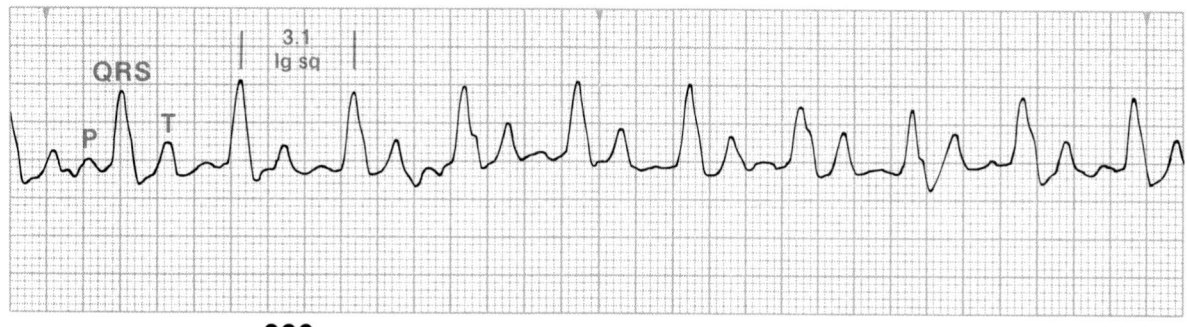

The heart rate $= \dfrac{300}{3.1 \text{ lg sq}} = 97.$

Fig. 18-26 R-R interval method 2.

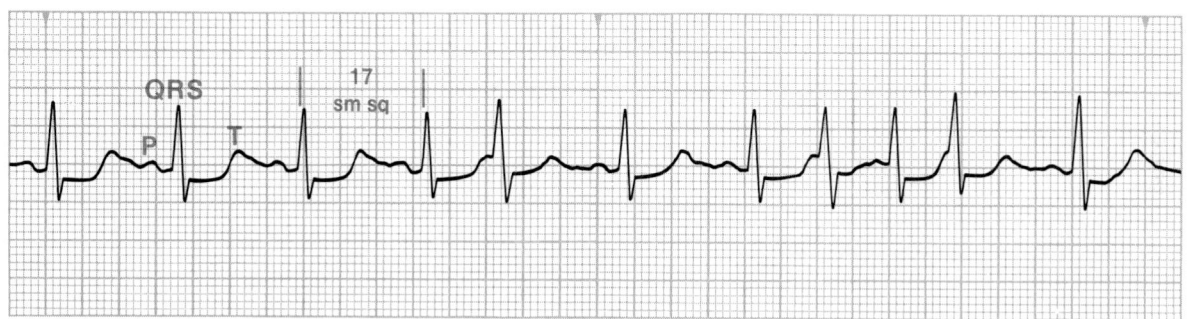

The heart rate $= \dfrac{1{,}500}{17 \text{ sm sq}} = 88.$

Fig. 18-27 R-R interval method 3.

Six-Second Count Method

The 6-second count method (Fig. 18-28) is the least accurate method of determining heart rate. It may be used, however, to obtain an approximate rate in regular and irregular rhythms.

As previously stated, the short vertical lines at the top of most ECG graph papers are divided into 3-second intervals when run at a standard speed of 25 mm/second. Two of these intervals equals 6 seconds. The heart rate is calculated by counting the number of QRS complexes in a 6-second interval and multiplying this number by 10.

Step 2: Analyze the Rhythm

To analyze the ventricular rhythm, the paramedic should compare the R-R intervals on the ECG tracing in a systematic way from left to right. This measurement may be taken using ECG cali-

pers or pen and paper. If calipers are used, one tip of the caliper is placed on the peak of one R wave, and the other tip is adjusted so that it rests on the peak of the adjacent R wave. The caliper is then used to map the distance of the R-R interval.

In the absence of calipers, a similar method of evaluating the R-R interval may be used using pen and paper. The straight edge of the paper is placed near the peaks of the R waves and the distance between the two consecutive R waves is marked off. This R-R interval is then compared with the other R-R intervals in the ECG tracing (Fig. 18-29).

If the distances between the R waves are equal or vary by less than 0.16 second (four small squares), the rhythm is "regular." If the shortest and longest R-R intervals vary by more than 0.16 second, the rhythm is "irregular". Irregular rhythms may be further classified as *regularly irregular* (patterned irregularity or "group beat-

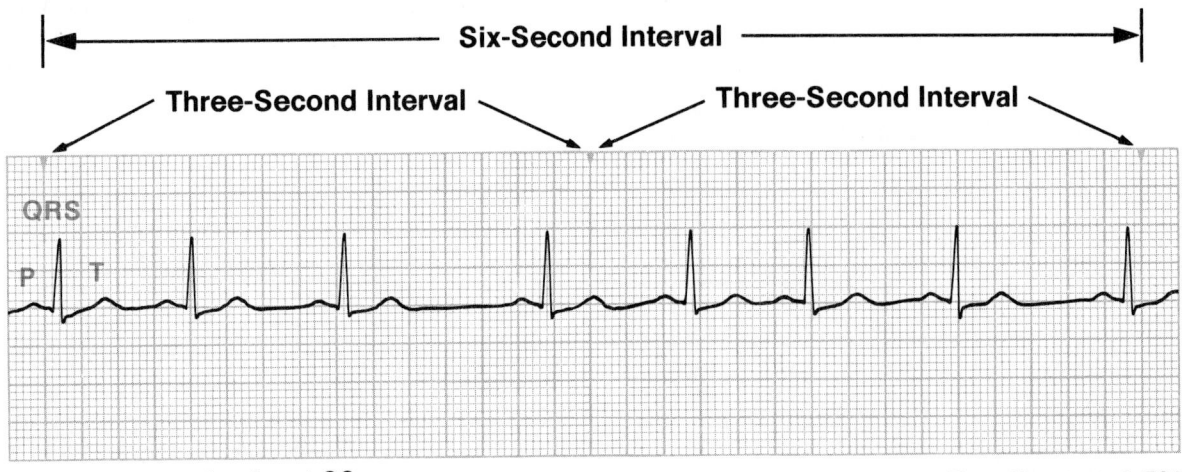

The heart rate is about 80.

(Actual heart rate is 72.)

Fig. 18-28 Six-second count method.

Fig. 18-29 Determining the rhythm.

The distances between the R waves are determined:

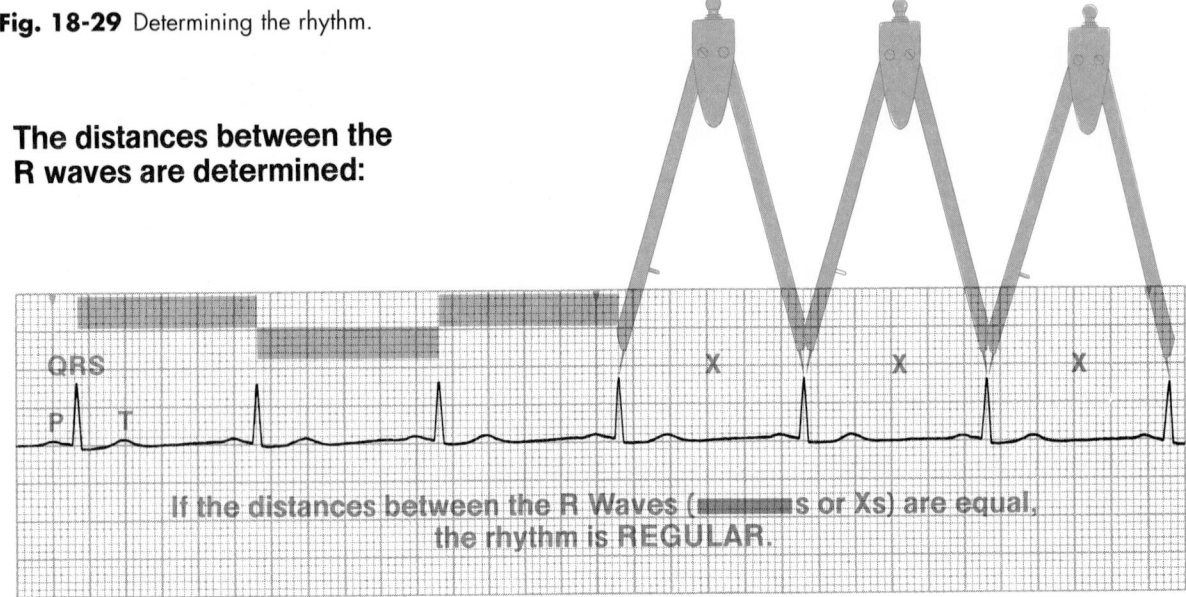

If the distances between the R Waves (▬▬▬s or Xs) are equal, the rhythm is REGULAR.

1. by estimating the R-R intervals,

2. by measuring the R-R intervals with ECG calipers,* or

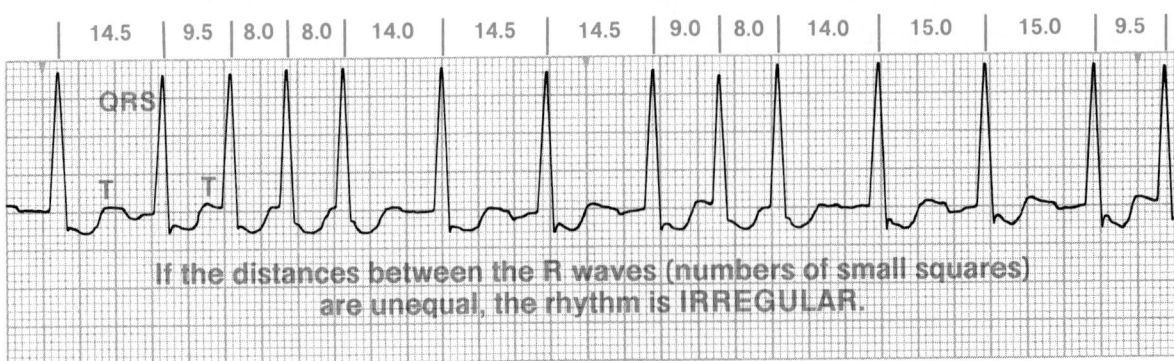

| 14.5 | 9.5 | 8.0 | 8.0 | 14.0 | 14.5 | 14.5 | 9.0 | 8.0 | 14.0 | 15.0 | 15.0 | 9.5 |

If the distances between the R waves (numbers of small squares) are unequal, the rhythm is IRREGULAR.

3. by counting the small squares between the R waves.

*If calipers are not available, mark off the distance between two R waves on a piece of paper and compare this distance with the other R-R intervals.

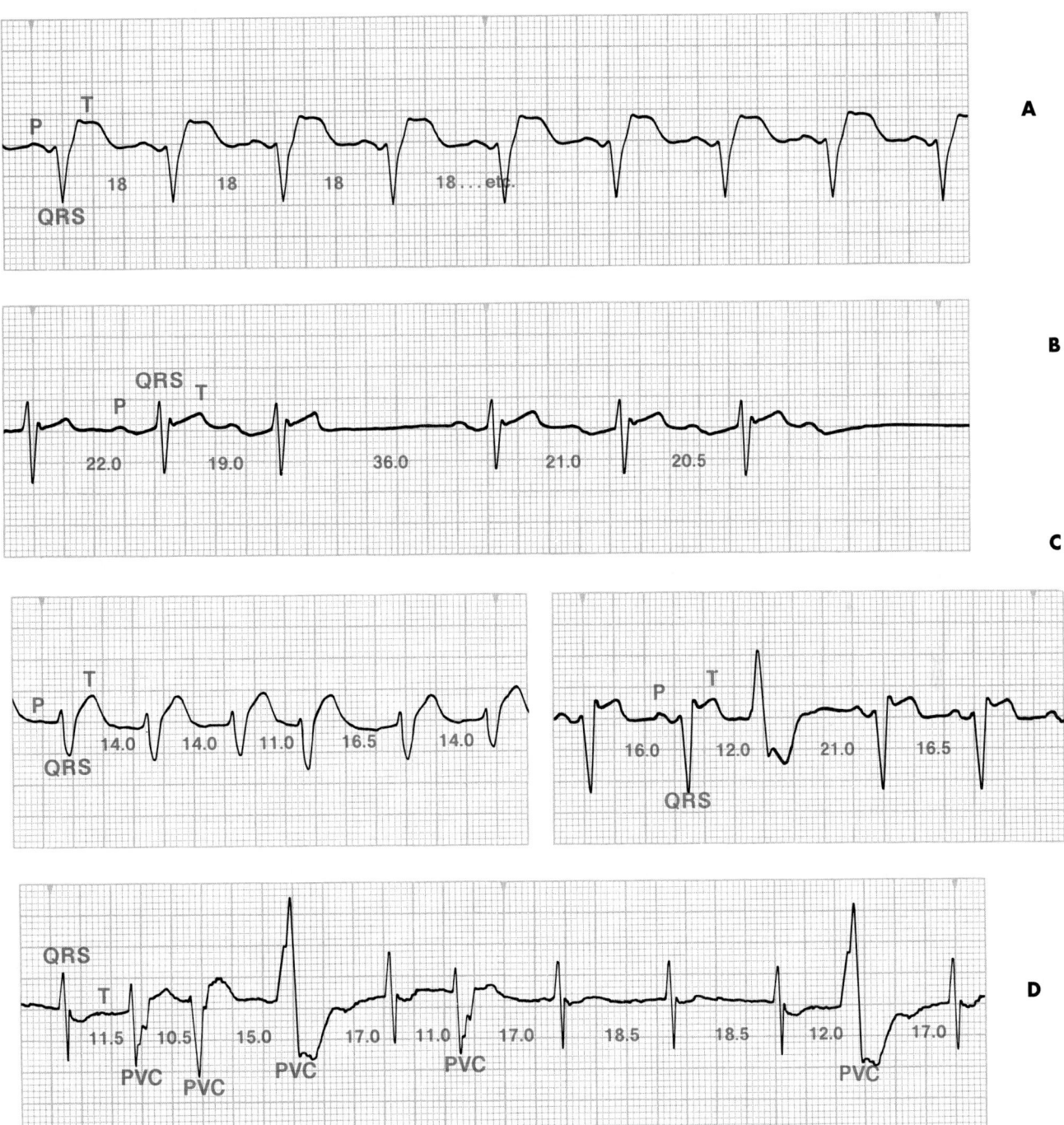

Fig. 18-30 A, Regular rhythm. **B,** Regularly irregular rhythm. **C,** Occasionally irregular rhythm. **D,** Irregularly irregular rhythm.

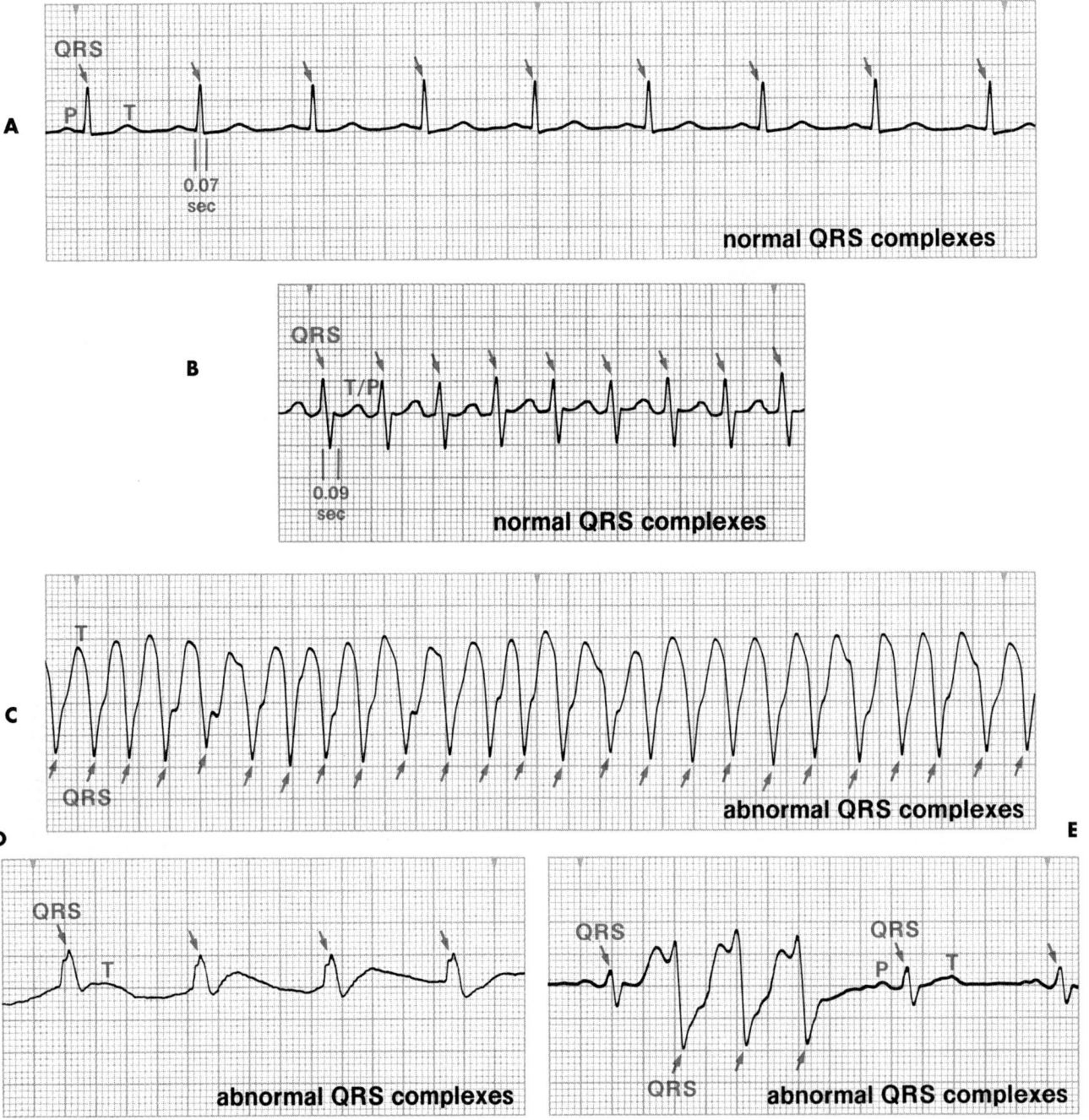

Fig. 18-31 A and **B,** Normal QRS complexes. **C** through **E,** Abnormal QRS complexes.

ing"), *occasionally irregular* (only one or two R-R intervals being unequal), or *irregularly irregular* (totally irregular in which there is no relationship between the R-R intervals) (Fig. 18-30).

Step 3: Analyze the QRS Complex

The QRS complex should be analyzed for regularity and width. QRS complexes less than or equal to 0.12 second wide (less than three small boxes) are supraventricular and normal. Complexes that are more than 0.12 second wide or that have a bizarre appearance indicate a conduction abnormality in the ventricles and are abnormal (Fig. 18-31). When evaluating an abnormal QRS width, identify the lead with the widest QRS complex because a portion of the QRS complex may be blended with the baseline in some leads.

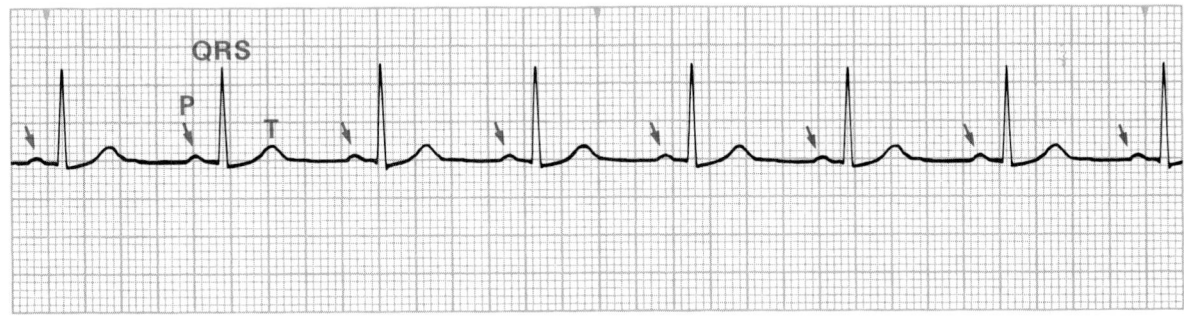

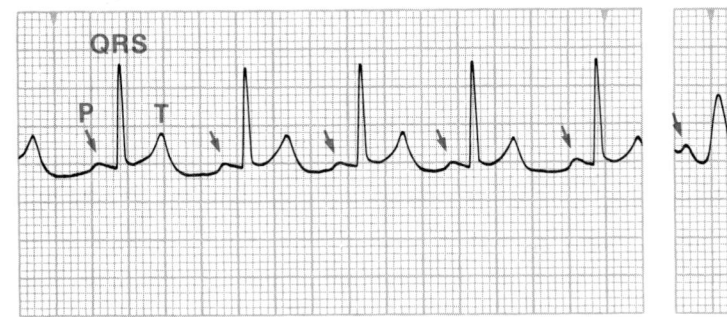

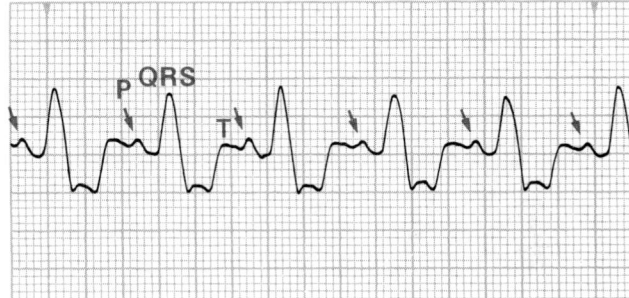

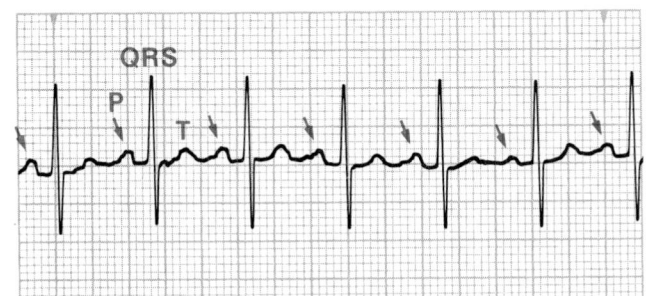

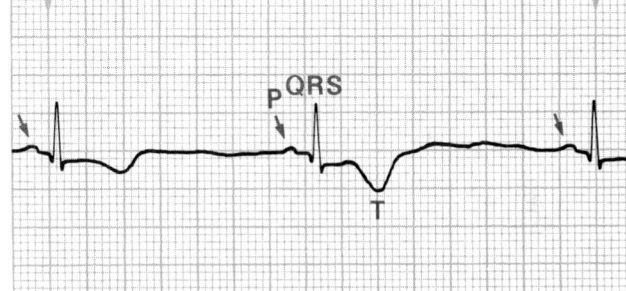

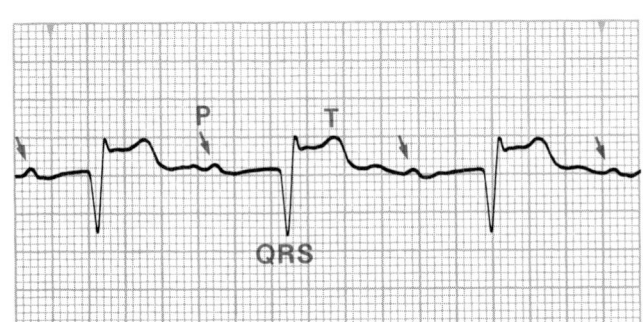

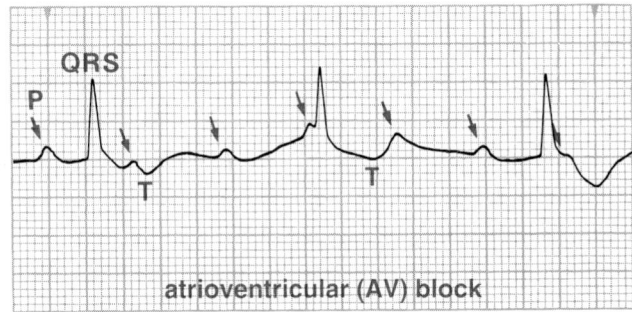

Fig. 18-32 Normal P waves.

Step 4: Analyze the P Waves

The normal P wave in lead II is positive and smoothly rounded and usually precedes each QRS complex, indicating that the pacemaker originates in the SA node (Fig. 18-32). Therefore the following four components should be observed when evaluating P waves:

1. Are the P waves regular (can they be mapped out similar to R-R intervals)?
2. Is there one P wave for each QRS complex?

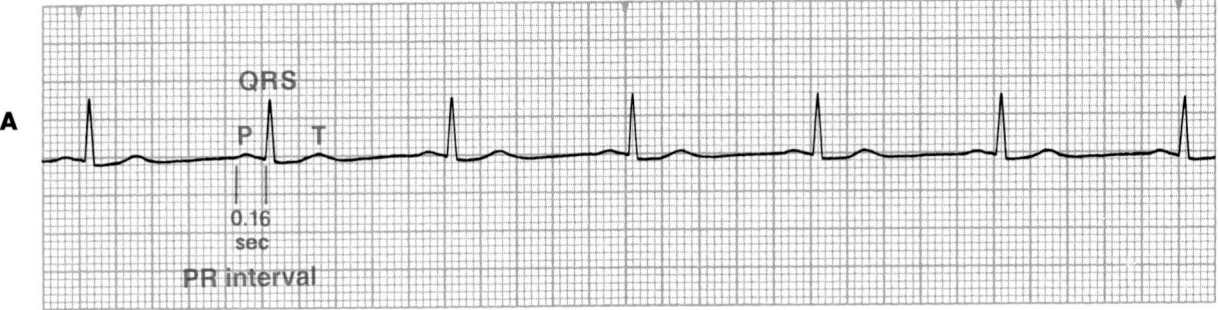

A

B

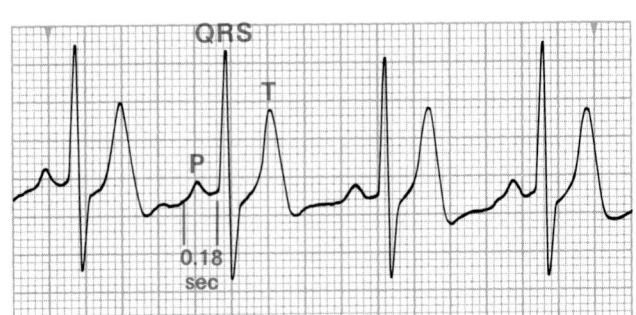

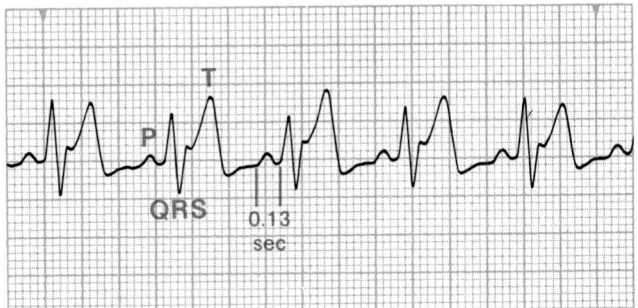

C

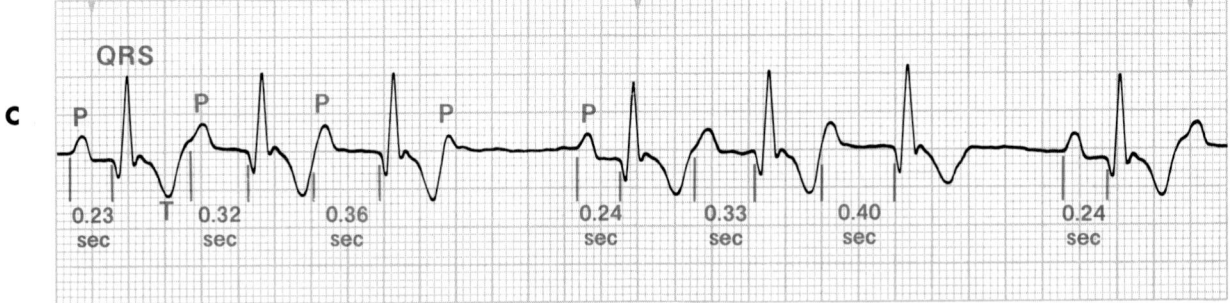

D

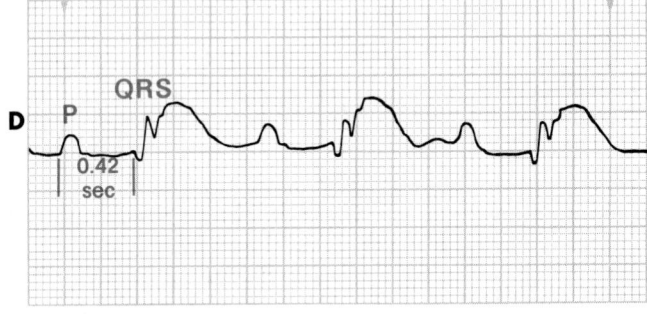

Fig. 18-33 A and **B,** Normal PR intervals. **C** and **D,** Abnormal PR intervals.

3. Are they upright or inverted?
4. Do they all look alike?

Step 5: Analyze the PR Interval

The PR interval indicates the time it takes for an electrical impulse to be conducted through the atria and AV node. It should be constant across the ECG tracing. A prolonged PR interval (greater than 0.20 second) indicates a delay in the conduction of the impulse through the AV node or bundle of His (AV block). A short PR interval (less than 0.12 second) indicates that the impulse progressed from the atria to the ventricles through pathways other than the AV node and bundle of His (Fig. 18-33).

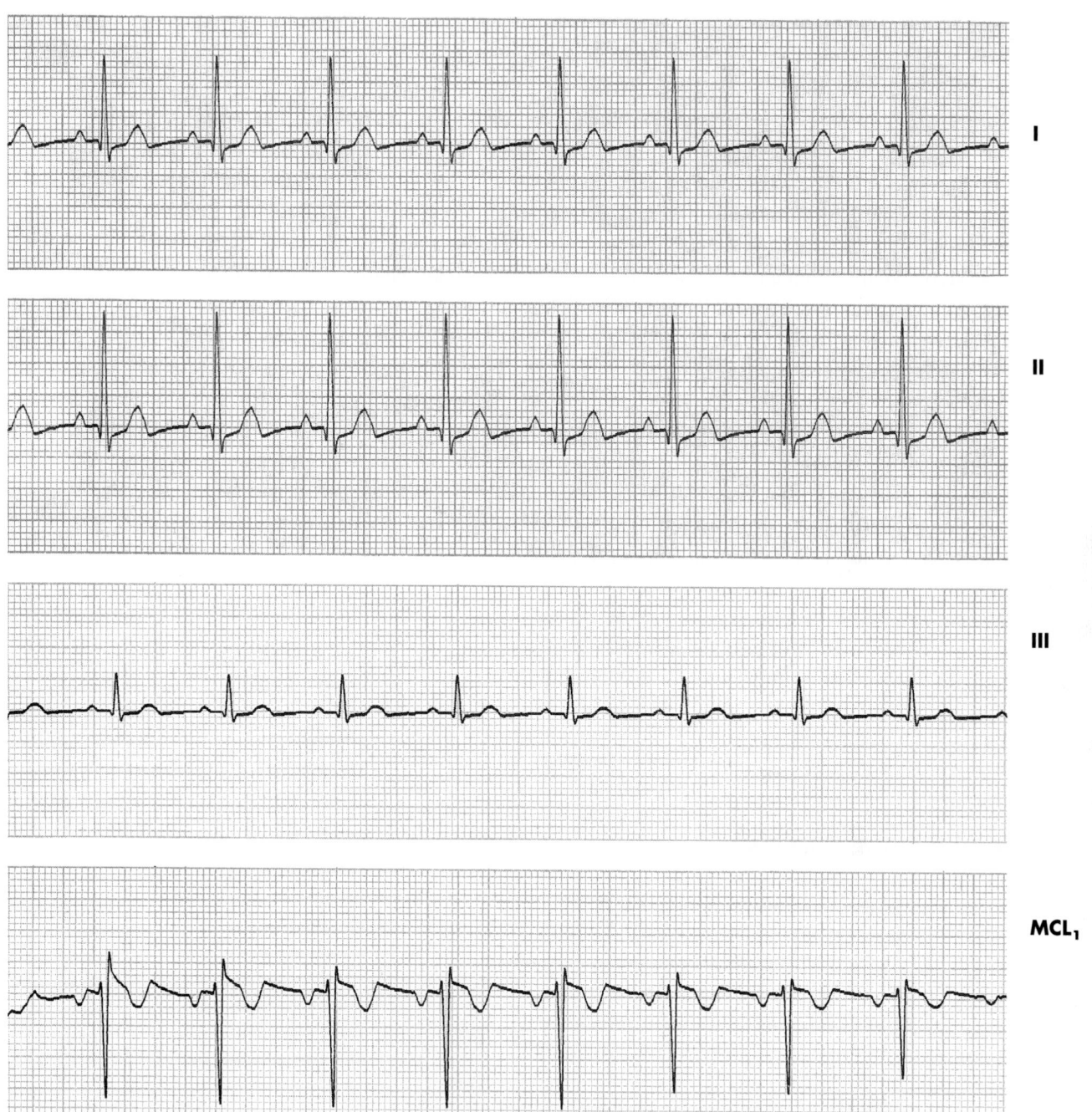

Fig. 18-34 Normal sinus rhythm.

Analyzing a Rhythm Using the Five Steps

To review, the normal sequence of atrial and ventricular activation as it relates to the ECG tracing is as follows: Each P wave is followed by a normal QRS complex and T wave. All QRS complexes are preceded by P waves; the PR interval is within normal limits, and the R-R interval is regular. The five steps in ECG rhythm interpretation can be applied to the rhythm in Fig. 18-34.

Section Five
Introduction to Dysrhythmias

Cardiac dysrhythmias can result from a number of physiological, pharmacological, and disease processes. Some conditions and abnormalities that can induce cardiac rhythm disturbances are:

- Myocardial ischemia or necrosis
- Autonomic nervous system imbalance
- Distention of heart chambers
- Blood gas abnormalities
- Electrolyte imbalance
- Drug effects or toxicity
- Electrocution
- Hypothermia
- Central nervous system injury

In addition to these potential causes of dysrhythmias, some cardiac rhythm disturbances are normal, even in patients who have healthy hearts (for example, sinus tachycardia from stress or anxiety). *Regardless of the etiology or type of dysrhythmia, treatment should focus on the patient, not merely the dysrhythmia.*

● CLASSIFICATIONS

The classification of dysrhythmias can be based on a number of factors, including changes in automaticity versus disturbances in conduction, major versus minor dysrhythmias, life-threatening versus non-life-threatening conditions, and site of origin. This text classifies rhythms by rate and pacer site (for example, ventricular tachycardia and sinus bradycardia) and includes the following five groups:

1. Dysrhythmias originating in the SA node
   a. Sinus bradycardia
   b. Sinus tachycardia
   c. Sinus dysrhythmia
   d. Sinus arrest
2. Dysrhythmias originating in the atria
   a. Wandering pacemaker
   b. PAC
   c. PSVT
   d. Atrial flutter
   e. Atrial fibrillation

3. Dysrhythmias originating in the AV junction
   a. PJC
   b. Junctional escape complexes or rhythms
   c. Accelerated junctional rhythm
4. Dysrhythmias originating in the ventricles
   a. Ventricular escape complexes or rhythm
   b. PVC
   c. Ventricular tachycardia
   d. Ventricular fibrillation
   e. Asystole
   f. Artificial pacemaker rhythm
5. Dysrhythmias that are disorders of conduction
   a. AV blocks
      First-degree AV block
      Second-degree AV block (Mobitz I or Wenckebach)
      Second-degree AV block (Mobitz II)
      Third-degree AV block
   b. Disturbances of ventricular conduction
   c. Pulseless electrical activity: electromechanical dissociation
   d. Preexcitation syndrome: Wolff-Parkinson-White syndrome

The text presents each dysrhythmia as it would appear in lead II monitoring. For comparison, the same dysrhythmia is also shown as it would appear in leads I, III, and MCL_1. We discuss the interpretation and emergency management, if required, of each dysrhythmia.

> **NOTE:**
> **All treatment modalities presented in this text follow the recommendations of the American Heart Association and are referenced to the appropriate treatment algorithm.**

Algorithms are illustrative methods used to summarize information, and some contain prehospital and in-hospital management recommendations. The following nine guidelines apply to all treatment algorithms[1]:

1. First, the paramedic should treat the patient, not the monitor.
2. Algorithms for cardiac arrest presume that the condition under discussion continually

persists, that the patient remains in cardiac arrest, and that CPR is always performed.

3. The paramedic should apply different interventions whenever appropriate indications exist.

4. The flow diagrams present mostly class I (acceptable, definitely effective) recommendations. The footnotes present class IIa (acceptable, probably effective), class IIb (acceptable, possibly effective), and class III (not indicated, may be harmful) recommendations.

5. Adequate airway, ventilation, oxygenation, chest compression, and defibrillation are more important than administration of medications and take precedence over initiating an intravenous line or injecting pharmacological agents.

6. Several medications *(epinephrine, lidocaine,* and *atropine)* can be administered via the endotracheal tube, but clinicians must use an endotracheal dose 2 to 2.5 times the intravenous dose.

7. With a few exceptions, intravenous medications should always be administered rapidly in bolus method.

8. After each intravenous medication, the paramedic should give a 20- to 30-ml bolus of intravenous fluid and immediately elevate the extremity. This enhances delivery of drugs to the central circulation, which may take 1 to 2 minutes.

9. The paramedic should treat the patient, not the monitor.

● DYSRHYTHMIAS ORIGINATING IN THE SA NODE

Most sinus dysrhythmias result from increases or decreases in vagal tone. The SA node generally receives sufficient inhibitory parasympathetic impulses from the vagus nerve to keep the heart rate well below the intrinsic discharge rate of the pacemaker cells. However, if vagal discharge increases, the heart rate becomes bradycardic; if vagal discharge decreases, sympathetic stimulation results in sinus tachycardia. Dysrhythmias that originate

in the SA node include sinus bradycardia, sinus tachycardia, sinus dysrhythmia, and sinus arrest. ECG features common to all SA node dysrhythmias include:

- Normal duration of QRS complex (in the absence of bundle branch block)
- Upright P waves in lead II
- Similar appearance of all P waves
- Normal duration of PR interval (in the absence of AV block)

Sinus Bradycardia

Description

Sinus bradycardia (Fig. 18-35) results from slowing of the SA node.

Etiology

- Intrinsic sinus node disease
- Increased parasympathetic vagal tone
- Hypothermia
- Hypoxia
- Drug effects (for example, digitalis, *propranolol, verapamil)*

Rules for Interpretation (Lead II monitoring)

Rate: Less than 60 beats per minute

Rhythm: Regular

QRS complex: Less than 0.12 second (normal), provided there is no ventricular conduction disturbance

P waves: Normal and upright; one P wave before each QRS complex

PR interval: 0.12 to 0.20 second and constant (normal), provided no AV block is present

Clinical Significance

Decreased rate may compromise cardiac output, resulting in hypotension, angina pectoris, or central nervous system symptoms (lightheadedness, vertigo, syncope). Sinus bradycardia may be associated with nausea and vomiting and is the cause of vasovagal syncope. Sinus bradycardia may follow the application of carotid sinus pressure (carotid sinus massage). The dysrhythmia is common during sleep and in well-conditioned athletes.

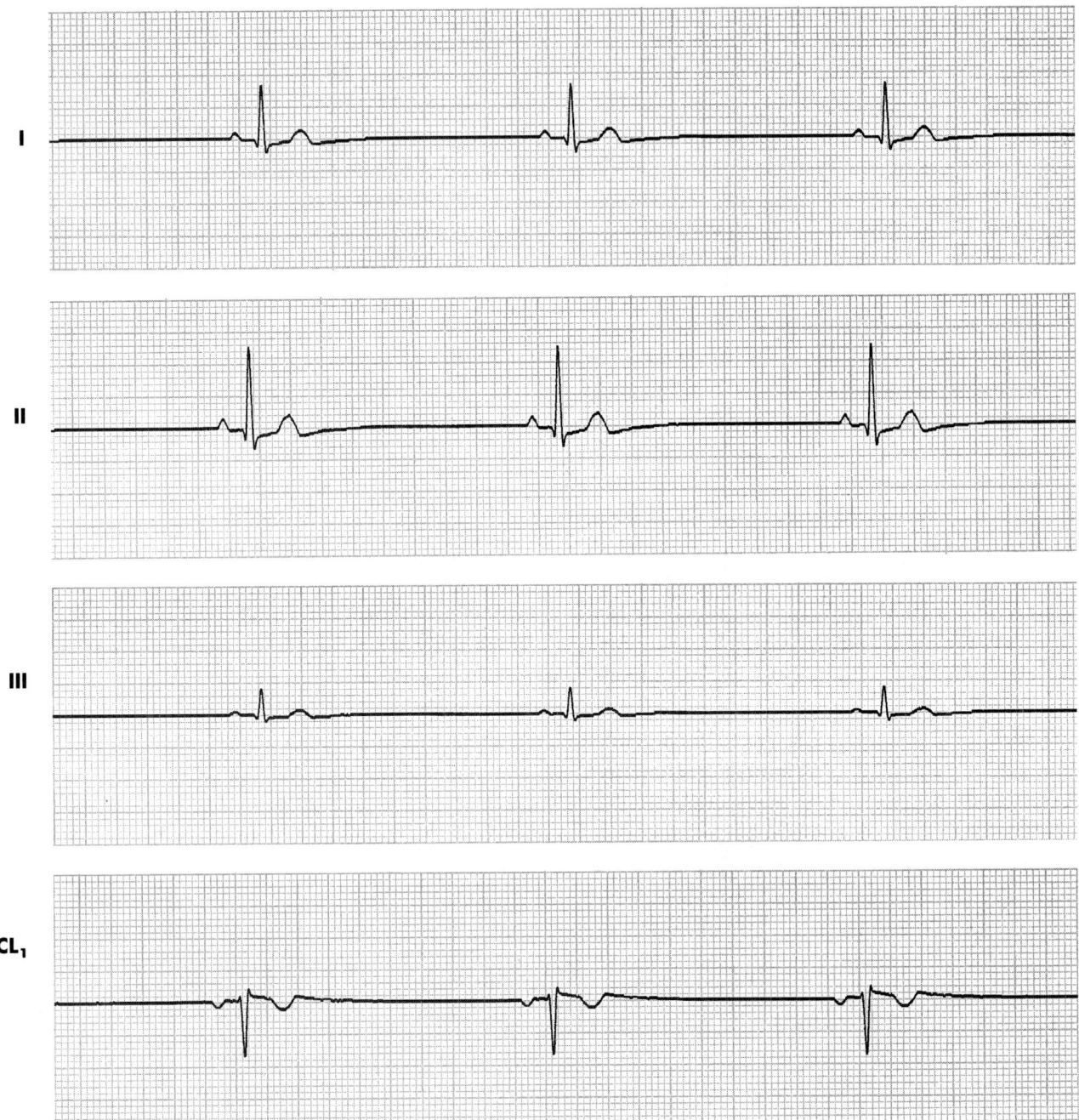

Fig. 18-35 Sinus bradycardia.

Management (Fig. 18-36)

Prehospital intervention is usually unnecessary unless hypotension or ventricular irritability is present (these are more common with rates below 50 beats per minute). If treatment is required, *atropine* is the drug of choice. If symptoms persist, transcutaneous pacing (TCP) should be considered. The use of *atropine* may exacerbate ischemia or induce ventricular tachycardia, ventricular fibrillation, or both, in patients with bradycardia associated with acute myocardial infarctions or second- and third-degree heart blocks. Therefore if the bradycardia is severe and the clinical condition unstable, TCP should be implemented immediately. In addition to external pacing, an *epinephrine* or *dopamine* infusion may be indicated for

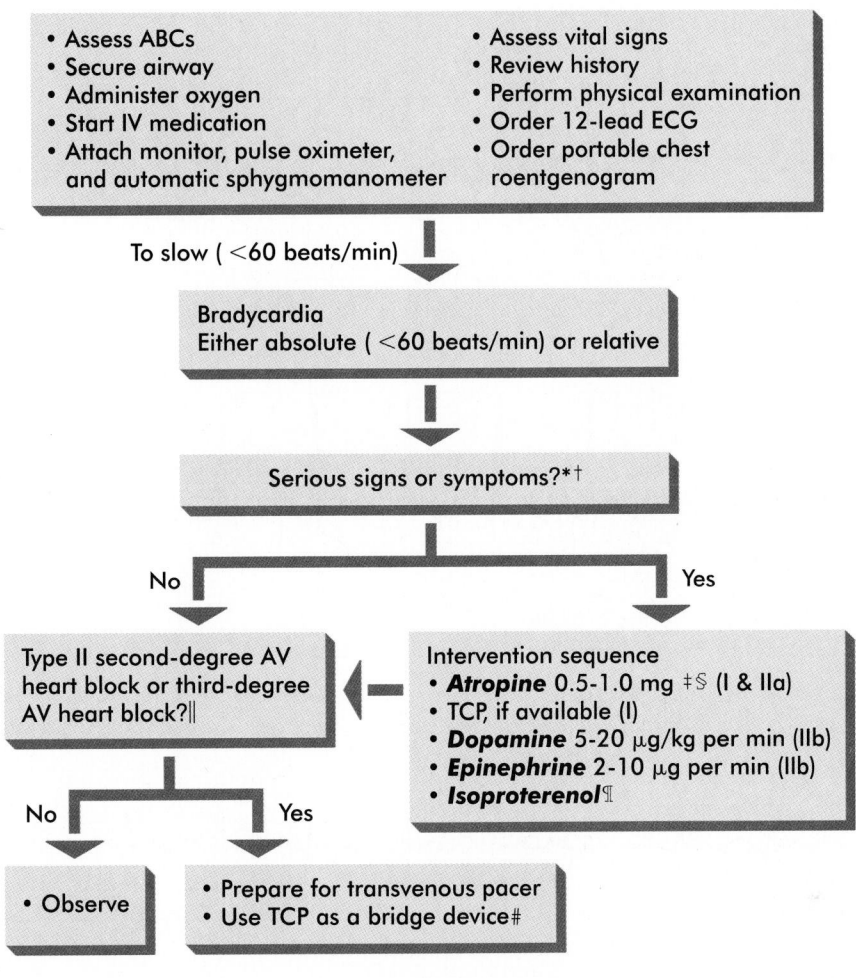

- Assess ABCs
- Secure airway
- Administer oxygen
- Start IV medication
- Attach monitor, pulse oximeter, and automatic sphygmomanometer

- Assess vital signs
- Review history
- Perform physical examination
- Order 12-lead ECG
- Order portable chest roentgenogram

To slow (<60 beats/min)

Bradycardia
Either absolute (<60 beats/min) or relative

Serious signs or symptoms?*†

No   Yes

Type II second-degree AV heart block or third-degree AV heart block?‖

Intervention sequence
- *Atropine* 0.5-1.0 mg ‡§ (I & IIa)
- TCP, if available (I)
- *Dopamine* 5-20 µg/kg per min (IIb)
- *Epinephrine* 2-10 µg per min (IIb)
- *Isoproterenol*¶

No   Yes

- Observe

- Prepare for transvenous pacer
- Use TCP as a bridge device#

*Serious signs or symptoms must be related to the slow rate. Clinical manifestations include: *symptoms* (chest pain, shortness of breath, decreased level of consciousness) and signs (low BP, shock, pulmonary congestion, CHF, acute MI).
†Do not delay TCP while awaiting IV access or for *atropine* to take effect if patient is symptomatic.
‡Denervated transplanted hearts will not respond to *atropine*. Go at once to pacing, *catecholamine* infusion, or both.
§*Atropine* should be given in repeat doses in 3-5 min up to 0.04 mg/kg. Consider shorter dosing intervals in severe clinical conditions. It has been suggested that atropine should be used with caution in atrioventricular (AV) block at the His-Purkinje level (type II AV block and new third-degree block with wide QRS complexes) (Class IIb).
‖Never treat third-degree heart block plus ventricular escape beats with *lidocaine*.
¶*Isoproterenol* should be used, if at all, with extreme caution. At low doses it is Class IIb (possibly helpful); at higher doses it is Class III (harmful).
#Verify patient tolerance and mechanical capture. Use analgesia and sedation as needed.

Fig. 18-36 Bradycardia algorithm (with the patient not in cardiac arrest). (Reproduced with permission. CPR Issue of *JAMA*, Oct 28, 1992. Copyright © American Medical Association.)

patients with severe bradycardia and hypotension.

Sinus Tachycardia

Description
Sinus tachycardia (Fig. 18-37) results from an increase in the rate of sinus node discharge.

Etiology
This dysrhythmia is common and may result from multiple factors, including:
- Exercise
- Fever
- Anxiety
- Ingestion of coffee, tea, or alcohol
- Smoking

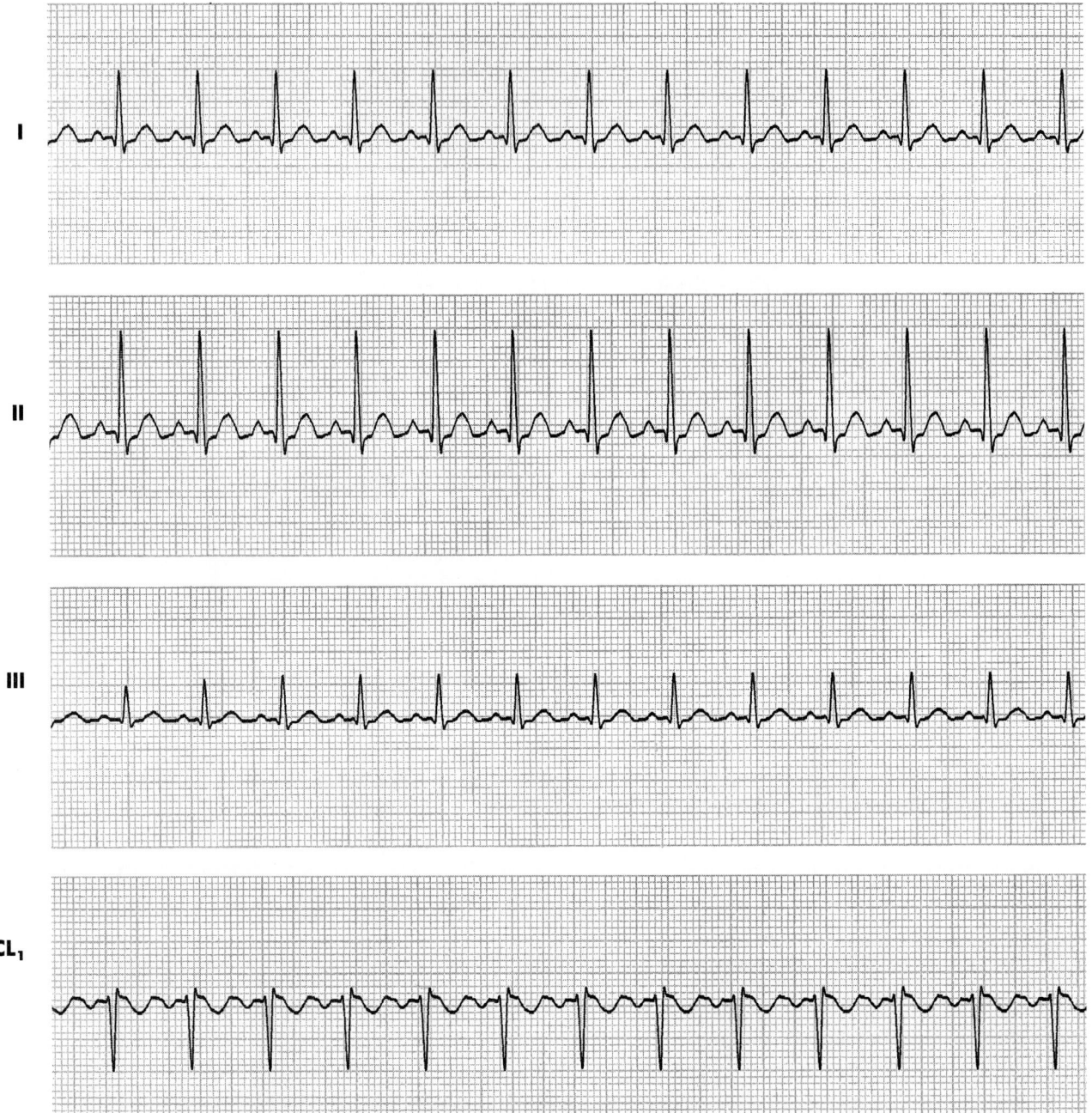

Fig. 18-37 Sinus tachycardia.

- Hypovolemia
- Anemia
- Congestive heart failure
- Excessive administration of *atropine* or any vagolytic or sympathomimetic drug (cocaine, phencyclidine, *epinephrine, isoproterenol*)

Rules for Interpretation (Lead II Monitoring)

Rate: Greater than 100 beats per minute

Rhythm: Regular

QRS complex: Less than 0.12 second (normal), provided there is no ventricular conduction disturbance

P waves: Normal and upright; one before each QRS complex

PR interval: 0.12 to 0.20 second (which is normal), provided that no AV conduction block is present

Clinical Significance

Sinus tachycardia in healthy individuals is a benign dysrhythmia. If associated with myocardial infarction, the tachycardia may increase the oxygen requirements of the heart, increase myocardial ischemia, and predispose the patient to more serious rhythm disturbances. The underlying etiology should be sought and corrected to avoid overlooking a serious cause of the dysrhythmia, such as hypoxia, hypovolemia, or congestive heart failure.

Management (Fig. 18-38)

Sinus tachycardia does not usually require treatment. When the underlying cause is removed, the tachycardia usually resolves gradually and spontaneously. If the rhythm is not sinus tachycardia and the ventricular rate is greater than 150 beats per minute, medical control may recommend a brief trial of medications and perhaps cardioversion.

Sinus Dysrhythmia

Description

Sinus dysrhythmia (Fig. 18-39) is present when the difference between the longest and shortest R-R intervals is greater than 0.16 second.

Etiology

Sinus dysrhythmia is normal. It is commonly related to the respiratory cycle and changes in intrathoracic pressure, which cause the heart rate to increase during inspiration and decrease during expiration. Another normal, although less common cause of sinus dysrhythmia is unrelated to respiration. It may occur in healthy individuals but is more common in patients with heart disease or myocardial infarction and in patients receiving certain drugs such as digitalis and *morphine.*

Rules for Interpretation (Lead II Monitoring)

Rate: Usually 60 to 100 beats per minute (varies with respiration)

Rhythm: Irregular (changes occur in cycles)

QRS complex: Less than 0.12 second (normal), provided no ventricular conduction disturbance is present

P waves: Normal and upright; one P wave before each QRS complex

PR interval: 0.12 to 0.20 second and constant (normal)

Clinical Significance

The dysrhythmia is common in children, young adults, and older adults and may be associated with palpitations, dizziness, and syncope (rare).

Management

Sinus dysrhythmia is usually of no clinical significance and requires no treatment.

Sinus Arrest

Description

Sinus arrest (Fig. 18-40) results from a marked depression in SA node automaticity. The failure of the sinus node causes short periods of cardiac standstill until lower-level pacemakers discharge (escape beats) or the sinus node resumes its normal function.

Etiology

Sinus arrest may be precipitated by an increase in parasympathetic tone on the SA node, hypoxia or ischemia, excessive administration of digitalis or *propranolol,* hyperkalemia, or damage to the SA node (acute myocardial infarction, degenerative fibrotic disease).

Rules For Interpretation (Lead II Monitoring)

Rate: Normal to slow, depending on the frequency and duration of sinus arrest

Rhythm: Irregular when sinus arrest is present

QRS complex: Less than 0.12 second (normal), provided there is no bundle branch conduction disturbance

P waves: Normal and upright (If the electrical impulse is not generated by the SA node or blocked from entering the atria, atrial depolarization does not occur, and the P wave is dropped.)

PR interval: PR intervals (when the P wave is present) of the underlying rhythm and are normal (0.12 to 0.20 second) in the absence of AV block. Junctional escape beats may occur with

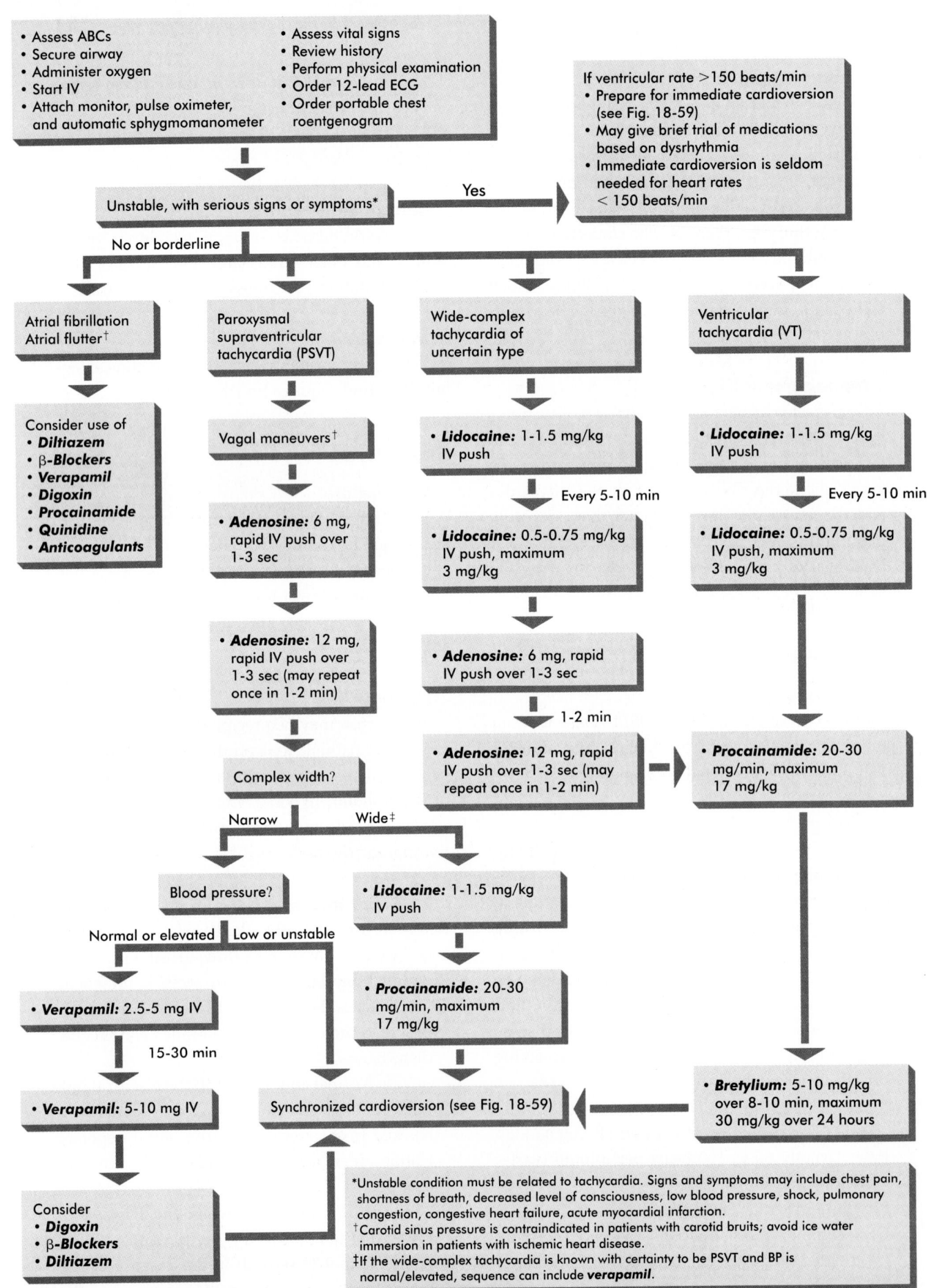

Fig. 18-38 Tachycardia algorithm. (Reproduced with permission. CPR Issue of *JAMA*, Oct 28, 1992. Copyright © American Medical Association.)

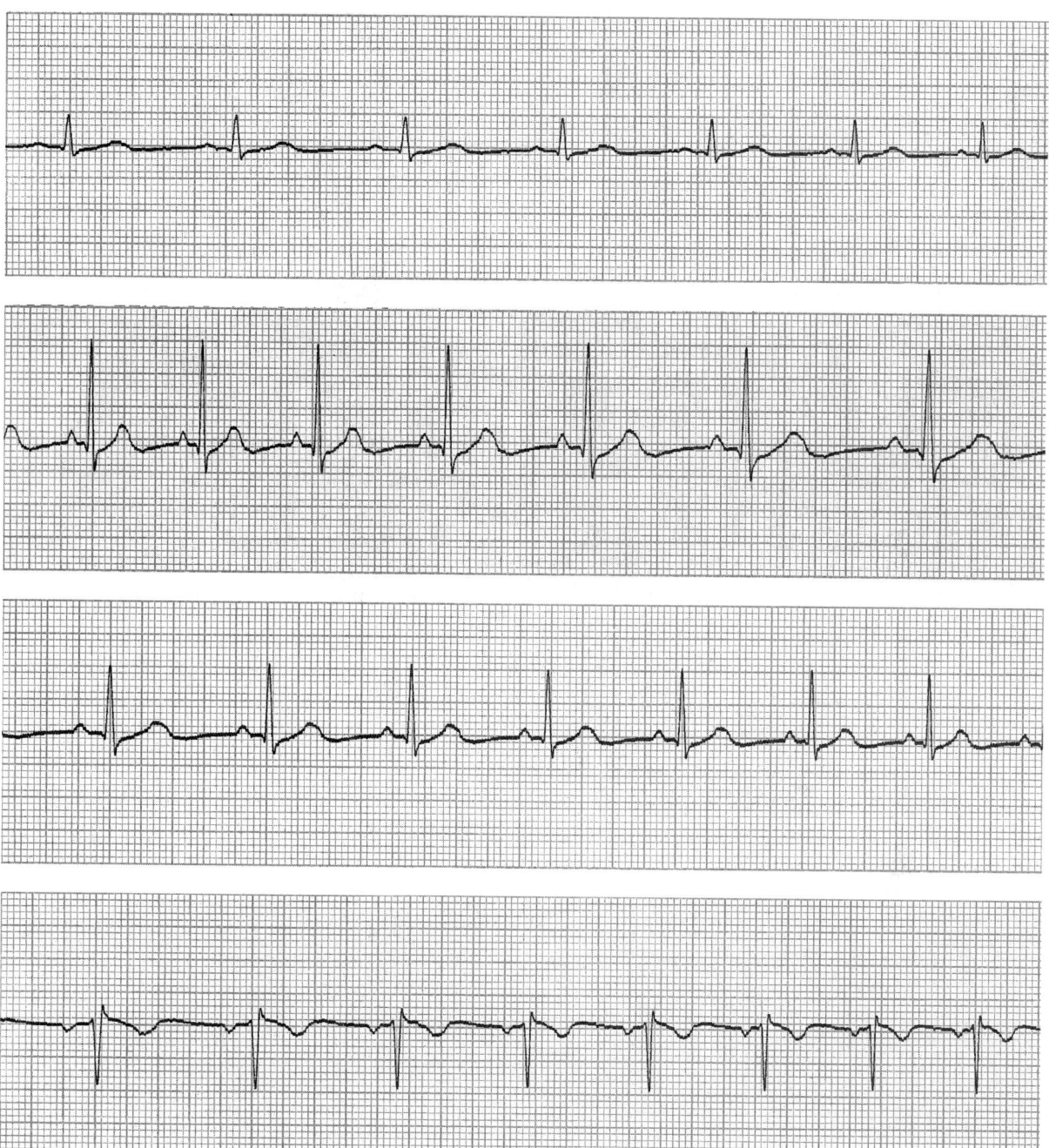

Fig. 18-39 Sinus dysrhythmia.

no P wave, a shortened PR interval, or a retro-grade P wave.

Clinical Significance

Frequent or prolonged episodes of sinus arrest may compromise cardiac output by decreasing heart rate and abolishing the atrial contribution to ventricular filling. If an escape pacemaker does not take over, ventricular asystole may result,

causing lightheadedness followed by syncope. With this dysrhythmia, there is danger that sinus node activity will completely cease.

Management

If the patient is asymptomatic, close observation is all that is required. In symptomatic patients with marked bradycardia, treatment may include the administration of *atropine.* If symptoms per-

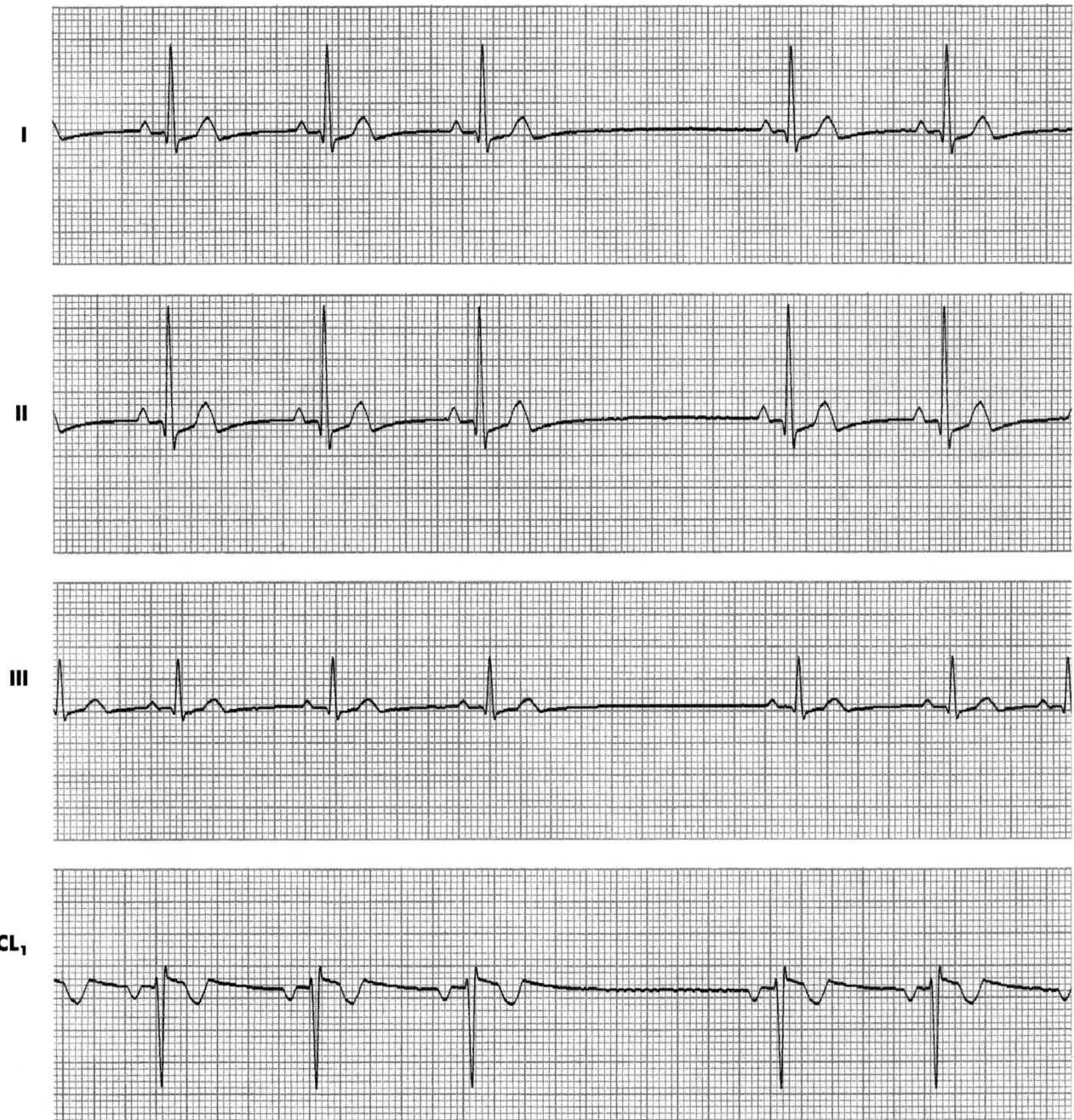

Fig. 18-40 Sinus arrest.

sist, TCP should be implemented if available (see Fig. 18-36).

● DYSRHYTHMIAS ORIGINATING IN THE ATRIA

Atrial dysrhythmias may originate in the tissues of the atria or in the internodal pathways. Com-mon causes of atrial dysrhythmias are ischemia, hypoxia, and atrial dilation caused by congestive heart failure or mitral valve abnormalities. Atrial dysrhythmias include wandering pacemaker PACs, PSVT, atrial flutter, and atrial fibrillation. ECG features common to all atrial dysrhythmias (provided there is no ventricular conduction dis-turbance) include:

• Normal QRS complexes

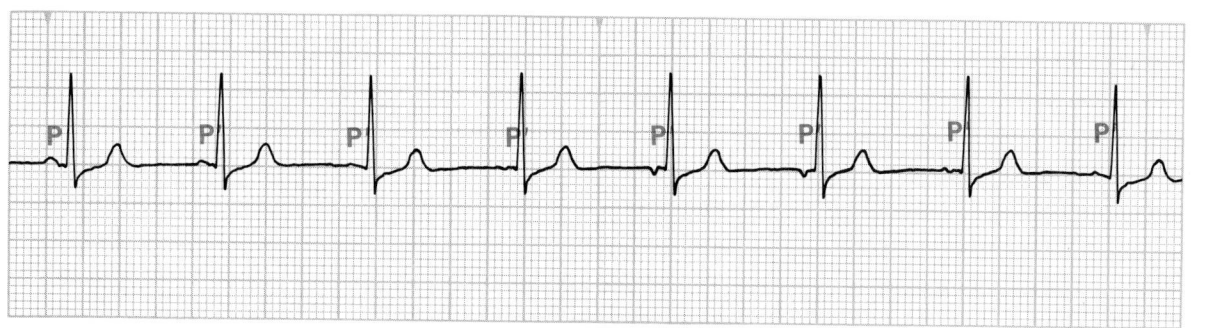

Fig. 18-41 Wandering atrial pacemaker.

- P waves (if present) that differ in appearance from sinus P waves
- Abnormal, shortened, or prolonged PR intervals

Wandering Pacemaker

Description

Wandering pacemaker (Fig. 18-41) (or wandering atrial pacemaker) is the passive transfer of pacemaker sites from the sinus node to other latent pacemaker sites in the atria and AV junction. The shift in the site is usually transient, back and forth along the SA node, atria, and AV junction.

Etiology

Wandering pacemaker is a variant of sinus dysrhythmia. It may be nonpathological in the very young, the older adult, and well-conditioned athletes. The dysrhythmia is generally caused by the inhibitory vagal effect of respiration on the SA node and AV junction. Other causes include associated underlying heart disease and the administration of digitalis. A variant of wandering atrial pacemaker is multifocal atrial tachycardia. This rhythm disturbance resembles wandering pacemaker, but it is associated with rates frequently in the 120 to 150 per minute range and is always considered pathological. Multifocal atrial tachycardia is most often found in patients with severe chronic obstructive pulmonary disease and may respond to treatment of this underlying disorder.

Rules for Interpretation (Lead II Monitoring)

Rate: Usually 60 to 100 beats per minute (The rate may gradually slow when the pacemaker site shifts from the SA node to the atria or AV junction and increase when the pacemaker site shifts back to the SA node.)

Rhythm: Usually slightly irregular

QRS complex: Usually less than 0.12 second (normal), provided no conduction block occurs in the bundle branches

P waves: Change in morphology from beat to beat. In lead II, the P waves may be upright, inverted, or buried in the QRS complex.

PR interval: Varies; may be less than 0.12 second as the pacemaker site shifts from the SA node to the atria or AV junction

Clinical Significance

A wandering pacemaker is not usually clinically significant and causes no detrimental effects. Other atrial dysrhythmias (such as atrial fibrillation) are occasionally associated with this dysrhythmia.

Management

In asymptomatic patients, no treatment is required. If the heart rate slows excessively, *atropine* may be indicated (see Fig. 18-36).

Premature Atrial Contraction

Description

A PAC (Fig. 18-42) is a single electrical impulse originating in the atria, outside the sinus node. The impulse creates a premature atrial complex (P wave) and, if conducted through the AV node, also causes a QRS complex before the next expected sinus beat. Since the PAC usually depolarizes the SA node prematurely, the timing of the

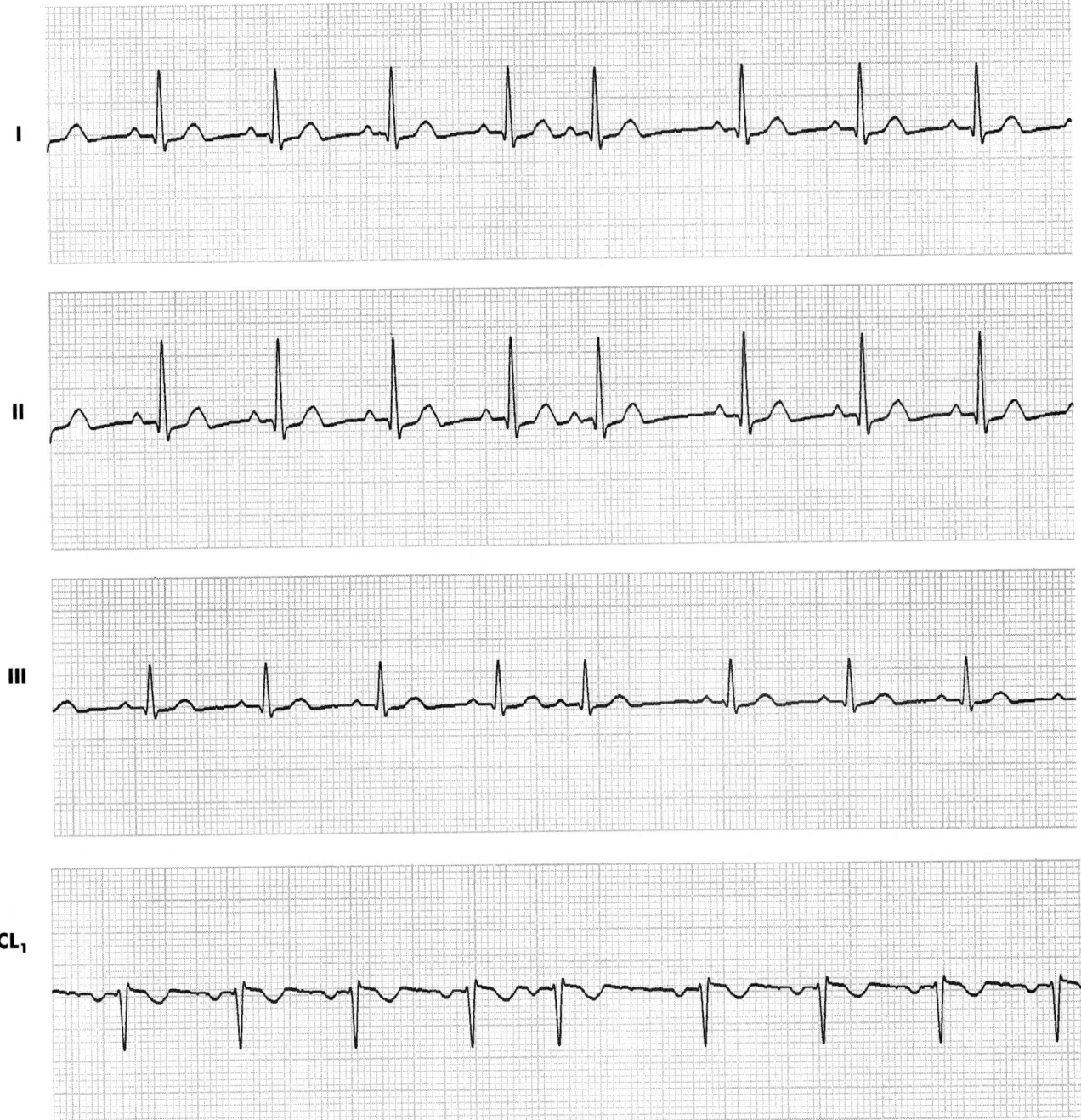

Fig. 18-42 PAC.

SA node is reset. The next expected P wave of the underlying rhythm appears earlier than it would have if the SA node had not been disturbed (noncompensatory pause). PACs may originate from a single ectopic pacemaker site or from multiple sites in the atria. The electrophysiological mechanism responsible for PACs is probably enhanced automaticity or a reentry mechanism.

Etiology

- Increase in catecholamines and sympathetic tone
- Use of caffeine, tobacco, or alcohol
- Use of sympathomimetic drugs (*epinephrine, isoproterenol, norepinephrine*)
- Electrolyte imbalance
- Hypoxia
- Digitalis toxicity

- Cardiovascular disease
- In some cases, no apparent cause

Rules for Interpretation (Lead II Monitoring)

Rate: Depends on underlying rhythm

Rhythm: Usually the underlying rhythm is sinus and regular with irregular premature beats when the PACs occur.

QRS complex: Usually less than 0.12 second. The QRS complex may be greater than 0.12 second and bizarre appearing if the PAC is abnormally conducted. It may be absent as a result of a temporary complete AV block (nonconducted PAC) (that is, a PAC that occurs during the refractory period of the AV node or ventricles).

> **NOTE:**
> PACs with aberrancy may resemble PVCs. It is important to distinguish between these two types of dysrhythmia so that the patient is not treated inappropriately.

P waves: The P wave of a PAC differs in shape from a sinus P wave. It occurs earlier than the next expected sinus P wave and may be so early that it is hidden in the preceding T wave.

PR interval: Usually in the normal range but differs from those of the underlying rhythm. The PR interval of a PAC varies from 0.20 second when the pacemaker site is near the SA node to 0.12 second when the pacemaker is near the AV junction.

Clinical Significance

Isolated PACs in patients with healthy hearts are not significant. Frequent PACs that occur in patients with heart disease may predispose the patient to serious supraventricular dysrhythmias such as atrial tachycardia, atrial flutter, atrial fibrillation, or PSVT.

Management

Prehospital care of asymptomatic patients usually requires only observation. If nonconducted PACs are frequent and the patient becomes symptomatic from bradycardia, TCP or *atropine* may be indicated (see Fig. 18-36).

Paroxysmal Supraventricular Tachycardia

Description

PSVT (Fig. 18-43) is commonly used to describe a paroxysmal tachycardia that originates in the atria (paroxysmal atrial tachycardia [PAT] or AV junction (paroxysmal junctional tachycardia [PJT]). The dysrhythmia results from rapid atrial or junctional depolarization that overrides the SA node. In most cases, PSVT is a reentry tachycardia in which the electrical impulses are caught in a cycle that continuously circulates around the AV node. The impulse reenters the AV node with each revolution at the same time as it divides into a branch that is conducted to the ventricles (to produce the QRS complex). The cycle and the tachycardia continue until the reentry pathway is interrupted. PSVT is characterized by repeated episodes (paroxysms) of atrial tachycardia, which often have a sudden onset (lasting minutes to hours) and an abrupt termination.

Etiology

PSVT may occur at any age and is commonly not associated with underlying heart disease. It is rare in patients with myocardial infarction. Precipitating factors include stress, overexertion, tobacco use, and caffeine consumption. PSVT is also common in patients who have accessory pathway conduction such as from Wolff-Parkinson-White syndrome.

Rules for Interpretation (Lead II Monitoring)

Rate: 150 to 250 beats per minute

Rhythm: Regular except at onset and termination

QRS complex: Less than 0.12 second (normal), provided no ventricular conduction disturbance is present

P waves: The ectopic P waves differ from the normal sinus P waves. In lead II, the P waves may be normal and upright if the pacemaker site is near the SA node but inverted if they originate near the AV junction. The P waves are frequently buried in preceding T or U waves or QRS complexes and therefore cannot be identified.

PR interval: If P waves are discernable, the PR interval is often shortened but may be normal or rarely prolonged.

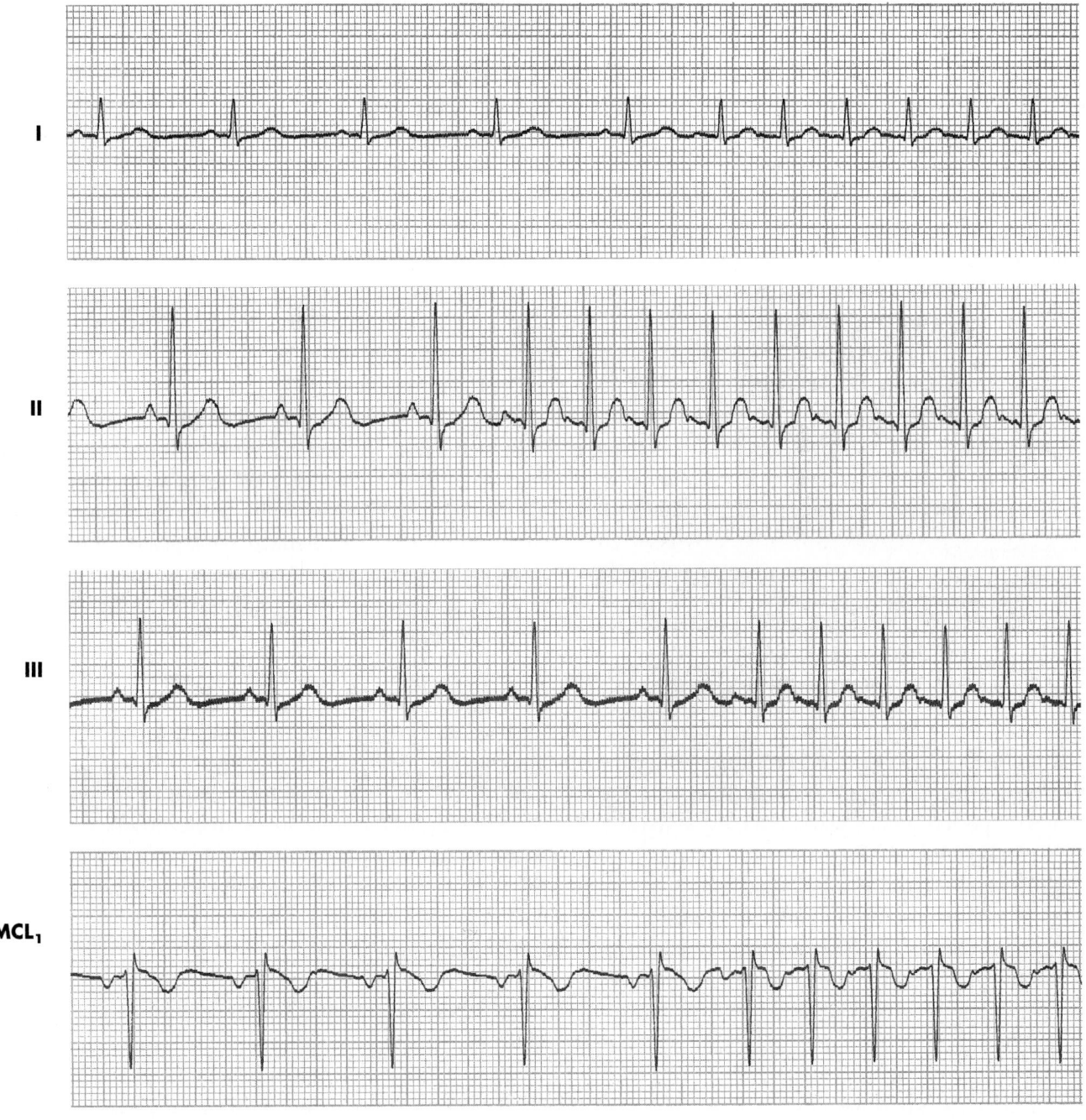

Fig. 18-43 PVST.

Clinical Significance

PSVT may occur in patients with healthy hearts and may be tolerated well for short periods. Frequently, the dysrhythmia is accompanied by palpitations, nervousness, and anxiety. Since a rapid ventricular rate may prevent the ventricles from filling completely during diastole, PSVT can significantly compromise cardiac output in patients with underlying heart disease. Decreased perfusion may cause confusion, vertigo, lightheadedness, and syncope and may precipitate angina pectoris, hypotension, or congestive heart failure. In addition, PSVT increases the heart's oxygen requirement, which may increase myocardial ischemia and the frequency and severity of the patient's chest pain.

> **NOTE:**
> The distinctions among sinus tachycardia, ventricular tachycardias, nonparoxysmal supraventricular tachycardias, and PSVT are difficult to make but are important. There are two critical points to remember: (1) If the patient displays serious signs and symptoms, particularly if the ventricular rate is greater than 150/min, prepare for immediate cardioversion; and (2) if the tachycardia complex appears wide, treat the rhythm as ventricular tachycardia. These two clinical rules should help treat the most difficult tachydysrhythmias.

Management (see Fig. 18-39)

Symptomatic PSVT should be treated promptly to reverse the consequences of the reduced cardiac output and increased workload on the heart. The paramedic should attempt the following techniques to terminate PSVT.

Vagal Maneuvers

Vagal maneuvers slow the heart and decrease the force of atrial contraction by stimulating postganglionic parasympathetic nerve fibers in the wall of the atria and specialized tissues of the SA and AV nodes via the vagus nerve. Vagal maneuvers may be used to terminate PSVT provided the patient is hemodynamically stable (conscious and normotensive without chest pain, congestive heart failure, or pulmonary edema).

> **NOTE:**
> The paramedic should only attempt vagal maneuvers with authorization from medical control. Continuous ECG monitoring and an intravenous line should be established before beginning these procedures. In addition, *atropine, lidocaine,* and airway equipment should be readily available.

Valsalva Maneuver

Place the patient in a sitting or semisitting position with his or her head tilted down. Instruct the patient to take in a deep breath and to "bear down" as if to have a bowel movement. The forced expiration against a closed glottis stimulates the vagus nerve and may terminate the tachycardia. The procedure may be repeated if unsuccessful.

Ice-Water Maneuver

Briefly immersing the patient's face in ice water may also stimulate the vagus nerve because of the mammalian diving reflex (see Chapter 25). To perform this procedure, the patient should sit up and hold his or her breath before immersion.

> **NOTE:**
> The ice-water maneuver requires a cooperative patient and should not be attempted if ischemic heart disease is present or suspected. The procedure may be repeated if unsuccessful.

Unilateral Carotid Sinus Pressure

Carotid sinus pressure stimulates the carotid bodies located in the carotid arteries. This localized pressure is interpreted by the body as an increase in blood pressure. This activates the autonomic nervous system and stimulates the vagus nerve, and the heart rate slows in an attempt to lower blood pressure. The carotids should be auscultated for the presence of a bruit (a pulse-related sound or murmur) before applying carotid sinus pressure. If bruits are present or if there is known carotid artery disease or cerebral vascular disease, carotid sinus pressure should not be applied. The procedure for carotid sinus massage is as follows:

1. Position yourself behind the patient, who is lying supine with neck extended and head turned away from the side of the applied pressure.
2. Gently palpate each carotid artery to confirm the presence of equal pulses. If pulses are unequal or one is absent, do not apply carotid sinus pressure.
3. Auscultate for the presence of bruits.
4. To apply carotid sinus pressure, place the index and middle fingers over the artery on the neck just below the angle of the jaw. Com-

press the artery firmly against the vertebral column while massaging the area. (The patient may experience some pain or discomfort.) Maintain pressure no longer than 5 to 10 seconds. Discontinue the massage immediately if bradycardia or signs of heart block develop or if the tachycardia breaks. Apply pressure to only one carotid sinus at a time.

5. Observe the ECG monitor during the procedure and obtain a tracing.

6. Repeat the procedure in 2 to 3 minutes if it is ineffective.

Pharmacological Therapy

If the vagal maneuvers fail and the patient remains stable, administration of *adenosine* (initial drug of choice) or *verapamil* may end PSVT (see Chapter 14 and the Emergency Drug Index).

> **NOTE:**
> If the complexes are wide, *lidocaine* or *procainamide* should be given rather than *verapamil* (see Fig. 18-38).

Patients who fail to respond to *adenosine* and *verapamil* may be treated (by physician order) by other means, including TCP, cardioversion, or a variety of other antidysrhythmics. Cardioversion should be reserved for patients with rapid rates (greater than 150 beats per minute) and serious signs or symptoms of clinical or hemodynamic instability. Cardioversion should commence with a synchronized shock of 50 joules. If this fails, the energy may be increased to 100, 200, 300, and finally 360 joules.

> **NOTE:**
> If synchronization cannot be performed when caring for a patient with a rapid tachycardia in whom the clinical situation is critical, then unsynchronized shocks should be delivered (see Fig. 18-38).

Electrical Therapy

If vagal maneuvers and pharmacological therapy fail to terminate PSVT or if the patient becomes hemodynamically unstable, synchronized cardioversion is indicated. The patient should be sedated before the cardioversion if time permits.

> **NOTE:**
> Cardioversion is relatively contraindicated in PSVT if digitalis toxicity is suspected because asystole may occur in this setting.

Atrial Flutter

Description

Atrial flutter (Fig. 18-44) is almost always the result of a rapid atrial reentry circuit. Atrial flutter not complicated by preexisting AV block usually manifests a 2:1 AV conduction ratio (that is, 50% of the atrial impulses are conducted through the ventricles). However, 3:1, 4:1, and greater conduction ratios are not uncommon, producing a discrepancy between atrial and ventricular rates. The conduction ratios may be constant or variable. Atrial flutter may be seen with atrial fibrillation ("atrial fib-flutter"). Rarely, particularly with accessory AV (bypass) tract, atrial flutter may conduct 1:1. This results in extremely rapid ventricular rates with rapid hemodynamic deterioration.

Etiology

Atrial flutter is generally seen in middle-aged and older patients with advanced cardiovascular disease. It also occasionally occurs in patients with healthy hearts. The dysrhythmia is commonly associated with:

- Preexcitation syndrome
- Cardiomyopathy
- Digitalis toxicity (rare)
- Hypoxia
- Cor pulmonale
- Congestive heart failure
- Damage to the SA node (pericarditis, myocarditis)

Rules for Interpretation (Lead II Monitoring)

Rate: Atrial rate 250 to 300 beats per minute; ventricular rate regular but often less than atrial rate

Rhythm: Atrial rhythm regular; ventricular rate usually regular but may be irregular if AV conduction ratio varies

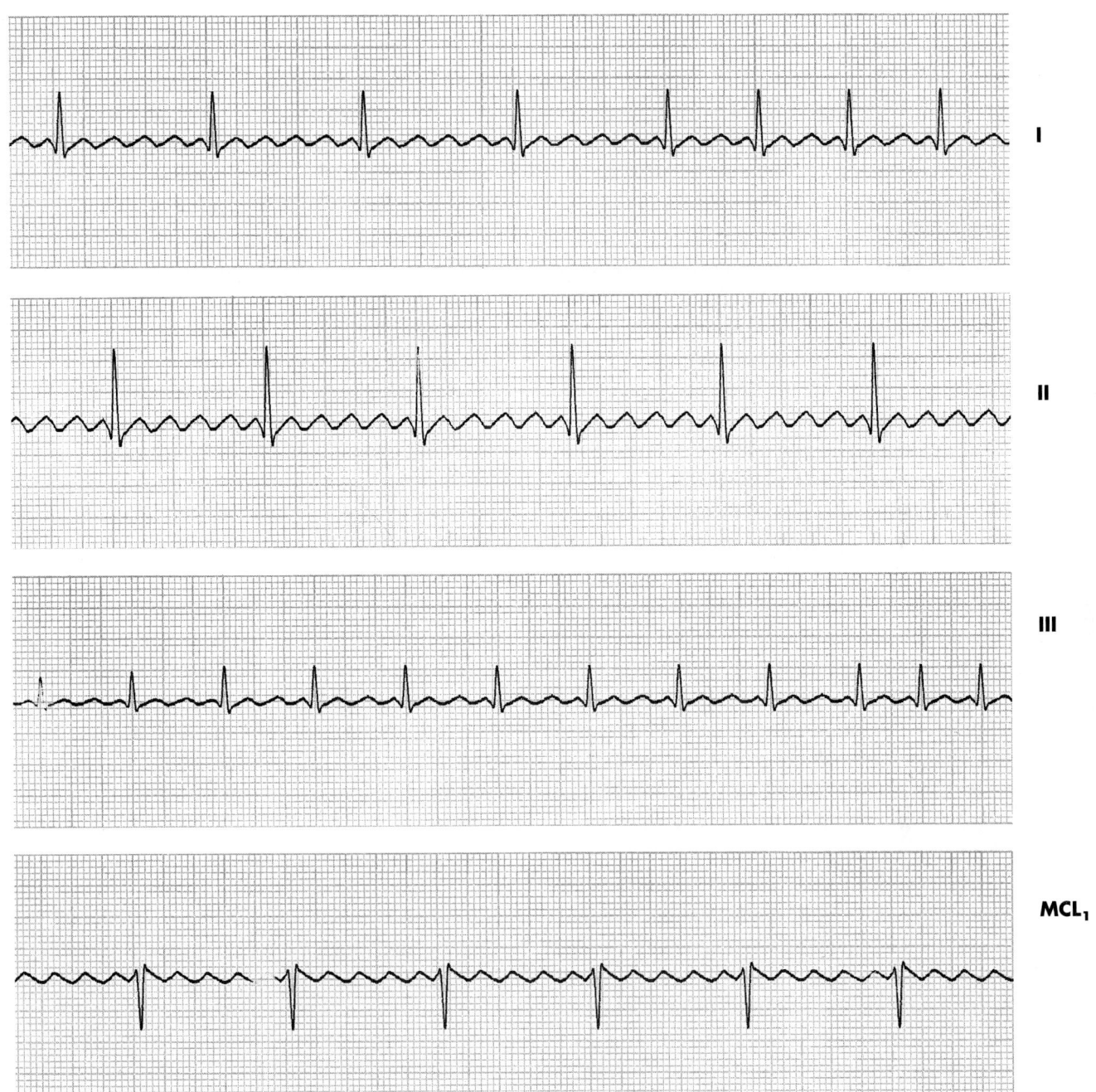

Fig. 18-44 Atrial flutter.

QRS complex: Less than 0.12 second (normal) unless ventricular conduction disturbance (aberrancy) is present

P waves: Normal P waves are absent. The flutter waves (f waves) usually resemble a "sawtooth" or "picket fence" pattern. The flutter waves represent atrial depolarization in an abnormal direction that is followed by atrial repolarization.

NOTE:
Flutter waves may be difficult to identify when there is a 2:1 ratio of atrial to ventricular complexes. The paramedic should suspect 2:1 flutter when the rhythm is regular and the ventricular rate is 150/min.

PR interval: The f-R interval is usually constant but may vary.

Clinical Significance

Provided there is a normal ventricular rate, atrial flutter is usually well tolerated by the patient. The signs and symptoms of decreased cardiac output from a rapid ventricular response are the same as those for atrial tachycardia. In addition, in some flutter rhythms (particularly a 2:1 atrial flutter), the atria do not regularly contract and empty before each ventricular contraction. The loss of the "atrial kick" results in incomplete filling of the ventricles and may further decrease cardiac output by as much as 25%.

Management

Vagal maneuvers rarely convert atrial flutter but may render flutter waves more apparent, thereby confirming the diagnosis. Patients who are hemodynamically stable require no immediate intervention. If the ventricular rate is 120 to 140 beats per minute and the patient does not show serious signs or symptoms of hemodynamic or clinical instability, medical control may prescribe the intravenous use of a beta blocker such as *propranolol*, calcium channel blockers such as *diltiazem* or *verapamil*, or *digoxin*. When ventricular rates exceed 150 beats per minute or when serious signs or symptoms of hemodynamic or clinical instability related to the tachycardia occur (chest pain, shortness of breath, decreased level of consciousness, low blood pressure), preparations should be made for immediate cardioversion. The initial attempt at cardioversion for atrial flutter should consist of a synchronized shock of 50 joules. If necessary, the energy may be increased to 100, 200, 300, and 360 joules.

Atrial Fibrillation

Description

Atrial fibrillation (Fig. 18-45) results from multiple areas of reentry within the atria or ectopic atrial pacemakers outside the SA node. (The activity of the SA node is completely suppressed by atrial fibrillation.) The electrical activity results in chaotic impulses too numerous to be conducted by the AV node through the ventricles. AV conduction is random, and ventricular response is irregular but usually rapid unless the patient is on medication to slow the ventricular rate.

Etiology

Paroxysmal atrial fibrillation, which occurs in young adults after heavy alcohol ingestion (the "holiday heart" syndrome) or as a result of acute stress, is a self-limited phenomenon, usually resolving without treatment. Chronic atrial fibrillation may be intermittent and is often associated with rheumatic heart disease, congestive heart failure (atrial dilation), and atherosclerotic heart disease. Chronic atrial fibrillation usually requires digitalis (or calcium channel or beta blocker) therapy to slow the ventricular rate to 80 to 100 beats per minute. Less commonly, atrial fibrillation may occur in cardiomyopathy, acute myocarditis and pericarditis, and chest trauma. It is rarely caused by digitalis toxicity, but a very slow, regular ventricular response with atrial fibrillation should raise suspicion of digitalis toxicity.

Rules for Interpretation (Lead II Monitoring)

Rate: Atrial rate 350 to 700 beats per minute (cannot be counted); ventricular rate varies greatly depending on conduction through AV node (average 150 to 180 beats per minute, if uncontrolled).

Rhythm: Irregularly irregular

QRS complex: Less than 0.12 second (normal), provided there is no ventricular conduction disturbance

P waves: P waves and organized atrial contractions are absent. Fibrillation waves (f waves) may be "fine" (less than 1 mm) or "coarse" (greater than 1 mm). Fine f waves may be so small that they appear as a wavy or flat (isoelectric) line. The f waves are irregularly shaped, rounded (or pointed), and dissimilar

PR interval: None

Clinical Significance

The "atrial kick" is lost in atrial fibrillation, which reduces cardiac output by as much as 25%. This, coupled with a rapid ventricular response, may cause cardiovascular decompensation (angina pectoris, myocardial infarction, congestive heart failure, or cardiogenic shock).

Management

If the rate of ventricular response is normal (often seen in patients taking digitalis), the dysrhyth-

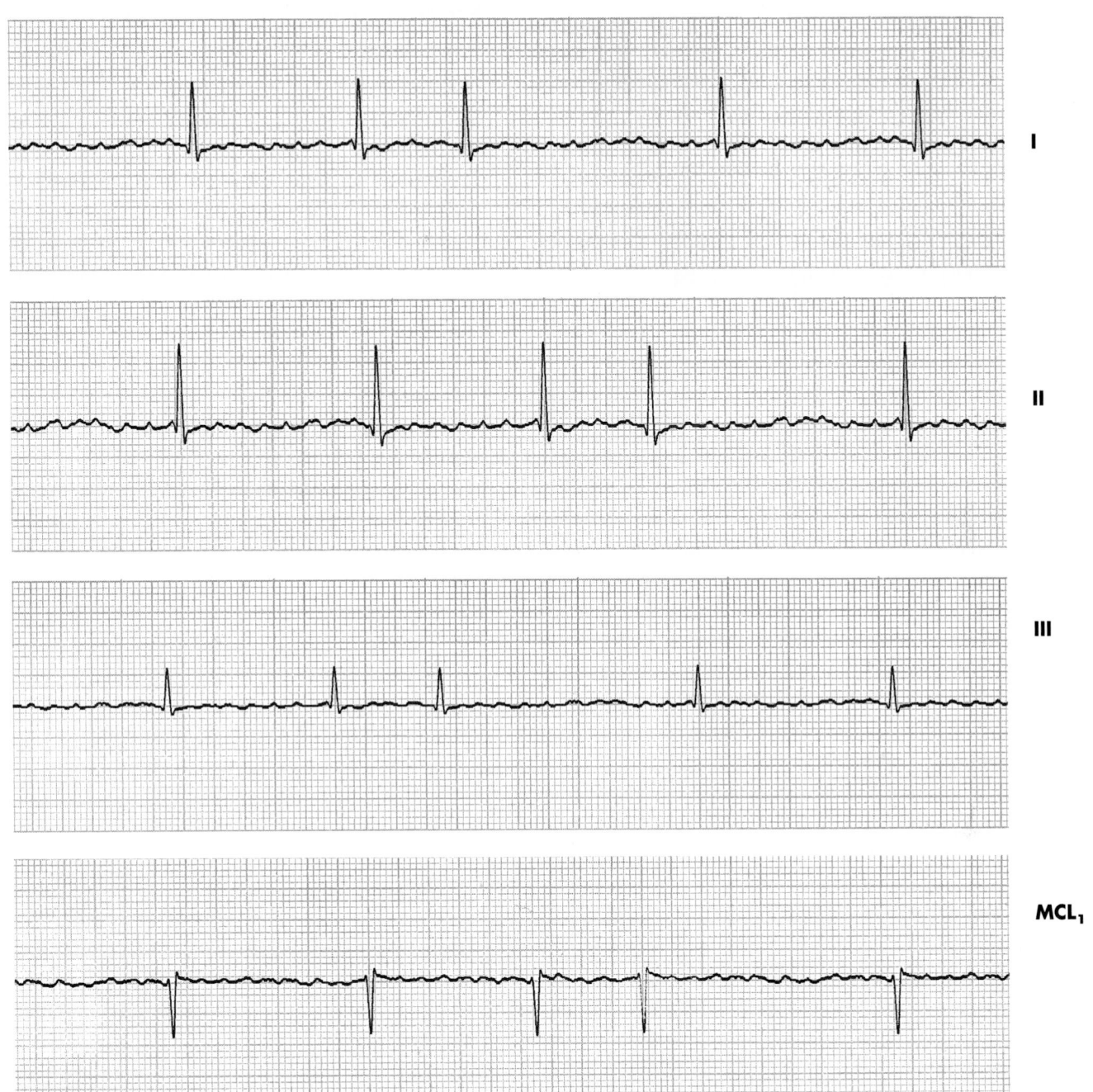

Fig. 18-45 Atrial fibrillation.

mia is usually well tolerated and requires no immediate intervention. If the ventricular response is rapid but less than 150 beats per minute and the patient does not show signs of hemodynamic or clinical instability, pharmacological therapy similar to that used for atrial flutter may be considered (see Fig. 18-38). For rates greater than 150 beats per minute, when serious signs or symptoms of hemodynamic or clinical instability re-

lated to the tachycardia occur, preparations for immediate cardioversion should be made. Since atrial fibrillation is a more difficult rhythm to cardiovert, recommendations are to initially use a synchronized shock of 100 joules, followed by 200, 300, and 360 joules if necessary.

Although calcium channel blockers such as *diltiazem* and *verapamil* are commonly used to treat atrial dysrhythmias, including PSVT, atrial flutter, and atrial fibrillation, *verapamil* is contraindicated in patients with known or suspected Wolff-Parkinson-White syndrome or when the QRS complex is abnormally wide (greater than 0.12 second).

● DYSRHYTHMIAS ORIGINATING IN THE AV JUNCTION

When the SA node and the atria cannot generate the electrical impulses needed to begin depolarization because of factors such as hypoxia, ischemia, myocardial infarction, and drug toxicity, the AV node or the area surrounding the AV node may assume the role of the secondary pacemaker. Rhythms that start in the AV node or AV junctional area are considered junctional rhythms. A junctional rhythm is not usually a lethal dysrhythmia, but it must be assessed to determine the patient's tolerance of the rhythm disturbance. Dysrhythmias that originate in the AV junction include the PJCs, the junctional escape complexes or rhythms, and the accelerated junctional rhythms.

In junctional rhythms, electrical impulses travel in a normal pathway from the AV junction through the bundle of His and bundle branches to the Purkinje fibers, ending in the ventricular muscle. Because conduction through the ventricles proceeds normally, the QRS complex is usually within normal limits of 0.04 to 0.12 second. However, the impulses that depolarize the atria travel in a backward or retrograde motion. The retrograde depolarization of the atria results in the following three P wave characteristics:

1. P waves are inverted in lead II (impulse moves toward negative electrode).
2. The relationship of the P wave to the QRS complex depends on the timing of atrial depolarization. Therefore the P wave may occur before the QRS complex (atria depolarized first), after the QRS complex (ventricles depolarized first), or during the QRS complex (atria and ventricles depolarize simultaneously).
3. The PR interval is frequently less than 0.12 second.

Premature Junctional Contraction

Description

A PJC (Fig. 18-46) results from a single electrical impulse originating in the AV junction, which occurs before the next expected sinus impulse. The pause that follows the PJC may be noncompensatory if the SA node is depolarized by the PJC or, more commonly, compensatory if the SA node discharged before the PJC reached it. If a compensatory pause occurs, the normal cadence of the myocardium is reestablished.

Etiology

Isolated PJCs may occur in healthy individuals without apparent cause. However, they are more commonly the result of intrinsic cardiac disease or pharmacological toxicity. The electrophysiological mechanism responsible for PJCs is thought to be enhanced automaticity or a reentry mechanism. PJCs have several causes:

- Digitalis toxicity
- Other cardiac medications (quinidine, *procainamide*)
- Increased vagal tone on the SA node
- Sympathomimetic drugs (*epinephrine, isoproterenol, norepinephrine*)
- Hypoxia
- Congestive heart failure
- Damage to the AV junction

Rules for Interpretation (Lead II Monitoring)

Rate: The heart rate is that of the underlying rhythm.

Rhythm: Usually regular, except when PJC is present

QRS complex: Usually less than 0.12 second (normal), provided there is no ventricular conduction disturbance

P waves: P waves may be associated with PJCs. P waves can occur before, during, or after the QRS complex or can be absent. If present, P waves are abnormal, differing in size, shape, and direction from normal P waves.

PR interval: Usually less than 0.12 second, if the P wave precedes the QRS complex. The PR interval may be somewhat prolonged (greater than 0.20 second) if there is any delay in the AV conduction.

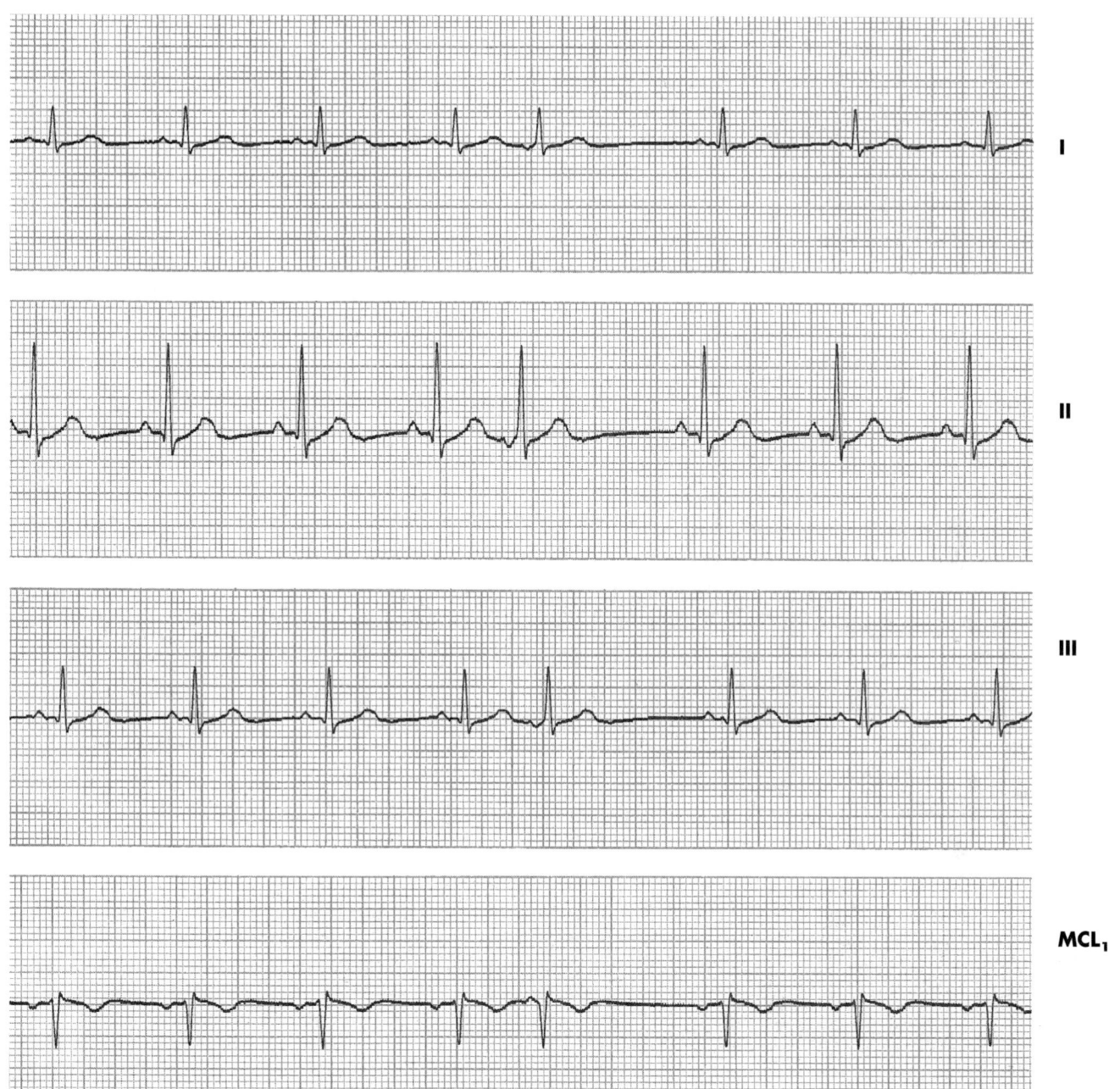

I

II

III

MCL₁

Fig. 18-46 PJCs.

Clinical Significance

Isolated PJCs are not usually significant. PJCs that occur more frequently than 4 to 6 per minute should alert the paramedic that more serious junctional dysrhythmias may develop.

Management

No management is required.

Junctional Escape Complex or Rhythm

Description

A junctional escape complex (isolated impulse) or rhythm (series of impulses) (Fig. 18-47) results when the rate of the primary pacemaker (usually the SA node) falls below that of the AV junctional area. The dysrhythmia may also occur when the electrical impulses from the SA node or atria fail

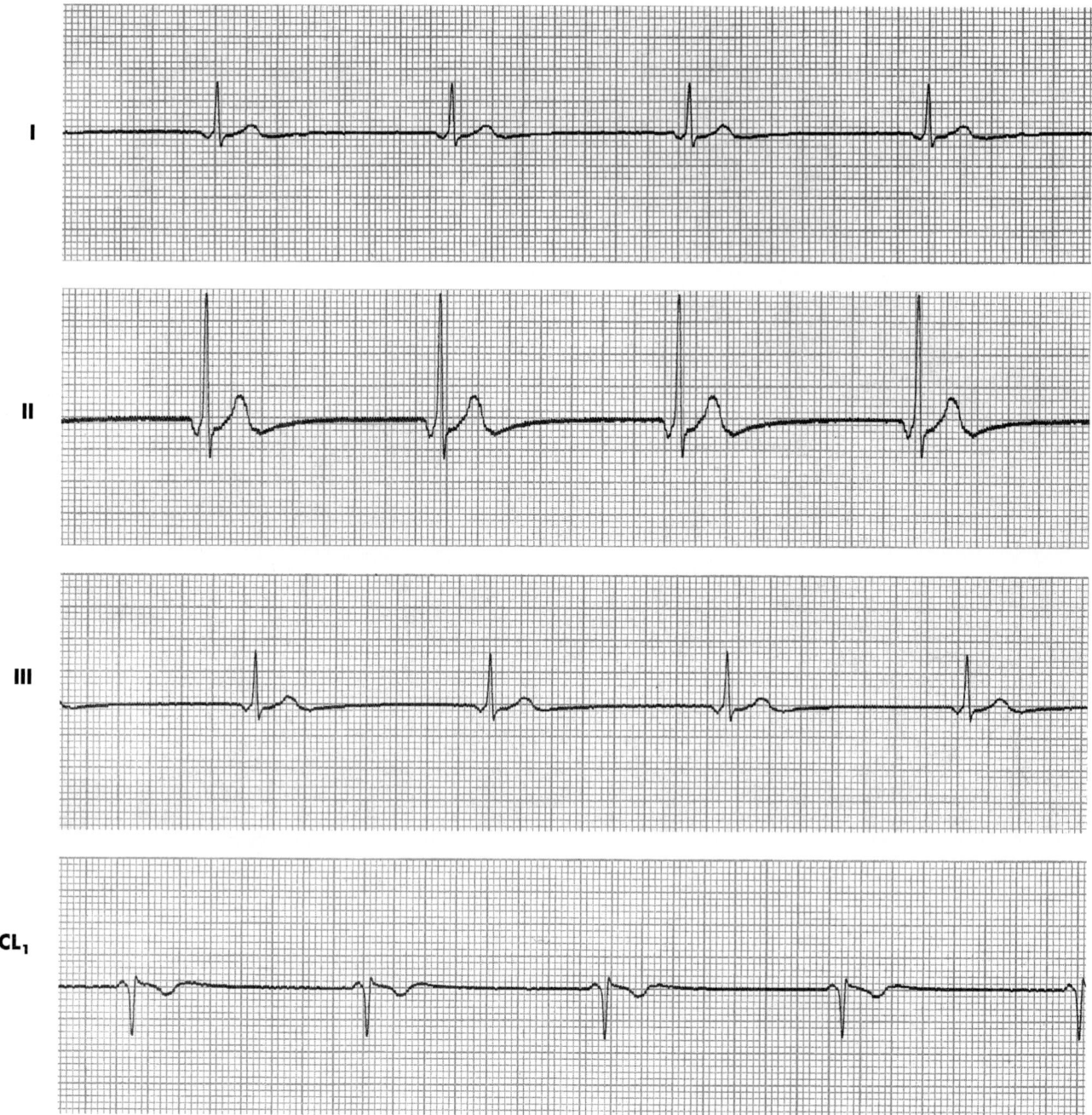

Fig. 18-47 Junctional escape complex or rhythm.

to reach the AV junction because of SA or AV block. The escape complex or rhythm provided by the AV junction serves as a safety mechanism to prevent cardiac standstill. The AV junction is likely to assume pacemaker duties at its inherent firing rate of 40 to 60 beats per minute when an electrical impulse fails to be transmitted to the pa-

tient's AV junction within approximately 1.0 to 1.5 seconds.

Etiology

A junctional escape complex or a junctional escape rhythm is a normal response that may result from an increased vagal tone on the SA node, a pathological slowing of the SA discharge, or a complete AV block.

Rules for Interpretation (Lead II Monitoring)

Rate: Usually 40 to 60 beats per minute but may be less

Rhythm: Ventricular rhythm is usually regular in junctional rhythm; may be irregular if an isolated junctional escape complex is present.

QRS complex: Usually less than 0.12 second (normal), provided no preexisting bundle branch block is present

P waves: May be present (with or without relationship to QRS complex) or absent. If P waves are present, they may occur before, after, or during the QRS complex. Depending on the pacemaker site, P waves may differ from normal P waves in size, shape, and direction and may be upright or inverted.

PR interval: If P waves precede the QRS complex, the PR interval is commonly shortened (less than 0.12 second) and constant.

Clinical Significance

Junctional bradycardias can cause decreased cardiac output. Therefore patients can exhibit signs and symptoms similar to those of other bradycardias (lightheadedness, hypotension, syncope). As a rule, the patient tolerates junctional rhythms of 50 beats per minute.

Management

Patients who are stable require no immediate intervention. If the patient is symptomatic or if ventricular irritability is present, pharmacological intervention (beginning with *atropine*) may be indicated. In severe cases and in patients unresponsive to *atropine,* external TCP may be necessary. If intrinsic disease is present in the SA node, the patient may ultimately require permanent pacemaker insertion (see Fig. 18-36).

Accelerated Junctional Rhythm

Description

Accelerated junctional rhythm (Fig. 18-48) results from increased automaticity of the AV junc-

tion, causing it to discharge faster than its intrinsic rate (40 to 60 beats per minute), overriding the primary (SA node) pacemaker. Technically, the rate of this dysrhythmia (usually 60 to 100 beats per minute) does not truly constitute a tachycardia, hence the term *accelerated junctional rhythm.* In this text, rapid junctional rhythms greater than 100 beats per minute (PJT or nonparoxysmal junctional tachycardia) and caused by a reentry mechanism are discussed with other supraventricular tachycardias.

Etiology

An accelerated junctional rhythm is commonly the result of digitalis toxicity. Other common causes of this problem include excessive catecholamine administration, damage to the AV junction, inferior-wall myocardial infarction, and rheumatic fever.

Rules for Interpretation (Lead II Monitoring)

Rate: Usually 60 to 100 beats per minute

Rhythm: Essentially regular

QRS complex: The QRS complex is usually less than 0.12 second (normal), provided there is no preexisting bundle branch block.

P waves: P waves may be present (with or without relationship to the QRS complex), absent (retrograde AV block), or buried in the QRS complex. If present, P waves are usually inverted and appear before or after the QRS complex.

PR interval: If the P wave occurs before the QRS complex, the PR interval will be less than 0.12 second. If the P wave follows the QRS complex, it is technically an R-P interval and is usually less than 0.20 second.

Clinical Significance

Accelerated junctional rhythm is usually well tolerated by the patient. However, the presence of myocardial ischemia may predispose the patient to more serious dysrhythmias.

Management

Accelerated junctional rhythm generally requires no immediate intervention.

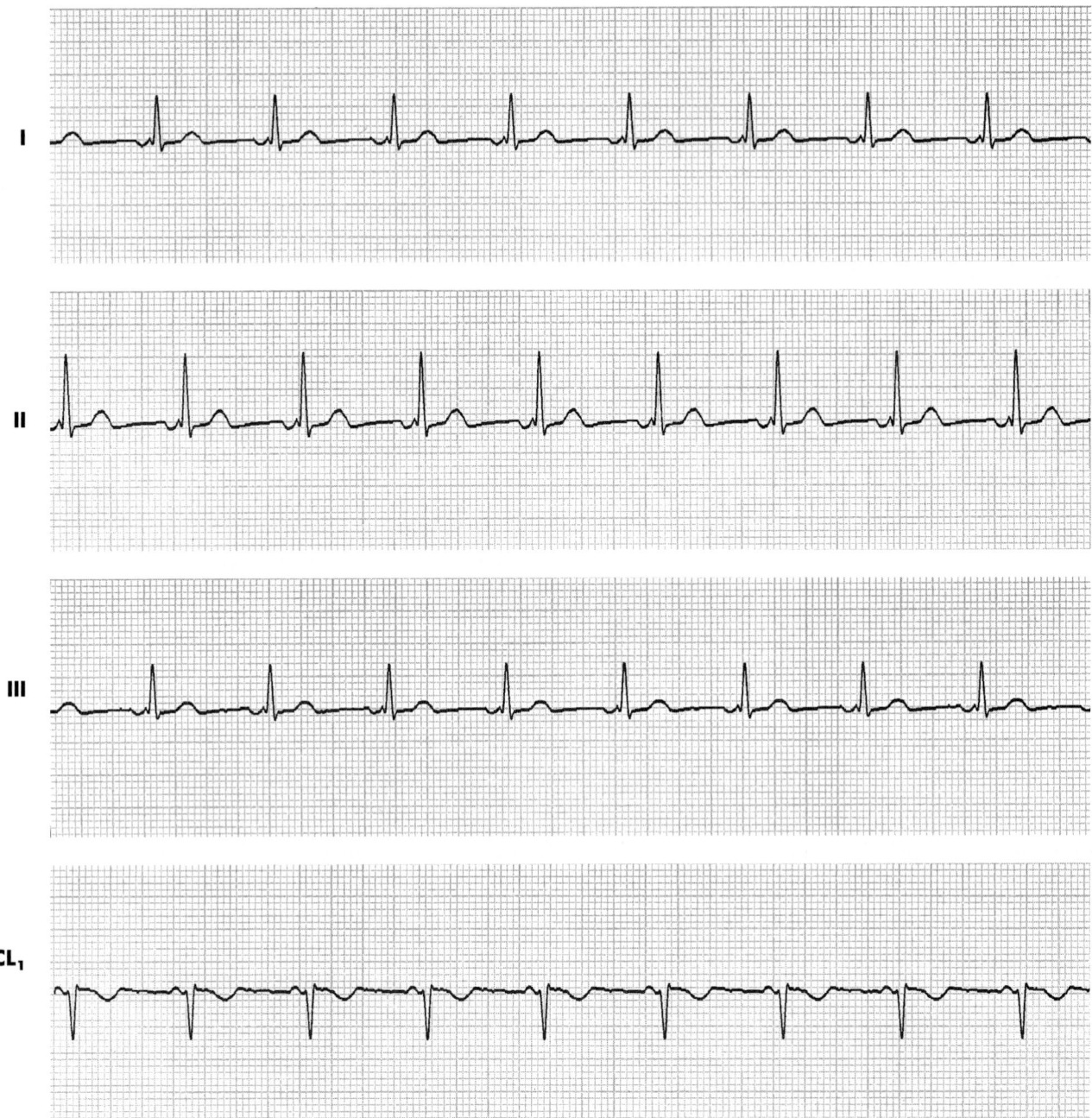

Fig. 18-48 Accelerated junctional rhythm.

● DYSRHYTHMIAS ORIGINATING IN THE VENTRICLES

Ventricular dysrhythmias are usually considered to be life threatening. Ventricular rhythm disturbances generally result from the failure of the atria, AV junction, or both, to initiate an electrical impulse (ventricular escape rhythms), or they are secondary to enhanced automaticity or reentry phenomena in the ventricles. The latter group leads to PVC, ventricular tachycardia, and even ventricular fibrillation and is often associated with myocardial ischemia or infarction. The ventricle is the least efficient pacemaker of the heart, usually generating only 20 to 40 electrical impulses per minute. However, the ventricle can develop in-

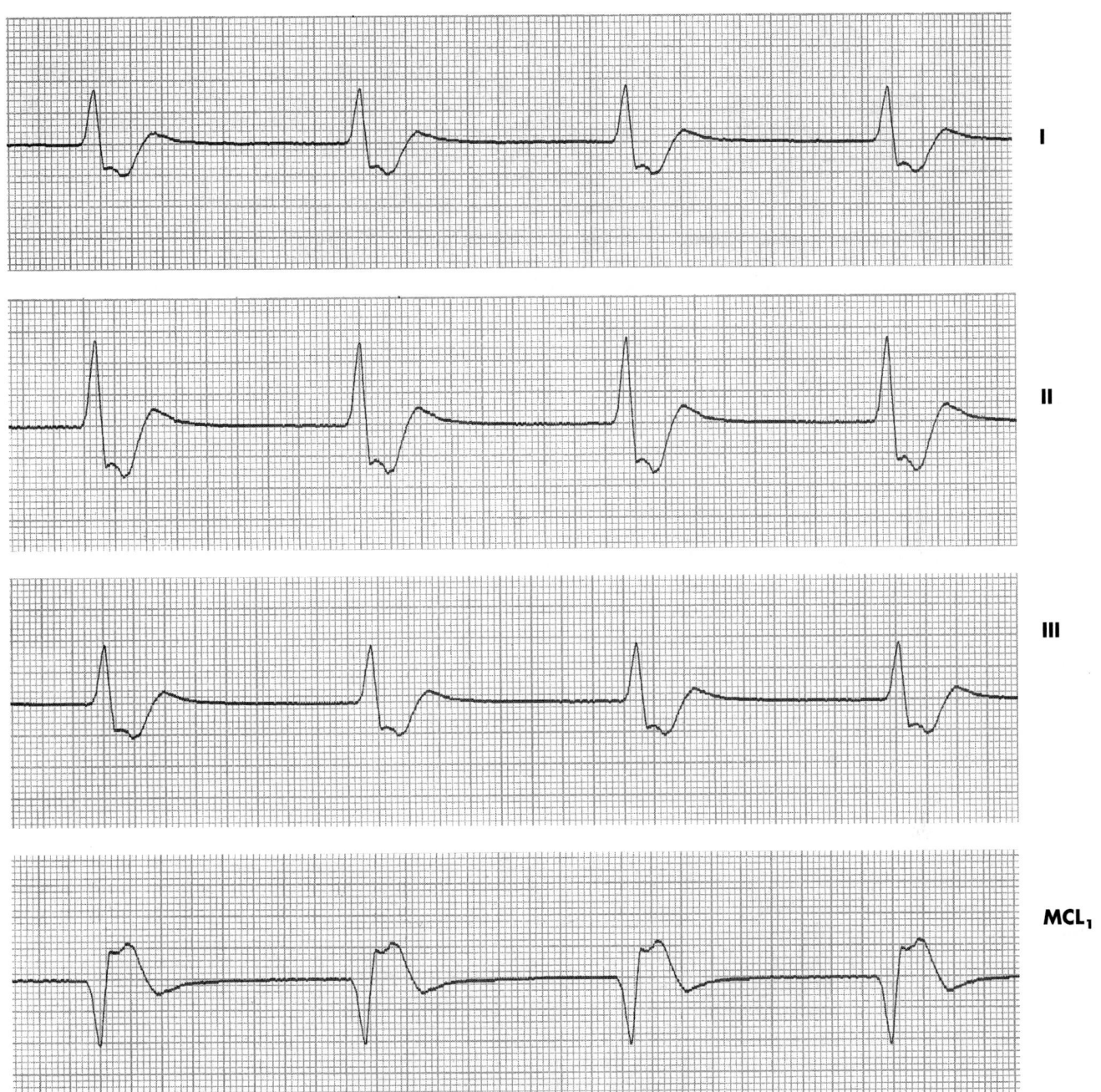

Fig. 18-49 Ventricular escape rhythm.

creased automaticity and may discharge at rates up to 100 impulses per minute (accelerated idioventricular rhythm) or even faster (ventricular tachycardia). Dysrhythmias originating in the ventricles include ventricular escape complexes or rhythms, PVCs, ventricular tachycardia, ventricular fibrillation, asystole, and artificial pacemaker rhythm.

Because electrical impulses of ventricular origin start in the lower portion of the heart (the ventricular muscle, bundle branches, or Purkinje fibers), the electrical impulse must travel in a retrograde conduction pathway to depolarize the atria. It may travel in an antegrade direction to depolarize the ventricles, depending on the site of initiation of the impulse. Regardless of the direction

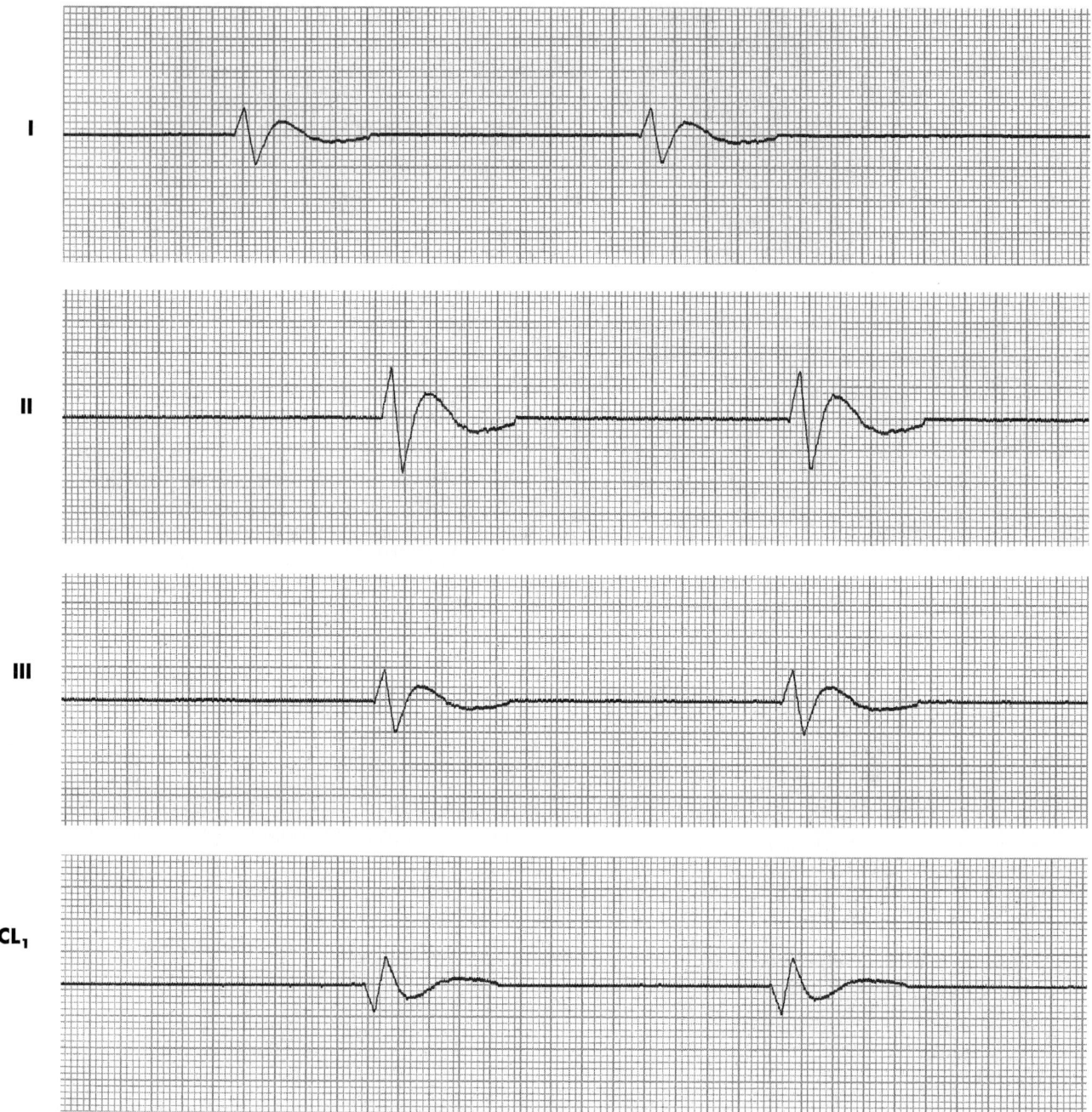

I

II

III

MCL₁

Fig. 18-50 "Dying heart" or agonal rhythm.

of depolarization, the normal, rapid conducting pathways are bypassed, producing the following two ECG features:

1. QRS complexes that are wide, bizarre in appearance, and 0.12 second or greater in duration
2. P waves that are hidden in the QRS complex (since the atria are depolarized at approximately the same time as the ventricles)

Ventricular Escape Complexes or Rhythms

Description

A ventricular escape complex (isolated impulse) or rhythm (series of complexes, also known as *idioventricular rhythm*) (Figs. 18-49 and 18-50) results when impulses from higher pacemakers fail to reach the ventricles or when the rate of discharge of higher pacemakers falls to less than that of the ventricles. Like the junctional escape complex or rhythm, this dysrhythmia serves as a safety mechanism to prevent cardiac standstill.

Etiology

Ventricular escape rhythms occur when the rate of impulse formation of the dominant pacemaker (usually the SA node) and the escape pacemaker in the AV junction fails or falls below that of the escape pacemaker in the ventricles. The escape complex or rhythm may also occur when the electrical impulses from the SA node, atria, or AV junction fail to reach the ventricles because of sinus arrest or a high degree of AV block. This dysrhythmia is frequently seen as the first organized rhythm after defibrillation as well as the last in an unsuccessful resuscitation (the "dying heart" or agonal rhythm).

Rules for Interpretation (Lead II Monitoring)

Rate: Usually 20 to 40 beats per minute; may be lower

Rhythm: The ventricular rhythm is usually regular, but may be irregular.

QRS complex: QRS complexes generally exceed 0.12 second and are bizarre in appearance. The shape of the QRS complex may vary in any given lead.

P waves: P waves may be present or absent. If present, they have no set relationship to the QRS complexes of the ventricular escape rhythm (appearing independently at a rate different from that of the QRS complexes).

PR interval: If P waves are present, the PR interval is variable and irregular.

Clinical Significance

A ventricular escape rhythm is generally symptomatic. This dysrhythmia is manifested by hypotension, decreased cardiac output, and decreased perfusion of the brain and other vital organs, often resulting in syncope and shock. Patient assessment is essential because the escape rhythm may be perfusing or nonperfusing (pulseless electrical activity).

Management (Fig. 18-51)

If the rhythm is perfusing, treatment must be directed at increasing the heart rate by administer-

ing *oxygen, atropine,* and TCP. Treating the escape rhythm with *lidocaine* may be lethal and is contraindicated. If the rhythm is nonperfusing, basic life-support measures should be initiated, and the treatment algorithm for pulseless electrical activity (electromechanical dissociation) should be followed.

Premature Ventricular Contraction

Description

A PVC (Fig. 18-52) is a single ectopic impulse arising from an irritable focus in either ventricle (bundle branches, Purkinje fibers, or ventricular muscle) that occurs earlier than the next expected sinus beat. It is a common dysrhythmia that can occur with any underlying cardiac rhythm and results from enhanced automaticity or a reentry mechanism.

When the ventricles initiate a PVC, the atria may or may not depolarize. If atrial depolarization does not occur, a P wave is not formed. If atrial depolarization does occur, the P wave is often hidden in the QRS complex because of the timing and large electrical force of ventricular depolarization compared with atrial depolarization. The altered sequence of ventricular depolarization results in a wide, bizarre QRS complex that may deflect in the opposite direction from the QRS complex in the underlying rhythm. The T wave that immediately follows the PVC is usually deflected in the opposite direction from the QRS complex of the PVC because of the altered sequence of repolarization. The ST segment of the PVC appears abnormal because of this opposite deflection.

A PVC does not usually depolarize the SA node or interrupt its rhythm (that is, the P wave of the underlying rhythm that follows the PVC occurs at its expected time but is obstructed by the PVC and finds the ventricles refractory). Therefore the ectopic impulse is usually followed by a full compensatory pause. Compensatory pauses are confirmed by measuring the interval between the R wave before the PVC and the R wave after it. If the pause is compensatory, the distance equals at least 2 times the R-R interval of the underlying rhythm. The combination of a full compensatory pause and a wide bizarre QRS complex of a

PEA includes
- EMD
- Pseudo-EMD
- Idioventricular rhythms
- Ventricular escape rhythms
- Bradyasystolic rhythms
- Postdefibrillation idioventricular rhythms

- Continue CPR
- Intubate at once
- Obtain IV access
- Assess blood flow using Doppler ultrasound

↓

Consider possible causes
(Possible therapies and treatments are within parentheses.)
- Hypovolemia (volume infusion)
- Hypoxia (ventilation)
- Cardiac tamponade (pericardiocentesis)
- Tension pneumothorax (needle decompression)
- Hypothermia (see *hypothermia algorithm, Section IV*)
- Massive pulmonary embolism (surgery, ***thrombolytics***)
- Drug overdoses such as tricyclics, digitalis, β-blockers, calcium channel blockers
- Hyperkalemia*
- Acidosis[†]
- Massive acute myocardial infarction (see Fig. 18-85)

↓

- ***Epinephrine:*** 1 mg IV push,*[‡] repeat every 3-5 min

↓

- If absolute bradycardia (< 60 beats.min) or relative bradycardia, give ***atropine*** 1 mg IV
- Repeat every 3-5 min up to a total of 0.04 mg/kg[§]

Class I, definitely helpful; *Class IIa,* acceptable, probably helpful; *Class IIb,* acceptable, possible helpful; *Class III,* not indicated, may be harmful.
*Sodium bicarbonate 1 mEq/kg is Class I if patient has known preexisting hyperkalemia.
[†]***Sodium bicarbonate*** 1 mEq/kg:
  Class IIa—if known preexisting bicarbonate responsive acidosis, if overdose with tricyclic antidepressants, to alkalinize the urine in drug overdoses
  ClassIIb—if intubated and long arrest interval, on return of spontaneous circulation after long arrest interval
  Class III: hypoxic lactic acidosis.
[‡]The recommended dose of ***epinephrine*** is 1 mg IV push ever 3-5 min. If this approach fails, several Class IIb dosing regimens can be considered:
  Intermediate: epinephrine 2-5 mg IV push, every 3-5 min
  Escalating: ***epinephrine*** 1mg-3mg-5mg IV push (3 min apart)
  High: ***epinephrine*** 0.1 mg/kg IV push, every 3-5 min
[§]Shorter ***atropine*** dosing intervals are possibly helpful in cardiac arrest (Class IIb).

Fig. 18-51 Algorithm for pulseless electrical activity (electromechanical dissociation). (Reproduced with permission. CPR Issue of *JAMA,* Oct 28, 1992. Copyright © American Medical Association.)

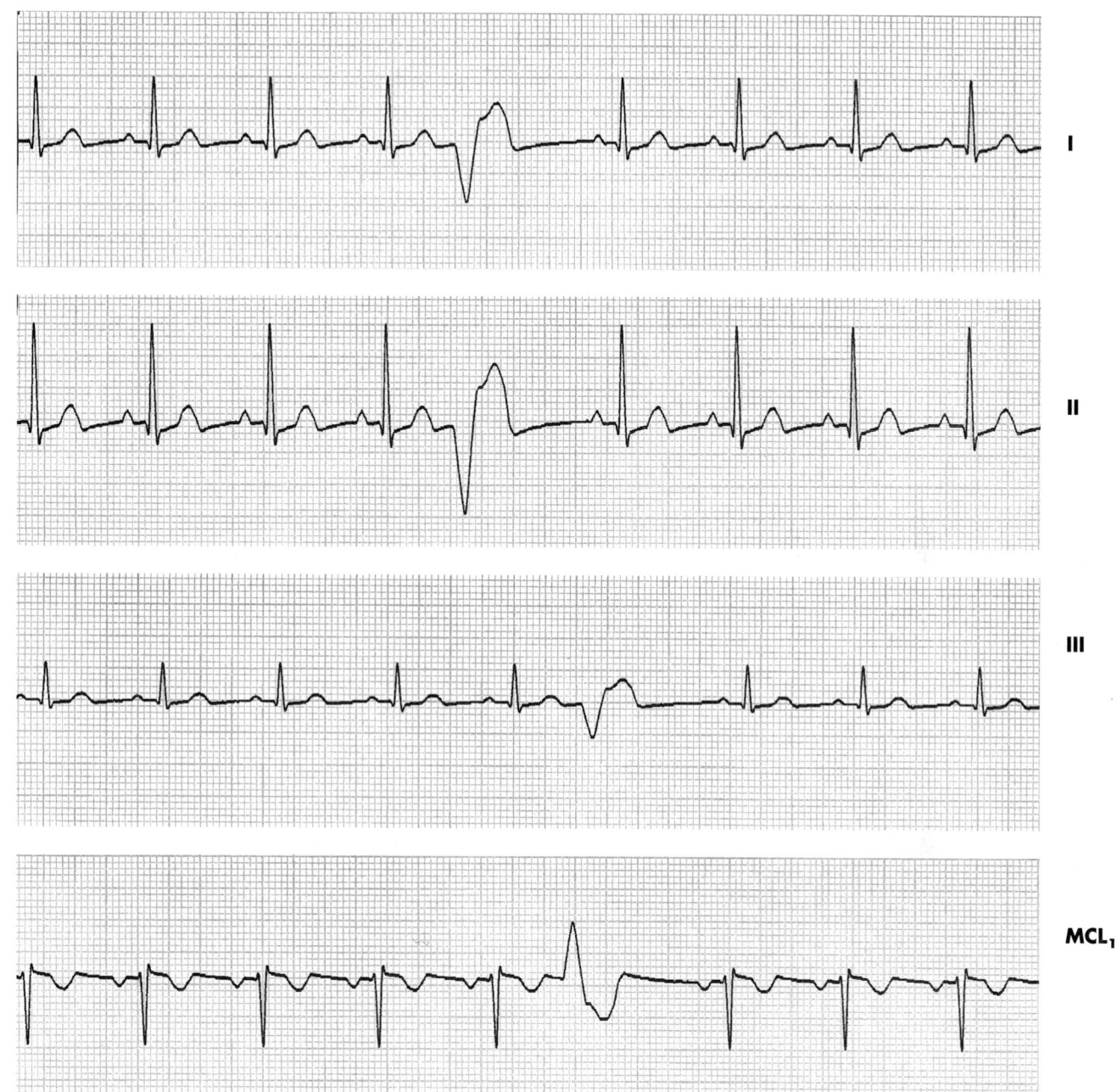

I

II

III

MCL₁

Fig. 18-52 PVCs.

premature impulse are diagnostic signs of PVC. Occasionally, a PVC falls between two sinus beats without interrupting the rhythm (called an *interpolated PVC*). This tends to occur when the underlying rhythm is relatively slow. The R-R interval that includes the PVC is often slightly greater than the underlying rhythm, but a full compensatory pause does not usually occur (Fig. 18-53).

PVCs may originate from a single ectopic pacemaker site (unifocal PVCs) or from multiple sites in the ventricles (multifocal PVCs) (Fig. 18-54). Unifocal PVCs that originate from a single site within the ventricles look alike. Multifocal PVCs that originate from different ventricular sites have varying shapes and sizes.

Multifocal PVCs are considered more dangerous than unifocal PVCs, perhaps because they are the result of a more global increased irritability within the ventricles. A PVC that occurs at approximately the same time that an electrical impulse of the underlying rhythm is activating the ventricles can cause ventricular depolarization to occur simultaneously in two directions. This fusion beat results in a QRS complex that has the characteristics of the PVC and the QRS complex of the underlying rhythm (Fig. 18-55). The pres-

ence of a fusion beat helps confirm that the ectopic impulse is ventricular in origin rather than supraventricular with aberrant ventricular conduction.

Frequently, PVCs occur in patterns of grouped beating: Bigeminy occurs when every other complex is a PVC, trigeminy occurs when every third complex is a PVC, and quadrigeminy occurs when every fourth complex is a PVC (Fig. 18-56). Consecutive PVCs that are not separated by a complex of the underlying rhythm can also occur on the ECG: Couplets or salvos are two PVCs in a row, and triplets are three PVCs in a row. (These terms may also be used to describe patterns of PACs and PJCs.)

Like multifocal PVCs, frequently occurring PVCs usually indicate that the ventricles are highly irritable. These grouped beatings can trigger life-threatening repetitive discharge of the ventricles (ventricular tachycardia or ventricular fibrillation), particularly if they occur during the relative refractory phase of the cardiac cycle. This

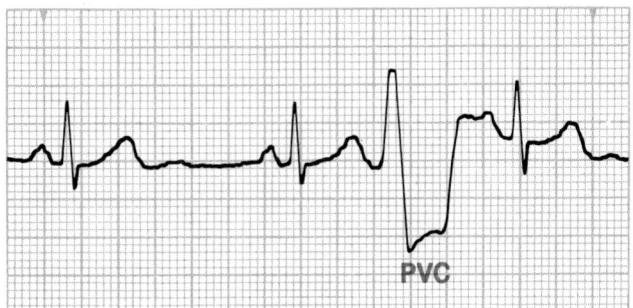

Fig. 18-53 Interpolated PVC.

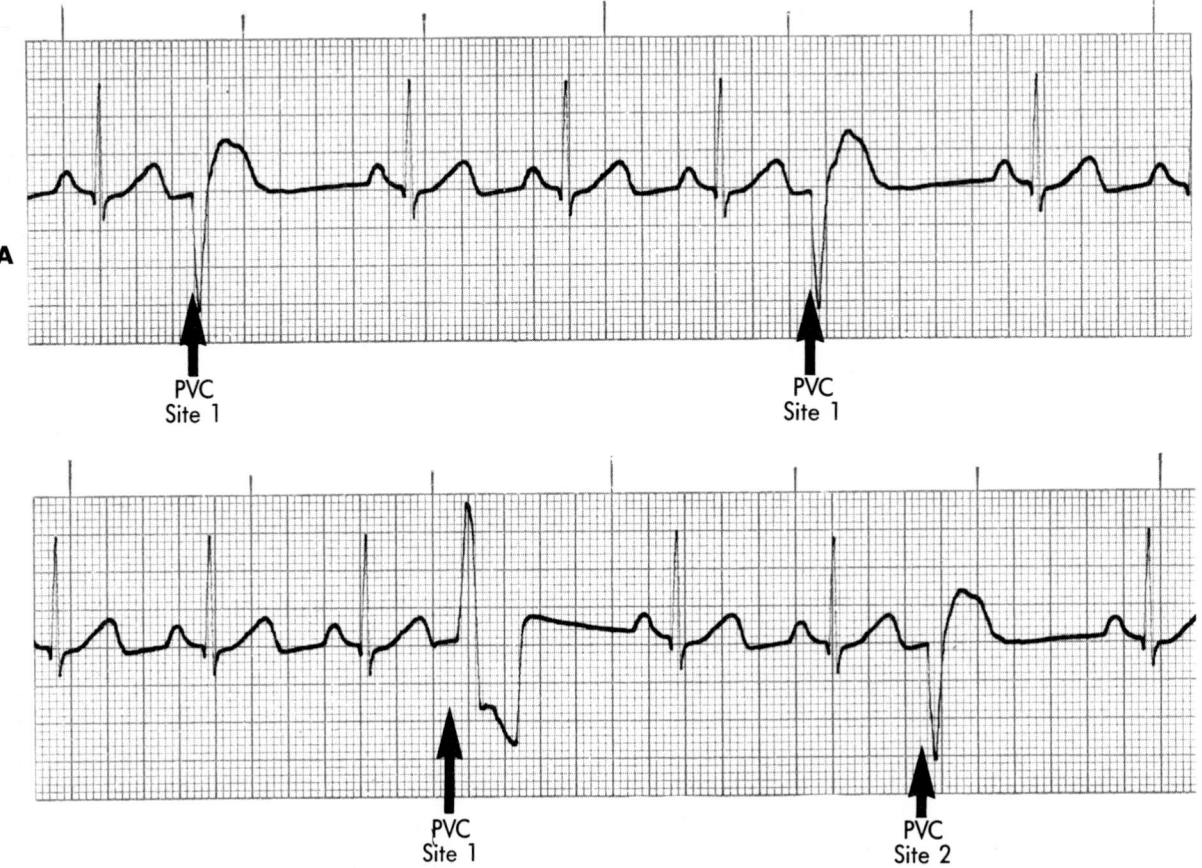

Fig. 18-54 A, Unifocal PVCs. **B,** Multifocal PVCs.

vulnerable period of ventricular repolarization is associated with the peak of the T wave. During this period, the heart muscle is at its greatest electrical nonuniformity.

Some of the ventricular muscle fibers may be partially repolarized; others may be completely repolarized, and still others may be completely refractory. Stimulation of the ventricles in the vulnerable period by an electrical impulse such as a PVC, cardiac pacemaker, or cardioversion may precipitate repetitive ventricular contractions, resulting in ventricular tachycardia or ventricular fibrillation. The occurrence of a ventricular depolarization during this vulnerable period of relative refractoriness is known as the *R-on-T phenomenon* (Fig. 18-57).

Etiology

PVCs may occur in healthy individuals without apparent cause but are usually a result of one or more of the following:

- Myocardial ischemia
- Hypoxia
- Acid-base and electrolyte imbalance
- Hypokalemia
- Congestive heart failure
- Increased catecholamine and sympathetic tone (as in emotional stress)
- Ingestion of stimulants (alcohol, caffeine, tobacco)
- Digitalis toxicity
- Sympathomimetic drugs (cocaine; stimulants such as phencyclidine, *epinephrine, isoproterenol*)

Rules for Interpretation (Lead II Monitoring)

Rate: Depends on underlying rhythm and number of PVCs

Rhythm: PVCs interrupt the regularity of the underlying rhythm.

QRS complex: Usually greater than 0.12 second; frequently distorted and bizarre

P waves: P waves may be present or absent. If they are present, they are usually of the underlying rhythm and have no relationship to the PVC.

PR interval: None

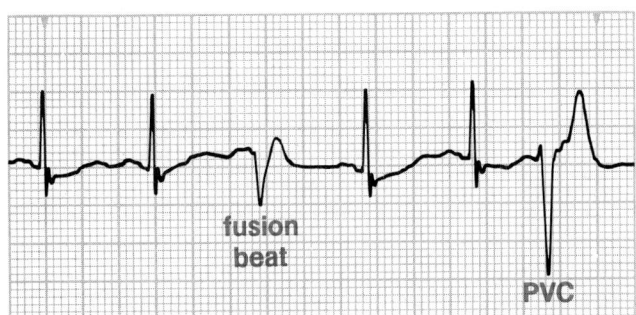

Fig. 18-55 Fusion beat with PVC.

A

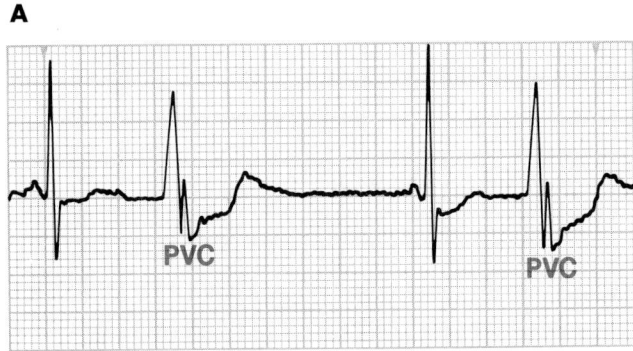

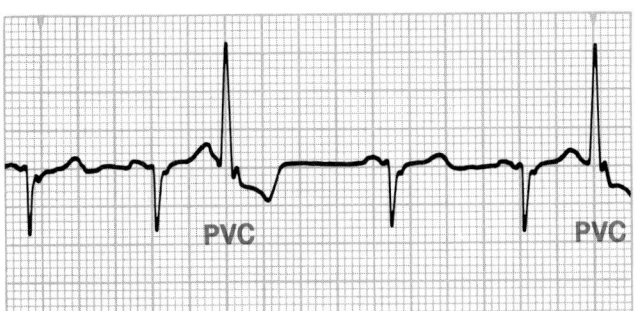

B **Fig. 18-56 A,** Bigeminy (unifocal PVCs). **B,** Trigeminy (unifocal PVCs).

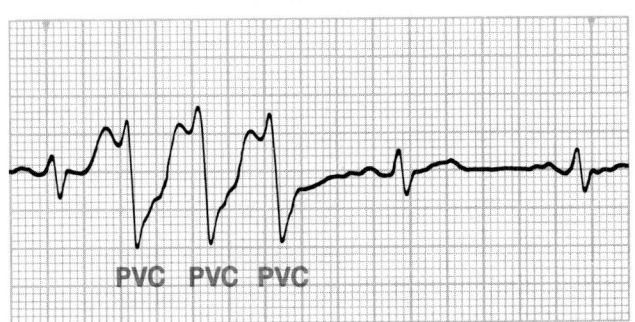

Fig. 18-57 R-on-T phenomenon (unifocal PVCs).

Clinical Significance

Isolated PVCs that occur in patients without underlying cardiovascular disease are usually of no significance. These patients frequently experience the sensation of "skipped beats." PVCs that occur with myocardial ischemia may indicate the presence of enhanced automaticity, a reentry mechanism, or both, and may trigger lethal ventricular dysrhythmias. PVCs do not permit complete ventricular filling and may produce a diminished or nonpalpable pulse (nonperfusing PVC). If the PVCs are frequent enough, cardiac output is compromised.

A number of warning signs of the potential development of serious ventricular dysrhythmias in patients with myocardial ischemia have been described. These include frequent PVCs (more than 6 per minute), the presence of multifocal PVCs, early PVCs (R-on-T), and patterns of grouped beating.

Management

PVCs that occur in asymptomatic patients without heart disease seldom require treatment. In patients with myocardial ischemia, frequent PVCs must be treated promptly with *oxygen* and antidysrhythmics (for example, *lidocaine, procainamide, bretylium*).

Ventricular Tachycardia

Description

Ventricular tachycardia (Fig. 18-58) is a dysrhythmia defined by three or more consecutive ventricular complexes occurring at a rate of more than 100 beats per minute, which overrides the primary pacemaker. The dysrhythmia generally starts suddenly, triggered by a PVC. During ventricular tachycardia, the atria and ventricles are asynchronous. If the rhythm disturbance is sustained, the patient's condition usually becomes unstable, often leading to unconsciousness and occasionally even to loss of a perfusing pulse. However, patients with an underlying rhythm of ventricular tachycardia may be able to walk and talk. The misconception that ventricular tachycardia cannot be associated with reasonable blood pressure may result in a patient's being inappropriately managed. The electrophysiological mechanism responsible for ventricular tachycardia is enhanced automaticity or reentry.

Etiology

Like PVCs, ventricular tachycardia usually occurs in the presence of myocardial ischemia or significant cardiac disease. Other causes of ventricular tachycardia include:

- Acid-base and electrolyte imbalance
- Hypokalemia
- Congestive heart failure
- Increased catecholamine and sympathetic tone (as in emotional stress)
- Ingestion of stimulants (alcohol, caffeine, tobacco)
- Medication toxicity (digitalis, tricyclic antidepressants)
- Sympathomimetic drugs *(epinephrine, isoproterenol,* cocaine, *norepinephrine)*
- Prolonged QT interval (may be caused by drugs or metabolic problems or be congenital)

Rules for Interpretation (Lead II Monitoring)

Rate: Usually between 100 and 250 beats per minute

Rhythm: Usually regular but may be slightly irregular

QRS complex: Greater than 0.12 second and usually distorted and bizarre. The QRS complexes are generally identical, but if fusion beats are present, one or more QRS complexes may differ in size, shape, and direction. Torsades de pointes ("twisting around a point") is a form of ventricular tachycardia characterized by QRS complexes that gradually change back and forth from one shape and direction to another over a series of beats. Torsades de pointes is usually caused by one of a number of conditions that prolong the QT interval, including hypokalemia, certain antidysrhythmic medications (quinidine or *procainamide*), and tricyclic antidepressant overdose.

P waves: P waves may be present or absent. If present, P waves have no set relation to the QRS complex, a situation known as *AV dissociation.* P waves may be positive or negative and are often difficult to detect if the ventricular rate is rapid.

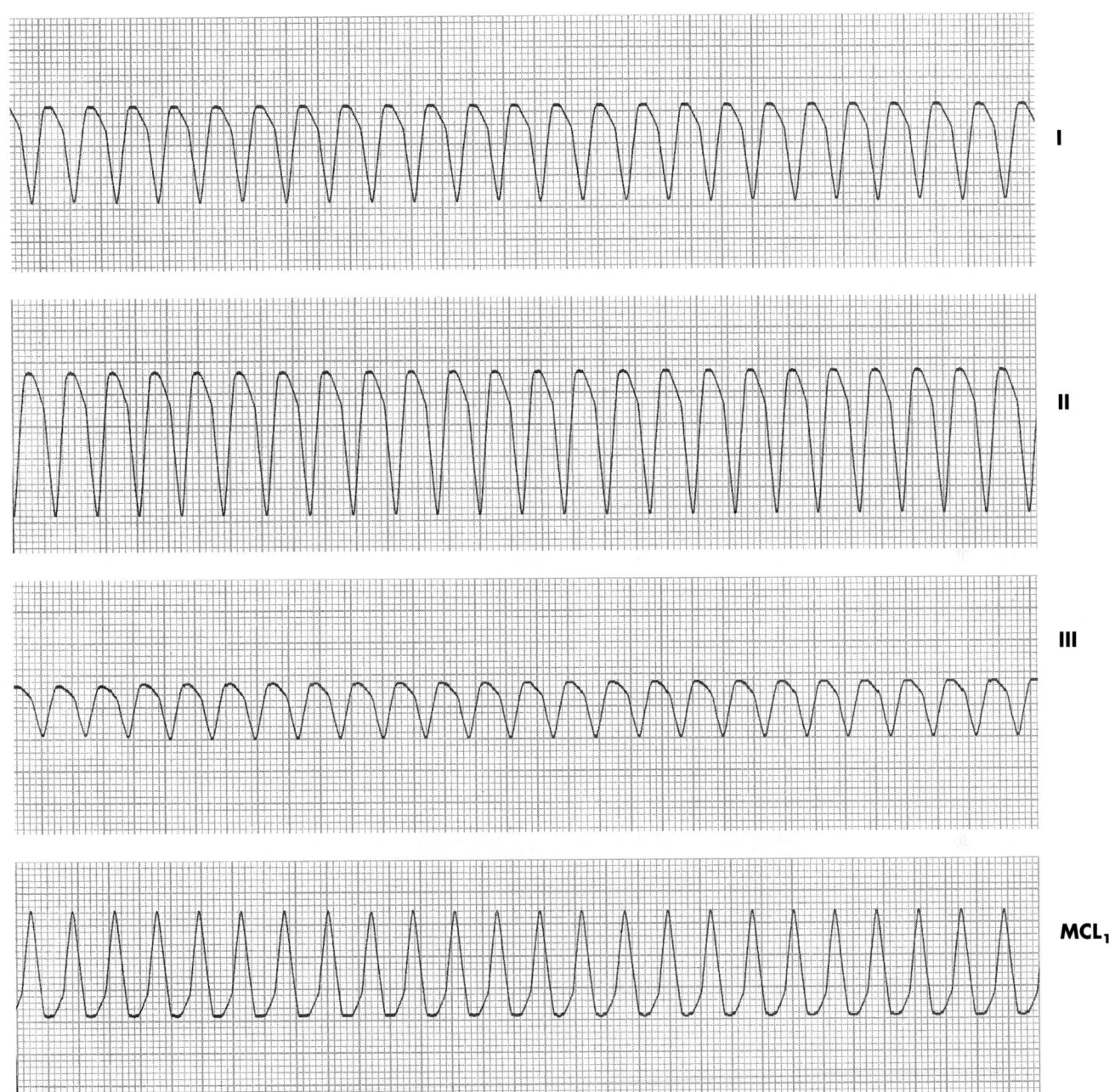

Fig. 18-58 Ventricular tachycardia.

PR interval: If P waves are present, the PR interval varies widely.

Clinical Significance

Ventricular tachycardia usually indicates significant underlying cardiovascular disease. The rapid rate associated with ventricular tachycardia and the concurrent loss of atrial kick result in compromised cardiac output and decreased coronary artery and cerebral perfusion. The severity of symptoms varies with the rate of the ventricular tachycardia and the presence or absence of underlying myocardial dysfunction. Ventricular tachycardia may be perfusing or nonperfusing, and it may initiate or degenerate into ventricular fibrillation.

Management

A conscious patient who has a perfusing rhythm and is not hypotensive, having ischemic

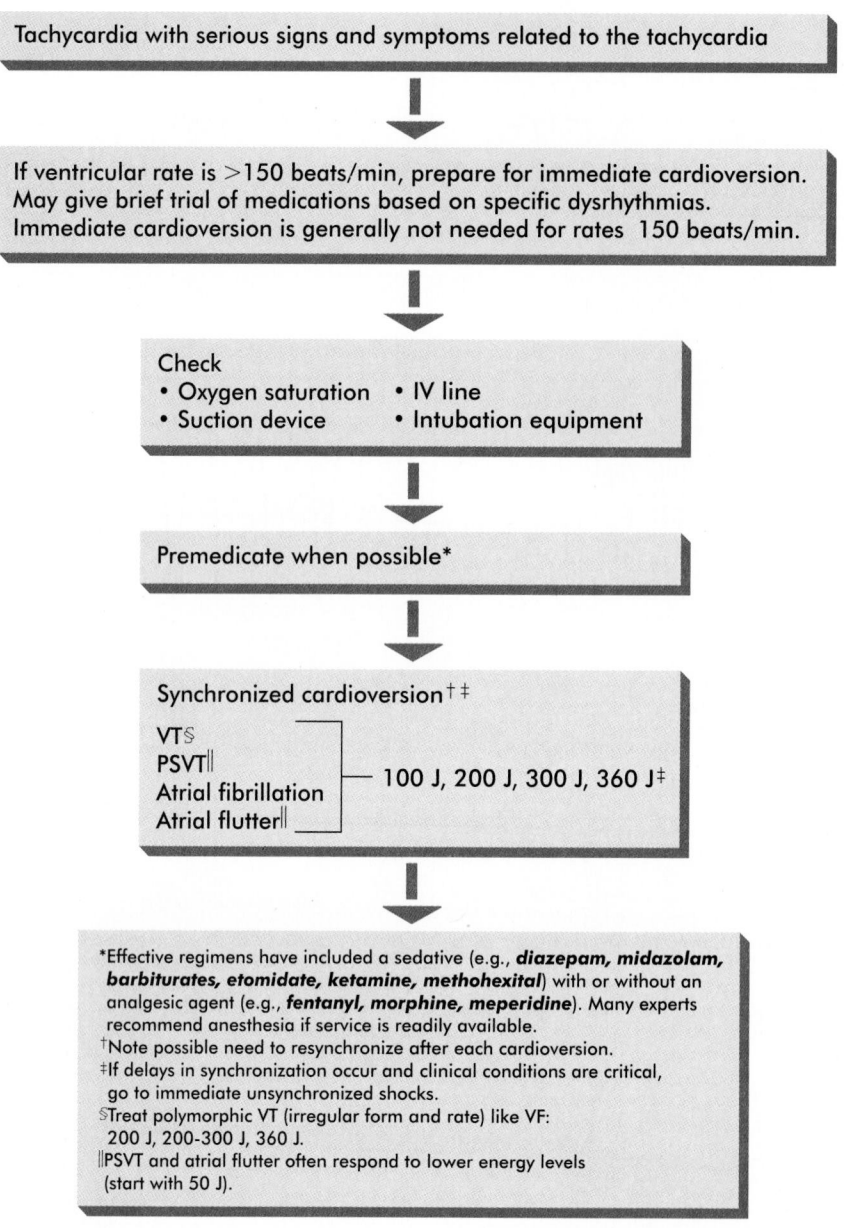

Tachycardia with serious signs and symptoms related to the tachycardia

↓

If ventricular rate is >150 beats/min, prepare for immediate cardioversion. May give brief trial of medications based on specific dysrhythmias. Immediate cardioversion is generally not needed for rates 150 beats/min.

↓

Check
• Oxygen saturation   • IV line
• Suction device   • Intubation equipment

↓

Premedicate when possible*

↓

Synchronized cardioversion†‡

VT§
PSVT‖   — 100 J, 200 J, 300 J, 360 J‡
Atrial fibrillation
Atrial flutter‖

↓

*Effective regimens have included a sedative (e.g., **diazepam, midazolam, barbiturates, etomidate, ketamine, methohexital**) with or without an analgesic agent (e.g., **fentanyl, morphine, meperidine**). Many experts recommend anesthesia if service is readily available.
†Note possible need to resynchronize after each cardioversion.
‡If delays in synchronization occur and clinical conditions are critical, go to immediate unsynchronized shocks.
§Treat polymorphic VT (irregular form and rate) like VF: 200 J, 200-300 J, 360 J.
‖PSVT and atrial flutter often respond to lower energy levels (start with 50 J).

Fig. 18-59 Electrical cardioversion algorithm (with the patient not in cardiac arrest). (Reproduced with permission. CPR Issue of *JAMA*, Oct 28, 1992. Copyright © American Medical Association.)

heart pain, or in pulmonary edema is considered clinically stable and should be treated with *oxygen,* antidysrhythmics *(lidocaine, procainamide, bretylium),* and synchronized cardioversion (as needed) to terminate the dysrhythmia (see Fig. 18-38). A patient who has a decreased level of consciousness, chest pain, shortness of breath, low blood pressure, shock, pulmonary congestion, heart failure, or acute myocardial infarction should be considered clinically unstable. These patients are initially treated with *oxygen* and im-

mediate cardioversion, followed by antidysrhythmics. If there is a delay caused by attempting synchronization and clinical conditions are critical, unsynchronized shocks should be delivered. The initial energy level for ventricular tachycardia is 100 joules, followed by 200, 300, and 360 joules. Polymorphic ventricular tachycardia (such as torsades de pointes) cannot be reliably synchronized and should be treated like ventricular fibrillation, with an initial unsynchronized shock of 200 joules (Fig. 18-59).

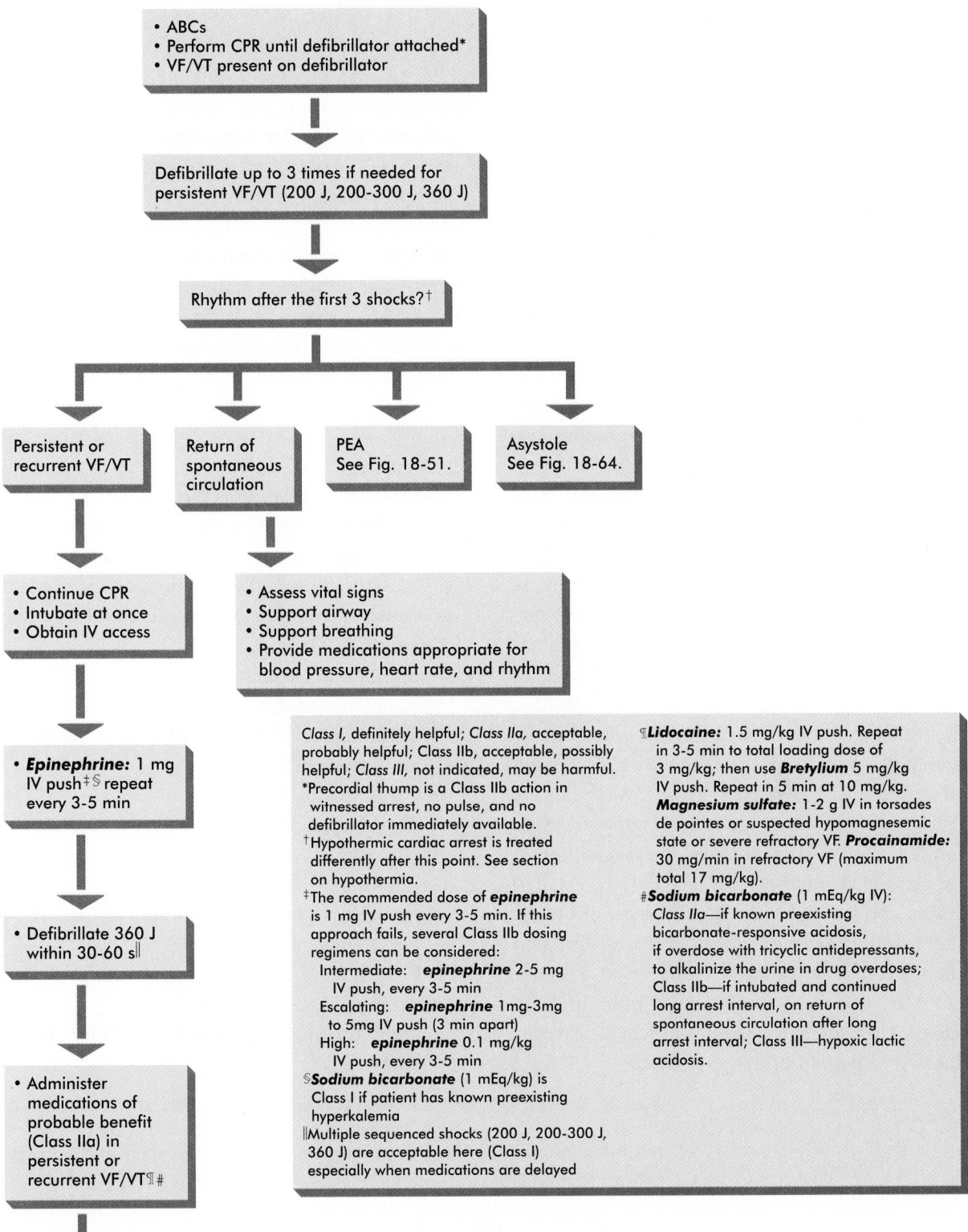

- ABCs
- Perform CPR until defibrillator attached*
- VF/VT present on defibrillator

Defibrillate up to 3 times if needed for persistent VF/VT (200 J, 200-300 J, 360 J)

Rhythm after the first 3 shocks?†

Persistent or recurrent VF/VT

Return of spontaneous circulation

PEA
See Fig. 18-51.

Asystole
See Fig. 18-64.

- Continue CPR
- Intubate at once
- Obtain IV access

- Assess vital signs
- Support airway
- Support breathing
- Provide medications appropriate for blood pressure, heart rate, and rhythm

- **Epinephrine:** 1 mg IV push‡§ repeat every 3-5 min

- Defibrillate 360 J within 30-60 s‖

- Administer medications of probable benefit (Class IIa) in persistent or recurrent VF/VT¶ #

- Defibrillate 360 J, 30-60 sec after each dose of medication‖
- Pattern should be drug-shock, drug-shock

Class I, definitely helpful; *Class IIa,* acceptable, probably helpful; *Class IIb,* acceptable, possibly helpful; *Class III,* not indicated, may be harmful.
*Precordial thump is a Class IIb action in witnessed arrest, no pulse, and no defibrillator immediately available.
†Hypothermic cardiac arrest is treated differently after this point. See section on hypothermia.
‡The recommended dose of **epinephrine** is 1 mg IV push every 3-5 min. If this approach fails, several Class IIb dosing regimens can be considered:
  Intermediate: **epinephrine** 2-5 mg IV push, every 3-5 min
  Escalating: **epinephrine** 1mg-3mg to 5mg IV push (3 min apart)
  High: **epinephrine** 0.1 mg/kg IV push, every 3-5 min
§**Sodium bicarbonate** (1 mEq/kg) is Class I if patient has known preexisting hyperkalemia
‖Multiple sequenced shocks (200 J, 200-300 J, 360 J) are acceptable here (Class I) especially when medications are delayed

¶**Lidocaine:** 1.5 mg/kg IV push. Repeat in 3-5 min to total loading dose of 3 mg/kg; then use **Bretylium** 5 mg/kg IV push. Repeat in 5 min at 10 mg/kg. **Magnesium sulfate:** 1-2 g IV in torsades de pointes or suspected hypomagnesemic state or severe refractory VF. **Procainamide:** 30 mg/min in refractory VF (maximum total 17 mg/kg).
#**Sodium bicarbonate** (1 mEq/kg IV): Class IIa—if known preexisting bicarbonate-responsive acidosis, if overdose with tricyclic antidepressants, to alkalinize the urine in drug overdoses; Class IIb—if intubated and continued long arrest interval, on return of spontaneous circulation after long arrest interval; Class III—hypoxic lactic acidosis.

Fig. 18-60 Algorithm for ventricular fibrillation and pulseless ventricular tachycardia. (Reproduced with permission. CPR Issue of *JAMA,* Oct 28, 1992. Copyright © American Medical Association.)

If the patient has a nonperfusing rhythm (that is, no palpable pulse), basic life support should be initiated, and treatment should proceed as though ventricular fibrillation were present (Fig. 18-60). Torsades de pointes is a special form of ventricular tachycardia that does not respond to the recommended antidysrhythmics *lidocaine, procainamide,* and *bretylium.* Although electrical pacing is the preferred treatment, at present it cannot be performed with transcutaneous units unless they are modified to pace more rapidly. *Isoproterenol* is sometimes useful in abolishing torsades de pointes by decreasing repolarization rates and causing a sinus tachycardia overdrive. Recent reports have also demonstrated that *magensium sulfate* can abolish runs of torsades des pointes.[1] With this dysrhythmia, it is important to search for an underlying cause and to institute corrective measures if possible.

Monitored adult patients whose rhythm is observed to be stable ventricular tachycardia (or ventricular fibrillation) may be treated with a solitary precordial thump, provided that a defibrillator and TCP are readily available. (A precordial thump may cause ventricular tachycardia to deteriorate to asystole, ventricular flutter, or electromechanical dissociation [EMD].[1]) A precordial thump may terminate a dysrhythmia by causing ventricular depolarization and the resumption of an organized rhythm. To deliver a precordial thump, the arm and wrist should be parallel to the long axis of the sternum to avoid rib fractures and other injury. The thump is delivered to the midsternum with the heel of the fist from 10 to 12 inches. The patient in stable ventricular tachycardia should be told of the procedure.

Ventricular Fibrillation

Description

Ventricular fibrillation (Fig. 18-61) is a chaotic ventricular rhythm that results in nonperfusing quivering ventricular movements, not actual contractions. The electrical impulses initiated by the multiple ectopic ventricular sites do not allow cardiac cells to fully depolarize and repolarize, so organized ventricular contraction does not occur. Ventricular fibrillation is the most common initial rhythm disturbance in sudden cardiac arrest. It probably results from enhanced automaticity or the presence of many reentry circuits in the ventricles.

Etiology

Ventricular fibrillation is most commonly associated with significant cardiovascular system disease. The dysrhythmias may also be precipitated by PVCs, the R-on-T phenomenon, or a sustained ventricular tachycardia. Other causes include the following:
- Myocardial ischemia
- Acute myocardial infarction
- Third-degree AV block with a slow ventricular escape rhythm
- Cardiomyopathy
- Digitalis toxicity
- Hypoxia
- Acidosis
- Electrolyte imbalance (hypokalemia, hyperkalemia, near-drowning)
- Cardiac trauma (blunt or penetrating)
- Accidental electrocution
- Drug overdose or toxicity (cocaine, tricyclics)

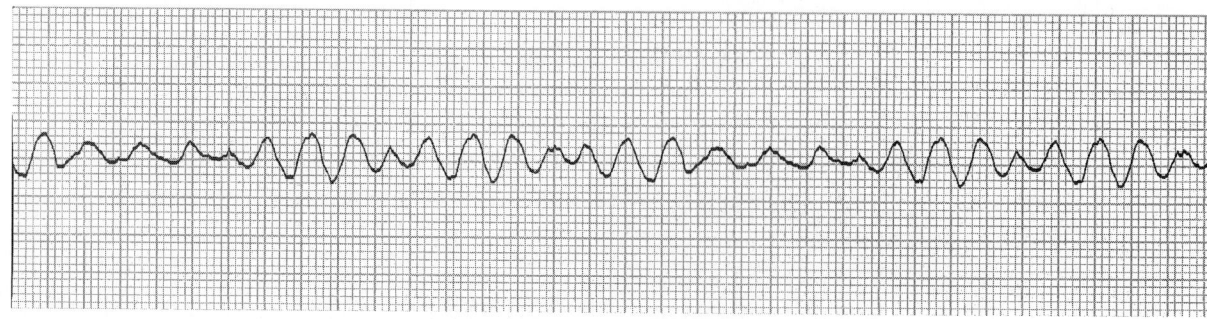

Fig. 18-61 Ventricular fibrillation.

Rules for Interpretation (All Leads)

Rate: No coordinated ventricular contractions are present. The unsynchronized ventricular impulses occur at rates from 300 to 500 beats per minute.

Rhythm: Irregularly irregular

QRS complex: Absent

P waves: Absent

PR interval: Absent

Because organized depolarizations of the atria and ventricles are absent, P waves, QRS complexes, ST segments, and T waves are absent. Ventricular fibrillatory waves (seen on the oscilloscope as bizarre, rounded or pointed, and markedly different, varying at random from positive to negative) represent haphazard depolarization of small individual groups of muscle fibers. Fibrillatory waves less than 3 mm in amplitude are considered **fine ventricular fibrillation,** and those greater than 3 mm are considered **coarse ventricular fibrillation** (Fig. 18-62). The fibrillatory waves may be so fine that they appear isoelectric, resembling ventricular asystole.

Clinical Significance

Ventricular fibrillation causes all life-supporting physiological functions to cease because of lack of circulating blood flow. The dysrhythmia may initially result in lightheadedness, followed within seconds by loss of consciousness, apnea, and if untreated, death.

Management

For adult resuscitation, treatment of ventricular fibrillation and ventricular tachycardia is the most important sequence, since most adult cardiac arrests result from these two rhythm disturbances and the vast majority of successful resuscitations result from the appropriate treatment of these two dysrhythmias.[1] Ventricular fibrillation and nonperfusing ventricular tachycardia are treated alike: basic life support (if a defibrillator is not immediately available), defibrillation, endotracheal intubation, and pharmacological therapy *(epinephrine, lidocaine, bretylium,* and perhaps *sodium bicarbonate)*. If the onset of ventricular fibrillation is witnessed (monitored), a solitary precordial thump may terminate the arrest.

Coarse ventricular fibrillation (indicating a recent onset of the dysrhythmia) is more apt to be reversed by defibrillation than fine ventricular fibrillation, indicating that the dysrhythmia has been present for a prolonged period. If the monitor appears to show asystole, fine ventricular fibrillation may still be the underlying rhythm. Asystole should be confirmed in two leads (90 degrees apart) to rule out fine ventricular fibrillation so that the patient is not inappropriately treated (see Fig. 18-60).

Ventricular Asystole

Description

Ventricular asystole (cardiac standstill) (Fig. 18-63) refers to the absence of all ventricular activity.

Etiology

Ventricular asystole may be the primary event in cardiac arrest. It may also occur in complete heart block when there is no functional escape pacemaker. The dysrhythmia is usually associated with global myocardial ischemia or necrosis and often follows ventricular tachycardia, ventricular fibrillation, electromechanical dissociation, or an idioventricular escape rhythm in the dying heart. When faced with an isoelectric line on the monitor, the paramedic should confirm asystole as the rhythm by changing placement of the defibrillation paddles by 90 degrees.

Rules for Interpretation (All Leads)

Rate: Absent

Rhythm: Absent

QRS complexes: Absent

P waves: Absent or present

PR Interval: Absent

Clinical Significance

Ventricular asystole produces complete cessation of cardiac output. It is an ominous dysrhythmia, often representing a confirmation of death in which the prognosis for resuscitation is dismal.

Management (Fig. 18-64)

The treatment for ventricular asystole is basic life support, endotracheal intubation, pharmaco-

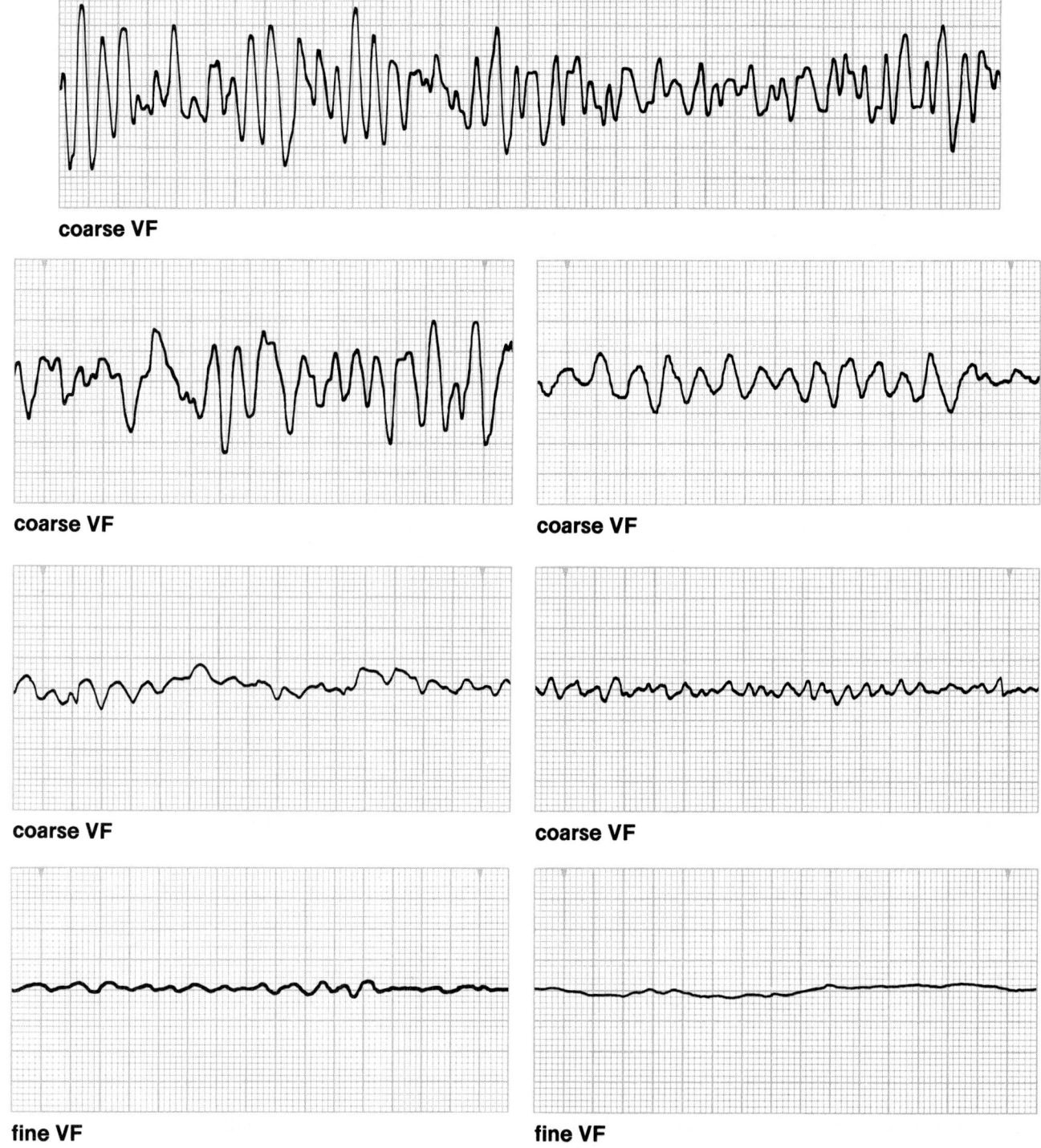

coarse VF

coarse VF

coarse VF

coarse VF

coarse VF

fine VF

fine VF

Fig. 18-62 Coarse and fine ventricular fibrillation.

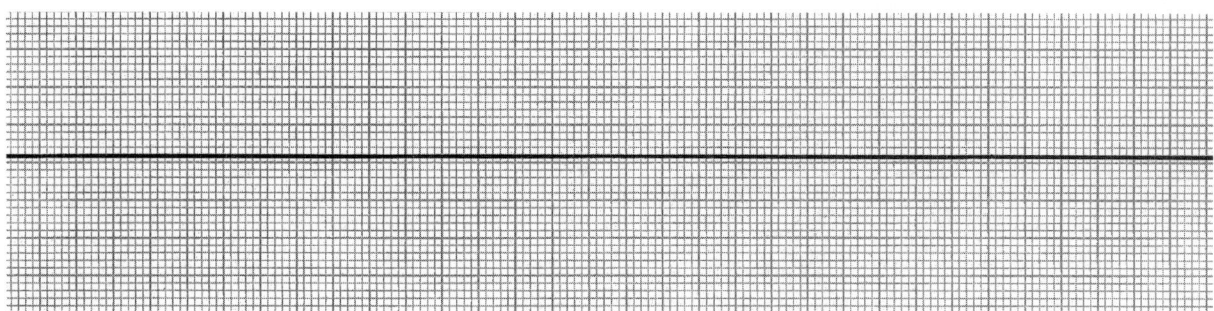

Fig. 18-63 Ventricular asystole.

- Continue CPR
- Intubate at once
- Obtain IV access
- Confirm asystole in more than one lead

↓

Consider possible causes
- Hypoxia
- Hyperkalemia
- Hypokalemia
- Preexisting acidosis
- Drug overdose
- Hypothermia

↓

Consider immediate transcutaneous pacing (TCP)*

↓

- *Epinephrine:* 1 mg IV push,†‡ repeat every 3-5 min

↓

- *Atropine* 1 mg IV, repeat every 3-5 min up to 0.04 mg/kg§‖

↓

Consider
- Termination of efforts¶

Class I, definitely helpful; Class IIa, acceptable, probably helpful; Class IIb, acceptable, possibly helpful; Class III, not indicated, may be harmful.
*TCP is a Class IIb intervention. Lack of success may result from delays in pacing. To be effective, TCP must be performed early with drugs. Evidence does not support routine use of TCP for asystole.
†The recommended dose of *epinephrine* is 1 mg IV push every 3-5 min. If this approach fails, several Class IIb dosing regimens can be considered:
  Intermediate: *epinephrine* 2-5 mg IV push, every 3-5 min
  Escalating: *epinephrine* 1mg-3mg to 5mg IV push (3 min apart)
  High: *epinephrine* 0.1 mg/kg IV push, every 3-5 min
‡*Sodium bicarbonate* 1 mEq/kg is Class I if patient has known preexisting hyperkalemia.
§Shorter *atropine* dosing intervals are Class IIb in asystolic arrest.
‖*Sodium bicarbonate* 1 mEq/kg: Class IIa— if known preexisting bicarbonate-responsive acidosis, if overdose with tricyclic antidepressants, to alkalinize the urine in drug overdoses; Class IIb—if intubated and continued long arrest interval, on return of spontaneous circulation after long arrest interval; Class III—hypoxic lactic acidosis.
¶If patient remains in asystole or other agonal rhythms after successful intubation and initial medications and no reversible causes are identified, consider termination of resuscitative efforts by a physician. Consider interval since arrest.

Fig. 18-64 Asystole treatment algorithm. (Reproduced with permission. CPR Issue of *JAMA*, Oct 28, 1992. Copyright © American Medical Association.)

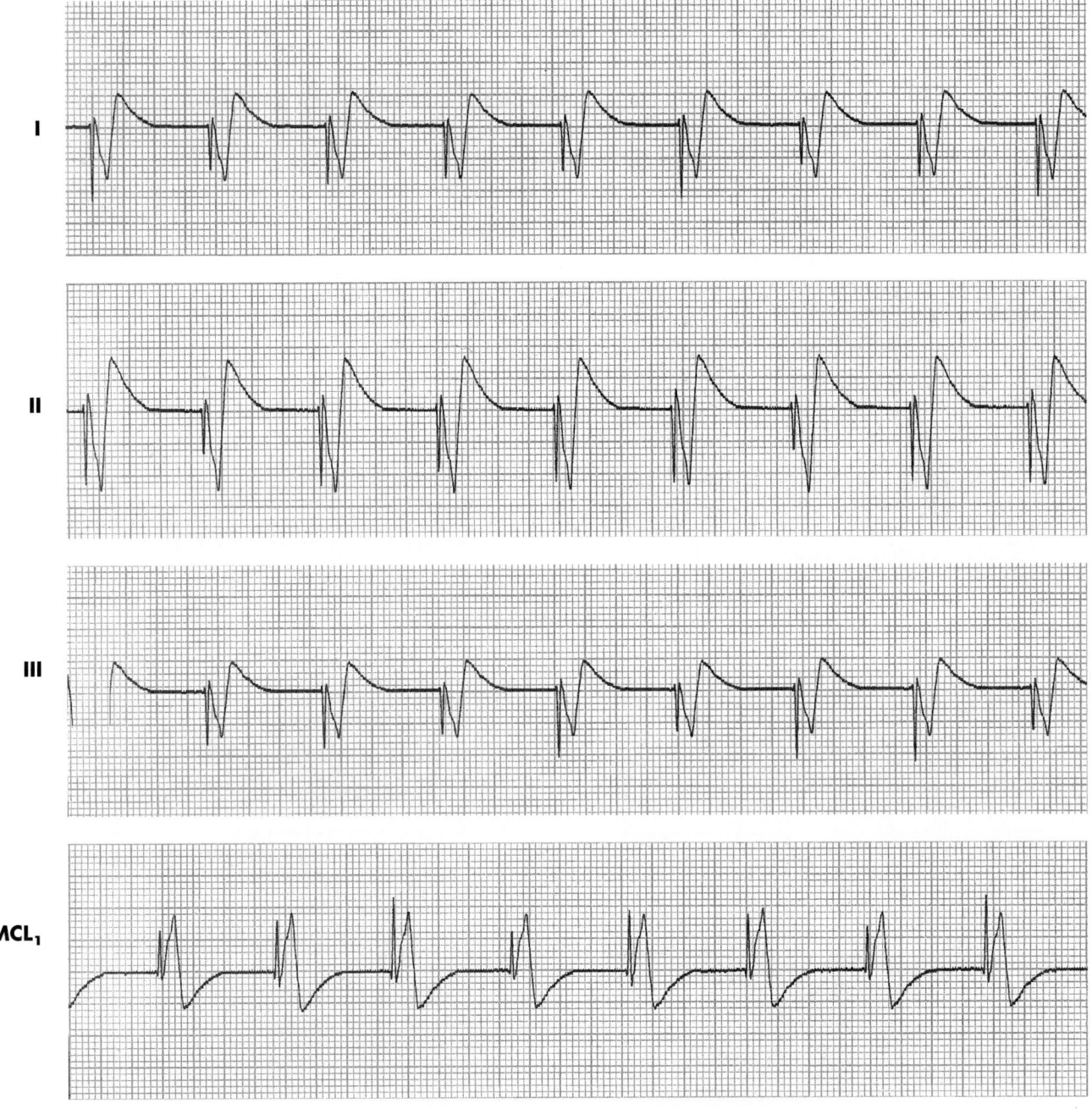

Fig. 18-65 Artificial pacemaker rhythms.

logical therapy *(epinephrine, atropine,* and *sodium bicarbonate),* and possibly TCP. (Studies suggest that very early use of external pacing may improve survival in patients with bradyasystolic arrests.) If fine ventricular fibrillation is suspected, defibrillation is indicated. However, defibrillating asystole "just in case" is no longer recommended.[1] Cessation of resuscitation efforts in the prehospital setting after system-specific crite-

ria and authorization from medical control is indicated in this scenario.[1]

Artificial Pacemaker Rhythms

Description

Artificial pacemakers generate a rhythm (Fig. 18-65) by regular electrical stimulation of the heart through an electrode implanted in the heart. The electrode is connected to a power source (a battery cell implanted subcutaneously in the right or left pectoral region). The tip of the pacemaker wire is commonly positioned in the apex of the right ventricle (ventricular pacemaker), in the right atrium (atrial pacemaker), or in both locations (dual-chamber pacemaker). These devices are implanted most frequently in patients with complete heart block and in those who have episodes of severe symptomatic bradycardia.

Pacemakers that fire continuously at a preset rate without regard to the patient's own electrical activity are known as *fixed rate* or *asynchronous pacemakers;* they are rarely used today. Pacemakers that fire only if the patient's own rate drops below the pacemaker's preset rate (acting as an escape rhythm) are known as *demand pacemakers.* Atrial and ventricular demand pacemakers "pace" the atria or ventricles when the intrinsic rate of the paced chamber drops dangerously low. Atrial synchronous ventricular pacemakers are synchronized with the patient's atrial rhythm. This type of pacemaker paces the ventricle at a preset time after the patient's intrinsic atrial depolarization. This pacemaker is useful in patients with normal sinus node activity but various degrees of AV block. AV sequential pacemakers pace the atria first and then the ventricles when spontaneous activity is absent or slowed in either or both. If intrinsic atrial activity is too slow, for example, then both chambers are paced sequentially to maintain the "atrial kick." If the atrial rate is adequate, the atrial pacer is suppressed. The ventricular pacemaker still fires if the ventricular rate is below a preset rate. This pacemaker is ideal for sick sinus syndrome, sinus arrest, and sinus pauses.

A class of newer pacemakers (rate-responsive pacemakers) can adjust their pacing rates to patient needs by sensing when cardiac output should be increased. Although there are several methods of sensing metabolic activity, the most popular rate-responsive pacers detect patient movement to determine the optimum firing rate. These devices are popular because they can increase cardiac output and increase tolerance of physical activity. These pacemakers occasionally increase the patient's pacing rate inappropriately if they sense muscle movement that is not caused by increased patient activity.

Rules for Interpretation (Lead II Monitoring)

Rate: Varies according to preset rate of pacemaker. Typically the rate is 60 to 80 beats per minute.

Rhythm: Regular if pacing is constant; irregular if pacing occurs only on demand.

QRS complex: If pacemaker induced, QRS complexes are 0.12 second or greater. Their appearance is usually bizarre, resembling a PVC. The pacemaker is said to be "capturing" if each pacemaker spike elicits a QRS complex. If only the atria are being paced, the QRS complexes are usually normal, provided no bundle branch block is present. With demand pacemakers, some of the patient's own QRS complexes may be present. These normal QRS complexes occur without pacemaker spikes.

P waves: P waves may be present or absent, normal or abnormal. The relationship of the P waves to the pacemaker (QRS) complex varies by type of artificial pacemaker. Pacemaker "spikes" precede QRS complexes induced by ventricular pacemakers, whereas dual-chambered pacemakers also produce an atrial spike followed by a P wave. The pacemaker spike is a narrow deflection on the oscilloscope and represents the electrical discharge of the pacemaker.

> **NOTE:**
> Pacemaker spikes only indicate that a pacemaker is discharging. They provide no information regarding ventricular contraction or perfusion.

PR interval: The presence and duration of PR intervals depend on the underlying rhythm and vary by type of artificial pacemaker.

Clinical Significance

Pacemaker spikes indicate that the patient's heart rate is being regulated by an artificial pacemaker. Pacemaker spikes followed by QRS complexes indicate electrical capture. If spikes do not elicit a QRS complex, the pacemaker is not capturing the ventricle electrically, and there will be no ventricular contraction. A large percentage of pacemaker failures occur within the first month after implantation. Four potential causes of pacemaker malfunction are:

1. Battery failure: Most implanted pacemakers today use a lithium-iodine cell power source that provides stable voltage output for approximately 80% to 90% of the life of the battery (5 to 10 years or more). Battery failure usually slows the pacemaker rate and decreases the spike amplitude. If the battery fails, the patient may have bradycardia or asystole.

2. Runaway pacemakers: Runaway pacemakers (pacemakers that develop very rapid discharge rates that may reach 300 beats per minute) occur rarely as the batteries decrease their voltage output. This type of failure is seldom seen in pacemakers used today because the newer power sources provide a gradual increase in rate as their batteries run low.

3. Failure of the sensing device in demand pacemakers: Demand pacemakers may fail to shut off when the patient has an adequate rate of his or her own. When this occurs, there is competition between the natural and artificial pacemakers of the heart, and the pacemaker may discharge during the vulnerable period of the cardiac cycle.

4. Failure to capture: Failure of the pacemaker to capture may result from a variety of causes, including battery failure, broken catheter electrode wires, inoperable electrodes, and a shift in the location of the catheter tip. In such cases, pacemaker spikes are usually present but are not followed by P waves or QRS complexes.

Management

Patients with artificial pacemakers require no special emergency care treatment. However, pacemaker failure is a *true emergency* that necessitates immediate recognition and transport for definitive care (battery replacement or temporary pacemaker insertion). Therefore prolonged in-field stabilization of these patients is contraindicated. The following five principles are also important in evaluating and managing patients with implanted pacemakers:

1. When examining an unconscious patient, be alert for battery packs implanted under the skin as well as any medical alert information.

2. Treat all dysrhythmias as usual.

3. Treat ventricular irritability with *lidocaine* without fear of suppressing ventricular response to a pacemaker rhythm.

4. Defibrillate the hearts of patients with artificial pacemakers in the usual manner, but do not discharge paddles directly over the implanted battery pack.

5. TCP, if indicated, may be used in the usual manner.

Besides pacemakers, automatic implantable cardioverter defibrillators are becoming more common today. The battery packs of these devices are located in the subcutaneous tissues of the abdominal wall. Emergency cardiac care may proceed in the usual manner. Medical personnel can wear rubber (latex) gloves to help avoid unpleasant sensations when the device discharges.

● DYSRHYTHMIAS THAT ARE DISORDERS OF CONDUCTION

Partial delays or complete interruptions in cardiac electrical conduction are called *heart blocks*. Heart blocks can occur anywhere in the atria, between the SA node and the AV node, or in the ventricles between the AV node and the Purkinje fibers. These dysrhythmias of conduction may be caused by pathology in the conduction system or by a physiological block, as occurs in atrial fibrillation or atrial flutter. Causes of heart blocks include AV junctional ischemia, AV junctional necrosis, degenerative disease of the conduction system, and drug toxicity, especially with digitalis toxicity.

Classifications

Conduction blocks may be classified on the basis of several characteristics: site of block (for example, left bundle branch block), degree of block (for example, second-degree AV block), or category of AV conduction disturbances (for example, Mobitz I). This text presents the dysrhythmias by degree as well as location. AV blocks are

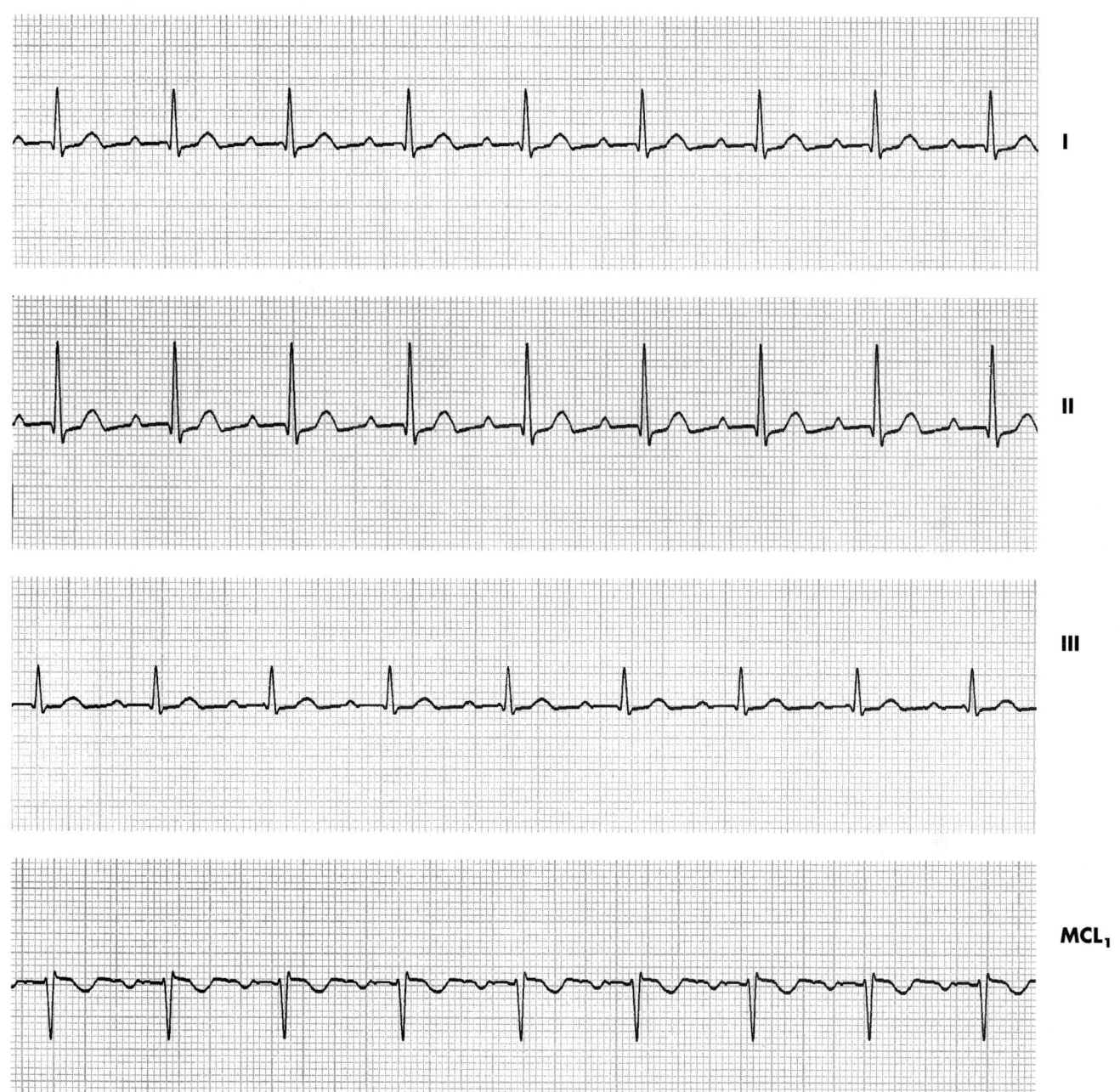

Fig. 18-66 First-degree AV block.

categorized by degree of block. It should be noted, however, that the term *degree* does not directly reflect gradients of clinical severity when applied to the classification of heart blocks. Any evaluation of heart block must consider the specific rates of the atria and ventricles, the patient's clinical presentation, and the findings of a complete history and physical examination before the clinical sever-

ity of AV conduction disturbances is determined. The dysrhythmias discussed in this section include first-degree AV block; second-degree AV block (Mobitz type I); second-degree AV block (Mobitz type II); third-degree AV block (complete heart block); ventricular conduction disturbances, including bundle branch blocks and hemiblocks; pulseless electrical activity; and preexcitation syndromes, including Wolff-Parkinson-White syndrome.

First-Degree AV Block

Description

First-degree AV block (Fig. 18-66) is not a true block but rather a delay in conduction, usually at the level of the AV node. First-degree AV block is not considered a rhythm in itself because it is usually superimposed on another rhythm. Therefore the underlying rhythm must also be identified (for example, sinus bradycardia with first-degree AV block).

Etiology

First-degree AV block may occur for no apparent reason. The dysrhythmia is commonly associated with myocardial ischemia, acute myocardial infarction, increased vagal (parasympathetic) tone, or digitalis toxicity.

Rules for Interpretation (Lead II Monitoring)

Rate: The rate is that of the underlying sinus or atrial rhythm.

Rhythm: The rhythm is that of the underlying rhythm.

QRS complex: Typically normal (less than 0.12 second), with an AV conduction ratio of 1:1 (a QRS complex follows each P wave)

P waves: Present, identical waves that precede each QRS complex

PR interval: A prolonged (greater than 0.20 second), constant PR interval is the hallmark of first-degree AV block and is often the only alteration in the ECG.

Clinical Significance

As a general rule, first-degree AV block in an asymptomatic patient has little or no clinical significance because all of the impulses are conducted to the ventricles. Rarely, however, a newly developed first-degree AV block progresses to a more serious AV block. Therefore all patients require careful monitoring and observation.

Management

No definitive treatment is required.

Second-Degree AV Block (Mobitz Type I or Wenckebach)

Description

Second-degree Mobitz type I AV block (Fig. 18-67) is an intermittent block that usually occurs at the level of the AV node. The conduction delay progressively increases from beat to beat until conduction to the ventricle is blocked. This dysrhythmia produces a characteristic cyclical pattern in which the PR intervals get progressively longer until a P wave occurs that is not followed by a QRS complex. By the time the SA node fires again, AV conduction has had time to recover, and the sequence starts over.

Etiology

Second-degree Mobitz type I AV block often occurs in acute myocardial infarction or acute myocarditis. Other causes include increased vagal tone, ischemia, drug toxicity (digitalis, *propranolol*, *verapamil*), and electrolyte imbalance.

Rules for Interpretation (Lead II Monitoring)

Rate: The atrial rate is that of the underlying sinus or atrial rhythm. The ventricular rate may be normal or slow but is always slightly less than that of the atria.

Rhythm: Atrial rhythm is regular; ventricular rhythm is irregular (characteristic group beating).

QRS complex: Usually less than 0.12 second (normal). Commonly, the AV conduction ratio (P waves to QRS complexes) is 5:4, 4:3, 3:2, or 2:1; the pattern may be constant or variable. A constant 2:1 block makes it difficult to distinguish between Mobitz I and Mobitz II blocks.

P waves: P waves are upright and uniform and precede the QRS complex when the QRS complex occurs.

PR interval: Progressively lengthens before the nonconducted P wave. The P-P interval is constant, but the R-R interval decreases until the dropped beat (producing grouping of QRS complexes).

Clinical Significance

Second-degree Mobitz type I AV block is usually a transient and reversible phenomenon but can progress to a more serious AV block. If

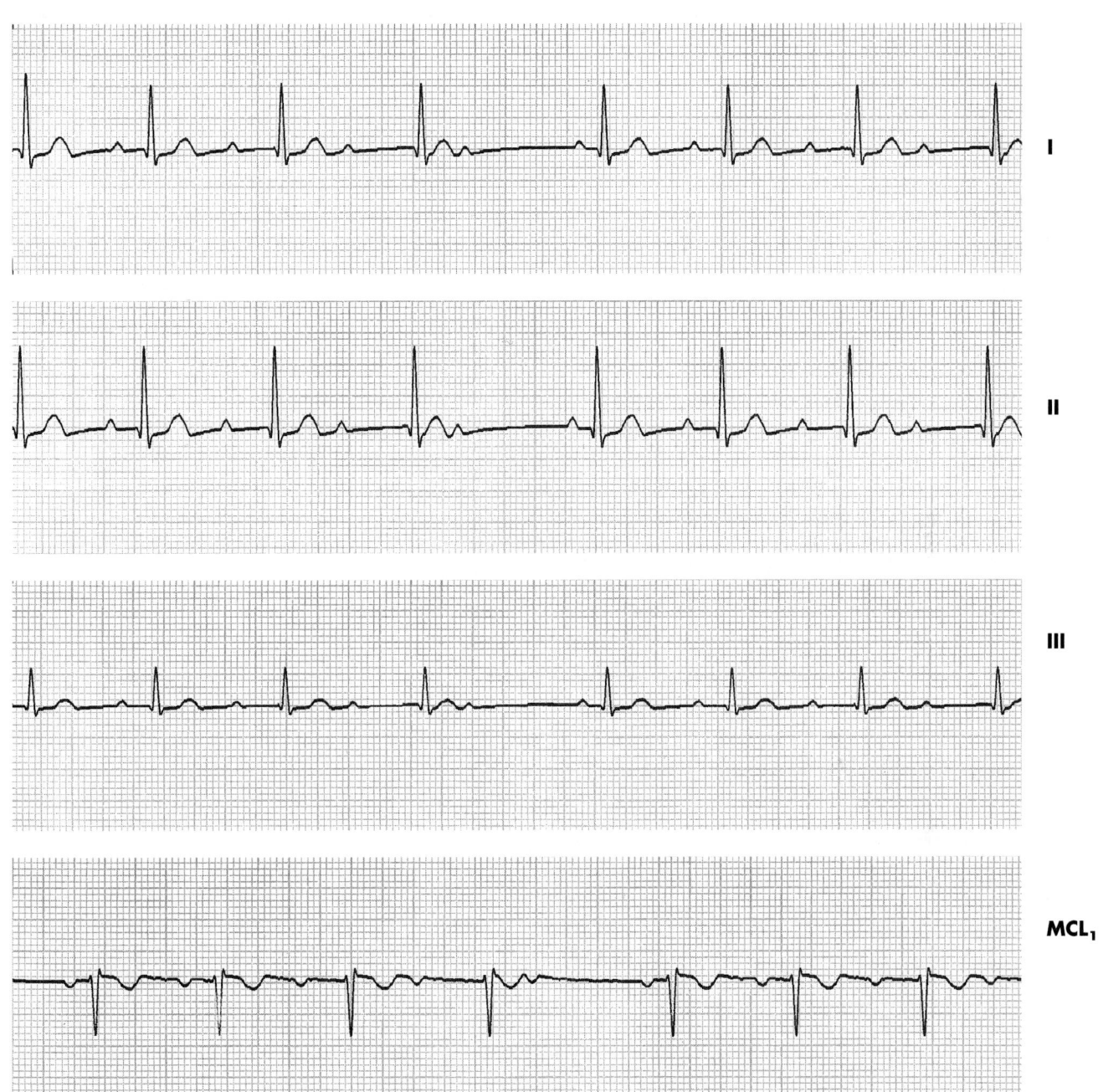

Fig. 18-67 Second-degree AV block, Mobitz type I.

dropped beats occur frequently, the patient may show signs and symptoms of decreased cardiac output.

Management

No management is required if the patient is asymptomatic. If the dropped beats compromise heart rate and cardiac output, *atropine* and TCP may be indicated (see Fig. 18-36).

Second-Degree AV Block (Mobitz Type II)

Description

Second-degree AV block Mobitz type II (Fig. 18-68) is an intermittent block that occasionally occurs when atrial impulses are not conducted to the ventricles. Unlike Mobitz type I, this block is characterized by consecutive P waves being conducted with a constant PR interval before a dropped beat.

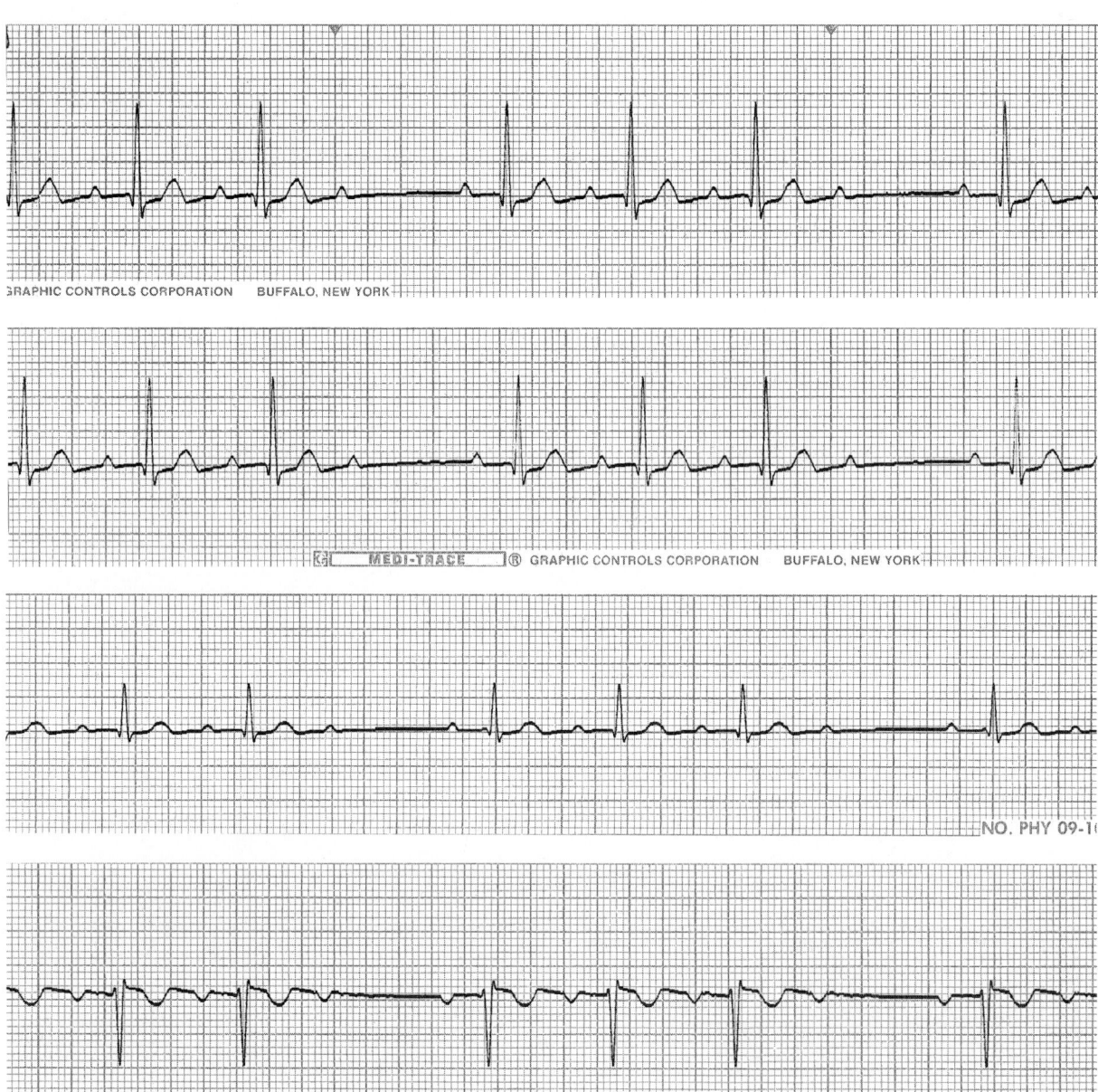

Fig. 18-68 Second-degree AV block, Mobitz type II.

This variation of AV block usually occurs in a regular sequence with the conduction ratios (P waves to QRS complexes) such as 2:1, 3:2, and 4:3 (Fig. 18-69). Second-degree AV block Mobitz type II usually occurs below the bundle of His. It represents an intermittent block of conduction of the electrical impulse through one bundle branch and a complete block in the other bundle branch.

When at least two consecutive AV impulses (atrial P waves) fail to be conducted to the ventricles, the AV block is referred to as a *high-grade AV block* (Fig. 18-70). Clinically malignant high-grade AV blocks and those with a more favorable prognosis are distinguished by the underlying atrial and ventricular rates. A 2:1 block might be considered high grade (and certainly is clinically significant) when the patient's underlying atrial rate is 60 beats per minute, but it is of much less

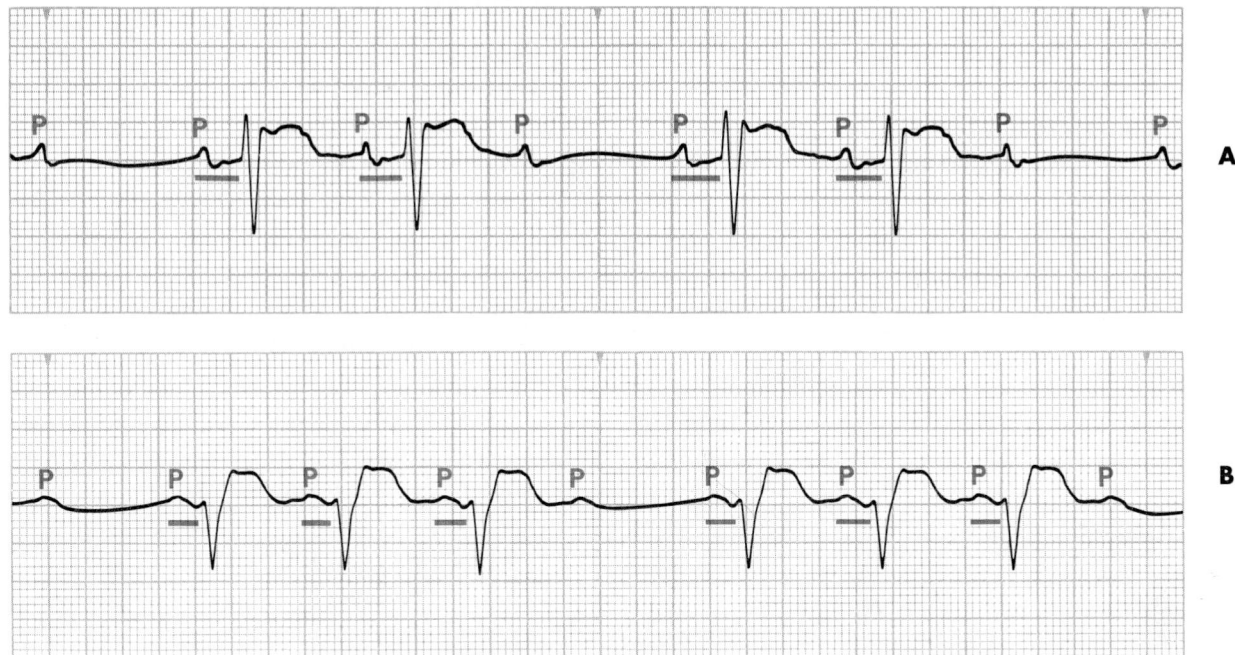

Fig. 18-69 A, 3:2 AV block. **B,** 4:3 AV block.

concern if the patient's atrial rate is 120 beats per minute.

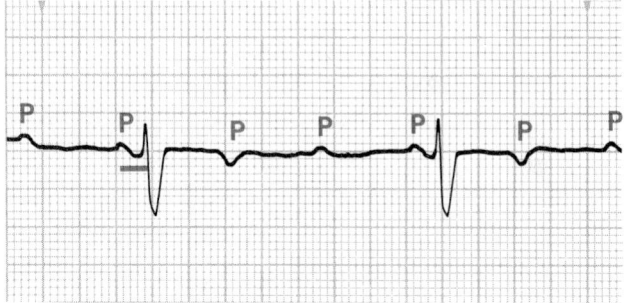

Fig. 18-70 3:1 high-grade AV block.

NOTE:
Mobitz type II, 2:1 AV block may be difficult to distinguish from Mobitz type I, 2:1 AV block. Therefore when assessing a patient who has two atrial complexes for each QRS complex, evaluate the conducted cycle (the cycle with the P wave and the QRS complex together). If the conducted cycle has a prolonged PR interval (greater than 0.20 second), a narrow QRS complex (less than 0.12 second, indicating the absence of bundle branch block), and an adequate escape rate, the patient probably has a 2:1 AV block, Mobitz type I. If the conducted QRS complex has a normal PR interval, a wide QRS complex (greater than 0.12 second, which indicates the presence of a bundle branch block), and an inadequate escape rate, a Mobitz type II, 2:1 AV block is most likely.

Etiology

Second-degree AV block Mobitz type II is usually associated with acute myocardial infarction and septal necrosis. Unlike second-degree Mobitz type I, Mobitz II does not normally result solely from increased parasympathetic tone or drug toxicity.

Rules for Interpretation (Lead II Monitoring)

Rate: Atrial rate is unaffected and is that of the underlying sinus, atrial, or junctional rhythm. The ventricular rate is usually less than that of the atria and is often bradycardic.

Rhythm: Regular or irregular, depending on whether the conduction ratio is constant or variable

QRS complex: May be abnormal (greater than 0.12 second) because of bundle branch block. The AV conduction ratio may be fixed or may vary throughout any given lead.

P waves: P waves are upright and uniform; some P waves may not be followed by QRS complexes.

PR interval: PR intervals are usually constant for conducted beats and may be greater than 0.20 second. (See Note, p. 621.)

Clinical Significance

Second-degree AV block Mobitz type II is a serious dysrhythmia usually considered malignant in the emergency setting (unlike type I AV blocks, which are usually considered benign). Slow ventricular rates may result in signs and symptoms of hypoperfusion. This dysrhythmia is likely to progress to a more severe heart block and even to ventricular asystole.

Management

Regardless of the patient's initial condition, pacemaker insertion is the definitive treatment. Prehospital care for symptomatic patients may consist of pharmacological therapy *(atropine, isoproterenol,* or *epinephrine),* and TCP (see Fig. 18-36).

> ### NOTE:
> A task force on the early treatment of patients with acute myocardial infarction consisting of members from the American Heart Association and the American College of Cardiology considered *atropine* to be class III (possibly harmful) for patients with third-degree heart block and wide complex ventricular escape beats and also for patients with Mobitz type II second-degree heart block.[4] Many of these patients cannot be effectively managed in the prehospital setting with only medication. Immediate transport is indicated.

Third-Degree Heart Block

Description

Third-degree AV block (Fig. 18-71) results from complete electrical block at or below the AV node. The dysrhythmia is said to be present when the opportunity for conduction between the atria and the ventricles is optimal but conduction does not occur (for example, when there is a slow ventricular rate of less than 45 beats per minute and numerous atrial impulses between the QRS complexes). In this condition, the SA node serves as the pacemaker for the atria, and an ectopic focus serves as a pacemaker in the ventricles. The result is that P waves and QRS complexes occur rhythmically, but the rhythms are unrelated to each other (AV dissociation).

Etiology

Common causes of third-degree AV block include increased vagal tone or septal necrosis (both of which may be associated with acute myocardial infarction), acute myocarditis, digitalis or *propranolol* toxicity, and electrolyte imbalance. The dysrhythmia may also occur in older adults from chronic degenerative changes in the conduction system (Lev's or Lenegre's disease) that are not usually associated with increased parasympathetic tone or drug toxicity.

Rules for Interpretation (Lead II Monitoring)

Rate: The atrial rate is that of the underlying sinus or atrial rhythm. The ventricular rate is typically 40 to 60 beats per minute if the escape focus is junctional and less than 40 beats per minute if the escape focus is in the ventricles.

Rhythm: The atrial and ventricular rhythms are usually regular. The rhythms are independent of each other.

QRS complex: May be less than 0.12 second if escape focus is junctional, 0.12 second or greater if escape focus is ventricular

P waves: P waves are present but have no relationship to the QRS complexes. In cases of atrial flutter or fibrillation, complete heart block is manifested by a slow, regular ventricular response.

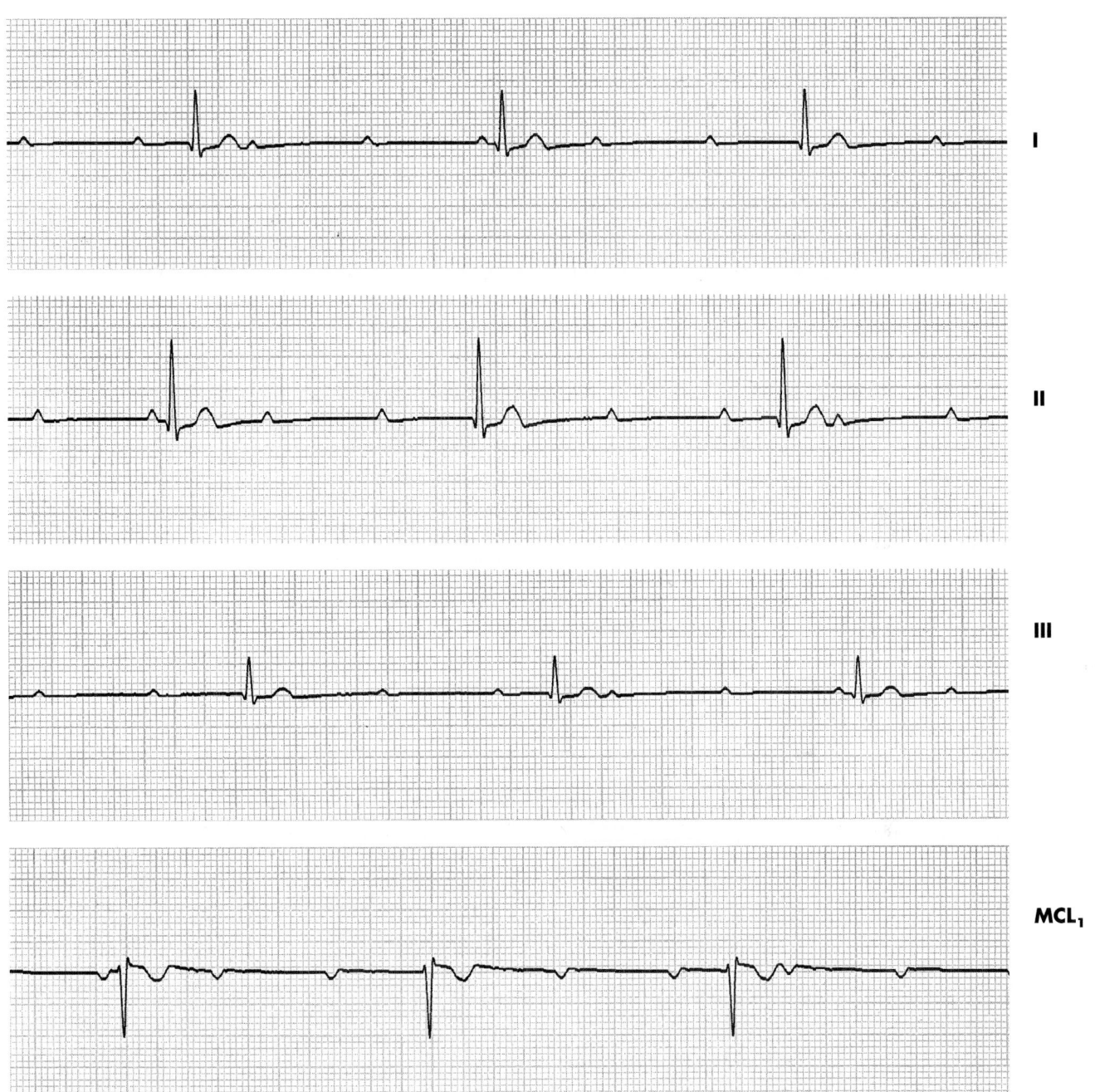

Fig. 18-71 Third-degree AV block.

PR interval: The PR interval varies with each complex because the atrial and ventricular rates are completely independent of each other. If the rates coincide for a period, the PR interval may appear constant (a phenomenon termed *parasystole*). In this situation, the paramedic should be alert for changes in the rhythm. P waves may be superimposed on QRS complexes or T waves (Fig. 18-72).

Clinical Significance

There may be signs and symptoms of severe bradycardia and decreased cardiac output because of the slow ventricular rate and asynchronous ac-

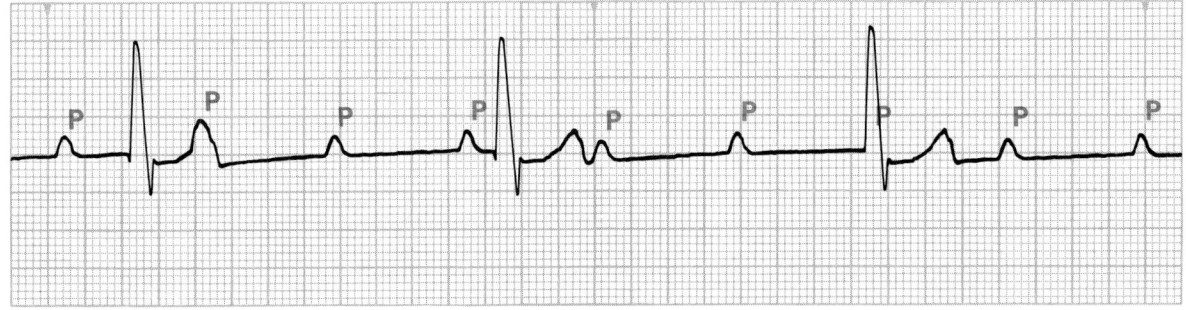

Fig. 18-72 Third-degree block demonstrating P waves superimposed on the QRS complex and T waves.

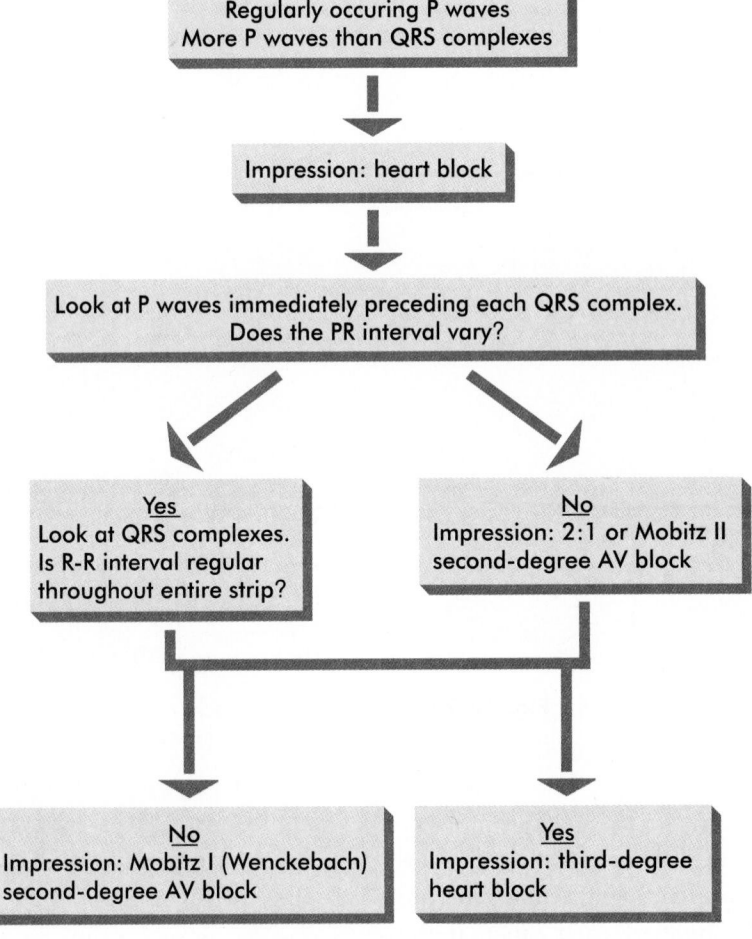

Fig. 18-73 Identifying heart blocks.

tion of the atria and ventricles. Third-degree AV block associated with wide QRS complexes is an ominous sign. The dysrhythmia is potentially lethal, and the patient may deteriorate rapidly (Fig. 18-73).

> **NOTE:**
> Complete AV block in the presence of atrial fibrillation is often caused by drug (usually digitalis) toxicity. There is almost always some AV block with atrial fibrillation or flutter, but complete AV block is recognized by a slow, regular ventricular response (usually less than 60 beats per minute). The QRS complex may be normal if the escape focus is junctional.

Management

Pacemaker insertion is the definitive treatment for symptomatic third-degree AV block and for asymptomatic third-degree block with bundle branch block. Initial prehospital care includes TCP, *dopamine* to increase the ventricular rate if needed, and possibly *atropine* to stimulate AV conduction or to increase the rate of a junctional escape rhythm if sanctioned by medical control.

> **NOTE:**
> *Atropine* is considered a class III (possibly harmful) drug for patients with third-degree heart block and wide complex ventricular escape beats. TCP is a class I intervention for all symptomatic bradycardias and should be implemented as soon as possible if the bradycardia is severe and the clinical condition is unstable (see Fig. 18-36).

● VENTRICULAR CONDUCTION DISTURBANCES

Ventricular conduction disturbances (bundle branch blocks and hemiblocks) are delays or interruptions in the transmission of electrical impulses that occur below the level of bifurcation of the bundle of His. Identifying these blocks can provide important information on a patient's being at increased risk of developing severe bradycardia and third-degree heart block (especially when combined with other forms of AV block). Common causes of bundle branch block include:

- Ischemic heart disease
- Acute heart failure
- Acute myocardial infarction
- Hyperkalemia
- Trauma
- Cardiomyopathy
- Aortic stenosis
- Infection

Bundle Branch Anatomy

To review, the bundle of His begins at the AV node and divides to form the left and right bundle branches (Fig. 18-74). The right bundle branch continues toward the apex and spreads throughout the right ventricle. The left bundle branch subdivides into the anterior and posterior fascicles and spreads throughout the left ventricle. Conduction of electrical impulses through the Purkinje fibers stimulates the ventricles to contract.

With normal conduction, the first part of the ventricle to be stimulated is the left side of the septum. The electrical impulse then traverses the septum to stimulate the other side. Shortly thereafter, the left and right ventricles are simultaneously stimulated. Because the left ventricle is normally much larger and thicker than the right ventricle, its electrical activity predominates over that of the right ventricle.

Common ECG Findings

When an electrical impulse is blocked from passing through either the right or left bundle branch, one ventricle depolarizes and contracts before the other. Because ventricular activation is no longer simultaneous, the QRS complex widens (often with a slurred or notched appearance). Therefore the hallmark of bundle branch block is a QRS complex that is 0.12 second or wider. (A widened QRS complex may also occur in Wolff-Parkinson-White syndrome.)

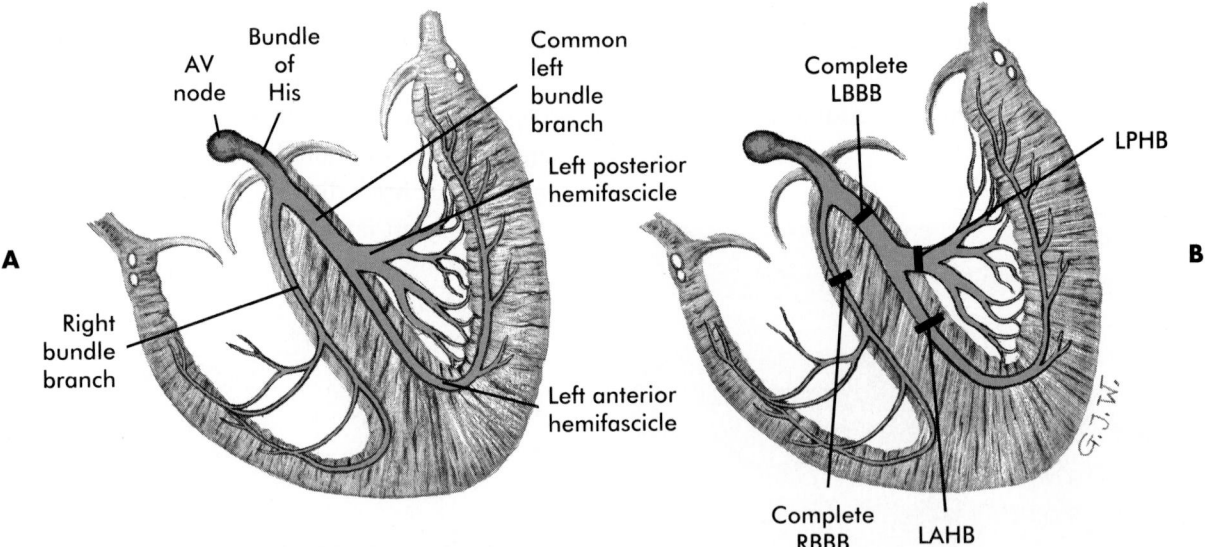

Fig. 18-74 A, Simplified illustration showing the major divisions of the ventricular conduction system. After passing through the AV node and the bundle of His, the electrical impulse is carried to the right and common left bundle branches. The latter structure divides into the left anterior and posterior hemifascicles. **B,** Possible sites of block and the conduction deficits that may be produced.

> **NOTE:**
> *Bundle branch block* and *hemiblock (fascicular block)* are terms used to describe aberrant conduction in ventricular complexes that originate above the ventricles. These patterns of aberrant conduction must be distinguished from beats of ventricular origin, which can have a similar QRS morphology.

Ventricular conduction disturbances are best identified by monitoring leads MCL_1 and MCL_6. These leads permit the easiest differentiation of the right and left bundle branch blocks. For ECG evaluation, the paramedic should ensure that the electrodes are placed properly for leads I, II, and III (on the arms and legs, not on the chest and abdomen). Lead MCL_1 should be run last and monitored during patient transport.[5]

Normal Conduction

In normal ventricular stimulation, the electrical impulse occurs first in the septum and then travels from the left endocardium through to the right endocardium of the septum (Fig. 18-75). This generates a small R wave in MCL_1. The remaining impulses are primarily conducted away from the MCL_1 electrode, yielding a negative deflection. During normal conduction therefore MCL_1 is predominantly negative, and the QRS complex is usually approximately 0.06 second wide.

Right Bundle Branch Block

In right bundle branch block, the left bundle branch performs normally, thus activating the left side before the right (Fig. 18-76). Initial stimulation of the heart remains unchanged. The impulses travel from the left to the right endocardium, generating a small R wave in MCL_1.

When the left ventricle is activated initially, the impulse travels away from the MCL_1 electrode, yielding a negative deflection (S wave). The electrical impulse then travels across the interventricular septum and activates the right ventricle. Since the impulse is coming back toward the MCL_1 electrode, a large positive deflection (R wave) occurs, resulting in the RSR-prime pattern seen in MCL_1 in patients with right bundle branch block. The QRS (or in this case, RSR) complex is at least 0.12 second.

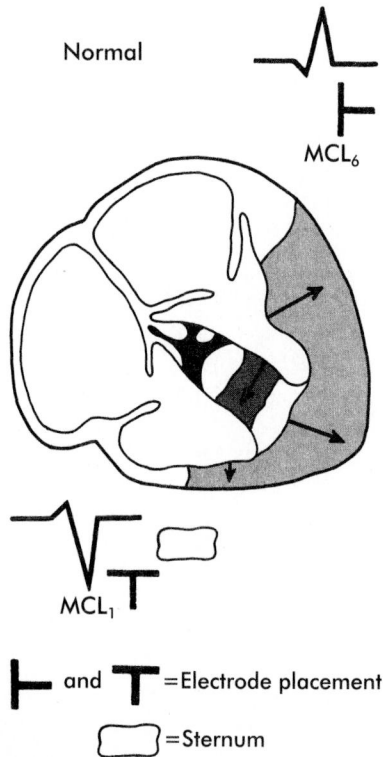

Fig. 18-75 Normal ventricular activation.

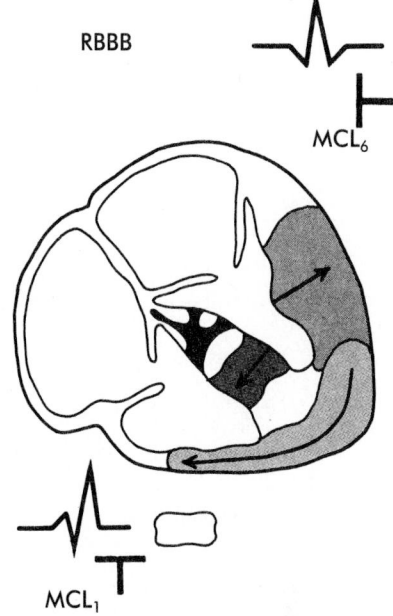

Fig. 18-76 Right bundle branch block.

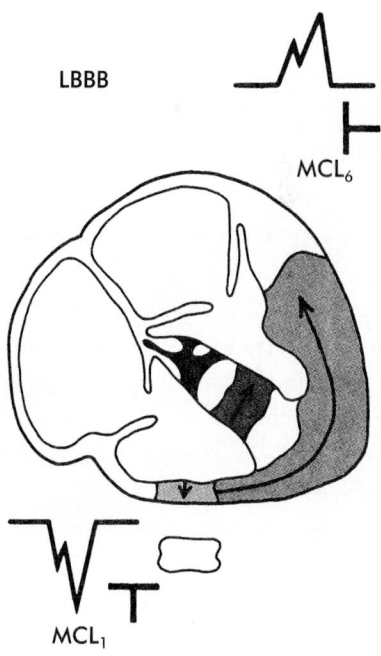

Fig. 18-77 Left bundle branch block.

Left Bundle Branch Block

In left bundle branch block, the fibers that usually fire the interventricular septum are blocked. This alters normal septal activation and sends it in the opposite direction (Fig. 18-77). This yields an initial Q wave in MCL$_1$ instead of the normal small R wave. The right ventricle is then activated, producing a positive deflection (R wave) in MCL$_1$; this impulse travels across the interventricular septum to the left ventricle. Since the impulse is leading away from MCL$_1$, it shows a deep, wide S wave. As with right bundle branch block, the activation takes at least 0.12 second.

Anterior Hemiblock

Anterior hemiblocks (anterior hemifascicle blocks) occur more frequently than posterior hemiblocks (posterior hemifascicle blocks). The anterior fascicle of the left bundle branch is a longer and thinner structure, and its blood supply comes primarily from the anterior descending coronary artery. Anterior hemiblock is characterized by left axis deviation (a QRS complex upright in lead I but negative in leads aV$_F$ and II) in a patient who has a supraventricular rhythm (Fig. 18-78). Other ECG findings associated with an anterior hemiblock include: a normal QRS complex (less than 0.12 second) or a right bundle branch

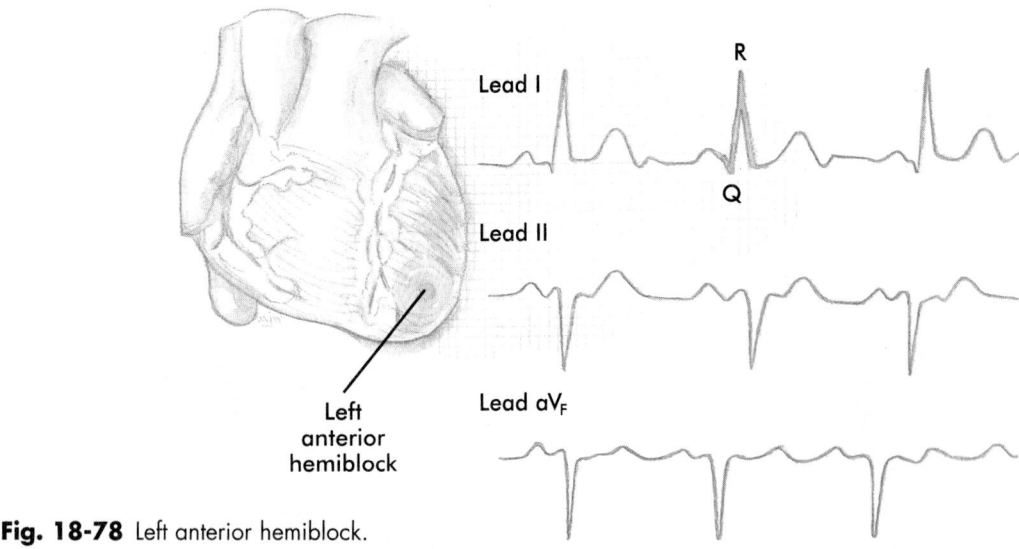

Fig. 18-78 Left anterior hemiblock.

Determining Right or Left Bundle Branch Block

When lead MCL₁ is monitored, the bundle branch blocked may be determined by the following procedure (Fig. 18-79):

1. Find a QRS complex that is at least 0.12 second wide.
2. Draw a line backward from the J point (the point at which the QRS complex ends and the ST segment begins) into the QRS complex.
3. Fill in the triangle that is created by this line and the last portion of the QRS complex.
4. If the triangle points up, it is a right bundle branch block.
5. If the triangle points down, it is a left bundle branch block.

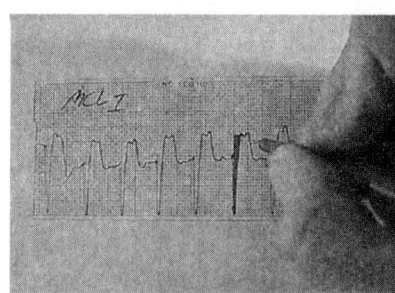

Fig. 18-79 To distinguish left from right bundle branch blocks, find the J point of the QRS complex, draw a line backward into the QRS complex, and fill in the triangle created by this line and the last portion of the QRS complex. The direction the triangle points distinguishes the two types of blocks.

block, a small Q wave followed by a tall R wave in lead I, and a small R wave followed by a deep S wave in lead III.

In a patient who has an anterior hemiblock with a right bundle branch block, impulses can only be conducted through the ventricles by way of the posterior fascicle of the left bundle branch. These patients are at high risk of developing complete heart block.

Posterior Hemiblock

The posterior fascicle of the left bundle branch is more difficult to block than the anterior fascicle, and consequently, posterior hemiblock occurs less frequently. Posterior hemiblock is identified by right axis deviation (a QRS complex negative in lead I and upright in lead aV_F), with a normal QRS complex or a right bundle branch block (Fig. 18-80). A definitive diagnosis for posterior hemiblock necessitates excluding right ventricular hypertrophy, which is difficult to do in the prehospital setting.

For practical purposes, posterior hemiblock can be assumed in patients with right axis deviation

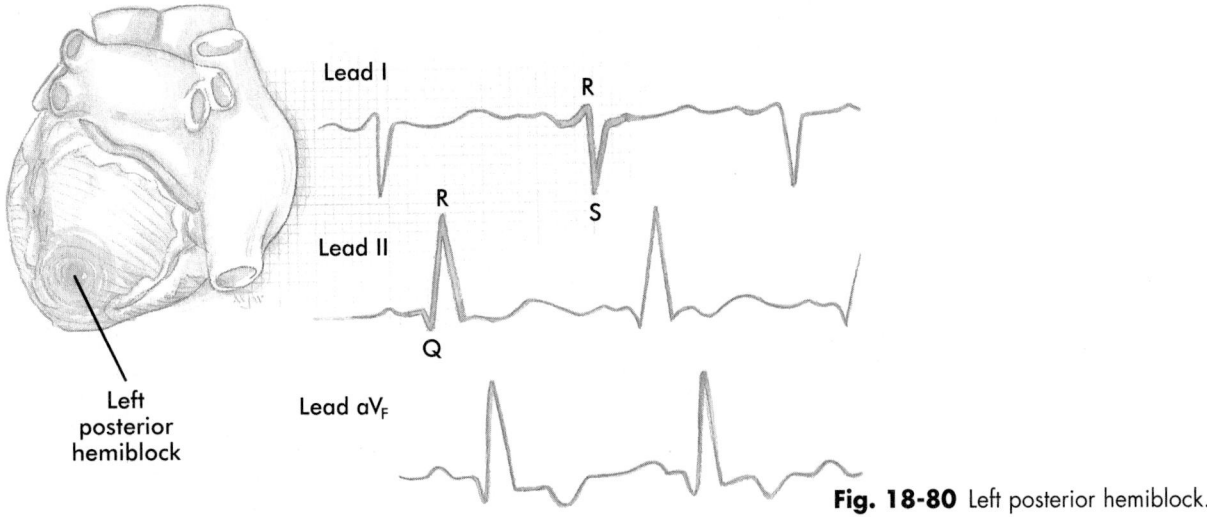

Fig. 18-80 Left posterior hemiblock.

Labels in figure: Lead I, Lead II, Lead aV_F, R, S, Q, R, Left posterior hemiblock.

and a QRS complex of normal width or with a right bundle branch block. Other ECG findings that indicate the presence of a posterior hemiblock include a small R wave followed by a deep S wave in lead I and a small Q wave followed by a tall R wave in lead III.

Management of Bundle Branch Blocks and Hemiblocks

Some emergency medications administered to cardiac patients (for example, *procainamide*, digoxin [Lanoxin], and morphine) can impede electrical impulse conduction through the AV node. Thus to safely administer these medications, the paramedic must ensure that the patient is not at high risk of developing complete heart block. Those at such risk include:

- Any patient with Mobitz type II AV block or high-grade AV block
- Any patient with evidence of disease in both bundle branches
- Any patient with two or more blocks of any kind (for example, prolonged PR interval and anterior hemiblock, right bundle branch block and anterior hemiblock, Mobitz type I AV block [Wenckebach] and left bundle branch block)

Prehospital care for these patients should include immediate transport (they will probably need pacemaker insertion), pharmacological ther-

apy to increase rate if needed, constant ECG monitoring, and anticipation of the need for external pacing. Emergent pacing has been recommended for the following four indications[1]:

1. Hemodynamically compromising bradycardias
2. Bradycardias with malignant escape rhythms unresponsive to pharmacological therapy
3. Overdrive pacing of refractory supraventricular or ventricular tachycardia unresponsive to pharmacological therapy or cardioversion
4. Bradyasystolic cardiac arrest (in rare situations)

Standby pacing has been recommended for the following indications[1]:

- Stable bradycardias
- Prophylactic pacing in acute myocardial infarction (for example, Mobitz II second-degree block and third-degree heart block)

● PULSELESS ELECTRICAL ACTIVITY

The term *pulseless electrical activity (PEA)* (Fig. 18-81) is defined as the absence of a detectable pulse and the presence of some type of electrical activity other than ventricular tachycardia or ventricular fibrillation. PEA incorporates electromechanical dissociation and a group of rhythms that

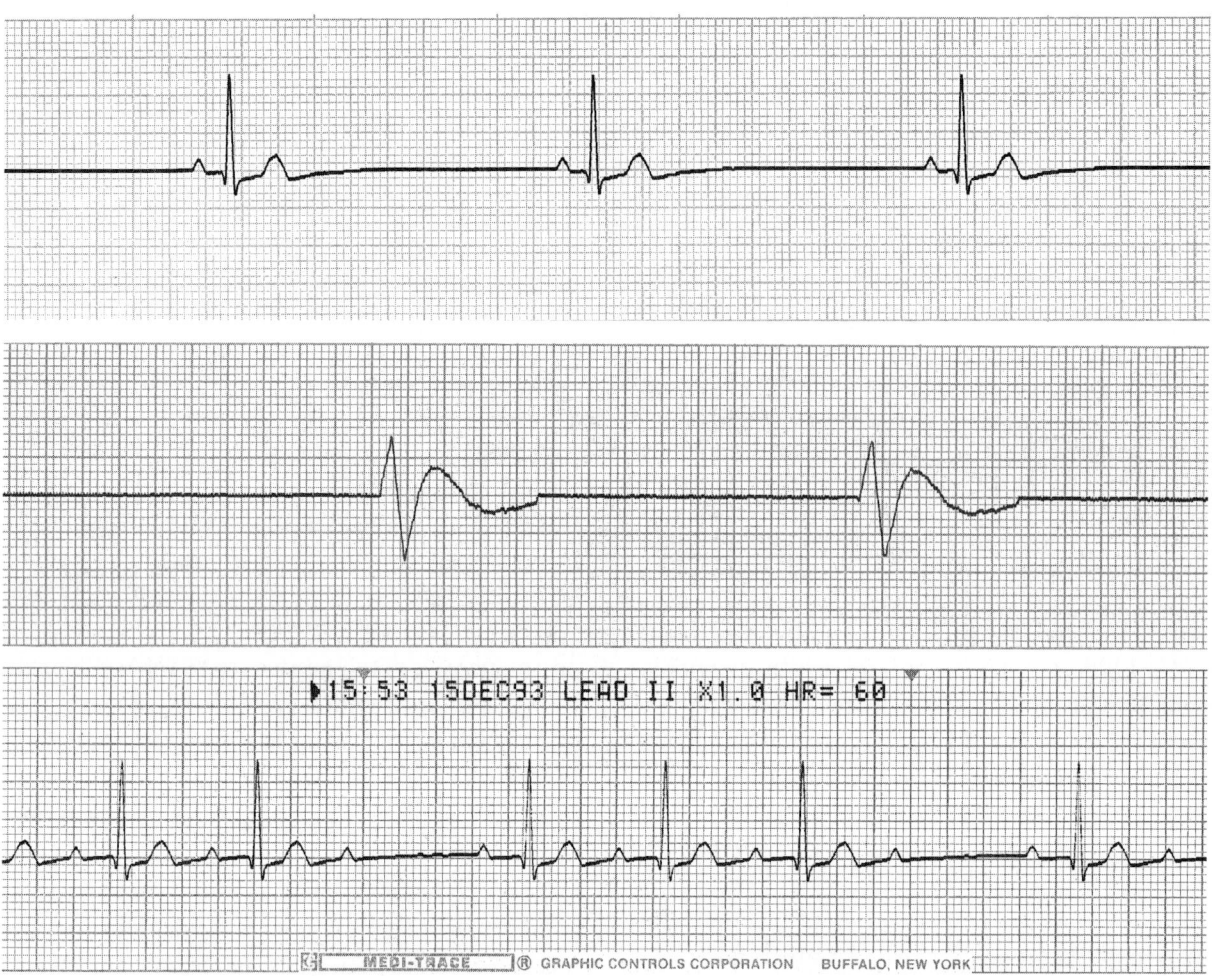

Fig. 18-81 Various PEA rhythms as seen in lead II.

includes pseudo–electromechanical dissociation (a rhythm that produces a pulse that can only be obtained with a Doppler), idioventricular rhythms, ventricular escape rhythms, postdefibrillation idioventricular rhythms, and bradyasystolic rhythms.[1] The prognosis for PEA is invariably poor unless an underlying cause can be identified and corrected. Therefore the highest priority of care is to maintain circulation for the patient with basic and advanced life support techniques while searching for a correctable etiology.

Correctable causes of PEA are hypovolemia, cardiac tamponade, tension pneumothorax, hypoxemia, acidosis, hyperkalemia, hypothermia, and overdoses of, for example, tricyclic antidepressants, beta blockers, and digitalis. Other less

correctable causes include massive myocardial damage from infarction, prolonged ischemia during resuscitation, and massive pulmonary embolism. Patients in profound shock of any type (including anaphylactic, septic, neurogenic, and hypovolemic) may present with PEA. If acute hypovolemia is present (secondary to hemorrhage), fluid resuscitation with volume expanders should be initiated. Tension pneumothorax should be treated with needle decompression; hypoxemia should be treated by improving oxygenation and ventilation. Acidosis should be treated by ensuring adequate CPR and hyperventilation; if preexisting acidosis or hyperkalemia is suspected, the use of **bicarbonate** may be indicated. **Calcium** is a specific therapy for hyperkalemia and calcium

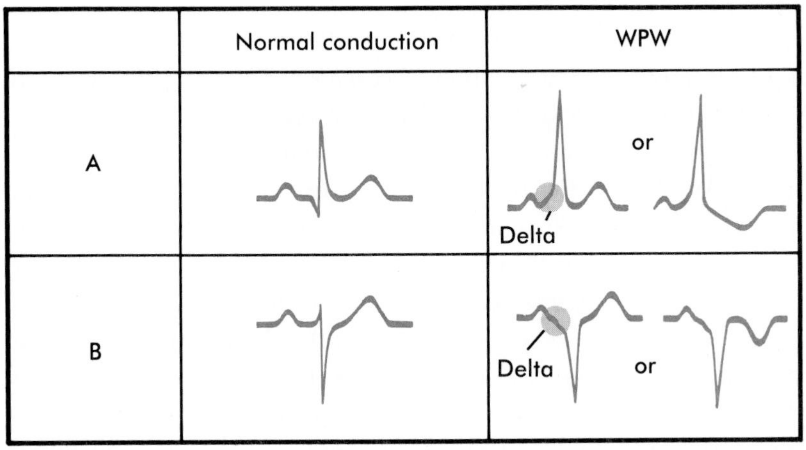

	Normal conduction	WPW
A		or
B		or

Fig. 18-82 The characteristic findings in WPW syndrome (short PR interval, QRS widening, and delta wave) compared with normal conduction. **A,** The usual appearance of WPW syndrome in leads where the QRS complex is predominantly upright. **B,** The appearance of WPW syndrome; the QRS complex is predominantly negative.

channel blocker toxicity, both of which can produce PEA. Besides calcium channel blockers, other drugs when taken in toxic amounts can produce broad-complex PEA. These overdoses can be treated with specific therapy, which may be effective in reestablishing a perfusing rhythm (see Fig. 18-51).

● PREEXCITATION SYNDROMES

Preexcitation syndrome (anomalous or accelerated AV conduction) is a clinical condition associated with abnormal conduction pathways between the atria and ventricles that bypass the AV node and bundle of His and allow the electrical impulses to initiate depolarization of the ventricles earlier than usual. This premature ventricular activation may occur through one of several accessory pathways. The most common preexcitation syndrome is Wolff-Parkinson-White (WPW) syndrome, which occurs in 3 out of every 1000 people.

Wolff-Parkinson-White Syndrome

Description
WPW syndrome occurs when the ventricular muscle is activated early by an accessory pathway known as the *bundle of Kent* or the *Kent fibers.* These fibers connect the atrial muscle to the ventricular muscle, bypassing the AV node. Kent fibers can be situated at any point where the atria

and the ventricles meet. They are usually found anteriorly connecting the right atrium and the right ventricle or posteriorly connecting the left atrium and the left ventricle. WPW syndrome is considered to be of minor clinical significance unless a tachycardia is present, in which case it can become life threatening.

Etiology
WPW syndrome may occur in young, healthy individuals (predominantly men) without apparent cause. Approximately 30% of these patients have associated cardiovascular disorders such as hypertension or coronary artery disease. The syndrome may occur in multiple members of a family and may be present in successive generations.

Rules for Interpretation (Lead II Monitoring)
Rate: Normal unless associated with rapid supraventricular tachycardia

Rhythm: Regular

QRS complex: Widened, often greater than 0.12 second; abnormal slurring or notching of the onset of the QRS complex (delta wave) indicates anomalous spread of the impulse and is a diagnostic finding. (Not all leads show the delta wave.)

NOTE:
QRS widening may simulate right or left bundle branch block.

P waves: Normal

PR interval: Usually less than 0.12 second, since the normal delay at the AV node does not occur

The three characteristic ECG findings in WPW (Fig. 18-82) are a short PR interval, a delta wave, and QRS widening.

Clinical Significance

Patients with WPW syndrome are highly susceptible to PVSTs. This is because the accessory pathway provides a ready-made reentry circuit that allows continued transmission of the impulse from the atria to the ventricles. The supraventricular tachycardia or atrial flutter and fibrillation that occur in patients with preexcitation syndrome may resemble ventricular tachycardia. True ventricular tachycardia, however, is not a part of WPW syndrome (although the two can occur in the same patient, particularly with underlying organic heart disease). Patients with WPW syndrome may have attacks of paroxysmal tachydysrhythmias for many years, but these attacks are not always benign. The AV node may be bypassed, and conduction rates can greatly exceed those in patients whose AV node is part of the reentry circuit. This leads to very rapid tachycardias, which can precipitate congestive heart failure and even death from ventricular fibrillation.

Management

It is important to recognize WPW syndrome and differentiate it from ventricular tachycardia and uncomplicated supraventricular tachycardia. Many emergency drugs used to treat other reentry tachycardias are contraindicated in WPW syndrome because they can paradoxically facilitate conduction over the accessory pathway. Treatment must be based on the patient's clinical presentation. If the patient's heart rate is normal, no emergency care is required. If the patient presents with a symptomatic rapid tachycardia, emergency intervention is indicated to restore a normal rhythm by blocking conduction through the accessory pathways from the atria to the ventricles.

Prehospital care may include pharmacological therapy for specific dysrhythmias, vagal maneu-

vers for PSVT, or cardioversion for severe clinical deterioration. *Verapamil* is contraindicated in wide QRS tachycardia because the drug may precipitate very rapid atrial-to-ventricular conduction down the accessory pathway (greater than 280 beats per minute) and may lead to ventricular fibrillation and sudden death. Therefore in patients with wide QRS tachycardia, the treatment of choice depends on the clinical impression and severity of symptoms. *Lidocaine* is the first drug of choice for presumed ventricular tachycardia, and *adenosine* and *procainamide* are the initial choices for uncertain or presumed supraventricular tachycardia. Cardioversion should be performed without delay in patients with rapid ventricular rates (greater than 150 beats per minute) who are unstable (see Fig. 18-38.)

Section Six
Assessment of the Cardiac Patient

● ASSESSMENT

A focused evaluation of any patient should identify a chief complaint, cover the history of the event and significant past medical history, and include a physical examination. These elements are important in determining the cause of the emergency event, directing initial patient care, and anticipating potential problems during patient transport to a medical facility. The following discussion of patient assessment serves as a framework for approaching a patient with a cardiovascular problem.

Chief Complaint

Cardiovascular disease may present with a variety of symptoms. It is the paramedic's responsibility to obtain an appropriate history of each symptom and apply the information to form a diagnostic impression in any patient with a possible coronary event. Common chief complaints include chest pain or discomfort, including shoulder, arm, neck, or jaw pain or discomfort; dyspnea; syncope; and abnormal heart beat or palpitations.

Chest Pain or Discomfort

Chest pain or discomfort is the most common chief complaint of patients with myocardial infarction. However, many causes of chest pain are unrelated to cardiac disease (for example, pulmonary embolus, pleurisy, and reflux esophagitis). Therefore a history of chest pain is important. As described in Chapter 11, the PQRST method (or a similar method) should be used to obtain the following information when possible:

P: What makes the pain better? What makes the pain worse? (for example, relief with rest or nitroglycerin, worsening with exercise or eating fried foods)

Q: Quality? Is the pain sharp or tearing, burning, heavy, or squeezing?

R: Region? Where does it hurt? (Try to localize it.) Does it radiate? (Where to?)

S: Severity? How badly does it hurt? Have you ever had pain like this before?

T: Time? When did the pain start? How long have you had it? When was the first time you experienced this pain?

Dyspnea

Dyspnea is often associated with myocardial infarction and is a primary symptom of pulmonary congestion caused by heart failure. Other common causes of dyspnea that may be unrelated to heart disease include chronic obstructive pulmonary disease, respiratory infection, pulmonary embolus, and asthma. Historical factors important in differentiating breathing difficulties include the following:

- Duration and circumstances of onset of dyspnea
- Anything that aggravates or relieves the dyspnea, including medications
- Previous episodes
- Associated symptoms
- Prior cardiac problems

Syncope

Syncope is caused by a sudden decrease in cerebral perfusion. Cardiac causes of syncope result from events that normally decrease cardiac out-

put. The most common cardiac disorders associated with syncope are dysrhythmias. Other causes of syncope in the medical patient include myocardial infarction, drug or alcohol intoxication, aortic stenosis, pulmonary embolism, and hypoglycemia. In the older patient, syncope may be the only symptom of a cardiac problem. Young, otherwise healthy people may have a syncopal episode resulting from increased vagal tone (vasovagal syncope) that produces hypotension and bradycardia. The history of a syncopal event should include:

- Presyncope aura (nausea, weakness, lightheadedness)
- Circumstances of occurrence (for example, patient's position before the event, severe pain, emotional stress)
- Duration of syncopal episode
- Symptoms before syncopal episode (palpitation, seizure, incontinence)
- Other associated symptoms
- Previous episodes of syncope

Abnormal Heart Beat and Palpitations

Many patients are aware of their own heartbeat, particularly if it is irregular ("skipping beats") or rapid ("fluttering"). Palpitations are sometimes a normal occurrence, but they should alert the paramedic to the possibility of a serious dysrhythmia. Important information to obtain from these patients includes:

- Pulse rate (if obtained)
- Regular versus irregular rhythm (if obtained)
- Circumstances of occurrence
- Duration
- Associated symptoms (chest pain, diaphoresis, syncope, confusion, dyspnea)
- Previous episodes, frequency
- Medication (drug stimulant or alcohol use)

Significant Past Medical History

Past medical history is an important aspect of any patient assessment. If possible, the paramedic should determine the following five points:

1. Is the patient taking prescription medications, particularly cardiac medications? Common medications that should alert the paramedic to a possible coronary event include:

a. *Nitroglycerin*
b. *Propranolol* (or other beta blockers)
c. Calcium channel blockers
d. Digitalis
e. Diuretics
f. Antihypertensives
g. Other antidysrhythmics

2. Is the patient being treated for any serious illness?
3. Has the patient ever had any of the following?
   a. Myocardial infarction or episodes of angina pectoris
   b. Coronary artery bypass procedure or angioplasty
   c. Heart failure
   d. Hypertension
   e. Diabetes mellitus
   f. Chronic lung disease
4. Does the patient have any allergies?
5. Are there any other associated risk factors for a cardiac event?
   a. Patient age
   b. Smoking
   c. Diabetes mellitus
   d. Family history
   e. Obesity
   f. Hypercholesterolemia (increased serum cholesterol level)
   g. Routine medications that may cause cardiac symptoms
   h. Cardiac effects from illicit drug use (for example, cocaine)

Physical Examination

The "classical presentation" of myocardial infarction is pain or discomfort beneath the sternum (often described as *crushing, pressure, squeezing,* or *burning*) that lasts more than 30 minutes. Associated symptoms may include apprehension, diaphoresis, dyspnea, nausea and vomiting, and a sense of impending doom (for example, the patient feels that he or she is going to die). Unfortunately, at times the presentation is atypical. The paramedic's skill in gathering a pertinent medical history and performing a thorough physical ex-

amination directs the focus of patient care and may greatly influence patient outcome. Patients with myocardial ischemia may deny chest "pain" and need to be questioned specifically about a tightness or squeezing sensation in the chest.

When caring for a patient with chest pain caused by a coronary event, the paramedic should remember that the patient is experiencing a devastating episode with life-threatening consequences. Throughout the patient encounter (physical examination, treatment, and patient transport), every effort should be made to calm and reassure the patient and to decrease his or her anxiety.

Primary Survey

As with any patient examination, attention must first be paid to the primary survey. In most medical emergencies involving conscious patients, the elements of the primary survey (airway, breathing, and circulation) can be assessed in the initial paramedic-patient encounter. Vital sign assessment and a quick neurological examination should evaluate the following:

- Pulse (rate, regularity)
- Level of consciousness (Alterations in the patient's level of consciousness may indicate decreased cerebral perfusion caused by poor cardiac output. If possible, determine the normal level of function for this patient.)
- Respirations
- Blood pressure

Secondary Assessment

The secondary survey of the cardiac patient should be systematic and complete, using a "look-listen-feel" approach.

Look
- Skin color and capillary refill
  ○ Indications of adequate hemoglobin level (amount)
  ○ Indications of adequate hemoglobin oxygenation
  ○ Indications of cardiac function (peripheral perfusion)
- Jugular vein distention (JVD)

- ° An increase in central venous pressure can produce engorgement of internal jugular veins. JVD should be evaluated with the patient's head elevated at 45 degrees.
  - ° JVD may be difficult to assess in obese patients
- Peripheral and presacral edema
  - ° Edema may be caused by chronic back-pressure in systemic venous circulation.
  - ° Edema is most obvious in dependent areas (ankles and sacral region in bedridden patients).
  - ° Edema may be mild or *nonpitting,* with minimal or no depression of tissue after removal of finger pressure, or pitting, when depression of tissue remains after removal of finger pressure.
- Additional indicators of cardiac disease
  - ° *Nitroglycerin* patch
  - ° Midsternal scar from coronary surgery
  - ° Implanted pacemaker or automatic implantable cardioverter defibrillator
  - ° Medical alert information

Listen
- Lung sounds
  - ° Assess for equality.
  - ° Assess for adventitious sounds that may indicate pulmonary congestion or edema.
- Heart sounds
- Carotid artery bruit: assessed if contemplating carotid sinus massage

Feel
- Peripheral or presacral edema
- Pulse
  - ° Rate
  - ° Regularity
  - ° Equality
  - ° Pulse deficit
- Skin
  - ° Diaphoretic pale skin is an indicator of peripheral vasoconstriction and sympathetic stimulation.
  - ° Cyanosis is an indicator of hemoglobin desaturation.
  - ° Fever is an indicator of infection.

Heart Sounds

Heart sounds can typically be auscultated with a stethoscope during ventricular systole and diastole. When the ventricles contract, both AV valves close nearly simultaneously. This closure causes a vibration of the valves and surrounding fluid and results in a low-pitched sound (often described as a "lubb" sound). Closing of the aortic and pulmonary semilunar valves at the end of ventricular systole produces a higher-pitched sound (described as "dubb"). These normal heart sounds are referred to as S_1 and S_2, respectively.

Rarely, a third heart sound can be heard near the end of the first third of diastole (S_3). The third heart sound (caused by turbulent flow of blood into the ventricles) may be normal but may be an indicator of congestive heart failure. A fourth heart sound (S_4) may be heard during the end of diastole. It is thought to result from turbulence and chamber stretching from the atrial contraction during this part of the cardiac cycle and is often a sign of congestive heart failure in adults.

NOTE: Both the S_3 and S_4 contribute to "gallop" rhythms, which are useful clinical indicators of congestive heart failure. Heart sounds are difficult to distinguish in the field. The evaluation of heart sounds should never delay emergency care or transportation; they do not alter prehospital patient management.

S_1: First heart sound occurs with closure of AV valves during ventricular systole.

S_2: Second heart sound occurs with closure of aortic and pulmonic valves and signifies the beginning of ventricular diastole.

S_3: Extra heart sound is heard after S_2 and is compatible with heart failure but not always present.

S_4: Extra heart sound is heard in late diastole (just before S_1); it is associated with atrial contractions and often heard in patients with congestive heart failure.

● PATHOPHYSIOLOGY AND MANAGEMENT OF CARDIOVASCULAR DISEASE

Many true medical emergencies are cardiovascular in nature; they often result from atherosclerosis of the coronary arteries or peripheral arteries. The specific medical conditions in this section are:

- Angina pectoris
- Myocardial infarction
- Left ventricular failure and pulmonary edema
- Right ventricular failure
- Cardiogenic shock
- Thoracic and abdominal aortic aneurysm
- Acute arterial occlusion
- Noncritical peripheral vascular conditions
- Hypertension

Pathophysiology of Atherosclerosis

Atherosclerosis is a disease process characterized by progressive narrowing of the lumen of medium and large arteries (for example, the aorta and its branches, cerebral arteries, coronary arteries). The process is thought to result in the development of thick, hard atherosclerotic plaques referred to as *atheromas* or *atheromatous lesions*. These lesions are most commonly found in areas of turbulent blood flow such as vessel bifurcations or in vessels with decreased lumen diameter.

Several theories have been proposed to explain the atherosclerotic process (lipogenic, thrombogenic, and others). It is currently believed that the disease process is a result of the endothelial cells' response to chronic mechanical or chemical injury.[6] This response includes platelet adhesion and aggregation (secondary to the release of certain chemical mediators) and proliferation and migration of smooth muscle cells from the media (where they are normally found) into the intima, forming the atheroma. The injured cell secretes a growth factor for smooth muscle cells and promotes attachment of monocytes to its surface. All of these factors can lead to development of atherosclerosis. The role of cholesterol in atherosclerosis is not completely known. Hypercholesterolemia may act

as a chronic chemical injury to the endothelium, and it also leads to increased incorporation of cholesterol into the atheromatous plaque.

According to the response-to-injury theory, the lesions begin to form within the intimal layer of the artery but extend into the media as the plaque enlarges. Over time, the atheromas become fibrotic and calcified, partially or totally obstructing the involved arteries. In most cases, some collateral circulation develops to compensate for the narrowed vessels.

Major Risk Factors

Atherosclerosis appears to be part of the aging process, occurring to some extent in all middle-aged and older people and in some young people. The condition seems to have a heritable component and is usually seen at a younger age in men than in women. Some risk factors, such as age, family history, and predisposing illness (diabetes mellitus), cannot be altered. Risk factors that can be reduced or eliminated include cigarette smoking, obesity, hypertension, and hypercholesterolemia. Some research has shown that plaque formation is not only preventable but reversible.[7]

Effects

Atherosclerosis has two major effects on blood vessels: (1) the disease disrupts the intimal surface, causing a loss of vessel elasticity and an increase in thrombogenesis, and (2) the atheroma reduces the diameter of the vessel lumen and thus decreases the blood supply to tissues. Both effects result in an insufficient supply of nutrients to the tissue, particularly under conditions of increased demand.

The severity of this insufficiency is related to the extent of narrowing (stenosis) in the blocked arterial segment, the time interval during which the occlusion develops, and the patient's inherent ability to develop collateral circulation around the obstruction. For example, a patient who gradually develops an atherosclerotic occlusion in a distal artery of a lower extremity may compensate well for the vascular insufficiency through collateral circulation. The patient may experience only mild, intermittent pain during periods of exercise. In contrast, sudden-onset occlusion in a coronary artery (secondary to an acute thrombus) almost always results in ischemia, injury, and necrosis to the area of the myocardium supplied by the affected artery.

Angina Pectoris

Angina pectoris is a symptom of myocardial ischemia; the term literally means "choking pain in the chest." It is caused by an imbalance between myocardial oxygen supply and demand. The result is an accumulation of lactic acid and carbon dioxide in ischemic tissues of the myocardium. These metabolites activate nerve endings that produce anginal pain. The most common cause of angina pectoris is atherosclerotic disease of the coronary arteries. A temporary occlusion caused by a spasm of a coronary artery with or without atherosclerosis (Prinzmetal's angina) can also cause angina pectoris. Precipitating events for development of angina, particularly in patients with atherosclerosis, include emotional stress and any activity that increases myocardial oxygen demand. Myocardial ischemia may, in turn, predispose the patient to dysrhythmias.

Angina pectoris is generally classified as *stable* or *unstable*. Stable angina is usually precipitated by physical exertion or emotional stress. The pain typically lasts 1 to 5 minutes but may last as long as 15 minutes and is relieved by rest, *nitroglycerin,* or *oxygen.* Stable angina "attacks" are usually similar in nature and are always relieved by the same mode of therapy.

Unstable angina (preinfarction angina) denotes an anginal pattern that has changed in its ease of onset, frequency, intensity, duration, or quality. It may occur during periods of light exercise or at rest. The pain usually lasts 10 minutes or more and is less promptly relieved with cessation of activity or *nitroglycerin* than the patient's stable anginal pattern. Unstable angina mimics acute myocardial infarction, and the two are sometimes difficult to differentiate in the prehospital setting. This phase of angina indicates severe atherosclerotic disease. These patients are at increased risk of acute myocardial infarction and sudden death.

The pain of angina is usually described by the patient as a pressure, squeezing, heaviness, or tightness in the chest. Although 30% of angina patients feel pain only in the chest, others describe the pain as radiating to the shoulders, arms, neck, and jaw and through to the back. Associated signs and symptoms include anxiety, shortness of breath, nausea or vomiting, and diaphoresis. The patient history often reveals previous angina attacks. Many times, the patient will have taken *nitroglycerin* before EMS arrival. If so, the paramedic should determine the age of the *nitroglycerin* prescription (*nitroglycerin* is unstable and quickly looses its strength), the amount of *nitroglycerin* taken, and its effect. If the pain is not relieved by rest and medication, a myocardial infarction should be suspected.

Management

All patients with chest pain should be treated as though an acute myocardial infarction is evolving. The goal of treatment is to increase the coronary blood supply, decrease the myocardial oxygen demand, or both. Management guidelines include the following:

1. Place patient at rest physically and emotionally.
2. Administer *oxygen.*
3. Initiate intravenous therapy for any drugs that may be needed.
4. If pain is present on EMS arrival, use pharmacological therapy, which may include *nitroglycerin* or, less commonly, *morphine.* Occasionally, calcium channel blockers are used, but these have not been shown to have a beneficial effect on mortality.
5. Monitor the ECG for dysrhythmias.
6. Transport patient for physician evaluation.

Myocardial Infarction

Acute myocardial infarction occurs when there is a sudden and total cessation of blood flowing through an affected coronary artery to an area of heart muscle. This results in ischemia, injury, and necrosis to the area of myocardium supplied by the affected artery. Acute myocardial infarction is most often associated with atherosclerotic heart disease (ASHD).

Precipitating Events

The process of myocardial infarction is dynamic and complex. Although the exact mechanism is not clearly understood, it is thought to begin with the formation of an atherosclerotic plaque involving the intimal layer of a coronary artery. The plaque disrupts the arterial lining and results in the formation of a thrombus on the surface of the plaque. Rupture of the plaque exposes the injured tissue to circulating platelets, resulting in the formation of a fibrin meshwork that may occlude the lumen. As the thrombus enlarges, it further reduces blood flow in the coronary vessel.

Acute thrombotic occlusion is generally accepted as the precipitating event in the vast majority of myocardial infarctions. Other factors that may lead to acute myocardial infarction include coronary spasm, coronary embolism, severe hypoxia, hemorrhage into a diseased arterial wall, and reduced blood flow after any form of shock, all of which may result in an inadequate amount of blood reaching the myocardium.

Types and Locations of Infarcts

Infarction of the myocardium develops distal to the occluded artery. The size of the infarct is determined by the metabolic needs of the tissue supplied solely or predominantly by the occluded vessel and by the duration of time until flow is reestablished. Therefore emergency care is directed at decreasing the metabolic needs of and reestablishing perfusion to the ischemic myocardium as quickly as possible after the onset of symptoms.

The majority of acute myocardial infarctions involve the left ventricle or interventricular septum, which is supplied by either of the two major coronary arteries, although some patients sustain damage to the right ventricle. If the occlusion is in the left coronary artery, the result is anterior, lateral, or septal wall infarcts. Inferior wall infarction (of the inferior-posterior wall of the left ventricle) is usually the result of right coronary artery occlusion. Infarction can also be classified as *transmural* or *subendocardial*. A transmural infarct extends through the full thickness of the myocardium, including the endocardium and epicardium. Patients who experience transmural infarcts are more likely to develop complications.

Muscle Death of the Myocardium

When blood flow to the myocardium ceases, a cascade of events begins. Cells go from aerobic to anaerobic metabolism with the release of lactic acid and increasing carbon dioxide tissue levels. This is thought to produce ischemic heart pain (angina). As cells lose their ability to maintain their electrochemical gradients, they begin to swell and depolarize. These initial changes are reversible, but within a few hours, if collateral flow and reperfusion are inadequate, much of the muscle distal to the occlusion dies. The periinfarction area surrounding the necrotic tissue usually survives because of collateral circulation, but it may become the origin of many dysrhythmias (Fig. 18-83).

Scar tissue replaces the infarcted area in a process that takes approximately 8 weeks, starting with deposition of connective tissue on approximately the twelfth day. Although scar tissue is durable, it lacks elasticity, prevents contraction, and conducts the depolarization wave front poorly in the damaged area of the myocardium. The left ventricle, however, can lose as much as 25% of its muscle and still function as an effective pump. Areas with poor perfusion after a large myocardial infarction may not develop strong scar tissue, resulting in an aneurysmal area that can markedly diminish the effectiveness of ventricular contractility and lead to the development of serious dysrhythmias.

It is during the first 1 to 2 weeks after a myocardial infarction that the damaged myocardium is most vulnerable to rupture, since the scar tissue has not attained adequate tensile strength. For this reason, minimal activity and the prevention of hypertension and excitement are usually necessary during this period. Nonetheless, over the last several years, the length of hospitalization in patients with uncomplicated myocardial infarctions has progressively decreased. Today, most patients resume activity within 2 to 3 days and leave the hospital within 7 to 10 days. Many patients get a submaximal stress test before discharge to determine whether there may be continued ischemia or a predisposition to dysrhythmias. The result of this test and clinical impression helps dictate what activities the patient may resume after discharge.

Fig. 18-83 Area of infarct.

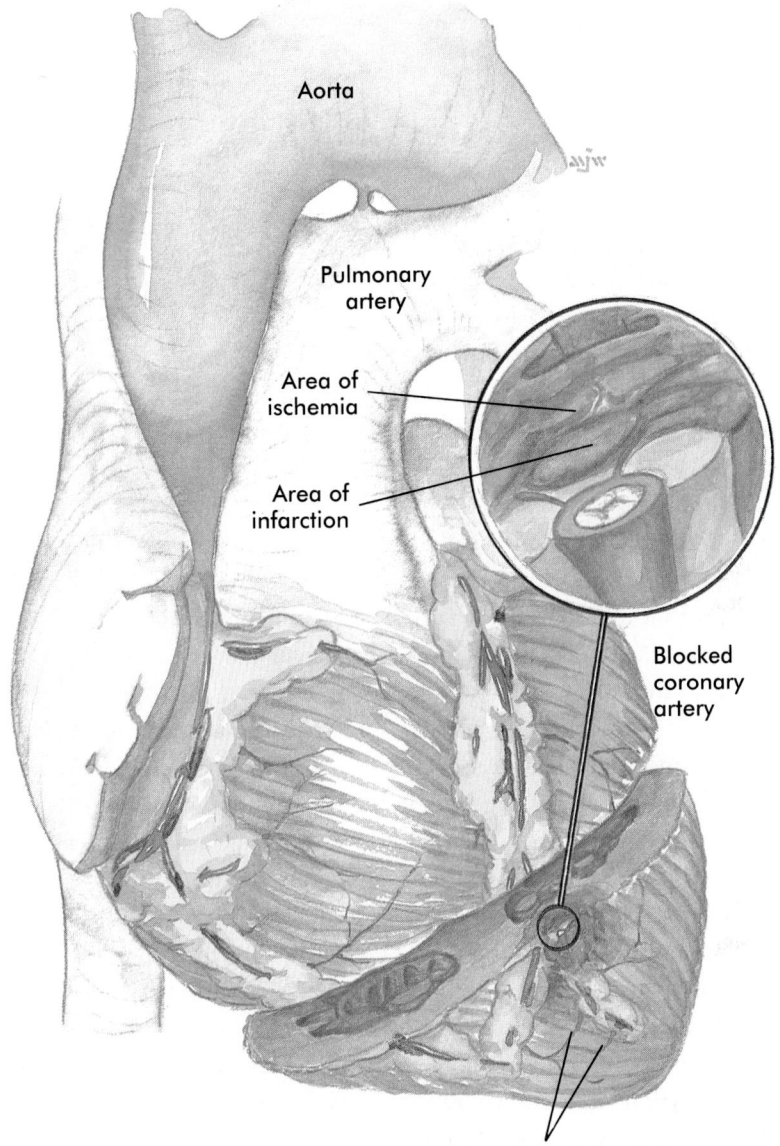

Aorta

Pulmonary
artery

Area of
ischemia

Area of
infarction

Blocked
coronary
artery

Areas of collateral circulation

Deaths Secondary to Myocardial Infarction

Deaths secondary to myocardial infarction usually result from lethal dysrhythmias (ventricular tachycardia, ventricular fibrillation, and cardiac standstill), pump failure (cardiogenic shock and congestive heart failure), or myocardial tissue rupture (rupture of the ventricle, septum, or papillary muscle). Fatal dysrhythmias are the most common cause of death from myocardial infarction. Deaths that occur within the first 24 hours after the onset of illness or injury are sudden deaths. Dysrhythmias are a major cause of all sudden deaths.[2] The majority of patients who suffer sudden death have no immediate premonitory symptoms.[3]

Signs and Symptoms

Although some patients with acute myocardial infarction, particularly those in the older age groups, have only symptoms of dyspnea, syncope, or confusion, substernal chest pain is usually present (70% to 90%) in patients with acute myocardial infarction. The pain generally has the same characteristics and locations as anginal pain and may radiate to the arms, neck, jaw, and back. The following signs and symptoms may accompany the pain and are occasionally present even in the absence of pain (in "silent myocardial infarction"):

- Dyspnea
- Anxiety

- Sense of impending doom
- Nausea and vomiting
- Diaphoresis
- Cyanosis
- Palpitations

The chest pain associated with acute myocardial infarction is often constant and is not altered or alleviated by *nitroglycerin* or other cardiac medications, rest, changes in body position, or breathing patterns. Unlike angina pectoris, which frequently occurs during periods of activity, the onset of pain in over half of all patients with acute myocardial infarction occurs during rest. Most patients have experienced warning anginal pains (preinfarction angina) hours or days before the attack. Many patients deny the possibility of an evolving myocardial infarction and attribute the chest pain or discomfort to unrelated causes such as fatigue or indigestion. This denial is a serious problem because it delays the request for EMS assistance during the most critical phase of the illness. According to the American Heart Association, more than 50% of deaths from ischemic heart disease occur outside the hospital, within the first 2 hours after the onset of pain.[2]

Vital signs vary, depending on the extent of pump damage and the degree and type of autonomic nervous system response. (Inferior myocardial infarctions frequently present with a predominantly parasympathetic autonomic response, whereas anterior myocardial infarctions commonly present with a predominantly sympathetic autonomic response.) For example, the patient's blood pressure may be normal, elevated (sympathetic discharge), or low (parasympathetic discharge or pump failure); the pulse rate (which depends on the presence or absence of dysrhythmias) may be normal, tachycardiac, bradycardic, regular, or irregular; and respirations may be normal or increased.

Common ECG Findings

When the heart muscle is damaged, the damaged area is unable to contract and remains in a constant depolarized state. The flow of current between the pathologically depolarized and normally repolarized areas produces abnormal ST-segment elevation on the ECG tracing (Fig. 18-84). ST-segment elevation greater than 0.1 mV in at

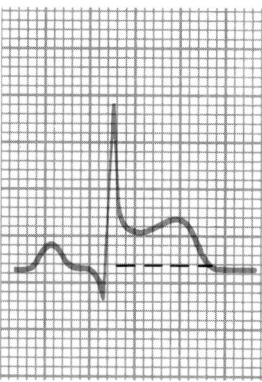

Fig. 18-84 ST-segment elevation likely to present with acute injury.

least two contiguous ECG leads indicates an acute myocardial infarction. Unfortunately, the initial ECG may not demonstrate ST-segment elevation in patients who are infarcting.

Management of the Uncomplicated Acute Myocardial Infarction (Fig. 18-85)

All patients with chest pain suggestive of angina are assumed to have an evolving myocardial infarction until proved otherwise. Any patient with chest pain should be transported to a medical facility for physician evaluation regardless of the apparent severity on EMS arrival, the patient's age, or associated complaints. The primary goals of prehospital care are to relieve pain and apprehension, to prevent the development of serious dysrhythmias, and to limit the size of the infarct.

A thorough patient history should be obtained while conducting the physical examination and during initial patient care interventions. Because time is of the essence, the following components of patient care are a high priority:

1. Place the patient physically at rest to decrease anxiety and heart rate, thereby decreasing oxygen demand.
2. Administer low-concentration *oxygen* (3 to 4 L/min) via nasal cannula. Patients with respiratory compromise need a higher *oxygen* concentration.
3. Consider use of pulse oximetry.
4. Obtain baseline vital signs and repeat them frequently. Vital sign assessment should include auscultation of lungs for indicators of heart failure (presence of crackles).

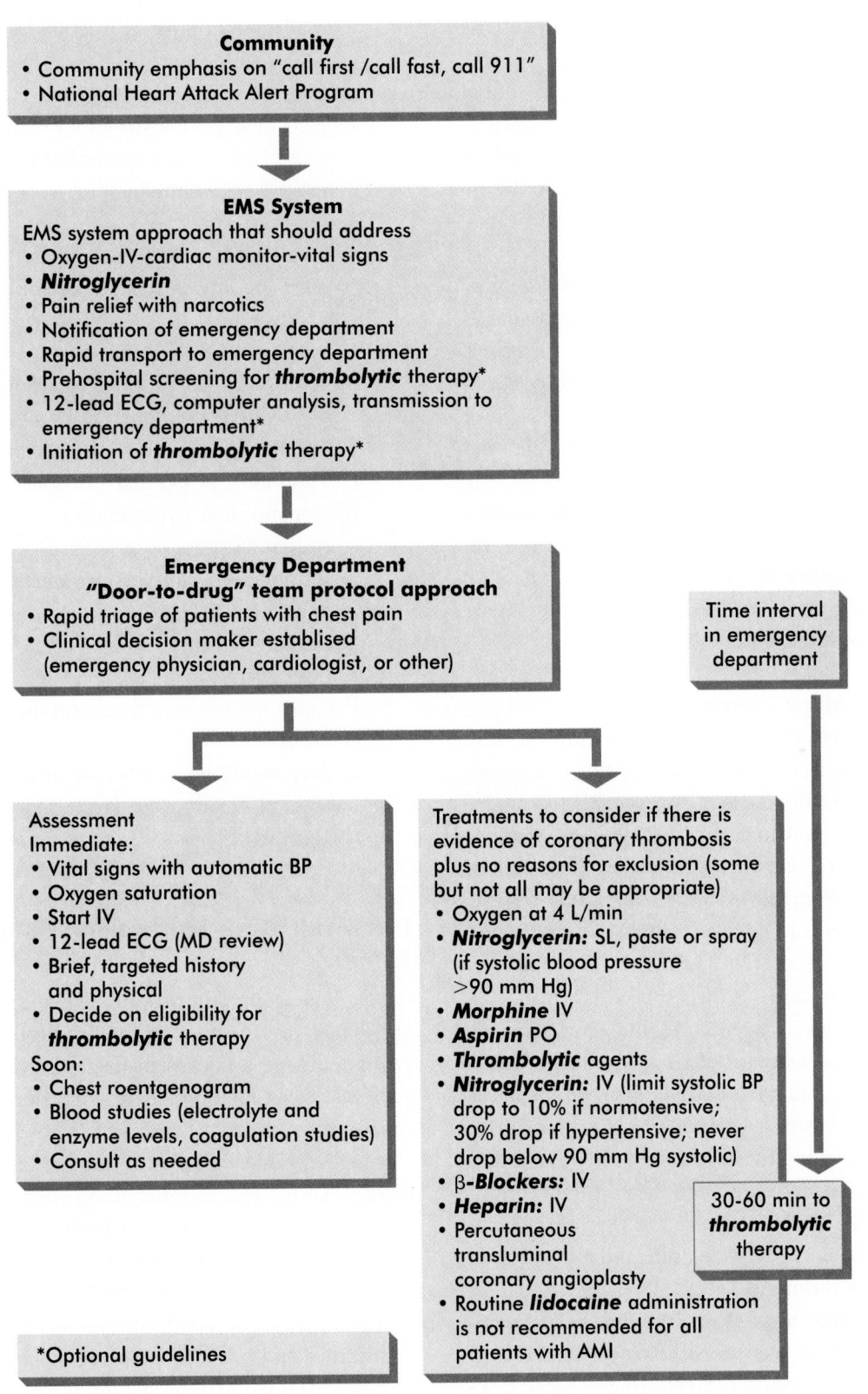

Community
- Community emphasis on "call first /call fast, call 911"
- National Heart Attack Alert Program

EMS System
EMS system approach that should address
- Oxygen-IV-cardiac monitor-vital signs
- *Nitroglycerin*
- Pain relief with narcotics
- Notification of emergency department
- Rapid transport to emergency department
- Prehospital screening for *thrombolytic* therapy*
- 12-lead ECG, computer analysis, transmission to emergency department*
- Initiation of *thrombolytic* therapy*

Emergency Department
"Door-to-drug" team protocol approach
- Rapid triage of patients with chest pain
- Clinical decision maker establised (emergency physician, cardiologist, or other)

Time interval in emergency department

Assessment
Immediate:
- Vital signs with automatic BP
- Oxygen saturation
- Start IV
- 12-lead ECG (MD review)
- Brief, targeted history and physical
- Decide on eligibility for *thrombolytic* therapy
Soon:
- Chest roentgenogram
- Blood studies (electrolyte and enzyme levels, coagulation studies)
- Consult as needed

Treatments to consider if there is evidence of coronary thrombosis plus no reasons for exclusion (some but not all may be appropriate)
- Oxygen at 4 L/min
- *Nitroglycerin:* SL, paste or spray (if systolic blood pressure >90 mm Hg)
- *Morphine* IV
- *Aspirin* PO
- *Thrombolytic* agents
- *Nitroglycerin:* IV (limit systolic BP drop to 10% if normotensive; 30% drop if hypertensive; never drop below 90 mm Hg systolic)
- β-*Blockers:* IV
- *Heparin:* IV
- Percutaneous transluminal coronary angioplasty
- Routine *lidocaine* administration is not recommended for all patients with AMI

30-60 min to *thrombolytic* therapy

*Optional guidelines

Fig. 18-85 Acute myocardial infarction algorithm. Recommendations for early treatment of patients with chest pain and possible acute myocardial infarction. (Reproduced with permission. CPR Issue of *JAMA*, Oct 28, 1992. Copyright © American Medical Association.)

5. Establish an intravenous line with normal saline or lactated Ringer's solution to keep the vein open.

6. Attach ECG electrodes, document initial rhythm, and monitor for dysrhythmias.

7. Administer medications (by order of medical control or according to protocol) for the relief of pain and for the management of dysrhythmias:

 a. Medications that may be used for analgesia, sedation, and to decrease preload and afterload include *nitroglycerin, nifedipine, morphine sulfate, nitrous oxide, diazepam,* and *nalbuphine.*

 b. Medications (partial list) that may be used to treat the various dysrhythmias include lidocaine, procainamide, *atropine sulfate, epinephrine, verapamil, adenosine,* and *bretylium tosylate.*

8. Calmly transport the patient without lights or sirens if the patient is stable.

Thrombolytic Therapy

Studies have shown that an acute intracoronary thrombus can be dissolved (thereby restoring blood flow to the ischemic area) with salvage of ischemic myocardium if a thrombolytic agent is administered within 6 hours after the onset of symptoms.[8] Some EMS services are authorized by medical control to administer these agents in the prehospital setting. (A 12-lead ECG is needed before administration of a thrombolytic agent.) Common thrombolytic agents include *streptokinase, urokinase, recombinant tissue plasminogen activator (t-PA),* and *anisoylated plasminogen streptokinase activator complex (APSAC).* All of these agents work through activation of the plasma protein plasminogen to dissolve the coronary thrombus. Plasminogen is converted to plasmin (the active form), which degrades fibrin, the basic component of a thrombus.

Thrombolytic agents can lyse beneficial hemostatic thrombi as well as pathological thrombi, so the drug is administered selectively. Most EMS systems using thrombolytic agents establish "inclusion-exclusion criteria" similar to the two listed below:

1. Patient inclusion criteria

 a. Alert and able to give informed consent

 b. Chest pain or symptoms of acute myocardial infarction for at least 30 minutes and less than 6 hours

 c. Less than 75 years of age

 d. ECG changes consistent with an acute anterior or inferior myocardial infarction (1-mV ST-segment elevation in two contiguous leads)

 e. Chest pain and ECG changes that persist after the administration of sublingual nitroglycerin

2. Patient exclusion criteria

 a. History of intracranial bleeding or cerebrovascular accident

 b. Ulcer or gastrointestinal bleeding

 c. Pregnancy or postpartum state

 d. Uncontrolled hypertension

 e. Recent surgery

 f. Intravenous catheters at noncompressible sites

 g. Intracranial tumor

 h. Aneurysm

 i. Cardiopulmonary resuscitation

 j. Trauma

 k. Any condition that would result in a significant bleeding hazard

 l. Terminal illness

Left Ventricular Failure and Pulmonary Edema

Left ventricular failure occurs when the left ventricle fails to function as an effective forward pump, causing a back-pressure of blood into the pulmonary circulation. This condition may be caused by a variety of forms of heart disease, including ischemic, valvular, and hypertensive heart disease. Untreated, significant left ventricular failure culminates in pulmonary edema.

In left ventricular failure, blood is delivered to the left ventricle but is not completely ejected from it. The increase in blood volume increases in left ventricular end-diastolic pressure, which is transmitted to the left atrium and subsequently to the pulmonary veins and capillaries. As pulmonary capillary hydrostatic pressure increases, the plasma portion of blood is forced into the alveoli and mixes with air, resulting in the characteristic finding in pulmonary edema: foamy, blood-tinged sputum. If left untreated, the progressive fluid accumulation can cause death from hypoxia. Since myocardial infarction is a common cause of left ventricular failure, all patients with pulmonary edema (particularly those with an abrupt onset) should also be suspected of having an acute myocardial infarction.

Left heart failure results in a reduction of SV, which initiates several compensatory mechanisms that act to restore cardiac output and organ perfusion (tachycardia, vasoconstriction, and activation of the renin-angiotensin-aldosterone system). These mechanisms often increase myocardial oxygen demand and thereby further decrease the functional capacity of the myocardium. Signs and symptoms of left heart failure and pulmonary edema are in Box 18-1.

Management (Fig. 18-86)

Pulmonary edema is an acute and critical emergency that may lead to death unless treated rapidly. Emergency management is directed at decreasing the venous return to the heart, improving myocardial contractility, decreasing myocardial oxygen demand, improving ventilation and oxygenation, and rapidly transporting the patient to a medical facility.

Emergency care entails patient positioning, oxygenation and ventilatory support, and pharmacological therapy. As in any other true emergency, a complete but focused patient history and examination should be obtained while initiating treatment. Although no characteristic ECG changes are associated with pulmonary edema, an initial tracing should be obtained and the patient's rhythm continuously monitored for evidence of myocardial infarction or dysrhythmias.

The patient should be placed in a sitting position with the legs dependent. This increases lung volume and vital capacity, diminishes the work of respiration, and decreases venous return to the heart.

High-concentration *oxygen* should be administered with a well-fitted face mask, preferably a nonrebreather to optimize the forced inspiratory oxygen (Fio₂). Cooperative patients may tolerate positive-pressure assistance to accelerate clearing of pulmonary edema and reduce the needed inspired oxygen concentration. If possible, a pulse

---

BOX 18-1

Signs and Symptoms of Left Ventricular Failure

- Severe respiratory distress
  Orthopnea
  Spasmodic cough that may produce foamy, blood-tinged sputum
  History of paroxysmal nocturnal dyspnea (a sudden episode of dyspnea that occurs after lying down)
- Severe apprehension, agitation, confusion
- Cyanosis (if severe)
- Diaphoresis
- Adventitious lung sounds
  Bilateral crackles that do not clear with coughing (usually present at the base of the lungs and up to the level of the scapulae)
  Rhonchi (fluid in upper airways)
  Wheezes (reflex airway spasm, sometimes referred to as *cardiac asthma*
- JVD (indicative of back-pressure through the right heart and into the venous system)
- Abnormal vital signs
  Blood pressure: possibly elevated
  Pulse rate: rapid to compensate for low stroke volume; possibly irregular if dysrhythmias are present
  Respirations: rapid, labored
- Level of consciousness (Patient may be anxious, agitated, uncooperative, or obtunded because of poor cerebral perfusion or hypoxia.)
- Chest pain
  Presence or absence of pain
  Possible masking by respiratory distress

---

oximeter should be used to ensure arterial oxygen saturation of at least 90% (corresponds to a oxygen pressure [Po₂] of approximately 60 mm Hg when pH and hemoglobin are normal). If this cannot be achieved with 100% *oxygen* or if there are signs of cerebral hypoxia or progressive hypercapnia, medical control may recommend intubation and mechanical ventilation.

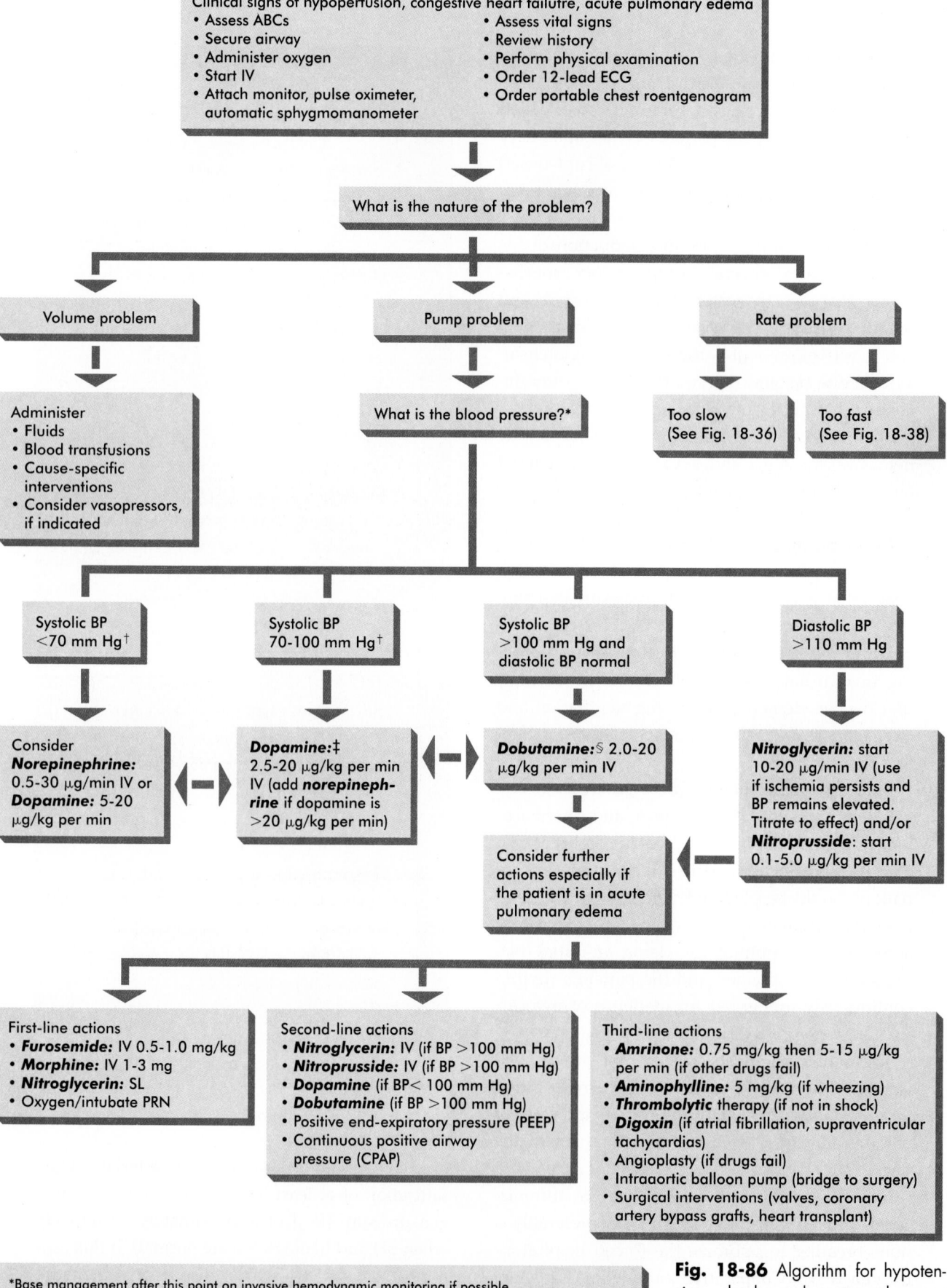

Fig. 18-86 Algorithm for hypotension, shock, and acute pulmonary edema. (Reproduced with permission. CPR Issue of *JAMA*, Oct 28, 1992. Copyright © American Medical Association.)

Pharmacological Therapy

The following three medications may be used to decrease venous return, enhance contractile function of the myocardium, and reduce dyspnea:

1. *Furosemide* (effect controversial)
   a. Direct relaxant effect on venous system within 5 minutes
   b. Diuretic effect that reduces intravascular volume
2. *Morphine sulfate*
   a. Decrease of venous return by dilation of the capacitance vessels of the peripheral venous bed (reduces preload)
   b. Reduction of myocardial work
   c. Reduction of anxiety
3. *Nitroglycerin* and *nifedipine*
   a. Induction of peripheral vasodilation
   b. Possible reduction of preload and after-load, thereby indirectly improving cardiac function.

> **NOTE:**
> Care must be taken in patients with pulmonary edema and hypotension (blood pressure less than 100 systolic), since any of these medications may lower blood pressure.

> ## BOX 18-2
>
> ### Signs and Symptoms of Right Ventricular Failure
>
> - Tachycardia
> - Venous congestion
>   Engorged liver, spleen, or both
>   Venous distention: distention and pulsation of the neck veins
> - Peripheral edema
>   Lower extremities or entire body (anasarca)
>   Sacral region in bedridden patients
>   Pitting edema
> - Fluid accumulation in serous cavities
>   Abdominal cavity (ascites)
>   Pericardium (pericardial effusion)
>
> **NOTE: Patients can often tolerate large quantities of effusion without compromise when the effusion develops over an extended period.**
>
> - History
>   Often previous myocardial infarction in patients with chronic congestive failure
>   Frequent medication history of digitalis and diuretics to control heart failure

---

Right Ventricular Failure

Right ventricular failure occurs when the right ventricle fails as an effective forward pump, causing back-pressure of blood into the systemic venous circulation. Right-sided heart failure can result from several diseases, including chronic hypertension (in which left-sided heart failure usually precedes right-sided heart failure), chronic obstructive pulmonary disease and cor pulmonale, pulmonary embolism, valvular heart disease, and infarction of the right ventricle. Right ventricular failure most commonly results from left ventricular failure.

Left ventricular failure produces elevated pressure in the pulmonary vascular system. This pressure causes resistance to pulmonary blood flow and an increase in the work load of the right heart to overcome the resistance. Over time, the right ventricle is unable to keep up with the venous return and begins to fail. As SV lessens, right atrial pressure rises and back-pressure is transmitted to the vena cava and the rest of the venous system. When the systemic venous pressure becomes too high, the plasma portion of the blood is forced out into the interstitial tissues of the body, resulting in edema, particularly in the dependent areas of the body (lower extremities and sacrum of patients who are bedridden).

Signs and symptoms of right ventricular failure are in Box 18-2. When both occur, signs and symptoms of each may be present.

Management

Right ventricular failure is not usually a medical emergency in itself unless it is associated with pulmonary edema or hypotension. The paramedic should be prepared to treat the patient for either complication. Patient management for right ventricular failure includes:

1. Placing the patient at rest in a sitting or semi-Fowler position (head elevated)
2. Administering high-concentration *oxygen* (except when the patient has a history of chronic obstructive pulmonary disease and there is no evidence of pulmonary edema)
3. Obtaining baseline vital signs and an ECG tracing
4. Initiating an intravenous line with D_5W to keep the vein open (unless the patient is hypotensive, in which case normal saline should be instituted)
5. Monitoring the ECG
6. Treating symptoms of left ventricular failure, if present

> **NOTE:**
> Pulmonary edema associated with right ventricular failure is treated the same as isolated pulmonary edema. Hypotension secondary to right ventricular failure (often seen in right ventricle infarcts) can mimic cardiogenic shock. It is treated like cardiogenic shock, except that fluid administration to help normalize left ventricular filling is crucial.

Cardiogenic Shock

Cardiogenic shock is the most extreme form of pump failure. It occurs when left ventricular function is so compromised that the heart cannot meet the metabolic needs of the body. The result is a marked decrease in SV (resulting from ineffective myocardial contraction), cardiac output, and blood pressure, all of which result in an inadequate supply of blood to the body's organs. Cardiogenic shock occurs in 5% to 10% of myocardial infarction patients.

By definition, cardiogenic shock is present when shock persists after correction of existing dysrhythmias, hypovolemia, or decreased vascular tone. It is usually caused by extensive myocardial infarction, often involving more than 40% of the left ventricle, or by diffuse ischemia. Even with aggressive therapy, cardiogenic shock has a mortality rate of 70% or higher.

In addition to the signs and symptoms of myocardial infarction, patients in cardiogenic shock show clinical evidence of hypoperfusion to vital organs and significant systemic hypotension similar to that found in other forms of shock. This evidence includes:

- Profound hypotension (systolic blood pressure usually less than 80 mm Hg)
- Pulmonary congestion
- Hypoxemia
- Acidosis
- Altered level of consciousness
- Sinus tachycardia or other dysrhythmias
- Cool, clammy, cyanotic, or ashen skin
- Tachypnea

Management

Patients in cardiogenic shock are severely ill and require rapid transport to a medical facility. (Prolonged in-field stabilization is not recommended.) Prehospital care should include airway management and ventilatory support with high-concentration *oxygen*, placement of the patient in a supine position (or semi-Fowler position, if the patient is dyspneic), insertion of an intravenous line with normal saline or lactated Ringer's solution to keep the vein open, ECG monitoring, correction of dysrhythmias, and frequent evaluation of vital signs (including auscultation of lungs and observation for jugular venous distention) (see Fig. 18-86).

Pharmacological therapy may include inotropic agents such as *dopamine* or *dobutamine* to improve cardiac output and vasodilators to increase forward flow by reducing afterload. If left-sided heart failure and pulmonary edema are also present, they should be treated concurrently. Pneumatic antishock garment use in cardiogenic shock is controversial, but it is definitely contraindicated if pulmonary edema is present.

Thoracic and Abdominal Aortic Aneurysms

Aneurysm is a nonspecific term meaning "dilation of a vessel." It may result from atherosclerotic disease (most common), infectious disease (primarily syphilis), traumatic injury, or certain ge-

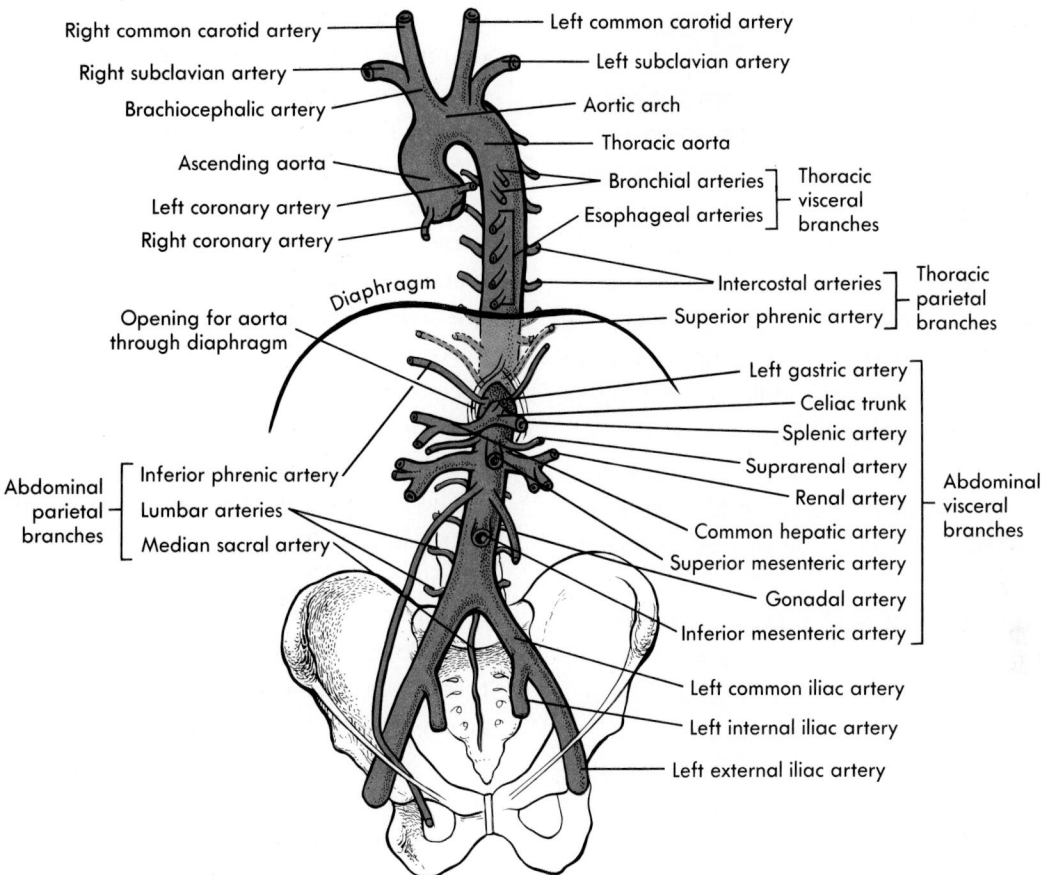

Fig. 18-87 Branches of the aorta. Aortic arch, thoracic aorta, abdominal aorta, and their branches.

netic disorders (for example, Marfan's syndrome). Fig. 18-87 illustrates the branches of the aorta. Although aortic aneurysms may occur in any portion of the aorta, this text limits discussion to abdominal aortic aneurysm and dissecting aneurysm of the aorta.

Most aneurysms develop at a weak point in the wall of an artery that results from degenerative changes in the medial layer. Weakening of the supportive elements of the vessel wall allows dilation, which causes turbulence and increasing lateral pressure. The aneurysm tends to enlarge over time as the lateral pressure increases in the dilated segment. Eventually the aneurysm may rupture, producing life-threatening hemorrhage.

Abdominal Aortic Aneurysm

Abdominal aortic aneurysms affect approximately 2% of the population. The most common site for an abdominal aortic aneurysm is below the renal arteries and above the bifurcation of the common iliac arteries. It is 10 times more common in men and is most prevalent between the ages of 60 and 70. An abdominal aneurysm is usually asymptomatic as long as it is stable. However, if the aneurysm begins to expand or leak, symptoms will indicate impending rupture (Box 18-3).

Rupture of an abdominal aortic aneurysm may begin with a small tear in the intima that allows blood to leak into the wall of the aorta. As the process continues with increasing pressure, the tear may extend through the outer layer of the vessel and cause bleeding into the retroperitoneal space. If bleeding is tamponaded by the retroperitoneal tissues, the patient may be normotensive on EMS arrival. If the rupture opens into the peritoneal cavity, however, massive fatal hemorrhage may follow. In either case, major blood loss results, and hypovolemic shock ensues.

BOX 18-3

Signs and Symptoms of a Leaking or Ruptured Abdominal Aortic Aneurysm

- Unexplained hypotension (that results from either hemorrhage or a compensatory vasovagal response mechanism)
- Unexplained syncope (As the aneurysm ruptures, blood pressure drops transiently to zero, producing sudden cerebral hypoperfusion and syncope.)
- Sudden onset of abdominal or back pain (described as *tearing* or *ripping*) from the physical trauma itself or from inflammation
- Low back or flank pain (radiating to the thigh, groin, testicle, or perineum) that is unrelieved by rest or changes in position
- Signs of peritoneal irritation
- Urge to defecate (caused by retroperitoneal leakage of blood)
- Pulsatile, tender mass that may be palpated when greater than 5 cm and that is usually located above the umbilicus, left of the midline
- Distal pulses (femoral artery and below) that may be present or absent, depending on the patient's blood pressure, the occurrence of a dissection, and the degree of peripheral vascular disease
- Possible presentation as bleeding in the gastrointestinal tract if the aneurysm erodes into it

Management

Patients with an expanding or a ruptured abdominal aneurysm usually appear acutely ill and require immediate operative repair of the vessel. A total of 20% of the patients with an abdominal aortic aneurysm rupture their aneurysm before reaching the hospital, and 80% of these patients die.[9] Therefore early recognition and prompt transport are imperative to avert a fatal outcome.

In most cases, prehospital care should be limited to gentle handling, *oxygen* administration, preparation of pneumatic antishock garments ac-cording to protocol, cardiac monitoring (myocardial infarctions may be associated with advanced aneurysms), initiation of volume-expanding intravenous fluids while en route to the receiving hospital, and alerting of the receiving facility to prepare for imminent surgery. Pulsatile masses (if present) are extremely fragile and in most cases membrane thin. The paramedic should avoid aggressive examination or deep palpation of the mass, which may cause rupture. Examination, if necessary, can be made by auscultation, which may reveal a sound similar to that of a systolic murmur or bruit.

The treatment of hypotension varies somewhat, depending on whether the aneurysm is leaking or ruptured. A patient with a suspected leaking aneurysm can be maintained with mildly hypotensive blood pressure to try to prevent frank rupture during transport. (The hypotension associated with small leaks is thought to be secondary to a compensatory vasovagal mechanism.) In these patients, fluid resuscitation should be minimal and less aggressive than in patients who have a ruptured aneurysm.

If rupture has occurred, hypotension, tachycardia, and loss of the pulsating mass may suddenly develop, and the patient may become unresponsive. This is often followed by full cardiac and respiratory arrest. These patients require rapid and aggressive resuscitation (intubation, ventilation, inflation of pneumatic antishock garments by protocol, fluid replacement, and rapid transport for surgical intervention).

Acute Dissecting Aortic Aneurysm

Acute dissection (separation of the arterial wall) is the most common aortic catastrophe, affecting 5 to 10 per million population each year (3 times as many as ruptured abdominal aortic aneurysm). Factors that can lead to the development of dissecting aneurysm are systemic hypertension, atherosclerosis, congenital abnormalities, degenerative changes in the connective tissue of the aortic media (cystic medial necrosis), trauma, and pregnancy. The syndrome affects men twice as often as women and is more common in African Americans.

A dissecting aneurysm of the aorta results from a small tear in the intimal layer of the vessel wall

(Fig. 18-88). After the tear, the process of dissection begins. The tear in the inner wall allows blood to move between the inner and outer layers, creating a false passage between the layers of the vessel wall. Blood that enters the false passage results in the formation of a hematoma, which can subsequently rupture through the outer wall (adventitia) at any time, usually into the pericardial or pleural cavity.

Although any area of the aorta may be involved, in 60% to 70% of cases the site of a dissecting aneurysm is in the descending aorta, just beyond the takeoff of the left subclavian artery (Fig. 18-89). Once begun, the aneurysm may extend distally or proximally to involve all of the thoracic and abdominal aorta as well as tributaries, coronary arteries, the aortic valve, and the carotid and subclavian vessels. Any vessels (including the carotid and other aortic arch vessels) bypassed by the dissection have their blood flow compromised. As a result, aortic dissection may cause:

- Syncope
- Stroke
- Absent or reduced pulses
- Heart failure resulting from sudden aortic valve regurgitation
- Pericardial tamponade
- Acute myocardial infarction

Signs and Symptoms

The signs and symptoms of a dissecting aortic aneurysm depend on the site of the intimal tear (ascending or descending aorta) and the extent of dissection. More than 70% of patients with acute dissecting aneurysm of the aorta complain of severe pain in the back, epigastrium, abdomen, or extremities, which they often describe as the most intense pain they have ever experienced. The pain is usually sudden in onset and may be characterized by the patient as "ripping," "tearing," and "sharp and cutting like a knife." It often originates in the back (between the scapulae) and possibly extends down into the legs. The patient with acute dissection may appear "shocky" with pallor,

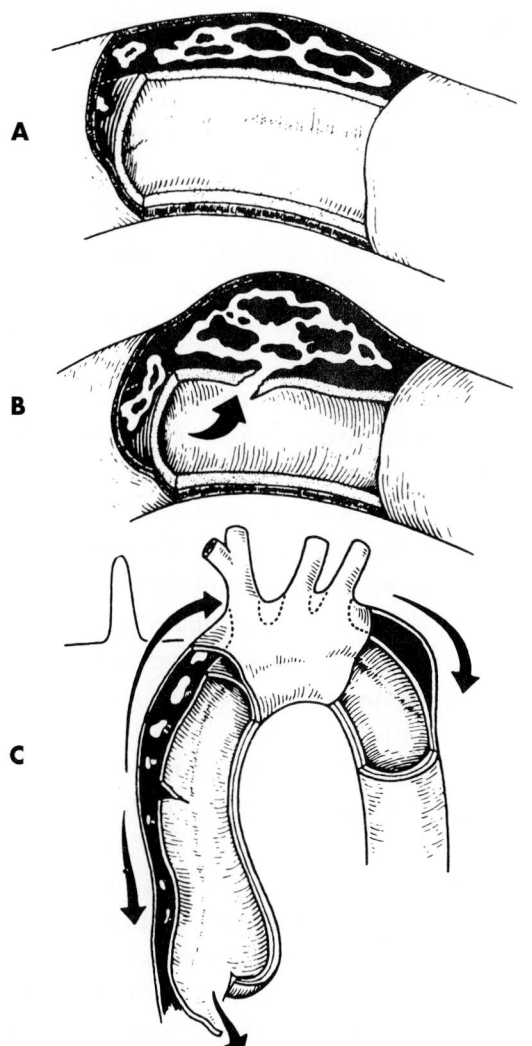

Fig. 18-88 Pathogenesis of dissecting aneurysms. **A,** Medial and intimal degeneration in anotic wall set stage. **B,** Hemodynamic forces acting on aortic wall produce intimal tear, directing bloodstream into diseased media. **C,** Resulting dissecting hematoma is propagated in both directions by pulse wave produced with each myocardial contraction.

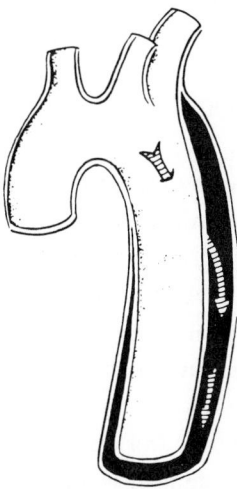

Fig. 18-89 Usual path of dissecting anerurysm originating in the descending aorta.

sweating, and peripheral cyanosis (from impaired perfusion), even when blood pressure is normal or elevated. If the patient is hypotensive, cardiac tamponade or aortic rupture should be suspected.

> **NOTE:**
> Blood pressure may differ in the two arms if the dissection bypasses the left subclavian artery, leading to factitious (artificial) hypotension in the left upper extremity.

Although it may be difficult to differentiate the pain of aortic dissection from that of myocardial infarction or pulmonary embolism in the prehospital setting, six distinctive features may help:

1. Severity of pain is maximal from the onset (compared with crescendo pain characteristic of acute myocardial infarction).
2. Pain may migrate from the anterior chest or interscapular area downward as dissection progresses.
3. Significant differences in blood pressure occur between the left and right arm or between the arms and the legs.
4. Peripheral pulses are unequal.
5. Neurological deficits result from occlusion of a cerebral vessel.
6. Signs of pericardial tamponade are found.

Management

The goals of managing suspected aortic dissection in the prehospital setting are relief of pain and immediate transport to a medical facility. The EMS crew should be prepared to initiate intubation and to assist ventilation in case the patient begins to decompensate. Other prehospital care measures include:

- Gently handling the patient
- Decreasing anxiety
- Administering high-concentration *oxygen*
- Beginning a large-bore intravenous line of crystalloid solution (Fluids should be kept to a minimum unless severe hypotension is present.)
- Giving analgesia (for example, *morphine sulfate*) if the diagnosis is strongly suspected

Definitive in-hospital care generally includes reducing the myocardial contractile force to stop progressive dissection (with antihypertensives and beta blockers), monitoring of intraarterial pressure, and possibly surgical repair.

Acute Arterial Occlusion

Acute arterial occlusion is a sudden blockage of arterial flow, most commonly caused by trauma, embolus, or thrombosis. The severity of the ischemic episode depends on the site of occlusion and the quality of collateral circulation around the blockage. Vascular occlusion caused by thrombosis is a complication of atherosclerosis. Occlusions secondary to emboli may indicate an underlying disturbance in cardiac rhythm, particularly atrial fibrillation.

Arterial occlusion may follow blunt or penetrating trauma; it is often associated with long bone fractures. These injuries vary from intimal disruptions to complete transection. The occlusion is usually evident from decreased circulation distal to the injury.

An embolism occurs when a blood clot breaks away and enters the arterial system. It travels until it reaches a point of luminal narrowing, often a bifurcation of an artery. Since 90% of peripheral emboli originate in the heart, a history of cardiac disease (for example, dysrhythmia, myocardial infarction, valvular heart disease) favors a diagnosis of embolic occlusion, particularly when the patient has an asymptomatic opposite extremity with normal pulses. The most common sites of embolic occlusion are the abdominal aorta, common femoral artery, popliteal artery, carotid artery, brachial artery, and mesenteric artery (Fig. 18-90).

Thrombosis usually results from atherosclerotic disease and occurs at a site of severe stenosis of a vessel. Unlike an embolus, thrombosis usually occurs gradually over a period of time. As the thrombosis propagates proximally, sources of collateral blood supply can become occluded, causing progressive ischemia. The location of the ischemic pain is often related to the site of occlusion:

- Terminal portion of abdominal aorta: pain in both hips or lower limbs
- Iliac artery: pain in buttocks or hip on involved side
- Femoral artery: pain and claudication in the involved leg

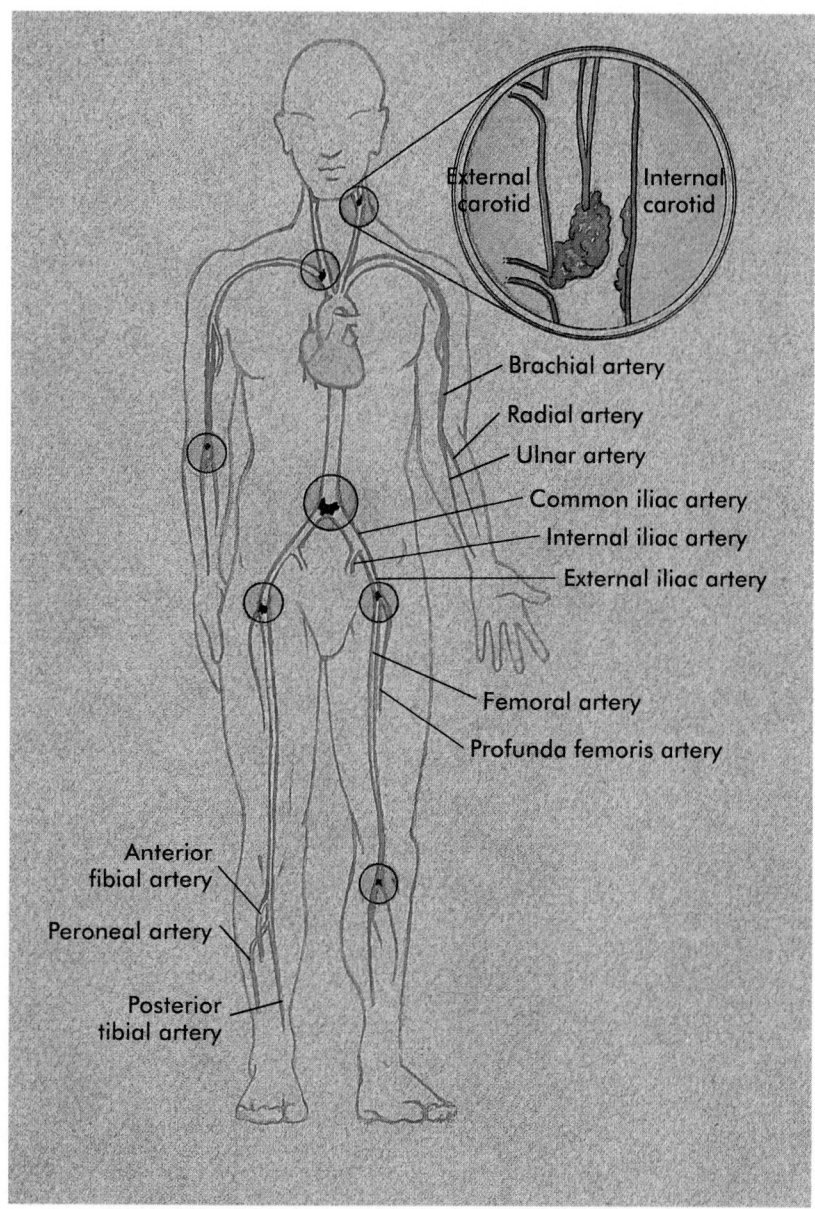

Fig. 18-90 Common sites of embolic arterial occlusion.

• Mesentery artery: severe abdominal pain

If severe ischemia persists, muscle necrosis occurs. Thrombotic occlusion is seen most often in men, smokers, and those over 60 years of age. Common sites of atherosclerotic (thrombotic) occlusions are depicted in Fig. 18-91.

Signs and Symptoms

Regardless of the origin of the occlusion, the signs and symptoms of ischemia are the same. These include:

• Pain in the extremity that may be severe and sudden in onset or be absent as a result of paresthesia
• Pallor (Skin may also be mottled or cyanotic.)
• Lowered skin temperature distal to occlusion
• Changes in sensory and motor function
• Diminished or absent pulse distal to the injury
• Slow capillary filling
• Sometimes, shock (particularly in mesenteric occlusion)

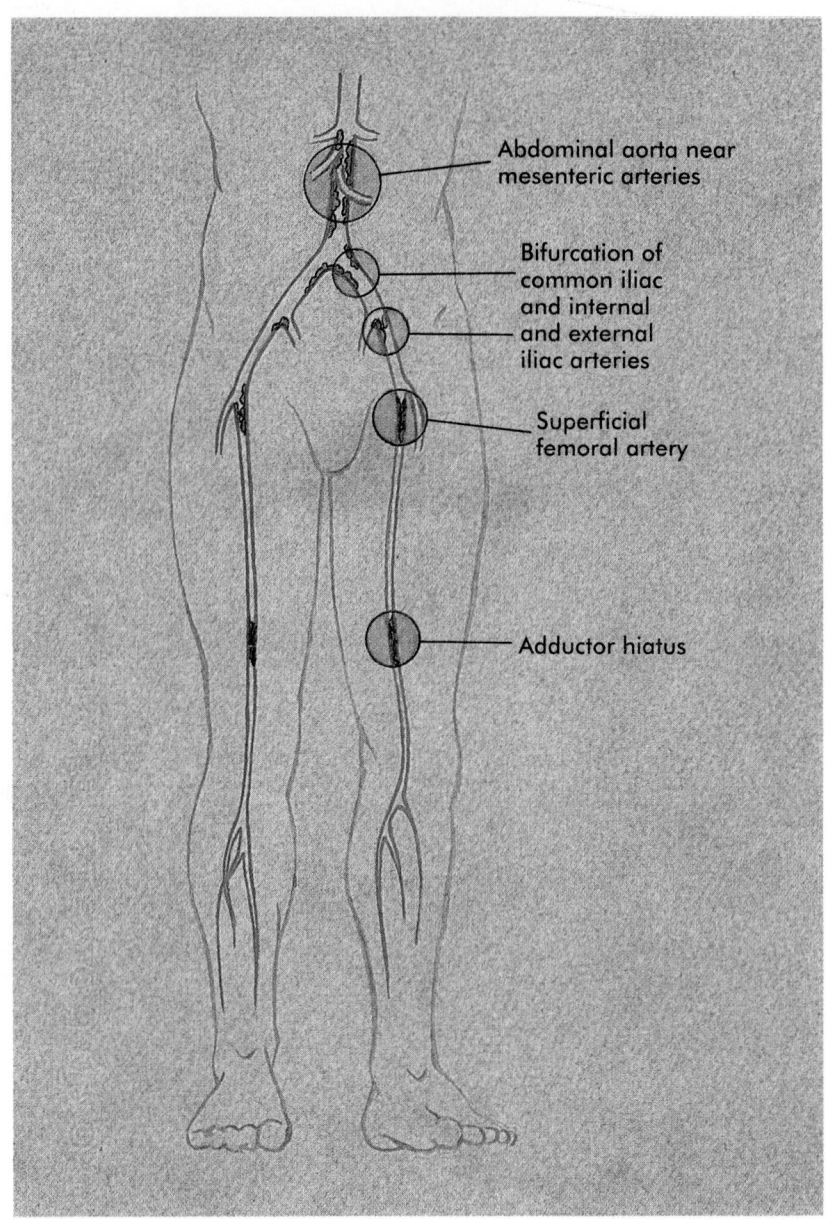

Fig. 18-91 Common sites of atherosclerotic occlusive disease.

Management

Arterial occlusion in an extremity is serious and painful but not usually limb or life threatening, provided that blood flow is reestablished within 4 to 8 hours. The affected limb should be immobilized and protected and the patient transported for physician evaluation. Patients with mesenteric occlusion should be treated for shock with *oxygen* and intravenous fluids. Analgesics may also be prescribed by medical control to relieve pain. Definitive care may include anticoagulant or thrombolytic therapy, transluminal arterial dila-

tion using a balloon catheter, embolectomy, or vascular reconstruction.

Noncritical Peripheral Vascular Conditions

Noncritical peripheral vascular conditions include varicose veins, superficial thrombophlebitis, and acute deep-vein thrombosis. Of these conditions, deep-vein thrombosis is the only one that can cause a life-threatening problem, pulmonary embolus. Thrombi in the large veins of the lower extremities may fragment and embolize, often ending up in the pulmonary circulation and leading to the constellation of signs and symptoms of pulmonary embolism (see Chapter 17). Predisposing factors to venous thrombosis include:

- History of trauma
- Sepsis
- Stasis or inactivity (for example, bedridden patients)
- Recent immobilization (for example, leg fracture)
- Pregnancy
- Birth control pills
- Smoking
- Varicose veins

Varicose Veins

The presence of varicose veins is usually a benign condition caused by chronic increased venous pressure with a resultant dilation of superficial veins. The syndrome is commonly associated with veins of the lower extremities but may also occur in other parts of the body as hemorrhoids, esophageal varices, and varicocele (collections of varicose veins in the scrotum). With the exception of esophageal varices, which can lead to exsanguinating gastrointestinal hemorrhage, varicosities are a nuisance but rarely a serious problem. The rest of this discussion is limited to varicose veins of the lower extremities.

Varicose veins are extremely common, affecting 15% of the adult population in the United States. The syndrome is more common in women than men and tends to be associated with genetic predisposition, hormonal changes during pregnancy or at menopause, obesity, and standing for long periods of time.

Etiology

There are two principal systems of veins in the legs: the deep veins that lie among the muscles and carry approximately 90% of the blood and the surface veins, which are often visible just under the skin and are less well supported. Valves in the veins prevent circulating blood from draining back down the leg under the force of gravity. These valves must support a high column of blood, and in many people become defective, causing pooling of blood in the superficial veins.

When this occurs, the veins become swollen and distorted.

Signs and Symptoms

The most common sites for varicose veins are the back of the calf and anywhere on the medial aspect of the leg. The veins are generally blue, prominent, swollen, and twisted. In some people, they cause no symptoms, but others experience a severe ache in the affected area (which is made worse by prolonged standing), swelling of the feet and ankles, and persistent itching of the skin. These symptoms may become progressively worse during the day and be relieved by sitting with the legs elevated. If backflow of blood is severe enough to cause ischemia of tissues, the skin may become thin, hard, dry, and scaly, and stasis ulcers may develop. This is rare with varicosities alone and is usually associated with deep venous valvular incompetence (a sequela of deep vein thrombosis). Minimal blunt trauma to a large varicose vein may cause rupture and severe bleeding.

Management

EMS assistance is seldom requested by these patients, unless bleeding occurs. Bleeding is usually controlled by direct pressure and elevation of the extremity. Stasis ulcers (if present) should be covered with a sterile dressing. In severe cases in which varicose veins are painful, ulcerated, or prone to bleeding, definitive care may include surgical removal of the veins (known as *stripping*).

Superficial Thrombophlebitis

Superficial thrombophlebitis results from chemical or mechanical injury to a vein (for example, intravenous therapy or injection) or from the development of a thrombus in a superficial vein. Redness and tenderness are usually present along the course of the involved vein. The inflammation is generally a minor condition that causes temporary discomfort without permanent consequence. Hospitalization is rarely necessary. Treatment is symptomatic and consists of:

- Removal of the causative agent (for example, birth control pills, intravenous line)
- Rest and elevation of the affected part
- Local, moist heat
- Analgesics as needed

Acute Deep-Vein Thrombosis

Occlusion of the deep veins is a serious, common problem. It may involve any portion of the deep venous system but is much more common in the lower extremities. Unlike superficial vein thrombosis, deep-vein thrombosis may have permanent consequences and is associated with a high mortality rate from pulmonary embolism and more rarely from systemic reactions (sepsis). Risk factors for deep-venous thrombosis include recent lower-extremity trauma, recent surgery, advanced age, recent myocardial infarction, inactivity, congestive heart failure, cancer, previous thrombosis, oral contraceptive therapy, and obesity. Signs and symptoms of acute deep-vein thrombosis include:

- Pain
- Edema
- Warmth
- Erythema or bluish discoloration
- Tenderness
- Palpable cord (occasionally)

Management

Patients with acute deep-vein thrombosis require hospitalization. Prehospital care is usually limited to immobilization and elevation of the extremity and transport for physician evaluation. Deep venous thrombosis in the calf of the leg is usually much less serious than deep venous thrombosis of the thigh, which has a higher incidence of associated pulmonary embolus. Definitive care includes bed rest, administration of anticoagulants or occasionally thrombolytic agents, and rarely, thrombectomy.

Hypertension

Hypertension is a common disorder, afflicting more than 60 million Americans, and is directly responsible for more than 30,000 deaths per year.[1] Hypertension is often defined by a resting blood pressure consistently greater than 140/90 mm Hg. There are several categories of hypertension based on level of blood pressure, symptomatology, and urgency of need for intervention. For our purposes, two general categories are presented: chronic hypertension and hypertensive emergencies (including hypertensive encephalopathy).

Chronic Hypertension

Chronic hypertension has an adverse effect on the function of the heart and blood vessels, requiring the heart to perform more work than normal, leading to hypertrophy of the cardiac muscle and left ventricular failure. It increases the rate at which atherosclerosis develops, which in turn increases the probability of cardiovascular, cerebrovascular, and peripheral vascular disease and the risk of aneurysm formation. Conditions commonly associated with chronic, uncontrolled hypertension are cerebral hemorrhage and stroke, myocardial infarction, and renal failure (secondary to vascular changes in the kidney).

Any hypertension-related problem, such as pulmonary edema, dissecting aortic aneurysm, toxemia of pregnancy, or cerebrovascular accident, requires stabilization and prompt, appropriate treatment. The hypertension associated with these situations is often the result of a primary problem. Treating the primary problem (for example, toxemia) often makes it easier to control the patient's blood pressure. However, the primary problem may not be easily correctable, and in situations such as dissecting aneurysm, controlling the blood pressure is essential to treating the primary problem. Any life-threatening problem that results from hypertension or is made significantly worse by coincidental hypertension can be considered a hypertensive emergency.

Hypertensive Emergencies

Hypertensive emergencies are conditions in which a blood pressure increase leads to significant, irreversible end-organ damage within hours if not treated. The organs most likely to be at risk are the brain, heart, and kidneys. This now uncommon condition is experienced by 1% of all hypertensives whose illness is poorly controlled or untreated. There is no predetermined criterion for the level of blood pressure necessary to induce a hypertensive emergency, although in 1984, the Joint National Committee on Hypertension defined *severe hypertension* as a "diastolic pressure greater than 115 mm Hg."[10] As a rule, the diagnosis is based on altered end-organ function and the rate of the rise in blood pressure, not the level of blood pressure (although diastolic blood pressure is usually greater than 100 mm Hg). All hypertensive emergencies require a 5% to 20% reduction of blood pressure within a few hours of discovery to avoid permanent organ damage.

Hypertensive emergencies include the following clinical conditions: (1) myocardial ischemia with hypertension, (2) aortic dissection with hypertension, (3) pulmonary edema with hypertension, (4) hypertensive intracranial hemorrhage, (5) toxemia, and (6) hypertensive encephalopathy. Although hypertension per se may not be the cause of the first five conditions, they all can be made worse by unremitting hypertension. The sixth condition, hypertensive encephalopathy, results solely from elevated blood pressure.

Hypertensive Encephalopathy

Unremitting hypertension produces hypertensive encephalopathy and cerebral hypoperfusion with loss of the integrity of the blood-brain barrier, which results in fluid exudation into the brain tissue. Two theories have been proposed to explain hypertensive encephalopathy. One holds that vessels vasoconstrict to the point of spasm, which causes ischemia, in an to attempt to protect the brain arterioles from high perfusion pressure. Continued maximal spasm produces ischemic brain damage recognizable as hypertensive encephalopathy. The other theory is that when autoregulation fails, vasoconstriction is overcome, allowing unchecked vasodilation of cerebral vessels and leakage of plasma into brain tissue driven by unchecked systolic blood pressure. This produces localized brain edema and hemorrhage recognized as hypertensive encephalopathy.

Hypertensive encephalopathy may progress over several hours from initial symptoms of severe headache, nausea, vomiting, aphasia, hemiparesis, and transient blindness to seizures, stupor, coma, and death. The condition is a true emergency that requires immediate transport to a medical facility for definitive care. The goal of therapy is to lower the mean arterial pressure over 30 to 60 minutes by approximately 10% or to 110 mm Hg, whichever is greater. The key is controlled but rapid lowering of blood pressure to normalize cerebral blood flow. If blood pressure is lowered too fast, infarction of end organs (heart, kidney, brain) may occur. Prehospital management of these patients includes:

- Supportive care
- Calming the patient
- *Oxygen* therapy
- Intravenous D_5W to keep the vein open
- ECG monitoring
- Rapid transport

In most circumstances, pharmacological therapy for hypertensive emergencies is not instituted in the prehospital setting. However, in severe cases of hypertensive encephalopathy or if transport is delayed, medical control may recommend administration of antihypertensives such as *labetalol* (an alpha and beta blocker) or *nifedipine* (a calcium channel blocker). Both of these agents result in arteriolar vasodilation.

Section Seven
Techniques of Managing Cardiac Emergencies

This section addresses various procedures, techniques, and equipment used in managing cardiac emergencies. These include basic life support, mechanical CPR devices, monitor defibrillators (manual, fully automated, and semiautomated), defibrillation, automatic implantable cardioverter defibrillators, synchronized cardioversion, and TCP. This section also provides an overview of managing a cardiac arrest as it applies to paramedics working within an advanced cardiac life-support (ACLS) system. The reader is encouraged to review the dysrhythmias and pharmacological therapy presented previously in this text.

● BASIC LIFE SUPPORT

Basic life support externally supports the circulation and respiration of a victim of cardiac arrest until advanced cardiac life support is available. According to the American Heart Association, "the highest hospital discharge rate—a measure of resuscitation success—is achieved in patients for whom CPR is initiated within 4 minutes of the time of the arrest and who, in addition, are provided with ACLS treatment within 8 minutes of

	OBJECTIVES	ACTIONS		
		Adult (over 8 yrs)	Child (1 to 8 yrs)	Infant (under 1 yr)
A—Airway	1. Assessment: Determine unresponsiveness.	Tap or gently shake shoulder.		
		Ask, "Are you okay?"		Observe.
	2. Position victim.	Turn on back as unit, supporting head and neck if necessary.		
	3. Open airway.	Open airway with head-tilt/chin-lift.		
B—Breathing	4. Assessment: Determine breathlessness.	Maintain open airway. Place ear over mouth, observing chest. Look, listen, feel for breathing (3-5 sec).		
	5. Give two rescue breaths.	Seal mouth-to-mouth with barrier device or bag-valve device.		Seal mouth-to-mouth/nose with barrier device.
		Give two rescue breaths 1½-2 sec each. Observe chest rise. Allow lung deflation between breaths.		
C—Circulation	6. Assessment: Determine pulselessness.	Feel for carotid pulse (5-10 sec); maintain head-tilt.		Feel for brachial pulse; maintain head-tilt.
	7. If pulseless, begin chest compressions. a. Landmark check	Run middle finger along bottom edge of rib cage to notch at center (tip of sternum).		Imagine line drawn between nipples.
	b. Hand placement.	Place index finger next to finger on notch:		Place 2-3 fingers on sternum, 1 finger's width below line. Depress ½-1 inch.
		Place two hands next to index finger. Depress 1½-2 inches.	Place heel of one hand next to index finger. Depress 1-1½ inches.	
	c. Compression rate.	Give 80-100 compressions per minute.	Give 100 compressions per minute.	
CPR Cycles	8. Compressions to breaths.	Give two breaths every 15 compressions.	Give 1 breath every 5 compressions.	
	9. Number of cycles.	4 (52-73 sec)	10 (60-87 sec)	20 (approx. 60 sec)
	10. Reassessment.	Feel for carotid pulse.		Feel for brachial pulse.
		If there is no pulse, resume CPR.		
Entrance of second rescuer	Second rescuer should perform one-rescuer CPR when first rescuer becomes fatigued. Compression rate for two-rescuer CPR is 80-100 per min; the compression ratio is 5 chest compressions to 1 breath.			
Option for pulse return	If no breathing, give rescue breaths.	Give 1 breath every 5 sec (12/minute).	Give 1 breath every 3 sec (20/minute).	

Fig. 18-92 CPR.

their arrest. The victim whose heart and breathing have stopped for less than 4 minutes has an excellent chance for recovery if CPR is administered immediately. After 4 to 6 minutes without circulation, brain damage may occur; after 6 minutes . . . brain damage will almost always occur."[11]

Physiology of Circulation via External Chest Compression

Two mechanisms are thought to be responsible for blood flow during CPR: (1) direct compression of the heart between the sternum and the spine, which increases pressure within the ventricles enough to provide blood flow to the lungs and body organs, and (2) increased intrathoracic pressure transmitted to all intrathoracic vascular structures, which produces an intrathoracic-to-extrathoracic pressure gradient that causes blood to flow out of the thorax. It is not known which mechanism contributes more to blood flow, and mechanisms not currently known may also be involved. Artificial circulation generates only approximately 20% to 30% of the normal output of the heart.[11]

Research has been conducted for many years on ways to improve CPR, including simultaneous chest compressions and ventilation, abdominal compression with synchronized ventilation, military antishock trousers–augmented CPR, interposed abdominal compression, continuous abdominal binding, and recently, a plunger mechanism for chest compression that causes active compression and active expansion. However, no alternative method has been shown to unequivocally improve survival or circulation. The standards of CPR as recommended by the American Heart Association and the American Red Cross are presented in Fig. 18-92.

Mechanical CPR Devices

A number of mechanical devices provide external chest compression, and others provide chest compression with a system for synchronized ventilation in the cardiac arrest patient (Fig. 18-93). These devices are designed to standardize CPR technique, eliminate rescuer fatigue, free other res-

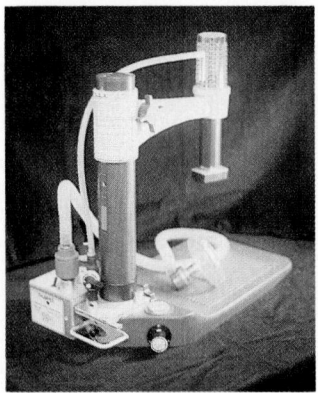

Fig. 18-93 Mechanical CPR device.

cuers to participate in ACLS procedures, and ensure adequate compression during patient transport. In addition, these devices permit acceptable ECG recordings during compressions and defibrillation without interruption of CPR. The American Heart Association recommends that use of mechanical CPR devices be limited to adult patients. The use of mechanical CPR devices requires special training and authorization from medical control. EMS providers should follow the recommendations of the equipment manufacturers.

● MONITOR-DEFIBRILLATORS

Cardiac monitor-defibrillators are classified as manual or automated external defibrillators (AEDs). The latter may be semiautomated or fully automated. The paramedic should be familiar with the monitor-defibrillators used in the local EMS system.

Manual Monitor-Defibrillator

Modern monitor-defibrillators, developed in the 1960s, are available from a number of equipment manufacturers and have a variety of designs and capabilities. All consist of:

- Paddle electrodes (with "quick look" capability)
- Defibrillator controls
- Synchronizer switch
- Oscilloscope
- Patient cable and lead wires
- Controls for monitoring

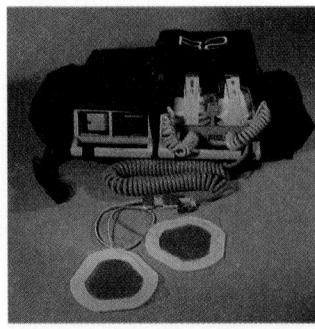

Fig. 18-94 R2 automated defibrillator.

In addition, some manual monitor-defibrillators contain special features such as data recorders and TCP capabilities.

Automated External Defibrillators

AEDs incorporate a rhythm analysis system (Fig. 18-94). They are designed to be used by individuals with minimal training, increasing the range of personnel who can use a defibrillator in a cardiac arrest emergency. The AED is widely used throughout much of the United States. The American Heart Association has recommended that all emergency personnel be familiar with AEDs and be able to interact with other emergency personnel equipped with these devices.[2]

All AEDs are attached to the patient by two adhesive monitor-defibrillatory pads (electrodes) and connecting cables. Like most other types of emergency equipment, AEDs are available from a number of equipment manufacturers; a variety of features and controls are available. Some units provide paper strip recorders, programmable modules, tape recorders, data cards, and voice messages to the operator. All users should familiarize themselves with the AED device used in their system and follow the recommendations of the manufacturer and the guidelines provided by medical control.

A fully automated defibrillator requires only that the operator attach the defibrillatory pads and turn on the device. The rhythm is analyzed in the internal circuitry of the AED. If a shockable rhythm is detected, the AED charges capacitors and delivers a shock.

A semiautomated defibrillator requires the operator to press an "analyze" control to interpret the rhythm and a "shock" control to deliver the shock. The shock control is pressed only when the AED identifies a shockable rhythm and "advises" the operator to press the shock control.

AEDs have five safety features:

1. They can analyze multiple features of electrical activity.
2. Built-in filters check for QRS-like signals, radio transmission waves, 60-cycle interference, and loose or poor electrode contact.
3. They are programmed to detect spontaneous patient movements, continued heartbeat and blood flow, and movement of the patient by others.
4. Multiple evaluations are made of the rhythm analysis before a shock advisory is made or a shock is delivered.
5. To date, there have been no reports of shocks delivered to conscious patients with perfusing ventricular or supraventricular dysrhythmias.

● DEFIBRILLATION

Defibrillation is the delivery of electrical current through the chest wall for the purpose of terminating ventricular fibrillation and certain other nonperfusing rhythms. The shock depolarizes a large mass of myocardial cells at once. If approximately 75% of these cells are in the resting state (depolarized) after the shock is delivered, a normal pacemaker may resume discharging.

The concept of electrical defibrillation was first introduced in animal experimentation in 1899. However, it was not until 1947 that the first successful human defibrillation by direct application of a 60-Hz alternating current (AC) to the heart during surgery was reported.[12] It was later discovered that direct current (DC) defibrillators were more effective and safer. This led to the development of the modern defibrillator in the 1960s.

As a result of the American Heart Association's 1985 Standards and Guidelines Conference, early defibrillation has become the standard of care for patients with prehospital or in-hospital cardiac arrest secondary to ventricular fibrillation.[2] This approach is preferred for four reasons:

1. The most frequent initial rhythm in sudden cardiac arrest is ventricular fibrillation.
2. The most effective treatment for ventricular fibrillation is electrical defibrillation.
3. The probability of successful defibrillation diminishes rapidly over time.
4. Ventricular fibrillation tends to convert to asystole within 4 to 8 minutes.

The modern defibrillator is designed to deliver an electrical shock via paddle electrodes to the patient's chest. The defibrillator accepts the electrical charge from the battery source, stores it in the capacitor, and releases the current into the patient in a short, controlled burst (within 5 to 30 ms).

Paddle Electrodes

Paddle electrodes are designated by location of use as "apex" or "sternum" to allow the operator to view an approximation of lead II though the "quick-look" function. (If the paddles are reversed in polarity or location, a negative QRS complex is noted.) With reference to defibrillation, however, reversal of the paddles is unimportant.

The position of the paddles on the chest wall is extremely important during shock delivery (Fig. 18-95). The paddles should be placed so that the heart (primarily the ventricles) is in the path of the current and the distance between the electrodes and the heart is minimized. This helps ensure adequate delivery of current through the heart. Bone is not a good conductor, and for that reason, the paddles should not be placed over the sternum. As recommended by the American Heart Association, one paddle should be placed to the right of the upper sternum below the right clavicle and the other to the left of the nipple in the midaxillary line.[2] Most manufacturers have both adult and pediatric paddles available. Adult paddles are usually 10 to 13 cm in diameter; pediatric paddles are 4.5 cm in diameter.

The resistance to current that is offered by the chest wall is called *impedance*. The greater the resistance, the less current delivered. Dry, unprepared skin has high impedance. To reduce resistance, electrode gel, gel pads, electrode paste, saline pads, or prepackaged self-adhesive monitor-defibrillatory pads should be placed between the paddles and skin. The electrodes should also be held firmly in place with approximately 20 to 25 pounds of pressure. Whichever method is chosen to decrease impedance, care should be taken to prevent contact (bridging) between the two conductive areas on the chest wall. If contact between the two areas is made, superficial burns of the skin may result and the effective current may bypass the heart (arcing). Even when gels or pads and proper techniques are used, minor skin damage may occur.

Stored and Delivered Energy

Electrical energy is commonly measured in joules (watt seconds). One joule of electrical energy is the product of one volt (potential) multiplied by one ampere (current) multiplied by one second. Delivered energy is approximately 80% of stored energy because of losses within the circuitry of the defibrillator and the resistance to the flow of current across the chest wall. As a rule, 80% of stored energy approximates the amount of joules delivered to the patient.

The American Heart Association recommends that initial defibrillation be attempted 3 times (200, 200 to 300, and 360 joules) and delivered in succession (see p. 656). The pediatric initial defibrillation

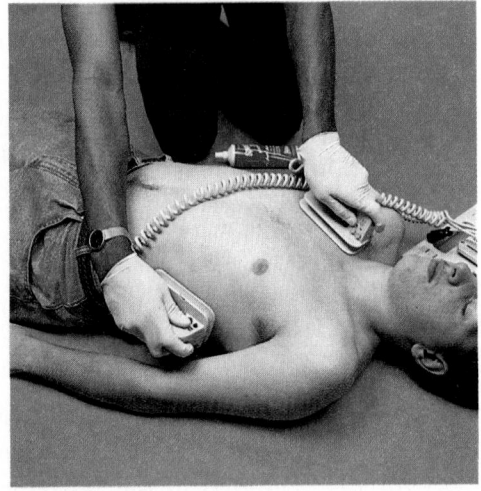

Fig. 18-95 Correct paddle placement for defibrillation.

is generally 2 joules/kg, followed by 4 joules/kg if needed.

Procedure

1. Apply conductive gel to the paddle electrodes (or place saline pads or defibrillatory pads on the patient's chest).
2. Turn the defibrillator power on (make certain that the defibrillator is not in the synchronized mode).
3. Select the energy to be delivered.
4. Charge the defibrillator to the desired energy level.
5. Place the gelled paddles on the patient's bare chest (or nongelled paddles on defibrillatory or saline pads if they are being used), one below the right clavicle near the sternum and one on the patient's lower left chest near the apex of the heart.
6. Make certain all personnel, including the operator, are clear of the patient, the bed, and any equipment that might be connected to the patient. Call *clear* and visually check the patient area from head to toe and from toe to head to ensure that the area is clear before discharge.
7. Press firmly on each paddle with 20 to 25 pounds of pressure. Do not lean over the patient because the paddles may slip.
8. Depress both paddle discharge buttons. Wait for discharge (which should occur within 1 second) and release the buttons.
9. Observe the patient (including palpating for a pulse) and monitor the ECG to determine results. The quick-look paddles are left in place for this purpose if monitoring leads have not been attached.

> ## NOTE:
> The 1992 American Hospital Association recommendation is to deliver the first three shocks in succession without stopping to check a pulse if the monitor clearly demonstrates ventricular fibrillation.[1]

10. If defibrillation fails, continue with the treatment algorithm.

Operator and Personnel Safety

The following ten guidelines are designed to ensure safe defibrillator use[12]:

1. Make certain that all personnel are clear of the patient, bed, and defibrillator before a defibrillation attempt.
2. Do not make contact with the patient except through the defibrillator paddle handles.
3. Do not use excessive gel or saline, which can become a contact between the patient's chest and the paddle handles. Do not discharge paddles over a pacemaker generator or nitroglycerin paste. Remove nitroglycerin patches before defibrillation.
4. To prevent gel from the patient's chest being transferring to the paddle handles, do not have one person perform CPR and defibrillation alternately.
5. Apply gel, paste, or saline pads before turning on the defibrillator.
6. Do not "open air" discharge the defibrillator to get rid of an unwanted charge. Turn the defibrillator off to "dump" the charge.
7. Do not fire the defibrillator with the paddles placed together. This can cause pits on the paddles that can increase the risk of burns to the patient.
8. Treat equipment with respect. It is safe when used properly. Do not touch the metal electrodes or hold the paddles to your body when the defibrillator is on.
9. Clean the paddles after use. Even dry gel presents a conductive pathway that could endanger the operator during a subsequent defibrillation attempt or equipment checkout procedure.
10. Routinely check the defibrillator (including batteries) to make sure the equipment is functioning properly. Follow the recommendations of the manufacturer.

Defibrillator Use in Special Environments

On occasion, a patient requires defibrillation in a special environment (for example, in inclement weather). Although the guidelines in operator and personnel safety always apply, additional precautions are taken in special situations.

A patient can be defibrillated in wet conditions, such as near water, in rain, or in snowy weather. The patient's chest should be kept dry between the defibrillator electrode sites, and the operator's hands and paddle handles should be kept as dry as possible. If in a rainstorm, it would be safest to find shelter.

Depending on the defibrillator and its equipment specifications, the device may not be guaranteed to work properly in nonpressurized aircraft at certain altitudes or pressures. In addition, some electrical interference may occur between the radio equipment in the aircraft and the monitor-defibrillator. This is affected by the distance and angle between the defibrillator and the radio equipment. Recent studies have demonstrated that defibrillation with current equipment in a medically equipped twin-engine helicopter is safe and would be expected to be safe in all types of rotary aircraft used for emergency medical transport.[13]

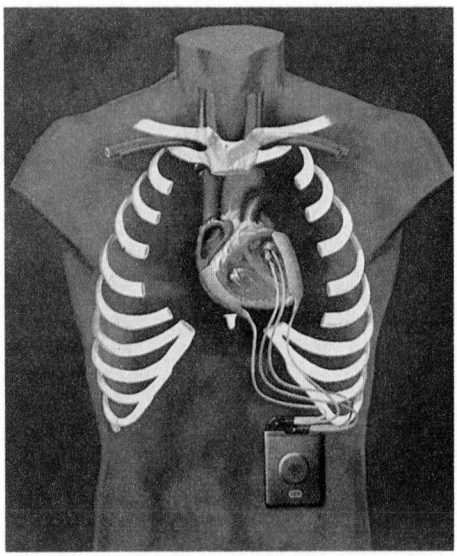

Fig. 18-96 AICD.

● AUTOMATIC IMPLANTABLE CARDIOVERTER DEFIBRILLATORS (AICDs)

The first human implantation of the AICD was performed on February 2, 1980, at Johns Hopkins Hospital in Baltimore, Maryland, by a team led by Dr. M. Mirowski. Since then, more than 35,000 devices have been implanted worldwide. AICDs are commonly implanted through a median sternotomy incision similar to that used for coronary artery bypass surgery, although left lateral thoracotomy, subcostal, and subxiphoid approaches are also used (Fig. 18-96).

During implantation, the two defibrillation patches of the AICD are placed on the epicardium, usually opposite each ventricle to optimize the effectiveness of the device, which is tested intraoperatively. A pair of epicardial sensors is also attached to the left ventricle to monitor cardiac rhythm. The leads are connected to the defibrillator device, which is surgically placed in the left upper quadrant of the abdomen. (An outline of the generator can usually be felt or seen under the patient's skin. The unit weighs approximately 240 g and measures 10 cm by 8 cm by 2 cm.)

The AICD functions by monitoring the patient's cardiac rhythm. When a monitored ventricular rate exceeds the preprogrammed rate, the AICD delivers a shock of approximately 700 volts (for delivered energy of 30 joules) through the patches to restore a normal sinus rhythm. The device requires 10 to 30 seconds to sense ventricular tachycardia or ventricular fibrillation and to charge the capacitor before delivering the shock. If defibrillation does not restore a normal sinus rhythm, the AICD will charge again and deliver up to four shocks. A complete sequence of five shocks, if required, may take up to 2 minutes. If the tachycardia or defibrillation persists after five shocks, no further shocks are delivered. Once a slower rhythm is restored (that is, sinus or idioventricular) for at least 35 seconds, the device can deliver another series of up to five shocks if ventricular tachycardia or ventricular fibrillation recurs.

It is important to treat patients with AICDs as if they did not have a device. Standard ACLS protocols should be followed if the patient is in cardiac arrest or in any other way medically unstable. The American Heart Association recommends the following three guidelines when caring for a patient with an AICD[2]:

1. If the AICD discharges while the rescuer has his or her hands on the victim's chest, the shock from the AICD is perceptible and possibly painful but is certainly not dangerous

to the rescuer. (Gloves protect against transmission of shocks.) The AICD shock is usually accompanied by patient muscle contractions.

2. AICDs are protected against internal damage from conventional external transchest defibrillation shock. Because the epicardial patches may block current, the standard positioning for defibrillation may be less effective, and modifying paddle positions (for example, anterior-lateral to anterior-posterior) should be considered.

3. If an unconscious patient with an AICD is found to be in ventricular tachycardia or fibrillation, external countershock should be applied. Do not wait for the AICD to fire; the device may have already delivered its five-shock sequence and be in the standby mode.

Since the AICD can be deactivated and activated with a magnet, patients with implantable defibrillators should be kept away from strong magnets to prevent accidental deactivation or reactivation of the device. The ability to use a magnet to deactivate and reactivate many of these devices can be useful when the unit is not functioning properly in the clinical situation. However, use of a hand-held magnet to turn the unit off or back on should only be considered with the advice and under the direction of medical control.

● SYNCHRONIZED CARDIOVERSION

Synchronized cardioversion (or countershock) is used to terminate dysrhythmias other than ventricular fibrillation and pulseless ventricular tachycardia. Unlike defibrillation, in which the current is delivered on the operator's command and with no regard as to where the shock occurs in the cycle of the underlying rhythm, synchronized cardioversion is designed to deliver the shock approximately 10 ms after the peak of the R wave of the cardiac cycle (thus avoiding the "vulnerable" relative refractory period). Synchronization may reduce the energy required to end the dysrhythmia and decrease the potential for development of secondary complicating dysrhythmias.

Procedure

When the defibrillator is placed in the synchronized mode, the ECG displayed on the oscilloscope shows a "marker" denoting where in the cardiac cycle the energy will be discharged. This marker should appear on the R wave; if it does not, another lead with a positive QRS complex should be selected. Adjustment of the ECG size may be needed if the marker does not appear. The procedure for synchronized cardioversion is as follows:

1. Turn on the defibrillator and select the synchronous mode.
2. Observe the oscilloscope to make certain the R wave coincides with the marker.
3. Prepare the paddles and place them on the patient's chest as previously described for defibrillation.
4. Set the energy level as prescribed by medical control or protocol.
5. Call *clear* and visually ensure that the patient area is clear.
6. Depress the discharge buttons simultaneously and hold them in. The defibrillator will fire on the next identified R wave. After discharge, release the buttons.
7. If synchronization fails, follow the treatment algorithm. If a repeat attempt is required, it may be necessary to reselect the synchronous mode (depending on the defibrillator).

● TRANSCUTANEOUS CARDIAC PACING

TCP (also known as *external cardiac pacing*) was first introduced in 1952 as a treatment for Stokes-Adams syndrome, a sudden loss of consciousness associated with complete AV block. However, because of the pain and ECG distortions secondary to muscular contractions, the device fell into disuse. In the 1980s, technological advances rendered external pacing an effective emergency therapy for bradycardia, complete heart block, asystole, and suppression of some malignant ventricular dysrhythmias. These devices have been recognized by the American Heart Association and included in the treatment algorithms for bradycardia and asystole (Figs. 18-36 and 18-64).

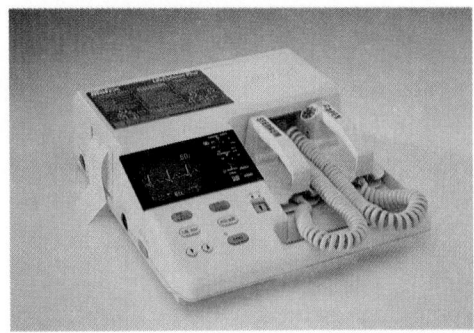

Fig. 18-97 Life Defense Plus defibrillator-pacer.

Artificial Pacemakers

Artificial pacemakers (Fig. 18-97) deliver repetitive electric currents to the heart, substituting for a natural pacemaker that has become blocked or dysfunctional. The patient with severe sinus bradycardia, heart block, or idioventricular rhythm who is capable of generating a pulse with cardiac contractions may respond to an external pacing device and produce a perfusing pulse. (However, the majority of patients in cardiac arrest do not respond to pacing because the heart is metabolically compromised from inadequate perfusion and is therefore incapable of effective contractions, even if it could be stimulated to depolarize by an externally applied electrical stimulus.)

The two modes of TCP are nondemand (asynchronous) pacing and demand pacing. Some devices provide both modes. An asynchronous pacemaker delivers timed electrical stimuli at a selected rate, regardless of the patient's intrinsic cardiac activity. These pacing devices are used less frequently than demand pacers because they have the potential to discharge during the vulnerable period of the cardiac cycle (producing the R-on-T phenomenon). The asynchronous mode is generally used only as a last resort and then usually in asystole. This mode may also be indicated when a significant artifact on the ECG signal interferes with the demand-mode sensing of intrinsic beats. Another use for asynchronous pacing is in overriding inherent symptomatic tachydysrhythmias. However, this should only be attempted if other means of controlling the dysrhythmia have failed and then only with authorization from medical control. This technique of "overdrive" pacing requires modification of most external pacing units.

Demand pacing is designed to sense the patient's inherent QRS complex, delivering electrical stimuli only when needed. It appears to be much safer to apply than the nondemand mode. When it senses an intrinsic beat, the pacemaker is inhibited. If no beats are sensed, the pacemaker delivers pacing stimuli at a selected rate. The device is usually set to discharge at a rate between 70 and 80 beats per minute. It is then increased in increments of 10 until the patient's clinical condition (blood pressure, level of consciousness, skin color, and temperature) improves.

The paramedic should ensure that each pacemaker spike on the oscilloscope is followed by a QRS complex. If not, the current should be gradually increased until there is consistent capture. Unfortunately, motion artifact often makes ECG confirmation of electrical capture quite difficult. The only definitive method of monitoring mechanical capture by the pacing device is the presence of a pulse with each QRS complex. Therefore the patient requires constant monitoring of perfusion status.

Procedure

1. Gather the required equipment.
2. Explain the procedure to the patient.
3. Connect the patient to a cardiac monitor and obtain a rhythm strip.
4. Obtain baseline vital signs.
5. Apply pacing electrodes (avoid large muscle masses) and attach the pacing cable and pacing device.
6. Select the pacing mode.
7. Select the pacing rate (usually 70 to 80 beats per minute) and set the current (begin with 50 milliamps).
8. Activate the pacemaker, oberving the patient and ECG.
9. Obtain rhythm strips as appropriate.
10. Continue monitoring the patient and anticipate further therapy.

Indications and Contraindications

The primary indications for TCP in the prehospital setting are symptomatic bradycardia, heart block associated with reduced cardiac output that is unresponsive to *atropine*, pacemaker failure, and asystole. As previously stated, cardiac pacing is seldom effective in cardiac arrest. It is also ineffective in pulseless electrical activity (for example, electromechanical dissociation) unless the underlying cause of pulseless electrical activity is corrected. Its use is contraindicated in patients with open wounds or burns to the chest and patients in a wet environment.

> **NOTE:**
> CPR may be performed during external pacing, but operator contact with the conductive surface of the electrodes should be avoided. The operator may experience an occasional tingling or muscle twitching in the hands during chest compressions. If the discomfort is great, pacing and CPR should not be performed simultaneously.

Electrode Placement

Proper electrode placement and polarity are important in providing effective external pacing (Fig. 18-98). The best electrode placement (anterior-posterior) is to apply the negative electrode anteriorly over the left hemithorax. The positive electrode is placed on the posterior chest, just beneath and medial to the left scapula and lateral to the spine. In rare situations in which posterior placement cannot be used, the positive electrode can be placed on the anterior right chest in the subclavicular area, with the superior margin of the electrode just below the clavicle. (Anterior-anterior placement may produce pronounced pectoral muscle twitching.) The electrodes should be applied to clean, dry skin without localized trauma or infection.

The conscious patient will probably experience some pain and discomfort during TCP, which is directly correlated to the intensity of muscle contractions and the amount of applied current. In severe cases, analgesia or sedation of the patient may be required.

● CARDIAC ARREST AND SUDDEN DEATH

It is becoming increasingly evident that patients who cannot be resuscitated in the prehospital setting rarely survive, even if they are resuscitated temporarily in the emergency department. The patient's best chance for survival is to have rapid and appropriate interventions in the field. However, if various procedures needed for appropriate intervention (endotracheal intubation, intravenous access) cannot be successfully completed in

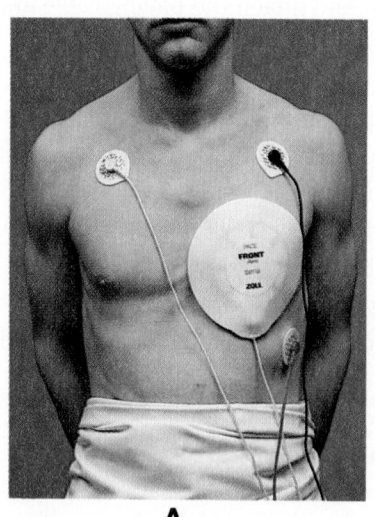
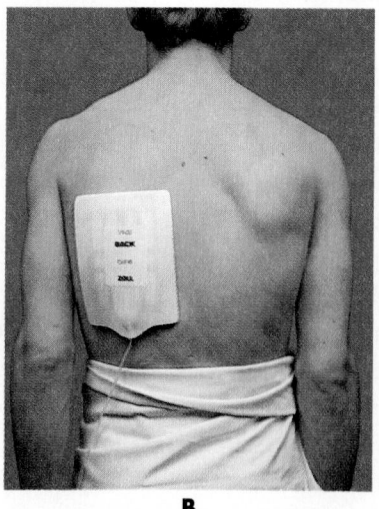
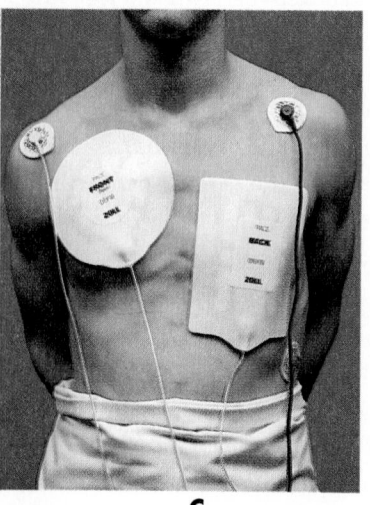

A   B   C

Fig. 18-98 Proper electrode attachment for external pacing. **A** and **B,** Preferred anterior-posterior placement. **C,** Alternative anterior-posterior placement.

a short period, maintaining ventilation and compressions and rapidly transporting the patient to the nearest medical facility should be considered. Initial defibrillation should always be attempted as soon as possible, but prolonged field resuscitation in the face of procedural difficulties is almost always destined to fail.

There is much active research in the area of emergency cardiac care. Some of this research deals with various drugs to improve cardiac or cerebral resuscitation. Because of the fairly large number of patients who regain cardiac function but never regain consciousness, tremendous interest has arisen in how to improve cerebral perfusion. Research in this area may lead to a variety of new medications to be used by paramedics during resuscitation in future years.

REFERENCES

1. Guidelines for cardiopulmonary resuscitation and emergency cardiac care, *JAMA* 268(16):2171, 1992.
2. American Heart Association: *Textbook of advanced cardiac life support*, ed 2, Dallas, 1990, The Association.
3. Grauer K: *A practical guide to ECG interpretation*, St Louis, 1992, Mosby.
4. Rapaport E et al: Guidelines for the early management of patients with acute myocardial infarction: a report of the American College of Cardiology/American Heart Association Task Force on Assessment and Diagnostic of Therapeutic Cardiovascular Procedures (Subcommittee to Develop Guidelines for the Early Management of Patients with Acute Myocardial Infarction), *J Am Coll Cardiol* 16:249, 1990.
5. Taigman M, Canan S: Reading bundle branch blocks, *JEMS* 15(5):41, 1990.
6. Lee G: *Flight nursing: principles and practice*, St Louis, 1991, Mosby.
7. Misinski M: Pathophysiology of acute myocardial infarction: a rationale for thrombolytic therapy, *Heart Lung* 17(6):743, 1980.
8. Tintinalli J et al, editors: *Emergency medicine: a comprehensive study guide*, ed 2, New York, 1988, McGraw-Hill.
9. Grubbs T: The ultimate emergency: managing aortic aneurysms, *JEMS* 16(10):56, 1991.
10. Callaham M: *Current practice of emergency medicine*, ed 2, Philadelphia, 1991, BC Decker.
11. American Heart Association: *Health care provider's manual for basic life support*, Dallas, 1988, The Association.
12. Higgins S: *Defibrillation: what you should know*, Redmond, Texas, 1978, Physio-Control.
13. Dedrick D et al: Defibrillation safety in emergency helicopter transport, *Ann Emerg Med* 18(1):69, 1989.

Summary

Cardiovascular emergencies are frequently encountered by paramedic crews in the prehospital setting. Unlike patients with traumatic injury, which often requires surgical intervention, patients with cardiovascular illness should often have much of their definitive and lifesaving care initiated at the scene. The chain of survival that emphasizes early emergency cardiac care is made possible by well-trained, skilled paramedics working within a sophisticated EMS system.

DIABETIC EMERGENCIES

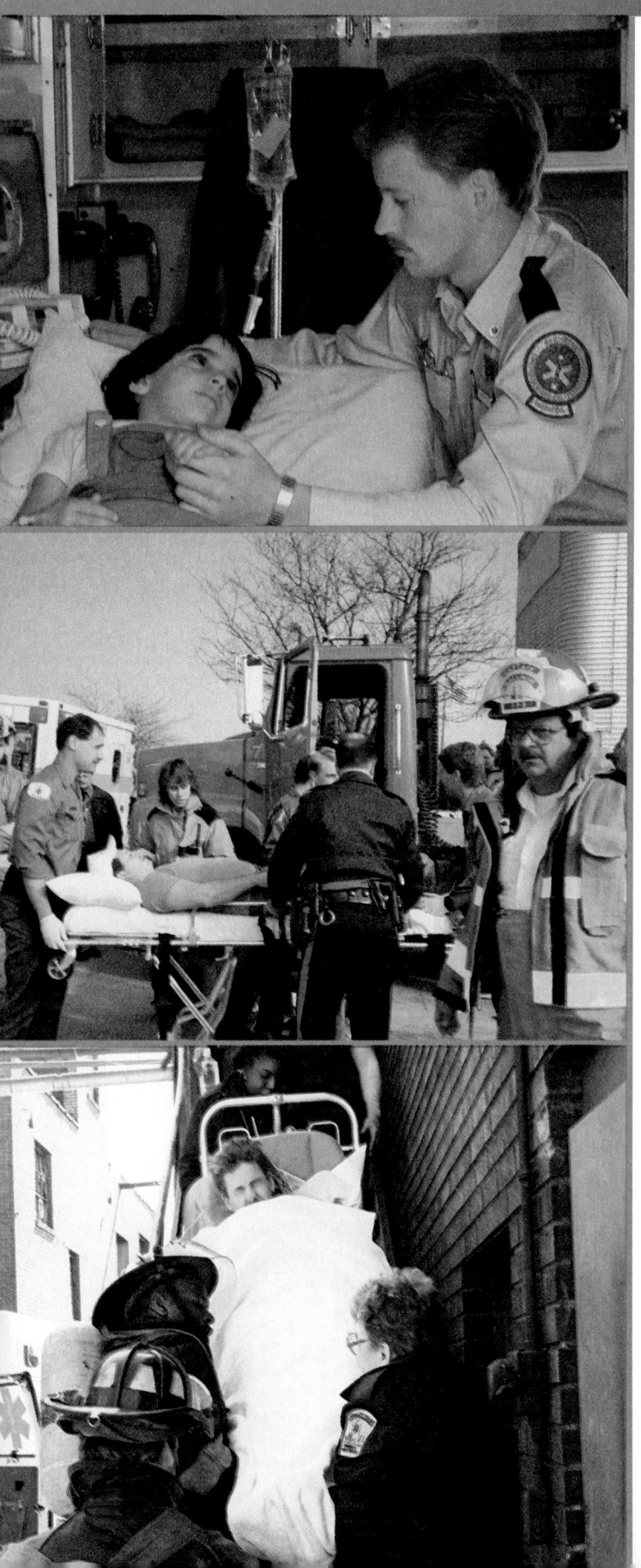

iabetes mellitus is a systemic disease of the endocrine system that usually results from pancreatic dysfunction. It is a complex disorder of fat, carbohydrate, and protein metabolism that affects approximately 5% of American adults, or 12 million people.[1] Diabetes mellitus is potentially lethal and predisposes the patient to several kinds of true medical emergencies.

As a paramedic, you should be able to:

1. Discuss the role of the pancreas in maintaining normal blood glucose.
2. Describe the mechanism of action of insulin and glucagon.
3. Outline how the process of digestion influences serum glucose levels.
4. Discuss the pathophysiology of diabetes as a basis for key signs and symptoms.
5. Describe the role of insulin and oral hypoglycemics in managing diabetes.
6. Discuss pathophysiology as a basis for key signs and symptoms, patient assessment, and patient management for diabetic emergencies of hypoglycemia, diabetic ketoacidosis, and hyperosmolar hyperglycemic nonketotic coma.

● ANATOMY AND PHYSIOLOGY OF THE PANCREAS

The pancreas is important in the absorption and use of carbohydrates, fat, and protein; it is a principal regulator of blood glucose concentration.

The pancreas is located retroperitoneally adjacent to the duodenum on the right and extending to the spleen on the left. The healthy pancreas has exocrine and endocrine functions. The exocrine portion consists of acini (glands that produce pancreatic juice) and a duct system that carries the pancreatic juice to the small intestine. The endocrine portion consists of pancreatic islets (islets of Langerhans) that produce hormones (Fig. 19-1).

Islets of Langerhans and Pancreatic Hormones

There are 500,000 to 1 million pancreatic islets dispersed among the ducts and the acini of the pancreas. Each islet is composed of **beta cells** (75%) that secrete insulin, **alpha cells** (20%) that secrete glucagon, and other cells of questionable function (5%), some of which are **delta cells** that secrete the hormone somatostatin. Nerves from both divisions of the autonomic nervous system innervate the pancreatic islets, and each islet is surrounded by a well-developed capillary network.

Insulin

Insulin is a small protein released by the beta cells when blood glucose levels rise. The primary functions of insulin are to increase glucose transport into cells, to increase glucose metabolism by cells, to increase liver glycogen levels, and to decrease blood glucose concentration toward normal levels. In many of these functions, insulin acts as an antagonist to glucagon.

KEY TERMS

alpha cell: A constituent of the islet of Langerhans that secretes glucagon.

beta cell: A constituent of the islet of Langerhans that secretes insulin.

delta cell: A constituent of the islet of Langerhans that secretes the hormone somatostatin.

diabetes mellitus: A complex disorder of carbohydrate, fat, and protein metabolism that is primarily a result of relative or complete lack of insulin secretion by the beta cells of the pancreas or of defects of the insulin receptors.

hyperosmolar hyperglycemic nonketotic (HHNK) coma: A diabetic coma in which the level of ketone bodies is normal and that is caused by hyperosmolarity of extracellular fluid and resulting in dehydration of intracellular fluid.

Fig. 19-1 Two pancreatic islets (of Langerhans) or hormone-producing areas are evident among the pancreatic cells that produce the pancreatic digestive juice.

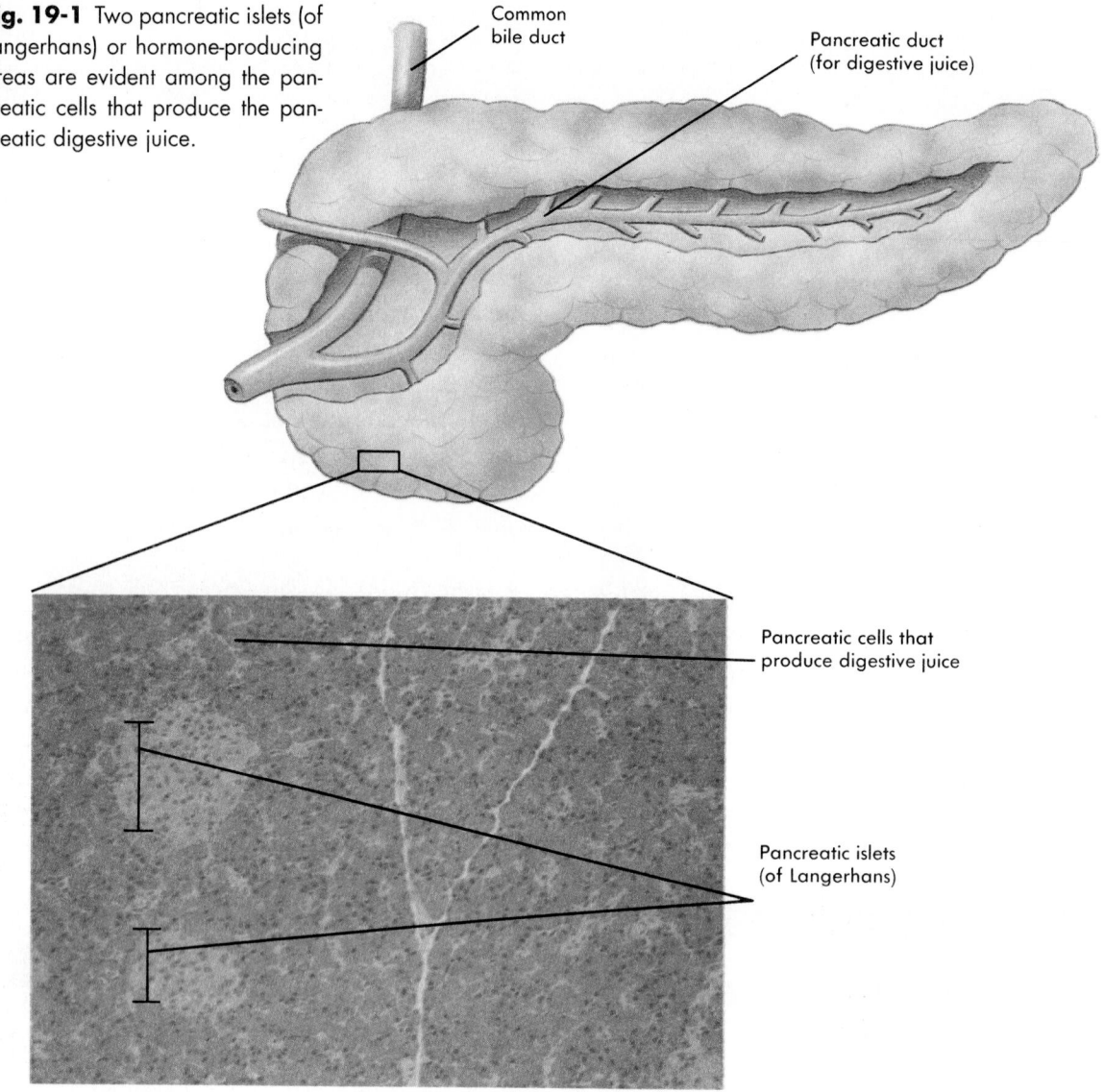

Glucagon

Glucagon is a protein released by the alpha cells when blood glucose levels fall. The two major effects of glucagon are to increase blood glucose levels by stimulating the liver to release glucose stores from glycogen and other glucose storage sites (glycogenolysis) and to stimulate gluconeogenesis (glucose formation) through the breakdown of fats and fatty acids, thereby maintaining a normal blood glucose level (Fig. 19-2).

Growth Hormone

Growth hormone (GH) is a polypeptide hormone produced and secreted by the anterior pituitary gland. GH secretion is triggered by many physiological stimuli, including exercise, stress, sleep, and hypoglycemia. Secretion is suppressed by a rising blood glucose level and is mediated by the hormone somatostatin. GH acts as an insulin antagonist by decreasing insulin actions on cell membranes, reducing the capacity of muscles and adipose and liver cells to absorb glucose.

● REGULATION OF GLUCOSE METABOLISM

Under normal conditions, the body maintains a range of serum glucose concentration that varies between 60 and 120 mg/dl. To understand glucose metabolism, one must understand food intake (food components) and digestion.

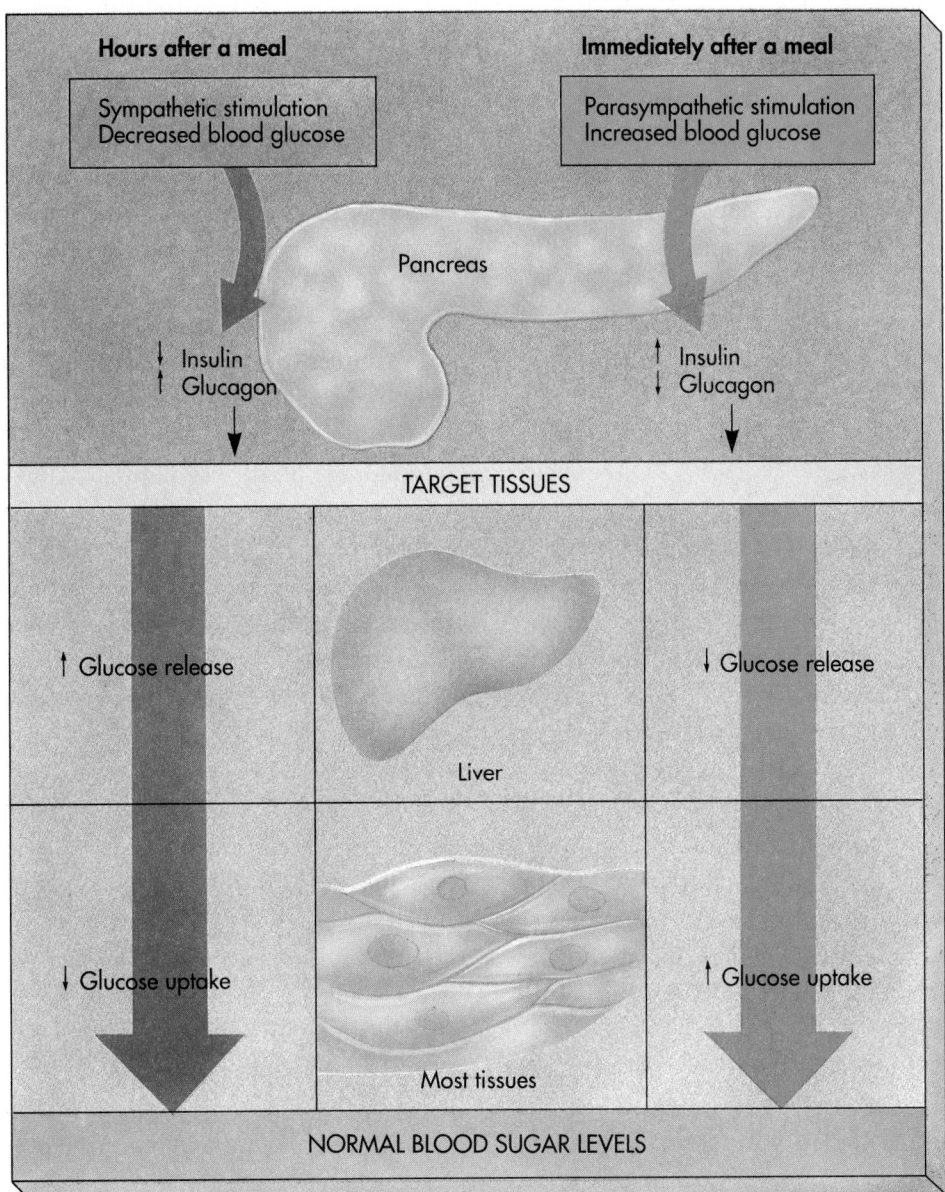

Fig. 19-2 Regulation of insulin and glucagon secretion. Sympathetic stimulation and decreasing concentrations of glucose increase the secretion of glucagon, which acts primarily on liver cells to increase the rate of glycogen breakdown and the secretion of glucose from the liver. The release of glucose from the liver helps maintain blood glucose levels. Increasing blood glucose levels have an inhibitory effect on glucagon secretion. Increasing concentrations of glucose and amino acids stimulate the beta cells of the islets to secrete insulin. In addition, parasympathetic stimulation causes insulin secretion. Insulin acts on most tissues to increase the uptake of glucose and amino acids. As the blood levels of glucose and amino acids decrease, the rate of insulin secretion also decreases.

Dietary Intake

There are three main organic components of food: carbohydrates, fats, and proteins. Food also contains vitamins and minerals. Carbohydrates, which are found in all sugary, starchy foods, are a ready source of near-instant energy and are the first food substances to enter the blood stream after a meal is ingested. Carbohydrates yield the simple sugar glucose. If not "burned" for immediate energy, glucose is stored in the liver and muscles as glycogen for short-term energy needs or converted into fat by adipose tissue and stored for intermediate and long-term needs. Fats in food are slow to convert to a usable form and must be broken down by enzymes into their component parts, fatty acids and glycerol, for uptake by the blood. Excess fat is stored in the liver or in fat cells, which lie mostly under the skin.

Ingested proteins are large molecules built from chains of 20 different subunits, the amino acids. Proteins, like fats and carbohydrates, consist mostly of carbon, hydrogen, and oxygen, along with nitrogen and sulfur.

Process of Digestion

Before food compounds can be used by body cells, they must be digested and absorbed into the blood stream. Digestion begins in the mouth and is accomplished by physical forces (chewing) and by chemical (enzymatic) forces (salivary amylase). This begins the process that reduces the food to soluble molecules and particles small enough to be absorbed. After food is swallowed, it enters the stomach, and various nutrients, including glucose, salts, water, and some other substances (alcohol and certain other drugs), are absorbed into the circulatory system. The remaining chyme is shunted from the stomach into the intestine for further digestion.

The duodenum signals the release of hormones that mobilize the pancreas to contribute its molecule-splitting enzymes and the gallbladder to release bile salts. These enzymes and salts neutralize acids and help emulsify fats. Carbohydrates are absorbed as simple sugars, fats as fatty acids and glycerol, and proteins as amino acids. These nutrients are then carried from the intestine to the liver by way of the portal vein. Water and remaining salts are absorbed from food residues reaching the colon. The liver synthesizes glycogen from the absorbed glucose, lipoproteins from the absorbed fatty acids, and many proteins required for health, including albumin, globulins, and coagulation factors, from absorbed amino acids.

Carbohydrate Metabolism

The secretion of insulin is under chemical, neural, and hormonal control. An increased concentration of blood glucose, parasympathetic stimu-

lation, and gastrointestinal hormones involved with regulation of digestion cause beta cells of the pancreas to release insulin after dietary intake of carbohydrates. Insulin travels through the blood to target tissues, where it combines with specific chemical receptors on the surface of the cell membrane to permit glucose to enter the cell (Table 19-1). This allows the body cells to use glucose for energy, prevents the breakdown of alternative energy sources (proteins and fat cells), and promotes the uptake of glucose into the liver, where it is converted to glycogen for storage. This rapid uptake and storage of glucose normally prevents a large increase in blood glucose levels, even just after a normal meal.

When the blood glucose begins to fall, the liver releases glucose back into the circulating blood. Thus the liver removes glucose from the blood when it is present in excess after dietary intake and returns it to the blood when it is needed between meals. Under normal circumstances, approximately 60% of the glucose in a meal is stored in the liver as glycogen and released later.

If the muscles are not exercised after a meal, much of the glucose transported into the muscle cells by insulin is stored as muscle glycogen. Muscle glycogen differs from liver glycogen in that it cannot be reconverted into glucose and released into the circulation. The stored glycogen must be used by the muscle for energy.

The brain is quite different from other body tissues with reference to glucose uptake. Insulin has little or no effect on the uptake or use of glucose by the brain; the cells of the brain do not have adequate storage capacities, and because the brain normally uses only glucose for energy, it cannot depend on stored supplies of glycogen. Therefore it is essential that serum glucose be maintained at a level that provides adequate energy to these tissues. When serum glucose falls too low, signs and symptoms of hypoglycemia can develop quickly. These include progressive irritability, fainting, convulsions, and even coma.

Fat Metabolism

Because only a limited amount of glycogen can be stored in the liver and skeletal muscles, a third of any glucose passing through the liver is con-

TABLE 19-1 Effects of Insulin and Glucagon on Target Tissues		
Target Tissue	**Response to Insulin**	**Response to Glucagon**
Skeletal muscle, cardiac muscle, cartilage, bone, fibroblasts, leukocytes, and mammary glands	Increased glucose uptake and glycogen synthesis; increased uptake of certain amino acids	Little effect
Liver	Increased glycogen synthesis; increased the use of glucose for energy (glycolysis)	Causes rapid increase in the breakdown of glycogen to glucose (glycogenolysis) and release of glucose into the blood
		Increased formation of glucose (gluconeogenesis) from amino acids and, to some degree, from fats
		Increased metabolism of fatty acids, resulting in increased ketones in the blood
Adipose cells	Increased glucose uptake, glycogen synthesis, fat synthesis, and fatty acid uptake; increased glycolysis	High concentrations cause breakdown of fats (lipolysis); probably unimportant under most conditions
Nervous system	Little effect except to increase glucose uptake in the satiety center	No effect

verted to fatty acids. Under the influence of insulin, fatty acids are converted to triglycerides (storable fats) and are stored in adipose tissue. In the absence of insulin, the stored fat is broken down, and the plasma concentration of free fatty acids rapidly increases. Thus relative insulin deficiency can result in a high circulating concentration of triglycerides and cholesterol (in the form of lipoproteins) in the plasma and is thought to contribute to the development of atherosclerosis in patients with serious diabetes.

If needed (as in the absence of insulin), fatty acids in the liver can be metabolized and used for energy. A byproduct of the breakdown of fatty acids in the liver is acetate, which is converted to acetoacetic acid and beta-hydroxybutyric acid. These products are released into the circulating blood as ketone bodies. The presence of these ketone bodies may cause acidosis and coma (diabetic ketoacidosis) in the diabetic patient.

Protein Metabolism

Insulin causes proteins as well as carbohydrates and fats to be stored. Amino acids (through the actions of GH and insulin) are actively transported into the various cells of the human body. Most amino acids are used as building blocks to form new proteins (protein synthesis), but some enter the metabolic cycle by being converted to glucose after their initial breakdown in the liver.

In the absence of insulin, protein storage stops, and protein breakdown (particularly in muscle) begins. This releases large quantities of amino acids into the circulation. The excess amino acids are used directly for energy or as substrates for gluconeogenesis. The degradation of the amino acids leads to increased urea excretion in the urine. This "protein wasting" has serious effects in diabetes mellitus because it leads to extreme weakness and dysfunction of many organs.

Glucagon and Its Functions

Glucagon has several functions that are opposite to those of insulin, the most important of which is to increase blood glucose concentration. The two major effects of glucagon on glucose metabolism are the breakdown of liver glycogen and increased gluconeogenesis.

As the serum glucose level returns to normal (several hours after dietary intake), insulin secretion is decreased with continued fasting, and the blood sugar level begins to drop. As a result, glucagon, cortisol, GH, and epinephrine (from sym-

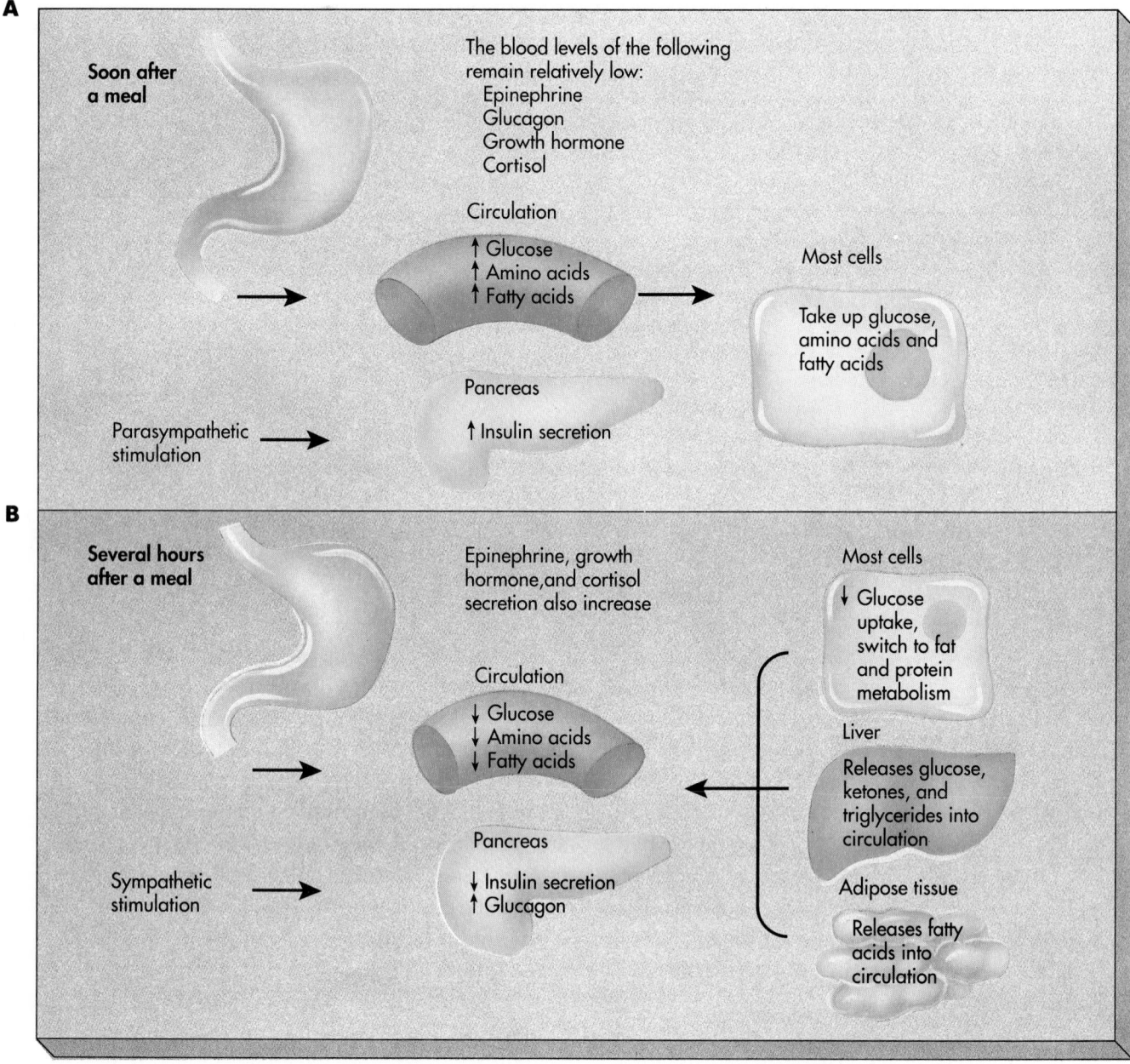

Fig. 19-3 A, Soon after a meal, glucose, amino acids, and fatty acids enter the blood stream from the intestinal tract. Glucose and amino acids stimulate insulin secretion. Cells take up the glucose and amino acids and use them in their metabolism. **B,** Several hours after a meal, absorption from the intestinal tract decreases, and blood levels of glucose, amino acids, and fatty acids decrease. As a result, insulin secretion decreases, and glucagon, epinephrine, and GH secretion increase. Cell uptake of glucose decreases, and usage of fats and proteins increases.

pathetic stimulation) are secreted, initiating the release of glucose from glycogen and other glucose-storage sites. Glycogen is converted back to glucose and released into the blood. Uptake of glucose by most tissues helps maintain blood glucose at levels necessary for normal function (Fig. 19-3).

In summary, the four mechanisms for achieving adequate blood glucose regulation are:

1. The liver functions as a blood glucose–buffer system, removing glucose from the blood when it is present in excess (and storing it as glycogen) and returning glucose to the blood when glucose concentration and insulin secretion decline.

2. Insulin and glucagon function as a feedback control system to maintain normal serum

glucose concentrations. When serum glucose levels rise, insulin is secreted to lower them toward normal levels. Conversely, when serum glucose levels fall, glucagon is secreted to raise serum glucose toward normal levels.

3. Low serum glucose levels stimulate the sympathetic nervous system to secrete epinephrine. Epinephrine and to a lesser degree norepinephrine have a glucagon-like effect that promotes liver glycogenolysis.

4. GH and cortisol play a role in less-immediate regulation of serum glucose levels. They are secreted in response to more prolonged hypoglycemic episodes (for example, late overnight fast) and tend to increase the rate of glucose production (gluconeogenesis) and to decrease the rate of glucose use.

● PATHOPHYSIOLOGY OF DIABETES MELLITUS

Diabetes mellitus is characterized by a deficiency of insulin or an inability of the body to respond to insulin. The disease is often associated with an increased intake of fluid (polydipsia), excretion of large quantities of urine-containing glucose (polyuria, glucosuria), and weight loss. Diabetes mellitus is generally classified as type I (insulin-dependent) or type II (noninsulin-dependent).

Type I Diabetes Mellitus

Type I diabetes is characterized by inadequate production of biologically effective insulin by the pancreas. This form of diabetes affects 1 in every 10 diabetics and may occur any time after birth, usually presenting in teenagers and young adults. Type I diabetes has a heritable component and appears to be an autoimmune phenomenon resulting from a genetic abnormality or susceptibility that causes the body to destroy its own insulin-producing cells. Type I diabetes requires lifelong treatment with insulin injections, exercise, and diet regulation. The symptoms of type I diabetes usually present suddenly and include polyuria, polydipsia, dizziness, blurred vision, and rapid, unexplained weight loss.

Type II Diabetes Mellitus

Type II diabetes is usually characterized by a decreased production of insulin by the beta cells of the pancreas and diminished tissue sensitivity to insulin. The disease occurs most often in adults over 40 years of age and in those who are overweight. (Obesity predisposes a person to this form of diabetes because larger quantities of insulin are required for metabolic control in obese individuals than in those with normal weight.)

Most patients with type II diabetes require oral hypoglycemic medications, exercise, and dietary regulation to control their illness. A small number of patients require insulin injection. Warning signs (if present) are gradual and include all of those associated with type I diabetes. Fatigue, changes in appetite, and tingling, numbness, and pain in the extremities are also indicators.

Effects of Diabetes Mellitus

Most effects of diabetes mellitus can be attributed to one of the following three effects of decreased insulin levels:

1. Decreased use of glucose by the body cells, with a resultant increase in serum glucose

2. Markedly increased mobilization of fats from the fat storage areas, causing abnormal fat metabolism, which may result in the short term in ketoacidosis and in the long term in severe atherosclerosis

3. Depletion of protein in the tissues of the body and muscle wasting

Loss of Glucose in the Urine

When the quantity of glucose entering the kidney tubules in the glomerular filtrate rises above the threshold for reabsorption of glucose by the tubules (typically 80 mg/dl), a significant portion of the glucose "spills" into the urine. The loss of glucose in the urine causes diuresis because the osmotic effect of glucose in the tubules prevents tubular reabsorption of fluid (osmotic diuresis). The effect is dehydration of the extracellular and intracellular spaces.

Acidosis in Diabetes

The shift from carbohydrate to fat metabolism results in the formation of ketone bodies (ketoacids). Ketone bodies are strong acids, and their continuous production leads to a metabolic acidosis, which is often at least partially compensated for by a respiratory alkalosis (manifested by Kussmaul's respirations). The body's mechanism for clearing the acid load by the kidneys is overwhelmed by the continuous production of ketone bodies, and profound acidosis eventually occurs. This acidosis, along with the usually severe dehydration secondary to the osmotic diuresis, can lead to death. The treatment of this condition can be lifesaving. Diabetes mellitus is a systemic disease with a number of long-term complications:

- Blindness
  - A total of 5000 diabetics loose their sight each year.
- Kidney disease
  - A total of 10% of all diabetics develop some form of kidney disease, including end-stage kidney failure, which requires dialysis or kidney transplant.
- Peripheral neuropathy that results in nerve damage to the hands and feet and increased incidence of foot infections
- Autonomic neuropathy that causes damage to nerves that control voluntary and involuntary functions and that may affect bladder and bowel control and blood pressure
- Heart disease and stroke
  - High blood glucose and blood fat contribute to atherosclerosis.
  - Diabetics are 2 to 4 times as likely to develop heart disease as nondiabetics and are 2 to 6 times as likely to have a stroke.

Management

The treatment of diabetes mellitus consists of pharmacological therapy (insulin or oral hypoglycemic agents), diet regulation, and exercise to enable the patient's metabolism to be as nearly normal as possible.

Insulin preparations that mimic the actions of the body's natural hormone were found to be effective in 1920. In the past, they were produced from pig (porcine insulin) or ox (bovine insulin) pancreas. More recently, genetic engineering has lead to human insulin (Humulin), which seems to

be associated with less antibody development. All of these forms of *insulin* are available in rapid-, intermediate-, and long-acting preparations. *Insulin* is administered by injection; it is a protein that would be digested if consumed orally.

Usually, an insulin-dependent diabetic self-administers a single dose of one of the long-acting *insulin* preparations each day and additional quantities of a rapid-acting *insulin* (lasting only a few hours) for those times of day when the serum glucose would be elevated (for example, at meal times).

Another means by which the patient self-administers *insulin* is via an *insulin*-infusion pump. These devices administer a continuous dose of *insulin* and are adjusted so that the level of blood glucose is constantly controlled. Regular monitoring by the patient of glucose levels (blood or urine testing) is necessary to ensure adequate medication control. Medication balance is delicate. The same dosage of *insulin* that appears correct on one occasion may be too much or too little on another occasion depending on various factors (for example, diet, exercise, and infection).

Oral Hypoglycemic Agents

Oral hypoglycemic agents stimulate the release of insulin from the pancreas. They are effective only in patients who have functioning beta cells. Commonly prescribed oral hypoglycemic agents include chlorpropamide (Diabinese), tolazamide (Tolinase), tolbutamide (Orinase), acetohexamide (Dymelor), Glucotrol, and glyburide (Micronase).

● DIABETIC EMERGENCIES

Three life-threatening conditions may result from diabetes mellitus: hypoglycemia (insulin shock), hyperglycemia (diabetic ketoacidosis [DKA]), and **hyperosmolar hyperglycemic nonketotic (HHNK) coma.**

Hypoglycemia

Hypoglycemia is a syndrome related to blood glucose levels below 80 mg/dl. Symptoms usually occur at levels less than 60 mg/dl or at slightly higher blood glucose levels if the fall has been rapid. The condition may occur in nondiabetic patients as well. It is usually a result of excessive response to glucose absorption, physical exertion, alcohol or drug effects, pregnancy and lactation, or decreased dietary intake. In diabetics, hypoglycemic reactions are usually caused by:

- Too much *insulin* (or oral hypoglycemic medication)
- Decreased dietary intake (a delayed or missed meal)
- Unusual or vigorous physical activity
- Emotional stress

Less common causes and predisposing factors include:

- Chronic alcoholism (Alcohol depletes liver glycogen stores.)
- Adrenal gland dysfunction
- Liver disease
- Malnutrition
- Tumor of the pancreas
- Cancer
- Hypothermia
- Sepsis
- Administration of beta blockers *(propranolol)*
- Administration of salicylates in ill infants or children
- Intentional overdose with *insulin*, oral hypoglycemic agents, or salicylates

Signs and Symptoms

The signs and symptoms of hypoglycemia are usually rapid in onset (often within minutes). In early stages, the patient may complain of extreme hunger and demonstrate one or more of the signs and symptoms secondary to decreased glucose availability to the brain:

- Nervousness, trembling
- Irritability
- Psychotic (combative) behavior
- Weakness and incoordination
- Confusion
- Appearance of intoxication
- Weak, rapid pulse
- Cold, clammy skin
- Drowsiness
- Seizures
- Coma (in severe cases)

> **NOTE:**
> Hypoglycemia should be suspected in any diabetic patient with behavioral changes, confusion, abnormal neurological signs, or unconsciousness. This condition is a true emergency that requires immediate administration of glucose to prevent permanent brain damage or death.

Diabetic Ketoacidosis

DKA results from an absence of or resistance to insulin. The low insulin level prevents glucose from entering the cells and causes glucose to accumulate in the blood. As a result, the cells become starved for glucose and begin to use other sources of energy (principally fat). The metabolism of fat generates fatty acids and glycerol. The glycerol provides some energy to the cells, but the fatty acids are further metabolized to form ketoacids, resulting in acidosis.

Because any acidosis increases transport of potassium from the intracellular space into the intravascular space, the subsequent diuresis results in hyperkaluria (high potassium concentration in the urine) and a total body potassium deficit (Box 19-1). In addition, the sodium concentration in the extracellular fluid usually decreases through osmotic dilution and is replaced by increased quantities of hydrogen ions, thus adding greatly to the

> **BOX 19-1**
>
> ## Common Causes of Diabetic Ketoacidosis
>
> - Too-small *insulin* dose
> - Failure to take *insulin*
> - Infection
> - Increased stress (trauma, surgery)
> - Increased dietary intake
> - Decreased metabolic rate
> - Other less common predisposing factors, including significant emotional stress, alcohol consumption (often associated with hypoglycemia), and pregnancy

acidosis. As blood sugar rises, the patient undergoes massive osmotic diuresis, which together with vomiting causes dehydration and shock. The associated electrolyte imbalances may cause cardiac dysrhythmias and altered neuromuscular activity (including seizures).

Signs and Symptoms

The signs and symptoms of DKA are usually related to diuresis and acidosis. They are usually slow in onset (over 12 to 48 hours) and include:

- Diuresis
  - Warm, dry skin
  - Dry mucous membranes
  - Tachycardia, thready pulse
  - Postural hypotension
  - Weight loss
  - Polyuria
  - Polydipsia
- Acidosis
  - Abdominal pain (usually generalized)
  - Anorexia, nausea, vomiting
  - Acetone breath odor (fruity odor)
  - Kussmaul's respirations in an attempt to reduce carbon dioxide levels
  - Decreased level of consciousness

> **NOTE:**
> DKA patients are seldom deeply comatose. Patients who are unresponsive should be assessed for another cause, such as head injury, stroke, and drug overdose.

Hyperosmolar Hyperglycemic Nonketotic Coma

HHNK coma is a life-threatening emergency that frequently occurs in older patients with type II diabetes or in undiagnosed diabetics. The syndrome differs from DKA in that residual insulin may be adequate to prevent ketogenesis and ketoacidosis but not enough to permit glucose use by peripheral tissues or decrease gluconeogenesis by the liver. The hyperglycemia produces a hyperosmolar state followed by an osmotic diuresis, dehydration, and electrolyte losses. Hence, these patients typically have greater hyperglycemia because they are more dehydrated and less ketone formation, since the presence of insulin in the liver directs free fatty acids into nonketogenic pathways, resulting in less acidemia than in patients with DKA (Fig. 19-4). Precipitating factors and signs and symptoms of HHNK coma include the following:

- Precipitating factors
  - Type II diabetes
  - Old age
  - Preexisting cardiac or renal disease
  - Inadequate insulin secretion or action
  - Increased insulin requirements (stress, infection, trauma, burns, myocardial infarction)
  - Medication use (thiazide, diuretics, glucocorticoids, *phenytoin*, sympathomimetics, *propranolol*, immunosuppressives)
  - Supplemental parenteral and enteral feedings

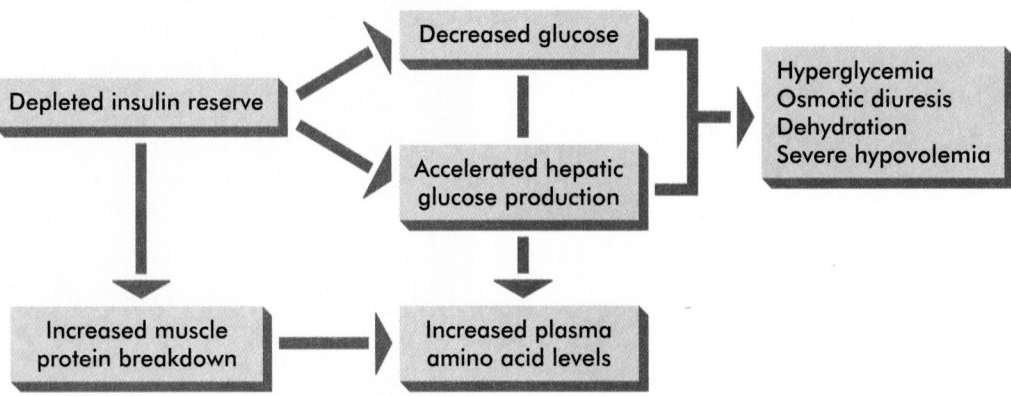

Fig. 19-4 Pathophysiology of HHNK coma.

- Signs and symptoms
  - Weakness
  - Thirst
  - Frequent urination
  - Weight loss
  - Extreme dehydration
    - Flushed, dry skin
    - Dry mucous membranes
    - Decreased skin turgor
    - Postural hypotension
    - Altered levels of consciousness
    - Tachycardia
    - Hypotension
    - Tachypnea

Assessment of the Diabetic Patient

A patient with a diabetic emergency may have a variety of signs and symptoms, many of which may mimic other more commonly encountered conditions. Therefore the paramedic must maintain a high degree of suspicion for diabetes-related illness.

In addition to the patient assessment measures appropriate for any emergency patient encounter (primary survey, secondary survey, and treatment of life-threatening illness or injury), the paramedic should be alert for medical alert information, the presence of insulin syringes, and diabetic medications (often kept in a refrigerator). Components of the patient history important in assessing diabetic patients include onset of symptoms, food intake, *insulin* or oral hypoglycemic use, alcohol or other drug consumption, predisposing factors (exercise, infection, illness, stress), and any associated symptoms.

Management of the Conscious Diabetic Patient

If the diabetic patient is conscious and able to converse, the paramedic should obtain a pertinent history while assessing the patient's airway, breathing, and circulation. High-concentration oxygen should be administered, and if appropriate, the patient should be given glucose.

Medical control may recommend drawing a blood sample for laboratory analysis before ad-

ministering glucose. Some EMS services use field glucose testing with Dextrostix, Chemstrips, or a glucometer (Fig. 19-5). Any patient with a glucose reading of less than 80 mg/dl and signs and symptoms consistent with hypoglycemia should receive *dextrose*. All patients who have experienced a diabetic reaction, regardless of severity, should be encouraged to be evaluated by a physician. During transport, the patient's level of consciousness, vital signs, and ECG should be continuously monitored.

Methods of glucose administration vary by protocol (Box 19-2). If the patient is alert with a gag reflex and able to swallow, sugar may be orally

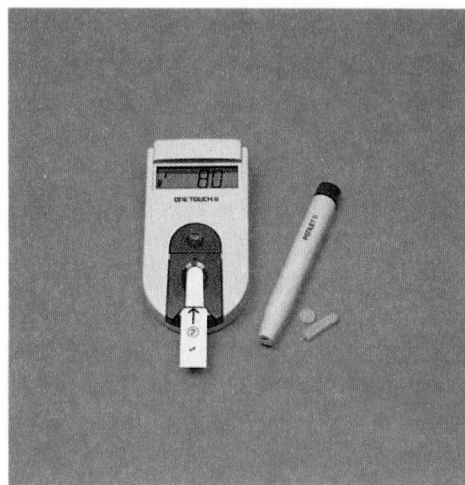

Fig. 19-5 Glucometer for measuring serum glucose levels.

BOX 19-2

Cautions for Administering Intravenous Glucose

- **Dextrose 50%** should not be administered to infants or young children.
- The administration of **dextrose 50%** may precipitate neurological complications in alcoholics and other patients with thiamine deficiency. Therefore **thiamine** administration before or concurrent with the administration of **dextrose** should be considered in patients with suspected thiamine deficiency.

administered in the form of a candy bar, a glass of orange juice mixed with sugar, or a nondiet soft drink or by sublingual or buccal administration of a glucose gel preparation. An alternate method is to slowly administer *dextrose 50%* through a stable peripheral vein. (This dose may be repeated by protocol.)

Management of the Unconscious Diabetic Patient

Prehospital management of any unconscious patient should be directed at airway management, high-concentration oxygen administration, and ventilatory support. Depending on protocol, an intravenous line of lactated Ringer's solution or a saline solution should be established to replenish fluids and electrolytes (flow rate to be indicated by patient's blood pressure and heart rate), and a blood sample should be drawn for laboratory analysis. If alcoholism or other drug abuse is suspected, medical direction may recommend administration of *thiamine naloxone* hydrochloride (Narcan), or both, before the administration of glucose.

TABLE 19-2 Differential Considerations in Diabetic Emergencies

Findings	Hypoglycemia	Hyperglycemia	HHNK Coma
History			
Food intake	Insufficient	Excessive	Excessive
Insulin dosage	Excessive	Insufficient	Insufficient
Onset	Rapid	Gradual	Gradual
Infection	Uncommon	Common	Common
Gastrointestinal tract			
Thirst	Absent	Intense	Intense
Hunger	Intense	Absent	Intense
Vomiting	Uncommon	Common	Uncommon
Respiratory system			
Breathing	Normal or rapid	Deep or rapid	Shallow/rapid
Breath odor	Normal	Acetone smell	Normal
Cardiovascular system			
Blood pressure	Normal	Low	Low
Pulse	Normal, rapid, or full	Rapid or weak	Rapid or weak
Skin	Pale or moist	Warm or dry	Warm or dry
Nervous system			
Headache	Present	Absent	Absent
Consciousness	Irritability	Restless	Irritable
	Seizure or coma	Coma (rare)	Seizure or coma
Urine			
Sugar level	Absent	Present	Present
Acetone level	Usually absent	Usually present	Absent
Serum glucose levels	Less than than 60 mg/dl	Greater than than 300 mg/dl	More than 600 mg/dl
Treatment response	Immediate (after glucose) (NOTE: If the hypoglycemic episode is prolonged or severe, the response may be delayed and may require more than one dose.)	Gradual (within 6-12 hours after medication and fluid replacement)	Gradual (within 6-12 hours after medication and fluid replacement)

NOTE:

If the patient's age (over 50) or clinical history suggests a transient ischemic attack or stroke, the administration of a concentrated glucose solution may exacerbate cerebral damage. (Consult with medical control.) Otherwise, *any patient in coma of unknown origin should receive dextrose*, particularly if hypoglycemia cannot be ruled out as a possibility.

If an intravenous line cannot be established, the administration of subcutaneous or intramuscular *glucagon* helps raise serum glucose levels by stimulating the breakdown of liver glycogen. However, *glucagon* is ineffective in chronic alcoholics and those with liver disease. As previously stated, all patients who experience a diabetic emergency should be transported for physician evaluation. Definitive treatment for patients with DKA requires administration of *insulin,* fluid replacement, and in-hospital observation.

Differential Diagnosis

Differentiating the origin of a diabetic emergency is sometimes difficult in the prehospital setting. When the paramedic is in doubt as to the cause, all diabetic patients should receive glucose. The findings in diabetic emergencies listed in Table 19-2 should assist in the differential diagnosis.

REFERENCE

1. A team approach to diabetes, *Barnes Health News* 8(4):9, 1989.

Summary

Diabetic emergencies are metabolic disorders frequently encountered in the prehospital setting. Although the illness may be life threatening, proper assessment, a thorough history, and appropriate pharmacological therapy can often reverse the immediate pathological process. Volume repletion is the initial primary therapeutic goal in DKA and HHNK coma, whereas administration of glucose is the primary goal of therapy in the hypoglycemic patient.

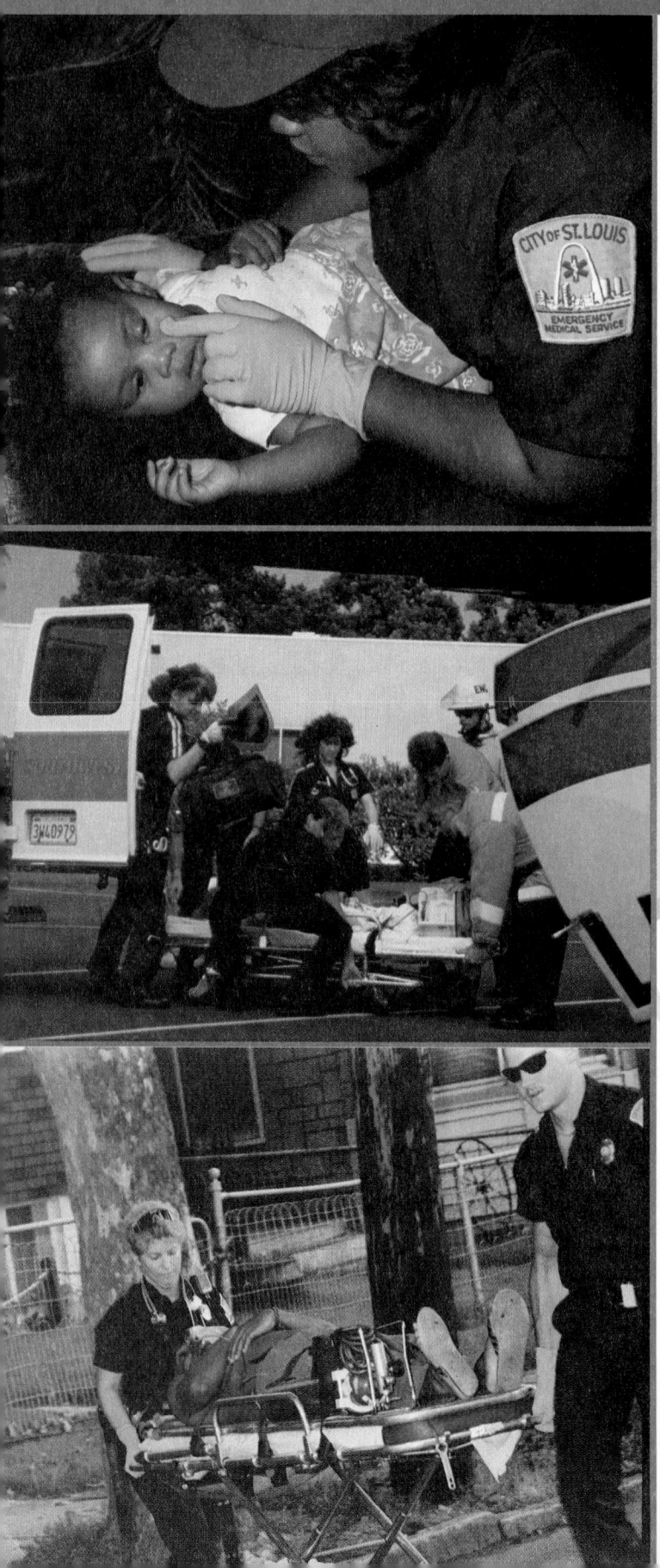

Acute disorders of the nervous system require rapid assessment and treatment. This chapter reviews the anatomy and physiology of the nervous system and explains the prehospital management of common nontraumatic neurological emergencies.

OBJECTIVES

As a paramedic, you should be able to:

1. Discuss the anatomy and function of nerve cells.
2. Describe impulse transmission in the nervous system.
3. Label a diagram of the brain and discuss the normal physiological functions of the blood vessels supplying the brain and the divisions and areas of specialization of the brain.
4. Describe the general assessment of a patient who has a nervous system disorder.
5. Discuss the specific neurological patient evaluation.
6. Describe the pathophysiology, assessment, and specific management techniques for each of the following neurological disorders: coma, seizure, and cerebral vascular accident.

● ANATOMY AND PHYSIOLOGY OF THE NERVOUS SYSTEM

As described in Chapter 10, the nervous system is divided into two parts: the central nervous system (CNS) and the peripheral nervous system (PNS). The human body's ability to maintain a state of homeostasis results primarily from the nervous system's regulatory and coordinating activities.

The CNS consists of the brain and spinal cord, both of which are encased in and protected by bone. A total of 43 pairs of nerves originate from the CNS to form the PNS: 12 pairs of cranial nerves originating from the brain and 31 pairs of spinal nerves originating from the spinal cord. Readers are encouraged to refer to Chapter 10 for a review.

Cells of the Nervous System

The cells of the nervous system include neurons (the fundamental units of the nervous system) and connective tissue cells known as *neuroglia* (specialized cells that protect and hold functioning neurons together). Each neuron consists of three main parts: a neuron cell body, which contains a single, relatively large nucleus with a prominent nucleolus; one or more branching projections called *dendrites;* and a single, elongated projection known as an *axon* (Fig. 20-1). Dendrites transmit impulses to the neuron cell bodies, and axons transmit impulses away from the cell bodies. Axons are surrounded by supportive and protective sheaths formed by the cytoplasmic extensions of neuroglial cells in the CNS (unmyelinated axons) and by the Schwann's cells in the PNS (myelinated axons).

Bundles of parallel axons with their associated sheaths are white in color and are called *white matter.* The action potential, which is initiated in the neuron body, is propagated through the axons via conduction pathways or **nerve tracts** from one

KEY TERMS

nerve: A bundle of nerve fibers and accompanying connective tissue located outside of the central nervous system.

nerve tract: Bundles of parallel axons with associated sheaths in the central nervous system.

postsynaptic neuron: The membrane of a nerve in close association with a presynaptic terminal.

presynaptic neuron: The nerve terminal that contains neurotransmitter vesicles.

reflex: An automatic response to a stimulus that occurs without conscious thought and that is produced by a reflex arc.

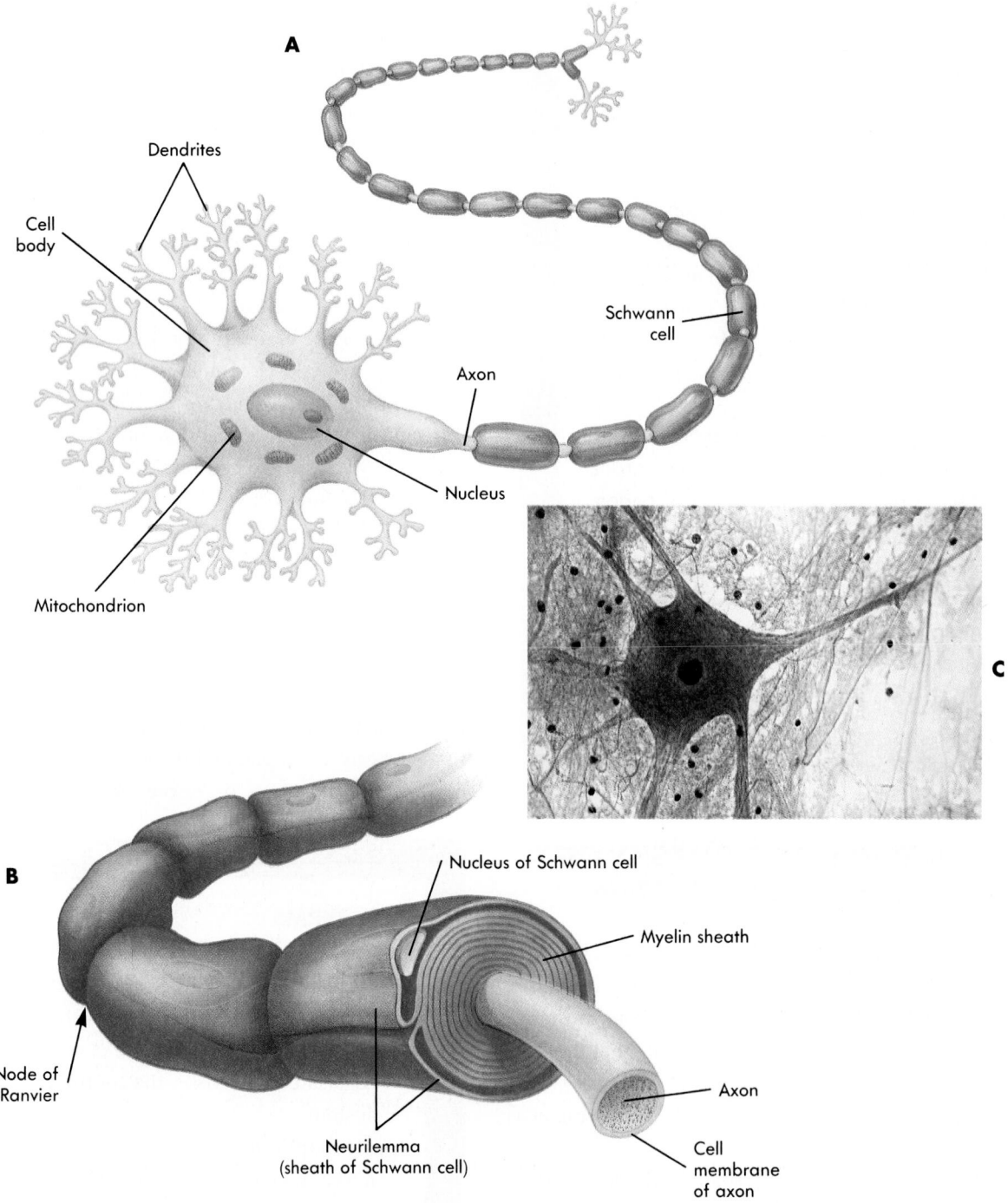

Fig. 20-1 Neuron. **A,** A typical neuron showing dendrites, a cell body, and an axon. **B,** Segment of a myelinated axon cut to show detail of the concentric layers of the Schwann's cell filled with myelin. **C,** Photomicrograph of a neuron.

area of the CNS to another. In the PNS, bundles of axons and their sheaths are called **nerves.** Collections of nerve cells are more gray in color and are called *gray matter.* Gray matter is the site of integration within the nervous system. The outer surface of the cerebrum and the cerebellum consists of gray matter comprising the cerebral cortex and cerebella cortex.

Types of Neurons

Based on the direction in which they transmit impulses, neurons are classified as sensory neurons, motor neurons, or interneurons. Sensory neurons transmit impulses to the spinal cord and brain from all parts of the body. Motor neurons transmit impulses in the opposite direction, away from the brain and spinal cord, and only to muscle and glandular epithelial tissue. Interneurons conduct impulses from sensory neurons to motor neurons. Sensory neurons are also called *afferent neurons,* motor neurons are called *efferent neurons,* and interneurons are called *central* or *connecting neurons.*

Impulse Transmission

The transmission of nerve impulses in the nervous system is similar to the conduction of electrical impulses through the heart. In its resting state, the neuron is positively charged on the outside and negatively charged on the inside. When stimulated by pressure, temperature, or chemical changes, the permeability of the neuron's membrane to sodium ions increases. As a result, positively charged sodium ions rush into the interior of the neuron. This inward movement begins a wave of depolarization that travels down the axon, resulting in the propagation of an action potential (Fig. 20-2).

In unmyelinated axons, action potentials are propagated along the entire axon membrane. Myelinated axons, however, have interruptions in the myelin sheaths known as *nodes of Ranvier.* These nodes allow nerve impulses to "jump" from one node to the next without propagation along the entire length of the cell (saltatory conduction). Therefore myelinated axons conduct action potentials more rapidly than unmyelinated axons.

Synapse

The membrane-to-membrane contact that separates the axon endings of one neuron **(presynaptic neuron)** from the dendrites of another neuron **(postsynaptic neuron)** is known as *synapse.* The structures that compose a synapse are the presynaptic terminal, the synaptic cleft, and the plasma membrane of the postsynaptic neuron. Within each presynaptic terminal are synaptic vesicles that contain neurotransmitter chemicals (Fig. 20-3).

Each action potential arriving at the presynaptic terminal initiates a series of specific events that results in the release of the neurotransmitter substance. The neurotransmitter chemical rapidly diffuses the short distance across the synaptic cleft and binds to specific receptor molecules on the postsynaptic membrane. After an impulse is generated and a conduction by postsynaptic neurons is initiated, neurotransmitter activity ends rapidly. Several substances have been identified as neurotransmitters, and others are suspected as neurotransmitters. Well-known neurotransmitters include acetylcholine, norepinephrine, epinephrine, and dopamine.

Reflexes

One type of route traveled by nerve impulses is known as a **reflex,** or *reflex arc.* A reflex is the basic functional unit of the nervous system that is capable of receiving a stimulus and generating a response. Reflexes allow unidirectional conduction of impulses and have several basic components: a sensory receptor, a sensory neuron, interneurons, a motor neuron, and an effector organ. Individual reflexes vary in their complexity. Some function to remove the body from painful stimuli or prevent the body from suddenly falling or moving as a result of external forces. Others are responsible for maintaining a relatively constant blood pressure, body fluid pH, blood carbon dioxide level, and water intake. All reflexes are homeostatic.

Action potentials initiated in sensory receptors are propagated along sensory axons within the PNS to the CNS, where they synapse with interneurons. Interneurons synapse with motor neurons in the spinal cord, which send their axons out

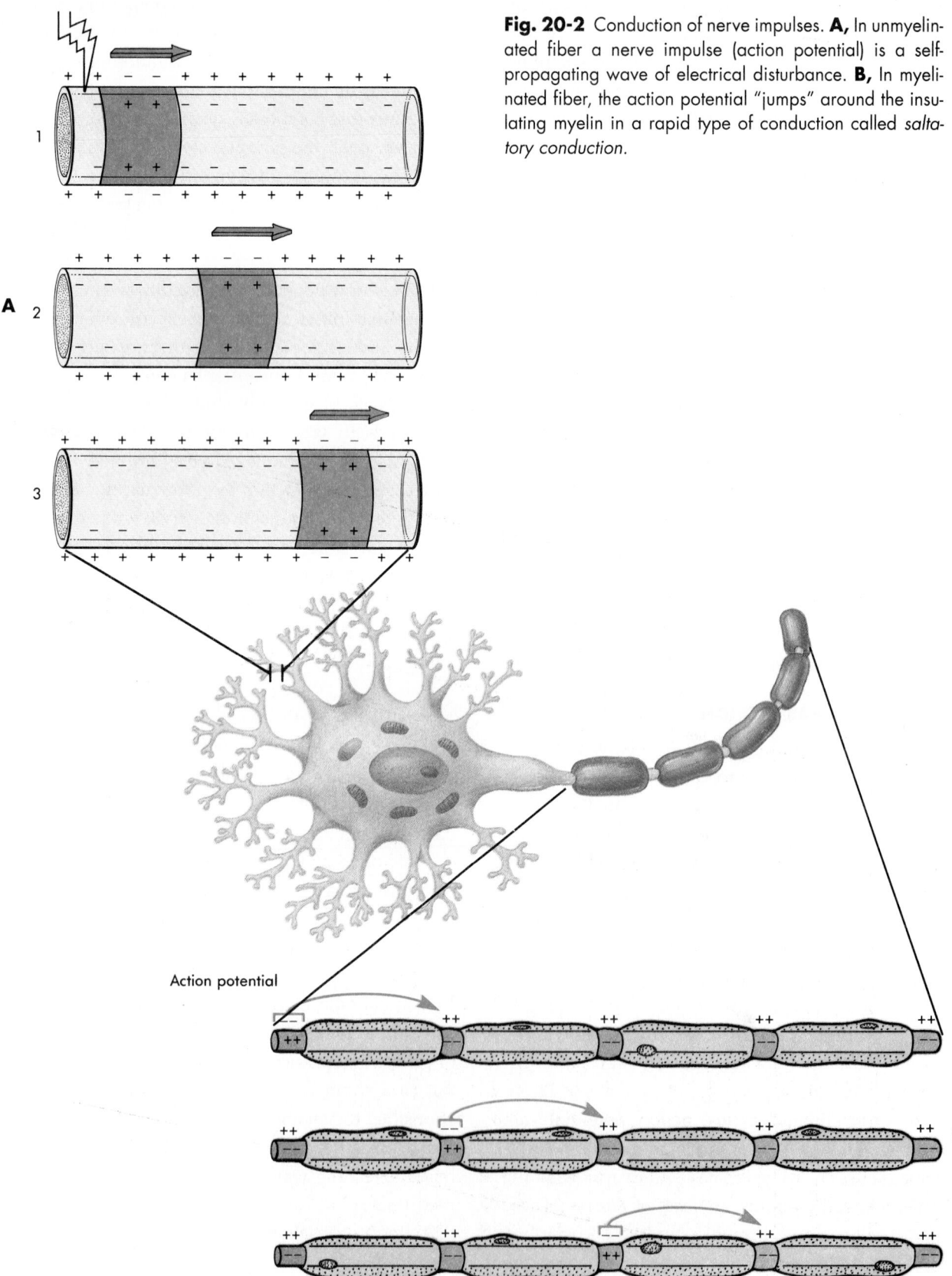

Fig. 20-2 Conduction of nerve impulses. **A,** In unmyelinated fiber a nerve impulse (action potential) is a self-propagating wave of electrical disturbance. **B,** In myelinated fiber, the action potential "jumps" around the insulating myelin in a rapid type of conduction called *saltatory conduction.*

Action potential

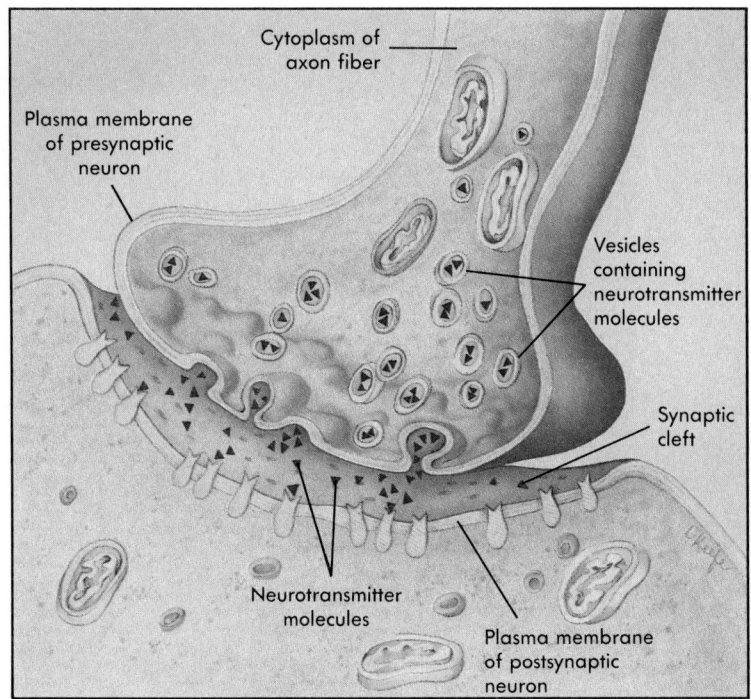

Fig. 20-3 Components of a synapse. Diagram shows axon terminal of presynaptic neuron and a synaptic cleft. When an action potential arrives at the axon terminal of a presynaptic neuron, neurotransmitter molecules are released from vesicles in the axon terminal into the synaptic cleft. Combining neurotransmitter and receptor molecules in the plasma membrane of the postsynaptic neuron initiates impulse conduction in the postsynaptic neuron.

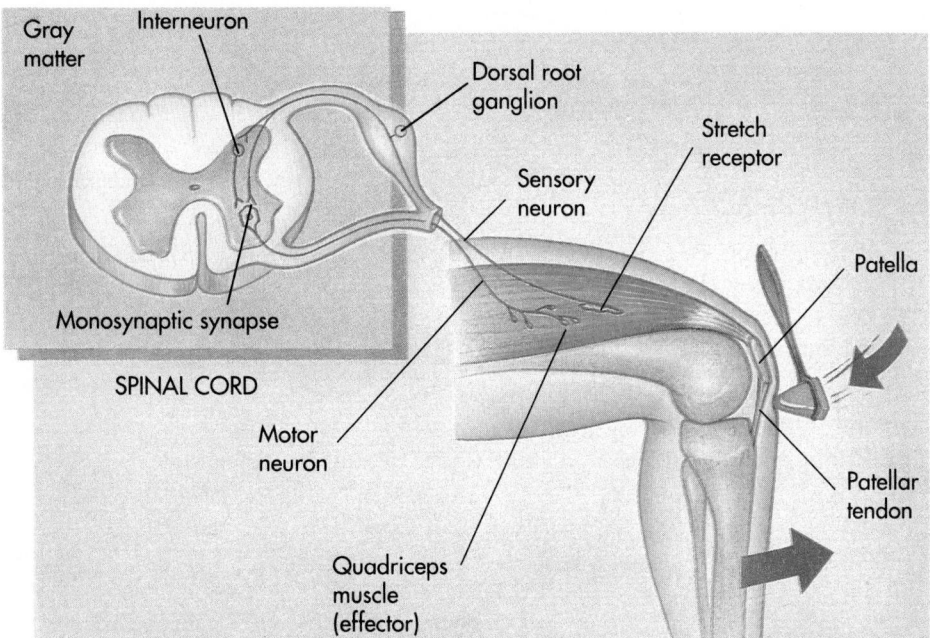

Fig. 20-4 The neural pathway involved in the patellar ("knee-jerk") reflex.

of the spinal cord and through the PNS to muscles or glands, causing the effector organ to respond. Fig. 20-4, which illustrates the neural pathway involved in the patellar reflex, shows the transmission of nerve impulses.

Blood Supply

The arterial blood supply to the brain comes from the vertebral arteries and the internal carotid arteries (Fig. 20-5). The right and left vertebral arteries (supplying the cerebellum) enter the cranial

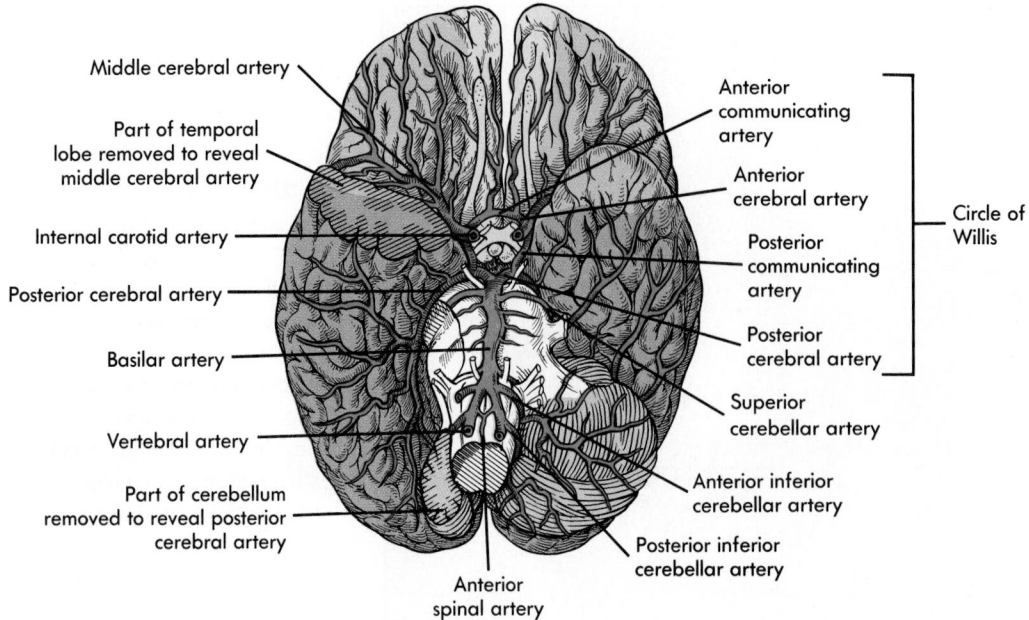

Fig. 20-5 Inferior view of the brain showing the vertebral, basilar, and internal carotid arteries and their branches.

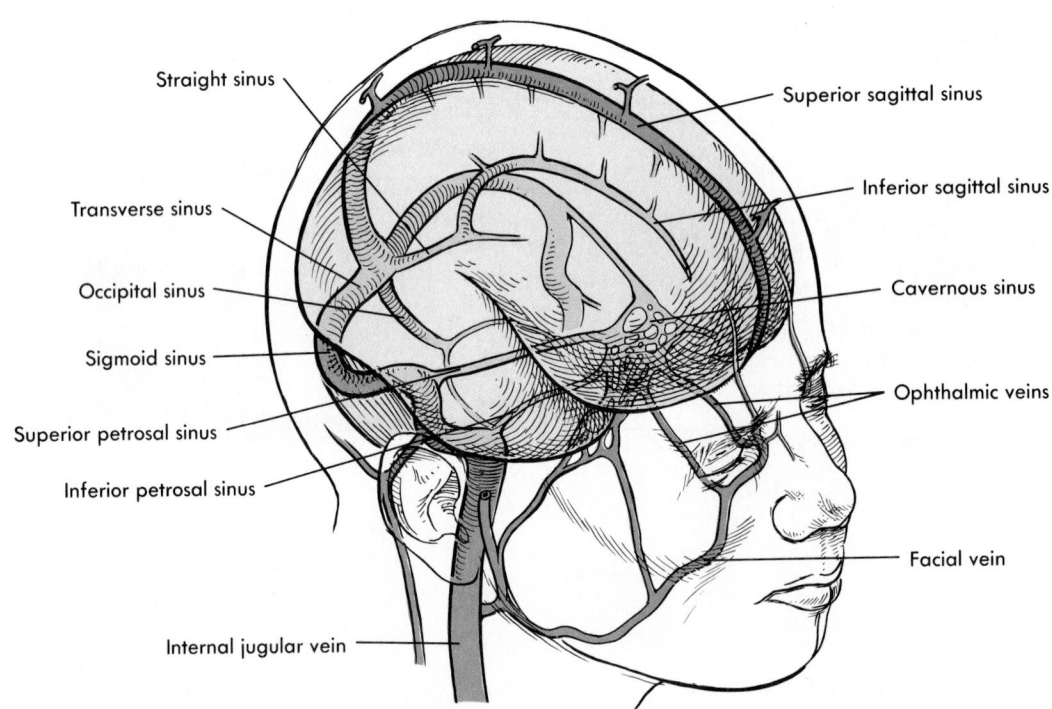

Fig. 20-6 Venous sinuses associated with the brain.

vault through the foramen magnum and unite to form the midline basilar artery. The basilar artery branches to supply the pons and cerebellum and bifurcates to form the posterior cerebral arteries, which supply the posterior portion of the cerebrum.

The internal carotid arteries enter the cranial vault through the carotid canals. These vessels give rise to the anterior cerebral arteries, which supply blood to the frontal lobes of the brain. They terminate by forming the middle cerebral arteries,

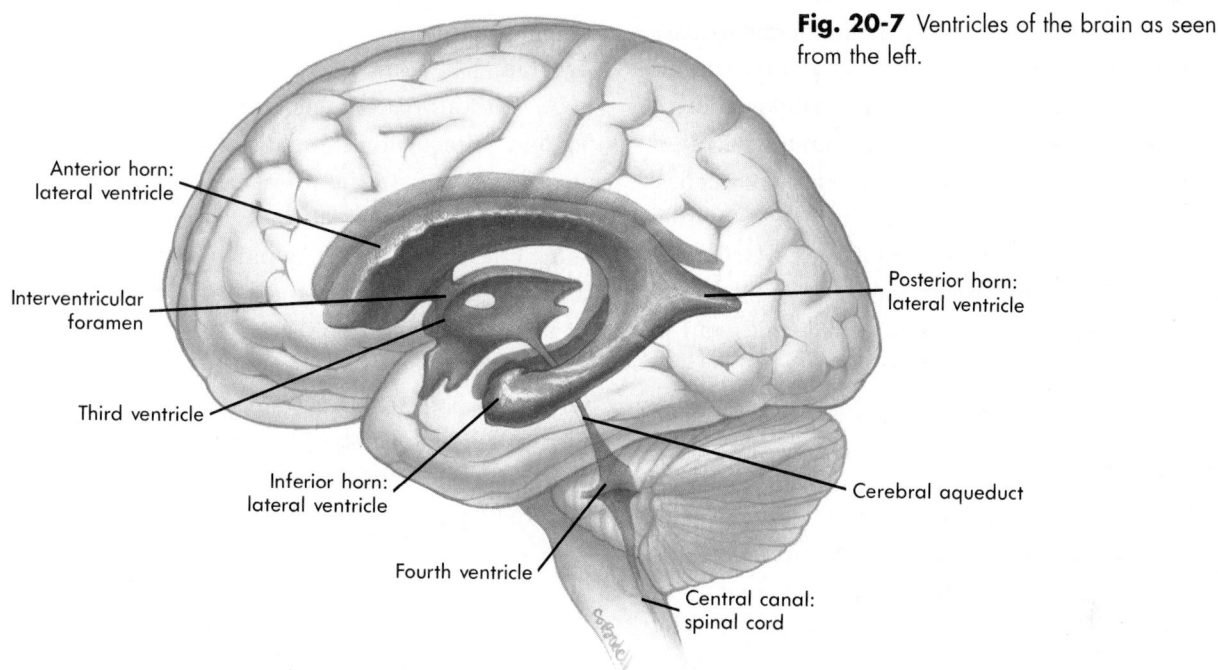

Fig. 20-7 Ventricles of the brain as seen from the left.

Anterior horn:
lateral ventricle

Interventricular
foramen

Third ventricle

Inferior horn:
lateral ventricle

Fourth ventricle

Posterior horn:
lateral ventricle

Cerebral aqueduct

Central canal:
spinal cord

which supply a large portion of the lateral cerebral cortex. A posterior communicating artery branches off each internal carotid artery and connects with the ipsilateral posterior cerebral artery. The two posterior cerebral arteries are connected at their common origin from the basilar artery. The anterior cerebral arteries are connected by an anterior communicating artery and thus complete a circle around the pituitary gland and the brain (circle of Willis). The circle of Willis provides an important safeguard to help ensure the supply of blood to all parts of the brain in the event of a blockage in the vertebral or internal carotid arteries.

The veins that drain blood from the head form the venous sinuses (spaces within the dura mater surrounding the brain) and eventually drain into the internal jugular veins (Fig. 20-6). These veins exit the cranial vault and receive several venous tributaries that drain the external head and face. The internal jugular veins join the subclavian veins on each side of the body.

Ventricles

Each cerebral hemisphere contains a large space filled with cerebral spinal fluid known as a *lateral ventricle*. The lateral ventricles are connected pos-

teriorly with the third ventricle located in the center of the diencephalon between the two halves of the thalamus. The two lateral ventricles communicate with the third ventricle through two interventricular foramina. The third ventricle communicates with the fourth ventricle (located in the superior region of the medulla) by way of a narrow canal known as the *cerebral aqueduct*. The fourth ventricle is continuous with the central canal of the spinal cord (Fig. 20-7).

Divisions of the Brain

As explained in Chapter 10, the major divisions of the adult brain are the brain stem (medulla, pons, midbrain, and site of the reticular formation), cerebellum, diencephalon (hypothalamus and thalamus), and cerebrum.

● NEUROLOGICAL PATHOPHYSIOLOGY

Some neurological emergencies are a consequence of structural changes or damage, circulatory changes, or alterations in intracranial pressure (ICP). Because the skull is a rigid closed space, any increase in volume of the intracranial contents causes a significant elevation in ICP. The three structures that occupy the intracranial space are brain tissue, blood, and water. Brain tissue contains mostly water, both intracellular and extracellular. Blood is contained within the major arteries in the base of the brain; in arterial branches, arterioles, capillaries, venules, and veins within the substance of the brain; and in the cortical veins and dural sinuses. Water is located in the ventricles of the brain, in cerebrospinal fluid, and in extracellular and intracellular fluid.

Intracranial Pressure

Normally, the volumes of brain tissue, blood, and water are such that the pressure inside the skull is maintained within a few millimeters of mercury above atmospheric pressure. (Normal ICP is 5.8 to 13 mm Hg, or 70 to 190 mm H_2O.) However, if a mass or cerebral edema develops, there must be an immediate reduction in the volume of one or more of these components to prevent the ICP from rising and compressing brain tissue. With mild-to-moderate elevation of ICP, mean arterial pressure (MAP) usually rises. As discussed in Chapter 15, MAP is the diastolic pressure plus one-third pulse pressure. MAP is proportional to cardiac output times peripheral resistance. The rise in MAP causes cerebral blood vessels to constrict and prevents the increase in blood volume and cerebral blood flow that would normally occur.

Conversely, if the MAP falls, the cerebral arteries dilate and increase cerebral blood flow. Thus between a MAP of approximately 60 and 140 mm Hg, cerebral blood flow may be maintained in a constant state. However, when ICP elevations are marked (greater than 22 mm Hg), perfusion of brain tissue often decreases despite a rise in systemic arterial pressure. Marked elevations in ICP can also lead to the catastrophic consequence of herniation of brain tissue. Both complications commonly result in brain death.

Assessment of the Nervous System

Although there are many similarities in the approaches to assessing traumatic and nontraumatic neurological deficits, the following discussion of patient assessment focuses on nontraumatic neurological emergencies. (Assessment of neurological trauma is addressed in Chapter 15.)

As with all patient encounters, initial care of a patient with a nontraumatic neurological emergency begins with the primary survey. The paramedic maintains a systematic approach in examining these patients to avoid overlooking signs and symptoms that may indicate the development of an urgent condition. Goals of emergency care are control of the airway, stabilization and support of the cardiovascular system, intervention to interrupt ongoing cerebral injury, and protection of the patient from further harm while at the scene and during transport to an appropriate medical facility.

Primary Survey

The primary survey should begin by determining the patient's level of consciousness and by ensuring an open and patent airway. If the patient is unconscious on EMS arrival and there is reason to suspect a cervical spine injury, the patient's airway should be opened with a chin-lift or modified jaw-thrust maneuver with spinal precautions, and the cervical spine should be immobilized. The paramedic should remember that unconscious patients are unable to maintain their airways. Therefore airway adjuncts (including tracheal intubation) may be indicated. The patient's airway should also be closely monitored for respiratory arrest, which may result from increased ICP and vomiting or aspiration of stomach contents. Suction should be readily available.

Ventilatory support and supplemental oxygen administration should be provided for any patient experiencing a neurological emergency. Increased carbon dioxide pressure (Pco_2) or decreased oxygen pressure (Po_2) results in dilation of the blood vessels, presumably in response to greater cerebral metabolic needs. As Pco_2 is lowered, blood volume and flow to the brain are reduced. Controlled hyperventilation should therefore be used to maintain Pco_2 at approximately 30 mm Hg and Po_2 at greater than 80 mm Hg.

Secondary Survey

The patient with neurological illness may be difficult to assess, particularly if the patient's mental function is impaired. Important elements of the secondary survey that may provide clues to the nature of the neurological emergency include patient history and history of the event, vital signs, and respiratory patterns.

History

After any life-threatening problems have been identified and corrected, the paramedic should attempt to gather a thorough history of the event from the patient or from family members or bystanders. Important elements of the patient history include the following six:

1. The patient's chief complaint
2. Details of the presenting illness
3. Pertinent underlying medical problems
   a. Cardiac disease
   b. Lung disease
   c. Neurological disease (for example, multiple sclerosis)
   d. Previous stroke
   e. Chronic seizures
   f. Diabetes
   g. Hypertension
4. Drug or alcohol use
5. Previous history of similar symptoms
6. Recent injury (particularly head trauma)

If loss of consciousness was involved, the paramedic should ascertain the events that preceded the unconscious state, such as patient position (sitting, standing, lying down), complaints of a headache, seizure activity, or a fall. When no history is available, the paramedic should assume that the onset of unconsciousness was acute and that an intracranial hemorrhage is likely. In addition, the paramedic should be alert to the presence of any environmental clues, such as evidence of current prescribed medications, medical alert identification, recreational drugs, or alcohol or drug paraphernalia.

Vital Signs

Vital signs should be checked and recorded frequently because they often change rapidly in patients with a neurological emergency. The patient's electrocardiogram (ECG) should also be monitored for dysrhythmias, which are common in these scenarios. In the early stages of increased ICP, there is an increase in systolic pressure, wid-ened pulse pressure, and a decrease in the pulse and respiratory rate (Cushing's triad). In the terminal stages, as ICP continues to rise and brain tissue is compressed, body temperature usually remains elevated, but the pulse rate generally decreases and the blood pressure falls, particularly after herniation occurs. Therefore hypotension is a late and ominous sign in patients with isolated neurological pathology.

Respiratory Patterns

The respiratory pattern of a patient with a neurological emergency may be normal or abnormal. In the absence of respiratory arrest caused by CNS dysfunction of the lower respiratory centers in the medulla, abnormalities of respiratory rate and rhythm may give clues to the mechanisms responsible and the level of neurological dysfunction. Although apnea can occur with loss of consciousness even with relatively minor head trauma, acute respiratory arrest usually results from involvement of the medullary respiratory center (brain stem compression or infarct). Neural pathway involvement (anywhere from the cortex down to the medulla) is more often associated with disturbances of respiratory rhythm, not with respiratory arrest. Abnormal respiratory patterns include the following:

- Cheyne-Stokes respiration
- Central neurogenic hyperventilation
- Ataxic respiration
- Apneustic respiration
- Diaphragmatic breathing

Neurological Evaluation

Some neurological complications are obvious (such as paralysis), whereas others may be subtle (for example, a decreasing sensorium). A sudden or rapidly worsening level of consciousness is the single most suggestive sign of a serious neurological condition.

Use of the mnemonic device AVPU and the Glasgow coma scale (see Chapters 11 and 15) are rapid, convenient ways to determine the patient's baseline neurological status and to allow comparisons during future treatment. Evaluation should be repeated and recorded frequently so that changes in the patient's mental state may be detected at the earliest possible time.

When evaluating a patient's neurological status, the paramedic should report and record patient information with descriptive terms specific to responses to certain stimuli (for example, "the patient has no recall of the event"; "the patient moves on command"; "the patient does not open his or her eyes to painful stimuli"). Using clear descriptions of the patient's response permits others involved in the patient's care to follow the patient's progression.

Posturing, Muscle Tone, and Paralysis

Significant neurological emergencies may be associated with abnormal or unusual posturing, paralysis of a limb or several limbs, or both. Generally, disturbances of posture result from flexor spasms, extensor spasms, or flaccidity. Abnormal flexor responses of one or both arms with extension of the legs is called *decorticate rigidity*. This abnormal posturing is thought to result from structural impairment of certain cortical regions of the brain. Abnormal extensor response of the arms with extension of the legs is called *decerebrate rigidity*. Decerebrate rigidity has a worse prognosis than decorticate rigidity and is thought to result from impairment of certain subcortical regions of the brain. Flaccidity is usually caused by brain stem or cord dysfunction and carries a dismal prognosis.

In addition to fixed, nonpurposeful posturing of the limbs, abnormal reflexes may also be present. These include Babinski's sign (see Chapters 11 and 15) and evacuation of the bowels and bladder.

Pupillary Reflexes

Examination of the pupils is an important evaluation in the unconscious patient. Often, the diagnosis of drug intoxication can at least be suspected based on pupillary appearance and reaction. For example, with opiate overdose, the pupils are usually small but reactive to light. If deviations from normal (in relative symmetry, size, and prompt reaction to light) are observed, it is important to note whether these deviations are unilateral or bilateral. If both pupils are dilated and do not react to light, the patient's brain stem has probably been affected, or the patient has suffered severe cerebral anoxia.

Pupillary constriction is controlled by parasympathetic fibers that originate in the midbrain and accompany the oculomotor nerve (cranial nerve III). Pupillary dilation involves fibers that descend the entire brain stem and ascend in the cervical sympathetic chains. Midbrain failure interrupts both pathways and generally results in fixed, midsize pupils. Third nerve compression interrupts parasympathetic tone and is manifested by a unilateral, fixed, dilated pupil. Any unconscious patient who suddenly develops a fixed, dilated pupil probably has a temporal lobe herniation, which requires immediate transport to an appropriate medical facility.

Extraocular Movements

Conscious patients should be able to move their eyes in full directional ranges. Extraocular movements can be evaluated by requesting that the patient follow the finger movements of the paramedic: to the extreme left and then up and down

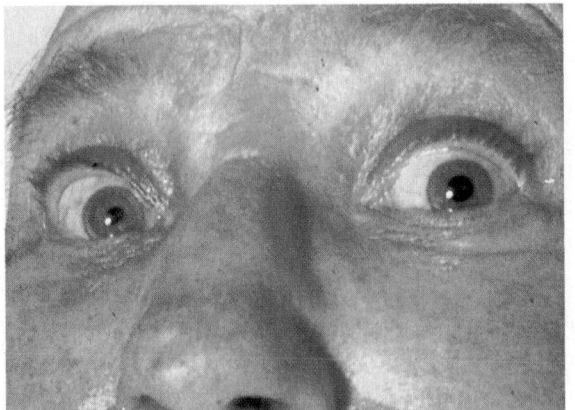

A

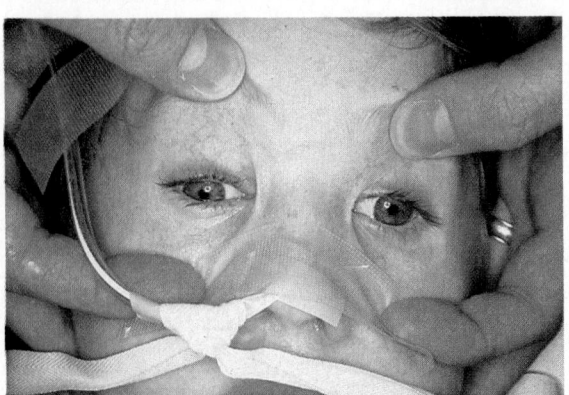

B

Fig. 20-8 A, Conjugate gaze. **B,** Dysconjugate gaze.

and to the extreme right and then up and down. Any deviations from normal should be recorded.

Deviation of both eyes to either side (conjugate gaze) at rest implies a structural lesion. The lesion may have an "irritative focus" in which the eyes look away from the lesion or a "destructive focus" in which the eyes look toward the lesion. Deviation of the eyes to opposite sides (dysconjugate gaze) at rest implies a structural brain stem dysfunction in the pathways that traverse the brain stem from the upper midbrain to at least the level of the lower pons (Fig. 20-8).

Management

Emergency care for patients with neurological emergencies is directed at controlling the airway, stabilizing and supporting the cardiovascular system, minimizing the potential for additional cerebral dysfunction, and protecting the patient from further harm while at the scene and during transport to an appropriate medical facility.

● PATHOPHYSIOLOGY AND MANAGEMENT OF SPECIFIC CNS DISORDERS

Although many CNS disorders can result in an altered level of consciousness, paramedics are most likely to encounter patients with abnormalities of the CNS who have coma, seizure, or cerebral vascular accident (CVA).

Coma

Coma is an abnormally deep state of unconsciousness from which the patient cannot be aroused by external stimuli. In general terms, only two mechanisms produce coma: (1) structural lesions that depress consciousness by destroying or encroaching on the ascending reticular activating system in the brain stem and (2) toxic metabolic states that involve the presence of circulating toxins or metabolites or the lack of metabolic substrate (for example, oxygen or glucose). Either mechanism may cause diffuse depression of both cerebral hemispheres, with or without depression of the ascending reticular activating system.

Within these two mechanisms there are six general causes of coma (Box 20-1).

In addition, coma states can be mimicked by certain psychiatric conditions (for example, "hysterical coma") in which the unconscious state has no organic origin. Patients who are experiencing a voluntary or involuntary psychogenic episode

---

BOX 20-1

Six General Causes of Coma

Structural Causes
- Intracranial bleeding
- Head trauma
- Brain tumor or other space-occupying lesions

Metabolic System
- Anoxia
- Hypoglycemia
- Diabetic ketoacidosis
- Thiamine deficiency
- Kidney and liver failure
- Postictal phase of seizure

Drugs
- Barbiturates
- Narcotics
- Hallucinogenics
- Depressants
- Alcohol

Cardiovascular System
- Hypertensive encephalopathy
- Shock
- Dysrhythmias
- Stroke

Respiratory System
- Chronic obstructive pulmonary disease
- Toxic inhalation (carbon monoxide poisoning)

Infection
- Meningitis
- Sepsis

often vigorously blink and move the eyes and generally respond to noxious physical or verbal stimuli, whereas patients with organic sources of coma are unresponsive. A mnemonic aid that may be useful in remembering the common causes of coma is AEIOU TIPS (Box 20-2).

Structural Versus Toxic-Metabolic Coma

Two major factors distinguish structural and toxic metabolic causes of coma. In patients with structural causes, there is a common association of focal (asymmetrical) neurological deficits, whereas in patients with coma of toxic metabolic origin the neurological findings are often symmetrical. In addition, coma of toxic metabolic origin is often slow in onset, whereas structural lesions occur acutely.

Perhaps the most important physical findings in helping distinguish structural and toxic metabolic causes of coma are the pupillary responses. Preserved pupillary responses suggest that the origin of coma is toxic metabolic, whereas unresponsive or asymmetrical pupillary responses point to a structural cause. The cerebral cortex is more sensitive to toxic metabolic disturbances than are other parts of the CNS. Management is principally medical. If toxic metabolic coma is associated with fever, bacterial meningitis should be suspected. Coma associated with very high fevers (body temperature greater than 40° C [105° F]) during the summer months suggests heat stroke. Cocaine, seizures (status or prolonged), and phenothiazines can also produce coma and fever.

Unlike metabolic coma, structural coma follows a progressive pattern of deterioration caused by focal pressure or compression. The syndrome is often sudden in onset with an asymmetrical secondary examination (for example, hemiparesis). As a rule, structural lesions affect the ascending reticular activating system by virtue of increased ICP and herniation and require rapid surgical correction. Distinguishing between toxic metabolic coma and structural coma can help prepare the paramedic to anticipate the course of the patient's condition.

Assessment and Management

Regardless of the cause of coma, prehospital care is directed at support of the patient's vital functions, prevention of further deterioration of the patient's condition, and administration of medications, intravenous fluids, or both, to treat potentially reversible causes of coma. As always, airway maintenance and ventilatory support with supplemental oxygen are the first priorities in patient stabilization.

If the patient's respirations are abnormally slow or shallow or if cerebral edema is suspected, the patient's lungs should be hyperventilated at 24 to 30 breaths per minute. The tracheas of unconscious patients who have no gag reflex should be intubated. After the airway is secured, management of a patient in coma of unknown origin includes the following:

1. Establish an intravenous line of D_5W to keep the vein open (or lactated Ringer's or normal saline if hypotension is present).
2. Monitor cardiac rhythm.
3. Per protocol, draw a blood sample for laboratory analysis. If hypoglycemia seems unlikely, medical control may recommend that a reagent strip be used for blood glucose determination before glucose administration to rule out hypoglycemia. If hypoglycemia is present (as evidenced by a reagent strip reading of 80 mg or less), treat the patient as described in Chapter 19. Per protocol, administer 100 mg *thiamine* (slow intravenous infusion), followed by 25 g of *50% dextrose.* *Thiamine,* which is used in carbohydrate metabolism, may prevent dextrose from precipi-

---

BOX 20-2

AEIOU Tips

A — Acidosis or alcohol
E — Epilepsy
I — Infection
O — Overdose
U — Uremia
T — Trauma
I — Insulin
P — Psychosis
S — Stroke

tating Wernicke's syndrome or Korsakoff's psychosis (an irreversible memory disorder) in alcoholic patients who have depleted thiamine stores.

4. If there is no response to glucose administration, administer *naloxone* (per protocol), 2 mg slow intravenous infusion, to rule out or reverse narcotic depression.

> **NOTE:**
> Patients who are physically dependent on narcotics may exhibit frank withdrawal symptoms. Therefore the paramedic should be prepared to restrain a patient who may become violent as the *naloxone* reverses narcotic effects. Repeated doses of *naloxone* may be necessary because the duration of some narcotics may be longer than that of *naloxone*. Doses should be titrated to keep the patient awake, responsive, and free from respiratory depression.

5. If alcohol is suspected as the cause of coma, *thiamine* administration should be considered. Thiamine is a B vitamin (B_1) usually found in adequate amounts in the normal diet. However, chronic alcoholism interferes with the intake, absorption, and utilization of *thiamine* and may result in the development of serious neurological disorders. *Thiamine* may be administered intramuscularly if an intravenous line is unavailable.

> **NOTE:**
> The incidence of these alcohol-related neurological syndromes varies markedly in different regions of the United States. Therefore administration of *thiamine* may be a local consideration. The paramedic should follow established protocols and consult with medical control.

6. If the patient remains in a comatose state, the patient's eyes should be protected from corneal drying by gently closing them and covering the lids with moist gauze pads.

7. If the patient's condition permits, the patient should be transported in a lateral recumbent position to facilitate drainage of secretions and to prevent the potential for aspiration of stomach contents. The patient's airway must be closely monitored and suction should be readily available.

Seizure

A seizure is a temporary alteration in behavior or consciousness caused by abnormal electrical activity of one or more groups of neurons in the brain. The annual incidence of seizure is estimated to be approximately half of 1% of the U.S. population, with the highest incidence among feverish children under 5 years of age. (Febrile seizures are further addressed in Chapter 27.)

Although the underlying neuropathophysiology of seizures is not well understood, it is generally believed to result from alterations in neuronal membrane permeability secondary to structural lesion or metabolic derangement. The increased membrane permeability to sodium and potassium ions enhances the ability of the neurons to depolarize and emit an electrical charge, sometimes resulting in seizure activity. Seizures may be caused by multiple factors, including:

- Stroke
- Head trauma
- Toxins, including alcohol or other drug withdrawal
- Hypoxia
- Hypoglycemia
- Infection
- Metabolic abnormalities
- Brain tumor
- Vascular disorders
- Eclampsia
- Drug overdose

In the prehospital setting, determining the origin of seizure activity is less important than managing the complications and recognizing whether the seizure is reversible with therapy (for example, resulting from hypoglycemia). A tendency toward recurrent seizures (excluding those that arise from correctable or avoidable circumstances [for example, alcohol withdrawal]) is called *epilepsy*.

Types of Seizures

All seizures are pathological. They may arise from almost any region of the brain and therefore have many clinical manifestations. The two most common seizure types are generalized and partial (focal).

Generalized Seizures

As the name implies, generalized seizures do not have a definable origin (focus) in the brain, although focal seizures may progress to a generalized seizure. This class includes petit mal (absence seizures) and grand mal (tonic-clonic) seizures. Petit mal seizures occur most often in children between the ages of 4 and 12. They are characterized by brief lapses of consciousness without loss of posture. Often there is no motor activity, although some children have eye blinking, lip smacking, or isolated clonic activity. These seizures usually last less than 15 seconds, during which the patient is unaware of the surroundings, followed by immediate return to normal environmental contact. Most patients have remission by age 20 but may subsequently develop grand mal seizures.

Grand mal seizures are common and are associated with significant morbidity and mortality. Grand mal seizures may be preceded by an aura (olfactory or auditory sensation), which is often recognized by the patient as a warning of the imminent convulsion. The seizure itself is characterized by a sudden loss of consciousness associated with loss of organized muscle tone and a tonic phase in which there is a sequence of extensor muscle tone activity (sometimes flexion) and apnea.

During the tonic phase of a grand mal seizure, tongue biting and bladder or bowel incontinence may occur. After the tonic phase (which lasts only seconds), the patient experiences a bilateral clonic phase (rigidity alternating with relaxation), which usually lasts 1 to 3 minutes. During this phase of the seizure, there is a massive autonomic discharge that results in hyperventilation, salivation, and tachycardia. After the seizure, the patient usually experiences a period of drowsiness or unconsciousness resolving over minutes to hours. On regaining consciousness, the patient is often con-fused and fatigued and may demonstrate a transient neurological deficit. This phase of the seizure is known as the *postictal phase*. Grand mal seizures may be prolonged or recur before the patient regains consciousness. When this occurs, the patient is said to be in *status epilepticus.*

Partial Seizures

In contrast to generalized seizures, in which a specific seizure focus is unknown, partial seizures arise from identifiable cortical lesions. Partial seizures may be classified as simple or complex. Simple partial seizures result mainly from seizure activity in the motor or sensory cortex. Simple motor seizures usually manifest in clonic activity limited to one specific body part (such as one hand, one arm or leg, or one side of the face). Simple sensory seizures result in symptoms such as tingling or numbness of a body part or abnormal visual, auditory, olfactory, or taste symptoms. Patients with partial seizures do not generally lose consciousness and maintain a relatively normal mental status. However, the seizure focus may subsequently spread and lead to a generalized tonic-clonic seizure. Partial seizure activity that spreads in an orderly fashion to surrounding areas is known as a *jacksonian seizure.*

Complex partial seizures arise from focal seizures in the temporal lobe (psychomotor) and manifest primarily as changes in behavior. The classic complex partial seizure is preceded by an aura, followed by abnormal repetitive motor behavior (automatisms) such as lip smacking, chewing, or swallowing, during which time the patient is amnestic. These seizures are typically brief (less than 1 minute), and the patient usually regains normal mental status quickly. Like simple partial seizures, complex partial seizures may also progress to a generalized tonic-clonic seizure.

Hysterical Seizures

A hysterical seizure can mimic a true seizure, but it stems from psychological causes. These seizures are not considered true seizures because they have no organic origin and do not respond to normal treatment modalities. Hysterical or pseudoseizures can usually be terminated by sharp commands or painful stimuli (for example, a sternal rub). These maneuvers may help provide a differential aid in distinguishing between pathological and psychogenic seizure activity.

Assessment

Prehospital assessment is determined by the patient's seizure status on EMS arrival. In most cases, the patient's seizure activity has ceased before the paramedic crew arrives. If possible, the assessment should include a thorough history and physical examination, including a neurological evaluation.

History

If the patient is postictal, information can be gathered from family members or bystanders who witnessed the event. Important components of the patient history include the following five:

1. History of seizures
   a. Frequency
   b. Compliance in taking prescribed medications (for example, *phenytoin, phenobarbital*)
2. Description of seizure activity
   a. Duration of seizure
   b. Typical or atypical pattern of seizure for patient
   c. Presence of aura
   d. Generalized or focal
   e. Incontinence
   f. Tongue biting
3. Recent or past history of head trauma
4. Recent history of fever, headache, nuchal rigidity (suggesting meningeal irritation)
5. Past significant medical history
   a. Diabetes
   b. Heart disease
   c. Stroke

Physical Examination

In conducting the physical examination, maintaining a patent airway is always of primary importance. The paramedic should also be alert to signs of trauma (head and neck trauma, tongue injury, oral lacerations) that may have occurred before or during the seizure activity. In addition, the patient's gums should be inspected for gingival hypertrophy (swelling of the gums), which is a sign of chronic *phenytoin* therapy. Three other components of the physical examination include:

1. Level of sensorium, including presence or absence of amnesia
2. Cranial nerve evaluation, particularly pupillary findings
3. Motor and sensory evaluation, including coordination (Abnormalities may be caused by metabolic disturbances, meningitis, intracranial hemorrhage, and drug use.)

Other aspects of the physical examination that may provide clues to the underlying disorder include the following three:

1. Presence of urine or feces (suggesting bladder or bowel incontinence)
2. Automatisms
3. Cardiac dysrhythmias

Syncope Versus Seizure

It may be difficult to determine whether the patient experienced a syncopal episode or a seizure because the main differentiating characteristics are in the symptoms before and after the event. The factors listed in Table 20-1 may aid in the determination.

Management

The first step in managing a patient with seizure activity is to prevent the patient from sustaining physical injury. This is best accomplished by removing obstacles in the patient's immediate area or, if necessary, moving the patient to a safe environment such as a carpeted or soft, grassy area. *At no time should a patient with seizure activity be restrained, nor should objects be forced between the patient's teeth to maintain an airway.* Restraining activity may harm the patient or paramedic crew. Forcing objects into the oral cavity in an effort to secure an airway or prevent the patient from biting his or her tongue may evoke vomiting, aspiration, or spasm of the larynx.

Most patients with an isolated seizure can be appropriately managed in the postictal phase by placing them in a lateral recumbent position to allow drainage of oral secretions and to facilitate suctioning (if needed). Supplemental oxygen should be administered via nonrebreather mask, and the patient should be moved to a quiet envi-

TABLE 20-1 Differentiating Characteristics of Syncope and Seizure

Characteristics	Syncope	Seizure
Position	The seizure usually starts in a standing position.	The seizure may start in any position.
Warning	There is usually a warning period of lightheadedness.	There is little or no warning.
Level of consciousness	The patient usually regains conscious immediately on becoming supine; fatigue, confusion, and headache last less that 15 minutes.	The patient may remain unconscious for minutes to hours; fatigue, confusion, and headache last longer than 15 minutes.
Clonic-tonic activity	Clonic movements (if present) are of short duration.	Tonic-clonic movements occur during unconscious state.
ECG analysis	Bradycardia is caused by increased vagal tone associated with syncope.	Tachycardia is caused by muscular exertion associated with seizure activity.

ronment (away from onlookers). Patients are commonly embarrassed or self-conscious after a seizure, particularly if incontinence has occurred. Therefore the paramedic should be sensitive to the physical and emotional needs of the patient.

All seizure patients should be transported to the emergency department for physician evaluation. Depending on the patient's status and seizure history, medical control may recommend that an intravenous lifeline be established in the event that anticonvulsant medication may become necessary. However, few patients who experience an isolated seizure require pharmacological therapy in the prehospital setting.

Status Epilepticus

Status epilepticus is continuous seizure activity lasting 30 minutes or longer or a recurrent seizure without an intervening period of consciousness. The condition is a true emergency; without immediate treatment, it can result in permanent neurological damage, respiratory failure, and death. Associated complications of status epilepticus include aspiration, brain damage, fracture of long bones and the spine, necrosis of heart muscle, and severe dehydration. The most common precipitating cause of this condition in adults is failure to take prescribed anticonvulsant medications.

Management

As in all patients with seizures, treatment priorities include managing the airway and provid-

ing ventilatory support, protecting the patient from injury, and transporting the patient to a medical facility for physician evaluation. In addition, treatment of a status seizure includes stopping the seizure activity with anticonvulsant medications (*diazepam, lorazepam*).

After securing of the airway with oral or nasal adjuncts (or intubating of the patient's trachea during the flaccid period between seizures), oxygen should be administered in high concentration and ventilation supported with a bag-valve device. An intravenous line should be established with normal saline to keep the vein open and secured well with tape and roller bandage. A sample of the patient's blood is drawn for laboratory analysis. With authorization from medical control, administration of the following medications may be considered:

- 25 grams of *50% dextrose* slow intravenous infusion (controversial unless hypoglycemia is suspected) to replace blood glucose lost during seizure activity or correct hypoglycemia that caused the seizure
- *Lorazepam* (Ativan) 1 mg intravenously or *diazepam* (Valium) 2- to 5-mg increments intravenously (maximum 10-mg total dose) to stop the spread of the seizure focus

While administering anticonvulsants, the paramedic should closely monitor the patient's blood pressure and respiratory status and be prepared for aggressive airway control and ventilatory assistance.

NOTE:
If the patient's blood pressure begins to fall or if the respiratory rate or effort decreases, discontinue pharmacological therapy and advise medical direction.

Cerebrovascular Accident

A CVA, or stroke, is a sudden interruption in blood flow to the brain that results in neurological deficit. Stroke is a serious disease that affects more than 500,000 Americans each year,[1] and it is associated with a 30-day mortality of approximately 10% to 15%. It is the third leading cause of death in the United States and frequently leaves its survivors severely debilitated. Patients more likely to suffer a CVA include those with the following six risk factors:

1. Hypertension
2. Diabetes mellitus
3. Atherosclerosis
4. Hyperlipidemia
5. Polycythemia
6. Cardiac disease

Pathophysiology

Blood reaches the brain through four major vessels: two carotid arteries (providing approximately 80% of cerebral blood flow) and two vertebral arteries, which combine to form the single basilar artery (supplying the remaining 20% of cerebral blood flow). These two systems are interconnected at various levels, the principal one being the circle of Willis. In addition, there are individual variations of extensive collateral blood flow supplied through facial anastomoses between scalp vessels and vessels of the dura and arachnoid. Beyond this, however, there is no collateral circulation in the depths of the brain. Therefore occlusion of any one of the more distal vessels may result in ischemia and infarction.

Normally, cerebral blood flow is maintained through autoregulation of cerebral vessels that constrict or dilate to preserve perfusion pressure even with systemic hypotension. Cerebral perfusion is also regulated at the arteriolar level by the level of oxygen glucose supplied (ischemia and ac-

idosis are profound vasodilators). The sudden cessation of circulation to a portion of the brain that results from vessel occlusion or hemorrhage cannot be readily corrected by these autoregulatory mechanisms. The uncorrected ischemia that results within a short period of time leads to neuronal dysfunction and death. The onset and symptoms of the stroke depend on the area of the brain involved.

Types

CVA is a general term that refers to the neurological manifestations of a critical decrease in blood flow to a portion of the brain, regardless of the cause. The most common causes of CVAs are cerebral thrombosis, cerebral embolus, and cerebral hemorrhage. Determining the origin of a CVA is often difficult and unnecessary in the prehospital setting. However, understanding the various signs and symptoms of each type of CVA better prepares the paramedic to anticipate the course of patient care. In addition, documenting a thorough history and physical examination helps others involved in the patient's care.

Cerebral Thrombosis

Approximately half of all strokes are caused by a cerebral thrombosis that occurs as a result of atherosclerotic plaques (see Chapter 18) or extrinsic pressure from a mass within the brain itself. The onset of stroke from cerebral thrombosis is usually associated with a long history of vessel disease. Therefore the majority of these patients are older and have evidence of atherosclerotic disease in other areas of the body (angina pectoris, claudication, previous strokes). Signs and symptoms of thrombotic stroke are usually slower to develop than those of embolic stroke or cerebral hemorrhage and include:

- Hemiparesis or hemiplegia on the side of the body opposite the lesion
- Numbness (or decreased sensation) on the side of the body opposite the lesion
- Aphasia
- Confusion or coma
- Convulsions
- Incontinence
- Double vision

- Numbness of the face
- Dysarthria (slurred speech)
- Headache
- Dizziness or vertigo

Cerebral Embolus

An embolic stroke results from an occlusion of any intracranial vessel by a fragment of a foreign substance arising outside of the CNS. Common sources of cerebral emboli include atherosclerotic plaques (originating from large vessels of the head and neck and the heart). Thrombi that develop on the valves or in the chambers of the heart are very common in patients with valvular heart disease and atrial fibrillation. Other rare causes of cerebral emboli include air embolism after thoracic injury and fat embolism after long bone injury. Bacterial and fungal endocarditis are also capable of causing stroke from embolization. Women taking oral contraceptives and patients with sickle cell disease are also at increased risk of developing a stroke (both by thrombotic and perhaps embolic origin). Signs and symptoms of cerebral embolus are similar to those of thrombotic stroke, but they usually develop more quickly and are often associated with an identifiable cause (atrial fibrillation, valvular heart disease).

Cerebral Hemorrhage

Cerebral hemorrhage accounts for 10% of all strokes. A hemorrhage may occur anywhere within the cranial vault, including the epidural, subdural, subarachnoid, intraparenchymal, and intraventricular spaces. The most common causes are cerebral aneurysms, arteriovenous malformations, and hypertension. Cerebral aneurysms and arteriovenous malformations are congenital anomalies that can be familial and often are asymptomatic until the time of rupture. Unlike thrombotic and embolic strokes, which have relatively high survival rates, cerebral hemorrhages are fatal in 50% to 80% of the cases.

Hemorrhagic strokes commonly occur during stress or exertion. Cocaine and other sympathomimetic amines may also contribute to intracranial hemorrhage by drug-induced rapid elevation of blood pressure. Presentation is abrupt and often begins with a headache (sometimes described as the worst headache of the patient's life) accompanied by nausea, vomiting, and progressive deterioration in mental status from alert to lethargic. Often, the patient loses consciousness or experiences a seizure at the time of the hemorrhage. As the hemorrhage expands and ICP increases, the patient becomes comatose, with increasing hypertension and bradycardia (Cushing's reflex).

Transient Ischemic Attacks

Transient ischemic attacks (TIAs) (often referred to as *little strokes)* are episodes of focal cerebral dysfunction that last from minutes to several hours from which the patient returns to normal within 24 hours without permanent neurological deficit. A TIA is thought to be the most important indication of impending stroke because it is often followed by a cerebral infarct within 2 years.

Signs and symptoms of a TIA are the same as those that characterize stroke and include weakness, paralysis, numbness of the face, and speech disturbances, all of which correspond to vascular occlusion of a specific cerebral artery. Most patients who experience a TIA are hospitalized for close observation, evaluation, and treatment of vascular disease.

Assessment

Initial examination of a patient who may have suffered a CVA (including TIA) follows the same sequence as for any other ill or injured patient in the emergency setting. Emergency care priorities are directed at maintaining a patent airway and providing adequate ventilatory support with supplemental oxygen. If the patient is conscious and able to converse, a thorough history should be obtained. Important components of the patient history are:

- Previous neurological symptoms (TIAs)
- Previous neurological deficits
- Initial symptoms and their progression
- Alterations in level of consciousness
- Precipitating factors
- Dizziness
- Palpitations
- Significant past medical history
  - Hypertension
  - Diabetes mellitus

○ Cigarette smoking
○ Oral contraceptive use
○ Cardiac disease
○ Sickle cell disease
○ Previous CVA

During the physical examination, special attention should be paid to the neurological component. To review, the neurological signs and symptoms that suggest the diagnosis of CVA include weakness (hemiparesis, hemiplegia); numbness; speech disturbances, including slurred speech (dysarthria) and difficulty naming objects correctly (aphasia); confusion; inappropriate laughing or crying; agitation; and visual disturbances. In addition, mobile patients may demonstrate gait disturbances or incoordination of fine motor movements.

The paramedic should remember that stroke patients have experienced a catastrophic event that may seriously affect their quality of life. They are often frightened, embarrassed, confused, and frustrated with their inability to move or communicate. These patients have special physical and emotional needs and deserve a compassionate and caring approach.

Management

Little specific therapy can be administered in the prehospital setting other than to prevent secondary problems that can further injure a damaged brain (hypoxia, hypercarbia, hypotension, acidosis). Therefore prehospital care of the stroke patient is largely supportive.

As previously stated, airway maintenance and ventilatory support with supplemental oxygen are of paramount importance. If the patient's condition permits, the patient should be kept supine with the head elevated 15 degrees to facilitate venous drainage. Seven other patient care measures are:

1. Initiate an intravenous line of lactated Ringer's solution or normal saline at 30 ml/hr.[2]
2. Draw a blood sample for laboratory analysis per protocol.
3. Perform serum glucose analysis and administer *50% dextrose* if indicated.
4. Monitor for cardiac dysrhythmias.
5. Protect paralyzed extremities.
6. Provide comforting measures and reassurance.
7. Provide gentle transportation to the receiving hospital.

REFERENCES

1. American Heart Association: *1990 heart and stroke facts,* Dallas, 1989, The Association.
2. Guidelines for cardiopulmonary resuscitation and emergency cardiac care, *JAMA* 268(16):2172, 1992.

Summary

Neurological emergencies may be potentially life threatening. The paramedic's knowledge and skills, combined with appropriate and aggressive intervention, can help reduce morbidity and mortality and produce maximal potential for rehabilitation and recovery.

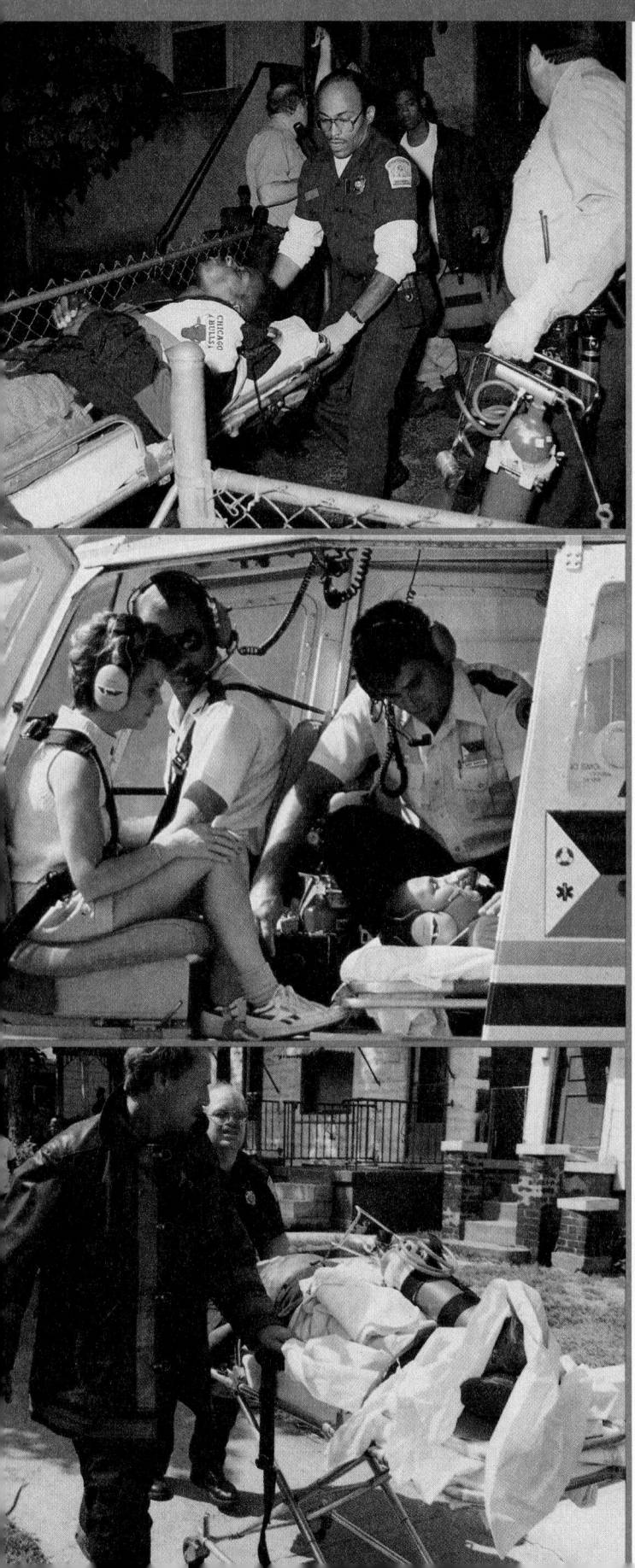

Acute abdominal pain is a common chief complaint in emergency care that may reflect serious illness. This chapter reviews gastrointestinal and genitourinary anatomy, disorders associated with these body systems that produce abdominal pain or gastrointestinal or genitourinary bleeding, and problems that may accompany renal failure and renal dialysis. Detailed evaluation and appropriate management of patients with acute abdominal emergencies may prevent the development of life-threatening complications.

OBJECTIVES

As a paramedic, you should be able to:

1. List the solid and hollow organs of the abdomen and retroperitoneal space.
2. Identify the location of abdominal organs by quadrant.
3. Label diagrams of female and male genitourinary anatomy.
4. Distinguish hemorrhagic and nonhemorrhagic gastrointestinal disorders.
5. Identify precipitating factors, signs and symptoms, and patient management techniques for selected gastrointestinal and genitourinary disorders.
6. Outline specific assessment techniques for evaluating the patient with acute abdominal pain.
7. Distinguish the following types of pain: visceral, somatic, and referred.
8. Outline general management techniques for care of the patient with acute abdominal pain.
9. Discuss the etiology of renal failure.
10. Distinguish between acute and chronic renal failure.
11. List the signs and symptoms of acute and chronic renal failure.
12. Describe hemodialysis.
13. Describe peritoneal dialysis.
14. Discuss the prehospital implications of emergencies that may be encountered in the dialysis patient.

● GASTROINTESTINAL AND GENITOURINARY ANATOMY

The organs and structures of the gastrointestinal system can be classified as primary or accessory. The primary gastrointestinal components in-

clude the mouth, pharynx, esophagus, stomach, small and large intestines, rectum, and peritoneum. The accessory gastrointestinal components are the salivary glands, teeth, liver, gallbladder, pancreas, and appendix. Fig. 21-1 reviews these structures.

The genitourinary anatomy includes the structures and organs of the urinary system and the male and female reproductive systems. The urinary system is composed of the kidneys, ureters, bladder, and urethra. Components of the male reproductive system include the testes, prostate, penile urethra, epididymis, and vas deferens. Female reproductive organs include the ovaries, fallopian

KEY TERMS

disequilibrium syndrome: A group of neurological findings that sometimes occurs during or immediately after dialysis and that are thought to result from a disproportionate decrease in osmolality of the extracellular fluid compared with that of the intracellular compartment in the brain or cerebral spinal fluid.

hemasite: A small, button-shaped indwelling vascular device usually placed in the upper arm or proximal, anterior thigh and similar to an arteriovenous graft but having an external rubber septum sutured to the skin through which a dialysis catheter is inserted for treatment.

melena: Abnormal black, tarry stools containing digested blood.

nocturia: Particularly excessive urination at night.

paralytic ileus: A decrease in or absence of intestinal peristalsis that may occur after abdominal surgery, illness, or injury and that is the most common cause of intestinal obstruction.

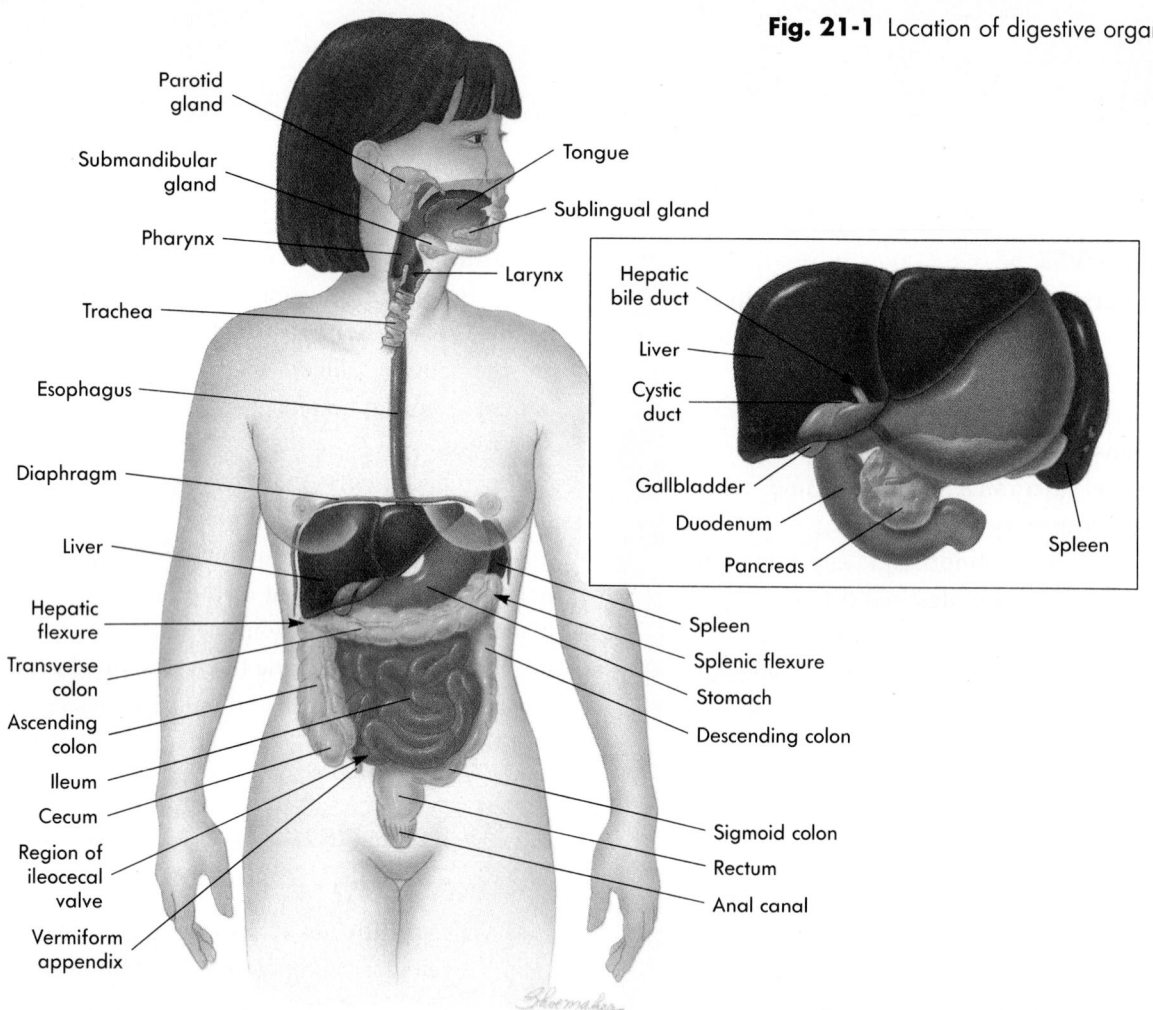

Fig. 21-1 Location of digestive organs.

tubes, uterus, vagina, and vulva. The male and female reproductive systems are explained and illustrated in Chapter 10. Readers are encouraged to refer to that section for a review.

● PATHOPHYSIOLOGY OF ACUTE ABDOMINAL PAIN

Acute abdominal pain is relatively sudden in onset and often severe in nature. An understanding of the pathophysiology of abdominal pain can help the paramedic direct patient assessment and recognize disorders that may be life threatening.

Gastrointestinal Disorders that Primarily Cause Abdominal Pain

The causes of acute abdominal pain can result from nonhemorrhagic etiologies (inflammatory

and obstructive conditions) and hemorrhagic etiologies. The specific gastrointestinal disorders discussed in this section include esophagitis, gastritis, appendicitis, pancreatitis, cholecystitis, intestinal obstruction, hernia, peptic ulcer, and diverticulitis. (Aortic aneurysm, which can also cause acute abdominal pain, is addressed in Chapter 18.)

Esophagitis

Esophagitis is inflammation of the distal (hiatal) esophagus usually caused by the regurgitation of gastric acid through the lower esophageal sphincter (reflux esophagitis). This condition can be associated with a gastric ulcer or hiatal hernia. Signs and symptoms of esophagitis include substernal pain (often described as burning in nature and commonly made worse by lying down or bending over), weight loss, bleeding, and presence of a foul breath odor. Bleeding from esophagitis produces an emesis similar in appearance and consistency to coffee grounds, indicating that blood has entered the stomach before regurgitation. Definitive treatment may involve dietary regulation (bland diet), medications (for example, antacids, histamine receptor antagonists), and sometimes surgery.

Gastritis

Gastritis is inflammation of the gastric mucosa that commonly results from hyperacidity, alcohol or drug ingestion, or bile reflux. Signs and symptoms of gastritis include epigastric pain, nausea and vomiting (which may be severe), mucosal bleeding, and epigastric tenderness on palpation. The patient with gastritis may be hypovolemic as a result of prolonged bleeding with or without **melena** (abnormal maroon-colored or tarry stools containing digested blood). The chronic use of alcohol, aspirin, and other nonsteroidal or antiinflammatory medications is probably the most common cause of this gastrointestinal illness. Gastritis is treated with diet regulation, medications (as listed for esophagitis), and fluid replacement or fluid resuscitation if hypovolemia or dehydration occurs.

Appendicitis

Appendicitis is a common abdominal emergency that occurs when the opening between the lumen of the appendix and the cecum is obstructed by fecal material (fecalith) or as a result of inflammation. If allowed to persist, the inflamed organ eventually becomes gangrenous and ruptures within the peritoneal cavity, resulting in peritonitis and shock, or the condition may evolve into a periappendiceal abscess.

The classic presentation of appendicitis is abdominal pain or cramping, nausea, vomiting, chills, low-grade fever, and anorexia. The pain is initially periumbilical and diffuse, later becoming intense and localized to the right lower quadrant just medial to the iliac crest (McBurney's point). On examination, the patient usually exhibits involuntary guarding. If the appendix ruptures, the patient's pain diminishes before the development of peritoneal signs. The goal of definitive care for appendicitis is surgical appendectomy before rupture.

> **NOTE:**
> Young children and older adults may have atypical illness caused by reduced inflammatory response associated with extremes of age; appendicitis is more difficult to diagnose in these age groups.

Pancreatitis

Inflammation of the pancreas may cause severe epigastric pain after the ingestion of alcohol or a large amount of food. It is frequently associated with nausea, vomiting, and abdominal tenderness and distention. The abdominal pain is often described as *severe*, radiating from midumbilicus to the patient's back and shoulders. In severe cases, the patient has fever, tachycardia, and signs of generalized sepsis and shock. These patients should be hospitalized and treated with intravenous fluids, pain medication, and placement of a nasogastric tube if vomiting.

Cholecystitis

Cholecystitis is inflammation of the gallbladder, which is most often associated with the presence of gallstones (75% of which are predominantly cholesterol stones). The disease is very common in the United States and occurs more often in women 30 to 50 years of age than in men. On occasion, the gallstones totally obstruct the neck or cystic duct of the gallbladder. This is followed by a large increase in pressure within the organ. The increased pressure causes a sudden onset of pain (gallbladder colic), which radiates from the epigastrium to the right upper quadrant. Patients with gallbladder disease commonly have their pain episodes at night, and it is generally associated with recent ingestion of fried or fatty foods.

Other associated hallmarks of cholecystitis include previous episodes, a family history of gallbladder disease, low-grade fever, nausea, vomiting that may be bile-stained and described as *bitter* (variable), and pain and tenderness on palpation in the right upper quadrant. Passage of stones into the common bile duct with subsequent obstruction may cause shaking chills, high fever, jaundice, and acute pancreatitis. Definitive treatment involves hospitalization, intravenous therapy, antibiotics, placement of a nasogastric

Nasogastric Tube Insertion

Nasogastric intubation may be indicated when the patient's stomach is severely distended or evacuation of gastric contents by lavage is necessary. This procedure should be attempted only in conscious patients with an intact gag reflex or in unconscious patients whose airway is protected with an endotracheal tube.

NOTE: Passage of a nasogastric tube is unpleasant under the most ideal of conditions and should be considered only as a prehospital procedure under unusual circumstances and after direction by medical control (Figs. 21-2 and 21-3).

Necessary Equipment
- Personal protective equipment (gloves, mask, face shield)
- Double-lumen Levin tube (large enough to evacuate desired material)
- Water-soluble lubricant
- Tape
- 50-ml irrigation syringe
- Cup of water or ice chips
- Emesis basin
- Intermittent suction equipment

Procedure
1. Explain the procedure to the patient.
2. Measure the length of tube to be inserted by placing the tip of the tube over the approximate area of the stomach and extending it to the patient's ear and from the ear to the tip of the nose. Note the marks on the tube used for measurement.
3. Lubricate the tip and the first 2 to 3 inches of the tube with a water-soluble lubricant.
4. Place the patient in a high Fowler's position and instruct the patient to lean forward and to flex his or her neck.
5. Instruct the patient to suck on ice chips or to take small sips of water (if not contraindicated) and to swallow on command during the procedure. This assists passage of the tube.
6. Insert the tube along the floor of an unobstructed nostril. If the patient has a deviated septum, choose the nostril with the most open channel.
7. Gently and slowly advance the tube while having the patient continue to swallow until the tube is at the level previously noted by the marks. It is common for the patient to choke and cough during the procedure. If this occurs, hold the tube in place and allow the patient to rest. If choking and coughing persist, remove the tube (it may have entered the trachea), and begin again.
8. After the tube has been fully inserted to its predetermined length, verify placement in the stomach by injecting 20 to 30 cc of air into the tube while auscultating the epigastric region for the sound of air movement. Leave the syringe attached to the tube until aspiration of stomach contents is initiated or intermittent suction is available.
9. Secure the tube with tape to the nose and forehead or cheek.
10. Lavage stomach contents by injecting 100- to 150-cc boluses of normal saline into the tube and allowing the return of gastric contents by aspiration or intermittent suction. Document the amount of fluid infused and returned by lavage.

Possible Complications
- Nasal hemorrhage
- Passage of the tube into the trachea
- Perforation of the esophagus
- Gastrointestinal bleeding
- Coiling of the tube in the posterior pharynx
- Obstruction of the passage resulting from septal deviation
- Passage of the tube intracranially (with cribriform plate fractures)

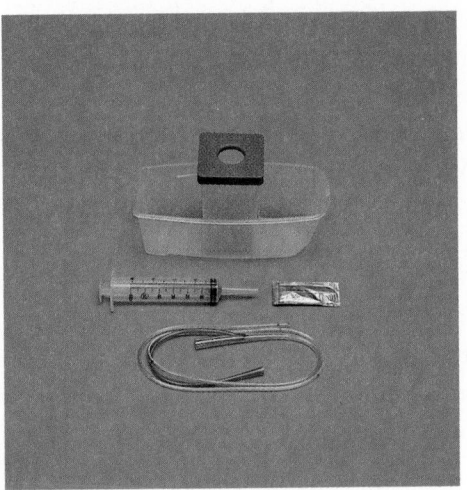

Fig. 21-2 Equipment for nasogastric tube insertion.

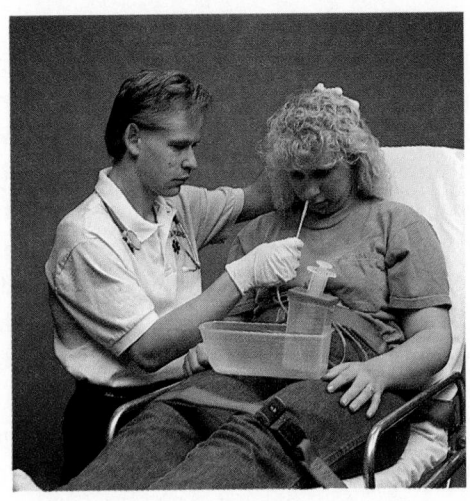

Fig. 21-3 Nasogastric tube insertion.

tube, and possible surgical removal of the gallbladder.

Intestinal Obstruction

Intestinal obstruction is an occlusion of the intestinal lumen that results in blockage of normal flow of intestinal contents. The condition may be caused by a number of factors, including adhesions, hernias, fecal impaction, polyps, and tumors. Obstructions can be closely mimicked by **paralytic ileus,** which may result from a number of localized or systemic conditions. Intestinal obstruction in the small bowel is most often caused by adhesions or hernia. Large bowel obstructions commonly result from tumors or impaction.

Signs and symptoms of intestinal obstruction include nausea and vomiting, abdominal pain, constipation, and abdominal distention. The speed of onset and degree of symptoms depend on the anatomical site of obstruction (small versus large bowel). The most significant danger of an obstructive condition is perforation with generalized peritonitis and sepsis. Usually the initial manifestation of intestinal obstruction is dehydration, which may result from vomiting, decreased intestinal absorption, and fluid loss into the lumen. As the affected portion of the bowel distends, its blood supply is attenuated and the segment becomes ischemic. The forces of distention and ischemia combine to produce perforation with secondary peritonitis. If the intestine be-

comes strangulated, blood or plasma may also be lost from the affected intestinal segment. Definitive care involves fluid replacement, antibiotics, placement of a nasogastric tube for decompression, and most often, surgery to correct the obstructing lesion.

Hernia

A hernia is a protrusion of viscus from its normal position through a congenital or acquired opening, most commonly in the groin or abdominal wall. Increases in abdominal pressure such as those associated with straining, coughing, or lifting can cause the peritoneum to push outward through a defect in the groin or abdominal musculature. When this occurs, a sac is formed into which various organs within the peritoneal cavity may enter.

Most hernias are uncomplicated and can be manually replaced or reduced into the peritoneal cavity by a physician. If they cannot, however, the incarcerated contents of the peritoneal sac (usually a portion of bowel) can become strangulated. These patients frequently have acute abdominal pain and systemic signs such as fever and tachycardia. Incarcerated or strangulated hernias can lead to serious complications, including intestinal obstruction, perforation, and peritonitis. Definitive care for complicated hernias is in-hospital observation, intravenous rehydration, pain medication, and surgical repair.

Peptic Ulcer

A peptic ulcer is an open wound or sore in an area of the digestive system (usually the stomach or duodenum) that results from a complex pathological interaction among the acidic gastric juice, the proteolytic enzymes, and the mucosal barrier. Ulcers cause disintegration and death of tissue as they erode the mucosal layers in the affected areas. If they are left untreated, massive hemorrhage or perforation may result. Perforation and exsanguination secondary to peptic ulcer disease are fairly uncommon. However, repeated small hemorrhages over long periods may result in anemia. The primary cause of peptic ulcer disease is probably related to prolonged hyperacidity.

The patient with a peptic ulcer is usually aware of the condition and often commonly uses over-the-counter antacids. The ulcer pain is often described as a burning or gnawing discomfort in the epigastric region or left upper quadrant that develops before meals (classically, early morning) or during stressful periods, when the production of gastric acids increases. The pain is usually sudden in onset and is commonly relieved by food intake, antacids, or vomiting. In addition to pain and vomiting of blood, the patient may experience melena as a result of hemorrhagic blood passing through the gastrointestinal tract.

Prehospital care for peptic ulcer disease includes obtaining a pertinent history, evaluating for hypotension, and providing circulatory support as needed. After physician evaluation, definitive care may involve antacids, H_2-receptor antagonists or other medications, and occasionally, diet regulation (the benefit of which is controversial). Some patients with acute peptic ulcer disease require hospitalization for fluid or blood replacement or surgery if medications are not effective.

Diverticulitis

A diverticulum is a sac or pouch that develops in the wall of the colon. It is a common development with advancing years and is associated with diets low in fiber. Diverticular outpouchings tend to develop at the weakest point in the colon wall where intraluminal vessels penetrate the circular muscular layer. Often there is a small artery or arteriole at the neck of the diverticulum from which subsequent bleeding may occur.

Most patients with diverticula are completely asymptomatic. However, up to 30% of these patients experience diverticulitis when one or more diverticulum becomes obstructed with fecal matter. Mild complications of diverticulitis include irregular bowel habits (alternating constipation and diarrhea), fever, and lower left quadrant pain ("left-sided appendicitis"). Recurrences of diverticulitis are common within the first 5 years after the onset of symptoms. Definitive care includes diet regulation, antibiotic therapy, and sometimes, surgical repair.

Gastrointestinal Disorders that Primarily Cause Bleeding

Gastrointestinal disorders that primarily cause bleeding include esophageal varices, diverticulosis, arteriovenous malformations, hemorrhoids, and peptic ulcer disease. As a rule, prehospital care for gastrointestinal bleeding is limited to securing a patent airway, high-concentration oxygen administration, fluid resuscitation, and rapid transport for physician evaluation.

Esophageal Varices

Esophageal varices are common with hepatic disease and often result from portal hypertension caused by cirrhosis of the liver. Obstruction to portal blood flow produced by the fibrosis in the liver increases portal pressure and dilates vessels that drain into the portal system. This subsequent dilation of thin-walled veins around the lower esophagus and upper end of the stomach produces esophageal varices. Varices are subject to rupture and life-threatening hemorrhage.

Other causes of esophageal bleeding include esophagitis (associated with chronic use of alcohol and antiinflammatory nonsteroidal medications); malignancy; and episodes of prolonged, violent vomiting that produce a tear or laceration in the mucosa of the upper esophagus (Mallory-Weiss syndrome).

The clinical presentation of a patient with esophageal bleeding is bright-red hematemesis and vomiting, which may be severe. If bleeding is profuse, melena may be evident, and the patient may manifest the classic signs of shock. Variceal bleeding is usually massive and generally difficult to control. Therapeutic intervention includes ensuring a patent airway and fluid resuscitation. (The placement of a nasogastric tube for gastric lavage is controversial.) Definitive care may include placement of a Sengstaken-Blakemore tube to tamponade bleeding vessels, surgical ligation of the bleeding varices, or transendoscopic injection of a sclerosing agent into the bleeding vessels. The mortality rate for patients with variceal bleeding is approximately 50%.

Diverticulosis

As previously discussed, diverticula are common in older patients. Serious complications of diverticular disease associated with perforation are massive, bright-red rectal bleeding, which can be brisk and commonly painless; peritonitis; and sepsis. Hemorrhage from a diverticulum is the most common cause of massive rectal bleeding in older patients.[1] If the hemorrhage does not cease spontaneously, emergency surgery may be necessary.

Arteriovenous Malformations

Arteriovenous malformations are small vascular abnormalities, especially of the intestinal tract. The lesions are most frequently found in the right colon but may be seen throughout the bowel. These malformations are more common in older patients with hypertension or aortic stenosis. The condition is characterized by painless bleeding, which may be mild to massive. Most bleeding episodes stop spontaneously. If bleeding is severe or prolonged, surgery may be necessary.

Hemorrhoids

Although hemorrhoids are present in 50% of all people by age 50, they most frequently present with blood streaking rather than life-threatening hemorrhage. Pain is infrequent unless thrombosis, ulceration, or infection is present. Slight bleeding is the most common symptom and usually occurs during or after defecation. Blood dripping into the toilet after defecation or blood-stained toilet tissue after wiping are common indications. Although blood loss is usually slight, recurrent episodes of bleeding may be significant enough to produce anemia. Definitive care includes conservative dietary management, tissue fixation techniques, and operative hemorrhoidectomy for severe cases.

Genitourinary Disorders that Cause Acute Abdominal Pain

Like gastrointestinal disorders, many genitourinary disorders can produce acute abdominal pain. These include urinary retention, urinary tract infection (UTI), pyelonephritis, urinary calculus, epididymitis, testicular torsion, and various gynecological and obstetrical conditions, such as pelvic inflammatory disease, ectopic pregnancy, and ruptured ovarian cyst (see Chapters 28 and 29).

Urinary Retention

Urinary retention is the inability to void. Possible causes include urethral stricture, an enlarged prostate (benign or malignant prostatic hypertrophy), central nervous system dysfunction, foreign body obstruction, and use of certain medications such as parasympatholytic or anticholinergic agents. Signs and symptoms include severe abdominal pain (except with central nervous system lesions) associated with an urgent need to urinate and a distended bladder, which is frequently palpable. Patients with a progressive obstruction, such as prostatic hypertrophy, often have a history of urinary hesitancy, a poor urinary stream, a sense of incomplete emptying of the bladder, and **nocturia.** In the emergency department, therapeutic intervention often requires passage of a urethral catheter to empty the bladder. Although urinary retention is often painful for the patient, prehospital care is primarily supportive. The cause of the retention should be sought, and if it is not easily correctable, the patient may require hospitalization.

Urinary Tract Infection

UTIs can involve the upper or lower urinary tract. Infections of the lower urinary tract involve the bladder and urethra and are common among young women because of the short length of the urethra. The disease also occurs in men and children, although urethritis in young men is most commonly a veneral disease rather than a true UTI.

Signs and symptoms of UTI include dysuria, urinary frequency, hematuria, and abdominal pain. In addition, fever, chills, and malaise may be present. Diagnosis is confirmed in the hospital through urinalysis and microscopic examination for blood cells, sediment, and bacteria. UTIs are generally treated with antibiotic therapy.

Pyelonephritis

Pyelonephritis is inflammation of the kidney parenchyma (upper urinary tract). The disease is associated with microbial infection that reaches the kidneys from the hematogenous route or by ascending the ureters from the lower urinary tract. Pyelonephritis is also more common in women than men and in patients who have obstructive lesions along the genitourinary tract. Signs and symptoms include fever, chills, flank pain, nausea, and vomiting. Urinary frequency and dysuria are often absent in pyelonephritis. Therapeutic intervention includes bed rest, hospitalization, fluid replacement, and antibiotic therapy. Pyelonephritis can progress to sepsis and also cause renal failure.

Urinary Calculus

It has been estimated that as many as 12% of people in the United States eventually form a urinary calculus.[2] These pathological concretions, which originate in the renal pelvis, result from supersaturation of the urine with insoluble salts (primarily calcium oxalate and uric acid). Kidney stones normally occur in patients between the ages of 30 and 50. The disease is recurrent and is more common in men than women.

Signs and symptoms of urinary calculus vary according to location. Most stones obstruct the ureter at points of ureteral narrowing in their passage from kidneys to bladder, producing acute pain that originates in the flank area and radiates to the right or left lower abdominal quadrant and groin. Renal or ureteral colic produces a most severe pain of a waxing-and-waning cyclical nature as the ureter attempts to use intensely forceful ureteral peristaltic contractions to push the stone into the bladder. It is often of the same nature and intensity as labor pain. The pain may be accompanied by restlessness, nausea, urinary urgency or frequency, diaphoresis, low-grade fever, hematuria, dysuria, and decreased blood pressure. Definitive care includes analgesics, fluid replacement, antiemetics, and possible hospital admission. If the calculus does not pass spontaneously, surgical intervention may be required.

Epididymitis

Epididymitis is inflammation of the epididymis, a tubular section of the male reproductive system that carries sperm from the testicle to the seminal vesicles. Epididymis is commonly caused by a bacterial infection associated with other structures of the genitourinary tract, and it tends to occur in sexually active young adults who are over the age of 20.

Signs and symptoms of epididymitis include a gradual onset of unilateral scrotal pain that radiates to the spermatic cord. Sometimes tender swelling of the scrotum and testicle occurs, producing orchitis. In addition, the patient may have a recent history of UTI, fever, and malaise. After physician evaluation, therapeutic intervention includes antibiotics, bed rest, analgesics, and elevation of the scrotum. The paramedic should attempt to differentiate epididymitis from the more serious testicular torsion.

Testicular Torsion

Testicular torsion is a true urological emergency in which a testicle twists on its spermatic cord, disrupting its own blood supply. It may result from blunt trauma to the scrotal area, but it is more commonly spontaneous. Testicular torsion usually affects young adolescents and men under age 30.

Like epididymitis, testicular torsion results in a tender epididymis and painful swelling of the scrotal sac. Unlike epididymitis, however, the patient is usually afebrile. The pain is sudden in onset (often preceded by strenuous physical activity or an athletic event), severe (sometimes radiating to the ipsilateral left quadrant), unrelieved by rest or scrotal elevation, and often associated with nausea and vomiting. Testicular torsion must be diagnosed and treated within 6 hours to prevent loss of the testis from ischemic infarction. Therapeutic intervention includes application of ice packs to the scrotum and manual manipulation by a physician to reduce the torsion. Because the patient must undergo surgical repair within 4 to 6 hours of onset of the torsion, rapid transport to the emergency department and efficient preoperative diagnosis are critical to a favorable outcome.

● ASSESSMENT OF ACUTE ABDOMINAL PAIN

After a primary survey to ensure adequacy of airway, breathing, and circulation, assessment of acute abdominal pain should begin with gathering of a thorough history focused on the patient's chief complaint. Baseline vital signs should be assessed and documented, and a systematic physical examination should be performed to help identify abdominal emergencies that may indicate the development of shock or the need for immediate transport for surgical intervention.

History

When obtaining a history of abdominal pain, the paramedic should attempt to identify the location and type of pain and any associated signs and symptoms. Using the mnemonic PQRST or a similar method may help in obtaining this information. Sample questions that might be included in the PQRST evaluation are listed below:

P (provocative)	What brought on the pain? What makes it better or worse?
Q (quality)	What does the pain feel like? Is it sharp, dull, burning, tearing?
R (region)	Where is the pain located? Does it radiate?
S (severity)	Is the pain mild, moderate, or severe? What is the degree of discomfort on a scale of 1 to 10?
T (time)	When did the pain begin? How long does it last?

Other important elements of a patient history include any recent illness, past significant medical history such as cardiac or respiratory disease that may manifest in abdominal pain, presence and character of penile or vaginal discharge, medication use, alcohol or other drug use, and previous abdominal surgeries. Women should

also be questioned regarding menstrual activity (including regularity and last menstrual period), the possibility of pregnancy, and use of oral contraceptives or an intrauterine device.

Location and Type of Abdominal Pain

Recalling the anatomical location of gastrointestinal and genitourinary organs and structures may provide a method to better assess a specific disorder. Location of abdominal pain and possible origins of illness are listed in Box 21-1.

The types of abdominal pain that may result from chronic or acute episodes may be classified as visceral, somatic, and referred.

Visceral Pain

Visceral pain is caused by the stimulation of autonomic nerve fibers that surround a hollow viscus or by the distention or stretching of hollow viscus organs or ligaments. It is usually described by the patient as *cramping* or *gas-type pain* that varies in intensity, increasing to a high degree of severity and then subsiding. Visceral pain is generally diffuse and therefore difficult to localize. Often it is centered at the umbilicus or lower in the midline.

Visceral pain is frequently associated with other symptoms of autonomic nerve involvement such as tachycardia, diaphoresis, nausea, or vomiting. Common causes of visceral abdominal pain include early appendicitis, pancreatitis, cholecystitis, and intestinal obstruction.

Somatic Pain

Somatic pain is produced by bacterial or chemical irritation of nerve fibers in the peritoneum (peritonitis). Unlike visceral pain, somatic pain is usually constant and localized to a specific area. It is often described by the patient as *sharp* or *stabbing*. A patient with somatic abdominal pain is generally hesitant to move about and lies on his or her back or side with legs flexed to prevent additional pain from stimulation of the peritoneal area. These patients often exhibit involuntary guarding of the abdomen and rebound tenderness during the physical examination. Common causes of somatic pain are appendicitis and an inflamed

BOX 21-1

Location of Abdominal Pain and Possible Origins

Right Upper Quadrant

Cholecystitis
Hepatitis
Pancreatitis
Perforated ulcer
Renal pain (right)

Left Upper Quadrant

Pancreatitis
Gastritis
Renal pain (left)

Right Lower Quadrant

Appendicitis
Abdominal aortic dissection or rupture
Ruptured ectopic pregnancy
Ovarian cyst (right)
Pelvic inflammatory disease
Urinary calculus
Hernia
Ovarian or testicular torsion

Left Lower Quadrant

Diverticulitis
Abdominal aortic dissection or rupture
Ruptured ectopic pregnancy
Ovarian cyst (left)
Pelvic inflammatory disease
Urinary calculus
Hernia
Ovarian or testicular torsion

Epigastric Pain

Gastritis
Esophagitis
Pancreatitis
Cholecystitis
Abdominal aortic aneurysm
Myocardial ischemia

Diffuse Pain

Intestinal obstruction
Perforation
Generalized peritonitis

or perforated viscus (ulcer, gallbladder, or small or large intestine).

Referred Pain

Referred pain is pain in a part of the body considerably removed from the tissues that cause the pain. This mechanism results from branches of visceral fibers that synapse in the spinal cord with the same second-order neurons that receive pain fibers from the skin. When these pain fibers are stimulated intensely, pain sensations spread, and the patient experiences the pain in areas distant from the original source.

A knowledge of referred pain is important because many visceral ailments cause no other symptoms except referred pain. For example, cardiac pain may be referred to the neck and jaw, shoulders, pectoral muscles, and down the arms; biliary pain to the subscapular area; renal calculus to the genitalia and flank area; uterine and rectal pain to the low back; and a leaking aortic aneurysm to the lower back or buttocks. Surface areas of referred pain from visceral organs are illustrated in Fig. 21-4.

Signs and Symptoms

Although numerous signs and symptoms may be associated with acute abdominal pain, the following are the most common:

- Nausea, vomiting, anorexia
  - Gastritis
  - Pancreatitis
  - Biliary tract disease
  - High intestinal obstruction
- Diarrhea
  - Inflammatory process (gastroenteritis, ulcerative colitis)
- Constipation
  - Dehydration, obstruction, medications (codeine, *morphine*)
- Stool color
  - Biliary tract obstruction (clay-colored stools)
  - Lower intestinal bleeding (black, tarry stools)
- Chills and fever
  - Bacterial infection

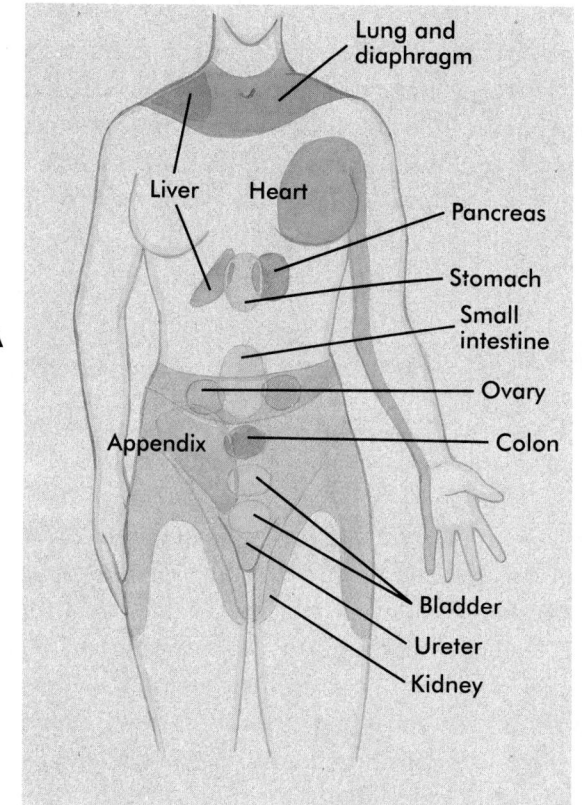 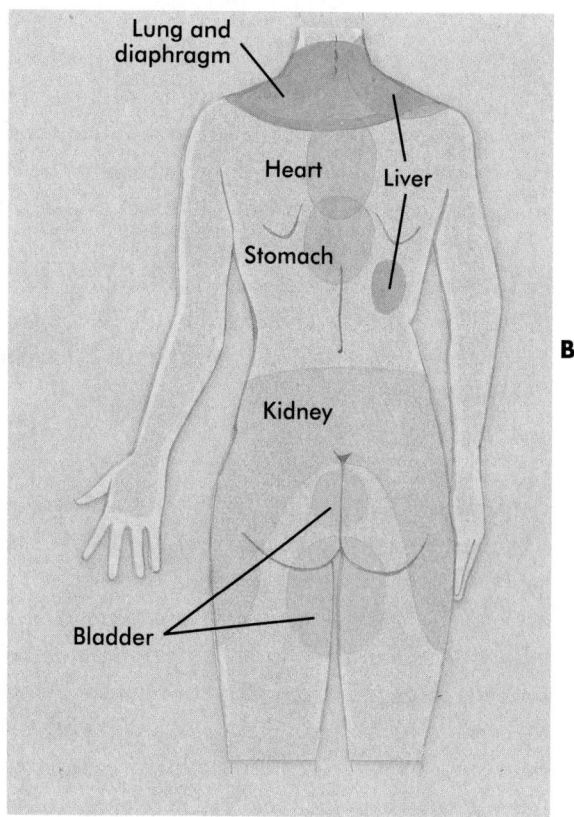

Fig. 21-4 Referred pain. **A,** Anterior view. **B,** Posterior view.

  ◦ Pyelonephritis
  ◦ Appendicitis
  ◦ Cholecystitis
• Urinary tract symptoms
  ◦ Dysuria
  ◦ Hematuria
  ◦ Urinary retention
• Gynecological symptoms
  ◦ Lower abdominal pain
  ◦ Vaginal discharge
  ◦ Pain with intercourse (dyspareunia)
  ◦ Vaginal bleeding

Vital Signs

Vital sign assessment should be complete, including evaluation and documentation of the patient's blood pressure, pulse rate, respiratory rate, skin color, moisture, temperature, and turgor. In addition, when possible, the presence or absence

of orthostatic changes in the patient's blood pressure should be noted by way of a tilt test. Relative hypovolemia, hemorrhage, or both, are indicated by a tilt test in which the patient's pulse rate increases 10 to 15 beats per minute or systolic blood pressure drops 10 to 15 mm Hg when the patient is moved from a supine to a sitting position.

Physical Examination

The physical examination of a patient with acute abdominal pain includes the skills of inspection, auscultation and palpation. If there is reason to suspect life-threatening illness requiring rapid stabilization and transportation of the patient, the examination should be completed en route to the receiving hospital. Physical examination of the patient's abdomen is described in Chapter 11, but the following discussion serves as a review.

Inspection

In the initial patient encounter, the paramedic should note the position in which the patient is lying. As previously stated, many patients with abdominal pain lie on their sides with their knees flexed and pulled in toward their chests. Other visual clues that may indicate abdominal pain are skin color, facial expressions such as grimacing, and the presence or absence of voluntary movement. The patient's clothing should be removed and the abdominal wall inspected for the presence of bruises, scars, ascites, abdominal distention, or abdominal masses.

Auscultation

Auscultation to confirm the presence or absence of bowel sounds is usually reserved for assessment in the emergency department. However, if auscultation is to be performed, it should be done in all four quadrants for a minimum of 1 to 2 minutes each and should always precede palpation, which may alter the intensity of bowel sounds. Bowel sounds that are increased in number, duration, or intensity indicate the possibility of gastroenteritis or intestinal obstruction. Bowel sounds that are markedly decreased in number and intensity or are absent may indicate peritonitis or ileus.

Palpation

Gentle palpation of the abdomen should begin by avoiding the painful area until the remainder of the abdomen is examined. The paramedic should be alert to rigidity or spasm, tenderness or masses, and the patient's facial expressions, which may provide clues about the severity of the pain. In addition, the paramedic should note whether the abdomen is soft and palpable or rigid.

● MANAGEMENT OF ACUTE ABDOMINAL PAIN

Patients with acute abdominal pain cannot be definitively managed in the prehospital setting. The majority require extensive evaluation in the emergency department, including laboratory analysis, radiological imaging, fluid and medication therapy, and perhaps surgical intervention.

The role of the paramedic (Box 21-2) is to support the patient's airway and ventilatory status; to perform and document an initial patient assessment, including a thorough history; to monitor vital signs and cardiac rhythm; to initiate intravenous therapy for fluid replacement or fluid resuscitation if needed; and to rapidly transport the patient for physician evaluation.

● RENAL FAILURE

The kidneys play a major role in maintaining homeostasis by controlling extracellular fluid volume, maintaining proper electrolyte composition and blood pH, and eliminating waste products. If this organ system malfunctions, serious systemic consequences develop, including uremia with subsequent encephalopathy or pericarditis, hyperkalemia, acidosis, hypertension, and volume overload with subsequent congestive heart failure. Depending on the duration of renal failure and its potential for reversibility, the disease can be classified as acute or chronic.

Acute Renal Failure

Acute renal failure is a clinical syndrome that results when there is a sudden and marked decrease in filtration through the glomeruli, leading

---

BOX 21-2

Emergency Care for Acute Abdominal Pain

1. High-concentration oxygen administration
2. Adequate intravenous access with a crystalloid solution (Application of pneumatic antishock garments for the treatment of shock with acute abdominal pain is controversial and should be authorized by medical control.)
3. Electrocardiogram monitoring
4. Rapid and gentle transport to an appropriate medical facility

to the accumulation of salt, water, and nitrogenous wastes (azotemia) within the body. Causes of acute renal failure are diverse and include trauma, shock, infection, urinary obstruction, and multisystem diseases. Acute renal failure can threaten the life of a patient, but if recognized early and treated appropriately, it may be readily reversible.

The pathophysiology of acute renal failure may be classified as prerenal, postrenal, or renal in origin. Prerenal failure results from inadequate perfusion of the kidneys, which can be caused by hypovolemia, impaired cardiac output, or vascular obstruction of renal arteries. Postrenal failure is caused by obstruction to urine flow from both kidneys. Postrenal failure may be caused by ureteral and urethral obstructions (bilateral calculus, prostatic enlargement, urethral strictures). Renal causes of acute renal failure include glomerular and other microvascular diseases, tubular diseases, and interstitial diseases that cause direct damage to the kidney parenchyma. Examples include hypertension, nephrotoxins, autoimmune diseases, and pyelonephritis.

Signs and Symptoms

The onset of acute renal failure can occur within hours. As normal kidney function rapidly deteriorates, urine output frequently decreases (oliguria) or stops completely (anuria). This results in generalized edema from water and salt retention, acidosis from failure of the kidneys to rid the body of normal acidic products, high concentrations of nonprotein nitrogens (especially urea) from failure of the body to excrete metabolic end products, and high concentrations of other products of renal excretion (such as uric acid and potassium). The resulting condition is often termed *uremia.*

If not recognized early and appropriately treated, renal dysfunction leads to the development of heart failure, hyperkalemia, and metabolic acidosis. Definitive care is directed at restoring the normal homeostatic environment (usually by dialysis) and treating the underlying condition that has precipitated the renal failure.

Chronic Renal Failure

Chronic renal failure is a progressive, irreversible systemic disease that develops over months to years. It may be caused by congenital disorders or prolonged pyelonephritis, but in the industrialized world, it more commonly results from diabetes and hypertension. This type of kidney dysfunction leads to progressive abnormality in blood counts and blood chemistry levels, which in its final stages commonly requires treatment with dialysis (hemodialysis or peritoneal dialysis) or renal transplantation for continued patient survival. In addition to oliguria, the patient with chronic renal failure may exhibit the following six systemic manifestations:

1. Gastrointestinal manifestations
   a. Anorexia
   b. Nausea
   c. Vomiting
2. Cardiopulmonary manifestations
   a. Hypertension
   b. Pericarditis
   c. Pulmonary edema
   d. Peripheral, sacral, and periorbital edema
3. Nervous system manifestations
   a. Anxiety
   b. Delirium
   c. Progressive obtundation
   d. Hallucinations
   e. Muscle twitching
   f. Seizures
4. Metabolic or endocrine manifestations
   a. Glucose intolerance
   b. Electrolyte disturbances
   c. Anemia
5. Personality changes
   a. Fatigue
   b. Mental dullness
6. Signs of uremia
   a. Pasty, yellow skin discoloration and thin extremities from protein wasting
   b. Uremic frost caused by urea crystals that form on the skin (late finding)

Renal Hemodialysis

Dialysis is a technique used to normalize blood chemistry in patients with acute or chronic renal failure and to remove blood toxins in some patients who have taken a drug overdose. The two dialytic techniques are hemodialysis and peritoneal dialysis, which bring the patent's blood into contact with a semipermeable membrane across which water-soluble substances diffuse into a dialyzing fluid (dialysate). After an interval, equilibration of the patient's blood with the dialysate normalizes the electrolyte composition, and waste products are eliminated.

The amount of substance that transfers during dialysis depends on the difference between the concentration on the two sides of the semipermeable membrane, the molecular size of the substance, and the length of time the blood and the dialysate remain in contact with the membrane. In patient's with end-stage renal disease, hemodialysis is usually performed 3 times a week for 4 to 5 hours each time.

Hemodialysis

In hemodialysis, the patient's heparinized blood is pumped through a surgically constructed arteriovenous fistula, which is an internal anastomosis between an artery and a vein, or an arteriovenous graft, which is a synthetic material grafted to the patient's artery and vein (Fig. 21-5). These "internal shunts" are usually located in the inner aspect of the patient's forearm or much less commonly in the medial aspect of the lower extremity. Other patients may have a small, button-shaped device **(hemasite)** usually located in the upper arm or proximal, anterior thigh. A hema-

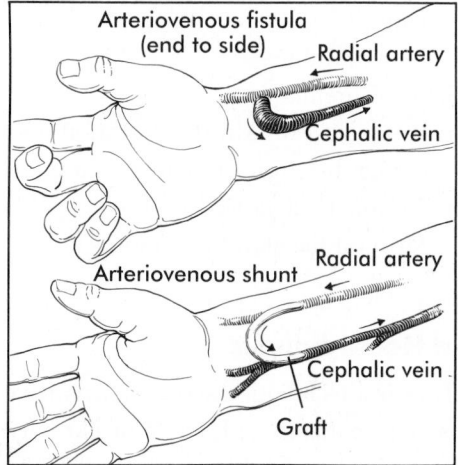

Fig. 21-5 Arteriovenous fistula.

site is similar to an arteriovenous graft but has an external rubber septum sutured to the skin through which a dialysis catheter is inserted for treatment.

Peritoneal Dialysis

In peritoneal dialysis, the dialysis membrane is the patient's own peritoneum. The dialysate is infused into the peritoneal cavity by a temporary percutaneous or permanently implanted catheter. Fluid and solutes diffuse from the blood in the peritoneal capillaries into the dialysate. After 1 to 2 hours, when equilibration has occurred, the dialysate is drained and fresh fluid is infused. Peritoneal dialysis works considerably more slowly than hemodialysis, but over time it is just as effective and does not require chronic blood access. A major complication of peritoneal dialysis is peritonitis, which usually results when the procedure is not performed with proper aseptic technique.

Dialysis Emergencies

Emergencies the paramedic may encounter when caring for a patient with acute or chronic renal failure may result from the disease process itself or from complications of dialytic therapy. For example, these patients may experience problems associated with vascular access, hemorrhage, hypotension, chest pain, severe hyperkalemia, disequilibrium syndrome, and the development of an air embolism. In addition, the paramedic should be aware of problems that may result from concurrent medical illness and its treatment. These include decreased ability to tolerate the stress of significant illness or trauma, inadvertent overadministration of intravenous fluid, and altered metabolism and unpredictable action of drugs.

Vascular Access Problems

Problems associated with vascular access are bleeding at the site of puncture for dialysis, thrombosis, and infection. Bleeding from the fistula or graft is usually minimal and can generally be controlled by direct pressure at the site. (However, excessive pressure can cause thrombosis in the graft or fistula.) A potential complication of an internal shunt is development of a pseudoaneurysm, which can rupture, causing a large hematoma and possible hypovolemia. If this occurs, direct pressure should be applied to the hematoma, and the patient should be assessed and treated for significant blood loss. This situation requires rapid transport for physician evaluation.

Fistulas and grafts that become occluded as a result of thrombus formation usually require surgical intervention or the administration of a thrombolytic agent to restore flow. Patients with a surgical anastomosis are instructed to periodically check for the presence of a bruit or "thrill" to verify unobstructed circulation. Attempts to clear the graft by irrigation or aspiration are not generally recommended. If thrombosis occurs while the patient is undergoing dialysis, the dialysis should be stopped and intravenous fluids initiated in an alternative site. Decreased blood flow is a common precipitating cause of thrombosis and is a main reason that blood pressure is not obtained in the arm with a vascular access.

Infection at the site of vascular access is usually the result of the puncture made during dialysis. Therefore meticulous sterile technique is mandatory when caring for these patients, and routine vascular access using this route should be discouraged. Vascular access infection should be considered when a dialysis patient has unexplained fever, malaise, or other signs of systemic infection.

Hemorrhage

Patients receiving dialysis have an increased risk of hemorrhage because of their regular exposure to anticoagulants and the decrease in their platelet function. Therefore a patient who experiences hemorrhage from trauma or a medical condition (for example, gastrointestinal bleeding) should be closely monitored for signs of hypovolemia. Most patients on dialysis have a baseline anemia that lowers their reserves when they have acute hemorrhage. Any significant blood loss (whether external or internal) may manifest as dyspnea or angina. If hemorrhage from trauma occurs in an extremity with a fistula or graft, bleeding should be controlled and the extremity immobilized in the normal fashion, using special

care to try to avoid obstructing circulation in the anastomosis.

Hypotension

Hypotension is not infrequently associated with hemodialysis. This may result from the rapid reduction in intravascular volume, abrupt changes in electrolyte concentrations, or vascular instability that may occur during the procedure. In addition, the patient's compensatory mechanisms to cope with these physiological alterations may be impaired, resulting in an inability to maintain normal blood pressure. Patients with hypotension caused by dialysis must be cautiously managed with the administration of volume-expanding fluids. The paramedic should be careful not to produce a fluid overload, which may manifest as hypertension and the classic signs of congestive heart failure (pulmonary edema, shortness of breath, crackles, engorged neck veins, liver congestion and engorgement, and pitting edema). Most patients respond to a relatively small (200- to 300-ml) fluid challenge. If they do not, other potentially serious etiologies should be considered.

Chest Pain

The episodes of hypotension and mild hypoxemia that commonly occur during dialysis may result in myocardial ischemia and chest pain. The patient may also complain of other symptoms associated with decreased oxygen delivery, such as headache and dizziness. Although these complaints may indicate an evolving myocardial infarction, they are often relieved with the administration of *oxygen,* fluid replacement, and antianginal medications. Regardless, all patients with chest pain should be treated as though a myocardial infarction has occurred.

Dysrhythmias resulting from myocardial ischemia may also be associated with dialysis. The most common ischemic rhythm disturbances are premature ventricular contractions, which generally respond well to the administration of supplemental *oxygen* and *lidocaine.* If dialysis is in progress, the procedure should be discontinued, and the paramedic should consult with medical control.

Indwelling Vascular Devices

Heparin Lock

A heparin lock is a peripheral intravenous cannula that has no attached intravenous tubing (Fig. 21-6). These vascular access devices are used to have ready access to peripheral veins for the brief administration of medications or for frequent intravenous therapy on an outpatient basis (for example, chemotherapy). The cannula is filled with 0.5 to 1.0 ml of a heparin solution to prevent clotting while it is not in use.

To gain access to the peripheral vein, 4 ml of normal saline should be drawn into a syringe. Aseptic technique is used; 2 ml of the normal saline is used to flush the heparin lock reservoir before and after the prescribed medication or intravenous fluid infusion. After intravenous therapy, 0.5 to 1.0 ml of heparin should be injected into the reservoir to keep the lock patent.

Atrial Catheters

An atrial catheter (Fig. 21-7) is a long, Silastic indwelling catheter sometimes used by patients with cancer, gastrointestinal dysfunction, or debilitating diseases and by those who need intermittent intravenous administration of antibiotics, nutritional supplements, or other intravenous medications. Patients are sometimes discharged from the hospital with the catheter in place and are taught to maintain it and to administer various medications and fluid therapies through the device.

The atrial catheter is approximately 90 mm long and 1.6 mm in diameter. It is surgically placed in the right atrium under fluoroscopy and local anesthesia. When seen on the patient's chest, the catheter looks like a thin, white cord with a Luer plug attached on the end. It protrudes from a small incision near the clavicle, which is usually covered with a dressing. Atrial catheters should only be used for venous access in emergency situations such as acute fluid loss, pulmonary edema, or cardiac arrest. Connecting intravenous lines to the catheter increases the chance of infection and embolism. Therefore the catheter should not be used in stable patients. When it is necessary to gain access to an atrial catheter, the following procedure should be followed[3]:

1. Gather needed material:
   20-ml, 5-ml, and 3-ml syringes
   18-gauge needle
   30-ml multidose vial of bacteriostatic 0.9% normal saline solution: povidone-iodine (Betadine) and intravenous administration set
2. Draw up 3 ml of normal saline and set it aside.
3. Apply gloves for patient and personal protection.

NOTE: Most patients with an atrial catheter are immunosuppressed or severely debilitated, so they are susceptible to routine pathogens. Special care should be taken by the paramedic to avoid contamination.

4. Explain the procedure to the patient.
5. Clamp the catheter with a padded smooth shunt clamp to prevent nicking or severing the catheter.

NOTE: Because the atrial catheter is a central line catheter, an air embolism is possible when changing tubing or changing syringes.

6. Remove and discard intermittent infusion device. (Connections are usually taped to avoid disconnection and air embolism.)
7. Wipe the connection site with povidone-iodine and allow it to dry.
8. Connect the 5-ml syringe. Remove the clamp and withdraw 5 ml of blood. (Do not use heparinized blood for the specimen.)
9. Replace the clamp.
10. Attach the 3-ml syringe of normal saline to the catheter, remove the clamp, and flush to prevent clot formation within the catheter.
11. Replace the clamp and remove the syringe.
12. Connect the intravenous tubing to the catheter, making sure that the tubing is free of air.
13. Remove the clamp and begin infusion.

Indwelling Vascular Devices—cont'd

14. Tape the connection site between the intravenous tubing and catheter. Use like any other peripheral intravenous line.

Implantable Ports

Implantable ports are venous access devices that are surgically implanted, with the distal end of the catheter inserted into a large central vein. An example of such a device is the Port-A-Cath (Fig. 21-8). The injection end of the catheter is implanted subcutaneously, often on the chest wall, and has a self-sealing septum over a small chamber or reservoir. The tubing extends from the side of the reservoir to the venous insertion point. Each time the implantable port is accessed, the skin must be punctured with a needle, but no daily cleansing is required as it is with partially implanted ports such as the Hickman catheter. Implantable ports should not be used in stable patients. To use implantable ports:

1. Locate the device and stabilize it with one hand.

2. Puncture the skin and septum with a Huber needle attached to a 3-ml syringe containing sterile saline. (Huber needles are special stainless-steel needles; they may be straight for injections or angled 90 degrees for intravenous infusion.)

3. Aspirate blood to determine patency and then inject the saline to flush the system.

4. Connect intravenous tubing to the reservoir, making sure that the tubing is free of air.

5. Tape the connection site between the intravenous tubing and reservoir.

6. After use, flush the device with a heparinized solution.

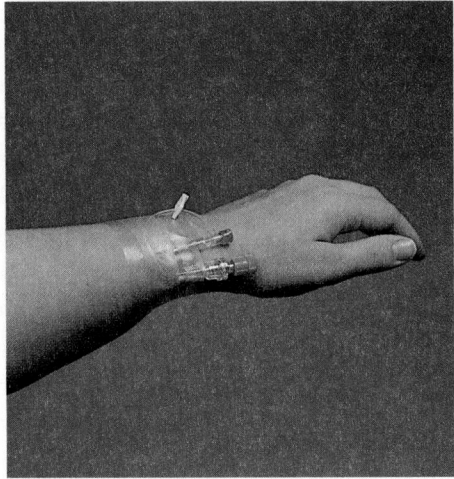

Fig. 21-6 Heparin lock.

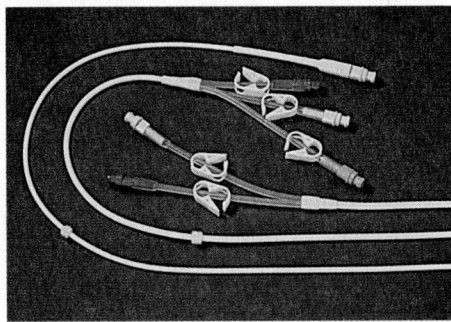

Fig. 21-7 Single-, dual-, and triple-lumen right atrial catheters.

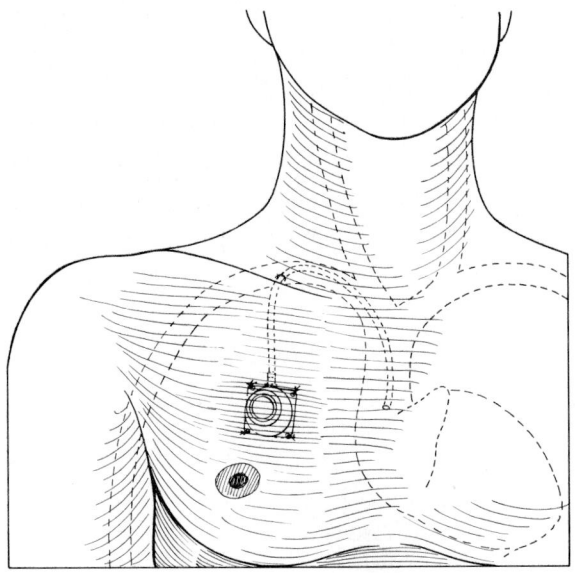

Fig. 21-8 Port-A-Cath.

Severe Hyperkalemia

Severe hyperkalemia is a life-threatening emergency that can occur rapidly in patients with acute renal failure. The condition frequently results from poor dietary regulation and missed dialysis treatments. Patients with severe hyperkalemia may have weakness, although they are frequently relatively asymptomatic. Typical electrocardiographic changes initially demonstrate a tall or tented T wave. As potassium levels rise above 6 to 6.5 mmol/L, conduction slows, resulting in a prolonged PR interval. Depressed ST segments and loss of P waves may occur after the potassium level rises above approximately 7 mmol/L. As levels rise even higher, the QRS complex widens, and delayed conduction in the interventricular conducting system can produce patterns resembling bundle branch blocks. Hyperkalemic disturbances may not become apparent until dangerous levels of potassium are present. Therefore any patient with renal failure who is in cardiac arrest should be suspected of having severe hyperkalemia. Based on patient history, medical control may recommend separate infusions of *calcium* and *sodium bicarbonate* during resuscitation.

Disequilibrium Syndrome

Disequilibrium syndrome refers to a group of neurological findings that sometimes occurs during or immediately after dialysis. Most often, these symptoms are mild (for example, headache, restlessness, nausea, and fatigue), but they may be severe (including confusion, seizures, and coma). The syndrome is thought to result from a disproportionate decrease in osmolality of the extracellular fluid compared with that of the intracellular compartment in the brain or cerebral spinal fluid. This results in an osmotic gradient between the blood and the brain, causing movement of water into the brain and subsequent cerebral edema and increased intracranial pressure. If seizures occur, *diazepam* may be indicated.

Air Embolism

Negative pressure on the venous side of the dialysis tubing or a malfunction in the dialysis machine can allow an air embolism to enter the patient's blood stream. If this occurs, the embolus may be carried to the right ventricle of the heart, blocking the passage of blood to the left myocardium. The patient may experience severe dyspnea, cyanosis, hypotension, and respiratory distress. A patient with an air embolus requires high-concentration oxygen administration and rapid transportation to a medical facility. In an effort to trap the embolism where it will be least likely to obstruct blood flow, the patient should be positioned on the left side and transported in the Trendelenburg position.

Management

To review, the prehospital management of patients with chronic or acute renal failure includes the following:

- Airway and ventilatory support with supplemental high-concentration oxygen administration
- Vascular access for fluid replacement, medication therapy (diuretics, antidysrhythmics), or fluid resuscitation if needed
- Meticulous aseptic technique
- Electrocardiogram and other vital sign monitoring
- Rapid transport to an appropriate medical facility

NOTE:

When it is necessary to obtain vascular access for drawing blood or infusing intravenous fluids in a patient with a surgical anastomosis, an alternative site should be chosen. In addition, blood pressure measurements and the use of tourniquets should be avoided in any extremity with an arteriovenous fistula or graft. As a last resort, medical control may recommend that the internal shunt be used to obtain vascular access. If so, the paramedic must be careful not to puncture the back wall of the vessel and to use careful aseptic technique throughout the procedure. Intravenous infusions must be closely monitored to avoid a "runaway IV," and the intravenous catheter should be taped securely in place.

REFERENCES

1. Tintinalli J et al, editors: *Emergency medicine: a comprehensive study guide*, ed 2, New York, 1988, McGraw-Hill.
2. Callaham M: *Current practice of emergency medicine*, ed 2, Philadelphia, 1992, BC Decker.
3. O'Keefe J: The hickman indwelling catheter in prehospital use, *JEMS* 11(6):51, 1986.

Summary

Management of the patient with acute abdominal pain or renal failure often begins in the prehospital setting, and success is often determined in large part by the assessment skills of the paramedic. Initial patient care measures include thorough evaluation of the patient's chief complaint, early management to provide stabilization, and rapid transport to an appropriate medical facility.

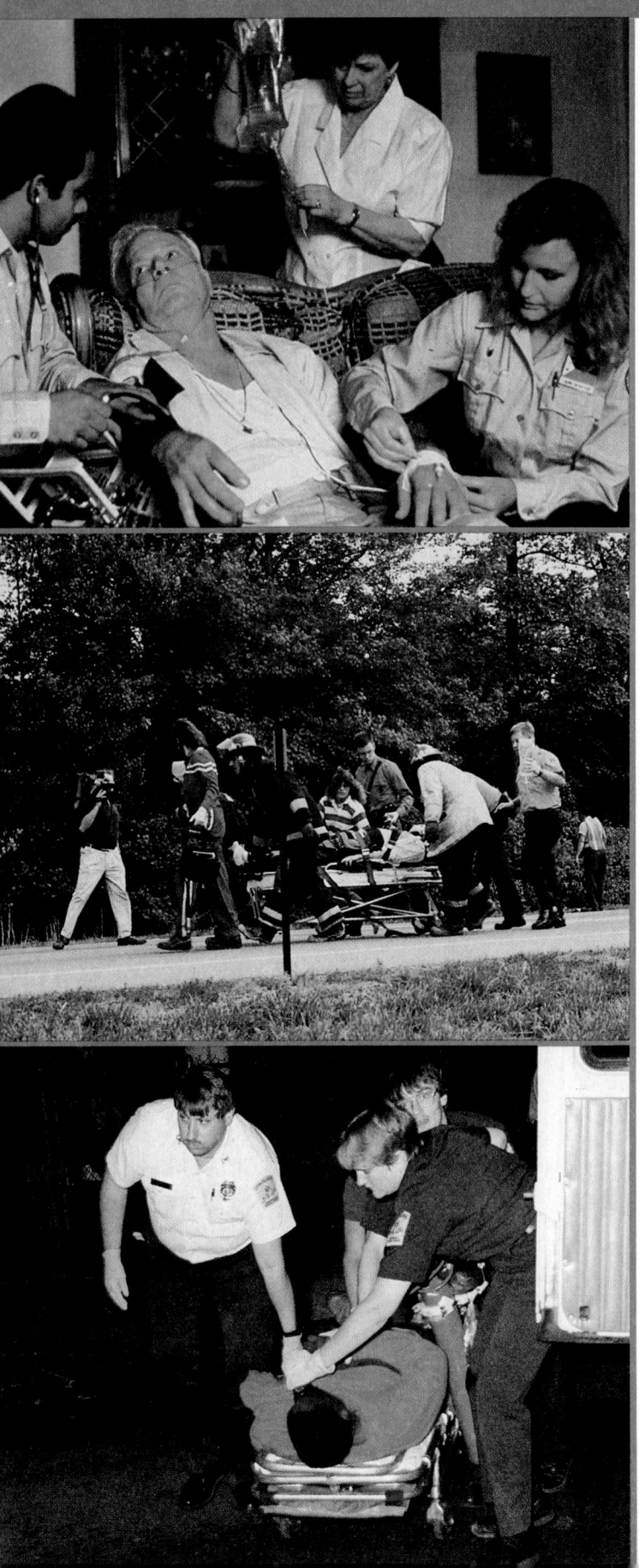

Anaphylaxis is an immediate, systemic, life-threatening reaction associated with major physiological changes in the cardiovascular, respiratory, and cutaneous systems. Prompt recognition and appropriate pharmacological therapy in the prehospital phase are crucially important to patient survival.

As a paramedic, you should be able to:

1. Describe how the lymphatic system, leukocytes, lymphocytes, immunoglobulins, and mediators work with other factors to provide the immune response.
2. Differentiate an allergic reaction and a normal immune response.
3. Define *anaphylaxis.*
4. Identify allergens associated with anaphylaxis.
5. Describe signs and symptoms of anaphylaxis.
6. Describe the pathophysiology, assessment, and management of anaphylaxis.

● ANTIGEN-ANTIBODY REACTION

An antigen is a substance that induces the formation of antibodies. Antigens may be introduced into the body by injection, ingestion, inhalation, or absorption. Examples of common antigens associated with anaphylactic reactions include drugs (penicillin, aspirin), envenomation (wasp stings), foods (seafood, nuts), and pollens.

Antibodies are protective protein substances developed by the body in response to antigens. Antibodies bind to the antigen that produced them and facilitate antigen neutralization and removal from the body. The normal reaction between antigens and antibodies protects the body from disease by activating the immune response.

● IMMUNE RESPONSE

The healthy body responds to an antigen challenge through a collective defense system known as *immunity.* Immunity may be natural, present at birth; acquired, resulting from exposure to a specific antigenic agent or pathogen; or artificially induced, such as that resulting from inoculation (**immunization**) against certain infectious diseases (for example, diphtheria and measles).

Immunization may be active or passive. In passive immunization, antibodies are injected and provide immediate but short-lived protection against specific disease-causing bacteria, viruses, or toxins. Active immunization primes the body to make its own antibodies against such microorganisms and confers longer-lasting immunity. Whether natural, acquired, or artificially induced, active immunity produces physiologically similar responses precipitated by the immune system. The components of the immune system are the lymphatic system, leukocytes, lymphocytes, immunoglobulins, and mediators.

Lymphatic System

Every tissue supplied by blood vessels (excluding the brain and placenta) also contains lymphatic vessels, which vary in size. Lymph fluid, which originates in the blood and enters the in-

---

KEY TERMS

allergen: A substance that can produce a hypersensitive reaction in the body but is not necessarily intrinsically harmful.

anaphylaxis: An exaggerated hypersensitivity reaction to a previously encountered antigen.

immunization: The process of rendering a person immune or of becoming immune.

immunoglobulin: Any of five structurally and antigenically distinct antibodies present in the serum and external secretions of the body, including immuglobulins A, D, E, G, and M.

terstitial spaces (by virtue of hydrostatic pressure in the capillaries), picks up microorganisms, cellular debris, or other foreign material in the tissues and carries it back through the lymphatic vessels to specialized lymphatic tissue, including lymph nodes. The foreign material is processed inside the nodes and presented to B or T lymphocytes, where an immune response to one or more specific antigens on the foreign material is activated. Lymph nodes are strategically clumped in areas that might be exposed to large amounts of antigen (for example, mesenteric nodes that monitor antigens arising from the gut). Fig. 22-1 shows the lymphatic system.

Leukocytes

Leukocytes are the blood component associated with the immune response. The majority of leukocytes in the peripheral blood consist of polymorphonuclear granulocytes, which are further divided into neutrophils, eosinophils, and basophils. Circulating lymphocytes account normally for approximately one third of the peripheral white cell count. (This may vary considerably with infections.) A third circulating leukocyte is the monocyte, which is essentially a circulating macrophage. The monocyte is capable of phago-

cytosis and is instrumental in processing antigens so that lymphocytes can recognize them and produce antibodies. Neutrophils and monocytes are the primary cells involved in phagocytosis and are capable of migrating out of blood vessels to sites where antigenic stimulation from a foreign body or infection has occurred.

Lymphocytes

Lymphocytes undergo a maturation process that depends on their lymphoid tissue of origin. The two classes of lymphocytes that are principal players in the immune response are T lymphocytes (T cells) and B lymphocytes (B cells).

T Lymphocytes

T lymphocytes compose 80% of all lymphocytes and are produced in the thymus. They help defend against foreign cells or viruses that enter the body. Each T lymphocyte possesses receptors for a specific antigen that allow it to "recognize" and

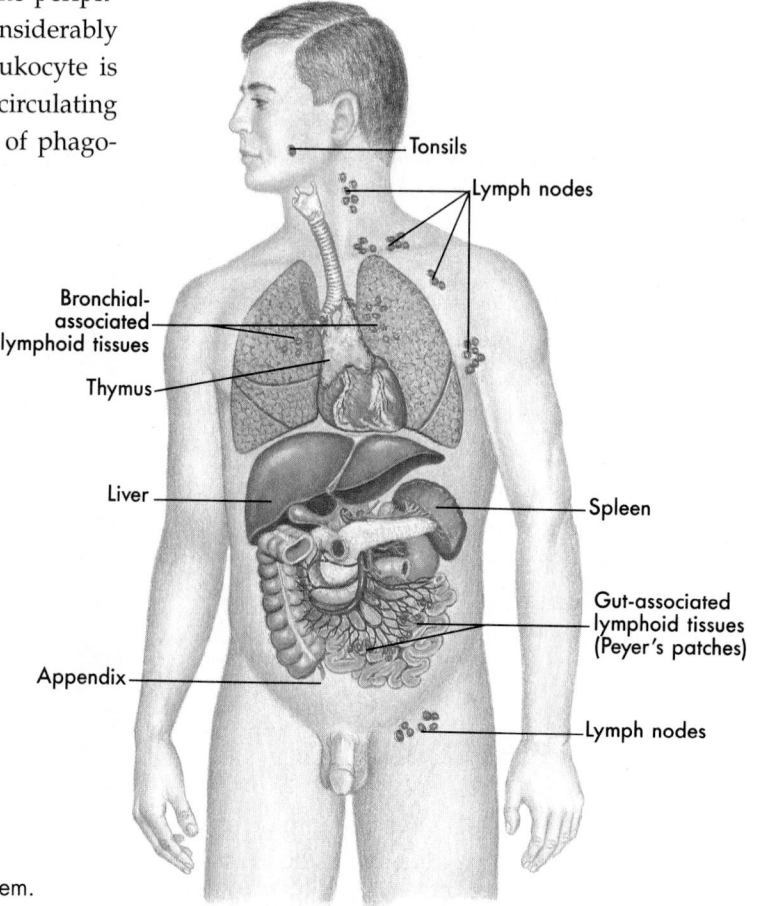

Fig. 22-1 Components of the lymphatic system.

attach to the antigen. Once stimulated by its specific antigen, the T lymphocyte proliferates and produces a large number of clone cells that contain identical antigen receptors. Within 48 hours, the clone cells further specialize with different receptors and travel to the designated site of action. Some of the clones (known as *killer T cells*) act directly to destroy the invading pathogens with enzymes. Others remain in lymph tissue as "memory cells" that facilitate a much more rapid response if a subsequent exposure to the same antigen occurs.

T lymphocytes can be further divided into helper and suppressor cells. A reduction in the ratio of helper to suppressor cells or a loss of T-lymphocyte function is the primary physiological alteration in the acquired immunodeficiency syndrome (AIDS) and is responsible for these patients' susceptibility to unusual infections and tumors (see Chapter 24).

B Lymphocytes

The remaining 20% of lymphocytes are B lymphocytes developed in the bone marrow. Like T lymphocytes, B lymphocytes are equipped with antigen-specific receptors. When activated, B lymphocytes clone to form two type of cells: antibody-secreting plasma cells and memory cells. The antibodies secreted by plasma cells bind to antigens on the organism and allow phagocytic cells and T lymphocytes to destroy the pathogen. Memory cells are reserved for future encounters with the same antigen and are the basis for developing acquired immunity.

Immunoglobulins

Antibodies, or **immunoglobulins** (Ig), are large glycoprotein molecules produced in large numbers by plasma cells (activated B lymphocytes) in response to antigenic stimulation. Five distinct classes of immunoglobulins are produced in humans; they consist of different subunits and perform different functions. Although the detailed structure of immunoglobulins is beyond the scope of this text, it is important to understand that there is a variable portion and a constant portion to each antibody (Box 22-1). The variable portion binds

---

BOX 22-1

Classes of Immunoglobulins

IgG

IgG accounts for 70% to 75% of antibodies in normal serum. IgG is most abundant in blood but is also found in lymph, cerebrospinal, synovial, and peritoneal fluid and breast milk. It is the major antibody involved in secondary immune responses and the only antitoxin antibody developed. IgG is also the only immunoglobulin that crosses the placenta, providing temporary immunity in neonates.

IgM

IgM accounts for approximately 5% to 10% of antibodies in normal serum and is the dominant antibody in ABO incompatibilities. IgM triggers the increased production of IgG in acute infections and the complement fixation required for an effective antibody response.

IgA

IgA accounts for approximately 15% of antibodies in normal serum. This immunoglobulin is found in blood, secretions such as tears and saliva, and the respiratory tract, stomach, and accessory organs. IgA combines with a protein in the mucosa and defends body surfaces against invading microorganisms.

IgE

IgE accounts for less than 1% of antibodies in normal serum. It is found in some tissues and on the surface membranes of basophils and mast cells; it is responsible for immediate hypersensitivity reactions.

IgD

IgD accounts for less than 1% of antibodies in normal serum. Its precise biological function is unknown.

the antigen, whereas the constant portion binds complement in some circumstances and phagocytic cells in others. Complement is a complex of at least 20 serum enzymatic proteins that mediate the inflammatory reaction and amplify a specific immune response.

Mediators

Mediators are proteins that cause a number of physiological responses. Most of these substances are present throughout the body and remain inactive until triggered by an immune response. Mediators have different properties, and most perform several functions. These substances are classified as follows:

- Vasoactive substances cause small vessels to dilate and become more permeable.
- Leukocytosis promoters stimulate the release of leukocytes from bone marrow and the production of new leukocytes.
- Chemotactic substances cause the attraction of phagocytic cells toward or away from the pathogenic agent.
- Leukotactic substances attract leukocytes to the pathogenic agent.
- Opsonins bind phagocytes to the invading microorganism, which promotes phagocytosis.

● ALLERGIC RESPONSE

The immune response is a normal, protective reaction between antigens and antibodies to guard the body against disease. Unfortunately, this response can become oversensitive or be directed toward harmless antigens to which we are often exposed. When this occurs, the response is termed *allergic.* The antigen causing the allergic response is called an **allergen.**

Allergic Reaction

Allergic reaction is marked by an increased physiological response to an antigen after a previous exposure (sensitization) to the same antigen. The allergic reaction is initiated when a circulat-

ing antibody (IgG or IgM) combines with a specific foreign antigen, resulting in type II and III hypersensitivity reactions (see Chapter 14), or to antibodies bound to mast cells or basophils (IgE). Type IV hypersensitivity is caused by T lymphocytes and is quite delayed in onset. Of these allergic or hypersensitivity reactions, type I or immediate hypersensitivity is the most dramatic.

This type of allergic reaction is mediated through IgE, which is bound to mast cells or basophils. When an antigen reacts with an IgE molecule, disruption of the mast cells or basophil membranes occurs, with prompt release of chemical mediators into the extracellular space. The target organs and the manifestations of the reaction are variable, ranging from hay fever to asthma to life-threatening anaphylaxis.

● ANAPHYLAXIS

The term **anaphylaxis** comes from Greek and means "against or opposite of protection." It is the most extreme form of an allergic reaction, accounting for 400 to 800 deaths per year. Anaphylaxis has a mortality rate of 3%.[1] Therefore rapid recognition and aggressive therapy are essential.

Causative Agents

Almost any substance can cause anaphylaxis (Box 22-2). The antigenic agents most frequently associated with anaphylaxis are penicillin (by ingestion or injection) and envenomation by stinging insects. Regardless of the offending antigen, the risk of anaphylaxis in sensitive individuals increases with the frequency of exposure and to a lesser extent the length of exposure.

Pathophysiology

A person must first be exposed to a specific antigen to develop type I hypersensitivity. In the first exposure, the antigen enters the body by ingestion, injection, inhalation, or absorption and activates the immune system. In susceptible individuals, large amounts of IgE antibody are produced.

IgE antibodies leave the lymphatic system and bind to the cell membranes of basophils circulating in the blood and to mast cells in tissues surrounding the blood vessels. They remain there, inactive, until the same antigen is introduced into the body a second time. With subsequent exposure to the specific antigen, the allergen crosslinks at least two of the cell-bound IgE molecules, resulting in degranulation of the mast cells and basophils and the onset of an anaphylactic reaction.

The degranulation of the target cell is associated with the release of pharmacologically active chemical mediators inside the affected basophils and mast cells. These chemicals include histamines, leukotrienes, eosinophil chemotactic factor of anaphylaxis, heparin, kinins, prostaglandins, and thromboxanes.

Histamines promote vascular permeability and cause dilation of capillaries and venules and contraction of nonvascular smooth muscle, especially in the gastrointestinal tract and bronchial tree. There is an associated increase in gastric, nasal, and lacrimal secretions, resulting in tearing and rhinorrhea. The increased capillary permeability allows plasma to leak into the interstitial space, decreasing the intravascular volume available for the heart to pump. The profound vasodilation that results further decreases cardiac preload, compromising stroke volume and cardiac output. These physiological effects lead to cutaneous flushing, urticaria, angioedema, and hypotension. The onset of action of the histamines is very rapid, but their effects are short lived as they are quickly broken down by plasma enzymes. The pathophysiology of anaphylactic shock is illustrated in Fig. 22-2.

Leukotrienes are the most potent bronchoconstrictors. These chemical mediators cause wheez-

---

BOX 22-2

Agents That May Cause Anaphylaxis

Drugs and Biological Agents

Antibiotics
Local anesthetics
Cephalosporins
Chemotherapeutics
Aspirin
Nonsteroidal antiinflammatory agents
Opiates
Muscle relaxants
Anticancer agents
Vaccines
Insulin

Insect Bites and Stings

Wasps
Bees
Fire ants

Foods

Peanuts, soybeans
Cod, halibut, shellfish (for example, shrimp)
Egg white
Strawberries
Food additives
Wheat and buckwheat
Sesame and sunflower seeds
Cottonseed
Milk
Mango

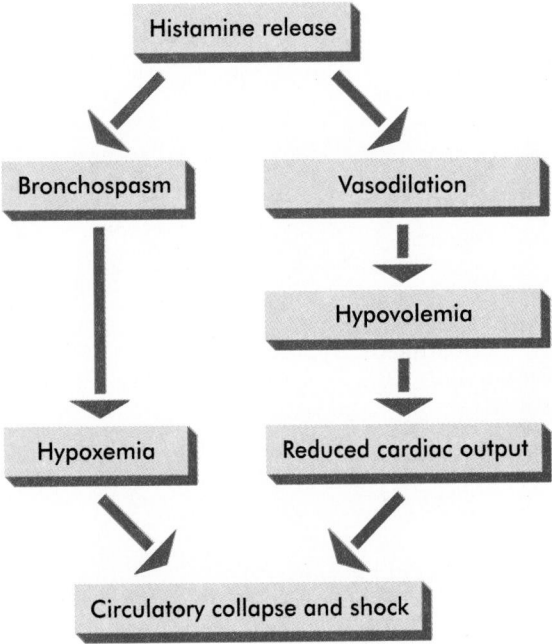

Fig. 22-2 Pathophysiology of anaphylactic shock.

BOX 22-3

Signs and Symptoms of Anaphylaxis

Upper Airway

Hoarseness

Stridor

Laryngeal or epiglottic edema

Rhinorrhea

Lower Airway

Bronchospasm

Increased mucus production

Accessory muscle use

Wheezing

Decreased breath sounds

Cardiovascular System

Tachycardia

Hypotension

Dysrhythmias

Chest tightness

Gastrointestinal System

Nausea

Vomiting

Abdominal cramps

Diarrhea

Neurological System

Anxiety

Dizziness

Syncope

Weakness

Headache

Seizure

Coma

Cutaneous System

Angioedema

Urticaria

Pruritus

Erythema

Edema

Tearing of the eyes

---

ing, coronary vasoconstriction, and increased vascular permeability. Leukotrienes were formerly known as *slow-reacting substances of anaphylaxis* because their effects were delayed relative to histamine. (However, the duration of action of these chemicals is much longer than that of histamines.)

The eosinophil chemotactic factor of anaphylaxis attracts eosinophils to the site of allergic inflammation. Its exact mechanism of action is unknown, but it is believed that eosinophils contain an enzyme that can deactivate leukotrienes. The remaining chemical mediators (heparin, neutrophil chemotactic factor, and kinins) exert varying effects that may include fever, chills, bronchospasm, and pulmonary vasoconstriction. These complex chemical processes can rapidly lead to upper airway obstruction and bronchospasm, dysrhythmias and cardiac ischemia, and circulatory collapse and shock.

Assessment

An accurate history and physical assessment are necessary to differentiate severe allergic reactions from other medical conditions that may mimic anaphylaxis. A flawed prehospital assessment in this group can have life-threatening consequences. Disease entities that may present with similar signs and symptoms of anaphylaxis include:

- Severe asthma with respiratory failure
- Upper airway obstruction
- Toxic shock
- Pulmonary edema (with or without myocardial infarction)
- Drug overdose
- Hypovolemic shock

Respiratory Effects

Initial signs of respiratory involvement associated with anaphylaxis may range from sneezing and coughing to complete airway obstruction (secondary to laryngeal and epiglottic edema) (Box 22-3). The patient may complain of throat tightness and dyspnea, and stridor or voice changes may be evident. Lower airway bronchospasm and associated hypersecretion of mucus caused by the actions of histamine, leukotriene, and prostaglandins may produce wheezing and significant respiratory distress. Symptoms can develop with startling rapidity.

Cardiovascular Effects

Cardiovascular manifestations of allergic reactions range from mild hypotension to vascular collapse and profound shock in anaphylaxis. Dysrhythmias are common and may be related to the severe hypoxia inherent in this situation. The patient may complain of chest pain if myocardial ischemia is present.

Gastrointestinal Effects

Nausea, vomiting, diarrhea, and severe abdominal cramping may occur in a patient with an anaphylactic reaction. The increased gastrointestinal activity is related to smooth muscle contraction, increased mucus production, and outpouring of fluid from the gut wall into the intestinal lumen, initiated by the chemical mediators.

Nervous System Effects

Nervous system responses are largely caused by the impaired gas exchange and shock associated with anaphylaxis. Initially the patient may be agitated and speak of a sense of impending doom. As hypoxia and shock worsen, neurological function may deteriorate, resulting in weakness, headache, syncope, seizures, and coma.

Cutaneous Effects

The physical findings on the skin are perhaps the most visible signs that distinguish anaphylaxis from other medical conditions. These signs are secondary to the vasodilation induced by histamine release from the mast cells. Initially the patient may complain of warmth and pruritus. Physical examination often reveals diffuse erythema and urticaria that result in well-circumscribed wheals of 1 to 6 cm, with raised erythematous margins and blanched centers (Fig. 22-3). Marked swelling of the face and tongue and angioedema may also be present, reflecting involvement of deeper capillaries of the skin and mucous membranes. As hypoxia and shock continue, cyanosis may be evident.

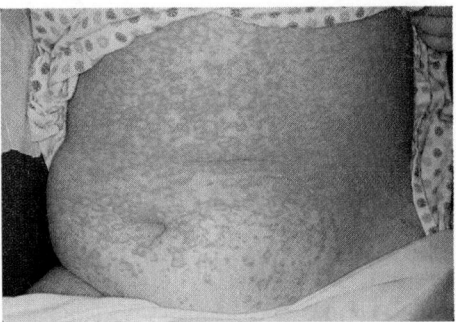

Fig. 22-3 Urticaria as a result of an allergic reaction.

Primary Survey

As in any critical emergency, initial patient care measures are directed at providing adequate airway, ventilatory, and circulatory support. However, pharmacological therapy is often the definitive treatment in anaphylaxis. Therefore drug administration should be expedited.

Airway assessment is critical because most deaths from anaphylaxis are directly related to upper airway obstruction. The conscious patient should be evaluated for voice changes, stridor, or a barking cough. Complaints of tightness in the neck and dyspnea should alert the paramedic to impending airway obstruction. If the patient is unconscious on EMS arrival, the airway should be evaluated and secured. If airflow is impeded, intubation should be attempted using direct observation (the orotracheal route). If there is severe laryngeal and epiglottic edema, needle cricothyrotomy may be indicated to provide airway access.

The patient should be closely monitored for signs of respiratory distress as indicated by skin color, accessory muscle use, wheezing, diminished breath sounds, and abnormal respiratory rates. Circulatory status may also deteriorate quickly. Therefore pulse quality, rate, and location should be frequently assessed. If available, pulse oximetry should be considered.

History

A history may be difficult to obtain but can be critical to rule out other medical emergencies that may mimic anaphylaxis. The patient should be questioned regarding the chief complaint and the rapidity of onset of symptoms. Signs and symptoms of anaphylaxis usually appear within 1 to 30 minutes of introduction of the antigen.

Significant medical history to be elicited includes previous exposure and response to the suspected antigen. In addition, the method of introduction of the antigen should be ascertained because injection frequently produces the most rapid and severe response. Other significant history includes chronic or concurrent illness and medication use. Preexisting cardiac disease or bronchial asthma should lead the paramedic to anticipate severe complications in these organ systems as a result of the allergic reaction. Use of certain drugs, such as beta-blocking agents, may diminish the patient's response to *epinephrine* and necessitate administration of other medications. The paramedic should also determine whether the patient has been prescribed an emergency *epinephrine* kit (for example, Epi Pen) and whether the medication was administered before the arrival of EMS personnel.

Secondary Survey

Vital signs should be assessed early in the patient encounter and reassessed frequently. In severe reactions, most patients are initially tachycardiac, tachypneic, and hypotensive if deterioration to cardiac arrest has not occurred. The patient's face and neck should be inspected for angioedema, hives, tearing, and rhinorrhea. The presence of erythema or urticaria on other body regions should be noted. Along with vital signs, lung sounds should be frequently assessed to evaluate the clinical progress of the patient and to monitor the effectiveness of interventions. Cardiac monitoring should also be instituted as soon as possible to aid in patient evaluation.

Pharmacological Therapy

Ventilatory support and the parenteral administration of *epinephrine* are the most specific interventions in the management of anaphylaxis. If manifestations are mild or moderate and the patient is alert, the subcutaneous administration of 0.3 to 0.5 ml of 1:1000 *epinephrine* is generally recommended. If the antigen was injected intradermally, medical control may recommend that 0.15 to 0.25 ml of 1:1000 *epinephrine* be injected into the site after the initial dose of *epinephrine*. Some experts also suggest that a constricting venous band be applied when possible at the site of injection (intradermal or intramuscular) of the presumed antigen to retard absorption. In addition, the affected limb should be splinted to limit movement.

If the patient has circulatory collapse, intravenous fluid therapy with a volume-expanding fluid should be initiated. This may need to be followed by slow intravenous administration of 0.1 to 0.2 mg (1 to 2 ml) of 1:10,000 *epinephrine*.

> **NOTE:**
> Complications of intravenous administration of *epinephrine* are significant and include the development of uncontrolled systolic hypertension, vomiting, seizures, dysrhythmias, and myocardial ischemia. This route should only be used in patients with a critical life-threatening condition. Intravenous administration of epinephrine is *rarely* performed in conscious patients. It is performed with *extreme* caution in *rare* circumstances and *only* at the direction of medical control.

The intravenous dose of *epinephrine* depends on the patient's size, medical history, and underlying condition. If the patient has a monitored rhythm but is pulseless, then intravenous administration of *epinephrine* is warranted. If intravenous access cannot be obtained during cardiac arrest, *epinephrine* may be administered via an endotracheal tube, but it should be diluted to 10 ml with normal saline. If no improvement is noted within 5 to 10 minutes after administration, continued rapid fluid infusion and a repeat dose of *epinephrine* are indicated.

Additional pharmacological therapy may be

helpful, but *epinephrine* is the only drug that can immediately reverse the life-threatening complications of anaphylaxis. Pharmacological agents that may be used with *epinephrine* include *diphenhydramine* to antagonize the effects of histamine, bronchodilators to improve alveolar ventilation, corticosteroids to prevent a delayed reaction, and perhaps *cimetidine* to relieve prolonged hypotension refractory to *epinephrine* or urticaria and pruritus.[2] After pharmacological therapy and stabilization, the patient should be rapidly transported to the receiving hospital.

REFERENCES

1. Tintinalli J et al, editors: *Emergency medicine: a comprehensive study guide,* ed 2, New York, 1988, McGraw-Hill.
2. Yarbrough J et al: Cimetidine in the treatment of refractory anaphylaxis, *Ann Allergy* 1989.

Summary

There are few situations in the prehospital environment in which a patient can be resuscitated from near death to a relatively stable hemodynamic state. Skilled and focused assessment techniques promoting recognition of anaphylaxis and appropriate pharmacological intervention can reverse the often lethal effects of this medical emergency.

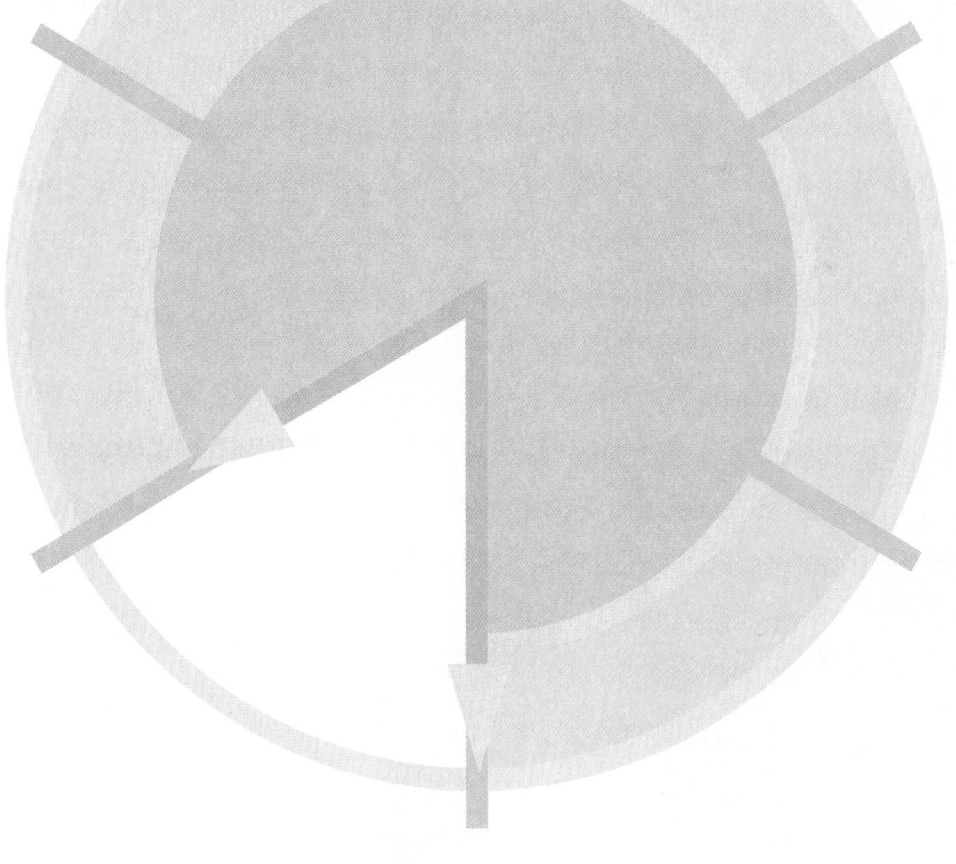

23 TOXICOLOGY, DRUG ABUSE, AND ALCOHOLISM

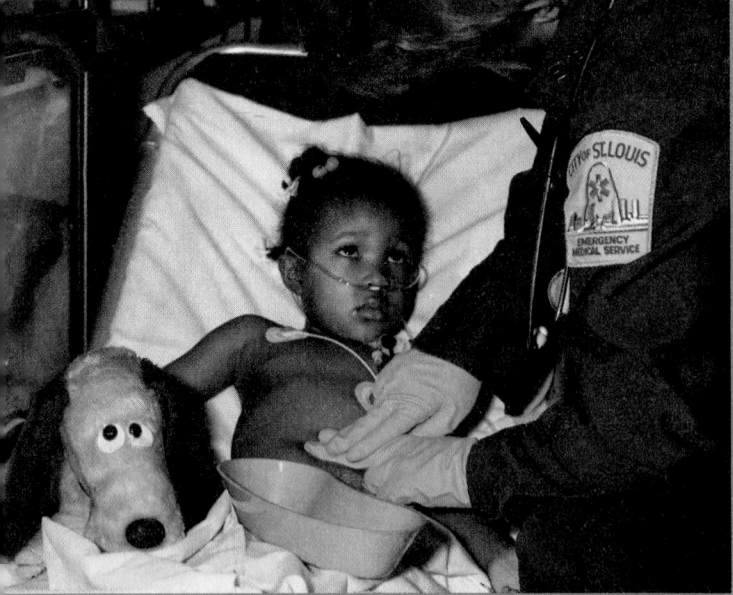

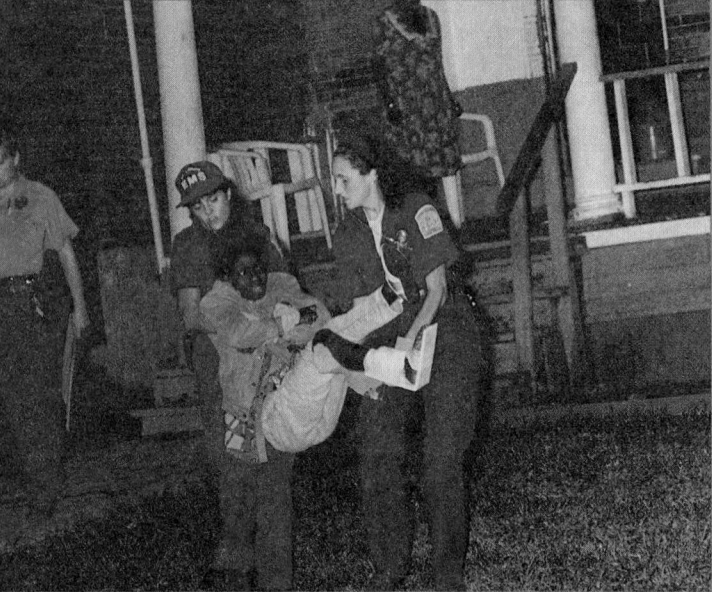

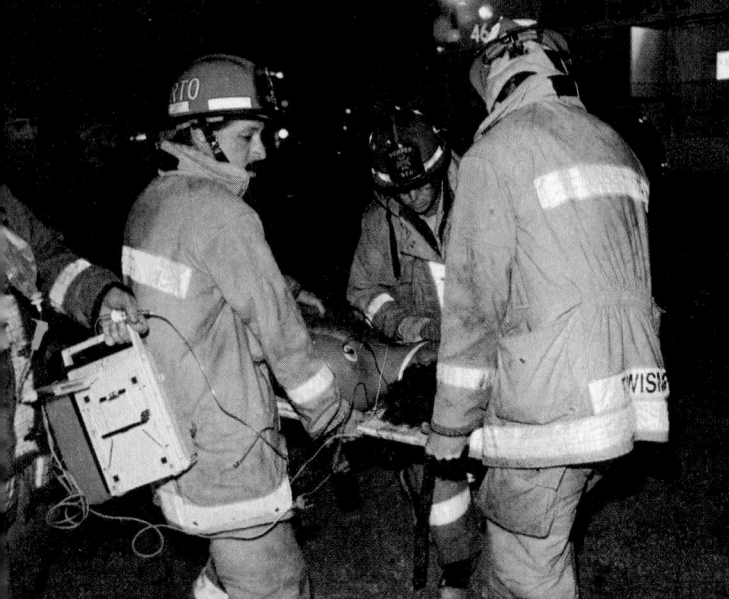

Our environment contains a large number of potentially harmful substances (natural and synthetic) that can be accidentally or deliberately introduced into the body. These include animal and plant toxins, industrial and household chemicals, therapeutic pharmaceuticals, and drugs of abuse. Early identification of these agents and prevention of systemic absorption are crucial to the successful management of patients with toxicological emergencies. The presentation of toxicological emergencies ranges from life-threatening situations to stable clinical conditions that can deteriorate over time.

OBJECTIVES

As a paramedic, you should be able to:

1. Define *poisoning*.
2. Discuss poison control centers.
3. Describe general principles of patient assessment and management of ingested poisons.
4. Describe the causative agents and pathophysiology of selected ingested poisons and management of patients who have taken them.
5. Distinguish among the three categories of inhaled toxins: simple asphyxiants, chemical asphyxiants and systemic poisons, and irritants or corrosives.
6. Describe general principles of managing the patient who has inhaled poison.
7. Describe the signs, symptoms, and management of patients who have inhaled ammonia or hydrocarbon.
8. Describe the signs, symptoms, and management of patients with organophosphate or carbamate poisoning.
9. Discuss key signs, symptoms, and management of patients injected with poison by insects, reptiles, and hazardous aquatic creatures.
10. List factors associated with drug and alcohol abuse.
11. Describe the common characteristics of drug and alcohol abuse.
12. Outline the general principles of managing patients with drug overdose.
13. Describe methods of administration, street names, signs, symptoms, and management for drug overdoses.
14. Describe the short- and long-term physiological effects of ethanol ingestion.
15. Describe signs, symptoms, and management of alcohol-related emergencies.

Section One
Poisonings

Emergencies involving a **poison** (any substance that produces harmful physiological or psychological effects) are a significant cause of morbidity and mortality in the United States. They are responsible for 10% of all emergency department visits, 9% of all ambulance patient transports, and 5% to 10% of all medical admissions to hospitals. According to the National Safety Council, poisoning by solids and liquids was the third leading cause of accidental death in the United States in 1988 and the second leading cause of accidental death for persons aged 24 to 48.[1]

Although it is estimated that as many as 5 million poisonings occur each year in the United States, more than half of these exposures are unreported. In 1990, the American Association of Poison Control Centers (AAPCC) reported 1.7 million exposures to toxic substances. Of these, 88.1% were classified as accidental (implying no harmful intent), 10% as intentional, and 0.5% as unknown.[2]

KEY TERMS

drug abuse: Self-medication or self-administration of a drug in chronically excessive amounts, resulting in psychological or physical dependence, functional impairment, and deviation from approved social norms.

poison: Any substance that produces harmful physiological or psychological effects.

withdrawal syndrome: Predictable set of signs and symptoms that occurs after a decrease in the amount of the usual dose of a drug or its sudden cessation.

Poison Control Centers

More than 120 poison control centers exist across the United States to help manage poisoning emergencies. Most are based in major medical centers or teaching hospitals, and each belongs to one of 35 AAPCC-designated regional poison control centers. Regional centers are staffed by medical professionals and offer 24-hour telephone access to population bases of at least 1 million.

By request, information and treatment advice is immediately provided through a comprehensive group of references on over 350,000 toxic substances, including drugs (legal, illicit, foreign, and veterinary), chemicals, plants, animals, insects, fish, snakes, cosmetics, and hazardous materials. Each request for patient care information is followed up to determine effectiveness and confirm desired outcome. In addition, the centers are responsible for the following six elements of an organized poison system:

1. Treatment information and toxicological consultation with health care providers (for example, hospitals, physicians, EMS services) and the public, using a toll-free number with linkage into various 911 systems
2. Professional education to train those involved in care of poisoned patients
3. Data collection on all poisonings in the region for epidemiological and evaluation purposes
4. Public education and prevention
5. Research
6. Regional EMS poison system development (for example, patient classification criteria, triage and treatment protocols, and regional transfer agreements)

Use by EMS Agencies

Regional poison control centers are a ready source of information for any toxicological emergency. Depending on local communications protocol, poison control centers may be contacted directly by EMS personnel through telephone, cellular phone, central dispatch, or medical control.

Definitive treatment can be initiated in approximately 85% of all poisoning incidents (if properly identified) in the prehospital phase of a poison system.[3] The immediate determination of potential toxicity is based on the specific agent or agents; amount ingested; time of exposure; age, weight, and medical condition of the patient; and any treatment rendered before EMS arrival. In addition, the poison control center can coordinate treatment protocol by notifying the receiving hospital while the ambulance is en route to the emergency department.

Poisons may be introduced into the body by ingestion, inhalation, surface absorption, and injection. Regardless of the route of entry, the basic principles of assessment and management include providing supportive care (maintenance of airway, breathing, and circulation), treating correctable life-threatening problems, obtaining a history of the event and any significant medical history of the patient, and preventing further absorption of the toxin. As always, crew safety must be kept in mind; a toxicological emergency response may involve hazardous materials or the possibility of unpredictable or violent behavior on the part of the patient.

● INGESTED POISONS

Some 80% of all accidental ingestions of poisons occurs in children aged 1½ to 3. The most common poison exposures in this group result from household products such as petroleum-based agents, cleaning agents, and cosmetics; medications; toxic plants; and contaminated foods. Poisoning in adults, on the other hand, is usually intentional, although accidental poisoning from exposure to chemicals in the workplace and at home is increasing. Deliberate poisonings are often a method or "gesture" of suicide or a result of recreational or experimental drug abuse.

The toxic effects of ingested poisons may be immediate or delayed, depending on the substance ingested. For example, corrosive substances such as strong acids and alkalis may produce immediate tissue damage, as evidenced by burns to the lips, tongue, throat, and upper gastrointestinal tract. Other substances, such as medications and toxic plants, usually require absorption through the blood stream to produce toxic effects. Because only minimal absorption occurs in the stomach, poisons may take several hours to enter the blood stream through the small intestine. Therefore early management of poisoning by ingestion focuses on removing the toxin from the stomach or binding it to prevent absorption before the poison enters the intestines.

Assessment and Management

The primary goal of physical assessment of poisoned patients is to identify effects on the three vital organ systems most likely to produce immediate morbidity and mortality: the respiratory system, the cardiovascular system, and the central nervous system. Five signs of major toxicity point to serious poisoning: coma, cardiac dysrhythmia, gastrointestinal disturbance, respiratory depression, and hypotension or hypertension. In addition, obtaining a detailed history of the event and of the patient's significant medical or psychiatric characteristics may direct patient management decisions in the field or emergency department.

Respiratory Complications

As in any patient care encounter, the first priority in managing a poisoned patient after ensuring scene safety is to secure a patent airway and provide adequate ventilatory support as needed. If there is any question about the integrity of the airway, aggressive airway management should be initiated to protect against potential compromise or aspiration. Other respiratory complications that may be associated with poisoning include the early development of noncardiogenic pulmonary edema or the later development of adult respiratory distress syndrome and bronchospasm, which may result from direct or indirect toxic effects.

Cardiovascular Complications

The most common cardiovascular complication of poisoning is cardiac rhythm disturbances. Therefore the patient's circulatory status should be assessed and continually monitored by electrocardiogram (ECG) and frequent blood pressure measurements. The presence of tachydysrhythmias or bradydysrhythmias may indicate serious metabolic disorders such as hypoxia and acidosis. Other cardiovascular complications include the development of hypotension (associated with decreased vascular tone) and, rarely, hypertension, which may lead to cerebral vascular hemorrhage.

Neurological Complications

If the patient has an altered level of consciousness, a baseline neurological examination should be performed and documented. Deviations from a normal sensorium may range from mild drowsiness and agitation to hallucinations, seizures, cardiopulmonary depression, and death. Neurological complications may result from the toxin itself, such as lead poisoning in children who have ingested paint chips, or be secondary to an underlying metabolic or perfusion problem.

History

A thorough history of the exposure and any significant medical history should be obtained from the patient, family members, or bystanders. Although this information may be unreliable (as in cases involving pediatric patients, drug abuse, suicide attempts), the following should be ascertained if possible:

- What was ingested? (Obtain the poison container and remaining contents [unless this poses a threat to rescuer safety].)
- When was the substance ingested? (This may affect the decision to induce emesis or to use gastric lavage, activated charcoal, or antidote administration.)
- How much of the substance was ingested?
- Was an attempt made to induce vomiting?
- Has an antidote or activated charcoal been administered?
- Does the patient have a psychiatric history pertinent to suicide attempts or episodes of recent depression?

Gastrointestinal Decontamination

The primary goal of treating serious poisonings by ingestion is to prevent the toxic substance from reaching the small intestine, thereby limiting its absorption. This may be accomplished by gastrointestinal decontamination through the use of *syrup of ipecac*, gastric lavage, or *activated charcoal.* Before attempting gastrointestinal decontamination, the paramedic should consult with medical control or a poison control center.

Syrup of Ipecac

Syrup of ipecac is the most widely used emetic in the United States. However, in recent years, the efficacy of *ipecac* in the treatment of ingested poisons has been seriously questioned, and it may no longer be considered the treatment of choice in preventing absorption. Studies have shown that *ipecac*-induced emesis only reduces absorption by approximately 30% and that its use may interfere with the efficacy of other methods of decontamination, such as *activated charcoal.*

If *syrup of ipecac* is administered, it should be given within the first 20 minutes after ingestion of a poison and only in patients who are alert with a gag reflex (Box 23-1). Potential complications of *ipecac*-induced emesis include Mallory-Weiss tear of the esophagus, pneumomediastinum, fatal diaphragmatic or gastric rupture, and aspiration pneumonitis. Contraindications include:

- Altered level of consciousness
- Ingestion of caustic substances (The esophagus would be exposed to the agent twice.)
- Loss of gag reflex
- Seizures
- Pregnancy
- Acute myocardial infarction
- Ingestion of:
  - Acids
  - Alkalis
  - Ammonia
  - Nontoxic agents
  - Petroleum distillates, unless advised otherwise by medical control or poison control
  - Rapidly acting central nervous system depressants (for example, cyanide, tricyclic antidepressants)
  - Rapidly acting central nervous system irritants (for example, strychnine)
  - Hydrocarbons (controversial)

Gastric Lavage

Gastric lavage is a method of gastrointestinal decontamination that may be superior to *ipecac*-induced emesis. Advantages include immediate recovery of a portion of gastric contents (if performed within 1 hour after ingestion), control of lavage duration, and direct access for administration of *activated charcoal.*

Current practice uses a large-bore orogastric tube (36 to 40 French in adults, 24 to 28 French in children) rather than a smaller nasogastric tube, which may be too narrow to empty the stomach if large particle or pill fragments are present. These large tubes should never be inserted nasally, since they may damage the mucosa or turbinates and result in epistaxis. The procedure for gastric lavage is:

1. Place the conscious patient in a left lateral Trendelenburg ("swimmer's") position to minimize the possibility of aspiration in case of emesis. Endotracheal intubation should precede gastric lavage in patients with a depressed level of consciousness or in those without an intact gag reflex.

BOX 23-1

Dosage of Ipecac

Patients 1 to 12 years

Contraindicated for patients less than 1 year old

15 ml of **ipecac** followed by two to three glasses of water

May be repeated in 20 minutes if vomiting does not occur

Patients Over 12 years

30 ml of **ipecac** followed by two to three glasses of water

May be repeated in 20 minutes if vomiting does not occur

2. Insert the tube through the mouth into the patient's esophagus and continue to advance the tube until it is placed in the stomach. If resistance to passage is noted, the procedure must cease.

3. Check tube placement before lavage by air insufflation into the stomach with a large syringe.

4. Infuse tap water or normal saline in amounts not to exceed 150 to 200 ml aliquots in adults or 50 to 100 ml aliquots in patients younger than 5 years of age.

> **NOTE:**
> To prevent water absorption and resultant fluid-electrolyte derangements in pediatric patients, only normal saline should be infused.

5. Gastric lavage should continue until the return fluid appears clear. The return fluid should be approximately the same amount as the fluid administered.

> **NOTE:**
> The first dose of *activated charcoal* is sometimes administered via lavage before actual lavage to allow immediate adsorption of toxins and before accidental passage of some stomach contents through the pylorus into the duodenum. In this case, the instilled *charcoal* may serve as a marker for lavage by continuing evacuation until *charcoal* clears (usually 2 to 3 L).

Gastric lavage is contraindicated in patients with altered levels of consciousness and those who have ingested low-viscosity hydrocarbons or caustic agents. Gastric lavage can be performed in patients with depressed consciousness, but the airway should be protected before the procedure. Potential complications include agitation of the patient (produced by the procedure), inadvertent tracheal intubation, esophageal perforation, aspiration pneumonitis, and as previously stated, fluid and electrolyte imbalances in pediatric patients.

Activated Charcoal

Activated charcoal is an inert, nontoxic product of wood material that has been heated to extremely high temperature. The surface characteristics of *activated charcoal* enable it to adsorb molecules of many chemical toxins while in the intestinal tract, thereby inhibiting absorption of the poison and preventing systemic toxicity. Some studies have suggested that when it is administered alone, the efficacy of *activated charcoal* may be equal to or greater than that of emesis or gastric lavage, particularly if the time from ingestion to treatment is greater than 1 to 2 hours. It may reduce absorption by as much as 50%. In addition, the administration of *activated charcoal* 20 to 30 minutes before gastric lavage or immediately after lavage shows a return of clear fluid has doubled the effectiveness of lavage. (If used with *ipecac*-induced emesis, *activated charcoal* should not be administered until gastric emptying is complete because it adsorbs and deactivates *ipecac*.)

Activated charcoal is considered a safe and effective treatment for most toxic ingestions (Box 23-2) and is administered in nearly all cases except when strong acid, strong alkali, or ethanol is the toxicant. Other agents not well adsorbed by *activated charcoal* include cyanide, ferrous sulfate, and methanol. If these substances have been ingested, *activated charcoal* should probably be withheld; consult with medical direction or a poison control center. It may also be withheld when specific oral antidotes (for example, acetaminophen) are available and when the ingestion occurred 4 or more hours before presentation.

Activated charcoal comes mixed in an aqueous solution with or without a cathartic (most com

> **BOX 23-2**
>
> ### Dosage of Activated Charcoal
> 1 to 2 g/kg body weight
> 30 to 100 g in adults
> 15 to 30 g in children
> Prepared in a slurry and administered orally or by gastric tube

monly sorbitol). Sorbitol can be harmful if aspirated, whereas *activated charcoal* is relatively harmless. Nonetheless, a cathartic is necessary to decrease the transit time and expel the *charcoal* within a short period. Complications of *activated charcoal* therapy include poor patient acceptance and vomiting (usually seen after *ipecac* administration). EMS personnel should protect themselves, the patient, and the immediate area from the staining properties of *activated charcoal* and should use personal protective measures when administering this agent.

Management of Specific Ingested Poisons

Specific ingested poisons to be discussed in this section include strong acids and alkalis, hydrocarbons, methanol, ethylene glycol, isopropanol, cyanide, and poisons from food and plants. Because there are very few effective antidotes that can be used in poisoning situations, supportive and symptomatic treatment and prevention of absorption are the primary approaches in caring for the poisoned patient. As previously stated, the paramedic should consult with medical control or a poison control center in any response involving a poisoning emergency.

Strong Acids and Alkalis

Strong acids and alkalis (such as those found in toilet bowl cleaners, rust remover, ammonia, and most liquid drain cleaners [Box 23-3]) may cause burns to the mouth, pharynx, esophagus, and sometimes the upper respiratory and gastrointestinal tracts. Perforation of the esophagus or stomach may result in vascular collapse, mediastinitis, or pneumoperitoneum. The frequency of caustic ingestions (most commonly lye) is highest in small children, accounting for 5000 to 8000 accidental exposures each year.

Ingestions of caustic and corrosive substances generally produce immediate damage to the mucosa and intestinal tract that is complete within 1 to 2 minutes after exposure. Therefore prehospital care is usually limited to airway and ventilatory support, intravenous fluid replacement, and rapid transport to an appropriate medical facility.

BOX 23-3

Common Acid and Alkali Substances

Acids
Hydrochloric acid
  Metal cleaners
  Swimming pool cleaners
  Toilet bowl cleaners
Sulfuric acid
  Battery acid
  Toilet bowl cleaners
Phenol
Acetic acid
Bleach disinfectants

Alkalis
Sodium or potassium hydroxide (lye)
  Washing powders
  Paint removers
Drainpipe and toilet bowl cleaners
Disk (button) batteries
Bleach
Ammonia
  Metal cleaners or polishes
  Hair dyes and tints
  Jewelry cleaners

In some situations, medical control may recommend attempts to dilute the acid or alkali in a conscious patient with oral administration of milk or water (200 to 300 ml in the adult, 15 ml/kg maximum in a child). Efforts to neutralize the ingested agent with other fluids, such as fruit juice, lemon juice, or vinegar, are contraindicated because of the potential for intense exothermic reactions, which may produce severe thermal burns.

Hydrocarbons

Hydrocarbons are a group of saturated and unsaturated compounds derived primarily from crude oil, coal, or plant sources. Mixtures vary in their viscosity, surface tension, and volatility, which with other factors (such as the presence of other chemicals in the product, total amount, and route of exposure) determine the toxic effects of these agents.

Hydrocarbons are found in many household products—cleaning and polishing agents (mineral seal oil or signal oil), spot removers, paints, cosmetics, pesticides, hobby and craft materials—and in petroleum distillates—turpentine, kerosene, gasoline, lighter fluids, and pine-oil products. In addition, there is a large group of halogenated hydrocarbons (carbon tetrachloride, trichloroethane, trichlorethylene, methyl chloride) and aromatic hydrocarbons (toluene, xylene, benzene). Hydrocarbon poisonings are common, accounting for 7% of all ingestions in children under 5 years of age. Most ingestions occur between May and September, when home use of petroleum products permits greatest exposure to children.

The most important physical characteristic in the potential toxicity of ingested hydrocarbons is its viscosity: the lower the viscosity, the higher the risk of aspiration and associated complications. For example, an ingested hydrocarbon product with a low viscosity, such as gasoline or turpentine, rapidly disperses over the pharyngeal and glottic surfaces, the more volatile components becoming gases on contact with the warm mucous membranes. This exposure causes irritation, coughing, and possible aspiration, which may allow a toxic amount of hydrocarbons to enter the tracheobronchial tree. Chemical characteristics (aromatic, aliphatic, or halogenated) and the presence of toxic additives are also important in determining toxicity.

The clinical features of hydrocarbon ingestion vary widely, depending on the type of agent involved (Box 23-4). If the patient is asymptomatic on EMS arrival, the chances of serious complications are usually minimal. These patients are generally observed in the emergency department for several hours and often require no treatment. However, any patient suspected of hydrocarbon ingestion who coughs, chokes, cries, or has spontaneous emesis on swallowing should be assumed to have aspirated until proven otherwise. Hydrocarbon ingestion may involve the patient's respiratory, gastrointestinal, and neurological systems; clinical features may be immediate or delayed in onset.

BOX 23-4

Clinical Features of Hydrocarbon Ingestion

Immediate: Up to 6 Hours

Gastrointestinal System
Mucous membrane hyperemia
Irritation
Abdominal pain
Nausea and vomiting
Belching

Respiratory System
Cough and choking
Inspiratory stridor
Tachypnea
Cyanosis
Dyspnea

Neurological System
Lethargy
Coma
Seizures

Systemic Factors
Fever
Malaise

Delayed: Days to Weeks

Gastrointestinal System
Diarrhea
Hepatic toxicity

Respiratory System
Bacterial pneumonia
Dyspnea
Sputum production
Atelectasis
Pulmonary edema

Systemic Factors
Spontaneous hemorrhage
Hemolytic and aplastic anemias

Emergency care for symptomatic patients who have ingested hydrocarbon products includes the following:

1. Ensure a patent airway and provide adequate ventilatory and circulatory support as needed.

2. Identify the substance and contact medical control or a poison control center.

3. As a rule, avoid gastric decontamination by *ipecac*-induced emesis or lavage to prevent potential aspiration pneumonitis. It is contraindicated with ingestion of mineral seal oil, signal oil, or polishing oils because of their low viscosity and the likelihood of aspiration. Medical control may recommend gastric emptying of a petroleum product containing significant amounts (greater than 1 ml/kg) of camphor, benzene and its derivatives, organophosphates, halogenated hydrocarbons, and heavy metals such as arsenicals, lead, and mercury. In these situations, the chance of systemic toxicity is greater than the risk of aspiration. The use of **activated charcoal** or diluents has not been shown to be effective in managing hydrocarbon ingestion.

4. Initiate intravenous fluid therapy.

5. Monitor cardiac rhythm.

6. Transport for physician evaluation.

Methanol

Methanol (wood alcohol) is a common industrial solvent obtained from distillation of wood. It is a poisonous alcohol found in a variety of products, such as gas line antifreeze, windshield washer fluid, paints, paint removers, varnishes, canned fuels such as Sterno, and many shellacs. Methanol is a colorless liquid that has an odor distinct from that of ethanol, the form of alcohol designed for consumption. Poisonings may result from intentional or accidental ingestions, absorption through the skin, or inhalation. Examples include deliberate use of the agent by chronic alcoholics to maintain an inebriated state, accidental ingestion resulting from misuse or distribution of methanol for ethanol (as in contraband liquor), and accidental ingestions in children.

Methanol itself is no more toxic than ethanol, but its metabolites are extremely toxic. (Death has been reported after the ingestion of 15 ml of a 40% solution.) As the alcohol is absorbed, it is rapidly converted in the liver to formaldehyde and in minutes to formic acid. The accumulation of formic acid in the blood results in a group of symptoms relating to the central nervous system (depression), the gastrointestinal tract (pain, nausea, vomiting), the eyes (as little as 4 ml causing blindness), and the development of metabolic acidosis. The onset of symptoms after ingestion ranges from 40 minutes to 72 hours. The symptoms of methanol poisoning correlate with the degree of acidosis and may include the following:

- Central nervous system depression
  - Lethargy
  - Confusion
  - Coma
  - Seizures
- Gastrointestinal tract
  - Nausea and vomiting
  - Abdominal pain
- Complaints relating to vision
  - Photophobia
  - Blurred or indistinct vision
  - Pupils that are dilated and sluggish to react to light
  - "Spots before the eyes"
  - "Snow-filled vision"
  - Blindness
- Metabolic acidosis
  - Shortness of breath
  - Tachypnea
  - Shock
  - Multisystem failure
  - Death

Emergency care for methanol poisoning is as follows:

1. Supportive care: Secure a patent airway and provide adequate ventilatory and circulatory support as needed. Adequate ventilation is essential to ensure adequate oxygenation, help correct the profound metabolic acidosis, and maximize respiratory excretion. An intravenous line should be established, and the patient should be placed on a cardiac monitor to detect rhythm disturbances.

2. Gastrointestinal decontamination: If the patient is seen within 4 hours after ingestion,

gastric lavage is indicated. The efficacy of *activated charcoal* in adsorbing methanol is controversial. Consult with medical control or a poison control center.

3. Correction of metabolic acidosis: Attempts to correct metabolic acidosis with *sodium bicarbonate* administration (1 mEq/kg) may be recommended by medical control. Larger or repeated doses may be necessary. Although serum formic acid may be neutralized with *bicarbonate* administration, hemodialysis will probably be necessary to remove toxic levels of methanol and formate.

4. Prevention of the conversion of methanol to formic acid: The conversion of methanol to formic acid may be prevented by the administration of ethanol. (Ethanol has a 9-times-greater affinity for the enzyme that converts methanol to formic acid.) If the patient is conscious, give 30 to 60 ml of 80-proof ethanol by mouth or gastric lavage tube. Unconscious patients should have their airway protected with an endotracheal tube before gastric tube administration of ethanol.

5. Transport: Rapidly transport the patient to an appropriate medical facility for definitive treatment.

Ethylene Glycol

Ethylene glycol is a colorless, odorless, water-soluble liquid commonly used in windshield de-icers, detergents, paints, radiator antifreeze, and coolants. Because of the brilliant coloring agents added to these preparations, their widespread availability, and the warm, sweet taste, accidental ingestion of ethylene glycol is common in young children. The agent is also commonly misused by alcoholics as a substitute for ethanol. The lethal dose of ethylene glycol is approximately 2 ml/kg (100 ml in adults).

Early signs and symptoms of central nervous system depression are usually caused by the ethanol-like effects of ethylene glycol. However, toxicity from ethylene glycol, as from methanol, is caused by the accumulation of intermediary metabolites, especially glycolic and oxalic acids after metabolism, which occurs primarily in the liver and kidneys. These metabolic intermediaries may affect the central nervous system and cardiopulmonary and renal systems and result in hypocalcemia (from the precipitation of oxalic acid as calcium oxalate). The signs and symptoms of ethylene glycol poisoning generally occur in three stages:

1. Stage 1: Central nervous system effects occurring 1 to 12 hours after ingestion
   a. Slurred speech
   b. Ataxia
   c. Somnolence
   d. Nausea and vomiting
   e. Focal or generalized convulsions
   f. Hallucinations
   g. Stupor
   h. Coma
2. Stage 2: Cardiopulmonary system effects occurring 12 to 36 hours after ingestion
   a. Rapidly progressive tachypnea
   b. Cyanosis
   c. Pulmonary edema
   d. Cardiac failure
3. Stage 3: Renal system effects occurring 24 to 72 hours after ingestion
   a. Flank pain
   b. Oliguria
   c. Crystalluria
   d. Proteinuria
   e. Anuria
   f. Hematuria
   g. Uremia

Emergency care for ethylene glycol poisoning is similar to that used in treating methanol poisoning and includes the following:

1. Ensure a patent airway and provide adequate ventilatory and circulatory support as needed. Monitor the patient for dysrhythmias.
2. Use gastric lavage if the patient is seen within 4 hours after ingestion. Administer *activated charcoal,* which has been shown to decrease gastrointestinal absorption of ethylene glycol by 50%.
3. Initiate intravenous fluid therapy with a volume-expanding fluid to maintain adequate urine output.
4. Administer intravenous *sodium bicarbonate* levels to correct acidosis.

5. Administer 80-proof ethanol (30 to 60 ml) by mouth or gastric tube to block the conversion of ethylene glycol into toxic metabolites. Unmetabolized ethylene glycol is excreted by the lungs and kidneys.

6. Rapidly transport the patient for definitive treatment, which may include hemodialysis and continued ethanol administration.

In addition, the paramedic should anticipate orders from medical control or a poison control center for the following medications:

- *Furosemide,* to promote renal clearance of ethylene glycol and oxalic acid
- *Thiamine,* an enzyme cofactor, to degrade glycolic acid to nontoxic metabolites
- *Calcium gluconate,* to treat hypocalcemia
- *Diazepam,* to control seizure activity

Isopropanol

Isopropanol (isopropyl alcohol) is a volatile, flammable, colorless liquid with a characteristic odor and bittersweet taste. Rubbing alcohol is the most common household source of this agent. It is also used in disinfectants, degreasers, cosmetics, industrial solvents, and cleaning agents. Common routes of toxic exposure to isopropanol include intentional ingestion as a substitute for ethanol, accidental ingestion, and inhalation of high concentrations of local vapor, as from alcohol sponging of febrile children (a harmful and inappropriate procedure). Isopropanol is more toxic than ethanol but less toxic than methanol or ethylene glycol. The lethal dose in adults is approximately 3 ml/kg. In children, any amount of ingestion should be considered potentially toxic.

After ingestion, the majority of isopropanol (80%) is metabolized to acetone. The rest is excreted unchanged by the kidneys. The acetone is excreted by the kidneys and to a lesser extent by the lungs. Isopropanol poisoning affects several body systems, including the central nervous, gastrointestinal, and renal systems. Signs and symptoms frequently occur within 30 minutes after ingestion and include central nervous system and respiratory depression (isopropanol is 2 to 3 times more potent a central nervous system depressant than ethanol), abdominal pain, gastritis, hematemesis, and hypovolemia. Although isopropanol

poisoning causes acetonemia and ketonuria, there is usually no associated metabolic acidosis unless the patient manifests hypotension.

Emergency care for isopropanol poisoning is primarily supportive and includes airway and ventilatory support to ensure adequate respiratory elimination of acetone, gastric lavage (isopropanol is also secreted by the salivary glands and stomach), fluid resuscitation as needed, and rapid transport to an appropriate medical facility, where dialysis may be necessary. Administration of ethanol has not proven to inhibit the toxic metabolite to the same degree as in methanol or ethylene glycol poisoning.

Cyanide

Cyanide refers to any of a number of highly toxic substances that contain the cyanogen chemical group. Because of its toxicity, cyanide has few applications. The agent is sometimes used in industry in electroplating, ore extraction, and fumigation of buildings and as a fertilizer. It has been used in gas chambers as a means of execution. Cyanide is one of the products of combustion from burning nylon and polyurethane and is therefore a potential hazard in fire environments.

Cyanide poisoning may result from the inhalation of cyanide gas; ingestion of cyanide salts, nitriles, or cyanogenic glycosides (for example, amygdalin, a substance found in the seeds of cherries, apples, pears, and apricots and the principal constituent of laetrile); or the infusion of nitroprusside. Cyanide can also be absorbed across the skin. Regardless of the route of entry, cyanide is a rapidly acting poison that combines and reacts with ferric ions (Fe^{3+}) of the respiratory enzyme cytochrome oxidase to inhibit cellular oxygenation. The cytotoxic hypoxia produces a rapid progression of symptoms from dyspnea to paralysis, unconsciousness, and death (Box 23-5). Large doses are usually fatal within minutes from respiratory arrest. Cyanide poisoning may produce a characteristic odor of bitter almonds on the patient's breath or body, but 20% to 40% of the population is unable to detect this odor.

After ensuring personal safety, emergency care for a patient with cyanide poisoning begins with securing a patent airway and providing adequate

---

BOX 23-5

Early and Advanced Signs and Symptoms of Cyanide Poisoning

Early Effects
Agitation
Anxiety
Confusion
Dyspnea
Hypertension with reflex bradycardia

Advanced Effects
Hypotension
Acidosis
Seizures
Pulmonary edema
Dysrhythmias
Intractable hypotension
Lactic acidosis
Coma

BOX 23-6

Cyanide Antidote Kit

Two *Amyl Nitrite* Inhalants in Gauze
Administer by inhalation 15 of every 30 seconds

3% Sodium Nitrite (Stop *Amyl Nitrite*)
Adults: 10-ml slow intravenous administration over 2 to 4 minutes
Children: 0.2 ml/kg (up to 10 ml) slow intravenous administration over 5 minutes

NOTE: If hypotension develops, stop nitrite, treat for shock, and consider administration of *dopamine* (per medical control).

25% Sodium Thiosulfate
Adults: 50-ml intravenous bolus
Children: 5 ml sodium thiosulfate per 1 ml sodium nitrite given

---

ventilatory support with high-concentration oxygen. Oxygen competitively displaces cyanide from cytochrome oxidase and enhances the efficacy of drug administration. After these measures, the principal treatment of cyanide poisoning is to convert (oxidize) ferrous ions in hemoglobin (Fe^{2+}) to ferric ions (Fe^{3+}), forming methemoglobin, hemoglobin with ferrous ion in the oxidized (Fe^{3+}) state. Cyanide, which has a greater affinity for iron in the ferric state, is released from the cytochrome oxidase and combines with methemoglobin, thus allowing cytochrome oxidase to resume its function in normal cellular respiration. Cyanide antidotes, such as those found in the Lily Cyanide Poison Kit, are thought to be effective because they induce methemoglobin (Box 23-6).

Methemoglobin cannot transport oxygen and must therefore be reconverted to hemoglobin by sodium thiosulfate. This is accomplished in a three-step process, which includes administration of (1) *amyl nitrite* by inhalation (converting approximately 5% of hemoglobin to methemoglobin); (2) sodium nitrite (300 mg intravenously),

which results in methemoglobinemia approaching 25% to 30%; and (3) sodium thiosulfate (12.5 mg intravenously).[3]

Prehospital care for patients with cyanide poisoning is:

1. Don personal protective equipment as needed to prevent rescuer contamination.
2. Remove the patient from the cyanide source. Rapid decontamination and removal of any contaminated clothing is essential.
3. Ensure a patent airway and provide adequate ventilatory support.
4. Administer high-concentration oxygen.
5. If using the Lily Cyanide Poison Kit, consult with medical control or a poison control center and follow the instructions provided by the manufacturer.
6. If an antidote kit is not available, a pearl of *amyl nitrite* should be crushed and held under the patient's nose for 15 of every 30 sec-

onds, followed by continuation of supplemental oxygen. If the patient's respirations are being assisted, place the crushed pearl under the intake valve of a bag-valve device.

> **NOTE:**
> Hypotension should be anticipated as a consequence of antidotal therapy. The patient should remain supine if possible, and the blood pressure must be closely monitored. If hypotension develops, medical control may recommend administration of vasopressors.

7. Initiate intravenous fluid therapy with a volume-expanding solution.
8. Monitor cardiac rhythm by ECG.
9. Rapidly transport the patient for physician evaluation.

Food Poisoning

Food poisoning is a term used for any illness of sudden onset (usually associated with stomach pain, vomiting, and diarrhea) suspected of being caused by food eaten within the previous 48 hours. Food poisoning can be classified as infectious, resulting from a bacteria or virus, or noninfectious, resulting from toxins or pollutants. Some foods can also cause poisoning of either type (for example, shellfish such as mussels, clams, and oysters, which may be contaminated by viruses or bacteria or by toxins or chemical pollutants in water).

Infectious (Bacterial) Types

One of the common types of bacteria responsible for food poisoning is salmonella, an organism found in many animals (especially poultry) as well as humans. Salmonella bacteria may also be transferred to food from the excrement of infected animals or humans and by food handling by an infected person. Other bacteria (for example, strains of staphylococcal bacteria) cause formation of toxins, which may be difficult to destroy even with thorough cooking. Other bacteria that commonly cause diarrhea are certain strains of *Escherichia coli* (traveler's diarrhea) and *Campylobacter* and *Shigella* organisms.

Botulism is a rare but life-threatening form of food poisoning that may result from eating improperly canned or preserved food contaminated with the bacterium *Clostridium botulinum. C. botulinum* is found in soil and untreated water in most parts of the world and is harmlessly present in the intestinal tracts of many animals, including fish. Its spore-forming properties resist boiling, salting, smoking, and some forms of pickling, allowing the bacterium to thrive in improperly preserved or canned foods. Although botulism is rare, the disease is more common in the United States than elsewhere in the world because of the popularity of preserving food in the home. Botulism is associated with severe central nervous system symptoms that appear in a characteristic head-to-toe progression: headache, blurred or double vision, dysphagia, respiratory paralysis, and quadriplegia. Death from respiratory failure occurs in some 70% of untreated cases. Another life-threatening form of diarrhea caused by *C. difficile* is pseudomembranous colitis. It is usually associated with long-term administration of certain antibiotics.

Infectious (Viral) Types

The viruses that most commonly cause food poisoning are Norwalk virus, a common contaminant of shellfish, and rotavirus. These agents may be responsible for illness when raw or partly cooked foodstuffs have been in contact with water contaminated by human excrement.

Noninfectious Types

Noninfectious types of food poisoning may result from consuming mushrooms and toadstools or from eating fresh foods and vegetables accidentally contaminated with large amounts of insecticide. Chemical food poisoning may also result from eating food stored in a contaminated container (for example, a container previously used to store poison) and from improperly preparing and cooking various exotic foods. Drugs or medications can also cause diarrhea. Quinidine, certain antacids, some antibiotics, and stool softeners or laxatives may all cause diarrhea.

Management Guidelines

The onset of signs and symptoms from food poisoning varies by cause and by how heavily the food was contaminated. As a rule, symptoms usually develop within 30 minutes in the case of chemical poisoning, in 1 to 12 hours in the case of bacterial toxins, and in 12 to 48 hours with viral and bacterial infections. General principles of management for patients with suspected food poisoning include the following:

- Ensure adequate airway, ventilatory, and circulatory support.
- Gather a complete history, including time and onset of symptoms, recent travel, the relation of symptoms to ingestion of a particular food, and effects on others who ate the same food. In addition, information on the consistency, frequency, and odor of stool (including the presence of mucus or blood) should be obtained, and fever should be noted. Any patient history should also include significant past medical history, allergies, and use of medications.
- Initiate intravenous therapy with a crystalloid solution to manage dehydration and electrolyte disturbances resulting from vomiting and diarrhea.
- Transport the patient for physician evaluation.
- Use precautions to avoid contamination of self (gloves, gown if appropriate) and equipment.

Plant Poisoning

The 1990 Annual Report of the AAPCC noted that over 100,000 plant and 9000 mushroom ingestions or exposures were reported to 72 poison control centers serving 191.7 million people and that plants and mushrooms represented 7.1% of total exposures reported that year.[2] Therefore toxic plant ingestion was a frequently reported category of poisonings, second only to ingestion of cleaning substances. Of these exposures, 8% resulted in treatment at a health care facility, with three deaths reported (one from mushroom poisoning and two from plant poisoning). Overall, 85% of plant ingestions reported involved children under 6 years of age.[1]

Signs and Symptoms

The toxic manifestations of major poisonous plant ingestions are predictable and are categorized by the chemical and physical properties of the plant. Most human physiological responses tend to be consistent with the type of major toxic chemical component in the plant, although some disparities exist. For example, anticholinergic crisis may result from ingestion of certain alkaloid components (jimsonweed and lantana), manifesting in tachycardia, dilated pupils, hot dry skin, decreased bowel sounds, altered vision, and abnormal mental status; cholinergic symptoms may result from ingestion of certain mushroom species, which is usually manifested by bradycardia, miosis, salivation, hyperactive bowel sounds, and diarrhea; and nicotinic alkaloids (poison hemlock and delphinium) may initially act as stimulants but are generally soon followed by depression and weakness. Most signs and symptoms appear within several hours after ingestion, but some symptoms may be delayed 1 to 3 days. Box 23-7 lists common poisonous plants and the symptoms associated with their ingestion. Paramedics should be familiar with common poisonous plant life in their response area.

Management

Several hundred species of green plants and more than 100 varieties of mushrooms in the United States contain toxic compounds. Many similar species of plants and mushrooms have widely varying potencies and combinations of toxins, and such factors as the age of the plant and soil conditions may influence the severity of toxic symptoms. Therefore management guidelines should be customized to the patient's symptoms rather than to a particular type of ingestion. Although it is important to identify the plant if possible, the inability to do so should not delay treatment. As always, the paramedic should consult with medical control or a poison control center regarding appropriate emergency care procedures. Principles in the management of toxic plant ingestion generally include the following:

1. Ensure adequate airway, ventilatory, and circulatory support.
2. In patients with a depressed gag reflex, unresponsiveness, or seizures, secure the airway with an endotracheal tube, and then use orogastric decontamination. Medical control or a poison control center may recommend

---

BOX 23-7

Common Poisonous Plants, Trees, and Shrubs

House Plants
Dieffenbachia
Hyacinth
Narcissus
Mistletoe
Oleander
Poinsettia

Flower-Garden Plants
Daffodil
Foxglove
Iris
Larkspur
Lily of the valley

Ornamental Plants
Azaleas
Daphne
Jessamine
Rhododendron
Wisteria

Other Plants
Buttercups
Jack-in-the-pulpit
Mayapple
Nightshade
Water and poison hemlock

Trees and Shrubs
Elderberry
Oaks
Wild and cultivated cherries

---

administration of *activated charcoal* in place of gastric emptying or after it.

3. Initiate intravenous fluid therapy with a volume-expanding solution.

4. Monitor the patient's vital signs and cardiac rhythm.

5. Transport the patient for physician evaluation. Most patients are hospitalized for observation and treatment as indicated for the toxin involved. Dialysis has not been shown to be effective in removing most plant toxins.

● INHALED POISONS AND INHALATION INJURY

Accidental or intentional inhalation of poisons can lead to a life-threatening emergency. The type and location of injury caused by toxic inhalation depend on the specific actions and behaviors of the chemical involved.[4]

Physical Properties

The concentration of a chemical in the air and the duration of exposure help determine the severity of inhalation injury. At low concentrations and with brief exposure, the chemical may be removed from the air before reaching the tracheobronchial tree, whereas large concentrations or prolonged exposure are more likely to cause contact with the lungs and damage to lung tissue. As a rule, increasing the concentration of the chemical or the duration of exposure increases the dose received.

Solubility also influences inhalation injury. For example, soluble chemicals such as chlorine and anhydrous ammonia can be converted to hydrochloric acid and ammonium hydroxide, respectively, when they contact moisture in the respiratory tract mucus, producing injury in the nasopharynx and conducting airways. In contrast, insoluble chemicals such as phosgene and nitrogen dioxide may have little impact on the upper airways but can produce severe damage to the alveoli and respiratory bronchioles.

Chemicals may be inhaled as gases and vapors, mists, fumes, or particles. Gases and vapors mix with air and distribute themselves freely throughout the lung and its airways. Mists are liquid droplets dispersed in air, their toxic effects depending on droplet size (the larger the size, the greater the exposure). Fumes contain fine particles of dust dispersed in air. Large particles are likely to be trapped in the nasopharynx and conducting airways, whereas small particles are more likely to penetrate the lower airways.

Chemical Properties

The ability of a chemical to interact with other chemicals and body tissue is called its *reactivity.* As a rule, highly reactive chemicals cause more severe and rapid injury than less-reactive chemicals. Four potential properties of chemicals that determine reactivity are:

1. Chemical pH: As the pH of an acid falls (pH less than 2.0) or the pH of an alkaline increases (pH greater than 11.5), the likelihood of severe injury from exposure increases.
2. Direct-acting potential of chemicals: Direct-acting chemicals are capable of producing injury without first being transformed or changed. An example is hydrofluoric acid, which causes severe corrosive burns on contact with mucous membranes of the upper airways.
3. Indirect-acting potential of chemicals: Indirect-acting chemicals must be transformed before they can produce injury. An example is phosgene, a gas that may cause acidic burns of the alveolar membranes after conversion to hydrogen chloride (a process that may take up to several hours).
4. Allergic potential of chemicals: Some reactive chemicals bind with proteins to form structures that stimulate allergic reactions. For example, formaldehyde can cause severe asthmatic and anaphylactic reactions after even a small exposure. In general, the allergic potential of a chemical is related to its reactivity.

Classifications

Toxic gases can be classified in three categories: simple asphyxiants, chemical asphyxiants and systemic poisons, and irritants or corrosives. Simple asphyxiants (methane, propane, and inert gases) cause toxicity by lowering ambient oxygen concentration. Chemical asphyxiants (carbon monoxide and cyanide) possess intrinsic systemic toxicity manifested after absorption into the circulation. Irritants or corrosives (chlorine and ammonia) cause cellular destruction and inflammation as they come into contact with moisture. Table 23-1 provides an overview of toxic gases and their clinical manifestations.

General Management

The general principles of managing inhaled poisons are the same as for any other hazardous materials incident. These include:

1. Scene safety
2. Personal protective measures: protective clothing and appropriate respiratory protective apparatus
3. Rapid removal of the patient from the poison environment
4. Surface decontamination
5. Adequate airway, ventilatory, and circulatory support
6. Primary and secondary survey
7. Irrigation of the eyes (as needed)
8. Intravenous line with a saline solution
9. Regular monitoring of vital signs and cardiac rhythm by ECG
10. Rapid transport to an appropriate medical facility

Management of Specific Inhaled Poisons

The specific inhaled poisons discussed in this section include ammonia and hydrocarbons. Carbon monoxide poisoning is described in Chapter 16.

Ammonia Inhalation

Ammonia is a toxic irritant that causes local pulmonary complications after inhalation. Exposure to ammonia vapors results in inflammation, irritation, and in severe cases, erosion of the mucosal tissue of all respiratory structures as the ammonia vapor combines with water, producing a

TABLE 23-1 Clinical Features of Toxic Gases and Fumes

Class of Toxin	Toxin	Source	Clinical Features	Treatment
Simple asphyxiants	Propane Methane Carbon dioxide Inert gases (nitrogen, argon)	Cooking gas Cooking gas All fires Industry (especially welding)	Displacement of normal air and lower fractional inspired oxygen concentration, symptoms of hypoxemia without airway irritation	Remove patient from source; give oxygen.
Chemical asphyxiants	Carbon monoxide	Fires	Formation of carboxyhemoglobin; inhibition of oxygen transport (Headache is earliest symptom.)	Give 100% oxygen.
	Hydrocyanic acid	Industry, burning plastics, furniture, fabrics	Highly toxic cellular asphyxiant	Use cyanide antidote.
	Hydrogen sulfide	Liquid manure pits, decaying organic materials	Highly toxic cellular asphyxiant similar to cyanide; sudden collapse; ability to smell characteristic odor of rotten eggs; rapid fatigue	Use sodium nitrite as for cyanide (makes sulmethemoglobin). *Do not* use thiosulfate.
Irritants				
High solubility in water	Chlorine gas Hydrochloric acid	Industry, swimming pool chemical, bleach mixed with acid at home	Early onset of lacrimation, sore throat, stridor, tracheobronchitis; with heavy exposure, pulmonary edema in 2 to 6 hours	Use humidified oxygen, bronchodilators, airway management.
	Ammonia	Industry, burning fabrics		
Low solubility in water	Nitrogen dioxide	Burning cellulose, fabrics Grain silos (acrid red gas)	Sweet "electric" smell; delayed onset (12-24 hours) of tracheobronchitis, pneumonitis, and pulmonary edema; late chronic bronchitis	Give oxygen: observe for 24 to 48 hours; give ateroids (controversial).
	Ozone	Inert gas arc welding industry		
	Phosgone	Burning of chlorinated organic material		
Allergenic	Toluene dilsocyanate	Manufacture of polyurethanes	Reactive bronchoconstriction; possible long-term effects (chronic obstructive pulmonary disease) in susceptible persons	Use bronchodilators.
Metal fumes	Zinc Copper Tin Teflon	Welding (especially galvanized metal welding)	"Metal fumes fever"; chills, fever, myalgias, headache, nonproductive cough, leukocytosis 4 to 8 hours after exposure	Self-limited (12-24 hours)
	Arsine	Burning arsenic-containing ores, electronics industry	Highly toxic effect; hemolysis, pulmonary edema, renal failure; chronic arsenic toxicity	Exchange transfusion; use dimercaprol (BAL) for chronic arsenic toxicity only.
	Mercury Lead	Industry, welding	See specific metals.	

highly caustic alkaline compound. Patients usually develop coughing, choking, congestion, burning and tightness in the chest, and a feeling of suffocation. These respiratory symptoms are often accompanied by burning of the eyes and lacrimation. In severe cases, bronchospasm and pulmonary edema may ensue. In addition to the general management principles, emergency care may include positive-pressure ventilation and the administration of diuretics and bronchodilators.

Hydrocarbon Inhalation

The hydrocarbons that pose the greatest risk for injury have a low viscosity, a high volatility, and a high surface tension or adhesion of molecules along a surface. These characteristics combine to allow hydrocarbons to enter the pulmonary tree, causing aspiration pneumonitis and the potential for systemic effects such as central nervous system depression and liver, kidney, or bone marrow toxicity.

Most hydrocarbon inhalations result from "recreational use" of halogenated hydrocarbons such as carbon tetrachloride and methylene chloride or aromatic hydrocarbons such as benzene and toluene. These agents may produce a state of inebriation or euphoria through "sniffing" or "huffing" (placing the solvent on a rag and inhaling the vapors through a plastic bag). The onset of these effects is usually rapid (occurring within seconds) and may be followed by central nervous system depression, respiratory failure, or cardiac dysrhythmias. Other signs and symptoms of hydrocarbon inhalation include:

- Burning sensation on swallowing
- Nausea and vomiting
- Abdominal cramps
- Weakness
- Anesthesia
- Hallucinations
- Changes in color perception
- Blindness
- Seizures
- Coma

Emergency care for hydrocarbon inhalation is generally supportive and includes airway, ventilatory, and circulatory support; intravenous fluid therapy; vital sign and ECG monitoring; and transport for physician evaluation.

● SURFACE-ABSORBED POISONS

Although many poisons may be absorbed through the skin, absorption of organophosphates and carbamates accounts for an estimated 3000 hospitalizations per year. The fatality rate is 50% in children and 10% in adults. A large number of these agents are available for commercial and public use in the form of flea collars and home and commercial insecticides. Organophosphates were also used in the development of military nerve agents (such as sarin and soman) during World War II. Because of their widespread availability, paramedics must be aware of the nature of these chemicals, necessary precautions for personal safety, and the immediate treatment that may be required before symptoms or signs of illness occur.

Organophosphates and carbamates are among the most toxic chemicals currently used in pesticides and are well absorbed by ingestion, inhalation, and dermal routes. Both classes of compounds have similar pharmacological actions, which inhibit the effects of acetylcholinesterase, the enzyme that degrades acetylcholine at the neuromuscular junction; however, organophosphates have a stronger bond to this enzyme than carbamates do. Thus carbamate poisoning is easier to treat than organophosphate intoxication. To review, acetylcholine is a cholinergic neurotransmitter for preganglionic autonomic fibers, postganglionic parasympathetic fibers, somatic nerves to skeletal muscle, and many synapses in the central nervous system. When acetylcholinesterase is inhibited, acetylcholine accumulates at the synapses, and a cholinergic "overdrive" occurs with resulting signs and symptoms characteristic of organophosphate and carbamate poisoning.

Signs and Symptoms

Early signs and symptoms of organophosphate or carbamate poisoning may be nonspecific, including headache, dizziness, weakness, and nausea. However, as overstimulation and subsequent disruption of transmission in the central and peripheral nervous systems occur, signs and symptoms begin to manifest in a spectrum of physi-

BOX 23-8

Signs and Symptoms of Organophosphate or Carbamate Poisoning

Cardiovascular System
Bradycardia
Variable blood pressure (usually hypotensive)

Respiratory System
Rhinorrhea
Bronchoconstriction
Wheezing
Dyspnea

Gastrointestinal System
Cramps
Emesis
Defecation
Increased bowel sounds

Vision
Miosis
Rapidly changing pupil size
Lacrimation
Blurred vision

Central Nervous System
Anxiety
Dizziness
Coma
Convulsions
Respiratory depression

Musculoskeletal System
Fasciculations
Flaccid paralysis

Skin
Diaphoresis

Other
Salivation
Urination

ological and metabolic derangements (Box 23-8). The rapidity and sequence in which these signs and symptoms develop depend on the particular compound and the amount and route of exposure. The onset of symptoms is probably quickest after inhalation and slowest (possibly delayed for several hours) after a primary skin exposure. A mnemonic aid that may help the paramedic recognize the signs of poisoning is *SLUDGE* (salivation, lacrimation, urination, defecation, gastrointestinal cramping, and emesis). The most specific findings, however, are miosis, rapidly changing pupils, and muscle fasciculation.

Management

Emergency care begins with scene safety, personal protection, and decontamination procedures (see Chapter 7). After these measures, patient care can be initiated. The general principles of management include respiratory support, drug administration, ECG monitoring, and gastrointestinal decontamination, including **activated charcoal.** Although organophosphates and carbamates produce similar physiological effects, carbamates have a shorter duration of action and therefore a more rapid decrement of effect.

Respiratory Support

Respiratory tract symptoms are usually first to appear after inhalation of organophosphates or carbamates, and respiratory paralysis may occur suddenly without clear warning signs. Therefore the need for aggressive airway management and ventilatory support should be anticipated throughout the patient care encounter. Copious bronchial secretions may require suctioning, and bronchoconstriction may necessitate positive-pressure ventilation and positive end-expiratory pressure.

Drug Administration

Drug therapy in organophosphate or carbamate poisoning is directed at inhibiting the release of acetylcholine, separating cholinesterase from the chemical compound, and suppressing seizure activity (if present). The drugs currently used as antidotes include *atropine sulfate, pralidoxime chloride* (2-PAM Chloride), and *diazepam.*

> **NOTE:**
> Medication therapy should be administered only if the patient exhibits two or more characteristic signs or symptoms of poisoning and only after consulting with medical control or a poison control center.

Atropine reverses the muscarinic effects (bradycardia, bronchoconstriction, respiratory secretions, and miosis) of moderate-to-severe organophosphate or carbamate poisoning. The drug competitively antagonizes the actions of acetylcholine, resulting in a decrease in the hyperactivity of smooth muscles and glands. The initial dose is 2 mg intravenous push every 5 to 15 minutes as required to induce relative tachycardia, flushing, and decreased secretions. The pediatric dose is 0.05 mg/kg, repeated every 15 minutes as necessary. (Medical control may recommend that *atropine* be administered intramuscularly during the decontamination process before establishing an intravenous line.) Because potentially hypoxic patients may require administration of large doses of *atropine,* ECG monitoring for signs of dysrhythmias (other than tachycardia) and provision of supplemental oxygen must be undertaken to minimize the risk of ventricular fibrillation. *Atropine* is the drug of choice for carbamate poisonings.

Pralidoxime is the treatment of choice for organophosphate poisoning and should be used for nearly all patients with clinically significant exposures, particularly those with muscular fasciculations and weakness. *Pralidoxime* is one of a few drugs that correct a biochemical lesion. It has three desirable effects in managing organophosphate poisoning: (1) the primary effect of clearing the phosphorylation-acetyl-cholinesterase bond, thus freeing and reactivating acetylcholinesterase; (2) directly reacting with and detoxifying the organophosphorus molecules; and (3) having an anticholinergic "atropine-like" effect.[5] The initial adult

dose of *pralidoxime* is 1 g intravenously over 15 to 30 minutes. The pediatric dose is 20 to 50 mg/kg intravenously over 15 to 30 minutes. Subsequent doses may be repeated within 1 to 2 hours.

Diazepam may be indicated if seizures are present. If the need for *diazepam* arises before decontamination is complete, the drug should be administered intravenously in titrated doses as necessary to control seizure activity. The paramedic should be alert to the possibility of respiratory and central nervous system depression.

ECG Monitoring

ECG monitoring may reveal a variety of abnormalities, including idioventricular rhythms, multifocal premature ventricular contractions, ventricular tachycardia, torsades de pointes, ventricular fibrillation, complete heart block, and asystole. These dysrhythmias usually occur in two phases, beginning with a transient episode of intense sympathetic tone that results in sinus tachycardia and followed by a period of extreme parasympathetic tone that may manifest as sinus bradycardia, atrioventricular block, and ST-segment and T-wave abnormalities. Significant ventricular bradydysrhythmias that do not respond to conventional therapy may need to be treated with overdrive pacing.

Gastrointestinal Decontamination

In addition to antidote therapy, gastrointestinal decontamination is indicated in organophosphate ingestion followed by *activated charcoal.* Airway protection before orogastric lavage is necessary for the patient who has an altered level of consciousness or who has lost the gag reflex.

> ### Section Two
> ### Injected Poisons

Human poisonings may result from arthropod bites and stings, reptile bites, and hazardous aquatic life. In contrast to most organic or inorganic compounds previously described, injected poisons are mixtures of many different substances, which may produce several different toxic reactions in humans. Therefore the paramedic must be prepared to manage reactions in many organ systems simultaneously.

● ARTHROPOD BITES AND STINGS

There are approximately 900,000 species of arthropods throughout the world. Some arthropods bite, some sting, and a few bite and sting. Hymenoptera (bees, wasps, and ants) and Arachnida (including spiders, scorpions, and ticks) cause the highest incidence of need for emergency care. Arthropod venoms are complex and diverse in their chemistry and pharmacology and may produce major toxic reactions such as anaphylaxis and upper airway obstruction in sensitized individuals. The various reactions to venoms are classified as local, toxic, systemic, and delayed (Box 23-9).[6]

Hymenoptera

Hymenoptera venom is used for defense and subjugation of prey. Medically important venoms are mixtures of protein or polypeptide toxins, enzymes, and other compounds such as histamines, serotonin, acetylcholine, and dopamine. Hymenoptera stings are most commonly inflicted on the head and neck followed by the foot, leg, hand, and arm. The mouth, pharynx, and esophagus may be stung when bees or yellow jackets in soft-drink or beer containers are accidentally ingested.

A single wasp, bee, or ant sting in an unsensitized individual usually causes instant pain followed by a wheal-and-flare reaction with variable edema. Large local reactions spread more than 15 cm beyond the sting site and persist for more than 24 hours. Anaphylaxis is the most serious complication of hymenoptera stings. An estimated 0.4% of the U.S. population has some degree of chemical allergy to insect venoms; 40 to 50 deaths caused by anaphylaxis from hymenoptera stings are reported annually.[6] In adults, there is a tendency toward more severe reactions with repeated single stings. In children 10 years and younger,

life-threatening reactions are less frequent than in adults, and there is no tendency toward more severe reactions with repeated sting episodes.[6] Individuals with a history of allergic reactions to stings often wear medical alert identification and carry an emergency kit containing a preloaded syringe of *epinephrine* (Epi-Pen).

The ant species of greatest concern in the United States is the imported fire ant, whose venom is primarily alkaloid. The fire ant is the only hymenopteran species whose venom results in necrotic activity, and sterile pustules at the sting site are not uncommon. Stings or bites from fire ants may produce systemic reactions and are managed like other hymenoptera stings. Secondary infection may occur (requiring antibiotic therapy), and scarring can be so extensive as to require skin grafts (rare).

Management

Prehospital care for mild hymenoptera stings includes application of ice packs (to help delay absorption and limit edema) and close observation for signs or symptoms of an allergic reaction. If an extremity is involved, immobilization and elevation can help limit the reaction's duration. If physician evaluation is warranted, as evidenced by signs of anaphylaxis or vigorous reaction, an antihistamine may be prescribed.

Honey bees frequently (and other hymenoptera rarely) leave their stingers in the wound. If a stinger is present, it should be scraped or brushed off. Stingers should not be removed with forceps, because squeezing the attached venom sac may worsen the injury. Severe allergic reactions should be managed as described in Chapter 22. Hypovolemia (if present) should be treated in the conventional manner with a volume-expanding crystalloid infusion.

Arachnida

Although there are eleven types of Arachnida, this discussion is limited to spiders, scorpions, and ticks.

Spider Bites

Approximately 20,000 species of spiders are found in the United States, and all, with the ex-

---

BOX 23-9

Types of Reactions to Venoms

Local Reaction

- Marked and prolonged edema at the sting site
- Possible involvement of one or more neighboring joints
- Possible occurrence in the mouth or throat, producing airway obstruction
- Severe local reactions that may increase the likelihood of future systemic reactions (controversial)
- Symptoms that usually subside within 24 hours

Toxic Reaction*

- Gastrointestinal disturbances:
  Vomiting
  Diarrhea
  Lightheadedness
- Other symptoms:
  Syncope (common finding)
  Headache
  Fever
  Involuntary muscle spasms
  Edema without urticaria
  Convulsions (rare)
- Symptoms that usually subside within 48 hours

Systemic (Anaphylactic) Reaction†

- Reactions that can progress to death within minutes
- Immediate symptoms:
  Itching eyes or generalized itching
  Facial flushing
  Generalized urticaria
- Subsequent symptoms:
  Respiratory failure, cardiovascular collapse, or both
  Hypotension
  Chest or throat constriction or both
  Wheezing
  Dyspnea
  Cyanosis
  Nausea and vomiting
  Chills and fever
  Laryngeal stridor
  Shock
  Loss of consciousness
  Loss of bowel or bladder control
  Bloody and frothy sputum production

Delayed Reaction‡

- Serum sickness symptoms:
  Fever
  Malaise
  Headache
  Urticaria
  Polyarthritis

*Should be considered with a history of 10 or more stings.
†May occur in response to single or multiple stings.
‡Usually occurs 10 to 14 days after a sting.

---

ception of two small groups (Uloboriade and Liphistiidae), have venom glands. Fortunately, only approximately 50 of these species have fangs long enough to pierce human skin or enough venom to cause significant injury. The two major types of reactions that occur from spider venom are neurotoxic reactions resulting from the black widow bite and local tissue necrosis from the bites of most other spiders.

The black widow is the most notorious spider in North America. Although there are a number of variations in the species, the typical mature female (who often devours her mate, thus the name *black widow*) is shiny black with a red hourglass marking on the undersurface of the abdomen (Fig. 23-1). The size of the female varies with age but rarely exceeds 2.5 cm overall. (The male is approximately half the size of the female, brown,

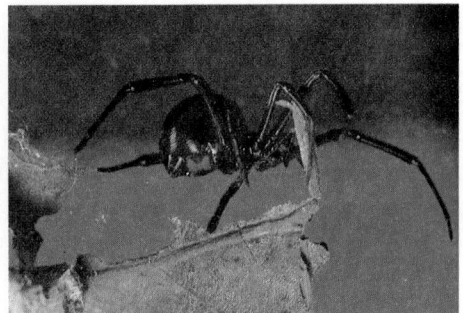

Fig. 23-1 Black widow spider.

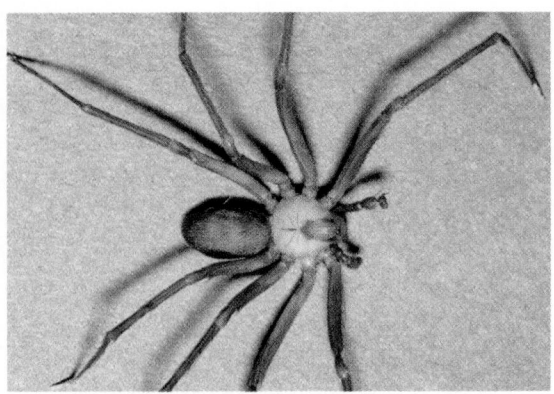

Fig. 23-2 Brown recluse spider.

and nonvenomous to humans.) The spider is generally found in undisturbed areas (under stones, logs, and clumps of vegetation) and rarely inhabits occupied dwellings. Most black widow bites occur in rural and suburban areas of southern and western states between April and October.

The bite of a black widow usually occurs when the spider has been disturbed. It is generally described by patients as a slight pinprick that is initially painless. As a rule, the only physical findings are two small fang marks approximately 1 mm apart surrounded by a small papule. Multiple bites usually rule out any type of spider envenomation, because spiders rarely bite more than once. Within 1 hour of envenomation, the neurotoxin produces characteristic muscle spasms and cramps, which may result in abdominal rigidity (in the absence of palpable tenderness) and intense pain.

Abdominal rigidity in the absence of palpable tenderness is an important finding that helps distinguish envenomation from an acute abdominal condition. Associated symptoms include paresthesia (frequently described as a burning sensation in the soles of the feet or entire body); pain in the muscles of the shoulders, back, and chest; headache; dizziness; nausea and vomiting; edema of the eyelids; and increased perspiration and salivation. Severe envenomation may cause hypertension and ECG abnormalities similar to those from digitalis. Emergency care for a patient with a black widow bite is primarily supportive and includes the following:

1. Ensure adequate airway, ventilatory, and circulatory support.

2. Clean the affected area with saline, cover with a sterile dressing, and intermittently apply ice. Obstruction tourniquets or suction devices are not helpful in delaying absorption. A commercially prepared antivenin is available but should only be administered in the emergency department and only after appropriate sensitivity testing.

3. Moderate-to-severe symptoms require aggressive treatment. Per medical control, muscle spasm, severe headache, vomiting, and paraesthesia may be managed with an intravenous infusion of 5 to 10 ml of 10% *calcium gluconate* solution or of 5 mg of *diazepam.* Severe hypertension may be managed with antihypertensive agents.

4. Transport the patient for physician evaluation. Most patients recover completely within 36 to 72 hours. Those at greatest risk for morbidity are the very young, older adults, and those with underlying hypertension.

The brown recluse spider, also known as the *fiddle-back spider,* is most prevalent in the Mississippi-Ohio-Missouri river basin and the southwestern United States. The species prefers hot, dry, and abandoned environments, such as vacant buildings; it is frequently found in clothing closets. The spider is fawn to dark brown in color and is between and 1 and 2 cm long (Fig. 23-2). Identifying characteristics of the brown recluse are six white eyes arranged in a semicircle on the head (versus the usual eight eyes of most other spiders) and the presence of a dark, violin-

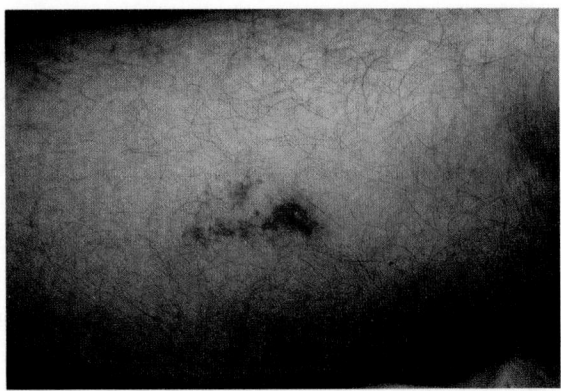

Fig. 23-3 Brown recluse spider bite at approximately 6 hours, with central hemorrhagic vesicle and gravitational pattern spread of venom.

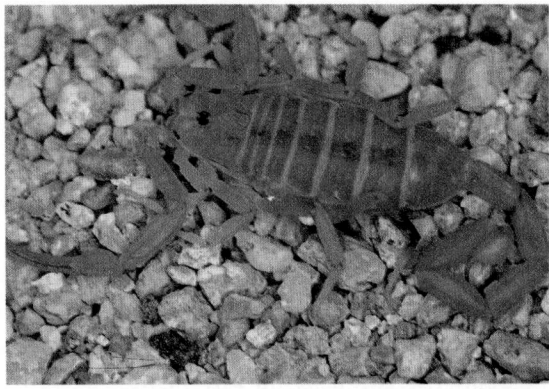

Fig. 23-4 The sculptured scorpion commonly found in the deserts of Arizona, New Mexico, and California.

shaped marking on the top of the cephalothorax (the combined head and thorax). The brown recluse is considered shy and does not generally attack unless threatened. Like black widows, these spiders are most active from April to October.

The venom of the brown recluse manifests in a broad spectrum of reactions. Initially the bite causes little pain and is often overlooked by the victim. Some 1 to 2 hours later, localized pain and erythema develop (Fig. 23-3). This transient irritation is often followed within 1 to 2 days by a blister or vesicle. The lesion may be surrounded by an ischemic ring that is further outlined by an irregular erythematous halo, producing the classical "bull's-eye" appearance. Over the next 24 to 72 hours, the area often becomes larger, and necrosis may occur, the center of the lesion yielding a purple or black eschar. The eschar eventually sloughs within 2 to 5 weeks, leaving an ulcer of variable size and depth. The tissue defect may extend to include underlying muscle and is typically slow to heal (often visible for months to years after the bite). Occasionally, excision and skin grafting are necessary. Systemic involvement may occur with signs and symptoms that include fever, chills, malaise, nausea and vomiting, generalized rash, and the development of hemolytic anemia, hemoglobinuria, and hypotension. Death occasionally occurs, usually from disturbance of the coagulation system or hepatic injury.

Emergency care for patients with a brown recluse bite is generally supportive. Cold compresses and sterile dressings should be applied to the lesion, and the patient should be transported for physician evaluation. As a rule, pharmacological therapy is not indicated in the prehospital setting. In-hospital therapy may include ice, antibiotics, and dapsone (a leukocyte inhibitor). Although an antivenin has been used in research, it is not widely clinically available. Most patients do well with outpatient management.

Scorpion Stings

There are over 650 species of scorpions, but only a few produce human envenomation. In North America, the sculptured or bark scorpion, found in the southwestern United States and Mexico, is the only species that is dangerous to humans. The scorpion is nocturnal and favors wooded areas along the edges of desert washes, where it generally clings upside down in its hideouts. It may be found under the bark of the eucalyptus and cottonwood trees. Occasionally the scorpion invades homes, especially adobe houses. The sculptured scorpion is small (2 to 7.5 cm) and yellow to brown in color, and some have tail stripes (Fig. 23-4). The species is most active from April to August, hibernating during the winter.

The scorpion's venom is delivered by a stinger on the telson (located on the abdomen) and is used for both defense and food acquisition. The venom is a mixture of proteins with complex effects on cellular sodium channels. It acts at the presynaptic terminal of the neuromuscular junction, releasing acetylcholine, which results in depolarization of the junction. The venom also stimulates sympathetic nerves, is directly cardiotoxic, and directly stimulates the central nervous system, causing hyperactivity and convulsions. This particular scorpion venom does not contain enzymes that cause tissue destruction, so local inflammation is not a feature. If swelling, ecchymosis, or erythema is present, the scorpion was not of the neurotoxic type. Signs and symptoms of sculptured scorpion envenomation are listed in Box 23-10.

Despite the potential for life-threatening systemic effects, the vast majority of scorpion envenomations, especially in adults, produce only minimal pain lasting less than 4 hours. As a rule, mild analgesics, cool compresses, and in-hospital observation are all that are required for these patients. If signs and symptoms of severe envenomation develop, sympathetic blocking agents such as *propranolol* may control effects on the cardiovascular system. In some cases, sedation is required to control convulsions. The use of antivenin for scorpion bites is controversial. Prehospital care is supportive, airway control being the highest priority. Ice should be applied to the wound to relieve pain, and the patient should be transported for physician evaluation.

BOX 23-10

Signs and Symptoms of Scorpion Envenomation

- Hyperesthesia at the site of bite
- Pain, tingling, and a burning sensation radiating along the nerves at the location of the bite
- SLUDGE: salivation, lacrimation, urination, defecation, gastrointestinal distress, and emesis
- Initial bradycardia followed by tachycardia
- Cardiac dysrhythmias
- Muscle twitching
- Convulsions
- Roving eye movements (cranial nerve dysfunction)
- Temporary blindness

Tick Bites

Although tick bites seldom require emergency care, ticks are capable of causing human disease by transmitting microorganisms or by secreting toxins or venoms. In North America, hard ticks are the most familiar type, although soft ticks are also common to western states. Hard ticks have a leathery exterior that makes them resistant to environmental stresses. They are relatively free of natural enemies. They can regenerate lost parts and have been known to survive without feeding for more than 4 years. Local reactions to tick bites vary from the formation of a small pruritic nodule to development of extensive areas of ulceration that may be accompanied by fever, chills, and malaise unrelated to infection. Some of the more important diseases for which ticks are vectors include Rocky Mountain spotted fever (RMSF), Lyme disease, and tick paralysis.

RMSF is an infectious disease transmitted from rabbits and other small mammals to humans by the bites of the wood tick and dog tick. The disease occurs more commonly on the Atlantic seaboard, and more than 1000 cases of the disease are reported annually. Signs and symptoms usually develop within 5 to 7 days of the tick bite and include headache, high fever, and loss of appetite. Usually within 2 to 3 days after the onset of symptoms, small pink spots appear on the wrists and ankles. Eventually the rash spreads over the entire body, and the spots darken and enlarge and become petechial. In mild cases, recovery occurs within 20 days. The mortality rate, if untreated, is between 8% and 20%.

Lyme disease has overtaken RMSF as the most commonly reported tick-borne disease in the United States. The disease was first described in the community of Old Lyme, Connecticut, in 1975. Lyme disease is caused by a spirochete transmitted by the bite of an *Ixodes* tick known to infect deer and dogs. The course of the disease follows several stages. Initially a red dot appears at the site of the tick bite. This gradually expands into a reddened annular rash, often with central clearing. During this stage, fever, lethargy, muscle pain, and general malaise may develop. This stage may be followed by a second stage approximately 4 to 6 weeks later, manifested by cardiac abnormalities (including various atrioventricular blocks) and neurological effects (including cranial nerve palsies). Approximately 10% of infected patients go on to the second stage. Still later, a third stage may develop, with arthritis as the primary symptom. Unless the disease is diagnosed and treated, symptoms may continue for several years, gradually declining in severity.

Tick paralysis results from a prolonged bite by a female wood tick. The disease occurs sporadically during the spring and summer months and is caused by a neurotoxin secreted from the tick's salivary glands during a blood meal. Tick paralysis develops in humans within 6 days after the tick attaches to the host. Initially the patient presents with restlessness and complaints of paresthesia in the hands and feet. Over the next 24 to 48 hours, an ascending, symmetrical flaccid paralysis may develop with loss of deep tendon reflexes. In severe cases, death may result from respiratory paralysis. Removal of the tick usually results in rapid improvement and complete resolution within several days. If undiagnosed, the disease may be fatal, particularly in young and older patients.

The principal treatment of tick bites is proper removal of the tick. The tick should be grasped as close to the skin surface as possible with forceps, tweezers, or protected fingers and pulled out with steady pressure. Care should be taken not to crush or squeeze the body of the tick, which can transmit disease from infective tick fluid. Other methods of tick removal, such as applying fingernail polish, isopropanol, or a hot match head, should be avoided. These traditional methods are ineffective and may induce the tick to salivate or regurgitate into the wound. After removal, the bite should be disinfected with soap and water and covered with a sterile dressing.

● REPTILE BITES

The AAPCC National Data Collection System listed a total 3726 bites from poisonous and nonpoisonous snakes in 1990.[2] Of these exposures, 979 were known to be poisonous, and 1712 were bites from unidentified snakes. According to these records, no deaths were reported, reflecting the high morbidity and low mortality rates associated with snake venom poisoning. Of the 115 species of snakes in the United States, only 19 are venomous. The two main families of venomous snakes indigenous to the United States are pit vipers and coral snakes.

Pit Vipers

The pit viper family that inhabits the United States consists of rattlesnakes (15 species), the cottonmouth (water) moccasin, the copperhead, the pigmy rattlesnake, and the massasauga. The vast majority of snakebites in the United States are caused by the rattlesnake family (Fig. 23-5).

The general term *pit viper* is derived from a depression or pit in the maxillary bone of these snakes, which is believed to be a heat-sensing organ that detects warm-blooded prey or enemies. The pit guides the direction of the strike and possibly determines the amount of venom released, based on the size and heat emission of the prey. Other identifying characteristics of the pit viper are vertical elliptical pupils and a triangular head that is distinct from the rest of the body. The rattlesnake is further characterized by "rattles" (interlocking horny segments formed on the tail) that sometimes vibrate in direct relation to environmental temperatures.

The venom apparatus of pit vipers consists of a gland and a duct connected to one or more elongated hollow fangs on each side of the head. The venom is composed of a variety of proteins designed to immobilize, kill, and digest prey. Depending on the species and the amount of venom injected, these proteins may be capable of producing various toxic effects on blood and other tissues, including hemolysis, intravascular coagula-

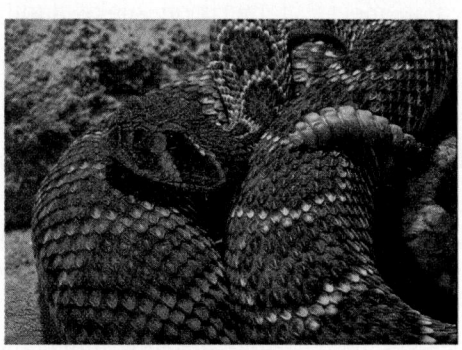

Fig. 23-5 Pit viper.

Signs and Symptoms of Pit Viper Envenomation

Mild Envenomation

Presence of one or more fang marks

Local swelling and pain

Lack of systemic symptoms

Moderate Envenomation

Presence of one or more fang marks

Pain and edema beyond the site

Systemic signs and symptoms

Weakness

Diaphoresis

Nausea and vomiting

Paresthesias

Severe Envenomation

Presence of one or more fang marks

Massive edema

Subcutaneous ecchymosis

Severe systemic symptoms

Shock

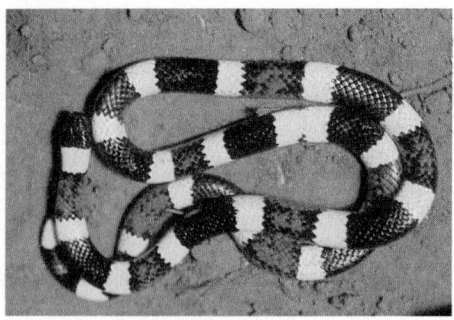

Fig. 23-6 Coral snake.

tion, convulsions, and acute renal failure (Box 23-11). Bleeding secondary to coagulation defects and massive swelling can lead to hypovolemic shock. On any given strike, the snake may release a quantity of venom varying from little or none to almost the entire content of the glands. (A total of 20% of bites do not result in envenomation.)

Coral Snakes

Two members of the coral snake family are found in the United States: the Arizona coral snake and the Eastern coral snake. In contrast to the pit viper, the coral snake has round pupils and small, fixed fangs located near the anterior end of the maxilla. Most coral snakes have a three-color pattern with red, black, and yellow or white bands that completely encircle the body, along with a black snout (Fig. 23-6). Many nonpoisonous snakes in the United States mimic the ap-

pearance of the coral snake. The coral snake is identified by the sequence of colors: red bands bordered by yellow indicate a venomous species. Thus "red on yellow, kill a fellow; red on black, venom lack."

Most coral snakes are shy and docile and seldom bite unless threatened. The snake's small mouth and fangs make it difficult to bite anything larger than a finger, toe, or fold of skin. The coral snake tends to hang on and chew rather than to strike and release like the pit viper. The venom of the coral snake is primarily neurotoxic and has a blocking action on acetylcholine receptor sites. The bite generally produces little or no pain and no necrosis or edema. Early signs and symptoms of a coral snake bite are slurred speech, dilated pupils, and dysphagia (usually delayed several hours after the bite). If untreated, the venom produces flaccid paralysis and death (within 8 to 24 hours) by respiratory failure, secondary to central nervous system inhibition.

Management of Snake Envenomation

Venom, like any drug or toxin, has absorption, distribution, and elimination characteristics. Tissue damage increases as venom spreads into the lymphatics and blood. Therefore emergency care is directed at retarding the systemic spread of the venom. Prehospital management of snake bites includes the following:

1. Stay clear of the snake's striking range (approximately the length of the snake), and move the patient to a safe area. If the snake

has been killed before EMS arrival, it should be transported in a closed container to the emergency department with the patient. No attempt should be made by EMS personnel to capture or destroy the snake—to do so may result in a second envenomation. It is not absolutely necessary to identify the snake to treat the patient appropriately.

2. Provide adequate airway, ventilatory, and circulatory support to the patient as needed. Continually monitor vital signs and the ECG and establish an intravenous line in an unaffected extremity with a volume-expanding fluid.

3. When practical, immobilize the bitten extremity in a dependent position. Immobilization by splinting may delay systemic absorption and diminish local tissue necrosis. Every effort should be made to keep the patient at rest.

4. Prepare the patient for immediate transport to an appropriate medical facility.

5. Additional measures in the management of snake envenomation, such as incision and suction or use of a lymphatic-venous constriction band or pressure device, are controversial. The paramedic should consult with medical control and follow local protocol. Application of ice or chemical cold packs should be avoided because their use may further tissue damage. In severe cases, in-hospital administration of antivenin to neutralize the venom may be required after appropriate sensitivity testing.

● HAZARDOUS AQUATIC LIFE

The marine animals most likely to be involved in human poisonings in U.S. costal waters are the Coelenterates, Echinoderms, and stingrays. The specialized venom apparatuses of these animals are used for defense and for capturing prey. In addition to venom produced by the animal, aquatic life may contain other poisonous substances as a result of toxic ingestions. Exposures to hazardous aquatic life result from recreational, industrial, scientific, and military oceanic activities.

Coelenterates

Coelenterates are a group of over 9000 species that may be encountered in the ocean (Fig. 23-7). Those that carry venomous stinging cells (nematocysts) are known as *cnidaria*. The nematocyst is venom filled and contains a long, coiled, hollow, threadlike tube that serves as a tiny hypodermic needle. There are many types of nematocysts; an individual coelenterate may have more than one type. The severity of envenomation is related to

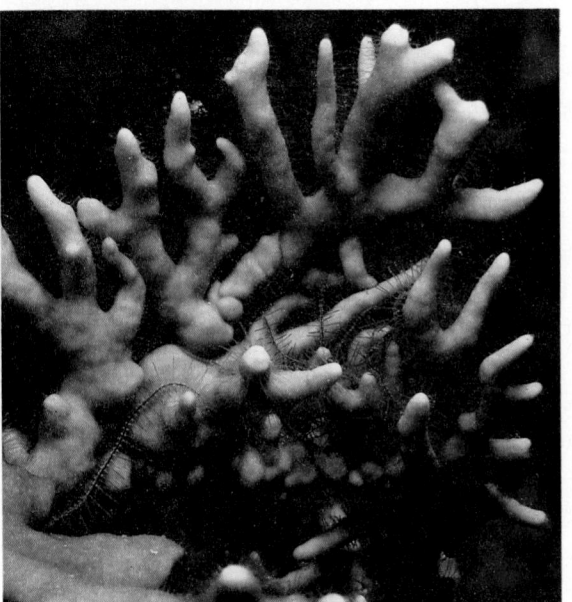

A

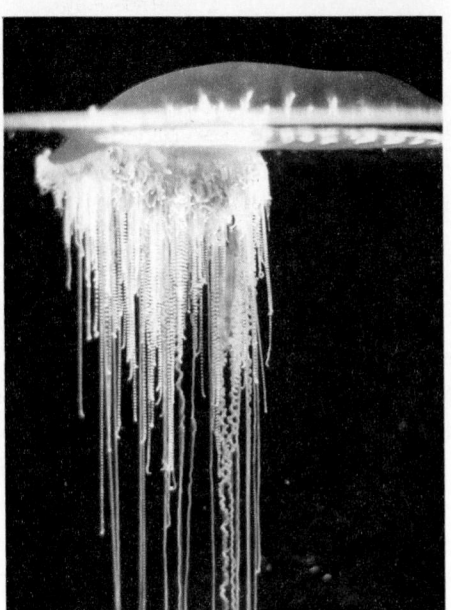

B

Fig. 23-7 Coelenterates. **A,** Fire coral. **B,** Man-of-war.

the toxicity of the venom (which may contain various fractions), the number of nematocysts discharged, and the physical condition of the victim.

Jellyfish, of which the Portuguese man-of-war is the largest and most dangerous, occur throughout the Atlantic and Pacific oceans, usually near the coastline. Their nematocyst-bearing tentacles may be up to 100 feet long, and a single envenomation may involve several hundred thousand nematocysts. A swimmer who comes into contact with the tentacles of the jellyfish may suffer sufficient envenomation to produce systemic signs and symptoms. Nematocysts frequently remain embedded in the tissues of the victim. Detached tentacle fragments can retain their potency for months.

Sea anemones are colorful bottom dwellers (sometimes found in tidal pools) that have a flowerlike appearance. They possess slender projections used to sting and paralyze passing fish. Their modifications of nematocysts are capable of producing mild-to-moderate pain in humans.

Fire corals are not true (stony) corals but rather ocean-bottom dwellers that are widely distributed in tropical waters. They are often mistaken for seaweed because they are frequently found attached to rocks, shells, and corals. These stinging corals may grow to 2 m in height and have a razor-sharp exoskeleton with thousands of protruding nematocyst-bearing tentacles.

Management

Coelenterate envenomation ranges in severity from irritant dermatitis to excruciating pain, respiratory depression, and life-threatening cardiovascular collapse. Envenomation is most often mild, characterized by stinging, paresthesias, pruritus, and reddish-brown linear wheals or "tentacle prints." If a potent venom or a large body surface area is involved, systemic symptoms may include nausea, vomiting, abdominal pain, headache, bronchospasm, pulmonary edema, and respiratory arrest. Emergency care is directed at stabilizing the patient and counteracting the effects of the venom.

1. Stabilize the patient.
   a. Provide adequate airway, ventilatory, and circulatory support as needed.

b. Continually monitor the patient's vital signs and the ECG. Be prepared to provide aggressive airway management if systemic reactions develop.
2. Counteract effects of the venom.
   a. Immediately rinse the patient's wound with seawater. (Wet sand or fresh water usually causes the nematocysts to discharge their venom and is therefore contraindicated.)
   b. Apply copious amounts of vinegar (preferred), isopropanol, a baking soda slurry, or household ammonia to inactivate the venom in intact nematocysts. A paste of unseasoned meat tenderizer may be recommended, but application to injured skin for more than 5 to 10 minutes may have deleterious effects.
   c. Remove visible tentacle fragments with forceps. Avoid self-contamination.
   d. Apply a lather of shaving cream and gently shave the affected area to remove invisible nematocysts. If shaving material is unavailable, use a knife or spatula to scrape away remaining tentacles.
   e. Rinse again until pain is largely alleviated. If necessary, consult with medical control regarding administration of analgesics.
   f. Transport the patient for physician evaluation.

Echinoderms

Echinoderms include the sea urchins, starfish, and sea cucumbers (Fig. 23-8). Sea urchins have a globular, dome-shaped body and are found on rocky bottoms or burrowed in sand or crevices. These animals have tiny spines, some of which are venomous. Between the spines of some sea urchins are small pincerlike organs that are also thought to discharge a poisonous substance. The spines are extremely dangerous to handle and may break off easily in the flesh, lodging deeply and making removal very difficult.

Starfish are covered with thorny spines of calcium carbonate crystals that secrete toxins. As the spine enters the skin, it carries venom into the wound with immediate pain, copious bleeding,

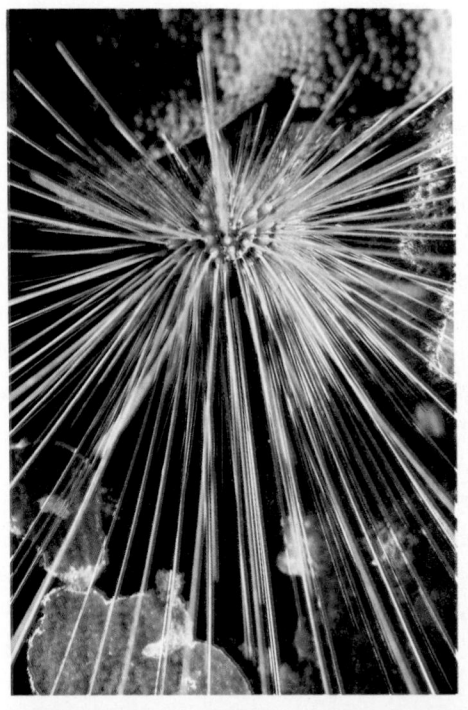

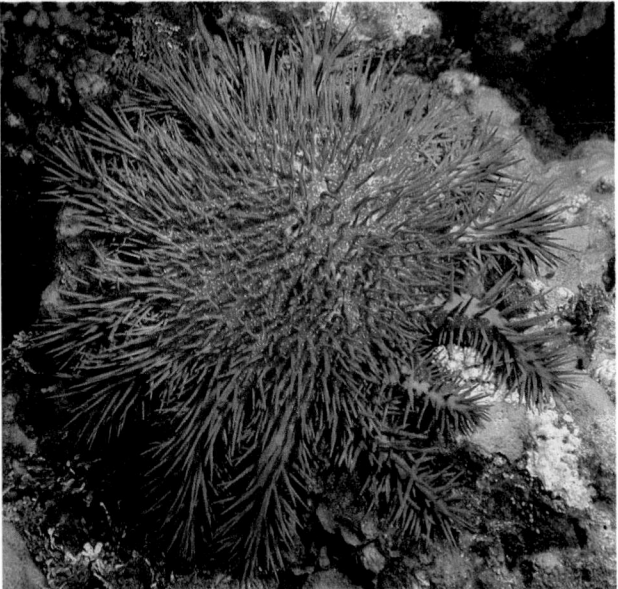

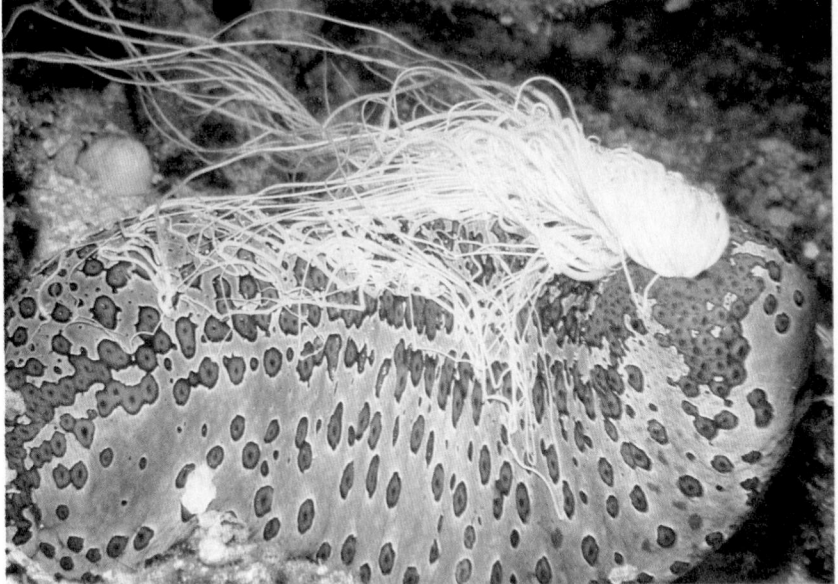

Fig. 23-8 Echinoderms. **A,** Black sea urchin. **B,** Crown-of-thorns starfish. **C,** Sea cucumber with extended tentacles.

and mild edema. Multiple puncture wounds may result in acute systemic reactions.

Sea cucumbers are sausage-shaped animals found in shallow and deep water. They produce a liquid toxin in a tentacle-shaped organ that can be projected and extended anally. Generally the substance is secreted into the surrounding ocean, producing only a minor dermatitis or conjunctivitis in swimmers and divers.

Management

Emergency management for echinoderm envenomation usually involves caring for puncture wounds caused by spines and inactivating the venom. Embedded spines should be removed with forceps. Protective gloves should be worn, and the paramedic should be careful to avoid self-contamination. Larger spines may require surgical removal by a physician.

Echinoderm toxins may cause immediate intense pain, swelling, redness, aching in the affected extremity, and nausea. Delayed toxic effects may include respiratory distress, paresthesia of the lips and face, and in severe cases, respiratory paralysis and complete atonia. Therefore the paramedic must be prepared to deal with a variety of physical reactions.

Most marine venoms lose their toxicity when exposed to changes in temperature or humidity. The recommended treatment for stable patients is to immerse the affected area (usually the foot or hand) in extremely hot water before and during transport. The water should be as hot as can be tolerated without scalding (45° to 50° C, 113° to 122° F). As a safety precaution, it is generally recommended that both hands or feet be immersed to protect against injury that may go unnoticed by the patient because of numbness or pain in the affected part.

Stingrays

Stingrays are responsible for approximately 1800 injuries each year in the United States. These marine animals vary in size from 2 inches to 14 feet and are often found half-buried in mud or sand in shallow water (Fig. 23-9). The venom organ of stingrays consists of two to four venomous stings on the dorsum of a whiplike tail. Envenomation generally occurs from stepping on the sand-buried ray, which causes the tail to thrust up and forward, driving the sting into the victim's leg or foot. The sting (which is purely defensive) produces a large, severe laceration, which may be more than 15 to 20 cm long. In addition to injecting venom into the wound, the entire spine tip of the venom apparatus is sometimes broken and embedded in the tissue.

Stingray venom has local and systemic complications. Locally, it produces a traumatic injury that causes immediate, intense pain; edema; variable bleeding; and necrosis. Systemic manifestations include weakness, nausea, vomiting, diarrhea, vertigo, seizures, cardiac conduction abnormalities, paralysis, hypotension, and death.

Management

Prehospital care is directed to life support, alleviation of pain, inactivation of venom, and prevention of infection.

1. Ensure adequate airway, ventilatory, and circulatory support. Continually monitor the patient's vital signs and ECG.
2. Copiously irrigate the wound with normal saline or fresh water. If the venom apparatus is visible, it should be removed. Avoid self-contamination.
3. If practical, immerse the affected part in very hot water as previously described. Immersion should continue until pain subsides or until the patient reaches the emergency department.
4. Medical control may recommend application of lymphatic-venous constricting bands (controversial) and administration of analgesics.
5. Transport the patient for physician evaluation.

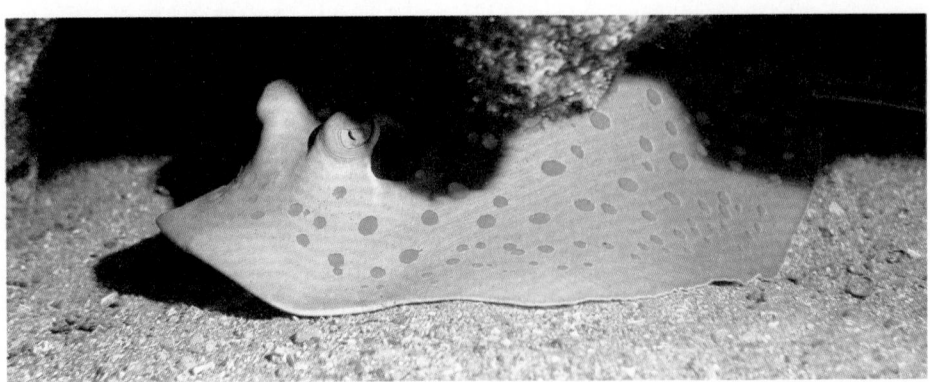

Fig. 23-9 Stingray.

Section Three
Drug Abuse

The term **drug abuse** refers to the use of prescription drugs for nonprescribed purposes or the use of drugs that have no prescribed medical use (Box 23-12). Emergencies resulting from drug abuse include adverse effects caused by the drug or impurities or contaminants mixed with the drug, life-threatening infections from intravenous or intradermal injection of drugs with unsterile equipment, accidents during intoxication, and drug dependence or **withdrawal syndrome** resulting from the habit-forming potential of many drugs.

BOX 23-12

Drug Abuse Terminology

Drug abuse: Self-medication or self-administration of a drug in chronically excessive amounts, resulting in psychological and/or physical dependence, functional impairment, and deviation from approved social norms

Drug dependence: Condition marked by an overwhelming desire to continue taking a drug for its desired effect, usually an altered mental activity, attitude, or outlook

Psychological dependence: Emotional reliance on a drug (Manifestations range from a mild desire for a drug to craving and drug-seeking behavior to repeated compulsive use of a drug for its subjectively satisfying or pleasurable effects.)

Physical dependence: An adaptive physiological state occurring after prolonged use of many drugs (Discontinuation causes withdrawal syndromes that are relieved by readministering the same drug or a pharmacologically related drug.)

Tolerance: A tendency to increase drug dosage to experience the same effect formerly produced by a smaller dose

Withdrawal syndrome: A predictable set of signs and symptoms that occurs after a decrease in the amount of the usual dose of a drug or its sudden cessation

● FACTORS THAT INFLUENCE DRUG ABUSE

No single cause or set of conditions clearly leads to drug abuse. It is widespread and common among all socioeconomic, cultural, and ethnic groups. Drug abuse is a major medical, social, and interpersonal problem that affects individuals from all backgrounds and of all ages. It has been conservatively estimated that 45 million Americans use drugs in a recreational way.[7] (This figure does not include the frequent use of legal drugs such as nicotine, caffeine in coffee and tea, ethanol, and over-the-counter medications such as sleeping aids.)

Because of the widespread use and misuse of drugs, the paramedic should maintain a high degree of suspicion and consider the possibility for a drug-related problem in any patient who has seizures, behavioral changes, stupor, or coma. In addition, consideration of the visibility, accessibility, and careful handling of all medications carried on an EMS vehicle should be a part of any EMS policy and procedure.

● COMMON DRUGS OF ABUSE

Common drugs of abuse may be classified into four major categories: narcotics, central nervous system depressants, central nervous system stimulants, and hallucinogens. Names for these drugs and their uses vary widely in different geographical areas and frequently change over time. Table 23-2 is a partial list of common drugs of abuse, their street names, and miscellaneous terminology relating to drug use.

● TOXIC EFFECTS OF DRUGS

In the field or emergency department, EMS personnel frequently encounter people suffering from

TABLE 23-2 Street Names for Common Drugs

Common Name	Classification	Chemical Names	Slang Names
Adipex-P	Anorexiant	Phentermine	Robin's eggs
Alcohol	Sedative and hypnotic	Ethanol, ethyl alcohol	Booze, juice
Amphetamines	Sympathomimetic	Benzedrine, Dexedrine, Methedrine (methamphetamine HCl)	Birds, cartwheels, crosses, leapers, white cross, whites, speed, pep pill, wake-ups, uppers, crank, crystal, meth
		Biphetamine (amphetamine and dextroamphetamine resin complex)	Black beauties (look alikes too), black cadillacs
		Benzedrine (amphetamine sulfate)	Beans, bennies, hearts, peaches, roses
		Dexedrine (dextroamphetamine sulfate)	Brown and clears (long acting), dexies, footballs, orange, orange hearts
Amyl nitrite	Vasodilator	Amyl nitrite; isobutyl nitrite	Aroma of men, Jac aroma, locker room, ames, amys, bolt, climax, hard-on, heart-on, pearls, poppers, snappers
Barbiturates	Sedative and hypnotic	Phenobarbital	Barbs, downers, goof balls, phennies, softballs, stumblers
		Nembutal	Nebbies, yellows, yellow jackets
		Seconal (secobarbital)	Red devils, reds
		Amytal (amobarbital)	Blue devils, blue heavens, blue angels, bluebirds, blues
		Tuinal	Rainbows, Christmas trees
Cocaine	Stimulant and local anesthetic	Cocaine HCl	Blow, candy, coke, flake, nose candy, snow, toot
		Cocaine sulfate or base	Crack, freebase, rock
Codeine	Narcotic	Methylmorphine	Schoolboy
DMT	Hallucinogen	Dimethyltryptamine	Businessman's trip
Doriden	Relaxant and sedative	Glutethimide	Cibas, D; doors
Hashish	Relaxant, euphoriant, and hallucinogen	*Cannabis sativa* (resin from the flowering tops)	Black Russian, hash; hemp
Heroin	Narcotic	Alpha methyl fentanyl	China white, pure Southeast Asian heroin
		Diacetylmorphine	H, horse, junk, smack, brown sugar, Mexican mud, Persian brown
Lidocaine	Anesthetic	Lidocaine	Florida snow
LSD	Hallucinogen	Lysergic acid diethylamide	Acid, sugar, cubes, trips, window panes, blotter, animal, barrels, blue bells, blue cheer, California sunshine, clowns, electric Kool-Aid acid, grape parfait, "Mickeys" (and other Disney characters), micro dots, paper acid, purple haze, royal blue, strawberry fields, twenty-five

Data from Budassi S: Street drugs. *Trauma Notebook*, 1982. Heidbreder G, Wolley B: Current street language for various drugs that are abused. *California Medicine*, February 1972. ISMA Ad Hoc Committee on Substance Abuse Education: *Substance Abuse Glossary*. Johnson NP, editor: *Dictionary of Street, Alcohol and Drug Terms*, School of Medicine, University of South Carolina, University Printing Office, 1986, Unknown Drug Names and Slang Terms.

TABLE 23-2 Street Names for Common Drugs—cont'd

Common Name	Classification	Chemical Names	Slang Names
Marijuana	Relaxant, euphoriant, and hallucinogen	*Cannabis sativa* (all parts)	African black, shit, pot, grass, tea, joint, weed, dope
[1]MDA	Stimulant	3,4-Methylenedioxyamphetamine	Love drug, Mellow Drug of America
[2]MDMA		3,4-Methylenedioxymethamphetamine	Adam, ecstacy, rhapsody, XTC
Mescaline	Hallucinogen	Mescaline	Buttons, beans, cactus
Methadone	Narcotic	Dolophine amidone	Dolly, dollies
Morphine	Narcotic	Morphine sulfate	M, white stuff
Noludar	Sedative and hypnotic	Methylprylon	Noodlars
PCP	Stimulant Analgesic Hallucinogen	Phencyclidine	Angel dust, hog, angel hair (mist), PeaCe Pill, sernyl, Shermans, tic or tac
Preludin	Stimulant and anorexiant	Phenmetrazine	Sweeties
Psilocybin	Hallucinogen	Psilocybin	Magic mushrooms, mushrooms, los niños, silly, silly putty
Quaaludes	Sedative and hypnotic	Methaqualone	Ludes, soaps, quacks, disco biscuits, Paris 400, Q, sopors
STP	Hallucinogen	Dimethoxymethylamphetamine	DOM, Serenity-Tranquility-Peace
Talwin and Pyribenzamine	Narcotic and antihistamine	Pentazocine Tripelennamine	T's & B's, T's & Blues
Tranquilizers	Sedative and hypnotic	Diazepam Chlordiazepoxide Meprobamate	Valium, Blues, Vals, yellows Librium Equanil, Miltown

Miscellaneous Terminology

357 magnums—combination of one to three drugs (caffeine, phenylpropanolamine, and ephedrine) in "look alikes."

ant—small-time dealer who sells to support a personal habit.

balling—sexual intercourse, with reference to placing an amphetamine (especially methamphetamine) in the vagina before intercourse.

base house—crack establishment.

baseballer—person who smokes freebase cocaine.

bazooka—mixture of coca paste and marijuana.

bike chemist—small-time, unqualified chemist

blue blood—person who injects drugs.

blue velvet—paregoric with Pyribenzamine or Elixir Terpin Hydrate with codeine with Pyribenzamine.

body packing—hiding drugs in body cavities for smuggling.

boys and girls—heroin (boys) and cocaine (girls) injected, usually in 2:1 ratio.

brown slime—mixture of nutmeg and cola syrup.

chasing the dragon—inhalation of vapors from heroin heated on aluminum foil.

four doors—Doriden with codeine (as Empirin No. 4 or Tylenol No. 4).

four way—LSD, STP, methedrine or cocaine, and strychnine.

ghost busting—smoking PCP and cocaine.

loads—Doriden with codeine (as Empirin No. 4 or Tylenol No. 4).

mules—transporters of drugs.

pineapple—heroin and Ritalin.

sinsemilla—unpollinated female *Cannabis* plants.

space basing—smoking PCP and cocaine (as crack) together.

steam burns—psychotic reaction from PCPA.

whited out—euphoria from inhaling typewriter correction fluid.

the toxic effects of drugs as the result of an overdose, a potential suicide, polydrug administration, or an accident (accidental ingestion, miscalculation, changes in drug strength). The drugs discussed in this chapter are narcotics, sedatives-hypnotics, stimulants, phencyclidine (PCP), tricyclic antidepressants, hallucinogens, salicylate, acetaminophen, and iron.

General Management Principles

As a rule, the general principles for treating drug overdose are the same as those described for ingestion of poisons. These include the following:

1. Ensure scene safety and be prepared for unpredictable patient behavior. (Consider the need for law enforcement assistance.)
2. Ensure adequate airway, ventilatory, and circulatory support as needed.
3. Obtain a history of the event (including the self-administration of other drugs that may have been taken by another route) and any significant past medical or psychiatric history.
4. Identify the substance and consult with medical control or a poison control center.
5. Perform a thorough secondary survey. Continually monitor the patient's vital functions and ECG.
6. Initiate intravenous therapy. Draw a blood sample for laboratory analysis and administer appropriate pharmacological antidotes such as *naloxone* if a narcotic overdose is suspected. Personal protective measures should be given special attention because many of these patients are at high risk of harboring hepatitis and the human immunodeficiency virus (HIV).
7. Prevent further absorption of an orally administered drug by gastrointestinal decontamination or the administration of *activated charcoal* (per protocol).
8. Rapidly transport the patient for physician evaluation.

Narcotic Overdose

Heroin accounts for approximately 90% of the narcotic abuse in the United States. Pure heroin is a bitter-tasting white powder that is usually adulterated or "cut" for street distribution with various agents such as lactose, sucrose, sodium bicarbonate (baking soda), powdered milk, starch, magnesium silicate (talc), procaine, or quinine. A typical "bag" is the single-dose unit of heroin and may weigh 100 mg, of which on average only 5% is pure. Other narcotic drugs include *morphine,* hydromorphone, methadone, *meperidine,* codeine, oxycodone, propoxyphene, and the newer "designer opiates" such as alpha methyl fentanyl ("China white").

Depending on the narcotic preparation, these drugs may be taken orally, injected intradermally ("skin popping") or intravenously ("mainlining"), taken intranasally ("snorted"), or smoked. All narcotics are central nervous system depressants and can cause life-threatening respiratory depression. In severe intoxication, hypotension, profound shock, and pulmonary edema may be present. Signs and symptoms of narcotic overdose include:

- Euphoria
- Arousable somnolence ("nodding")
- Nausea
- Pinpoint pupils (except with *meperidine,* hypoxia, or in combination with other types of drugs)
- Coma
- Seizures

Antidotal Therapy

As described in Chapter 14, *naloxone* is a pure narcotic antagonist effective for virtually all narcotic and narcotic-like substances. The drug reverses the triad of symptoms of narcotic overdose (respiratory depression, coma, and miosis) and should always be administered when narcotic intoxication is suspected or when a coma of unknown origin is present. The EMS crew should be prepared to restrain the patient, whose behavior may be unpredictable when the effects of the narcotic are reversed. Medical control may recommend that the *naloxone* administration be titrated to keep the patient responsive and free from respiratory depression but somewhat docile during transport.

Some narcotics have a longer duration than *naloxone.* Therefore the patient must be closely monitored during antidotal therapy, and repeated

BOX 23-13

Signs and Symptoms of Narcotic Withdrawal

Gooseflesh
Tachycardia
Diaphoresis
Irritability
Insomnia
Abdominal cramps
Tremors
Nausea and vomiting
Anorexia
Cold sweats or chills
Fever
Diarrhea
General malaise

doses of *naloxone* may be necessary. *Naloxone* can also precipitate a withdrawal syndrome in narcotic-dependent patients. Narcotic withdrawal is seldom life threatening and can usually be managed by symptomatic and supportive care. Signs and symptoms of narcotic withdrawal are listed in Box 23-13.

Sedative-Hypnotic Overdose

Sedative-hypnotic agents include benzodiazepines and barbiturates. These drugs are usually taken orally but may be diluted and injected intravenously. Use with alcohol markedly increases their effects. Sedative-hypnotic drugs are commonly known as *downers.*

Benzodiazepines are among the best-known and most widely prescribed drugs used to control symptoms of anxiety, stress, and insomnia. In addition, these drugs are sometimes used to manage alcohol withdrawal and control epilepsy. Benzodiazepines promote sleep and relieve anxiety by depressing brain function; they are frequently abused for their sedative effects. Individually, these drugs are relatively nontoxic, but they may accentuate the effects of other sedative-hypnotic agents. Common benzodiazepines are Valium and Librium.

Barbiturates are general central nervous system depressants that inhibit impulse conduction in the ascending reticular activating system. These drugs were once widely used to treat anxiety and insomnia. Their addictive properties and potential for abuse have led to their replacement by benzodiazepines and other nonbarbiturate drugs. Commonly prescribed barbiturates include *phenobarbital,* amobarbital, and secobarbital.

Signs and symptoms of sedative-hypnotic overdose are chiefly related to the central nervous and cardiovascular systems. Adverse effects include excessive drowsiness, staggering gait, and in some cases, paradoxical excitability. In cases of severe toxicity, the patient may become comatose, with respiratory depression, hypotension, and shock. Pupils may be constricted but often become fixed and dilated even in the absence of significant brain damage. Airway control and ventilatory management are the essential points in treating significant sedative-hypnotic overdose. Recently a benzodiazepine antagonist, *flumazenil* (Mazicon), has been approved for clinical use (see Emergency Drug Index).

Stimulant Overdose

Commonly abused stimulant drugs are those of the amphetamine family (for example, Benzedrine, Dexedrine, cocaine, methamphetamine).

Amphetamine drugs are frequently used to produce general mood elevation, improve task performance, suppress appetite, and prevent sleepiness. Structurally, the amphetamines are similar to the endogenous catecholamines (epinephrine and norepinephrine) but differ in their more pronounced effects on the central nervous system. Adverse effects include tachycardia, increased blood pressure, tachypnea, agitation, dilated pupils, tremors, and disorganized behavior. In severe intoxication, the patient may exhibit psychosis and paranoia and experience hallucinations. Sudden withdrawal or cessation of amphetamine use may result in a "crash" stage in which the patient becomes depressed, suicidal, incoherent, or near coma. As a rule, these agents are taken orally, but they may also be smoked for a rapid onset of action. Amphetamines are commonly known as *speed* or *uppers.*

Cocaine

Cocaine is one of the most popular illegal drugs in the United States. It is estimated that 25 million Americans have had some experience with the agent; 3000 to 4000 people each day are initiated into its use, and 4 million use the drug regularly.[8] Cocaine-related deaths are the third leading cause of drug-related fatalities, preceded only by heroin and drug-alcohol combinations.

Cocaine is most commonly used as a fine, white crystalline powder. Like heroin, street forms of cocaine are usually adulterated and vary in purity from 25% to 90%; doses vary from near 0 to 200 mg. This form of cocaine is generally taken intranasally by snorting a "line" containing 10 to 35 mg of the drug (depending on purity). After absorption through the mucous membranes, the effects of the drug begin within minutes. Peak effects occur 15 to 60 minutes after use, with a half-life of 1 to 2½ hours. Cocaine is also used parenterally by the subcutaneous, intramuscular, and intravenous routes; the intravenous route provides immediate absorption and intense stimulation (peak occurs within 5 minutes and half-life within approximately 50 minutes).

Freebase or "crack" cocaine has also become very popular. This more potent formulation is prepared by mixing powdered street cocaine with an alkaline solution and then adding a solvent such as ether. The combination separates into two layers, the top layer containing the dissolved cocaine. Evaporation of the solvent results in pure cocaine crystals, which are smoked and absorbed via the pulmonary route. Cocaine in this form is called *rock* or *crack* because of the popping sound produced when the crystals are heated. Freebase cocaine is generally combined with marijuana or tobacco and smoked in a water pipe or a cigarette. The reactions are similar to those experienced in intravenous use, with equal intensity and pleasure.

Cocaine is a major central nervous system stimulant that causes profound sympathetic discharge. The increased levels of circulating catecholamines result in excitement, euphoria, talkativeness, and agitation. The effects of the drug can precipitate significant cardiovascular and neurological complications such as cardiac dysrhythmias, myocardial infarction, seizures, cerebrovascular accidents (intracranial hemorrhage), hyperthermia, and psychiatric disturbances. Cocaine overdose can occur with any form of the drug and any route of administration. The adult fatal dose is thought to be approximately 1200 mg, but fatalities from cocaine-induced cardiac dysrhythmias have been reported with single doses of as little as 25 to 30 mg.

Prehospital management of the cocaine-intoxicated patient may be complex; the toxicity may range from minor symptoms to life-threatening overdose. Emergency care may require a full spectrum of basic and advanced life-support measures, including aggressive airway management, ventilatory and circulatory support, pharmacological therapy, and rapid transport to an appropriate medical facility.

Phencyclidine Overdose

PCP is a dissociative analgesic (originally used as a veterinary tranquilizer) with sympathomimetic and central nervous system stimulant and depressant properties. It is a potent psychoactive drug illegally sold in tablet or powder form to be taken orally, intranasally, or with other drugs to be smoked. It is rarely taken intravenously. Most tablets contain approximately 5 mg of PCP. As a rule, PCP in its powder form is relatively pure (50% to 100% PCP). Chronic use results in permanent memory impairment and loss of higher brain functions. The pharmacological effects are dose related and can be divided into low-dose and high-dose toxicity.

Low-Dose Toxicity

In low doses (less than 10 mg), PCP intoxication produces an unpredictable state that can resemble drunkenness; the user may have a sense of euphoria or confusion, disorientation, agitation, or sudden rage. An intoxicated patient often has a blank stare and a stumbling gait and is in a dissociative state. The patient's pupils are generally reactive; the patient may experience flushing, diaphoresis, facial grimacing, hypersalivation, and vomiting. Nystagmus with a burstlike quality is characteristic of low-dose PCP use. In this range of toxicity, death is usually related to behavioral disturbances resulting from spatial disorientation, drug-induced immobility, and insensitivity to pain.

Low-dose toxicity is best managed by keeping sensory stimulation to a minimum (verbal and physical stimuli exacerbate the clinical symptoms). Violent and combative patients require protection from self-injury while safeguards are provided for the emergency crew and bystanders. Vital signs and level of consciousness should be closely monitored, and the patient should be observed for increasing motor activity and muscle rigidity, which may precede seizures.

High-Dose Toxicity

Patients with high-dose PCP intoxication (more than 10 mg) may be in a coma, which may last from hours to several days, and are thus often unresponsive to painful stimuli. Respiratory depression, hypertension, and tachycardia may also be present, depending on the dosage. In severe cases, a hypertensive crisis causing cardiac failure, hypertensive encephalopathy, seizures, and intracerebral hemorrhage may result. Prehospital care is directed at managing life-threatening complications such as respiratory and cardiac arrest and status epilepticus and rapidly transporting the patient for physician evaluation.

Phencyclidine Psychosis

Phencyclidine psychosis is a true psychiatric emergency that may mimic schizophrenia. The psychosis is usually of acute onset and may not become apparent until several days after ingestion. It can occur after a single low-dose exposure to PCP and may last from several days to weeks. The clinical syndromes range from a catatonic and unresponsive state to bizarre and violent behavior. The patient frequently appears agitated and suspicious and often experiences auditory hallucinations and paranoia. Appropriate management usually requires involuntary hospitalization, control of violent behavior, and administration of antipsychotic agents. When dealing with these patients in the prehospital setting, personal safety is of paramount importance, so consider law enforcement for assistance.

Tricyclic Antidepressant Overdose

Tricyclic antidepressants (TCAs) are commonly prescribed in the treatment of depression. These drugs work by blocking the uptake of norepinephrine, serotonin, or both, into the presynaptic neurons and by altering the sensitivity of brain tissue to the actions of these chemicals. TCA toxicity is thought to result from central and peripheral atropine-like anticholinergic effects and direct depressant effects on myocardial function. Commonly prescribed antidepressant drugs include the TCAs amitriptyline, imipramine, and nortriptyline, as well as newer agents such as trazodone and fluoxetine, which are chemically unrelated but may manifest some similar signs and symptoms to TCAs in overdoses.

Early symptoms of TCA overdose are dry mouth, blurred vision, confusion, inability to concentrate, and occasionally visual hallucinations. More severe symptoms include delirium, depressed respirations, hypertension, hypotension, hyperthermia, hypothermia, seizures, and coma. Cardiac effects may range from tachycardia to bradycardia and various dysrhythmias secondary to atrioventricular block. A prolonged QRS complex, a Glasgow coma scale less than 8, or both, are characteristic findings that should alert the paramedic to a major toxicity with potentially serious complications. Sudden death from cardiac arrest may occur several days after an overdose.

There is little effective prehospital management for major toxicity of a TCA overdose. Basic supportive care and rapid transport should be instituted. A total of 25% of patients who ultimately die as a result of the overdose are alert and awake, and 75% have normal sinus rhythm when EMS personnel arrive.[9] Tachycardia, especially with a wide QRS complex greater than 100 ms, is an early sign of toxicity. *Sodium bicarbonate*, 44 mEq given intravenously per medical control, may begin to reverse cardiac toxicity. Any patient with a history of TCA ingestion should receive airway, ventilatory, and circulatory support; intravenous access; ECG monitoring; and rapid transport for physician evaluation. More definitive treatment for specific problems (for example, seizures, ventricular dysrhythmias) is complex, using a combination of alkalinization, anticonvulsants, and *physostig-*

mine when appropriate. Rapid transport to the emergency department is the most appropriate course of action.

Hallucinogen Overdose

Hallucinogens are substances that cause perceptual distortions. The most common hallucinogens in use today are PCP and lysergic acid diethylamide (LSD). Other hallucinogens include mescaline, found in the buttons of peyote cactus, which can be used legally in some religious settings; psilocybin mushrooms, found in the United States and Mexico; marijuana, the active agent of the plant *Cannabis sativa;* jimsonweed plant; morning glory plant; nutmeg; mace; and some amphetamines, such as MDMA ("Ecstasy") and MDEA ("Eve").

Depending on the agent, the effects of hallucinogens may range from minor visual illusions and classic anticholinergic syndromes resembling TCA toxicity to more serious complications (associated with LSD use) such as permanent psychosis, flashbacks, and respiratory and central nervous system depression. Prehospital management is usually limited to supportive care, minimal sensory stimulation, calming measures, and transportation to a medical facility. After arrival at the emergency department, these patients are generally observed in a quiet environment. Pharmacological agents may be administered to counteract the anticholinergic effects of the drug.

Salicylate Overdose

Salicylates are widely available in prescription and over-the-counter products such as acetylsalicylic acid (aspirin), many cold preparations, and oil of wintergreen (methyl salicylate) and in combination with some analgesics such as propoxyphene and oxycodone. At one time, ingestion of colorful and tasty children's aspirin was the most common cause of pediatric poisoning. In response to this problem, the number of tablets is now limited to 25 per container. Table 23-3 contains general guidelines for salicylate toxicity.

The mechanism of toxicity with salicylate poisoning is complex and includes direct central nervous system stimulation, interference with cellu-

TABLE 23-3 Toxicity Guidelines to Salicylate

Toxicity	Amount Ingested
Mild	Less than 150 mg/kg
Moderate to severe	150 to 300 mg/kg
Severe	Greater than 300 mg/kg
Fatal	Greater than 500 mg/kg

lar glucose uptake, and inhibition of Krebs cycle enzymes that affect energy production and amino acid metabolism. The volume of distribution is dose dependent and usually small; with toxic ingestion, however, redistribution of the drug into the central nervous system occurs and prolongs elimination of the drug from the body. Complications that may result from chronic or acute ingestion of salicylates include central nervous system stimulation, gastrointestinal irritation, glucose metabolism, fluid and electrolyte imbalance, neurological symptoms, and coagulation effects.

Central Nervous System Stimulation

Salicylates initially produce direct stimulation of the respiratory center in the central nervous system, causing an increased rate and depth of respiration. This early respiratory alkalosis is followed by a compensatory elimination of bicarbonate ions by the kidneys and a subsequent compensatory metabolic acidosis. After this period, there is an accumulation of intermediate acids involved in energy metabolism, leading to profound metabolic acidosis. Confusion, lethargy, convulsions, respiratory arrest, coma, and brain death can all occur in severe salicylate poisoning.

Gastrointestinal Irritation

Salicylates have irritant effects on the gastric mucosa, which can lead to nausea, vomiting, and hematemesis.

Glucose Metabolism

Interference with cellular glucose uptake causes accumulation of serum glucose. Eventually, cellular glucose is depleted, and the patient can demonstrate tissue effects of hypoglycemia (particularly in central nervous system tissue). Patients who die from salicylate poisoning frequently demonstrate primary central nervous system tissue toxicity and severe cerebral edema.

Fluid and Electrolyte Imbalance

Total body fluids are adversely affected by hypermetabolism. Fluid and electrolyte losses occur via gastrointestinal fluids, emesis, and renal clearance. Acid-base disturbances may result in hypokalemia and hypocalcemia. Cardiac dysrhythmias, including premature ventricular contractions, ventricular tachycardia, and ventricular fibrillation, are possible.

Neurological Symptoms

Mild neurological effects such as tinnitus (a symptom of salicylism on the cranial nerve VIII) and lethargy are common. Severe intoxication may result in hallucination, seizure, and coma.

Coagulation Effects

Salicylates alter normal platelet function and often lead to coagulation disorders when taken in toxic amounts. Therefore these patients are at increased risk of significant bleeding. Patients who take anticoagulants are at even greater risk for hemorrhage after salicylate ingestion.

In addition to general supportive measures, prehospital care for salicylate poisoning may include administration of *activated charcoal* for gastric emptying and glucose intravenously to manage hypoglycemia. Salicylates are weak acids excreted by the kidney. Therefore medical control may recommend the administration of *sodium bicarbonate* to produce an alkaline urine. Definitive care includes intensive care observation, continued support of vital functions, and perhaps hemodialysis.

Acetaminophen Overdose

Acetaminophen is a commonly prescribed analgesic and antipyretic agent available in many prescription and nonprescription preparations. Its widespread availability accounts for its high incidence in accidental and intentional poisoning. Acetaminophen overdose can cause life-threatening hepatic toxicity from formation of a hepatotoxic intermediate metabolite if not managed within 16 to 24 hours of ingestion. As few as 30 standard-size (325 mg) acetaminophen tablets are toxic in an average adult.

The toxic effects of acute acetaminophen ingestion (doses of 140 mg/kg or greater) can be classified in four stages (Box 23-14). The course of toxicity begins with mild symptoms that may be overlooked or masked by more dramatic effects of other agents followed by transient clinical improvement and finally peak liver abnormalities. (If acetaminophen was the sole ingestant and a dangerously high dose was ingested, there may be no symptoms in the first two stages.) If antidote treatment is started within 16 to 24 hours of ingestion, complete recovery should occur.

Emergency care includes respiratory, cardiac, and hemodynamic support in critically ill patients. If ingestion is recent (within 4 hours) and the patient is alert, medical control may recommend gastric decontamination and the administration of *activated charcoal* (controversial). Definitive care for patients with progressive acetaminophen toxicity is in-hospital administration of the antidote, *N*-acetylcysteine (Mucomyst).

Iron Overdose

Approximately 10% of the ingested iron (mainly ferrous sulfate) is absorbed each day from the small intestine. After absorption, the iron is converted, stored in iron storage protein, and transported to the liver, spleen, and bone marrow for incorporation into hemoglobin. When ingested iron exceeds the body's ability to store it, the free iron circulates in the blood and is deposited into other tissues.

Accidental or intentional ingestion of iron is a common poisoning that may have lethal complications. Ingested iron is corrosive to gastrointestinal tract mucosa and may produce bloody vomitus, painless bloody diarrhea, and dark stools. Prehospital care includes supportive measures and the prevention of further absorption by gastrointestinal decontamination. The administration of *activated charcoal* is not generally recommended, since it adsorbs iron poorly.

BOX 23-14

Stages of Acetaminophen Poisoning

Stage I: Gastrointestinal Irritability (0 to 24 hours)

Anorexia

Nausea

Vomiting

General malaise

Pallor

Diaphoresis

Stage II: Abnormal Laboratory Findings (24 to 48 hours)

Resolution of stage I symptoms

Possible abdominal pain and tenderness in the right abdominal quadrant

Stage III: Hepatic Damage (72 to 96 hours)

Hepatotoxicity, with significant increase in hepatic enzymes

Vomiting

Lethargy

Jaundice

Hypoglycemia

Dysrhythmias

Stage IV: Recovery (4 to 14 days) or Progressive Hepatic Failure

Resolution of hepatic dysfunction

Lack of permanent effects in patients who recover

NOTE: The percentage of patients who recover in stage IV depends on the amount of acetaminophen ingested and whether effective therapy (*charcoal,* acetylcysteine [Mucomyst], or both) was given. Patients with serum levels in the hepatotoxic range have mortality rates up to 25% if untreated.

Section Four
Alcoholism

It has been conservatively estimated that more than 10 million Americans suffer from alcohol-related problems and that the disease contributes to more than 200,000 deaths annually.[9] The mortality rate of alcoholism is exceeded only by that of heart disease and cancer. In addition, alcohol is involved in more than half of all vehicular trauma fatalities, most homicides, and one third of all suicides. One fifth of the total national expenditure for hospital care is related to alcohol abuse.[7]

● ALCOHOL DEPENDENCE

Alcohol dependence is a disorder characterized by chronic, excessive consumption of alcohol that results in injury to health or in inadequate social function and the development of withdrawal symptoms when the patient stops drinking suddenly. It is estimated that there are 5 million alcohol-dependent persons in the United States (1 in 50) and another 7 million who have difficulty controlling their consumption of the drug. Alcohol dependence should be considered a chronic, progressive, potentially fatal disease characterized by remissions, relapses, and cures.

Although there is no single cause of alcohol dependence, it is believed that three causative factors interact in development of the illness: personality, environment (widespread social acceptance and availability of alcohol), and the addictive nature of the drug. In some cases, genetic and hormonal factors may also play a role in causing dependence. However, it is generally believed that any person, regardless of environment, genetic background, or personality traits, can become dependent on alcohol when the drug is consumed for long periods.

The development of alcohol dependence can be divided into four main stages, which merge imperceptibly. The time frame of these stages may range from 5 to 25 years, but the average is approximately 10 years. In the first stage, tolerance of the drug develops in the heavy social drinker, allowing the individual to consume larger quantities of alcohol before experiencing its ill effects. On entering the second stage, the drinker experiences memory lapses relating to events occurring during the drinking episodes. The third stage is characterized by loss or lack of control over alcohol; the drinker can no longer be certain of discontinuing alcohol consumption at will. The final stage begins with prolonged binges of intoxication with associated mental and physical complications. Some drinkers halt their consumption temporarily or permanently during one of the first three stages.

● ETHANOL

The active ingredient in all alcoholic beverages is ethanol, a colorless, flammable liquid produced from the fermentation of carbohydrates by yeast. All alcoholic drinks are rated based on their ethanol percentage. The alcohol content of beer and wine is measured as a percentage by weight or volume. United States beers contain 2.3% to 5.1% alcohol by volume. Wines vary in content up to 14% to 16%. Distilled liquors are subjected to a rating process called *proof.* Proof was initially based on a test in which gunpowder moistened with a distilled product was ignited. Ignition was "proof" that the alcohol content of the product was at least 50%. Although the ignition test has been replaced with modern techniques to determine alcohol percentage, the term has been retained. A product containing 50% alcohol is considered 100 proof.

Metabolism

A total of 80% to 90% of ingested alcohol is absorbed within 30 minutes (20% in the stomach, the remainder in the small intestine). Once absorbed, the drug is rapidly distributed throughout the vascular space and reaches virtually every organ system. Approximately 3% to 5% of alcohol is excreted unchanged via the lungs and kidneys; the rest is metabolized in the liver to carbon dioxide and water. The actual rate at which alcohol is me-

tabolized depends on individual variation (for example, physical and mental state, body weight and size) and whether the drinker is alcohol dependent. Alcohol is generally metabolized at a constant rate of approximately 20 mg/dl per hour (in nonalcoholics), regardless of its concentration. However, the rate of metabolism may be increased in alcoholics.

Blood Alcohol Content

The alcohol content of blood is measured in terms of weight (milligrams) of alcohol per given volume of blood (deciliter). The time it takes for the alcohol concentration to peak in the blood depends on a number of factors, including the rate at which the alcohol is consumed, the amount of food present in the stomach before drinking, and physical characteristics of the drinker. Although blood alcohol content is widely used to evaluate the central nervous system status of an intoxicated person, there is marked individual variation in blood alcohol content and degree of intoxication. In many states the legal limit of intoxication is 100 mg/dl (equivalent to 0.10%).

> **NOTE:**
> Some states have legislation that allows paramedics to assist in conducting breathalyzer or blood tests to detect alcohol or drug intoxication. EMS personnel should be well versed in the laws of their state before assisting with the detection of alcohol or drug intoxication and should carefully follow established protocols.

● MEDICAL CONSEQUENCES OF CHRONIC ALCOHOL INGESTION

Because alcohol affects nearly every organ system, people who consume large quantities of alcohol are susceptible to numerous physical and mental disorders. Through a variety of direct and indirect mechanisms, alcohol causes multiple systemic effects, including neurological disorders, nutritional deficiencies, fluid and electrolyte imbalances, gastrointestinal disorders, cardiac and skeletal muscle myopathy, and immune suppression. In addition, alcohol may affect a patient's ability to tolerate traumatic injury.

Neurological Disorders

Alcohol is a potent central nervous system depressant. When consumed in moderate amounts, the drug reduces anxiety and tension and provides most drinkers with a feeling of relaxation and confidence. The clinical manifestations of alcohol are dose dependent and progress predictably as the level of consumption increases and blood alcohol content rises (Table 23-4). Initial feelings of well-being give way to impaired judgment and discrimination, prolonged reflexes, and incoordination and drowsiness, which may ultimately progress to stupor and coma. The long-term neurological effects of chronic alcohol abuse are similar to those of the aging process and include short-term memory deficit, problems with coordination, and difficulty with concentration and abstraction.

Nutritional Deficiencies

Although alcohol may temporarily satisfy the body's caloric requirements, the drug decreases a

TABLE 23-4 Alcohol Intake and Its Behavioral Effects

Alcohol Content (oz)	Beverage Intake in 1 hr*	Blood Alcohol Level (mg/dl) in a 150-lb Man	Behavioral Effects
½	1 oz 100-proof spirits 1 glass wine 1 can beer	0.025	No noticeable effect
1	2 oz 100-proof spirits 2 glasses wine 2 cans beer	0.050	Lower alertness, impaired judgment, good feeling, and less inhibition
2	4 oz 100-proof spirits 4 glasses wine 4 cans beer	0.100	Slow reaction time, impaired motor function, and less cautious; should not drive; may activate vomiting reflex
3	6 oz 100-proof spirits 6 glasses wine 6 cans beer	0.150	Large increase in reaction times
4	8 oz 100-proof spirits 8 glasses wine 8 cans beer	0.200	Marked depression of sensory and motor abilities
5	10 oz 100-proof spirits 10 glasses wine 10 cans beer	0.250	Severe depression of sensory and motor abilities
6	12 oz 100-proof spirits 12 glasses wine 12 cans beer	0.300	Stuporous and unconscious of surroundings
7	14 oz 100-proof spirits 14 glasses wine 14 cans beer	0.350	Unconscious
8	16 oz 100-proof spirits 16 glasses wine 16 cans beer	0.400	Lethal dose in 50% of the population
12	24 oz 100-proof spirits 24 glasses wine 24 cans beer	0.600	Lethal dose in 95% of the population

*Since only ¼ to ⅓ oz of alcohol is metabolized each hour, alcohol rapidly accumulates.

drinker's appetite through an irritant effect on the stomach, and it has little or no nutritious content. Therefore alcohol-dependent individuals have a potential for decreased dietary intake and malabsorption, leading to multiple vitamin and mineral deficiencies. Clinical manifestations associated with these deficiencies include:

- Altered immunity
- Anorexia
- Cardiac dysrhythmias
- Coma
- Irritability and disorientation
- Muscle cramps
- Paresthesias
- Poor wound healing
- Seizures
- Tremor and ataxia

Wernicke-Korsakoff Syndrome

Alcohol-dependent persons are at particular risk of developing Wernicke-Korsakoff syndrome, a disease that results from chronic thiamine (vitamin B_1) deficiency combined with an inability to utilize thiamine from a heritable disorder or from a reduction in intestinal absorption and metabolism of thiamine by alcohol. Wernicke-Korsakoff syndrome affects the brain and nervous system by disrupting central and peripheral nerve function. The disease may consist of two stages: Wernicke's encephalopathy, Korsakoff's psychosis, or a combination of the two.

Wernicke's encephalopathy usually develops suddenly with the clinical manifestations of ataxia, ocular changes (nystagmus), disturbances of speech and gait, signs of neuropathy (paresthesias, impaired reflexes), stupor, or coma (rare). Since the body uses up thiamine stores to metabolize sugar, the syndrome may be precipitated in the malnourished patient by the intravenous administration of glucose or glucose-containing fluids. Wernicke's encephalopathy is also the cause of coma in 1% of all alcoholics. Therefore intravenous administration of *thiamine* should always precede the intravenous administration of glucose in patients with altered mental status or coma of unknown origin.

After administration of *thiamine*, patients with Wernicke's encephalopathy usually become more alert and attentive, but gait and mental difficulties often persist for days or months; fewer than half of the affected patients recover completely. Many chronic alcoholic patients also display signs of Korsakoff's psychosis, a mental disorder often found with Wernicke's encephalopathy. These signs include apathy, poor retentive memory, retrograde amnesia, confabulation (invention of stories to make up for gaps in memory), and dementia. Korsakoff's psychosis is usually considered irreversible, leaving the patient permanently handicapped by memory loss and in need of continual supervision.

Fluid and Electrolyte Imbalances

Urinary output increases (over and above that expected from the amount of fluid ingested) after alcohol consumption. This diuresis results from an inhibition of antidiuretic hormone secretion, which can lead to dehydration as well as electrolyte imbalances.

Gastrointestinal Disorders

The effects of alcohol on the gastrointestinal system can produce several types of alcohol-related illnesses and diseases. The alcohol-related gastrointestinal disorders most likely to initiate an EMS response include gastrointestinal hemorrhage, cirrhosis, and acute or chronic pancreatitis.

Gastrointestinal Hemorrhage

The three primary causes of gastrointestinal hemorrhage in patients who drink alcohol are gastritis, esophageal tear (Mallory-Weiss syndrome), and variceal hemorrhage. Gastritis results from the toxic effects of ethanol on the gastric mucosa, which leads to diffuse or localized areas of erosion. In the chronic form of gastritis, blood may ooze continually from the mucosal lining.

Esophageal tears of the gastroesophageal junction, stomach, or esophagus usually follow severe or protracted vomiting or retching. The injury results when gastric contents are forced against an unrelaxed gastroesophageal junction, which produces a sudden increase in pressure and a mucosal tear with subsequent bleeding. The bleeding can be exacerbated by clotting abnormalities, which are common in patients with alcoholic liver disease.

Varices are a result of portal hypertension caused by cirrhosis. Any of these thin-walled esophageal veins are subject to rupture and hemorrhage, although the most common site is the varices of the esophagus. Bleeding esophageal varices remain one of the most difficult conditions to treat.

Cirrhosis

Cirrhosis of the liver is caused by chronic damage to liver cells that results in inflammation and eventually necrosis. In this disease process, bands of fibrosis (scar tissue) develop and break up the normal structure of the liver. The distortion and fibrosis of the liver lead to portal hypertension, with the resultant complications of ascites, splenomegaly, and bleeding esophageal and gastric varices. In addition, cirrhosis may lead to hepatic encephalopathy caused by the accumulation of toxic metabolic waste products, which would normally be detoxified by a healthy liver and which have an adverse effect on the brain. In the United States, it is estimated that 1 in 70 people dies as a direct result of chronic liver disease and cirrhosis, accounting for some 30,000 deaths each year.

Acute or Chronic Pancreatitis

Alcohol is the most common cause of acute and chronic pancreatitis. Although the exact mechanism by which alcohol produces pancreatic inflammation is not clear, it may be caused at least in part by activation of pancreatic proenzymes, obstruction of pancreatic ducts, and stimulation of enzymatic secretion. There may also be a direct toxic effect, as has been demonstrated for the liver. Chronic pancreatitis usually produces the same symptoms as the acute form (see Chapter 21). However, the pain may last from several hours to several days, and the attacks become more frequent as the condition progresses. Other effects of chronic pancreatitis include malabsorption (a result of a deficiency of pancreatic enzymes), electrolyte imbalances such as hypocalcemia, and diabetes mellitus (caused by insufficient insulin production). Hemorrhagic pancreatitis, sepsis, and pancreatic abscess usually cause mortality.

Cardiac and Skeletal Muscle Myopathy

Cardiac and skeletal muscle myopathy is thought to result from a direct toxic effect of alcohol or its metabolites. The pathological changes associated with these alcoholic muscle syndromes include intracellular edema, formation of lipid droplets, excessive cellular glycogen, and deranged sarcoplasmic reticula and mitochondria. In heart muscle, these changes result in a decreased force of contraction (negative inotropic effect), dysrhythmias, and a tendency to develop congestive heart failure. In skeletal muscle, the major symptoms are weakness and muscle wasting. The clinical prevalence of cardiac and skeletal myopathy has been estimated at between 50% and 60% of all chronic alcoholics.

Immune Suppression

Long-term alcohol abuse renders the immune system less effective by suppressing bone marrow production of white blood cells; red blood cells and platelet production are also often decreased. Alcohol has direct, specific effects on lung tissue, which impair macrophage mobilization and mucociliary function. As a result, the body's ability to fight pulmonary infection is altered, making the alcoholic more susceptible to viral and bacterial pneumonia, which may occur secondary to aspiration during alcoholic stupor or for other reasons. Although the exact mechanism is unknown, there is an increased incidence of cancer in alcoholic patients, which may also be related to immune suppression.

Trauma

Alcohol suppresses 11 of the 12 blood clotting factors produced in the liver. This blood clotting deficiency makes alcoholics susceptible to bruising and internal hemorrhage and adds to the frequency of subdural bleeding, even after relatively minor head trauma. There is also evidence that alcohol causes increased myocardial irritability and a decrease in tidal and minute volume, which may alter the trauma patient's ability to compensate for the metabolic acidosis seen in shock.

● ALCOHOL EMERGENCIES

In addition to the clinical conditions previously described, several other conditions caused by consumption or abstinence from alcohol may require emergency care. These include acute alcohol intoxication, alcohol withdrawal syndromes, and disulfiram-ethanol reaction. Alcohol-induced ketoacidosis and hypoglycemia are covered in Chapter 19.

Acute Alcohol Intoxication

The ingestion of alcohol may cause acute poisoning if consumed in sufficiently large amounts over a relatively short period. The clinical features are similar to those induced by sedative-hypnotic agents and can be correlated to a degree with blood alcohol content. At toxic levels, hypoventilation (including respiratory arrest), hypotension, and hypothermia may develop. The patient who has signs and symptoms of acute alcohol intoxication should be carefully considered for occult trauma and coexisting medical conditions such as hypoglycemia, cardiac myopathy and dysrhythmias, gastrointestinal bleeding, polydrug abuse (particularly barbiturates or tranquilizers), and ethylene glycol or methanol ingestion. Because of the patient's susceptibility to injury and potential for numerous secondary disease processes, the paramedic should never assume that an intoxicated patient is merely inebriated.

Management

A patient who is mildly intoxicated should be transported for physician evaluation. In most cases, treatment only requires patient observation in the emergency department until he or she is sober. The patient's vital signs and level of consciousness should be carefully monitored en route. A thorough secondary survey is warranted to rule out illness or injury masked by alcohol ingestion.

Treatment of the acutely intoxicated patient is directed at protecting the patient from further injury and maintaining vital functions. If the patient is conscious and agitated, it may be necessary to use restraints to protect the patient and various health care providers from bodily harm. If physical restraint becomes necessary, police should be summoned. After scene safety has been established, initial assessment and resuscitation should include the following:

1. Rapidly evaluate airway patency with spinal precautions and ventilatory and hemodynamic status while obtaining a patient history. The patient's account of the history of the event may be unreliable as a result of alcohol ingestion.
2. Initiate intravenous therapy. Draw blood samples for laboratory analysis. Per protocol, administer *thiamine, 50% dextrose* (if hypoglycemia is likely or confirmed), and *naloxone* (if opiate overdose is suspected) intravenously.
3. Continually monitor the patient's airway and provide adequate ventilatory and circulatory support as needed. Be prepared to provide suction and aggressive airway management.
4. Monitor ECG for dysrhythmias.
5. Rapidly transport the patient for physician evaluation.

Alcohol Withdrawal Syndromes

A period of relative or absolute abstinence from alcohol may cause withdrawal in an alcoholic. The severity of these syndromes depends on the magnitude of blood alcohol content (serum ethanol level), the length of time the level was maintained, the abruptness of cessation, the tissue tolerance to alcohol, and the general physical and psychological condition of the patient. Although the pathophysiological mechanism of alcohol withdrawal remains largely undefined, it is thought to result from central nervous system hyperexcitability (as the central nervous system depressant is removed) and from biochemical changes such as respiratory alkalosis and hypomagnesemia. Alcohol withdrawal syndromes can be divided into four general categories: minor reactions, hallucinations, alcohol withdrawal seizures, and delirium tremens.

Minor Reactions

Minor reactions begin approximately 6 to 8 hours after cessation or reduction of alcohol intake. These symptoms peak within 24 to 36 hours and may persist for 10 to 14 days. When alcohol withdrawal is confined to minor reactions, the prognosis for full recovery is excellent with appropriate management. Minor reactions include:

- Sudden and unexpected startle
- Flushed face and diaphoresis
- Anorexia
- Nausea and vomiting
- Insomnia
- General muscle weakness
- Slight disorientation
- Generalized tremor (worsened by agitation)
- Mild tachycardia, hypertension, hyperreflexia

Hallucinations

Hallucinations usually occur 24 to 36 hours after cessation of alcohol. Disorders of perception are common and may vary from auditory and visual illusions to frank hallucinations, which can produce agitation, fear, and panic. During this period, the patient may show signs of suicidal and homicidal tendencies, and minor reactions may be more pronounced. The prognosis for hallucinations is the same as for minor reactions with appropriate management.

Alcohol Withdrawal Seizures

Alcohol withdrawal seizures (or rum fits) usually occur 7 to 48 hours after ethanol cessation, with a peak incidence between 13 and 24 hours. These seizures may occur singly or in groups of two to six. They are most often grand mal of short duration; status seizures are rare. Alcohol withdrawal seizures are associated with varying degrees of tremor, anorexia, hallucinations, and autonomic hyperactivity. This category of withdrawal may be self-limiting or may progress to delirium tremens with or without a lucid interval.

Because of the drug tolerance level of the alcoholic patient, seizure activity may require intravenous administration of large doses of *diazepam* (5 mg every 5 minutes up to 30 mg). *Diazepam* may synergistically interact with any ethanol still in the patient's system, so vital signs, respirations, and mental status should be closely monitored.

Delirium Tremens

Delirium tremens (DTs) is the most dramatic and serious form of alcohol withdrawal. It affects approximately 5% of all alcoholics hospitalized for withdrawal. It usually occurs 72 to 96 hours after cessation of alcohol but may be delayed up to 14 days. The syndrome is characterized by psychomotor, speech, and autonomic hyperactivity; profound confusion; disorientation; delusion; vivid hallucinations; tremor; agitation; and insomnia. A single episode may last 1 to 3 days and, with multiple recurrences, may last up to 1 month.

Autonomic hyperactivity is the most distinguishing feature of DTs. It is characterized by tachycardia, fever, hypertension, dilated pupils, and profuse diaphoresis. In severe cases, cardiovascular collapse may be present. DTs is a true medical emergency with a mortality rate as high as 15%. Associated alcohol-related illnesses such as pneumonia, pancreatitis, and hepatitis are frequent contributing causes of death.

Management

Prehospital care for patients experiencing alcohol withdrawal syndromes is primarily supportive. After scene safety is ensured, the patient's airway, ventilatory, and circulatory status should be carefully monitored. Intravenous therapy should be initiated with a saline solution for rehydration. Pharmacological therapy may be indicated for an altered level of consciousness, dysrhythmias, or seizure activity. In addition, these patients need calm reassurance and frequent reorientation. All patients with signs and symptoms of alcohol withdrawal syndrome require physician evaluation.

Disulfiram-Ethanol Reaction

Disulfiram (tetraethylthiuram disulfide or Antabuse) is a medication prescribed to some alcoholic patients to help them abstain. The drug works by inhibiting ethanol metabolism and by allowing the accumulation of the metabolite acetaldehyde. Acetaldehyde produces ill effects on the gastrointestinal, cardiovascular, and autonomic nervous systems and is the metabolic product thought to be responsible for the common "hangover." Patients who take disulfiram and then ingest ethanol experience an unpleasant and potentially life-threatening physiological response. A disulfiram-like reaction can also occur in patients taking metronidazole (Flagyl) for trichomonas and other types of vaginitis.

The disulfiram-ethanol reaction begins 15 to 30 minutes after ingestion of 2 to 5 alcoholic drinks and continues for 1 to 2 hours. The reaction causes the patient to experience vertigo, headache, vomiting, flushing (which may give the skin a "lobster-red" appearance), dyspnea, diaphoresis, abdominal pain, and sometimes chest pain. More serious reactions include hypotension, shock, and dysrhythmias. Sudden death, myocardial and cerebral infarction, and cerebral hemorrhage have also been reported after as little as one drink of ethanol in patients taking disulfiram.

Management

Prehospital care for a disulfiram-ethanol reaction involves airway, ventilatory, and circulatory support; the administration of intravenous fluids to treat hypotension; pharmacological therapy as needed to manage dysrhythmias; and rapid transport for physician evaluation. Most episodes are self-limiting. Supportive care and in-hospital observation are usually all that are required.

REFERENCES

1. National Safety Council: *Accident facts,* 1991 ed, Chicago, 1990, The Council.
2. Litovitz T et al: 1990 Annual report of the American Association of Poison Control Centers national data collection system, *Am J Emerg Med* 9:461, 1991.
3. Bayer M, Rumack B, editors: Poisonings and overdose, *Top Emerg Med* 1(13):30, 1979.
4. Borak J et al: *Hazardous material exposure,* Englewood Cliffs, NJ, 1991, Brady.
5. Maddad L, Winchester J: *Clinical manifestations of poisoning and drug overdose,* ed 2, Philadelphia, 1990, WB Saunders.
6. Auerbach P, Geehr E, editors: *Management of wilderness and environmental emergencies,* ed 2, St Louis, 1989, Mosby.
7. Moore E et al: *Early care of the injured patient,* ed 4, Philadelphia, 1990, BC Decker.
8. Heckman J, editor: *Emergency care and transportation of the sick and injured,* ed 5, Chicago, 1992, American Academy of Orthopaedic Surgeons.
9. Callaham M: *Current practice of emergency medicine,* ed 2, Philadelphia, 1991, BC Decker.

Summary

Emergencies involving toxicological agents, drug abuse, and alcoholism can be a challenge to the EMS professional. The widespread use and accessibility of these agents requires the paramedic to maintain a high degree of suspicion in any emergency response. A systematic approach to patient care that focuses on airway, ventilatory, and circulatory support and rapid transportation to an appropriate medical facility can play a major role in decreasing complications and mortality from prevalent health care problems.

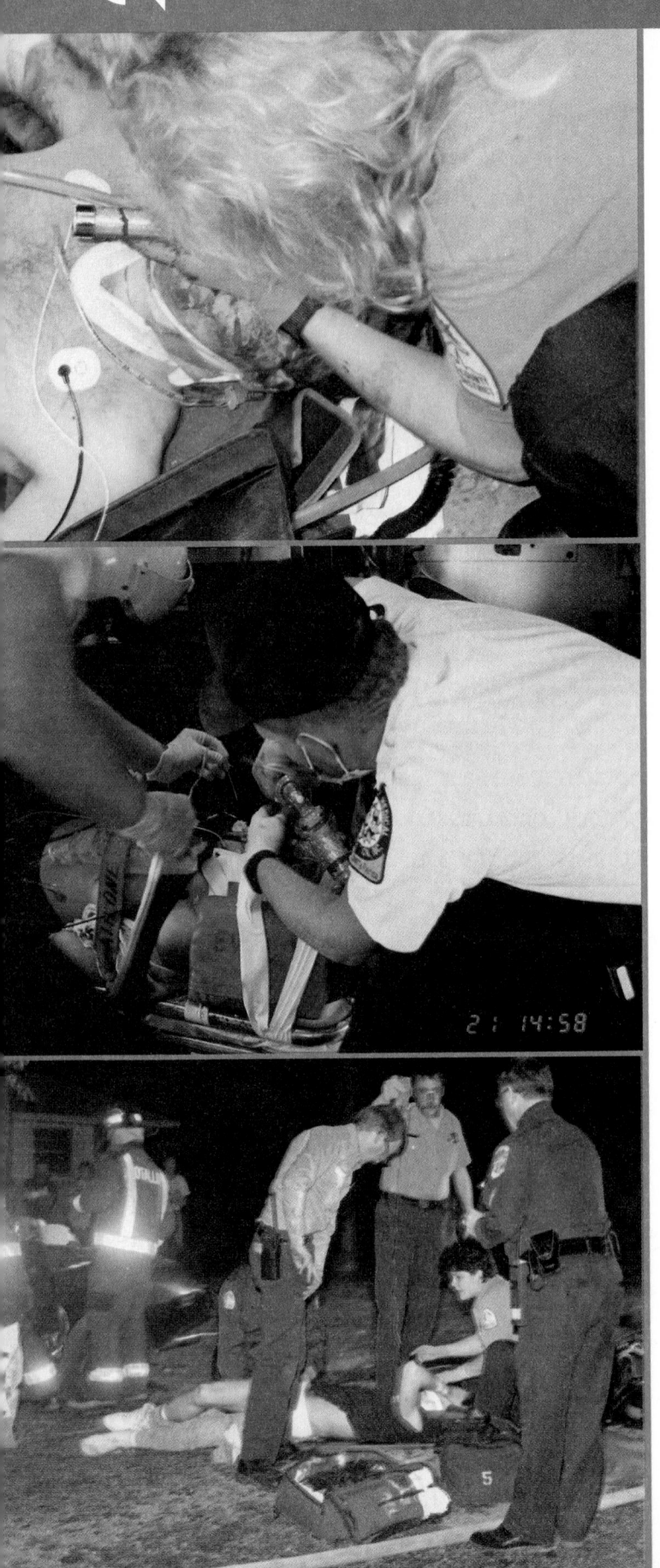

Emergencies involving infectious diseases are common in the prehospital setting, and some can pose a significant health risk to EMS providers. This chapter addresses the pathophysiology of infectious disease, special aspects of providing emergency care to patients with infectious diseases, and the responsibility of the paramedic in ensuring personal protection.

As a paramedic, you should be able to:

1. Describe the chain of elements necessary for an infectious disease to occur.
2. Explain how internal and external barriers decrease susceptibility to infection.
3. Outline the inflammatory response.
4. Distinguish among the four stages of infectious disease: the latent period, the incubation period, the communicability period, and the disease period.
5. Given specific patient scenarios, describe the Centers for Disease Control recommendations for personal protection.
6. Describe mode of transmission, pathophysiology, prehospital interventions, and personal protective measures to be taken for selected infectious diseases.
7. List signs, symptoms, and potential secondary complications of selected childhood infectious diseases.

● PATHOPHYSIOLOGY OF INFECTIOUS DISEASE

Infectious diseases rank as the fifth most common cause of death in the United States. The causative microorganisms can afflict healthy patients and lead to complications in patients who have other primary disorders, causing significant morbidity. For an infectious disease to occur, there must be an intact "chain of elements" (Fig. 24-1), including[1]:

- The pathogenic agent
- A reservoir
- A portal of exit from the reservoir
- An environment conducive to transmission of the pathogenic agent
- A portal of entry into the new host

- Susceptibility of the new host to the infectious disease

Pathogenic Agent

Pathogens are organisms that create pathological processes in the human host. They are classified according to morphology, chemical composition, growth requirements, and viability. Regardless of the classification, pathogens cannot synthesize their own amino acids and must rely on a host to supply their nutritional requirements.

Some pathogens (such as certain bacteria) are metabolically equipped so that they can survive outside a host, whereas others (such as viruses) can only survive in the human cell. Most bacteria are susceptible to certain drugs (antibiotics) that kill them or inhibit their growth. Viruses, however, are more difficult to treat because they reside in cells for most of their life cycle and become intricately enmeshed in the host cell's deoxyribonucleic acid (DNA). Factors affecting any pathogen's ability to create pathological processes are:

KEY TERMS

communicability period: A stage of infection that begins when the latent period ends and continues as long as the agent is present and can spread to other hosts.

disease period: A stage of infection that follows the incubation period; the duration varies with the disease.

incubation period: A stage of infectin during which an organism reproduces and that begins with invasion of an agent and ends when the disease process begins.

latent period: A stage of infection that begins with pathogenic invasion of the body and ends when the agent can be shed or communicated.

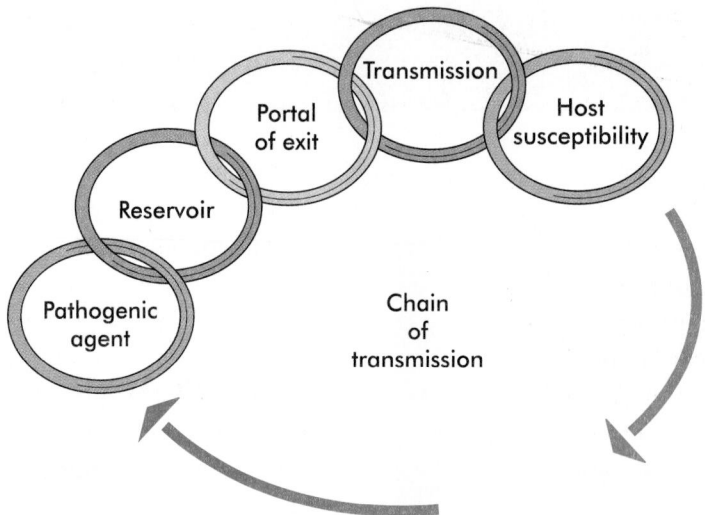

Fig. 24-1 Chain of transmission for infection. The chain must be intact for an infection to be transmitted to another host. Transmission can be controlled by breaking any link in the chain.

- Its ability to invade and reproduce within a host and the mode in which it does so
- Its speed of reproduction, ability to produce a toxin, and the extent of tissue damage that it causes
- Its potency
- Its ability to induce an immune response in the host

Reservoir

The environment in which a pathogen lives and reproduces may be a human or other animal host, an arthropod, a plant, soil, water, food, or some other organic substance or a combination of these reservoirs. When infected, the human host may exhibit signs of clinical illness or be an asymptomatic carrier, transmitting the pathogen to others.

Portal of Exit

The mechanism or method by which a pathogenic agent leaves one host to invade another involves a "portal of exit." The portal of exit from the human host depends on the agent. It may be single or multiple, involving the genitourinary (GU) tract, intestinal tract, oral cavity, respiratory tract, an open lesion, or any wound through which blood escapes. The period of time over which an actively infectious pathogen can escape to produce disease in another organism coincides with the period of communicability, which varies with each disease.

Transmission

The portal of exit determines the mode of transmission, which may be direct or indirect. Direct transmission occurs when there is physical contact between the source and the victim. Examples of direct transmission include oral transmission and transmission by airborne mucus droplets, fecal contamination, and sexual contact.

In indirect transmission, the organism survives on animate or inanimate objects for a period without a human host. Diseases can be indirectly transmitted by air, food, water, soil, or biological matter.

Portal of Entry

The means by which the pathogenic agent enters a new host is called the *portal of entry*. The portal of entry may be by ingestion, inhalation, per-

Factors that Influence Host Susceptibility

Human characteristics

    Age

    Gender

    Ethnic group

    Heredity

General health status

    Nutrition

    Hormonal balance

    Presence of concurrent disease

    History of previous disease

Immune status

    Prior exposure to disease (conferring resistance)

    Effective immunization against disease (conferring host immunity)

Geographical and environmental conditions

Cultural behaviors

    Eating habits

    Personal hygiene

Sexual behaviors

cutaneous injection, crossing of a mucous membrane, or crossing of the placenta. The duration of exposure to the pathogen and the number of organisms required to initiate the infectious process vary with the disease and host susceptibility. Exposure to an infectious agent does not always produce infection.

Host Susceptibility

Host susceptibility is influenced by a person's immune response (see Chapter 22) and by several other factors (Box 24-1).

● PHYSIOLOGY OF THE HUMAN RESPONSE TO INFECTION

The human body is constantly exposed to pathogens capable of producing illness; yet most people do not succumb to infectious disease. This protection is provided by external and internal barriers that serve as lines of defense against infection.

External Barriers

The first line of defense against infection is the surface of the body that is exposed to the environment. These surfaces, inhabited by an indigenous flora (agents that could produce disease if allowed to access to the interior of the body), include the skin and the mucous membranes of the digestive, respiratory, and GU tract. These surfaces form a continuous closed barrier between the internal organs and the environment (Fig. 24-2).

Flora

Nearly the whole body surface is inhabited by normal microbial flora, which enhance the effectiveness of the surface barrier by interfering with the establishment of pathogenic agents in several ways. Indigenous flora compete with pathogens for space and nutrients. They maintain a pH optimal for their own growth, which can be incompatible with that needed for many pathogenic agents to survive. Some flora also secrete germicidal substances and are thought to stimulate the immune system.

Although resident (normal) flora play an important role in defense, some indigenous flora can be pathogenic under certain conditions. For example, flora can be responsible for infection when the skin or mucous membranes are interrupted or when flora are displaced from their natural habitat to another area of the body (a common cause of urinary tract infection after catheterization of the bladder).

Skin

Intact skin defends against infection by preventing penetration and by maintaining an acidic pH level that inhibits growth of pathogenic bacteria. In addition, microbes are sloughed from the skin's surface with dead skin cells, and oil and sweat wash microorganisms from the skin's pores.

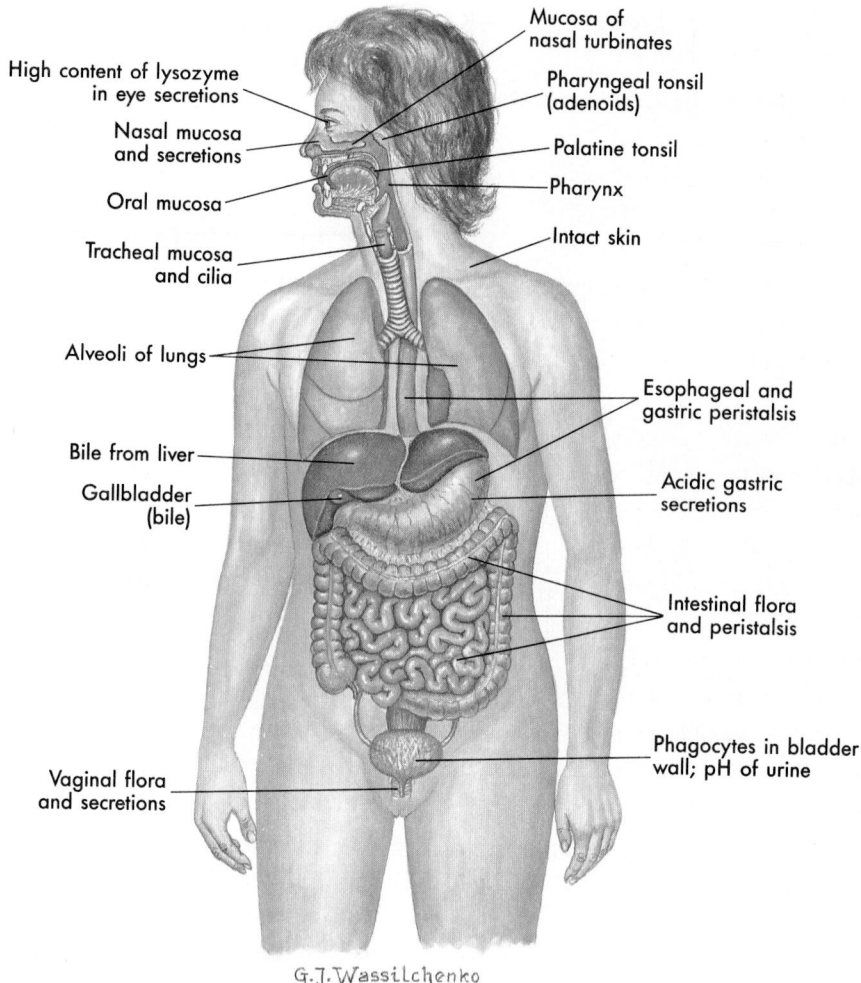

High content of lysozyme in eye secretions

Nasal mucosa and secretions

Oral mucosa

Tracheal mucosa and cilia

Alveoli of lungs

Bile from liver

Gallbladder (bile)

Vaginal flora and secretions

Mucosa of nasal turbinates

Pharyngeal tonsil (adenoids)

Palatine tonsil

Pharynx

Intact skin

Esophageal and gastric peristalsis

Acidic gastric secretions

Intestinal flora and peristalsis

Phagocytes in bladder wall; pH of urine

G.J. Wassilchenko

Fig. 24-2 First line of defense: external barriers.

Upper Respiratory Tract

The sticky membranes of the upper airway protect against pathogens by trapping large particles, which may then be swallowed or expelled by coughing or sneezing. Coarse nasal hairs and cilia also trap and filter foreign substances in inspired air and thereby prevent the pathogens from reaching the lower respiratory tract. In addition, the lymph tissues of the tonsils and adenoids permit a rapid local immunological response to pathogenic organisms that may enter the respiratory tract.

Genitourinary Tract

The natural process of urination and the bacteriostatic properties of urine help prevent the establishment of microorganisms in the GU tract.

Antibacterial substances in prostatic fluid and the presence of vaginal flora also help to prevent infection in the GU system.

Internal Barriers

Internal barriers protect against pathogenic agents when the external lines of defense are breached. Internal barriers include the inflammatory response and the immune response, which share many of the same processes and cellular components.

Inflammatory Response

Inflammation is a local reaction to cellular injury. The response may be initiated by physical, thermal, or chemical damage or by microbial infection. When invasion occurs, this line of defense is activated to prevent further invasion of the pathogen by isolating, destroying, or neutralizing the microorganism (Fig. 24-3). As a rule, the inflammatory response is protective and beneficial. However, if the response is sustained or directed toward the host's own antigens, healthy tissue may be destroyed. The inflammatory response may be divided into three separate stages: cellular response to injury, vascular response to injury, and phagocytosis.

Cellular Response to Injury

Metabolic changes occur with any type of cell injury. The most common primary effect of injury on the cell's aerobic respiration and oxidative phosphorylation leads to decreasing energy reserves. When the energy sources are depleted, the sodium-potassium pump can no longer function effectively and the cell swells because of the accumulation of sodium ions. The organelles within the cell also swell. This swelling, along with increasing acidosis, leads to further impairment of enzyme function and further deterioration in the integrity of membranes. Eventually the membranes of the cellular organelles begin to leak. Release of hydrolytic enzymes by the lysosomes contributes further to cellular destruction and autolysis. As the cellular contents are dissolved by enzymes, the inflammatory response is stimulated in surrounding tissues.

Vascular Response to Injury

After cellular injury, localized hyperemia develops as the surrounding arterioles, venules, and capillaries dilate. The associated increase in filtration pressure and capillary permeability causes fluid to leak from the vessels into the interstitial space, producing edema. Leukocytes (particularly neutrophils and monocytes) begin to collect along the vascular endothelium and, as a result of release of chemotactic factors, eventually migrate to the injured tissue.

Phagocytosis

Phagocytosis is the process by which leukocytes engulf, digest, and destroy pathogens. The circulating macrophages are also responsible for clearing the injured area of dead cells and other debris. Intracellular phagocytosis (ingestion of bacteria and dead cell fragments) occurs at the site of tissue invasion and may extend into the general circulation if the infection becomes systemic. Intracellular phagocytosis stimulates the release of chemicals that induce lysis of the leukocytes. These leukocytes combine with dead organisms and fluid to form an inflammatory exudate, commonly known as *pus*.

Immune Response

The first two lines of defense against infection respond to all infectious agents using the identical nonspecific mechanism, but the immune response is specific to individual pathogens. Four unique characteristics of the immune system are:

1. It possesses "self-nonself" recognition and therefore normally responds only to foreign antigens.
2. It produces antibodies that are antigen specific and can produce new antibodies in response to new antigens.
3. Some of the antibody-producing lymphocytes become "memory cells" that allow a more rapid response to subsequent invasions by the same antigen.
4. It is self-regulated to activate itself only when there is an invading pathogen. This ability to activate or deactivate the immune response prevents the destruction of healthy tissues. When this regulatory function goes awry, autoimmune disease (for example, rheumatoid arthritis, active glomerulonephritis, and systemic lupus erythematosus) can occur. The immune system may require extrinsic regulation (as much as possible) with certain medications in patients with transplanted organs or severe autoimmune diseases.

The immunological response to an invading pathogen depends somewhat on the size and antigenic properties of the pathogen. Often, peripheral phagocytic cells encounter a pathogen first, but circulating B and T lymphocytes also play a reconnaissance role. The interactions among neutrophils, macrophages, and B and T lymphocytes are complex. The various cellular components assist each other in processing antigen so that it

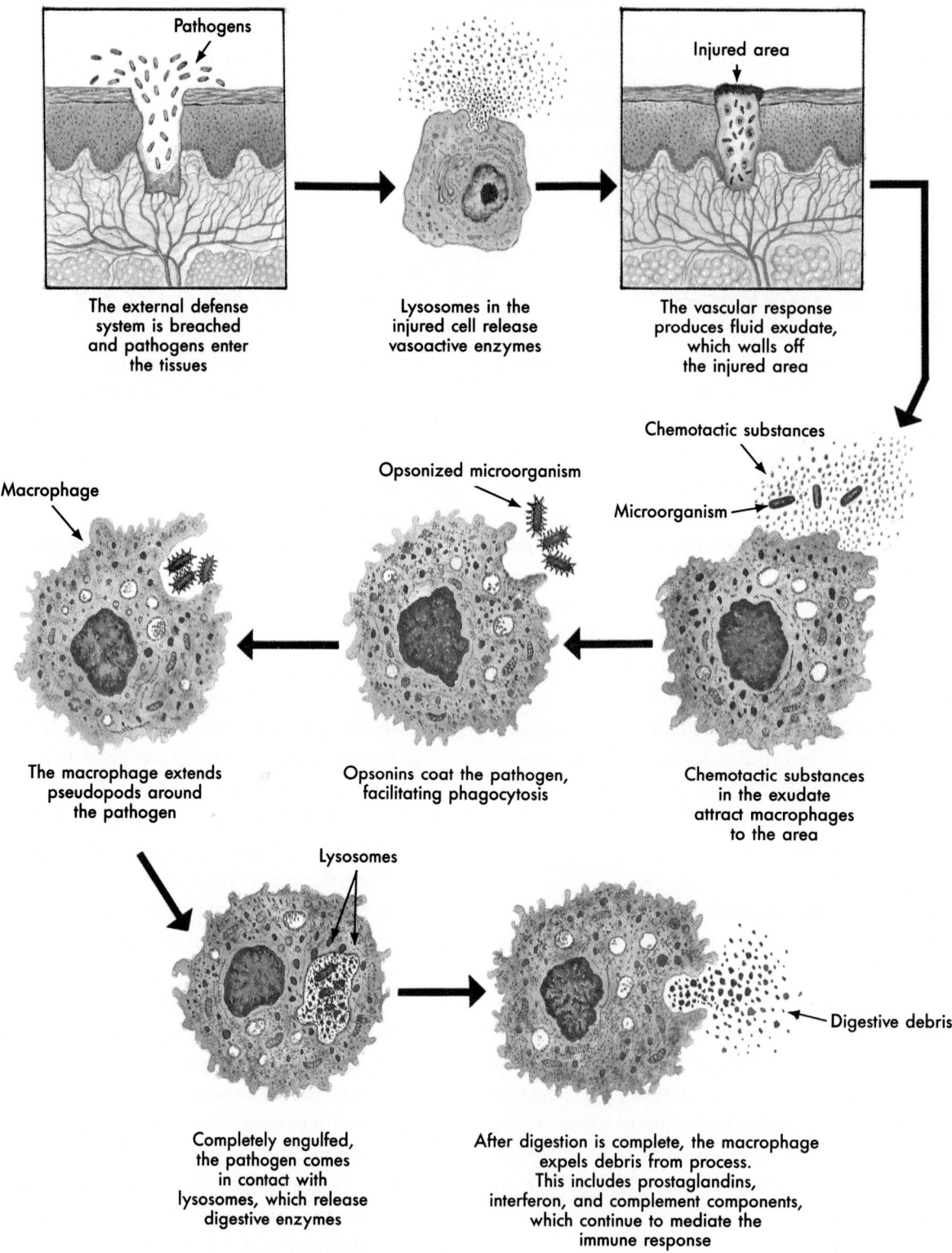

Fig. 24-3 Second line of defense: inflammatory response.

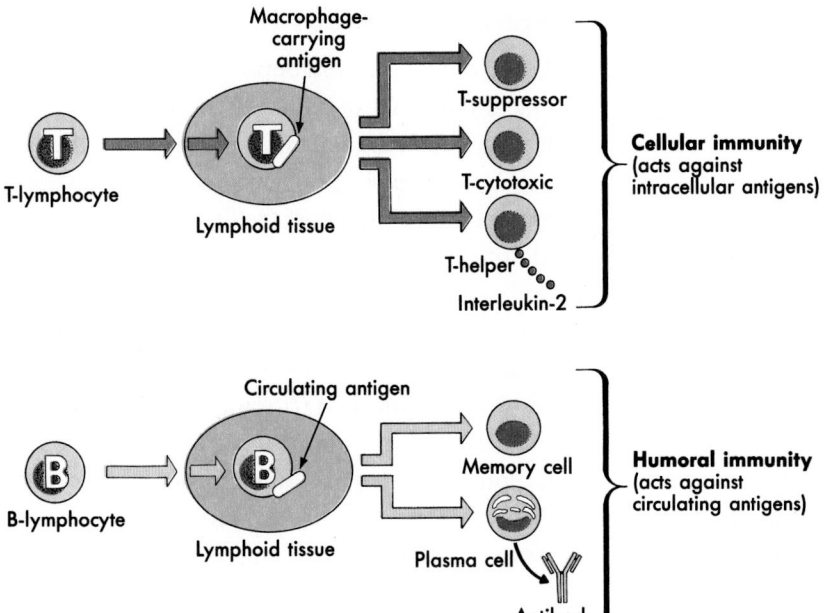

Fig. 24-4 Cellular and humoral immunity. Cellular immunity results from activation of T lymphocytes by contact with intracellular organisms. Activated T lymphocytes differentiate and proliferate. Humoral (antibody-mediated) immunity results from activating B lymphocytes.

is recognizable and in neutralizing the invading organism.

The B lymphocyte's role is to produce antibody (humoral immunity), which coats the pathogen and makes phagocytosis easier. Antibody can also fix complement, a protein cascade that often results in the death of the organism and in the production of chemotactic factors. The T lymphocyte not only processes antigen for the B lymphocyte, but also has a subpopulation of "killer cells," which are a major component of cell-mediated immunity (Fig. 24-4).

Drugs to Treat Infection, Inflammation, Mild Pain, and Fever

Infections are usually accompanied by various defense mechanisms and numerous reactions of body tissues, including inflammation, mild pain, and fever. Although these reactions do not necessarily depend on the presence of infection, the drugs used to treat infections, inflammation, mild pain, and fever are presented here.

Infections

Drugs used to treat infectious diseases are antiinfective agents. Antiinfective agents may be classified as antibiotics and antiviral drugs.

Antibiotics are drugs that are selectively effective against specific organisms. They may be broadly categorized as bacteriocidal or bacteriostatic. Bacteriocides directly kill the bacterial cell. Bacteriostatic drugs may not kill the bacterial cell but halt its growth and reproduction. Examples of bacteriocidal antibiotics are penicillin G (Crystipen, others), penicillin V (Pen-Vee-K, V-Cillin K), and dicloxacillin (Dycill, Dynapen). Bacteriostatic antibiotics include erythromycin base (E-Mycin, others), and tetracycline hydrochloride (Achromycin, others).

To date, no effective drugs exist to treat minor viral infections such as colds. In fact, very few drugs exist for use in any viral infections. This is due in part to the relative delay in symptoms that occurs in viral diseases; drug therapy is difficult once the disease is established.

Many agents have been tested as antiviral drugs. Few, however, have proven effective against specific virus-infected cells without producing toxic effects on uninfected cells. Examples of specific antiviral drugs include acyclovir (Zovirax), which is effective against herpes infection; vidarabine (Vira A), used for more serious herpes infections; and zidovudine (Retrovir, azldothymidine [AZT]), which is currently used to treat human immunodeficiency virus (HIV) infection.

Inflammation, Mild Pain, and Fever

Drugs used to treat inflammation or its symptoms are classified as analgesic-antipyretic drugs or nonsteroidal antiinflammatory drugs. A number of medications have both properties.

An antipyretic drug reduces fever. The body's thermoregulatory mechanism, the body's "thermostat," is located in the anterior hypothalamus. Normally, the "set point" of this hypothalamic center is approximately 98.6° F (37° C). When there is an inflammatory response in the body, endogenous pyrogens are released by the phagocytic leukocytes, producing fever. Analgesic-antipyretic drugs work by reversing the effect of the pyrogen on the hypothalamus so that the set point of the hypothalamus is returned to normal. The analgesic effects of these drugs block activation of peripheral pain receptors. Examples of these drugs include acetaminophen (Datril, Tylenol, Panadol, others), aspirin or acetylsalicylic acid (A.S.A, Aspergum, Bayer Aspirin, others), and buffered aspirin (Aluprin, Bufferin, Alka-Seltzer, others).

Aspirin is the prototype of the nonsteroidal antiinflammatory drugs. During the past several years, new drugs have been developed that, like aspirin, are analgesic, antipyretic, and antiinflammatory. These drugs are often prescribed for patients with various inflammatory conditions such as rheumatoid arthritis and especially for those who cannot tolerate aspirin. In addition, these drugs may be used to treat painful joint disorders (with or without inflammation) such as osteoarthritis, low back pain, and gout. Like aspirin, the other nonsteroidal antiinflammatory agents may decrease platelet activity and cause gastrointestinal bleeding.

Nonsteroidal antiinflammatory drugs are thought to act by inhibiting specific enzymes so that prostaglandins (substances that promote inflammation and pain) are not formed. Examples of these drugs are:

- aspirin (Bayer Timed-Release, Bufferin, others)
- diflunisal (Dolobid)
- ibuprofen (Advil, Motrin, Nuprin, others)
- indomethacin (Indocid, Indocin, others)
- naproxen (Anaprox, Naprosyn)
- sulindac (Clinoril)
- *ketorolac* (Toradol)

Stages of Infectious Disease

The progression from exposure to an infectious agent to the onset of clinical disease follows specific stages. The duration of each stage and the potential outcomes vary, depending on the infectious agent and individual host factors. These stages include the latent period, the incubation period, the communicability period, and the disease period.

The **latent period** begins with pathogenic invasion of the body and ends when the agent can be shed or communicated (communicability period). The **incubation period** (during which the organism reproduces) begins with invasion of the agent and ends when the disease process begins. The **communicability period** begins when the latent period ends and continues as long as the agent is present and can spread to other hosts. This stage is variable and is often the major determining factor in ease of transmission. The communicable period and the method of transmission can be altered in some diseases (for example, tuberculosis, syphilis, gonorrhea), depending on the stage of the disease and the primary site of infection.

The **disease period** follows the incubation period and is of variable disease-specific duration. This stage may be subclinical or produce overt symptoms, which can arise directly from the invading organism or from the host's physiological responses. During the disease period, the pathological process may resolve completely, or the organism may become incorporated and quiescent inside certain cells. The infection is then considered to be in a latent stage. A number of viruses can lead to latent infection.

Infectious Disease Protection for Health Care Providers

National concerns regarding communicable disease and infection control have resulted in the development of public law, standards, guidelines, and recommendations to protect health care providers and emergency responders from infectious diseases. Federal and national organizations have been involved in this process, including the:

- U.S. Congress (public law)
- U.S. Department of Labor, Occupational Safety and Health Administration (OSHA regulations)

TABLE 24-1 Personal Equipment for Protection Against Transmission of HIV and Hepatitis B Virus

Activity	Disposable Gloves	Gown	Mask	Protective Eyewear
Bleeding control (spurting blood)	Yes	Yes	Yes	Yes
Bleeding control (minimal blood)	Yes	No	No	No
Emergency childbirth	Yes	Yes	Yes*	Yes*
Intravenous therapy	Yes	No	No	No
Endotracheal intubation	Yes	No	Yes*	Yes*
Oral or nasal suctioning	Yes	No	No	No
Administration of an injection	No	No	No	No

*If splashing is likely.

Guidelines for Prevention of Transmission of HIV and Hepatitis B Virus to Health Care and Public Safety Workers

The general principles presented here have been developed from existing principles of occupational safety and health in conjunction with data from studies of health care workers in hospital settings. The basic premise is that workers must be protected from exposure to blood and other potentially infectious body fluids in the course of their work activities. There is a paucity of data concerning the risks these worker groups face, however, which complicates development of control principles. Thus the guidelines presented here are based on principles of prudent public health practice.

Fire and emergency medical services personnel are engaged in delivery of medical care in the prehospital setting. The following guidelines are intended to assist these personnel in making decisions concerning use of personal protective equipment and resuscitation equipment, as well as for documentation, disinfection, and disposal procedures.

Personal Protective Equipment

Appropriate personal protective equipment should be made available routinely by the employer to reduce the risk of exposure. For many situations, the chance that the rescuer will be exposed to blood and other body fluids to which universal precautions apply can be determined in advance. Therefore if the chance of being exposed is high (for example, cardiopulmonary resuscitation, intravenous line insertion, trauma, and childbirth), the worker should put on protective attire before beginning patient care (Table 24-2). (This list is not intended to be all-inclusive.)

1. Gloves: Disposable gloves should be a standard component of emergency response equipment and should be donned by all personnel before initiating any emergency patient care tasks involving exposure to blood or other body fluids to which universal precautions apply. Extra pairs should always be available. Considerations in the choice of disposable gloves should include dexterity, durability, fit, and the task being performed. Thus there is no single type or thickness of glove appropriate for protection in all situations. For situations in which large amounts of blood are likely to be encountered, it is important that gloves fit tightly at the wrist to prevent blood contamination of hands around the cuff. For multiple trauma victims, gloves should be changed between patient contacts, if the emergency situation allows.

Greater personal protective equipment measures are indicated for situations in which broken glass and sharp edges are likely to be encountered, such as extricating a person from an automobile wreck. Structural firefighting gloves that meet the federal OSHA requirements for firefighter gloves (as contained in 29 Code of Federal Register (CFR) 1910.156 or National Fire Protection Association Standard 1973, *Gloves for Structural Fire Fighters*) should be worn in any situation in which sharp or rough surfaces are likely to be encountered.

Continued.

Guidelines for Prevention of Transmission of HIV and Hepatitis B Virus to Health Care and Public Safety Workers—cont'd

While wearing gloves, avoid handling personal items, such as combs and pens, that could become soiled or contaminated. Gloves that have become contaminated with blood or other body fluids to which universal precautions apply should be removed as soon as possible, taking care to avoid skin contact with the exterior surface. Contaminated gloves should be placed and transported in bags that prevent leakage and should be disposed of or, in the case of reusable gloves, cleaned and disinfected properly.

2. Mask, eyewear, and gowns: Mask, eyewear, and gowns should be present on all emergency vehicles that respond or potentially respond to medical emergencies or victim rescues. These protective barriers should be used in accordance with the level of exposure encountered. Minor lacerations or small amounts of blood do not merit the same extent of barrier use as required for exsanguinating victims or massive arterial bleeding. Management of the patient who is not bleeding and who has no body fluids present should not routinely require use of barrier precautions. Masks and eyewear (for example, safety glasses) should be worn together, or a face shield should be used by all personnel before any situation in which splashes of blood or other body fluids to which universal precautions apply are likely to occur. Gowns or aprons should be worn to protect clothing from splashes with blood. If large splashes or quantities of blood are present or anticipated, im-

pervious gowns or aprons should be worn. An extra change of work clothing should be available at all times.

3. Resuscitation equipment: No transmission of hepatitis B virus or HIV infection during mouth-to-mouth resuscitation has been documented. However, because of the risk of salivary transmission of other infectious diseases (for example, herpes simplex, *Neisseria meningitidis*) and theoretical risk of HIV and hepatitis B virus transmission during artificial ventilation of trauma victims, disposable airway equipment or resuscitation bags should be used. Disposable resuscitation equipment and devices should be used once and disposed of or, if reusable, thoroughly cleaned and disinfected after each use according to the manufacturer's recommendations.

Mechanical respiratory assist devices (for example, bag-valve masks, oxygen demand-valve resuscitators) should be available on all emergency vehicles and to all emergency response personnel who respond or potentially respond to medical emergencies or victim rescues.

Pocket mouth-to-mask resuscitation masks designed to isolate emergency response personnel (that is, double-lumen systems) from contact with victims' blood and blood-contaminated saliva, respiratory secretions, and vomitus should be provided to all personnel who provide or potentially provide emergency treatment.

- National Fire Protection Association (NFPA standards)
- U.S. Department of Health and Human Services, Centers for Disease Control (CDC guidelines)
- Federal Emergency Management Agency and U.S. Fire Administration (infection control program guidelines)

To protect against infection, OSHA requires that personal protective equipment be available to all employees considered to be at high risk for exposure to infectious diseases and that all employees

be offered preexposure prophylaxis to hepatitis by inoculation with hepatitis vaccines.[2] The CDC and NFPA have established similar guidelines, recommendations, and standards regarding the protection of health care workers and emergency providers from blood-borne pathogens, including regular testing for tuberculosis and vaccination for measles in nonimmune individuals.

The Ryan White Comprehensive AIDS Resources Emergency Act of 1990 (PL 101-381) lists notification requirements that emergency responders be advised if they have been exposed to

TABLE 24-2 Reprocessing Methods for Equipment Used in the Prehospital Health Care Setting¹

Organisms Destroyed	Methods	Use
Sterilization All forms of microbial life including high numbers of bacterial spores	Steam under pressure (autoclave), gas (ethylene oxide), dry heat, or immersion in EPA-approved chemical "sterilant" for prolonged period (for example, 6 to 10 hours or according to manufacturer's instructions. NOTE: liquid chemical sterilants should be used *only* on instruments impossible to sterilize or disinfect with heat.)	For instruments or devices that penetrate skin or contact normally sterile areas of the body (for example, scalpels, needles) (Disposable invasive equipment eliminates the need to reprocess these types of items. When indicated, however, arrangements should be made with a health care facility for reprocessing of reusable invasive instruments.)
High-Level Disinfection All forms of microbial life *except* high numbers of bacterial spores	Hot water pasteurization (80° to 100° C, 30 minutes) or exposure to an EPA-registered sterilant chemical, except for a short exposure time (10 to 45 minutes or as directed by the manufacturer)	For reusable instruments or devices that come into contact with mucous membranes (for example, laryngoscope blades, endotracheal tubes)
Intermediate-Level Disinfection *Mycobacterium tuberculosis,* vegetative bacteria, most viruses, and most fungi but *not* bacterial spores	EPA-registered "hospital disinfectant" chemical germicides that have a label claim for tuberculocidal activity, commercially available hard-surface germicides or solutions containing at least 500 ppm free available chlorine (a 1:100 dilution of common household bleach—approximately ¼ cup bleach per gallon of tap water)	For surfaces that come into contact only with intact skin (for example, stethoscopes, blood pressure cuffs, splints) *and* have been visibly contaminated with blood or bloody body fluids (Surfaces *must* be precleaned of visible material before the germicidal chemical is applied for disinfection.)
Low-Level Disinfection Most bacteria, some viruses, some fungi but not *Mycobacterium tuberculosis* or bacterial spores	EPA-registered hospital disinfectants (*no* label claim for tuberculocidal activity)	For routine housekeeping or removal of soiling in the *absence* of visible blood contamination
Environmental Disinfection —	Any cleaner or disinfectant agent intended for environmental use	For environmental surfaces that have become soiled and that should be cleaned and disinfected (for example, floors, woodwork, ambulance seats, countertops)

Important: To ensure the effectiveness of any sterilization or disinfection process, equipment and instruments must first be thoroughly cleaned of all visible soil.
*EPA, Environmental Protection Agency.

infectious diseases, including hepatitis, tuberculosis, bacterial (meningococcal) meningitis, rubella (German measles), and HIV. It also requires that employers name a designated officer to coordinate communications between the hospital and emergency response organization in case there is an exposure.

It is part of the professional responsibility of the paramedic to be familiar with laws, regulations, and national standards that address issues of infectious disease and to take personal protective measures against exposure to these pathogens.[3] Table 24-1 is an overview of recommended guidelines established by the CDC to help prevent the transmission of infectious disease to public safety and emergency response workers. (For a more complete discussion regarding personal protection as recommended by the CDC, see the sidebar on p. 787.) The paramedic should follow local protocol regarding similar or additional precautions concerning personal protection.

● VIRAL HEPATITIS

Hepatitis is the sudden onset of malaise, weakness, anorexia, intermittent nausea and vomiting, and dull right-upper-quadrant pain, usually followed within 1 week by the onset of jaundice, dark urine, or both. Although many viruses can infect the liver, the three classes of viruses that are of main concern as causes of acute hepatitis are hepatitis A virus (HAV), hepatitis B virus (HBV) and hepatitis C virus (HCV), formerly known as *non-A/non-B hepatitis virus*. All types produce similar pathological alterations in the liver and stimulate an antibody response specific to the type of virus causing the disease.

Hepatitis A Virus

Hepatitis A (also known as *infectious hepatitis*) is the most common type of viral hepatitis in the United States; 45% of the U.S. population has hepatitis A antibodies. The disease is acquired by the ingestion of HAV-contaminated food or drink or by the fecal-oral route. The virus localizes in the liver, reproduces, enters the bile, and is carried to the intestinal tract, where it is shed in the feces. Fecal shedding occurs late in the incubation period, usually before the onset of clinical symptoms. Antibodies (anti-HAV) develop during acute disease and later during convalescence. HAV is the only hepatitis virus that does not lead to chronic liver disease or a chronic carrier state (Box 24-2).

Although there is no vaccine for HAV, preventive medications may be used for preexposure prophylaxis against HAV for those traveling to high-risk areas outside tourist routes. The duration of this passive immune state is approximately 2 months (Table 24-3). Once infected with the virus, the person is immune to HAV for life. It should be noted that many infections are subclini-

---

> **BOX 24-2**
>
> ### Signs and Symptoms of HAV Infection of Variable Severity
>
> Fever
> Weakness
> Loss of appetite
> Nausea
> Abdominal pain
> Jaundice
> Dark-colored urine
> Light-colored stools

---

cal and often present with influenza-like symptoms.

Hepatitis B Virus

Infectious HBV particles are found in blood and in secretions containing serum (for example, oozing, cutaneous lesions) or in secretions derived from serum (for example, saliva, semen, vaginal secretions). Like other viral types of hepatitis, HBV affects the liver and causes the signs and symptoms previously described. The virus may produce chronic infection that can lead to cirrhosis as well as other complications. HBV usually lasts less than 6 months, but the carrier state may persist for years (see Table 24-3).

The effects of HBV vary from low-grade fever and malaise (influenza-like illness) with complete resolution of symptoms to extensive liver necrosis that may lead to death. Other complications associated with HBV include coagulation defects, impaired protein production, impaired bilirubin elimination, pancreatitis, and hepatic cancer. Exposure generally occurs in one of five ways:

1. Direct percutaneous inoculation of infectious serum or plasma by needle or transfusion of infected blood or blood products
2. Indirect percutaneous introduction of infective serum or plasma through skin cuts or abrasions
3. Absorption of infective serum or plasma through mucosal surfaces, such as those of

TABLE 24-3 Incubation and Communicability Periods

Incubation Period	Communicability Period
Hepatitis Virus	
HAV	
15 to 50 days (28 to 30 days average)	Usually occurs in the latter half of the incubation period and continues for several days after the onset of jaundice
HBV	
45 to 180 days (60 to 90 days average)	Occurs during incubation period and throughout clinical course (Carrier state may persist for years.)
HCV	
2 weeks to 6 months (average 6 to 9 weeks)	Occurs 1 or more weeks before symptom onset and indefinitely during chronic and carrier states
HIV	
Variable (4 weeks to 6 months from exposure to seropositivity, up to 20 years for symptomatic immune suppression and to diagnosis of AIDS)	Is lifelong from presence of HIV in serum until death (The degree of communicability may vary during the course of the HIV infection.)
Tuberculosis	
4 to 12 weeks after exposure or any time the disease is in a latent stage	Occurs as long as bacilli are in the sputum, sometimes intermittently for years
Meningitis	
2 to 10 days	Is variable: lasts as long as infectious agents remain in the nasal and oral secretions (Microorganisms disappear from the upper respiratory tract within 24 hours of antibiotic therapy.)
Sexually Transmitted Diseases	
Syphilis	
10 days to 10 weeks (average 3 weeks)	Is variable: occurs during primary and secondary stages and in mucocutaneous recurrences (2 to 4 years if untreated)
Gonorrhea	
2 to 7 days	Occurs for months if disease is untreated
Chlamydia	
5 to 10 days	Is unknown
Herpesvirus	
HSV-1: 2 to 12 days	Occurs when lesions are present (Virus is found in saliva as long as 7 weeks after recovery of lesions; transient shedding of virus is common.)
HSV-2: 2 to 12 days (average 6 days)	Occurs in 7 to 12 days with lesion (Transient shedding of virus in the absence of lesions probably occurs.)
Childhood Diseases	
Rubella	
14 to 23 days (average 16 to 18 days)	Occurs from 1 week before and 4 days after appearance of rash (Infants with congenital rubella syndrome may shed virus for months after birth.)
Rubeola	
Commonly 10 days, 8 to 13 days until fever, 14 days until rash	Occurs a few days before the fever to 4 days after the appearance of the rash
Mumps	
2 to 3 weeks (average 18 days)	Occurs 6 days before parotid symptoms to 9 days after (Disease is most communicable 48 hours after parotid swelling.)
Chickenpox	
2 to 3 weeks (average 13 to 17 days)	Occurs 1 to 2 days before the onset of rash and until lesions have crusted over and not more than 6 days after the appearance of vesicles

AIDS, Acquired immunodeficiency syndrome.

the eyes or mouth, or transplacentally or through contamination from the mother's infective blood at birth

4. Absorption of infective secretions (such as saliva or semen) through mucosal surfaces, as might occur during vaginal, anal, or oral sexual contact, but never fecal transmission (Sexual transmission accounts for 30% of the estimated 300,000 HBV infections that occur annually.[3])

5. Transfer of infective serum or plasma via inanimate environmental surfaces or possibly vectors

Preexposure Prophylaxis

The exposure risk for health care providers to HBV-positive patients is estimated to be between 6% to 30%; approximately 12,000 health care personnel acquire HBV through their occupations each year. Of these, 700 to 1200 become carriers, and 250 die as a result of the infection.[4] Therefore HBV is a serious concern to all health care workers.

Blood is the most important potential source of HBV in the workplace. The risk of infection is directly proportional to the probability that the blood contains hepatitis B virus, the immunity status of the recipient, and the efficacy of transmission. HBV vaccinations are available that provide protection for 5 to 7 years in those who respond to the inoculation. The HBV vaccination schedule generally requires three intramuscular (deltoid) doses over 6 months. For optimal protection against HBV infection, the vaccination series should be completed before an exposure occurs. HBV vaccinations currently available include Recombivax HB and Engerix-B. The CDC and OSHA recommend that all EMS personnel be vaccinated.[5]

Postexposure Prophylaxis

If a nonvaccinated person or an individual who has not completed the vaccination schedule is exposed to HBV, postexposure prophylaxis may be indicated. Before treatment, a blood test is usually performed to determine immunity to HBV. If the candidate is seronegative, he or she generally receives the HBV vaccine and hepatitis B immune globulin, an antibody used in postexposure patients to provide passive immunity to HBV.

Hepatitis C Virus

HCV is a blood-borne virus that causes a disease similar to HBV. The virus is often associated with receipt of contaminated blood during transfusion (accounting for more than 90% of posttransfusion hepatitis in the United States) but recently has been implicated in sexually transmitted disease. It is estimated that more than 150,000 new cases of HCV occur in the United States each year and that 4% to 8% of identified health workers develop this disease through an occupational exposure.

Although signs and symptoms of the disease, when they occur, are similar to those of other types of hepatitis, 75% of persons infected with HCV are asymptomatic[6] (see Table 24-3). According to the National Institutes of Health, approximately one half to two thirds of those infected with HCV develop chronic hepatitis; one in five suffer severe liver disease such as cirrhosis and liver cancer.[7]

● HUMAN IMMUNODEFICIENCY VIRUS

The HIV causes disease with a wide clinical spectrum, ranging from the asymptomatic to acquired immunodeficiency syndrome (AIDS), a debilitating illness that is manifested by various opportunistic infections and malignancies and that is almost always fatal. Since the disease was first identified in 1981, it has become a global health problem, affecting between 5 and 10 million people worldwide.

HIV is present in blood and serum-derived body fluids (semen, vaginal, or cervical secretions) in individuals infected with the virus. The disease is directly transmitted person to person through anal or vaginal intercourse, across the placenta, or by contact with infected blood or body fluids on mucous membranes or open wounds. HIV may also be indirectly transmitted by transfusion with contaminated blood or blood products, transplanted tissues and organs, and use of contaminated needles or syringes. Occurrence is highest in persons with the following risk factors[8]:

- High-risk sexual behavior
- Intravenous drug abuse
- Transfusion recipient between 1978 and 1985
- Hemophilia or other coagulation disorders requiring blood products
- Infant born of HIV-positive mother

Pathophysiology

HIV is a retrovirus that converts genetic ribonucleic acid (RNA) to DNA after entering the host cell. Once it is inside the cell, the cell's genetic material is altered into a hybrid that is part virus, part cell. The virus essentially commandeers the cell's machinery to make more virus particles. When sufficient quantities of the virus are produced, the host cell ruptures, destroying the cell and releasing the virus into the blood to seek new target cells. The cell receptor sought by HIV is called *CD4+ T lymphocyte*. It is found on the surface of T-4 lymphocytes (T helper cells, T-4 cells), certain nerve cells, and monocytes and macrophages which probably carry the virus to other parts of the body. Even though the body develops antigen-specific antibodies to HIV, they are not protective.

Classification and Categories

The average time from HIV transmission to serious complications in the absence of treatment is approximately 10 years, although there is considerable variation (see Table 24-3). The CDC has devised a classification system for HIV infection that uses three categories of CD4+ T cell counts[9]: category 1, 500 or more per microliter; category 2, 200 to 499 per microliter; and category 3, less than 200 per microliter. (As the number of CD4+ T lymphocytes decreases, the risk and severity of opportunistic illness increase.) After viral transmission of HIV (which occurs almost always through sexual intercourse or exposure to contaminated blood), the progression of the disease in adolescents and adults can be divided into three clinical categories.

Category A

- Acute retroviral infection: This syndrome generally occurs 2 to 4 weeks after exposure. Clinical features are those of an infectious mononucleosis-like illness with fever, adenopathy, and sore throat. The febrile illness is self-limited, usually lasting 1 to 2 weeks. During this stage, there is a transient decrease in CD4+ T cell counts.
- Seroconversion: The serological response with antigen-specific antibodies to HIV generally takes place between 6 and 12 weeks after transmission. This is accompanied by a return of CD4+ T lymphocyte counts to normal levels.
- Asymptomatic infection: The person with HIV infection may have persistent generalized lymphadenopathy (enlarged lymph nodes involving two noncontiguous sites other than inguinal nodes) and a gradual decline in the CD4+ T lymphocyte count.

Category B

1. Early symptomatic HIV infection: The usual CD4+ T-cell count in this group is 100 to 300 per microliter. Common complications at this stage include localized *Candida* infections (thrush, *Candida* esophagitis, *Candida* vaginitis), oral lesions, shingles, pelvic inflammatory disease, peripheral neuropathy, and constitutional symptoms such as fever or diarrhea lasting more than 1 month.

Category C

1. Late symptomatic HIV infection: This stage represents all AIDS-defining diagnoses found primarily with CD4+ T-lymphocyte counts of 0 to 200 per microliter, including severe opportunistic infections; bacterial pneumonia (*Pneumocystis carinii* pneumonia); pulmonary tuberculosis; debilitating diarrhea; tumors in any body system, including Kaposi's sarcoma (Fig. 24-5); HIV-associated dementia; and neurological manifestations.
2. Advanced HIV infection: This stage applies to individuals with CD4+ T-lymphocyte counts of 0 to 50 per microliter. This group

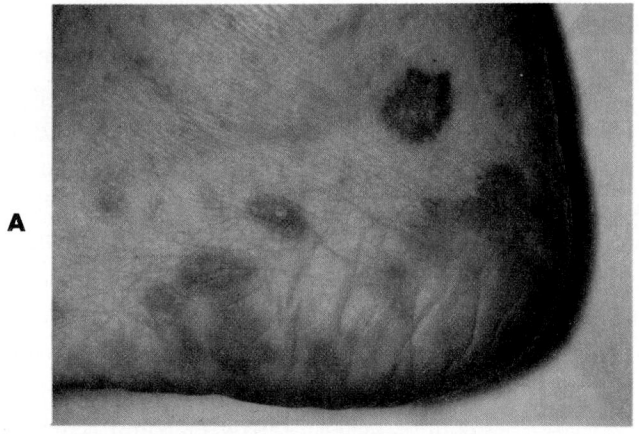
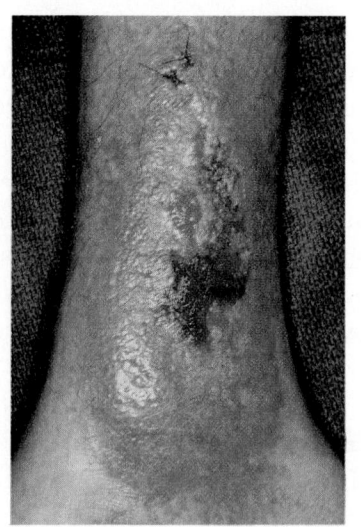

Fig. 24-5 A, Karposi's sarcoma of the heel and lateral foot. **B,** Karposi's sarcoma of the distal leg and ankle.

of patients has a limited life expectancy and most die from AIDS-related complications.

Personal Protection

Strict compliance with universal precautions is the only known prophylactic measure that health care workers can take to protect themselves against HIV infection. However, the chance of EMS personnel acquiring this disease by exposure to infected blood appears to be low (HBV poses a much greater occupational hazard). If a possible exposure occurs (for example, an accidental needle stick injury), the paramedic should be tested for HIV within 2 to 3 weeks after the exposure and again at 6 weeks, 3 months, 6 months, and 1 year. Paramedics should follow local protocol regarding reporting and notification of significant exposures to any infectious disease.

Psychological Reactions to HIV Infection

HIV infection is almost invariably a progressive disease with morbid late consequences. Throughout the course of the infection, HIV-infected persons are likely to feel and express anger about many aspects of their illness, including pain, dying prematurely and without dignity, and the social rejection and prejudice that they may experience. An important aspect of patient care is to help

these patients feel that they can obtain acceptance and compassion from health care workers. New developments in treatment are evolving rapidly, and despite current limitations, progression of the illness can be delayed, permitting access to new therapeutic options in the future.

● TUBERCULOSIS

Although reports of tuberculosis (TB) in the United States declined continually after the turn of the century, in 1985 this trend reversed. The reversal is attributed to the epidemic of HIV infection. (It has been estimated that up to 40% of all patients with active TB have HIV infection.[8])

As described in Chapter 17, TB is a chronic pulmonary disease acquired by inhalation of a dried-droplet nucleus containing a tubercle bacilli (*Mycobacterium tuberculosis, M. bovis,* or a variety of atypical mycobacteria). The infection is transmitted primarily from infected persons coughing or sneezing the bacteria into the air or from contact with sputum that contains virulent TB bacilli. Less commonly, transmission may occur by ingestion or invasion of the skin or mucous membranes.

The pathology of tuberculosis is related to the production of inflammatory lesions throughout the body and to the TB bacilli's ability to break through the body's natural defenses, leading to the formation of caseating granulomas (necrotic inflammatory cells) and TB cavities, which may cause chronic and debilitating lung disease. Susceptibility to mycobacterial infection is generally highest in children less than 3 years of age, in those older than 65, and in chronically ill, malnourished, and immunosuppressed or immunocompromised individuals. The disease is characterized by stages of early infection (frequently asymptomatic), latency, and a potential for recurrent postprimary disease (see Table 24-3). Signs and symptoms of tuberculosis include cough, fever, night sweats, weight loss, fatigue, and hemoptysis.

Personal Protection

As with any other infectious disease, universal precautions (including respiratory barriers for patient and paramedic) should be taken during the patient care encounter. Although the signs and symptoms of initial infection may be minimal, early infection can be detected with a tuberculin skin test (purified protein derivative [PPD]) and a chest x-ray examination. A positive reaction to the PPD test indicates past infection and the presence of antibodies. Treatment for acute disease as well as prophylactic therapy includes a lengthy course of antibiotic administration and careful physician follow-up. A negative immune response does not preclude reinfection with subsequent exposure. Therefore health care providers should have periodic PPD skin tests to ascertain their TB exposure status.

● MENINGITIS

Meningitis (inflammation of the membranes that surround the spinal cord and brain) can be caused by a variety of different bacteria, viruses, and other microorganisms. Despite considerable therapeutic advances in treating this infection, meningitis is a serious disease that should always be considered a true medical emergency. A primary goal of emergency treatment is administration of an appropriate antibiotic agent within 30 to 60 minutes of arrival to the emergency department.

The risk of bacterial meningitis is most significant in neonates and children between 2 months and 4 years of age but should also be suspected in any patient with fever, headache, stiff neck, altered mental status, or underlying health problems (such as recent neurosurgery, trauma, or immunocompromise). Common pathogens that cause bacterial meningitis include *Streptococcus pneumoniae, Haemophilus influenza,* and *Neisseria meningitides.* The usual mode of transmission is direct contact with upper respiratory secretions (discharge from the nose and throat) from an infected person or carrier. Once inhaled, the bacteria invade the respiratory passages and travel by way of blood to the brain and spinal cord. As the infecting agent spreads to additional organs, it causes toxic manifestations in the involved organ system. Bacterial meningitis is considered more communicable than viral meningitis.

Viral meningitis (aseptic meningitis) is a syndrome generally associated with an existing systemic viral disease (for example, mumps). Toxic and meningeal symptoms are similar to those of bacterial meningitis but are usually less severe. In most cases, viral meningitis is self-limited with complete recovery. The patient may experience muscle weakness and malaise during prolonged convalescence.

Signs and Symptoms

Signs and symptoms of meningitis depend on the age and general health of the patient. In infants, for example, signs of meningeal irritation may be absent or include only irritability, poor feeding or vomiting, a high-pitched cry, and fullness of the fontanelle. In older infants and children, signs of meningitis may include the presence of malaise, low-grade fever, headache, and stiff neck (from meningeal irritation). If there is extensive meningeal involvement in a toxic or debilitated patient, the illness may be accompanied by convulsions, coma, and shock. Severe cases of meningitis may result in cranial nerve damage that can lead to blindness and deafness. Arthritis, myocarditis, pericarditis, and ultimately death may ensue from overwhelming infection. Health care workers exposed to patients with bacterial meningitis may be required to take prophylactic antibiotics for a time to protect themselves and to avoid transmitting the infection to others (see Table 24-3).

● SEXUALLY TRANSMITTED DISEASES

Sexually transmitted diseases (STDs) are a group of disease syndromes that can be transmitted sexually, whether or not the disease has genital pathological manifestations. More than 20 etiological agents have been identified as belonging to this group of diseases (including HBV and HIV infections). Other common STDs include syphilis, gonorrhea, chlamydia, and herpesvirus infections.

A number of pathogenic agents are responsible for the host of STDs, including bacteria, viruses, protozoa, fungi, and ectoparasites. Many of these pathogens can produce multiple disease syndromes, and patients with STD syndromes frequently have multiple STDs. These infections usually result in a short-lived cellular immune response and a longer-lasting humoral antibody response, neither of which protects against future exposures.

Syphilis

Syphilis is a systemic disease characterized by a primary lesion, a secondary eruption involving skin and mucous membranes, long periods of latency, and late seriously disabling lesions of the skin, bone, viscera, central nervous system, and cardiovascular system. The disease is caused by penetration of *Treponema pallidum* into intact mucous membranes or abraded skin. Common modes of transmission include direct contact with exudate from lesions on skin and mucous membranes, blood transfusions (rare), and congenital transmission. After penetration, the organisms travel (within hours) to lymph nodes, where they are disseminated throughout the body. After the initial infection, syphilis follows well-defined stages of disease (see Table 24-3). Syphilis is treatable with antibiotic therapy.

Primary Stage

Within 10 to 90 days after exposure, a primary lesion or chancre develops at the site of initial invasion (Fig. 24-6). The surface of the chancre is usually crusted or ulcerated and varies in size from 1 to 2 cm in diameter. The lesion is usually single and painless, and it generally heals spontaneously within 1 to 5 weeks. During this stage, syphilis is highly communicable.

Secondary Stage

The secondary stage begins approximately 2 to 10 weeks after the appearance of the primary lesion and lasts 2 to 6 weeks. This stage is heralded by systemic symptoms, including headache, malaise, anorexia, fever, sore throat, and lymphadenopathy. In addition, the patient may develop a rash, which is usually bilaterally symmetrical and frequently involves the palms and soles (Fig. 24-7).

Latency

A period of latency (ranging from 1 to 40 years or more) follows the secondary stage in untreated persons. During latency, there may be recurrent episodes of secondary-stage symptoms with subclinical infection. In some individuals, the infection produces progressive involvement, especially in the central nervous system and cardiovascular systems (tertiary syphilis). Central nervous system manifestations include paresis, tabes dorsalis (spinal column degeneration characterized by

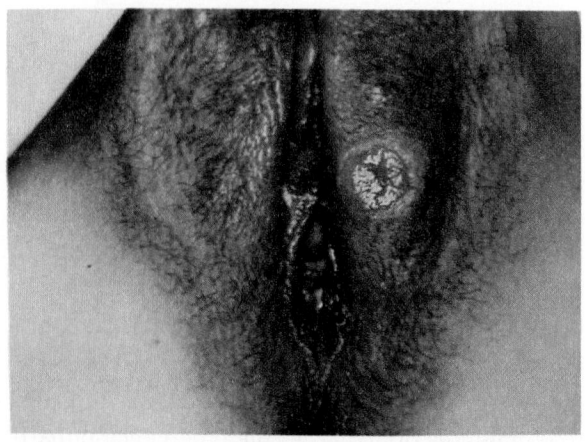

Fig. 24-6 Primary syphilis chancre on the labia.

wide gait and ataxia: "syphilitic shuffle"), and psychosis. Cardiovascular injury may result in myocardial insufficiency and aortic necrosis, which can lead to aortic rupture and death.

Gonorrhea

Gonorrhea is caused by the sexually transmitted bacterium *N. gonorrhoeae,* which is communicated by a purulent exudate from mucous membranes of an infected person. Other modes of transmission include maternal infection during pregnancy and transmission of the pathogen during birth. The disease occurs in men and women but differs in course, severity, and ease of recognition. As a rule, gonorrhea is treatable with antibiotics, but some strains brought into the United States from other countries have been resistant to conventional antibiotic therapy (Fig. 24-8).

Affected areas of the male anatomy are the urethra, Littre's gland, Cowper's gland, prostate gland, seminal vesicles, and epididymis. Several days after exposure, there is usually a sudden onset of dysuria, urgency, and frequency (see Table 24-3). The associated discharge rapidly becomes purulent and profuse. Direct spread of the infection may result in prostatitis, epididymitis, and seminal vesiculitis. Primary gonorrheal infections may also affect the pharynx, conjunctivae, and anus.

Affected areas of the female anatomy are the Bartholin glands, Skene glands, urethra, cervix, and fallopian tubes. More than 50% of infected women remain asymptomatic; others have a mucopurulent discharge that varies from scant to profuse. Contiguous spread of the disease may lead to endometritis, salpingitis, and parametritis (pelvic inflammatory disease) and the formation of tuboovarian abscesses. Complete or partial occlusion of the fallopian tubes may result in sterility and increased risk for ectopic pregnancy.

Between 1% and 3% of gonococcal infections become disseminated in the blood. This extension of the disease may produce septicemia, arthritis, endocarditis, meningitis, and skin lesions. In the bacteremic stage, the patient may complain of fever, chills, and malaise. Erythematous lesions are common, especially on the extremities, and may occur in groups or singly.

Chlamydia

Chlamydia trachomatis is a major cause of sexually transmitted nonspecific urethritis (NSU) or nongonococcal genital infection. The disease is

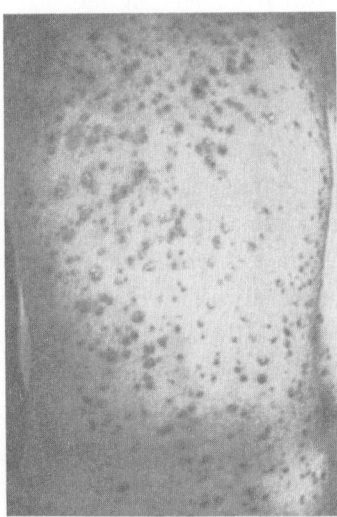

Fig. 24-7 Secondary syphilis rash on the back.

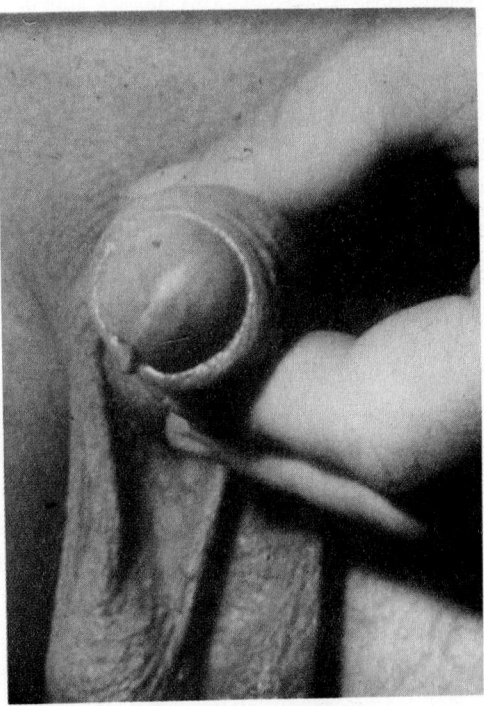

Fig. 24-8 Symptomatic gonococcal urethritis.

prevalent worldwide and is the most common sexually transmitted disease in the United States.

In men, NSU may cause a penile discharge and complications such as swelling of the testes, which if untreated may lead to infertility. In women, NSU is usually symptomless but may cause a vaginal discharge or pain with urination, salpingitis, and cervicitis. Transmission occurs from direct contact with exudates, either sexually or during birth (see Table 24-3). Chlamydial infections are treated with antibiotics.

Herpesvirus Infections

The herpes simplex virus (HSV) is one of four herpes viruses. The others are the cytomegalovirus, which is associated with mononucleosis, hepatitis, and severe systemic disease in the immunosuppressed host; the Epstein-Barr virus, which causes mononucleosis; and the varicellazoster virus, which causes chickenpox and shingles. This section of the text addresses only the HSVs associated with STDs.

Herpes Simplex Virus

The two antigenically distinct herpes simplex viral agents responsible for STDs are herpes simplex virus type 1 (HSV-1) and herpes simplex virus type 2 (HSV-2). Both pathogens may lead to herpes infection, and both can produce infection anywhere in the body. As a rule, HSV-1 is most often associated with herpes above the waist, whereas HSV-2 is generally associated with genital herpes. However, either type can cause disease in the genital area.

HSV is common in the United States, producing 300,000 to 500,000 new infections each year. (It is estimated that 70% to 90% of adults have antibodies against HSV-1.) The mode of transmission for HSV is strictly by skin-to-skin contact with an infected area of the body. The virus enters through a break in the skin or through mucous membranes. Sexual contact is not required for transmission. For example, many young children who experience oral herpes (HSV-1) probably contract the virus from a casual kiss from a parent or relative. The virus may also be spread to other external body sites by autoinoculation (for example, lip to

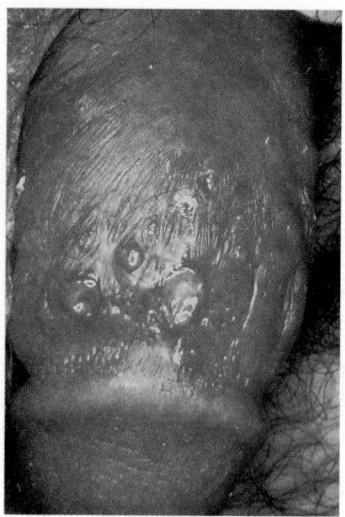

Fig. 24-9 HSV-2 infection: herpes corona.

finger to genitalia). Initial HSV-1 transmission usually occurs by 4 years of age and is manifested by gingivostomatitis ("cold sores" or "fever blisters"). Initial HSV-2 transmission (Fig. 24-9) generally occurs during sexual activity and is manifested by painful vesicular lesions in the genital area.

Once the virus is present in tissue, HSV produces an acute infection with self-limited tissue destruction. This "primary infection" produces a vesicular lesion (blister) that heals spontaneously from the periphery without residual scarring. However, the virus remains viable in the body despite circulating antibodies (see Table 24-3).

After the primary infection, the HSV enters the nervous system (nearest the site of initial infection) and travels along sensory nerve pathways to a sensory nerve ganglion, where it remains in a latent stage until it is reactivated. When triggered by another infectious disease, menstruation, emotional stress, trauma, or immunosuppression, the virus reaches the epidermis by way of peripheral nerves and reproduces a recurrent infectious disease state that usually lasts from 4 to 10 days. The lesions generally appear in the area of initial inoculation. The number of lesions a person might experience during any given episode varies considerably. The disease is manifested by clusters of painful vesicles that become pustular and dry or rupture, leaving shallow, painful ulcers. Genital

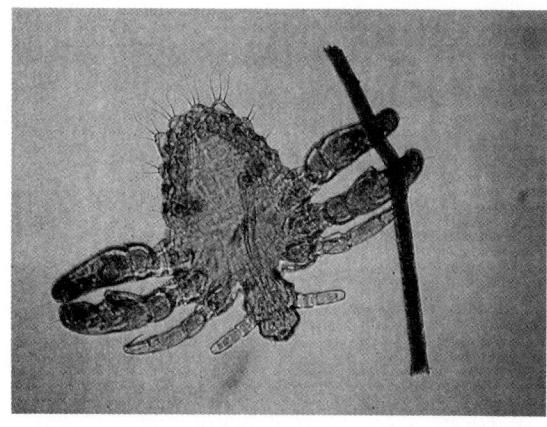
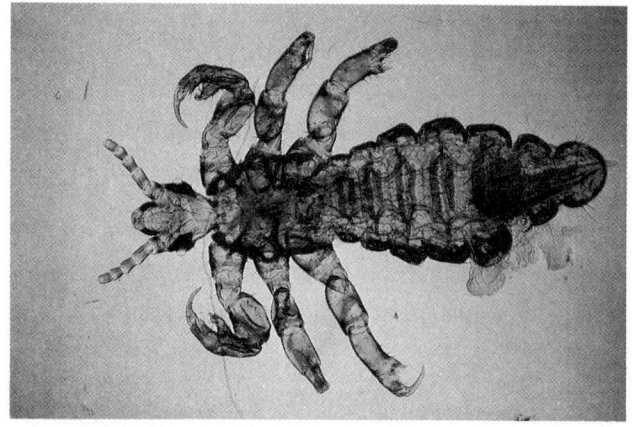

A   B

Fig. 24-10 A, The pubic or crab louse. **B,** Male of the human head louse.

herpes in women may involve all of the vulvar tissue, the perianal skin, and the vaginal mucosa. As a rule, genital herpes in men is a milder disease, affecting the glans penis and sometimes the penile shaft.

The HSV can remain dormant indefinitely. It is unknown why many infected people never exhibit the disease, whereas others experience a lifetime of periodic outbreaks. Acyclovir (Zovirax), an antiviral agent, may shorten the disease episode, and it is useful as a prophylactic agent in instances of frequent recurrence.

● LICE AND SCABIES

Lice and scabies are potential health hazards for all emergency care providers. Both are medically important as potential vectors of communicable skin disease and systemic illness, as well as dermatitis and discomfort.

Lice

Lice are small, wingless insects that are ectoparasites of birds and mammals. Most are host specific. Two of the species are human parasites: *Phthirus pubis,* the pubic or crab louse, and *Pediculus humanus,* with two varieties, *P. h. capitis,* the head louse, and *P. h. corporis,* the body louse (Fig. 24-10). Lice subsist on blood from the host and have mouths modified for piercing and sucking.

During biting and feeding, secretions from the louse cause a small, red macule and pruritus. Long periods of infestation may bring a decrease in pruritus and often impart a thick, dry, scaly appearance to the skin. In severe cases, oozing and crusting may be present. If sensitization to lice saliva and feces occurs, inflammation may develop. Secondary infection may develop from scratching of lesions. Lice spread through close personal contact and sharing of clothing and bedding.

Pubic lice have a distinctive appearance, suggestive of a miniature crab. Grayish-blue spots may be observed on the abdomen and thighs of infested patients. The eggs (nits or ova) are often evident on the shaft of pubic hairs and sometimes in eyelashes, eyebrows, and axillary hairs. Pubic lice are usually acquired during sexual activity or from unchanged bedding where egg-infested pubic hairs have been shed. Primary bite lesions are seldom evident, but the patient normally complains of intense pruritus and pubic scratching.

Head lice have an elongated body with a head that is slightly narrower than the thorax. Each louse has three pairs of legs that possess delicate hooks at the distal extremities. The white ova of head lice (usually one nit to a shaft) are easily mistaken for dandruff, but the nits cannot be brushed out. These parasites most frequently affect children.

Body lice are slightly larger than head lice and concentrate about the waist, shoulders, axillae, and neck. Body lice and their nits are usually found in seams and on fibers of clothing. The lesions from their bites begin as small, noninflammatory red spots that quickly become papular wheals that resemble linear scratch marks (parallel scratch marks on the shoulders are a common finding). Head lice and body lice interbreed.

The treatment of all types of lice is aimed at eradicating the parasites and nits and at preventing reinfestation. Patients are usually advised to thoroughly wash all clothing, bedding, and personal articles in hot water and to wash the infected body area with gamma benzene hexachloride shampoo (Kwell), crotamiton (Eurax), Rid, or Nix.

Scabies

The human scabies mite (*Sarcoptes scabiei* var. *hominis*) is a parasite that completes its entire life cycle in and on the epidermis of its host. Scabies infestation resembles that of lice, but scabies bites are generally concentrated around the hands and feet, especially between the webs of the fingers and toes. Other common areas of infestation include the face and scalp of children, the nipples in females, and the penis in males. The scabies mite is usually passed by intimate contact or from infested bedding, furniture, and clothing.

Scabies infestation is often manifested by severe nocturnal pruritus (although it takes 4 to 6 weeks for sensitization to develop and itching to begin). The adult female mite is responsible for symptoms. After impregnation, she burrows into the epidermis to lay her eggs and remains in the burrow for a life span of approximately 1 month. Vesicles and papules form at the surface, but they are often disguised by the results of scratching. In severe cases, oozing, crusting, and secondary infection may result.

Treatment is similar to that prescribed for lice infestation. Symptoms may persist for over a month until the mite and mite products are shed with the epidermis. Reinfestation is common. Therefore if the itching has not been abated within several weeks, the patient should be reexamined. Antibiotic therapy may be required to treat secondary infection.

● INFECTIOUS DISEASES OF CHILDHOOD

The childhood infectious diseases to be presented in this chapter include rubella (German measles), rubeola (red measles or hard measles), mumps (parotitis), and chickenpox (varicella). With the exception of chickenpox, these infectious diseases are preventable with the triple immunization (MMR vaccine). With widespread immunization of children, the incidence of these childhood infectious diseases has decreased.

Rubella

Rubella is a mild, febrile, and highly communicable viral disease characterized by a diffuse punctate macular rash (Fig. 24-11). The disease is usually transmitted by direct contact with nasopharyngeal secretions or droplet spray from an infected person. It may also be transmitted transplacentally (producing active infection in the fetus) and by contact with articles contaminated with blood, urine, or feces. After inoculation, the virus invades the lymph system. From there, it enters the blood and produces an immune response that initiates the development of a rash. After the rash appears, the patient is no longer infectious. Complications from the disease are rare.

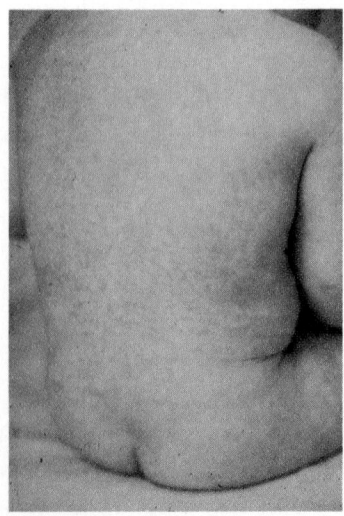

Fig. 24-11 Acquired rubella (German measles) in an 11-month-old infant.

Congenital rubella syndrome is a serious manifestation that affects approximately 25% of infants born to women who were infected with rubella during the first trimester of pregnancy. The disease is associated with multiple congenital anomalies, mental retardation, and an increased risk of death from congenital heart disease and sepsis during the first 6 months of life. The CDC recommends that all health care providers receive immunization if they are not immune from previous rubella infection to reduce the risk of exposure to themselves and those they treat. As a precaution, pregnant EMS providers should not be exposed to these patients (see Table 24-3).

Rubeola

Rubeola is an acute, highly communicable viral disease characterized by fever, conjunctivitis, cough, bronchitis, and a blotchy red rash (Fig. 24-12). The virus is found in the blood, urine, and pharyngeal secretions. The disease is usually transmitted directly or indirectly through contact with infected respiratory secretions. After exposure, the virus invades the respiratory epithelium and spreads via the lymph system. Rubeola may predispose to secondary bacterial complications such as otitis media and pneumonia.

Patients with rubeola usually have white spots on the buccal mucosa (Koplik's spots) and a dermal rash a few days after respiratory tract involvement (see Table 24-3). The onset of rash coincides with the production of serum antibodies. Uncomplicated cases of rubeola last 7 to 10 days.

Mumps

Mumps is an acute, communicable systemic viral disease characterized by localized unilateral or bilateral edema of one or more of the salivary glands (usually the parotid), with occasional involvement of other glands (Fig. 24-13). The virus is transmitted through direct contact with the saliva droplets of an infected person.

The virus invades and multiplies in the parotid gland or epithelium of the upper respiratory passages. From there, it enters the blood and localizes in glandular or nervous tissue. The parotid, testes, and pancreas are the glands most frequently involved (see Table 24-3). When mumps occurs past the age of puberty, it may cause a painful inflammation of the testicle (orchitis) and testicular atrophy; however, sterility is rare. The intensity of symptoms in mumps is variable; 30% of infections are asymptomatic. Immunity after clinical and subclinical disease is lifelong. Placental transfer of antibodies sometimes occurs.

Chickenpox (Varicella)

Chickenpox is a common childhood disease for which no routine preventative vaccine is available

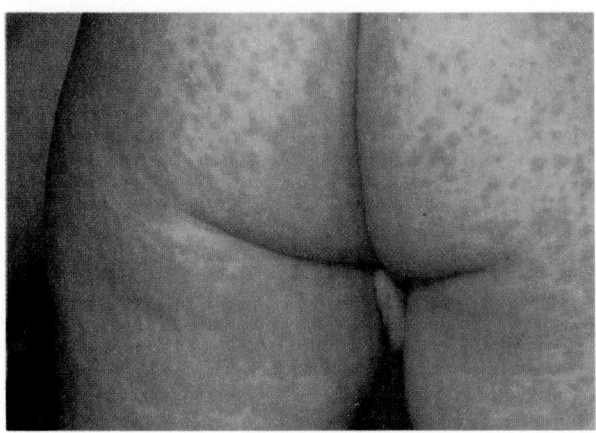

Fig. 24-12 Rubeola (measles) rash on the third day.

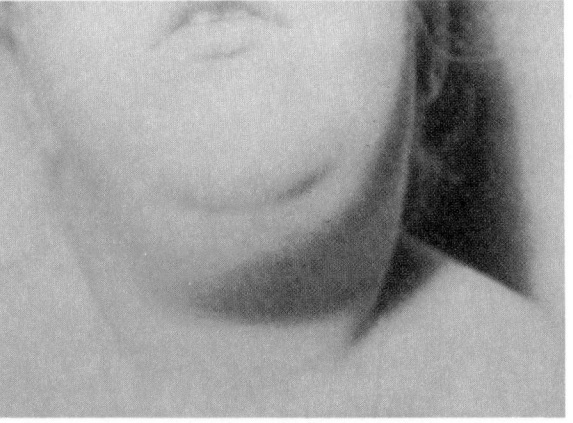

Fig. 24-13 Submaxillary mumps in an infant.

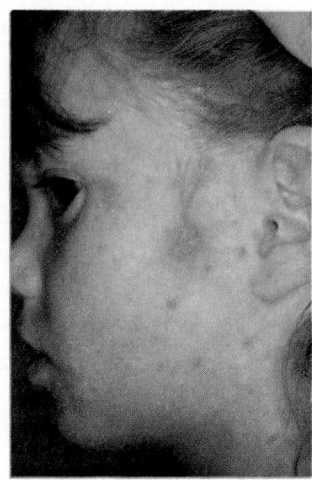

Fig. 24-14 Chickenpox skin lesions.

in this country. The disease is caused by the varicella-zoster virus (a member of the herpesvirus family) and is transmitted by direct and indirect contact with droplets from respiratory passages of an infected person.

Chickenpox is highly communicable (see Table 24-3) and is characterized by a sudden onset of fever, mild malaise, and a skin eruption that is maculopapular for a few hours and vesicular for 3 to 4 days, leaving a granular scab (Fig. 24-14). Initially the skin lesions appear on the trunk and usually move to the extremities. The crops of skin eruptions (each associated with itching) are generally more abundant on covered areas of the body; the scalp, conjunctivae, and upper respiratory tract may be affected. The appearance of crops of vesicles (fresh vesicles appearing while other lesions are scabbed) differentiates chickenpox from smallpox, which has vesicles of the same age. Treatment is symptomatic, and the disease is self-limited. Complications are rare but may include secondary bacterial infections, aseptic meningitis, mononucleosis, and Reye syndrome.

After recovery, the virus is believed to remain in the body in an asymptomatic latent stage (possibly localized in the dorsal root ganglia). The virus may reactivate during periods of stress or immunosuppression, producing an illness known as *shingles.* The vesicles associated with shingles are restricted to the skin area supplied by the sensory nerves of a single group or associated groups of dorsal root ganglia. Unlike chickenpox, shingles is not transmitted through respiratory droplets, but it can cause chickenpox in susceptible individuals who are in contact with skin lesions.

REFERENCES

1. Grimes D: *Infectious diseases*, St Louis, 1991, Mosby.
2. *Title 29 code of federal regulations* (CFR), Part 1910.1030, December 1991.
3. US Department of Health and Human Services, Centers for Disease Control, National Institute of Occupational Safety and Health: *Guidelines for prevention of transmission of human immunodeficiency virus and hepatitis B virus to health-care and public-safety workers*, vol 38, No. S-6, Washington, DC, 1989, DHHS, CDC, NHOSH.
4. US Department of Health and Human Services: *Curriculum guide for public-safety and emergency response workers*, Washington, DC, 1989, DHHS.
5. US Department of Labor, Occupational Safety and Health Administration. *Occupational exposure to bloodborne pathogens: precautions for emergency responders*, OSHA 3130, Washington, DC, 1992, OSHA.
6. West K: Assessing the risks, *Emerg Mag* 24(30):30, 1992.
7. Sexual transmission of hepatitis C linked to HIV, *Emerg Mag* 24(3):10, 1992.
8. Bartlett J: *The Johns Hopkins Hospital guide to medical care of patients with HIV infection*, ed 3, Baltimore, 1993, Williams & Wilkins.
9. US Department of Health and Human Services, Centers for Disease Control and Prevention: 1993 revised classification system for HIV infection and expanded surveillance case definition for AIDS among adolescents and adults, *MMWR* 41(RR-17):1, 1992.

Summary

Paramedics are called to assist in the care of patients with infectious diseases. This chapter presented the more common types of infectious processes and the protective measures that should be used while rendering emergency care. Although those involved in health care cannot be provided with a totally risk-free environment, simple measures of protection greatly reduce exposure to pathogenic agents.

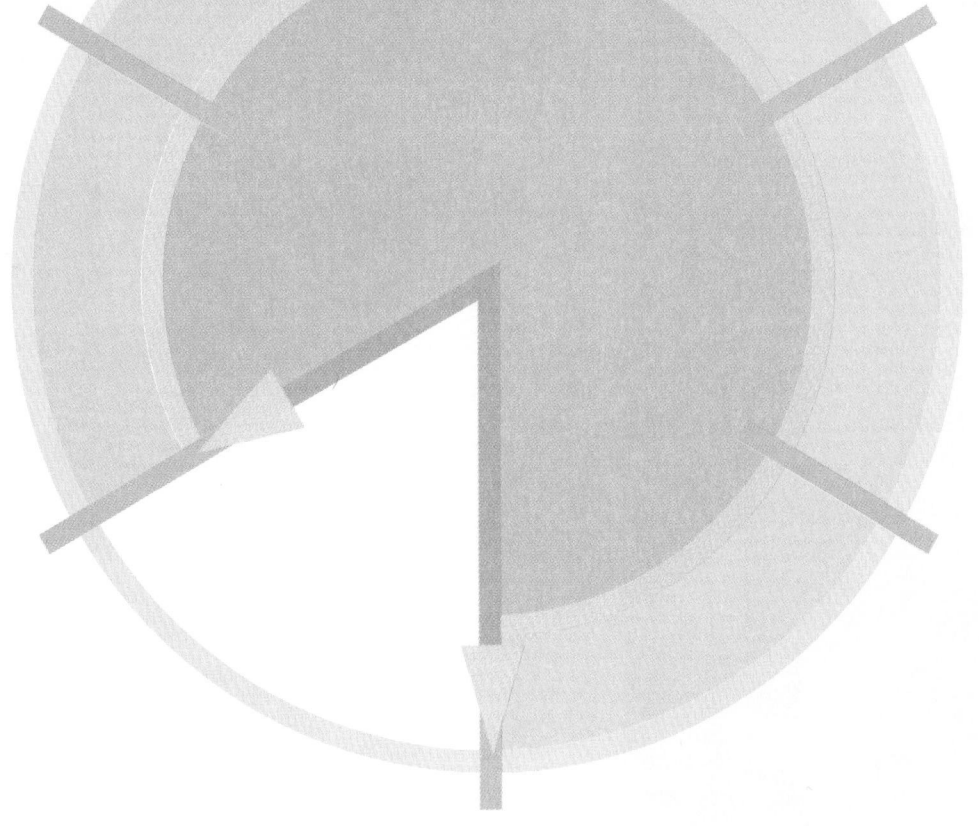

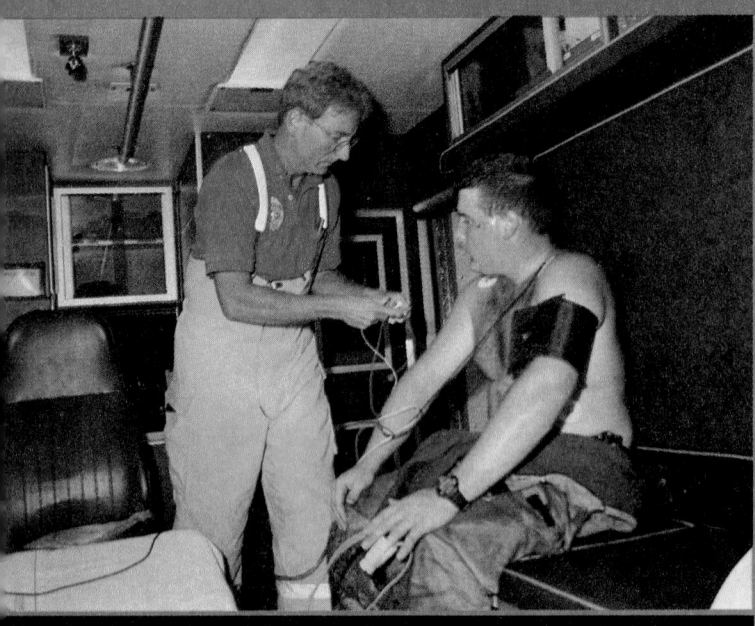

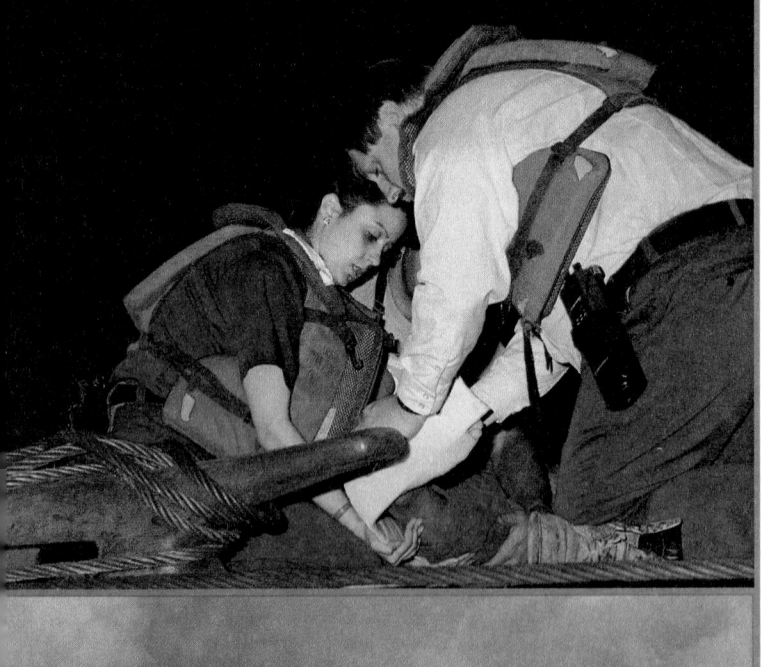

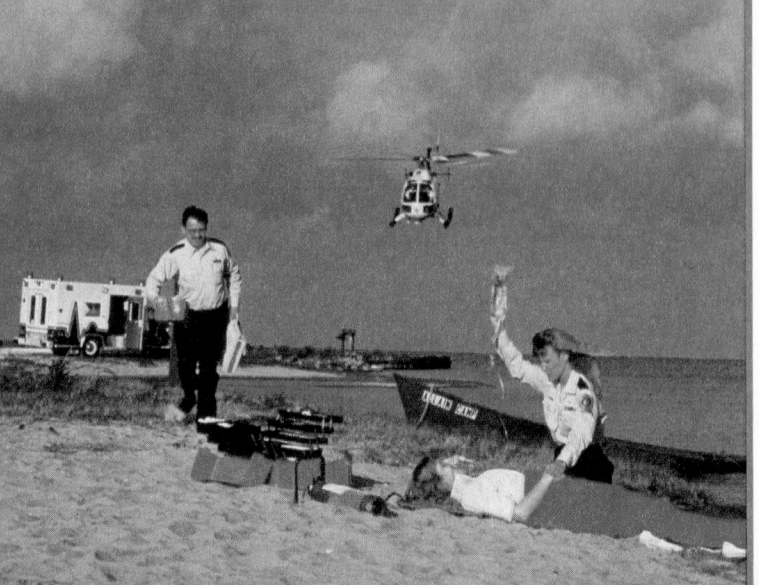

A number of medical emergencies can result from physical exposure to environmental elements. The paramedic must be prepared to recognize and manage these conditions by understanding their causative factors and distinctive underlying pathophysiology.

OBJECTIVES

As a paramedic, you should be able to:

1. Describe the physiology of thermo-regulation.
2. Discuss the pathophysiology, assessment findings, and management of specific hyperthermic conditions, hypothermia, and frostbite.
3. Distinguish between hyperthermia syndrome and fever.
4. Describe patient management of fever.
5. Identify patients at increased risk for hypothermia.
6. List factors that predispose to frostbite.
7. Distinguish between drowning and near-drowning.
8. Discuss the pathophysiology, assessment, and prehospital management of near-drowning and pressure-related diving emergencies.
9. Identify factors that influence patient survival of a near-drowning episode.
10. Differentiate the pathophysiology of saltwater and fresh-water drowning.
11. Outline properties of gas that affect pressure-related diving emergencies.
12. Discuss the pathophysiology, assessment, and prehospital management of high-altitude illness.

● THERMOREGULATION

Body temperature is regulated by a thermoregulatory center in the posterior hypothalamus. This center receives input from central thermoreceptors in or near the anterior hypothalamus and from peripheral thermoreceptors located in the skin and some mucous membranes. Peripheral thermoreceptors are nerve endings usually categorized as cold receptors, which are stimulated by a lower skin-surface temperature, and warm receptors stimulated by higher temperatures. There are up to 10 times as many cold receptors as warm ones in many parts of the skin. Information from these receptors is transmitted via afferent nerves and ascending pathways to the posterior hypothalamus,

KEY TERMS

classic heat stroke: A severe, sometimes fatal condition that results from failure of temperature-regulating capacity and that is caused by prolonged exposure to the sun or to high temperatures.

deep frostbite: A cold injury that results in significant tissue loss even with appropriate therapy and that is associated with subdermal layers and deep tissues.

drowning: Death by asphyxia after submersion.

exertional heat stroke: An abnormal condition that is characterized by weakness, vertigo, nausea, muscle cramps, and loss of consciousness and that is caused by depletion of body fluid and electrolytes resulting from exposure to intense heat or the inability to acclimatize to heat.

frostnip: The mildest form of cold injury that may be treated without tissue loss.

near-drowning: Submersion with at least temporary survival.

superficial frostbite: A cold injury usually involving the dermis and shallow subcutaneous layers, with at least some minimal tissue loss.

thermogenesis: Production of heat, especially by the cells of the body.

thermolysis: Dissipation of body heat by radiation, evaporation, conduction, or convection.

which responds with appropriate efferent output to decrease heat loss and increase heat production (cold-receptor stimulation) or increase heat loss and decrease heat production (warm-receptor stimulation).

Central thermoreceptors are temperature-sensitive neurons that react directly to alterations in the temperature of blood. Via descending pathways, these neurons innervate skeletal muscle through somatic motor nerves. They affect vasomotor tone, sweating, and metabolic rate via sympathetic nerve output to skin arterioles, sweat glands, and the adrenal medulla.

As discussed in Chapter 24, the thermoregulatory center has an inherent set point, which maintains a relatively constant temperature (core temperature) of 98.6° F (37° C). To maintain an optimum environment for normal cell metabolism, it is necessary to keep the core temperature fairly constant, notwithstanding the external and internal conditions that tend to raise or lower it. The body temperature can be increased or decreased in two ways: through regulation of heat production (**thermogenesis**) and regulation of heat loss (**thermolysis**).

Regulating Heat Production

Heat can be generated by the body in response to cold through chemical, metabolic, and endocrine activities. The direction and magnitude of these compensatory responses are affected by a number of physiological and biochemical factors, such as the individual's age, general health, and nutritional status.

Heat production is controlled chemically by cellular metabolism (the oxidation of food). Every tissue contributes to this type of heat production, but

TABLE 25-1 Cooling Power of Wind on Exposed Flesh Expressed as an Equivalent Temperature (Under Calm Conditions)

Estimated Wind Speed (in mph)	Actual Thermometer Reading (°F)											
	50	40	30	20	10	0	−10	−20	−30	−40	−50	−60
	Equivalent Chill Temperature (°F)											
Calm	50	40	30	20	10	0	−10	−20	−30	−40	−50	−60
5	48	37	27	16	6	−5	−15	−26	−36	−47	−57	−68
10	40	28	16	4	−9	−24	−33	−46	−58	−70	−83	−95
15	36	22	9	−5	−18	−32	−45	−58	−72	−85	−99	−112
20	32	18	4	−10	−25	−39	−53	−67	−82	−96	−110	−124
25	30	16	0	−15	−29	−44	−59	−74	−88	−104	−118	−133
30	28	13	−2	−18	−33	−48	−63	−79	−94	−109	−125	−140
35	27	11	−4	−21	−35	−51	−62	−82	−98	−113	−129	−145
40	26	10	−6	−21	−37	−53	−69	−85	−100	−116	−132	−148

(Wind speeds greater than 40 mph have little additional effect.)

Little danger. In < 5 hr with dry skin. Maximum danger of false sense of security.

Increasing danger. Danger from freezing of exposed flesh within 1 minute

Great danger Flesh may freeze within 30 seconds.

Trenchfoot and immersion foot may occur at any point on this chart.

INSTRUCTIONS

Measure local temperature and wind speed if possible. If not, *estimate*. Enter table at closest 5° F interval along the top and with appropriate wind speed along left side. Intersection gives approximate equivalent chill temperature (that is, the temperature that would cause the same rate of cooling under calm conditions). Note that regardless of cooling rate, you do not cool below the actual air temperature unless wet.

in humans, skeletal muscles produce the largest amount of heat, particularly when shivering occurs. Along with shivering, which is often associated with chattering of teeth, the body undergoes vasoconstriction and piloerection ("goose pimples") to conserve as much heat as possible. Shivering is the body's best defense against cold and may increase heat production by as much as 400%.

Endocrine glands also regulate heat production through the release of hormones from the thyroid gland and adrenal medulla. Sympathetic discharge of epinephrine and norepinephrine and the activity of sympathetic nerves that lead to adipose tissue are thought to increase the basal metabolic rate and thereby augment heat production.

Regulating Heat Loss

Heat is lost from the body to the external environment through the skin, lungs, and excretions. The most important of these in regulating heat loss is the skin. Radiation, conduction, convection, and evaporation are the major sources of heat loss.

The surface of the human body constantly emits heat in the form of infrared rays, as do all other warm objects. The rate of emissions is determined by the temperature of the radiating surface. Thus if the surface of the body is warmer than the average of the various surfaces in the environment, net heat is lost, the rate depending directly on the temperature difference between the environment and the body (thermal gradient).

Conduction is the exchange of heat that occurs simply by the transfer of thermal energy. Heat, like any other entity, moves down a concentration gradient from higher to lower temperature. Therefore the body surface loses or gains heat by direct contact with cooler or warmer surfaces, including air. If ambient air temperature is lower than skin temperature, body heat is lost to the surrounding air by conduction.

Convection is the process whereby air (or water) next to the body is heated, moves away, and is replaced by cool air (or water), which repeats the same pattern. Convection can be greatly facilitated by external forces such as wind or fans and aids conductive heat exchange by continuously maintaining a supply of cool air. Factors that con-

tribute to the cooling effects of convection are the velocity of air currents and the temperature of the air. The windchill chart was developed to calculate the cooling effects of the ambient temperature based on thermometer readings and the wind speed (Table 25-1).

Evaporation of any fluid absorbs heat from surrounding objects and air. Evaporative heat loss from moisture on the skin or lining membranes of the respiratory tract is greatly affected by ambient temperature and relative humidity. (The relative humidity is the ratio of the actual amount of moisture in the air to the greatest amount it can hold at a specified temperature. When at a given temperature the air is fully saturated with moisture, the relative humidity is 100%.) Diaphoresis can markedly increase evaporative heat loss provided that the relative humidity is low enough that the sweat can evaporate. At humidity levels

---

BOX 25-1

Hyperthermic and Hypothermic Compensation

Hyperthermic Compensation
Increased Heat Loss
Vasodilation of skin vessels
Sweating

Decreased Heat Production
Decreased muscle tone and voluntary activity
Decreased hormone secretion
Decreased appetite

Hypothermic Compensation
Decreased Heat Loss
Peripheral vasoconstriction
Reduction of surface area by body position (or clothing)
Piloerection (not effective in humans)

Increased Heat Production
Shivering
Increased voluntary activity
Increased hormone secretion
Increased appetite

above 75%, evaporation decreases; at levels approaching 90%, evaporation essentially ceases.

Maintenance of Thermoregulation

The balance between heat loss and heat production is constantly changing because of changes in metabolic rate or changes in the external environment. The extent to which the hypothalamus initiates and integrates physiological activity to maintain body temperature is not fully understood. However, several hyperthermic and hypothermic compensatory responses are thought to be the basis for maintaining thermoregulation (Box 25-1).

● HYPERTHERMIA

Heat illness results from one of two basic causes: (1) The normal thermoregulatory mechanisms are overwhelmed by environmental conditions such as heat stress (exogenous heat load) or, more commonly, by excessive exercise in moderate-to-extreme environmental conditions (endogenous heat load) and (2) failure of the thermoregulatory mechanisms, as may be encountered in older adults or ill or debilitated patients. Either cause may result in heat illness such as heat cramps, heat exhaustion, or heat stroke.

Heat Cramps

Heat cramps are brief, intermittent, and often severe muscular cramps that frequently occur in muscles fatigued by heavy work or exercise. They are believed to be caused primarily by a rapid change in extracellular fluid osmolarity resulting from sodium and water loss.

Heat cramps are suffered by persons who sweat profusely and subsequently drink water without adequate salt. During environmental heat stress, 1 to 3 L of water per hour may be lost through sweating. Each liter contains between 30 and 50 mEq of sodium chloride. The water and sodium deficiency combine to cause muscle cramping, which normally occurs in the most heavily exercised muscles, including the calves and arms (al-

though any muscle may be involved). These patients are usually alert with hot, sweaty skin; tachycardia; and normotension; they have a normal core temperature. Heat cramps are easily treated by removing the patient from the hot environment and replacing sodium and water. In severe cases, medical control may recommend intravenous infusion of a saline solution.

Heat Exhaustion

Heat exhaustion is a more severe form of heat illness characterized by minor aberrations in mental status (irritability, poor judgment), dizziness, nausea, headache, and mild-to-moderate core temperature elevation (less than 103° F [39° C]). In severe cases, orthostatic dizziness and syncope may occur.

Like heat cramps, heat exhaustion is more commonly associated with hot ambient temperature; it results in profuse sweating. With water and salt deficiency, electrolyte imbalance and vasomotor regulatory disturbances contribute to inadequate peripheral and cerebral perfusion, the signs of which are characteristic of this illness. Rapid recovery generally follows fluid administration. Patients with significant fluid abnormalities or orthostatic hypotension may require intravenous administration of a saline solution. Left untreated, heat exhaustion may progress to heat stroke.

Heat Stroke

Heat stroke is a syndrome that occurs when the thermoregulatory mechanisms normally in place to meet the demands of heat stress break down entirely. This failure results in body temperature elevated to extreme levels (usually greater than 105.8° F [41° C]), producing multisystem tissue damage and physiological collapse. Heat stroke is a true medical emergency. The syndrome may be classified into two types: classic heat stroke and exertional heat stroke.

Classic heat stroke occurs during periods of sustained high ambient temperatures and humidity. The illness commonly affects the young, older adults, and those who live in poorly ventilated homes without air conditioning. Examples include young children left in an enclosed automobile on a hot afternoon and older persons confined to a hot room during a heat wave. Classic heat stroke victims also frequently suffer from chronic diseases such as diabetes, heart disease, alcoholism, or schizophrenia, which predispose them to the syndrome. Many of these patients take prescribed medications such as diuretics, antihypertensives, tranquilizers, and anticholinergics, which further impair their ability to tolerate heat stress. In these patients, the illness develops from poor dissipation of environmental heat.

In contrast to patients with classic heat stroke, patients with **exertional heat stroke** are usually young and healthy. Commonly afflicted groups include athletes and military recruits who exercise in hot and humid conditions. In these situations, heat accumulates more rapidly in the body than it can be dissipated into the environment.

Clinical Manifestations

Body temperature is controlled in the hypothalamic thermoregulatory centers. These centers receive their information largely from the temperature of circulating blood and from peripheral thermoreceptors in the skin. In response to hypothalamic stimulation, the respiratory rate quickens to increase heat loss via exhaled air, cardiac output expands to provide increased blood flow through skin and muscle to enhance heat radiation, and sweat gland activity increases to enhance evaporative heat loss. These compensatory mechanisms require a normally functioning central nervous system to integrate thermal inputs and initiate appropriate thermoregulatory responses and an intact cardiovascular system to transport excess heat from the core to the periphery. Dysfunction in either or both of these systems leads to rapidly increasing core temperatures.

Central Nervous System Manifestations

The central nervous system manifestations of heat stroke vary. Some patients may be in frank coma; others exhibit confusion and irrational behavior before collapse. Convulsions are common and can occur early or late in the course of the illness. Since the brain stores little energy, it depends on a constant supply of oxygen and glucose. De-

creased cerebral perfusion pressure results in cerebral ischemia and acidosis, and increased temperatures markedly increase the metabolic demands of the brain. The extent of cerebral damage depends on the severity and duration of the hyperthermic episode.

Cardiovascular Manifestations

A rise in skin temperature reduces the thermal gradient between the core and the skin and evokes an increase in skin blood flow (peripheral vasodilation) that results in cutaneous flushing. Although in the classic form of heat stroke sweating is usually absent (because of dehydration, drug use that impairs sweating, direct thermal injury to sweat glands, or sweat gland fatigue), 50% of exertional heat stroke cases have persistent sweating that results from increased catecholamine release. Therefore the presence of sweating does not preclude the diagnosis, and cessation of sweating is not the cause of heat stroke.

As the illness progresses, peripheral vasodilation results in decreased vascular resistance and shunting. High-output cardiac failure is common, manifested by extreme tachycardia and hypotension. Cardiac output may initially be 4 to 5 times that of normal, although as temperatures continue to rise, myocardial contractility begins to decrease and patients can demonstrate an elevated central venous pressure. In any age group, the presence of hypotension and decreased cardiac output indicates a poor prognosis.

Other Systemic Manifestations

Other systemic manifestations that may be associated with heat stroke include pulmonary edema (plus concomitant systemic acidosis, tachypnea, hypoxemia, and hypercapnia), myocardial dysfunction, gastrointestinal bleeding, aberrations in renal function (secondary to hypovolemia and hypoperfusion), hepatic injury, clotting disorders, and electrolyte abnormalities.

Management

If untreated, heat stroke almost invariably culminates in death. The factors most important to a successful outcome are initiation of basic and advanced life-support measures, rapid recognition of the heat illness, and rapid cooling of the patient. After ensuring adequate airway, ventilatory, and circulatory support, the patient with heat stroke should be managed as follows:

1. Move the patient to a cool environment and remove all clothing. If available, use hyperthermic thermometers such as rectal probes or tympanic membrane devices to monitor core temperature. Take and record the temperature at least every 5 minutes during the cooling process to ensure adequate rates of cooling and to avoid rebound hypothermia. Rebound hypothermia can best be avoided by stopping the cooling measures when the patient's core temperature reaches approximately 102° F (39° C).

2. Begin cooling by fanning the patient while keeping the skin wet and massaging the patient with bags of ice or commercial cold packs. Lowering the body temperature by this method should be continued en route to the receiving hospital. If transport is to be delayed, medical control may recommend complete immersion or spraying of tepid water (60° F [16° C]) over the body surface. Ice-water submersion or cold-water cooling should be avoided because these methods may precipitate shivering, frank shaking, peripheral vasoconstriction, and convulsions as the body temperature is being lowered.

3. If hypovolemia is present, give the patient an initial fluid challenge of 500 ml over 15 minutes. In the majority of patients, the blood pressure rises to a normal range during the cooling process as large volumes of blood in the cutaneous vessels shift back to the central circulation (rapid cooling improves cardiac output directly). Therefore be extremely cautious with fluid replacement and closely monitor the patient for signs of fluid overload. Vigorous fluid administration may precipitate pulmonary edema, especially in the older adult.

4. Administer pharmacological agents as prescribed by medical control. Depending on the patient's status and response to cooling methods, these drugs may include *diazepam* for sedation and seizure control, *mannitol* to promote renal blood flow and diuresis, and glucose to treat hypoglycemia.

● ACCIDENTAL HYPOTHERMIA

Hypothermia (core temperature less than 95° F [35° C]) may result from a decrease in heat production, an increase in heat loss, or a combination of the two factors. Although hypothermia may result from metabolic, neurological, traumatic, toxic, and infectious causes, it is most commonly seen in cold climates and during periods of exposure to extreme environmental conditions. Failure to recognize and properly treat hypothermia can lead to significant morbidity and mortality.

Pathophysiology

Cold exposure produces a cascade of physiological events to conserve core heat. Initially there is immediate vasoconstriction in the peripheral vessels and a simultaneous increase in sympathetic nervous discharge, catecholamine release, and basal metabolism. In addition, the heart and respiratory rates increase dramatically, as does the blood pressure. As cold exposure continues, preshivering muscle tone increases, and the body generates heat in the form of shivering. Shivering continues until the core temperature reaches approximately 86° F (30° C), glucose or glycogen is depleted, or insulin is no longer available for glucose transfer. When shivering stops, cooling is rapid, and there is a general decline in all physiological responses.

With continued cooling, respirations decline slowly, pulse and blood pressure decrease, and there are significant decreases in blood pH and commonly electrolyte imbalances. Hypovolemia can develop from a shift of fluid out of the vascular space, with increased loss of fluid through urination (cold diuresis). After early tachycardia, progressive bradycardia develops that is often refractory to *atropine.* Significant electrocardiographic (ECG) changes occur, including prolonged PR, QRS, and QT intervals; obscure or absent P waves; and ST-segment and T-wave abnormalities. In addition, the J wave (Osborn wave) may be present at the junction of the QRS complex and ST segment. These events are generally followed by cardiac and respiratory arrest as the core temperature approaches 68° F (20° C).

The progression of clinical signs and symptoms of hypothermia may be divided into three classes[1]: mild (core temperature between 93.2° and 96.8° F [34° and 36° C]), moderate (core temperature between 86.0° and 93.0° F [30° and 34° C]), and severe (core temperature below 86.0° F [30° C]). Characteristics of the three classes of hypothermia are listed in Table 25-2.

Those at increased risk for developing accidental hypothermia are outdoor enthusiasts (for example, campers, hikers, hunters, fisherman), older adults, the very young, and individuals with concurrent illness. Thermoregulatory mechanisms may also be impaired by brain damage resulting from trauma, hemorrhage, hypoxia, and central nervous system depression from drug overdose or intoxicants. Drugs known to impair thermoregulation include alcohol, antidepressants, antipyretics, phenothiazines, and sedatives. Acid-base imbalances such as those that occur during ketoacidosis may also affect thermostability by decreasing heat production or increasing heat loss.

Management

The first step in managing accidental hypothermia is to maintain a high degree of suspicion for its presence. When the exposure is obvious (for example, a victim involved in an avalanche), diagnosis is simple. However, in some situations, signs and symptoms may be subtle, (for example, hunger, nausea, chills, and dizziness). When hypothermia is suspected, the paramedic's immediate action is to extricate and evacuate the patient to a site of shelter, prevent a further drop in the victim's core temperature, survey for traumatic injuries, and rapidly transport the patient for definitive care. Fig. 25-1 presents a treatment algorithm for hypothermia.

Mild-to-Moderate Hypothermia

In mild-to-moderate cases of hypothermia, removal of the victim from the cold environment and passive rewarming may be all that are necessary to manage the cold exposure. This may be accomplished by removing wet clothing (wet clothes allow 5 times as much heat loss as dry clothes) and wrapping the victim in a dry blanket to prevent further chilling and help retain endogenously produced heat. If the victim is conscious, warm drinks and sugar sources may support a gradual rise in core temperature and help correct any dehydration present. Alcoholic beverages (which produce peripheral vasodilation and increase heat loss from the skin) and coffee and tea (which may cause vasoconstriction and diuresis) should be avoided. These patients may be lethargic and somewhat dulled mentally but are generally oriented with no marked mental derangements.

External application of hot packs (covered with towels to avoid burns) to the neck, armpits, and groin is considered a safe and effective way to re-

TABLE 25-2 Progression of Clinical Signs and Symptoms of Hypothermia

Class	Core Temperature °C	°F	Signs and Symptoms
Mild	36°	96.8°	Increased metabolic rate, maximum shivering, thermogenesis
	34°	93.2°	Impaired judgment, slurred speech
Moderate	30°	86.0°	Respiratory depression, myocardial irritability, bradycardia, atrial fibrillation, Osborne waves
Severe	<30°	<86.0°	Basal metabolic rate that is 50% of normal, loss of deep tendon reflexes, fixed and dilated pupils, spontaneous ventricular fibrillation

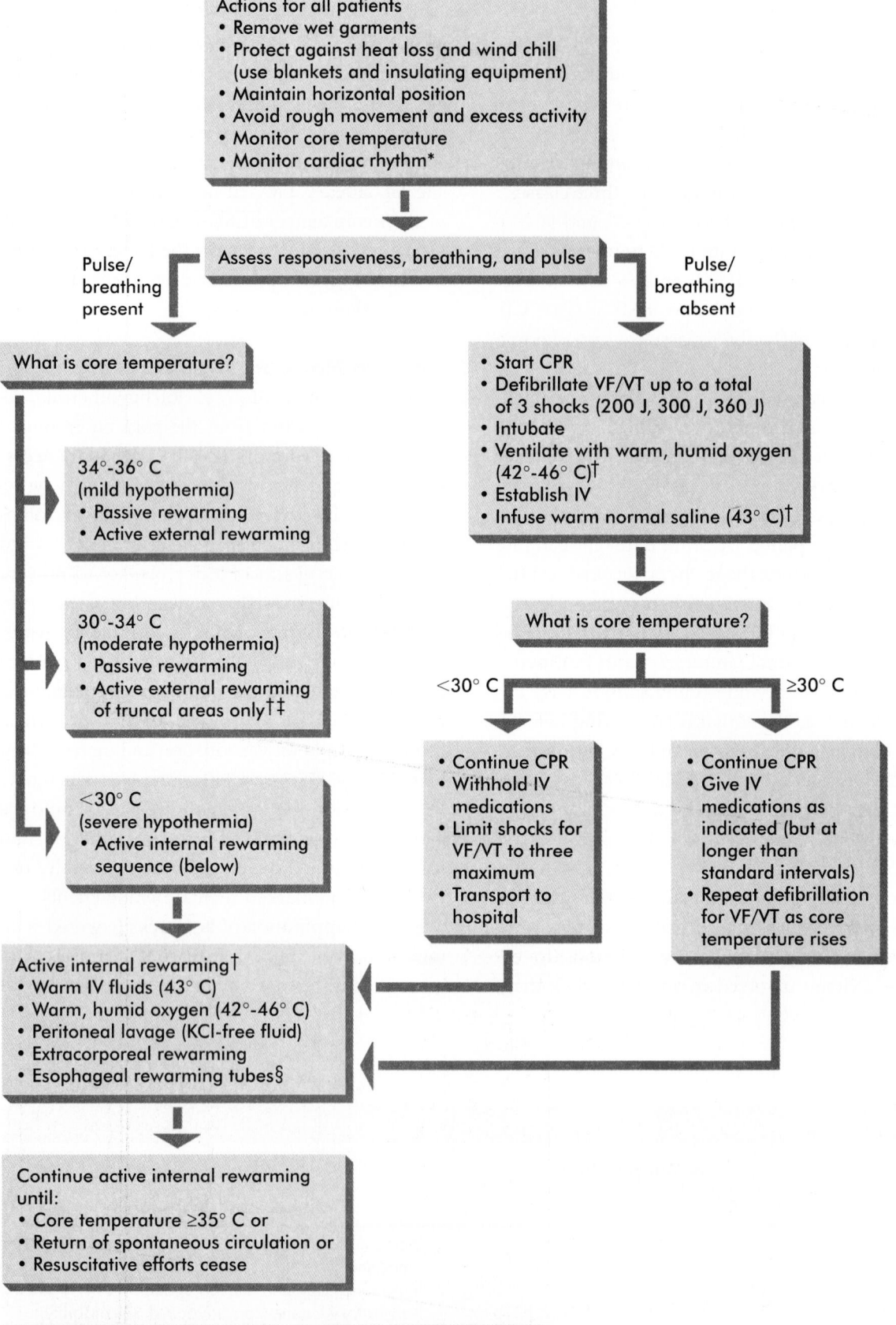

Fig. 25-1 Algorithm for the treatment of hypothermia. (Reproduced with permission, CPR Issue of *JAMA*, Oct 28, 1992. Copyright © American Medical Association.)

warm these patients. (Intravenous fluid therapy may be warranted to correct a drop in blood pressure caused by heat-stimulated peripheral vasodilation.) If possible, heated, humidified oxygen should be administered. Patients with mild-to-moderate hypothermia generally improve rapidly with proper treatment. However, close monitoring and transportation for physician evaluation are indicated.

Moderate-to-Severe Hypothermia

At core temperatures below 90° F (32° C), mental derangements are invariably present and may include disorientation, confusion, and lethargy proceeding to stupor and coma. These patients have usually lost their ability to shiver, and their uncoordinated physical activity renders them unable to perform meaningful tasks.

Treatment for these patients begins with ensuring adequate airway, ventilatory, and circulatory support and maintaining body temperature. These patients should not be permitted to move about independently or physically exert themselves. Even minor physical activity can bring about dysrhythmias, including ventricular fibrillation. Moderate hypothermia should be managed with external heat application; heated, humidified oxygen administration; intravenous fluid therapy; and rapid and gentle transport for definitive care. Careful monitoring of the patient's mental status, ECG, and vital functions is imperative. If low-reading thermometers are available, they should be used to measure the patient's core temperature at 5-minute intervals.

If core temperature is below 82.4° F (28° C), the patient is usually unconscious. If vital signs are present, the patient should be gently moved to a warm environment. Passive external rewarming and heated, humidified oxygen administration should be instituted during transport to a medical facility. Airway management should be limited to basic manual procedures (head-tilt, chin-lift) and slow ventilatory assistance. The use of oral or nasal adjuncts, including intubation, may induce ventricular dysrhythmias, and overzealous ventilatory assistance can induce hypocapnia and resultant ventricular irritability. However, when indicated, these procedures should not be withheld.

Medical control may recommend the administration of *thiamine, 50% dextrose, naloxone,* and an initial fluid challenge of 250 to 500 ml of D_5W or normal saline. (Lactated Ringer's solution should be avoided because the cold liver may not be able to metabolize the lactate.)

Severely hypothermic patients have no vital signs, including respiratory effort, pulse, and blood pressure. Depending on core temperature, cyanosis, fixed and dilated pupils, and stiff and rigid muscles (simulating rigor mortis) may be present. Prolonged resuscitation may be beneficial in severely hypothermic patients, and cardiopulmonary resuscitation (CPR) is indicated even if signs of death are present. Hypothermic patients cannot be presumed dead until a core temperature of 89.6° F (32° C) has been achieved and resuscitation efforts are still unsuccessful. A nonperfusing rhythm (ventricular fibrillation, pulseless ventricular tachycardia, or asystole) should be confirmed by ECG monitor for a minimum of 30 to 45 seconds, and CPR should only be instituted if there are absolutely no vital signs.

If the patient in cardiac arrest fails to respond to initial defibrillation attempts, subsequent defibrillations or additional cardiac life support medications should be avoided until the patient has been rewarmed in the emergency department. These patients need to be rapidly transported to a facility that can institute internal core rewarming techniques. In patients with vital signs, the rewarming technique of choice is to place the patient on cardiopulmonary bypass (active core rewarming) to sustain perfusion and to rewarm the patient concurrently. Peritoneal and pleural lavage have also been used to successfully treat patients with profound hypothermia and cardiac arrest.

Most authorities agree that active rewarming methods other than the administration of heated, humidified oxygen are inappropriate field care for severe hypothermia. Rewarming methods such as hot water immersion may cause hypotension from peripheral vasodilation (rewarming shock) and a sudden return of cold blood and waste products to the body's core (afterdrop phenomenon). Therefore active field rewarming techniques should generally be avoided unless patient transport is to be delayed.

● FROSTBITE

Frostbite is a localized injury that results from environmentally induced freezing of body tissues. It frequently occurs in the lower extremities (particularly the toes and feet) and less commonly in the upper extremities (particularly the fingers and hands). Frostbite may also occur in the ears, nose, and other body areas that are unprotected from environmental extremes.

Pathophysiology

Frostbite is thought to occur as ice crystals form in tissue, producing macrovascular and microvascular abnormalities as well as direct cellular injury. The freezing depth depends on the intensity and duration of cold exposure. In addition, severe freezing can occur in tissue exposed to volatile hydrocarbons at low temperatures.

Under most conditions of frostbite, ice crystals form in the extracellular tissue. This draws water out of the cells into the extravascular spaces, allowing the electrolyte concentration within the cell to reach toxic levels. These crystals can also expand and cause direct mechanical destruction of tissue. This phenomenon leads to damage of blood vessels (particularly the endothelial cells), partial shrinkage and collapse of the cell membrane, loss of vascular integrity, local edema, and disruption of nutritive blood flow. Ischemia often produces the most damaging effects of frostbite.

When frozen tissue thaws, capillary patency is initially restored, but blood flow declines within minutes after thawing through vasoconstriction of arterioles and venules and the release of emboli that course through microvessels. Ultimately, there is progressive tissue loss from thrombosis and hypoxia. This vascular injury damages the endothelium and results in deterioration of the microvasculature and dermal necrosis. Thawing and refreezing is more dangerous to tissue than allowing the frostbitten part to remain frozen until it can be warmed with minimal risk of refreezing.

In addition to extreme temperature, wind, and humidity, predisposing factors to frostbite include:
- Lack of protective clothing
- Poor nutrition
- Preexisting injury or illness
- Fatigue
- Decrease in local tissue perfusion
  ◦ Tobacco
  ◦ Atherosclerosis
  ◦ Tight constrictive clothing
- Increase in vasodilation
  ◦ Alcohol
  ◦ Medications
- History of previous cold injury

Classifications and Symptoms

There are numerous classifications for cold injury. A common one separates cold injury into three categories: frostnip, superficial frostbite, and deep frostbite. **Frostnip,** the mildest form of cold injury, may be treated without loss of tissue. In superficial frostbite there is at least some minimal tissue loss; with deep frostbite there is significant tissue loss even with appropriate therapy. Superficial frostbite usually involves the dermis and shallow subcutaneous layers, whereas deep frostbite is associated with subdermal layers and deep tissues.

The initial evaluation of severity is difficult because the injury does not always reflect underlying vascular changes. Regardless of the depth of injury, the area may appear to be frozen; palpation may distinguish between superficial and deep injury. With superficial injury, the underlying tissue feels resilient on compression, whereas in deep injury the underlying tissue is hard and not compressible.

Superficial Frostbite

In most patients with **superficial frostbite,** the initial symptoms are coldness and numbness in the affected area. This is followed by extreme pain (tingling and throbbing) during rewarming. After rewarming, edema usually appears within 3 hours, followed by the formation of vesicles within 3 to 24 hours (Fig. 25-2). These blisters begin to resolve within a week, after which the skin blackens into a hard eschar. Eventually, the blackened tissue peels away (demarcation), revealing shiny, red skin beneath. This tissue is sensitive to heat and cold and for unknown reasons remains unusually susceptible to repeated frostbite injury.

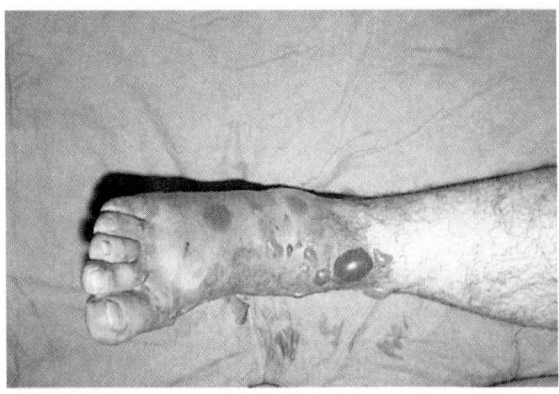

Fig. 25-2 Edema and blister formation 24 hours after frostbite injury in an area covered by a tightly fitted boot.

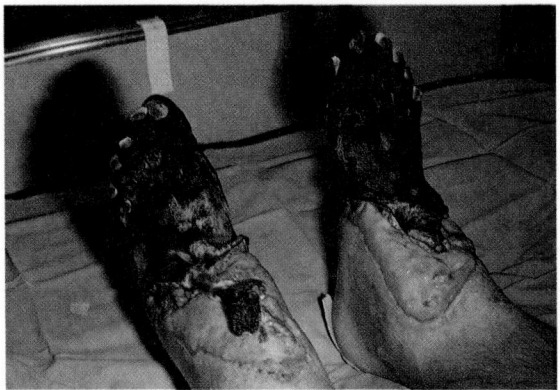

Fig. 25-3 Gangrenous necrosis 6 weeks after a frostbite injury.

Deep Frostbite

In **deep frostbite,** the disrupted nutritional capillary flow is never restored to the patient's damaged tissue. The affected area remains cold, mottled, and blue or gray after rewarming. During the first 9 to 15 days, severely frostbitten skin forms a black, hard eschar. In contrast to superficial frostbite, edema is slow to develop. Deep blisters with purple blood-containing fluid may appear within 1 to 3 weeks. Within 22 to 45 days, definite lines of demarcation between the eschar and viable tissue develop. Eventually, nonviable skin and deep structures mummify and slough (Fig. 25-3).

Management

Prehospital care for frostbite is limited to supporting the patient's vital functions, elevation and protection of the affected extremity, and rapid transport to a medical facility. Vigorous rubbing is ineffective and potentially harmful, and partial, slow rewarming with blankets or other warm objects is injurious. If frostbite involves the patient's lower extremities, he or she should not be permitted to walk. During transport, change all of the patient's restrictive and wet clothing to guard against hypothermia. Consumption of alcohol and tobacco smoking should be prohibited. Rapid rewarming of the frozen part is the most effective therapeutic measure for preserving viable tissue. This should not be attempted in the prehospital setting because the risk of refreezing is present.

● NEAR-DROWNING

According to the National Safety Council, drowning was the fifth leading cause of accidental death in the United States in 1991, accounting for more than 4600 deaths. In addition, there are approximately 80,000 near-drownings reported each year. Of these, 85% of near-drowning victims are male, and two thirds of the victims are nonswimmers.[2]

Classifications

There are numerous classifications of submersion incidents. For the purposes of this text, **drowning** is defined as death by asphyxia after submersion. **Near-drowning** is submersion with at least temporary survival. Victims of submersion incidents usually fall into one of two categories. The first category includes conscious victims such as exhausted swimmers, river canoeists who become trapped by roots or strong currents, persons who have fallen overboard or off a dock, and motor vehicle crash victims trapped in submerged vehicles. The second category includes unconscious patients, such as those who have suffered a stroke or cardiac arrest while swimming and those who have fallen into water and succumbed to hypothermia.

Pathophysiology

Drowning begins with intentional or accidental submersion. After submersion, the victim realizes

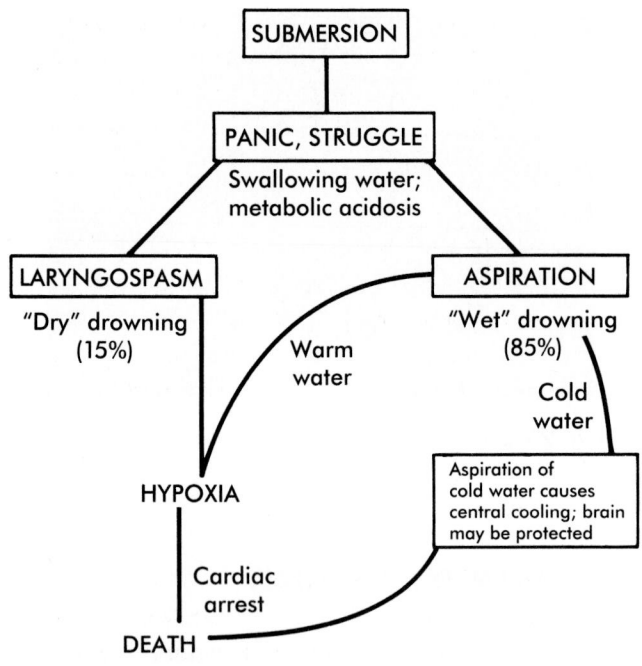

Fig. 25-4 Progression of the drowning incident.

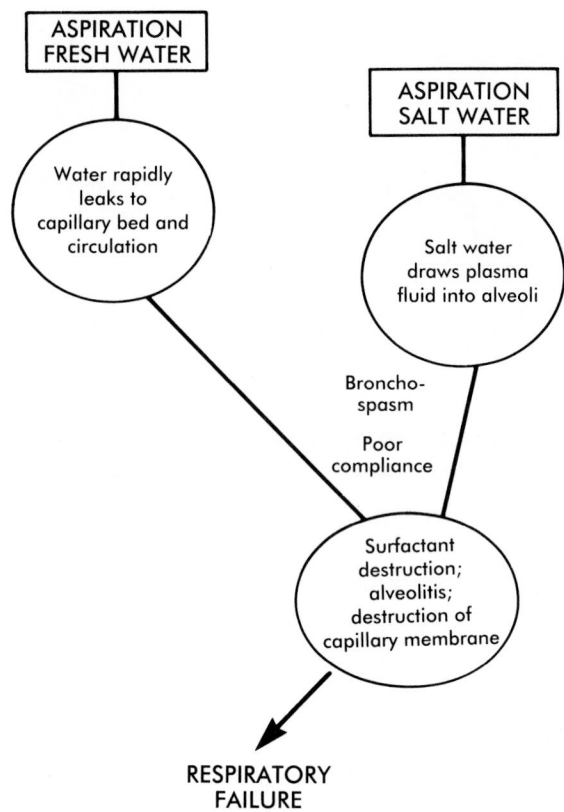

Fig. 25-5 Pulmonary effects of water aspiration.

that a near-drowning event may ensue (for example, a nonswimmer who panics or a swimmer who tires). The sequence of events that leads to drowning begins with the conscious victim taking in several deep breaths in an attempt to store oxygen before breath-holding (Fig. 25-4). The victim holds the breath until reflex inspiratory efforts override the breath-holding effort. As water is aspirated, laryngospasm occurs. Laryngospasm and aspiration produce severe hypoxia. The resultant profound hypoxemia and acidosis lead to cardiac dysrhythmias and central nervous system anoxia. In 10% of drownings, the laryngospasm is severe enough that very little fluid is aspirated ("dry drowning"); in the remaining 90% of drownings, fluid enters the lungs ("wet drowning"). The physiological events that follow are determined by the type and amount of water aspirated. Regardless of the type of water aspirated, the pathophysiology of drowning is characterized by hypoxia, hypercapnia, and acidosis, which result in cardiac arrest.

Drowning may occur in almost any type of water. Victims of submersion may aspirate saltwater or fresh water, tap water, or contaminated water (such as water containing sewage, chemicals, algae, bacteria, or sand). Although the type of water is not important in the initial management of near-drowning, saltwater drowning can produce different pathophysiological responses than those seen in fresh-water drowning, which may affect patient outcome (Fig. 25-5).

Saltwater is a hypertonic fluid that tends to cause a rapid shift of plasma and fluid into the alveoli and interstitial spaces of lung parenchyma. This fluid shift results in pulmonary edema, poorly ventilated alveoli, and hypoxia.

Fresh water is hypotonic to plasma and passes readily out of the alveoli into the circulation. If sufficient volume is aspirated (over 20 ml/kg, an amount found in only 15% of drowning victims), blood volume can increase and hemolysis can result. In addition, fresh water leads to surfactant destruction ("washout"), producing reduced compliance, alveolar collapse, and hypoxia. If enough fresh water is absorbed, hemolysis may result in subsequent hyperkalemia and anemia. Dangerous electrolyte abnormalities may also occur in this setting.

Pulmonary Pathophysiology Secondary to Near-Drowning

Respiratory failure and ischemic neurological injury from hypoxia and acidosis are the life-threatening complications of submersion. Hypoxia may result from the following factors: fluid in the alveoli and interstitial spaces, loss of surfactant, contaminant particles in the alveoli and tracheobronchial tree, and damage to the alveolar-capillary membrane and vascular endothelium. Poor perfusion and hypoxemia lead to metabolic acidosis in the majority of patients. In those who survive the incident, acute respiratory failure may follow, with a reduction in compliance and an increase in ventilation-perfusion mismatching and intrapulmonary shunting. The onset of symptoms may be delayed for as long as 24 hours after the submersion.

In addition to having pulmonary effects, near-drowning may affect other body systems. For example, cardiovascular derangements may occur secondary to hypoxia and acidosis, resulting in dysrhythmias and decreased cardiac output. Central nervous system dysfunction and neuronal damage are commonly caused by cerebral edema and anoxia. One must also be suspicious of concurrent spinal injury in near-drowning victims. Renal dysfunction is unusual but may progress to acute renal failure as a result of hypoxic injury or hemoglobinuria, leading to acute tubular necrosis.

Factors that Affect Clinical Outcome

Four factors that can affect clinical outcome after a submersion incident include the following:

1. Temperature of the water: Submersion in cold water can have beneficial as well as deleterious effects on survival. The rapid development of hypothermia can serve a protective function, particularly regarding brain viability in patients with prolonged submersion. (The survival of a child submerged for 66 minutes in a creek with a water temperature of 37° F (5° C) is the longest documented submersion with good neurological outcome.[3]) The exact mechanism of this phenomenon is not understood; in the past it was attributed to a "mammalian diving reflex" found in seals and lower mammals. Hypothermia itself also contributes to neurological recovery after prolonged submersion, probably by decreasing the metabolic needs of the brain. The relative contributions of these two mechanisms are not clear. The adverse effects of cold water submersion include the occurrence of severe ventricular dysrhythmias.

2. Length of submersion: The longer the duration of submersion, the less likely the patient is to survive. When rescue operations have been in progress for more than 30 minutes, victims retrieved from warm water in summer months or in warm southern waters are usually considered nonviable. Because cold water submersion for up to 60 minutes has been associated with neurological recovery, most patients rescued from cold-water drowning should receive resuscitative life-support measures. Resuscitation is not indicated if there is evidence of putrefaction or submersion for more than 1 hour.

3. Cleanliness of the water: Contaminants in water have an irritant effect on the pulmonary system, leading to bronchospasm and an increased tendency toward poor gas exchange. They can also cause a secondary pulmonary infection with delayed severe respiratory compromise.

4. Age of the victim: The younger the patient, the better the chance for survival.

Management

Safety at the scene and of the EMS crew are of paramount importance at the site of a submersion incident, and only personnel trained in water rescue should attempt emergency intervention. Depending on the type and duration of submersion, patients may vary from an asymptomatic presentation to cardiac arrest. After gaining access to the victim, spinal precautions should be taken while the victim is still in the water (see Chapter 15), and rescue breathing (if needed) should be initiated as soon as possible.

After extrication from the water, the patient should be evaluated to ensure an adequate airway and ventilatory and circulatory support. Other initial patient care management includes high-concentration oxygen administration, ECG monitoring, and establishment of an intravenous line. Patients who are in cardiac arrest should be managed with standard basic and advanced life-support protocols and rapid transport to the receiving hospital.

Victims of submersion incidents are often at risk from immersion hypothermia; heat loss in water may be up to 32 times greater than in air. Hypothermia can make resuscitation more difficult and requires special consideration with reference to gentle handling, use of pharmacological agents, and defibrillation. As with all other hypothermic patients, wet clothes should be removed and the patient dried and wrapped in blankets to maintain body heat. External warming and the administration of heated, humidified oxygen should be considered at the scene and during transport.

Asymptomatic patients also require transport for physician evaluation. These patients should receive oxygen and be carefully monitored to guard against aspiration pneumonia and undetected hypoxia that may result from the submersion incident. Oxygen is the most important treatment required by near-drowning victims.

● DIVING EMERGENCIES

It is estimated that there are more than 3 million recreational scuba divers in the United States and over 300,000 new sport divers certified each year. The medical emergencies unique to pressure-related diving include those caused by the mechanical effects of pressure (barotrauma), air embolism, and breathing compressed air (decompression sickness and nitrogen narcosis).[4]

Mechanical Effects of Pressure

When a scuba diver submerges under water, the ambient pressure to which the diver is exposed in-

creases because of the weight of the water. Water is much denser than air, so pressure changes are greater under water, even at reasonably shallow depths (a depth of 33 feet is equal to 2 atmospheres (2 atm) of pressure). Since body tissues are composed mostly of water (which is not compressible), they are not directly affected by pressure changes. However, gases are compressible, and gas-filled organs of the body are directly affected by pressure changes.

Basic Properties of Gases

The laws pertaining to the basic properties of gas responsible for all pressure-related diving emergencies are Boyle's law, Dalton's law, and Henry's law.

Boyle's law states that the volume of gas is inversely related to its pressure at a constant temperature. This is expressed by $PV = K$, where P is pressure, V is volume, and K is a constant. Thus when the pressure is doubled, the volume of gas is halved, and vice versa. This principle is the basic mechanism for all types of barotrauma.

Dalton's law states that the pressure exerted by each individual gas in a mixture of gases is the same as it would exert if it alone occupied the same volume; alternatively, the total pressure of a mixture of gases equals the sum of the partial pressures of the component gases. This law is expressed by the equation $P_t = P_{O_2} + P_{N_2} + P_x$ where P is the total pressure, P_{O_2} is the partial pressure of oxygen, P_{N_2} is the partial pressure of nitrogen, and P_x is the partial pressure of the remaining gases in the mixture. The principles of this law explain problems caused by breathing compressed air.

Henry's law states that the amount of gas dissolved in a given volume of fluid is proportional to the pressure of the gas with which it is in equilibrium. The law is expressed by the equation $\%X = P_x/P_t \times 100$, where $\%X$ is the amount of gas dissolved in a liquid, P_x is the partial pressure of gas X, and P_t is the total atmospheric pressure. This law explains why more nitrogen (which makes up almost 80% of air) dissolves in the diver's body as ambient pressure increases with descent. This dissolved nitrogen is then released from tissues on ascent.

Barotrauma

Barotrauma is tissue damage that results from compression or expansion of gas spaces when the gas pressure in the body (or its compartments) differs from ambient pressure. The type of injury produced by barotrauma depends on whether the diver is in descent or ascent. Barotrauma is the most common affliction of scuba divers.

Barotrauma of Descent

Barotrauma of descent (also known as *squeeze*) results from the compression of gas in enclosed spaces as the ambient pressure increases with descent under water. Air trapped in noncollapsible chambers is compressed, leading to a vacuum-type effect that results in severe, sharp pain caused by the distortion; vascular engorgement; edema; and hemorrhage of the exposed tissue (Box 25-2). As a rule, squeeze usually results from a blocked eustachian tube or from failure of the diver to clear the eustachian tube with exhalation during descent. The ears and paranasal sinuses are most likely to be affected. Squeeze may occur in the ears, sinuses, lungs and airways, gastroin-

---

BOX 25-2

Signs and Symptoms of Diving-Related Conditions

Squeeze
Pain
Sensation of fullness
Headache
Disorientation
Vertigo
Nausea
Bleeding from the nose or ears

POPS
Gradually increasing chest pain
Hoarseness
Neck fullness
Dyspnea
Dysphagia
Subcutaneous emphysema

Air Embolism
Focal paralysis or sensory changes (strokelike symptoms)
Aphasia
Confusion
Blindness or other visual disturbances
Convulsions
Loss of consciousness
Dizziness
Vertigo
Abdominal pain
Cardiac arrest

Decompression Sickness
Shortness of breath
Itch
Rash
Joint pain
Crepitus
Fatigue
Vertigo
Paresthesias
Paralysis
Seizures
Unconsciousness

Nitrogen Narcosis
Impaired judgment
Sensation of alcohol intoxication
Slowed motor response
Loss of proprioception
Euphoria

testinal tract, thorax, teeth (pulp decay, recent extraction sockets or fillings), or added air spaces (face mask or diving suit).

Management of barotrauma of descent begins with the diver performing a gradual ascent to shallower depths. Prehospital care is largely supportive. After physician evaluation, definitive care may include bed rest with the head elevated, avoidance of strain and strenuous activity, use of decongestants and possibly antihistamines and antibiotics, and perhaps surgical repair.

Barotrauma of Ascent

Barotrauma of ascent occurs through the reverse process of descent ("reverse squeeze"). Assuming that the air-filled cavities of the body have equalized pressure during the diver's descent, air trapped in those spaces expands as ambient pressure decreases with ascent (Boyle's law). If air is not allowed to escape because of obstruction, the expanding gases distend the tissues surrounding them. The most common cause of this type of barotrauma is breath-holding during ascent because of running out of air at depth or of panic.

Although problems from reverse squeeze are rare, pulmonary overpressurization syndrome (POPS) resulting from expansion of trapped air in the lungs occurs. POPS may lead to alveolar rupture and extravasation of air into extraalveolar locations (see Box 25-2). The clinical syndromes associated with barotrauma of ascent include pneumomediastinum, subcutaneous emphysema, pneumopericardium, pneumothorax, pneumoperitoneum, and systemic arterial air embolism. Except for pneumothorax (rare), which may call for management by needle decompression (see Chapter 15), and air embolism, POPS usually requires only oxygen administration, observation, and transport for physician evaluation.

Air Embolism

Air embolism is the most serious complication of pulmonary barotrauma and is a major cause of death and disability among sport divers. Divers risk this injury when they ascend too rapidly or when they hold their breath during ascent.

Air embolism results as high-pressure air is forced into the circulatory system through ruptured pulmonary veins. The air bubbles pass through the heart and become lodged in small arteries, occluding distal circulation. The syndrome usually presents as the diver surfaces and exhales, releasing the high intrapulmonic pressure that resulted from lung overexpansion. With the decrease in intrathoracic pressure, bubbles return to the left side of the heart, resulting in a dramatic presentation, with clinical manifestations that depend on the site of systemic arterial occlusion (see Box 25-2).

Air embolism should be suspected when a diver suddenly loses consciousness immediately on surfacing. Basic and advanced life-support measures should be instituted, and the patient should be rapidly transported for recompression treatment. If endotracheal intubation is necessary, the balloon should be filled with normal saline, not air, to avoid inadvertent extubation during recompression. In addition, the patient should be thoroughly evaluated for signs of POPS such as a pneumothorax.

A patient with a suspected air embolism should be transported in a left lateral recumbent position with a 15-degree elevation of the thorax if not contraindicated by injury. Some medical-control agencies recommend that the patient be transported in a supine position to avoid aggravating cerebral edema that may develop. (The paramedic should follow local protocol.) If air transportation is to be used, the diver should be transported by aircraft pressurized to sea level so that existing intraarterial air bubbles do not expand further. The flight altitude must be as low as possible, never over 1000 feet above sea level.

Recompression

Recompression is accomplished in a hyperbaric chamber. Treatment consists of rapidly increasing ambient pressure (recompression) to reduce intravascular bubble volume and restore tissue perfusion. In addition, oxygen-enriched breathing mixtures are used to enhance bubble resolution and to supply oxygen to partially ischemic and hypoxic nervous tissue. Slow decompression is calculated to avoid the re-formation of bubbles. The paramedic should be familiar with the location of the nearest hyperbaric treatment facility and follow protocol established by medical control.

Decompression Sickness

Decompression sickness is also known as *the bends, dysbarism, caisson disease,* and *diver's paralysis.* It is a multisystem disorder that results when nitrogen in compressed air dissolved into tissues and blood (because of the increase in its partial pressure at depth) converts back from solution to gas, forming bubbles in the tissues and blood. The syndrome occurs when the ambient pressure decreases (Henry's law) and results from too rapid ascent, in which equilibrium between the dissolved nitrogen in tissue and blood and the partial pressure of nitrogen in the inspired gas cannot be established.

The most significant mechanical effect of bubbles is vascular occlusion that impairs venous return. Since the bubbles can form in any tissue, lymphedema, cellular distention, and cellular rupture can also occur (see Box 25-2). The net effect of all these processes is poor tissue perfusion and ischemia. The joints and the spinal cord are the anatomical areas most often affected.

Decompression sickness should be suspected in any patient who has symptoms within 12 to 36 hours after a scuba dive that cannot be adequately explained by other conditions. Prehospital care includes support of vital functions, high-concentration oxygen administration, fluid resuscitation, and rapid transport for recompression. The patient transport and air evacuation guidelines described for air embolism should also be used when caring for these patients.

Nitrogen Narcosis

Nitrogen narcosis ("rapture of the deep") is a condition in which nitrogen becomes dissolved in solution as a result of greater-than-normal pressures. Dissolved nitrogen produces neurodepressant effects similar to those of alcohol and may impair the diver's judgment and discrimination (see Box 25-2). Symptoms of nitrogen narcosis usually become evident at depths between 75 and 100 feet.

At depths over 300 feet, unconsciousness ensues. Nitrogen narcosis affects all divers but tends to be better tolerated by experienced divers.

The narcotic effects of nitrogen are reversed with ascent. The syndrome is a common precipitating factor in diving accidents and may be responsible for memory loss about events before the episode. Prehospital care is primarily supportive. The patient should be assessed for injuries that may have occurred during the diving episode and transported for physician evaluation.

● HIGH-ALTITUDE ILLNESS

High-altitude illness is attributed directly to exposure to reduced atmospheric pressure, resulting in hypobaric hypoxia. Activities associated with these syndromes include mountain climbing, aircraft or glider flight, and use of hot-air balloons and low-pressure or vacuum chambers. The high-altitude syndromes discussed in this chapter are acute mountain sickness (AMS), high-altitude pulmonary edema (HAPE), and high-altitude cerebral edema (HACE). Emergency care for all forms of high-altitude illness includes airway, ventilatory, and circulatory support and descent to a lower altitude. In addition, all patients with high-altitude illness should be evaluated by a physician.

Acute Mountain Sickness

AMS is a common high-altitude illness that results from rapid ascent of an unacclimatized person to altitudes of 8000 feet or more. The illness in susceptible individuals usually develops within 4 to 6 hours of reaching high altitude, attains maximal severity within 24 to 48 hours, and abates on the third or fourth day after exposure (Box 25-3).

Physical findings are variable and may include tachycardia, bradycardia, postural hypotension, and ataxia (the most useful sign for recognizing the progression of the illness). As AMS becomes severe, the victim may experience alterations in consciousness, disorientation, and impaired judgment. Coma may ensue within 24 hours after on-

---

BOX 25-3

Signs and Symptoms of High-Altitude Illness

AMS

Headache (most common symptom) attributed to subacute cerebral edema or to spasm or dilation of cerebral blood vessels secondary to hypocapnia or hypoxia
Malaise
Anorexia
Vomiting
Dizziness
Irritability
Impaired memory
Dyspnea on exertion

HAPE

Shortness of breath
Dyspnea
Cough (with or without frothy sputum)
Generalized weakness
Lethargy
Disorientation

HACE

Headache
Ataxia
Altered consciousness
Confusion
Hallucinations
Drowsiness
Stupor
Coma

---

set of ataxia. Emergency care includes oxygen administration and descent to as low an altitude as necessary to achieve relief. Definitive treatment after physician evaluation may involve the use of diuretics to treat fluid retention associated with AMS, steroids to reduce associated cerebral edema, and hyperbaric therapy.

High-Altitude Pulmonary Edema

HAPE is thought to be caused at least in part by increased pulmonary artery pressure that develops in response to hypoxia. The increased pressure results in the release of leukotrienes, which increase pulmonary arteriolar permeability, and in leakage of fluid into extravascular locations. Initial symptoms of HAPE usually begin 24 to 72 hours after exposure to high altitudes and are often preceded by strenuous exercise (see Box 25-3).

Physical findings in patients include hyperpnea, crackles, rhonchi, tachycardia, and cyanosis. Emergency care includes oxygen administration to increase arterial oxygenation and reduce pulmonary artery pressure and descent to lower altitude. After physician evaluation, the patient may be hospitalized for observation.

High Altitude Cerebral Edema

HACE is the most severe form of acute high-altitude illness. It is characterized by a progression of global cerebral signs in the presence of AMS that are probably related to increased intracranial pressure. Therefore the distinctions between AMS and HACE are inherently blurred. The progression from mild AMS to unconsciousness associated with HACE may be as fast as 12 hours but usually requires 1 to 3 days of exposure to high altitudes (see Box 25-3).

Management of HACE must be prompt because the syndrome rapidly progresses to stupor, coma, and death without treatment. Like other forms of high-altitude illness, emergency care is focused on airway, ventilatory, and circulatory support and descent to a lower altitude.

REFERENCES

1. Guidelines for cardiopulmonary resuscitation and emergency cardiac care, *JAMA* 268(16):2172, 1992.
2. National Safety Council: *Accident facts,* Chicago, 1992, The Council.
3. Callaham M: *Current practice of emergency medicine,* ed 2, Philadelphia, 1991, BC Decker.
4. Tintinalli J et al: *Emergency medicine: a comprehensive study guide,* ed 2, New York, 1988, McGraw-Hill.

Summary

Exposure to environmental elements may produce life-threatening emergencies. The paramedic should be familiar with specific exposures likely to occur in the immediate response area, exercise caution, and use personal protection during rescue attempts and while providing emergency care.

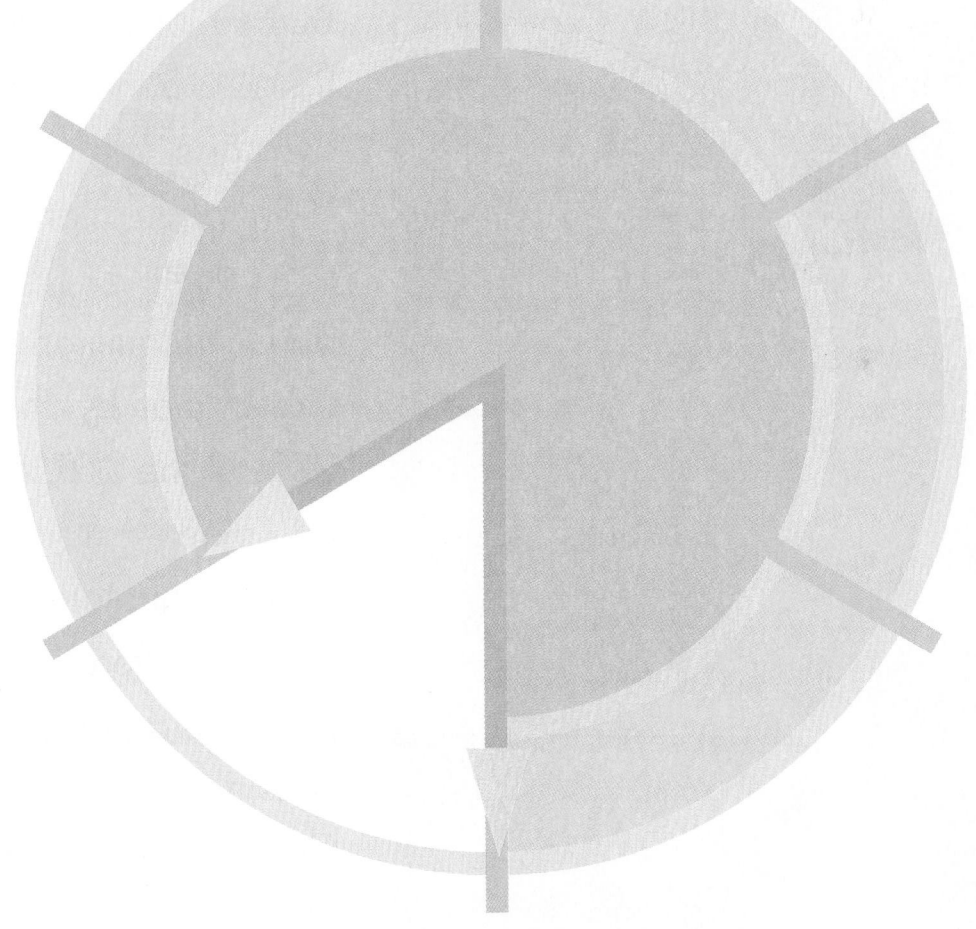

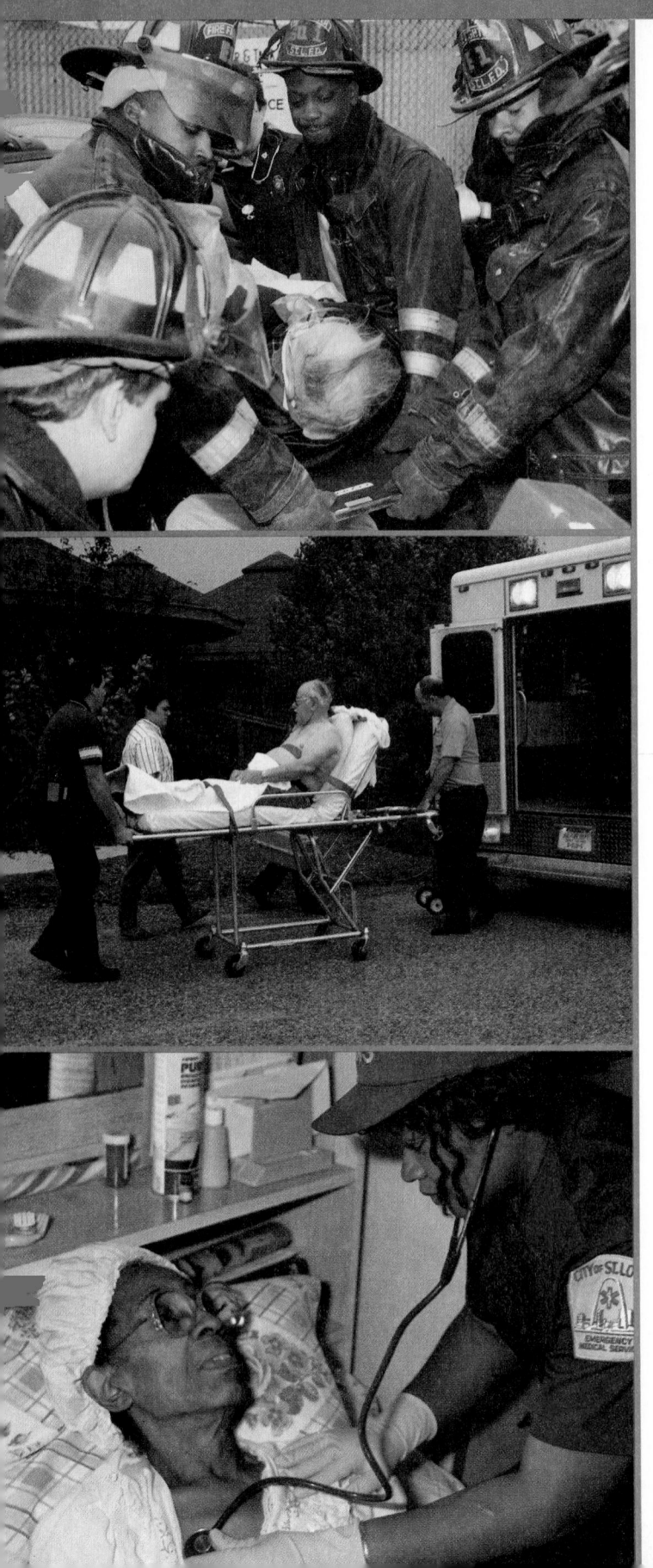

The progressive "graying" of American society carries with it the prospect that the health care needs of older adults will continue to increase in all areas, including prehospital care. In 1983, the U.S. Department of Commerce Bureau of the Census reported that 26.5 million people were over age 65 (some 11% of the U.S. population). Since then, that number has climbed to about 40 million, and it is estimated that by the year 2050, 20% of the U.S. population will be older.[1] This chapter addresses anatomical and physiological alterations that accompany the aging process, special considerations in assessing and managing the older patient, and common medical emergencies that may result from normal aging and chronic illness.

As a paramedic, you should be able to:

1. Describe the pathophysiology of the aging process as it relates to major body systems and homeostasis.
2. Describe physical assessment techniques specific to older adults.
3. Discuss the effects of aging as they relate to the physiological response to trauma.
4. Describe management techniques specific to older patients who have sustained trauma.
5. Discuss incidence and unique features of selected medical problems in the older patient.
6. Distinguish between delirium and dementia.
7. Discuss the incidence and symptoms of depression in the geriatric population.
8. Identify factors that contribute to drug toxicity in the older adult.

● PHYSIOLOGICAL CHANGES OF AGING

Gerontology is the study of the problems of all aspects of aging. The aging process proceeds at different rates in different people and among various organs. In certain areas, however, predictable functional declines occur in all people with increasing age. As a rough guideline, these changes begin to occur at a rate of 5% to 10% for each decade of life after the age of 30. Although all body systems are affected by the aging process, the effects on specific organ systems particularly relevant to the older adult are those that occur in the respiratory system, cardiovascular system, renal system, nervous system, and musculoskeletal system.

Respiratory System Changes

Respiratory function in the older adult is generally compromised as a result of changes in pulmonary physiology that accompany the aging process. Reduced pulmonary capacity is related to alterations in lung and chest wall compliance. With aging, the chest wall becomes increasingly stiff as the bony thorax becomes more rigid, and lung elastic recoil decreases. Despite the loss of elastic recoil, which would tend to increase total lung capacity, total lung capacity remains unchanged because of the opposing loss of chest wall compliance and weakened respiratory muscles. Variable increases in alveolar diameter and the tendency for distal airways to collapse on expiration lead to an increase in residual volume and a decrease in vital capacity. Consequently, by age 75, vital capacity may decrease by as much as 50%, maximum breathing capacity by as much as 60%, and maximum work rate and maximum oxygen uptake by as much as 70%.

Arterial oxygen pressure (Pa_{O_2}) also slowly decreases with age, but arterial carbon dioxide pressure (Pa_{CO_2}) remains unchanged (probably related to the much greater reserve in carbon dioxide elimination than in oxygen absorption). At age 30, the Pa_{O_2} of a healthy person breathing ambient air at sea level is approximately 90 torr, whereas at age 70, the expected Pa_{O_2} is 70 torr. These findings, combined with the normal decline in central

KEY TERMS

elder abuse: The infliction of physical pain, injury, debilitating mental anguish, unreasonable confinement, or willful deprivation by a caretaker of services necessary to maintain the mental and physical health of an older patient.

gerontology: The study of the problems of all aspects of aging.

and peripheral chemoreceptor function, produce a diminished ventilatory response to hypoxic as well as hypercapnic challenge.

Other factors affecting the respiratory system are the loss of cilia in the airways and a diminished cough reflex, which may impair the body's defense against inhaled bacteria and particulate matter. The decline in pulmonary defense mechanisms makes infectious pulmonary diseases of the older adult more common and more difficult to eradicate.

Cardiovascular System Changes

Cardiac function declines with age as a result of nonischemic physiological changes and the high incidence of atherosclerotic coronary artery disease. It is difficult to sort out changes due solely to aging from those associated with ischemia, since coronary artery disease is so prevalent in the older adult. However, it appears that even with aging alone, structural and physiological changes occur in the cardiovascular system that limit cardiac function. These changes include a diminished ability to raise the heart rate even in response to exercise or stress, a decrease in compliance of the ventricle, a prolonged duration of contraction, and a decreased responsiveness to catecholamine stimulation. Between the ages of 30 and 80, resting cardiac output decreases approximately 30%. This, combined with the progressive increase in peripheral vascular resistance that occurs after age 40, yields a significant drop in organ perfusion. Myocardial hypertrophy, coronary artery disease, and hemodynamic changes predispose the geriatric patient to dysrhythmias, heart failure, and sudden cardiac arrest when the cardiovascular system is placed under unexpected stress.

Changes also occur in the heart's electrical conduction pathways as functional cells are lost in the sinoatrial and atrioventricular nodes and the rest of the conduction system. These physiological changes often lead to dysrhythmias, including chronic atrial fibrillation, sick-sinus syndrome, and various types of bradycardias and heart blocks, all of which can contribute to the decline in cardiac output.

Renal System Changes

In the kidneys, structural and functional changes occur during the aging process. For example, renal blood flow falls an average of 50% between the ages of 30 and 80. This reduction in renal blood flow is associated with a proportional decrease in the glomerular filtration rate of approximately 8 ml/min per decade. Renal mass decreases by approximately 20% between the ages of 40 and 80. The steady decline in kidney function places the older patient at greater risk of renal failure from trauma, obstruction, infection, and vascular occlusion.

As decades pass, significant impairment develops in renal concentrating ability, sodium conservation, free water clearance (diuresis) and glomerular filtration, and renal plasma flow. Hepatic blood flow also decreases, limiting the effectiveness of liver metabolism. These decreases in renal and hepatic function, combined with changes in lean body mass and body water, make the older person more susceptible than young adults to electrolyte abnormalities or toxic manifestations in response to medications or drugs.

Nervous System Changes

Although it was long thought that mental dysfunction in the older adult was caused solely by senility, it is now well known that intellectual functioning deteriorates selectively and may result from many organic causes. For example, beginning at approximately age 30, the total number of neurons in certain cortical areas decreases gradually, so by age 70, a 10% reduction in brain weight has occurred. These factors, decreased cerebral blood flow, and alterations in the location and amounts of specific neurotransmitters probably contribute to alterations in the central nervous system. With aging, the velocity of nerve conduction in the peripheral nervous system also decreases. This may lead to changes in motor or position sense and delays in reaction time and motor responses. Other gradual alterations in the patient's nervous system can result in decreased visual and auditory acuity and changes in sleep patterns.

Toxic or metabolic factors that can affect mental functioning include the use of medications (for example, anticholinergics, antihypertensives, antidysrhythmics, analgesics); electrolyte imbalances; hypoglycemia; acidosis; alkalosis; hypoxia; liver, kidney, and lung failure; pneumonia; congestive heart failure; and cardiac dysrhythmias.

Musculoskeletal System Changes

As the body ages, there is muscle shrinkage, calcification of muscles and ligaments, and thinning of the intervertebral disks. Osteoporosis (decreased bone density) is common in older adults (especially women); an estimated 68% of older patients show some degree of kyphosis, an increase in the curvature of the thoracic spine ("humpback posture"). These musculoskeletal changes result in a decrease in total muscle mass, a decrease in height of 2 to 3 inches, widening and weakening of certain bones, and a posture that impairs mobility and alters the body's balance. As a result, falls are common and are often associated with significant morbidity and mortality.

Other Physiological Changes

Other physiological changes that occur with aging include alterations in body mass and total body water, a decreased ability to maintain internal homeostasis, a decrease in the function of immunological mechanisms, and possible nutritional disorders.

As an individual approaches age 65, lean body mass may decrease as much as 25%, and fat tissue may increase as much as 35%. These changes in body composition can influence the dosage and frequency of administration of fat-soluble drugs because there is more drug per weight of metabolically active tissue and a larger reservoir for accumulation of the drug. Similarly, the decrease in total body water is likely to increase the concentration of water-soluble drugs.

The body's ability to maintain internal homeostasis through normal thermoregulatory mechanisms declines over time in a linear fashion beginning at about age 30. This and other factors predispose the older adult to cold- and heat-related conditions such as hypothermia, heat exhaustion, and hyperthermia. Several factors contribute to the increased risk of thermoregulatory disorders, including impaired sympathetic nervous system function causing decreased capacity for peripheral vasoconstriction, lowered metabolic rate, poor peripheral circulation, and chronic illness. Because of the progressive decline in homeostatic control, including blood pressure, cardiac output, and temperature regulation, specific illness or injury often puts the patient "over the edge," presenting as a generalized deterioration in the patient's condition.

Aging causes a decrease in primary antibody response and cellular immunity and elevations in the amount of abnormal immunoglobulins and immune complexes. These physiological changes increase the risk of infection, autoimmune disorders, and perhaps cancer.

Numerous studies have demonstrated that older adults frequently consume less than the minimum daily requirement of most vitamins. This may be a result of loneliness and depression, decreased sensitivity to taste, decreased appetite, physical infirmity, decreased vision, or a combination of these elements, all of which may act to reduce the motivation to shop for and prepare fresh food. Other factors associated with poor nutrition are poor dentition and reduced mastication, decreased esophageal motility, frequent hypochlorhydria, and decreased intestinal secretions that tend to reduce absorption.

● ASSESSMENT OF THE GERIATRIC PATIENT

Normal physiological changes and underlying acute or chronic illness may make evaluation of an ill or injured older person a challenge. In addition to the components of a normal physical assessment (see Chapter 11), the paramedic should consider special characteristics of older patients that can complicate the clinical evaluation:

- Geriatric patients are likely to suffer from concurrent illness.

○ Chronic problems can make assessment for acute problems difficult.

○ Signs or symptoms of chronic illness may be confused with signs or symptoms of an acute problem.

• Aging may affect an individual's response to illness or injury.

○ Pain may be diminished or absent.

○ The patient or paramedic may underestimate the severity of a condition.

• Social and emotional factors may have greater impact on health than in any other age group.

○ The patient fears losing autonomy.

○ The patient fears the hospital environment.

○ The patient has financial concerns about health care.

History Taking

Gathering a history from an older patient usually requires more time than with younger patients. In addition to a longer medical history because of the patient's age, chronic illness, and medication use, there may be physical impediments such as hearing loss and visual impairment. Questioning a patient who is fatigued or easily distracted may also lengthen the interview process. The following techniques should be used when communicating with older patients:

• Always identify yourself.

• Talk at eye level to ensure that the patient can see you as you speak.

• Speak slowly and distinctly.

• Listen closely.

• Be patient.

Physical Examination

When conducting the physical examination of an older patient, the paramedic should consider the following five points:

1. The patient may fatigue easily.

2. Patients commonly wear many layers of clothing for warmth, which may hamper the examination.

3. Explain actions clearly before examining all patients, especially those with diminished sight.

4. Be aware that the patient may minimize or deny symptoms through fear of being bedridden or institutionalized or losing self-sufficiency.

5. Try to distinguish symptoms of chronic disease from acute immediate problems. For example, the patient may have nonpathological crackles in the lung fields, loss of skin elasticity and mouth breathing may give a false appearance of dehydration, and dependent edema may be secondary to venous insufficiency and inactivity rather than congestive heart failure.

If time permits, the patient's immediate surroundings should be evaluated for evidence of alcohol or legal or illegal medication use (for example, insulin syringes, "vial of life," medical-alert information), presence of food items, general condition of housing, and signs of adequate personal hygiene. If available, ask friends or family members about the patient's appearance and responsiveness *now* versus his or her normal appearance, responsiveness, and other characteristics. These and other observations may provide information to the physician regarding the patient's general health and ability for self-care after release from the hospital.

● TRAUMA IN THE OLDER PATIENT

Trauma is the fifth leading cause of death for persons over age 65.[2] One third of traumatic deaths in people aged 65 to 74 are secondary to vehicular trauma, and 25% result from falls. In those older than 75, falls account for 50% of injury-related deaths.[1]

Vehicular Trauma

It is estimated that more than 13 million licensed drivers are over age 65; in 1990, more than 7600 deaths in this age group were attributed to motor vehicle crashes.[2] According to the American College of Surgeons, the majority of these vehicle collisions are not related to high speed or alcohol but rather to errors in perception or judgment or to delayed reaction time. In addition, although a large number of older patients are injured as drivers or passengers in moving vehicles, more than 2000 pedestrian fatalities among older adults occur each year in the United States, accounting for 20% of all pedestrian deaths from trauma.

The risk of fatality from multiple trauma is estimated to be 3 times greater at age 70 than at age 20. This is largely because the older patient is more susceptible to serious injury from equivalent degrees of trauma and less capable of an appropriate, protective physiological response. Prompt identification of injuries and sources of hemorrhage is critical in any trauma patient, especially the older patient, who has much less cardiac reserve and who will succumb more quickly to shock.

Head Trauma

Head injury with loss of consciousness in older patients is often associated with poor outcome. Two thirds of head-injured patients over age 65 who are unconscious on arrival at the emergency department do not survive. Among other physiological changes, the aging process is often associated with cerebral atrophy that produces a notable distance between the surface of the brain and the inner tables of the skull. As bridging veins stretch across this subdural space, they are more easily torn, resulting in subdural hematomas. The extra space within the cranial vault often allows an older person to sustain a significant amount of internal hemorrhage before the volume-pressure relationship of the cranium is exceeded and symptoms are manifested.

Older patients are also particularly susceptible to injuries of the cervical spine because of progressive arthritic and degenerative changes (cervical spondylosis) associated with aging. These structural alterations lead to increased stiffening and decreased flexibility of the spine with narrowing of the spinal canal, which renders the spinal cord much more susceptible to damage from relatively minor trauma.

Chest Injuries

A mechanism of injury that suggests thoracic trauma in an older patient must be considered potentially lethal. The aged thorax is less elastic and more susceptible to injury; the pulmonary system has marginal reserve because of a reduced alveolar surface area, decreased patency of small airways, and diminished chemoreceptor responses.

Injuries to the heart, aorta, and major vessels are a greater risk to older patients than younger adults, again because of decreased functional reserve and anatomical alterations that make significant injury in these areas more likely. Myocardial contusion may be a complication of blunt injury to the chest and, if severe, may result in pump failure or life-threatening dysrhythmias. Rarely, cardiac tamponade is seen after blunt thoracic trauma. Cardiac rupture, valvular injury (for example, flail valves), and aortic dissection may also occur with significant blunt chest injury. The first two entities are rare but rapidly fatal. Dissecting aortic aneurysms should always be considered when the mechanism of injury produced rapid deceleration. Aortic dissections are often not immediately fatal, and proper evaluation and treatment can be lifesaving.

Because of impaired coronary response to increased oxygen demands and commonly occurring underlying conduction disturbance, older patients may develop ischemia and dysrhythmias from significant trauma, even if the heart has not been directly affected. These patients need meticulous attention given to their oxygenation and circulatory status.

Abdominal Injuries

Abdominal injuries in older adults have more serious sequelae than those in any other anatomical site, producing a death rate 4.7 times higher than in other age groups. Abdominal injuries are often less apparent (requiring a high degree of suspicion). The older patient is also less likely to tolerate surgery and is more susceptible to postoperative pulmonary and septic complications.

Musculoskeletal Injuries

The osteoporotic bones of older patients are vulnerable to fracture with even mild trauma. Pelvic fractures are highly lethal in this age group, causing severe hemorrhage and associated soft tissue injury. When evaluating for skeletal trauma, the paramedic should remember that the older patient may have decreased pain perception and often surprisingly little tenderness with major fractures. Even with appropriate care, the mortality rate for older patients with musculoskeletal injury is increased by delayed complications such as adult respiratory distress syndrome, sepsis, renal failure, and pulmonary embolism.

Falls

Falls are a major cause of morbidity and mortality in older adults, accounting for approximately 9500 deaths each year. It has been estimated that one third of the older population living at home falls each year, and 1 in 40 of these persons is hospitalized. Of older patients who are hospitalized as a result of a fall, 50% die within 12 months.[3] A major cause of falls in older adults is use of prescribed sedative-hypnotics that affect balance and postural control, such as alprazolam (Xanax), *diazepam* (Valium), chlordiazepoxide (Librium), and flurazepam (Dalmane). Older patients taking these medications are 2 to 3 times as likely to fall.[4]

Fractures are the most common fall-related injuries, the hip being the fracture that most commonly results in hospitalization. In those who survive hip fracture, 60% have significant mobility problems, and another 25% become more functionally dependent.[5] Falls that do not result in physical injury may lead to self-imposed immobility resulting from the fear of falling again. When immobility is strict and prolonged, joint contractures, pressure sores, urinary tract infection, muscle atrophy, depression, and functional dependency may result.

Assessment

The paramedic should assume that any fall indicates an underlying problem until proved otherwise. Attempts should be made to uncover the multitude of medical, psychological, and environmental factors that may have been responsible for the fall. So that as much information as possible is obtained about the falling episode, the patient history should include a comprehensive review of all medical problems and medications and a precise recounting of the fall (previous history of falling, time of fall, location, symptoms experienced, activity in which the victim was engaged, use of devices, and presence of witnesses). Evaluating the patient's cardiovascular, neurological, and musculoskeletal systems should be emphasized.

Trauma Management Considerations

Priorities of trauma care for older patients are similar to those for all trauma patients (see Chapter 15).

Cardiovascular System

- Recent or past myocardial infarction contributes to the risk of dysrhythmias and congestive heart failure.
- Adjustment of heart rate and stroke volume may be decreased in response to hypovolemia.
- Older patients may require higher arterial pressures than younger patients for perfusion of vital organs because of atherosclerotic peripheral vascular disease.
- Rapid intravenous fluid administration to older patients may precipitate volume overload. Care must be taken not to overhydrate these patients, since older adults as a group are more susceptible to congestive heart failure; however, hypovolemia and hypotension are also poorly tolerated. The paramedic should consider hypovolemia in any older person whose systolic blood pressure is less than 120 mm Hg. Tachycardia may be an unreliable sign if the patient takes beta blockers. The paramedic should monitor lung sounds and vital signs carefully and frequently during fluid administration.

Respiratory System

- Physical changes decrease chest wall compliance and movement and thus diminish vital capacity.
- Pao_2 decreases with age.

- Lower P_{O_2} at the same fractional inspired oxygen concentration occurs with each passing decade.
- All organ systems have less tolerance to anoxia.
- Chronic obstructive pulmonary disease (common in older patients) requires that airway management and ventilation support be carefully adjusted for appropriate oxygenation and carbon dioxide removal. High-concentration oxygen may suppress hypoxic drive in some patients, but this therapy should never be withheld from a patient with clinical signs of cyanosis.

Renal System

- The kidneys have decreased ability to maintain normal acid-base balance and to compensate for fluid changes.
- Any preexisting renal disease may further decrease renal ability to compensate.
- Decreased renal function (along with decreased cardiac reserve) places the injured older patient at risk for fluid overload and pulmonary edema secondary to intravenous fluid therapy.

Transport Strategies

- Positioning, immobilization, and transport of an older trauma patient may require modifications to accommodate physical deformities (for example, arthritis, spinal abnormalities).

● MEDICAL EMERGENCIES OF OLDER PATIENTS

In addition to the various medical emergencies presented in this text, several are unique to older patients and warrant special consideration in assessment and management. These include acute myocardial infarction, pulmonary embolism, bacterial pneumonia, cancer, acute abdominal pain, delirium and dementia, and depression.

Acute Myocardial Infarction

Chest pain as a symptom of myocardial infarction becomes less frequent by age 70, and only 45% of patients over age 85 with myocardial infarction have this complaint. Lack of typical chest pain can cause myocardial infarction to go unrecognized in the older patient.

Studies have shown that 55% of older patients have chest pain or discomfort, but a significant percentage (13%) complain only of vague symptoms such as dyspnea, abdominal or epigastric distress, and fatigue. In the remaining 32%, the event is completely "silent," which may be a result of decreased visceral sensory function or higher incidence of mental deterioration in this age group.[6] Silent myocardial infarctions are almost always marked by an atypical complaint such as fatigue, breathlessness, nausea, or abdominal pain. The paramedic must maintain a high index of suspicion for myocardial infarction in patients with unusual or absent warning signs.

Pulmonary Embolism

Pulmonary embolism is associated with venous stasis, heart failure, chronic obstructive pulmonary disease, malignancy, and immobilization, all of which are common in older adults. Most pulmonary emboli in the geriatric age group arise indirectly from the leg veins with propagation to the iliofemoral veins. The clinical presentation of pulmonary embolism, like myocardial infarction, is often misleading in older adults.

Signs and symptoms of pulmonary embolism may range from a presentation of left ventricular failure with sudden tachypnea, unexplained tachycardia, and atrial fibrillation to signs and symptoms solely of the underlying venous thrombosis (calf discomfort without tenderness, mild calf or ankle edema, increased warmth, and dilation of superficial veins in one foot or leg). Pulmonary embolism may precipitate congestive heart failure and may also masquerade as pneumonia in this age group.

Bacterial Pneumonia

The incidence and mortality rate of lower respiratory tract infection increase with age. Unlike in younger patients with bacterial pneumonia, the usual clinical picture of pyrexia, productive cough, pleurisy, and signs of pulmonary consolidation is often absent in the older patient. With the atypical presentation, it takes 7 to 9 days from onset of symptoms to the diagnosis in a geriatric patient, compared with 2 to 3 days in a younger person. Because of the decreased pulmonary reserve in older patients, pneumonia may commonly be associated with respiratory failure.

Cancer

Approximately one in eight deaths in older adults results from cancer. Unlike younger patients, in whom cancer is often the main or only disease, older adults frequently have concurrent disease processes and disabilities. Therefore signs and symptoms such as a change in bowel habits, rectal bleeding, malaise, fatigue, weight loss, and anorexia may be attributed to other maladies. Treatment with chemotherapy frequently results in immunosuppression. This not only increases the risk of infection but also often masks the typical signs and symptoms associated with infection.

Acute Abdominal Pain

Older patients with abdominal emergencies (for example, appendicitis, perforation) often fail to exhibit the usual signs and symptoms, such as guarding, rigidity, localized pain, and fever. This may result from a number of factors, including an inability to communicate fully because of auditory impairment, mental deterioration, increased tolerance to pain, and an inability to localize or describe the pain adequately. Many older patients reach advanced stages of acute abdominal conditions with sepsis and shock before the diagnosis is apparent. Diffuse peritonitis is fatal in more than 12% of patients over age 60 and in more than 30% of those over age 70. Several causes of acute abdominal pain in the older patient are cholecystitis, colonic diverticular disease, appendicitis, aortic abdominal aneurysm, acute mesenteric artery occlusion, and mesenteric vein thrombosis.

Delirium and Dementia

Delirium is a mental state associated with an acute organic brain syndrome that is sudden in onset and of self-limited duration. It is manifested by an attention deficit, rambling or incoherent speech, a fluctuating course, and other indications of impaired cognition. The symptoms of delirium may change over the course of a day. The patient may exhibit emotional lability, as well as hyperactivity (restlessness and screaming) alternating with hypoactivity (quietness, inactivity, and stuporousness). Patients with delirium may have preexisting dementia. Mild delirium may be subtle and be elicited only through careful questioning, but delirium that is evident from the signs and symptoms previously listed should be considered a true emergency.

A number of factors can precipitate delirium, including infection, trauma, various medications, and even a change in the patient's surroundings. Studies indicate that delirium occurs in 10% to 15% of all hospitalized medical and surgical patients ("ICU psychosis"). Acute delirium carries a grave prognosis, with fatality rates of 15% to 30%. Mechanisms that have been proposed to trigger the onset of delirium are listed in Box 26-1.

Dementia is the result of a diffuse neurological process that produces chronic global impairment (either reversible or progressive) in which the patient has been symptomatic for a year or longer. Unlike delirium, which is acute, dementia is a chronic mental status change in the patient's usual level of functioning. Recent memory loss is almost universal in this condition, and there are usually associated mental defects such as loss of language, reasoning, judgment, the ability to calculate, spatial orientation, and the ability to move about safely. Reversible dementia may result from certain systemic illnesses (hypothyroidism, Cushing syndrome), vitamin deficiencies (particularly *thiamine* and vitamin B_{12}), and certain primary central nervous system disorders (hydrocephalus). There is a much longer list of irreversible causes of dementia, but in the United States, the most common cause of progressive dementia is Alzheimer's disease.

Alzheimer's disease is a degenerative disorder of unknown cause in which nerve cells of the cerebral cortex die and the cortex becomes atrophic. Although the deterioration in mental function does not directly cause death, patients ultimately stop eating and become malnourished and immobilized, so they are prone to infections. Of all older patients with chronic dementias, approximately two thirds are victims of Alzheimer's disease.

Depression

Depression is the most common psychiatric disorder in older patients. It usually begins insidiously and frequently stems from stress associated with multiple chronic illnesses, environmental changes, bereavement, and social rejection. Manifestations of depression include lack of energy, loss of appetite and libido, low self-esteem, and negative feelings.

When depression becomes more severe, older adults become high risks for suicide; 25% of all suicides occur in persons over age 65. Paramedics should be alert to the signs and symptoms of depression and advise medical control of any suspicions that a patient may have suicidal tendencies. Depression and other psychiatric disorders are further described in Chapter 29.

● PHARMACOLOGY FOR THE OLDER PATIENT

Older patients are at increased risk for adverse drug reactions, because of age-related alterations in body composition and drug distribution, metabolism, and excretion and because multiple drugs are often prescribed to them. It is estimated that more than 80% of geriatric patients take at least one prescription drug, and one third take three to four different drugs daily.

Drug-Induced Illness

Accidental drug overdose and medication noncompliance account for approximately 30% of all hospital admissions related to drug-induced illness in older people. The most problematic drugs are primarily cardiovascular agents, antibiotics, and anticoagulants. Common reasons for these medication mishaps include:
- Noncompliance
- Confusion
- Vision impairment
- Self-selection of drugs

BOX 26-1

Organic Causes of Delirium

Intoxication
Medications
Alcohol
Poisons

Withdrawal Syndromes
Alcohol
Sedatives and hypnotics

Metabolic Factors
Electrolyte imbalance
Hypoglycemia or hyperglycemia
Acid-base imbalance (acidosis or alkalosis)
Hypoxia
Failure of vital organs (liver, kidneys, or lungs)
Wernicke encephalopathy

Infections
Encephalitis
Meningitis
Pneumonia
Septicemia

Neurological Factors
Tumors
Subdural hematoma
Aneurysm
Cerebral vascular disease
Epilepsy

Endocrine Factors
Thyroid disorders

Cardiovascular Factors
Congestive heart failure
Cardiac dysrhythmias
Myocardial infarction

- Forgetfulness
- Multiple prescriptions from more than one physician
- Improper resumption of old medications in addition to newly prescribed ones

- Sedative and hypnotic drugs
- Phenothiazines
- *Propranolol*
- Theophylline
- Narcotic analgesics and acetaminophen
- Antiparkinsonian drugs
- Quinidine
- *Lidocaine*

- Excessive dosing of an over-the-counter drug with synergistic or cumulative effects
- Changes in habits regarding alcohol, diet, and exercise that may affect drug metabolism
- Dispensing error

Drugs Commonly Causing Toxicity

Although most any drug can produce toxic effects in an older person, the prescription drugs that most commonly cause toxicity are:

- Anticoagulants
- Diuretics
- Digitalis
- Tricyclic antidepressants

● ELDER ABUSE

Elder abuse is the "infliction of physical pain, injury, debilitating mental anguish, unreasonable confinement, or willful deprivation by a caretaker of services which are necessary to maintain mental and physical health of an elderly patient." Elder abuse and neglect have become increasingly recognized as a growing problem in the United States, occurring in 1 of every 25 older persons (making it slightly less common than child abuse).[3] Elder abuse has been classified into four major categories: physical abuse, psychological abuse, financial or material abuse, and neglect (both active and passive) (Box 26-2).

Recognizing Elder Abuse

Abuse of the older adult can be subtle and difficult to recognize in the prehospital setting. The average victim is 80 years old with multiple chronic health conditions that make the patient dependent on others for care. (Widows over age 75 carry the greatest risk of elder abuse.) Unexplained trauma is the primary finding (Box 26-3).

Recent evidence suggests that elder abuse is associated more with the personality of the abuser or the caretaker than with the burden of caring for a sick, dependent person. Most often the abuser is a relative (86%) and lives with the victim (75%). Children or grandchildren are implicated in 50% of cases and spouses in 40% of cases. Abusers have frequently been abused as children. In addition to those who live in noninstitutional settings, more than 1.5 million people are currently residents in nursing homes and other health care facilities. These individuals are also at risk for intentional harm, physical violence, verbal aggression, or neglect.

All 50 states have elder abuse statutes, and in most states, reporting of suspected elder abuse is mandatory under law. If abuse or neglect of an older patient is suspected, the paramedic should advise medical control and follow the procedures established by local protocol.

REFERENCES

1. Kaudner D, Schwab W: Trauma in the elderly, *Emerg Mag* 23(2):22, 1991.
2. National Safety Council: *Accident facts*, Chicago, 1991, The Council.
3. Rose C, editor: Emergency care of the elderly, *Emerg Med Clin North Am* May 1990.
4. Buchner D: Falls and syncope in the elderly, *Audio Dig Emerg Med* 8(10):36, 1991.
5. Bosker G et al: *Geriatric emergency medicine,* St Louis, 1990, Mosby.
6. Bayer A: Changing presentation of myocardial infarction with increasing old age, *J Am Geriatr Soc* 34:263, 1986.

Summary

Advances in medical care and technology, along with a decline in the birth rate, are causing a rapid and profound shift in the age distribution of the U.S. population. Therefore emergency health care teams will continue to have an increasing number and percentage of older patients. Numerous age-related physiological factors can disguise the severity of illness in this age group and present a variety of challenges in assessment and management. The paramedic must always suspect serious illness and provide appropriate care with consideration for the special needs of the geriatric patient.

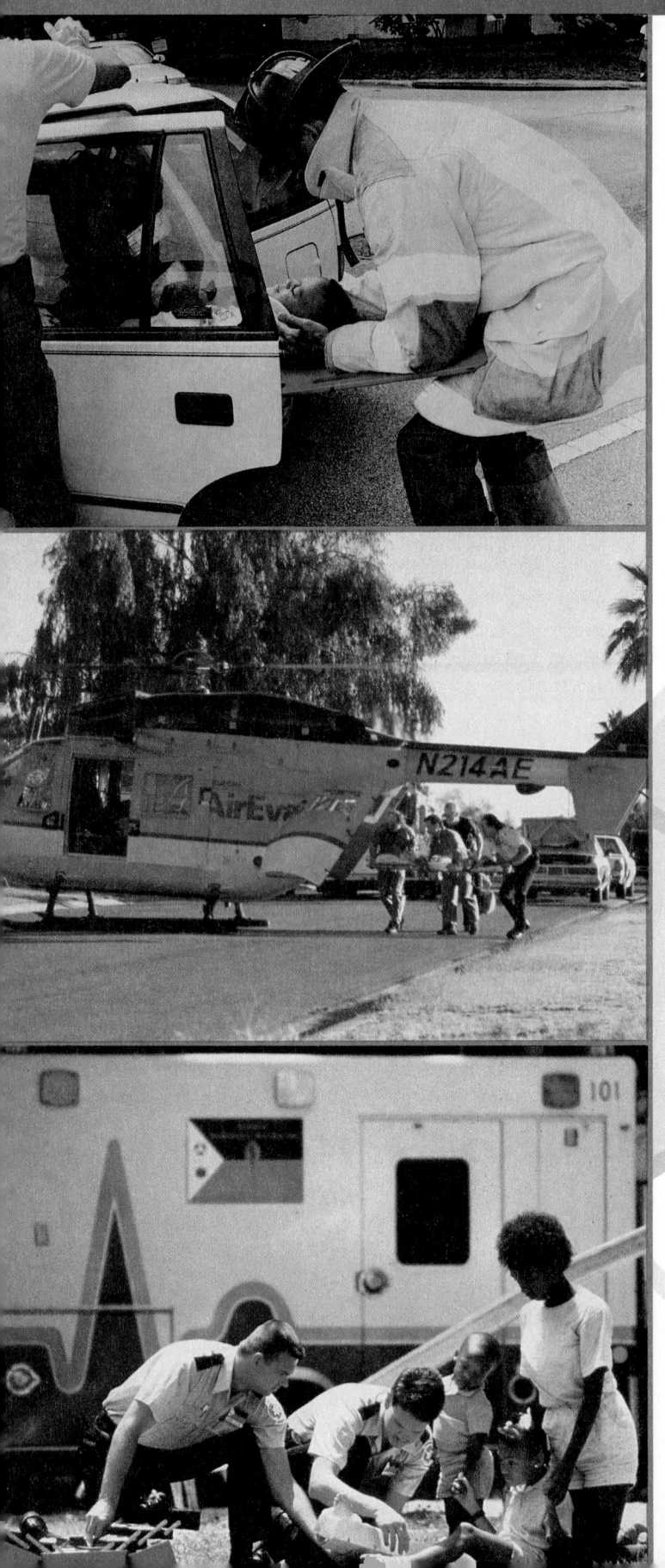

Emergencies involving pediatric patients account for 10% to 20% of all EMS responses.[1] Caring for these patients presents unique challenges that relate to size, physical and intellectual maturation, and diseases specific to neonates, infants, and children. This chapter addresses the anatomical and physiological mechanisms of growth and development, medical emergencies common to pediatric patients, and initial assessment and management strategies that are often critical factors in the patient's survival.

As a paramedic, you should be able to:

1. Distinguish among patient assessment techniques appropriate for patients at different developmental levels.
2. Identify common age-related illnesses in pediatric patients.
3. Discuss common historical and physical findings of the sudden infant death syndrome patient.
4. Describe common features in the profile of an abusive situation.
5. Describe abnormal physical findings that have a high index of suspicion for child abuse.
6. Discuss appropriate interventions in cases of suspected child abuse.
7. Discuss the pathophysiology, assessment, and management of seizures and dehydration in children.
8. Describe the pathophysiology, assessment, and management of children with selected respiratory illnesses.
9. Outline the correct pediatric drug dosage, cardioversion energy levels, and sequence for specific pediatric resuscitation situations.
10. Select the correct endotracheal blade and tube for a given age group.
11. Interpret vital sign values as normal or abnormal for selected age groups.
12. For a seriously injured child, identify considerations for blood volume, hypothermia, cardiac reserve, respiratory fatigue, and vital sign assessment.
13. Describe special considerations for intravenous fluid therapy and intraosseous infusion in children.

● EMERGENCY MEDICAL SERVICES FOR CHILDREN

In 1985, the Emergency Medical Services for Children (EMSC) Demonstration Program was established through grants provided by the Department of Health and Human Services, Maternal and Child Health Bureau, and the Department of Transportation, National Highway Traffic Safety Administration. This program was designed to

KEY TERMS

bronchiolitis: An acute viral infection of the lower respiratory tract that occurs primarily in infants under 18 months of age and that is characterized by expiratory wheezes, respiratory distress, inflammation, and obstruction at the level of the bronchioles.

child abuse: The physical, sexual, or emotional maltreatment of a child.

croup: An acute viral infection of the upper and lower respiratory tract that occurs primarily in infants and young children 3 months to 3 years old and that is characterized by hoarseness; fever; harsh, brassy cough; inspiratory stridor; and varying degrees of respiratory distress (also known as *laryngotracheobronchitis*).

epiglottitis: Severe inflammation of the epiglottis, which is characterized by fever, sore throat, stridor, croupy cough, and an erthymatous epiglottis.

febrile seizure: A seizure that results from fever.

sudden infant death syndrome: The unexpected and sudden death of an apparently normal and healthy infant that occurs during sleep and with no physical or autopsic evidence of disease.

enhance and expand emergency medical services for acutely ill and injured children. Between 1985 and 1990, 20 states received funding for grant projects addressing the seven basic components of an effective EMSC system:

1. System description
2. Education
3. Prevention
4. Research and data collection
5. Medical direction and supervision
6. Quality assurance and improvement
7. Ongoing funding

Through the funding of EMSC grants and the efforts of organizations dedicated to improving emergency care for children, specific programs targeted to prehospital care providers have been developed. These include continuing education programs such as the American Heart Association's *pediatric advanced life support* course and other educational resources for instructors, equipment guidelines, protocols for prehospital management, quality improvement procedures for evaluating pediatric prehospital care, and designation of facilities with special capabilities for pediatric care. As stated in *Emergency Medical Service for Children: A Report to the Nation*, "The lives of many infants, children, and young adults . . . can be saved through implementation of emergency medical services for children (EMSC). Outcomes for critically ill and injured children can be influenced by the provision of timely care by health care professionals who are well trained and equipped for pediatric emergency and critical care."[2]

BOX 27-1

Pediatric Age Classifications

Neonate: Birth to 1 month
Young infant: 1 to 5 months
Infant: 6 to 12 months
Toddler: 1 to 3 years
Preschooler: 3 to 5 years
School age: 6 to 12 years
Adolescent: 12 to 15 years

● DEVELOPMENTAL STAGES

Children have unique characteristics in their anatomical, physiological, and psychological makeup, which change during their development (Box 27-1). The sidebar describes the developmental stages and the special considerations that must be taken into account when caring for the pediatric patient.

● PEDIATRIC EMERGENCIES

Some childhood diseases and disabilities are predictable by age group. Illnesses and accidents in the following seven age groups are frequently encountered by prehospital providers:

1. *Neonate*
   a. Respiratory distress
   b. Sepsis and meningitis
   c. Jaundice
   d. Vomiting
   e. Fever
2. *1- to 5-month-old infant*
   a. Respiratory distress
   b. Fever
   c. Sudden infant death syndrome (SIDS)
   d. Vomiting and diarrhea with dehydration
   e. Meningitis
   f. Child abuse
3. *6- to 12-month-old infant*
   a. Fever, febrile seizures
   b. Vomiting and diarrhea with dehydration
   c. Bronchiolitis
   d. Croup
   e. Meningitis
   f. Respiratory distress (bronchiolitis, foreign body aspiration, croup)
   g. Child abuse
   h. Ingestions
   i. Foreign body airway obstruction
   j. Falls
   k. Injuries from motor-vehicle crashes
4. *1- to 3-year-old child*
   a. Fever, febrile seizure
   b. Vomiting and diarrhea with dehydration
   c. Respiratory distress (bronchiolitis, foreign body aspiration, croup)

Developmental Stages and Approach Strategies for Pediatric Patients

Infants
Major Fears
Separation and strangers

Approach Strategies
Provide consistent caretakers.
Decrease parent's anxiety, since it is transmitted to infant.
Minimize separation from parents.

Toddlers
Major Fears
Separation and loss of control

Characteristics of Thinking
Primitive
Inability to recognize views of others
Little concept of body integrity

Approach Strategies
Keep explanations simple.
Choose words carefully.
Let toddler play with equipment (stethoscope).
Minimize separation from parents.

Preschoolers
Major Fears
Bodily injury and mutilation
Loss of control
The unknown and the dark
Being left alone

Characteristics of Thinking
Highly literal interpretation of words
Inability to abstract
Primitive ideas about their bodies (fearing that all blood will "leak out" if a bandage is removed)

Approach Strategies
Keep explanations simple and concise.
Choose words carefully.
Emphasize that a procedure will help the child be more healthy.
Be honest.

School-Age Children
Major Fears
Loss of control
Bodily injury and mutilation

Failure to live up to expectations of others
Death

Characteristics of Thinking
Vague or false ideas about physical illness, and body structure and function
Ability to listen attentively without always comprehending
Reluctance to ask questions about something they think they are expected to know
Increased awareness of significant illness, potential hazards of treatments, lifelong consequences of injury, and the meaning of death

Approach Strategies
Ask children to explain what they understand.
Provide as many choices as possible to increase the child's sense of control.
Assure the child that he or she has done nothing wrong and that necessary procedures are not punishment.
Anticipate and answer questions regarding long-term consequences (for example, what the scar will look like, how long activities may be curtailed).

Adolescents
Major Fears
Loss of control
Altered body image
Separation from peer group

Characteristics of Thinking
Ability to think abstractly
Tendency toward hyperresponsiveness to pain (reactions not always in proportion to event)
Little understanding of the structure and workings of the body

Approach Strategies
When appropriate, allow adolescents to be a part of decision making about their care.
Give information sensitively.
Express how important their compliance and cooperation are to their treatment.
Be honest about consequences.
Use or teach coping mechanisms such as relaxation, deep breathing, and self-comforting talk.

    d. Meningitis

    e. Child abuse

    f. Ingestions

    g. Foreign body airway obstruction

    h. Falls

    i. Injuries from motor-vehicle crashes

5. *3- to 5-year-old child*

    a. Croup

    b. Asthma

    c. Epiglottitis

    d. Febrile seizures

    e. Meningitis

    f. Burns

    g. Drowning, near-drowning

    h. Child abuse

    i. Injuries from motor-vehicle crashes (occupant and pedestrian)

6. *6-to 12-year-old child*

    a. Drowning, near-drowning

    b. Injuries from motor-vehicle crashes

    c. Injuries from bicycle accidents

    d. Fractures

    e. Falls

    f. Sports injuries

    g. Child abuse

    h. Burns

7. *12- to 15-year-old adolescent*

    a. Asthma

    b. Injuries from motor-vehicle crashes

    c. Sports injuries

    d. Drug or alcohol use

    e. Suicide gestures

    f. Sexual abuse

    g. Pregnancy

Seizures

A seizure is an episode of sudden abnormal electrical activity in the brain that results in abnormalities in motor, sensory, or autonomic function usually associated with abnormal behavior, alterations in level of consciousness, or both. The most common cause of seizure in adult and pediatric patients is noncompliance with a drug regimen for the treatment of epilepsy, head trauma, intracranial infection, metabolic disturbance, or poisoning. The most common cause of new onset of seizure in children is fever. It has been estimated that

febrile seizures account for 8% of all pediatric prehospital transports.[3]

Febrile Seizures

A **febrile seizure** is a seizure associated with fever but without evidence of intracranial infection or other definable cause; it usually occurs between the ages of 6 months and 5 years of age. Approximately 1 of every 20 children under the age of 7 years experiences a febrile seizure, and 30% to 50% of those who have one will experience a recurrence. More than half of febrile seizures occur in children aged 9 to 20 months. There is a family history of febrile seizures in 20% of cases.

Febrile seizures are usually associated with an underlying viral infection (most frequently of the upper respiratory tract), gastroenteritis, roseola, otitis media, or another febrile illness. The seizures generally occur in vulnerable patients during a rapid rise in body temperature, but the intensity of the seizure is not related to the severity of the fever.

Febrile seizures may present with generalized tonic-clonic activity or be of more subtle presentation. As a rule, classic febrile seizures are of short duration (usually lasting less than 5 minutes) and have an uncomplicated and short postictal period. (Seizures that last longer than 5 minutes require extensive investigation and should never be considered benign.) Regardless of the suspected etiology, all pediatric patients who have suffered a seizure should be transported for physician evaluation per protocol.

Assessment and Management

In most cases, the febrile seizure has ceased before EMS arrival, and in many instances, the patient is in a postictal state. As in any emergency, the first priorities are airway management and ventilatory and circulatory support. This should include airway positioning, suctioning the airway, and administering oxygen. Repeated assessment of the adequacy of ventilation is necessary, with special emphasis on respiratory rate and depth. If the airway cannot be maintained with manual maneuvers, airway adjuncts should be used.

After initial stabilization of the patient, vital signs should be obtained and a history should be performed. Important elements of the history include:

- Previous seizures
- Number of seizures in this episode
- Description of seizure activity
- Presence of vomiting during the seizure (aspiration risk)
- Condition of the child when first found
- Recent illness
- Potential for toxic ingestion
- Previous head injury
- Significant medical problems
- Recent headache or stiff neck
- Medication use and compliance with anticonvulsant medication

During transport to the emergency department, the patient should be continuously monitored, and the paramedic should be alert for recurrent seizures. Medical control may recommend that a febrile patient be cooled with tepid water to reduce the fever en route to the receiving hospital.

Status Epilepticus

Status epilepticus is a true emergency that can lead to hypotension and cardiovascular, respiratory, and renal failure as well as permanent brain damage. Pediatric patients in status epilepticus should be managed with the following initial interventions:

1. Provide adequate airway, ventilatory, and circulatory support. Intubation for airway protection or mechanical ventilation is seldom necessary and should be withheld unless the child fails to respond to initial management.
2. Attach a cardiac monitor and observe for rhythm or conduction abnormalities that may suggest hypoxia.
3. Per protocol, obtain vascular access through an intravenous (IV) or intraosseous (IO) route and check the blood glucose level with a Chemstrip test to screen for hypoglycemia. If the Chemstrip value is below 60 mg/dl, administer **25% dextrose** (2 to 4 ml/kg/dose IV push for children 2 years of age or younger) or **50% dextrose** (1 ml/kg/dose for children older than 2 years of age). If seizures do not stop, consult with medical control for

use of the anticonvulsants **diazepam** or **lorazepam.**

Diazepam

Diazepam breaks active seizures in 80% to 90% of cases. The initial dose is 0.1 to 0.3 mg/kg via slow IV or IO infusion at a rate not to exceed 1 mg/min (maximum dose is 5 mg for children under 5 years, 10 mg for those over 5 years). **Diazepam** has a short duration of action (15 minutes) and may require repeat administration to a maximum of three doses. In addition, the paramedic should be prepared for unpredictable sudden respiratory depression or hypotension associated with use of this drug. If IV or IO access cannot be obtained, **diazepam** may be administered rectally (Box 27-2).

Lorazepam

An alternative to IV or IO diazepam is **lorazepam,** which is preferred over **diazepam** by some physicians because of its longer half-life. **Lorazepam** may be injected intramuscularly, intravenously, or intraosseously (0.1 mg/kg, up to 4 mg), or rectally (0.1 to 0.2 mg/kg). Side effects resemble those of **diazepam** in terms of cardiorespiratory and central nervous system depression. Therefore the paramedic should be alert to these complications.

Dehydration

Profound fluid and electrolyte imbalances can occur in pediatric patients as a consequence of diarrhea, vomiting, poor fluid intake, fever, or burns. Dehydration compromises cardiac output and systemic perfusion if the infant or child loses the fluid equivalent of 7% to 10% total body weight or if the adolescent loses 5% to 7% of total body weight. If allowed to progress, dehydration can result in renal failure, shock, and death.

The severity of the dehydration and fluid volume deficit can be estimated from a history of the child's weight loss and the physical examination. Physical findings depend on the type of dehydration (isotonic, hypotonic, hypertonic [see Chapter 13]). Table 27-1 provides guidelines for assessing dehydration in a child with isotonic fluid losses.

BOX 27-2

Procedure for Administration of Rectal Diazepam

1. Carefully restrain the child. If possible, place the child in a knee-chest position or decubitus with legs flexed at hip and knee.
2. Draw the calculated diazepam dose into a syringe. A higher dose of 0.5 mg/kg is required because absorption is incomplete.
3. Introduce a lubricated 1-ml syringe just beyond the external sphincter (aiming just above the junction of the skin and mucous membranes and directed toward the rectal wall).
4. Inject the solution into the rectum and clear the syringe with 1 ml of normal saline.
5. Facilitate drug retention by squeezing the buttocks together with manual pressure.
6. Transport the patient for physician evaluation. Remove excessive clothing and cool the patient with tepid water if he or she is febrile. En route, continually monitor the patient for recurrent seizures and the need for airway, ventilatory, and circulatory support.

Management

After provision of airway and ventilatory support, the initial management of dehydration in the pediatric patient is directed at restoring and maintaining intravascular volume and systemic perfusion. Regardless of the type of dehydration, IV infusion should be initiated with isotonic crystalloids such as lactated Ringer's solution or normal saline. A fluid bolus of 20 ml/kg should be administered and may be repeated until the patient's systemic perfusion improves and an appropriate blood pressure has been obtained. After physician evaluation and initial shock resuscitation, the fluid administration rate and type of fluid replacement are determined by the volume and type of fluid deficit and the patient's response to therapy.

Reye Syndrome

Reye syndrome (first described in 1963) is a disorder of unknown etiology that produces a disease process in multiple organ systems. It is characterized by encephalopathy secondary to disruption of mitochondrial function and is associated with fatty infiltration of the liver and hepatic dysfunction. Other organ systems, including the heart, kidneys, and musculature, are also involved. The striking features of the disease are development of cerebral edema with increases in intracranial pressure, significant hepatic dysfunc-

TABLE 27-1 Assessment of Degree of Dehydration in Isotonic Fluid Loss

Clinical Parameters	Mild	Moderate	Severe
Body weight loss			
Infant	5% (50 ml/kg)	10% (100 ml/kg)	15% (150 ml/kg)
Adult	3% (30 ml/kg)	6% (60 ml/kg)	9% (90 ml/kg)
Skin turgor	Slightly ↓	↓↓	↓↓↓
Fontanelle	Possibly flat or depressed	Depressed	Significantly depressed
Mucous membranes	Dry	Very dry	Parched
Skin perfusion	Warm with normal color	Cool (extremities)	Cold (extremities)
		Pale	Mottled or gray
Heart rate	Mildly tachycardic	Moderately tachycardic	Extremely tachycardic
Peripheral pulses	Normal	Diminished	Absent
Blood pressure	Normal	Normal	Reduced
Sensorium	Normal or irritable	Irritable or lethargic	Unresponsive

tion, and liver enlargement. In-hospital differential diagnosis includes central nervous system infection of bacterial or viral cause, such as meningitis or encephalitis; septicemia; and drug or isopropyl alcohol ingestion.

Reye syndrome is an acute, noninfectious, life-threatening condition that has worldwide distribution. The disease primarily affects children and adolescents (with a peak incidence in those 5 to 15 years of age) and rarely occurs in young adults. More cases are reported in the winter and spring, and there appears to be a higher incidence after 1 year of age in suburban and rural populations. Although no single etiological factor has been identified, Reye syndrome is known to be associated with many viruses, especially influenza B (epidemic Reye syndrome) and varicella (20% of sporadic cases). Studies also suggest a strong association between the development of Reye syndrome and the ingestion of salicylate-containing medications during viral illness.

Signs and Symptoms

The course of Reye syndrome is biphasic. The first phase is characterized by a viral prodromal illness for 5 to 7 days with apparent recovery. The second phase is associated with unexpected, recurrent vomiting and a progressive disturbance in level of consciousness (ranging from lethargy and combative behavior to flaccid coma). The disease can have various stages, and a number of staging systems based on neurological findings have been proposed.

Reye syndrome cannot be diagnosed in the prehospital setting because the disease is usually confirmed through liver biopsy and other laboratory findings. However, the disease should be suspected in any child or adolescent who repeatedly vomits and has an altered mental status after a presumed viral illness. Signs and symptoms vary depending on the progression of the disease and may include rapid, deep, and irregular respirations; dilated, sluggish pupils; right upper-quadrant tenderness; cardiac dysrhythmias; and other signs associated with increased intracranial pressure. Respiratory failure is common in these patients, and death may ensue rapidly.

Management

Prehospital management of a patient with suspected Reye syndrome is primarily supportive and usually limited to airway, ventilatory, and circulatory management and rapid transport to an appropriate medical facility. Early diagnosis and maintenance of normoglycemia and cerebral perfusion account for current survival rates of 70% to 90% in children with Reye syndrome.

Poliomyelitis

Poliomyelitis is an infectious disease caused by *Poliovirus hominis*. The virus attacks with variable severity ranging from inapparent infection to a febrile illness without neurological sequela to aseptic meningitis and finally to paralytic disease (including respiratory paralysis) and possible death. Although the incidence of poliomyelitis has declined since the Salk and Sabin vaccines have been available, it may affect nonimmune adults and indigent (particularly immigrant) children.

Signs and symptoms of poliomyelitis differ in the nonparalytic and paralytic forms:

- Nonparalytic
  ◦ Fever
  ◦ Malaise
  ◦ Headache
  ◦ Nausea and vomiting
  ◦ Abdominal pain
  ◦ Neck pain
- Paralytic
  ◦ Fever
  ◦ Malaise
  ◦ Headache
  ◦ Generalized pain, weakness, and muscle spasms
  ◦ Paralysis of limbs and other muscles

Prehospital care is primarily supportive and should be directed at ensuring adequate ventilation and oxygenation and transporting the patient for physician evaluation.

Respiratory Emergencies

Four of the most important conditions that manifest chiefly as respiratory distress in pediatric patients are asthma, bronchiolitis, epiglottitis, and croup. The majority of cardiac arrests in children are secondary to respiratory insufficiency. Therefore respiratory emergencies require rapid prehospital assessment and management.

Asthma

As described in Chapter 17, asthma is termed *reactive airway disease* and is characterized by bronchoconstriction that results from autonomic dysfunction or sensitizing agents. The hallmarks of an asthmatic attack are dyspnea, tachypnea, and audible expiratory wheezes. Asthma is common among children and affects 5% to 10% of those under 10 years of age. The etiology of asthma may be allergic or infectious.

The goals of prehospital management include ventilatory assistance, humidified oxygen administration, reversal of the bronchospasm, and rapid transport for physician evaluation. Severe asthma attacks may be life threatening and can rapidly progress to respiratory failure. The paramedic should be prepared to initiate aggressive airway management and ventilatory and circulatory support. Depending on local protocol, prior medication use, and the recommendations of medical control, pharmacological therapy may include aerosolized bronchodilators, *epinephrine*, and occasionally corticosteroids during prolonged transports (Box 27-3).

Bronchiolitis

Bronchiolitis is a viral disease frequently caused by respiratory syncytial virus (RSV) that usually affects children aged 6 to 18 months. It is generally associated with an upper respiratory infection and presents similarly to asthma, with tachypnea and wheezing. Unlike some asthma, however, bronchiolitis results from infection, and the resulting inflammation of the distal airway is sometimes unresponsive to therapy aimed at relieving bronchospasm (beta-agonists usually work fairly well). Important features that may aid in differential diagnosis are listed in Table 27-2.

Bronchiolitis is generally benign and self-limiting, but it may become life threatening when the airway obstruction is significant. The infant is also at greater risk for developing respiratory fail-

---

BOX 27-3

Pharmacological Treatment of Asthma

Oxygen (Preferably Humidified)
- Simple face mask (6 L/min)
- Nonrebreather (15 L/min)

Aerosolized Beta₂-Adrenergic Agonist
- *Albuterol* (0.5% solution): 0.15 mg/kg up to 5 mg in 3 ml of normal saline by nebulizer
- *Terbutaline* (1% solution): 0.02-0.03 mg/kg up to 0.5 mg in 2 ml of normal saline by nebulizer

Subcutaneous Beta₂-Adrenergic Agonist
- *Terbutaline* (1 mg/ml solution): 0.01 mg/kg up to 0.25 to 0.30 mg every 15 minutes as needed
- *Epinephrine* (1 mg/ml 1:1000 solution): 0.01 mg/kg up to 0.3 mg every 15 minutes as needed

Corticosteroids
- *Methylprednisolone* (IV solution in 40-, 125-, and 500-mg vials): 1 to 2 mg/kg IV bolus
- *Hydrocortisone* (IV solution in 100- and 250-mg vials): 4 to 6 mg/kg IV bolus

---

ure because of the relatively small diameter of the bronchioles. Prehospital care for a child with bronchiolitis is aimed at providing ventilatory support with humidified oxygen and rapid transport for physician evaluation. Although no medication treats the cause of the illness, a therapeutic trial of *epinephrine* or *albuterol* via nebulizer may greatly decrease respiratory distress.

Epiglottitis

Epiglottitis is a rapidly progressive, life-threatening bacterial infection that most often affects

TABLE 27-2 Differentiation of Bronchiolitis and Asthma

Clinical Features	Bronchiolitis	Asthma
Occurrence	Usually <18 months	Any age
Season	Winter, spring	Any time
Family history of asthma	Usually absent	Usually present
Etiology	Virus	Allergy, infection, exercise
Response to drugs	Some reversal of bronchospasm with beta agonists	Reversal of bronchospasm

children between 3 and 7 years of age. The disease is usually associated with *Haemophilus influenza* type B, but *Streptococcus, Pneumococcus,* and *Staphylococcus* organisms have also been implicated. The bacterial infection causes edema and swelling of the epiglottis and supraglottic structures (pharynx, aryepiglottic folds, and arytenoid cartilage). Epiglottitis is a true emergency that requires prompt, expert airway management.

Epiglottitis usually begins suddenly. Commonly, the child goes to bed asymptomatic and wakens within a few hours complaining of a sore throat and pain on swallowing. The child may also be febrile, have a muffled voice because of edema of the mucosa covering of the vocal cords, and may be drooling from the presence of pooled saliva secondary to dysphagia (an ominous sign of impending airway obstruction).

On EMS arrival, the child with epiglottitis is typically found sitting upright and leaning forward with the head hyperextended to facilitate breathing (tripod position). The patient's mouth is often open with the tongue protruding. Audible inspiratory stridor may be present. These children are not usually crying or struggling because all available attention and energy is being expended to maximize air exchange. Inspiratory stridor with a characteristic "rattle" is often present, and the patient may be gasping or gulping for air. Classic signs of respiratory distress are usually present. Definitive care for epiglottitis is in-hospital intubation and parenteral antibiotic therapy.

Children with acute epiglottitis are in danger of progressing to complete airway obstruction and respiratory arrest. Occlusion can occur suddenly and may be precipitated by minor irritation of the throat, aggravation, and anxiety. Therefore it is very important that a child with suspected epiglottitis be handled gently. The following guidelines in prehospital management should be observed:

- Make no attempt to lay the child down or to change his or her position of comfort.
- Make no attempt to visualize the airway if the child is still ventilating adequately.
- Advise medical control of the suspected epiglottitis so that appropriate personnel and resources can be made available.
- Administer 100% humidified oxygen by mask unless it provokes agitation.
- Do not attempt vascular access.
- Have appropriate-sized emergency airway equipment selected and immediately available.
- Transport the child to the receiving hospital in the position of comfort.

If the patient progresses to respiratory arrest before arrival at the emergency department, field intubation must be attempted. The child's lungs should be hyperventilated and preoxygenated with a bag-valve device before intubation. After the airway has been established, an IV access should be obtained if time permits.

The paramedic should be prepared for a difficult intubation, since the vocal cords are likely to be obscured by the swollen supraglottic tissues. An uncuffed endotracheal tube (one to two sizes smaller than normal) should be used. The paramedic should locate the laryngeal inlet by looking for mucus bubbles appearing in the cleft between the edematous aryepiglottic folds and the swollen epiglottis. If intubation cannot be achieved and the child cannot be adequately ventilated via bag-valve device (rare), medical control may recommend needle cricothyrotomy.

Croup

Croup (laryngotracheobronchitis) is a common inflammatory respiratory illness in pediatric patients. It is usually a viral infection of the upper airway that occurs in children between the ages of 3 months and 3 years, frequently during the late fall and early winter months. The responsible organism is usually the parainfluenza virus, although RSV, rubeola, and adenovirus have also been implicated. Croup may involve the entire respiratory tract, but the symptoms are caused by inflammation at the level of the larynx extending to the cricoid cartilage.

The child with croup usually has a history of recent upper respiratory tract infection and a low fever. The patient may be hoarse and have respiratory stridor from subglottic edema and a "barking" cough produced by edematous vocal cords as an expiratory sound. Wheezing may also be present if the lower airways are involved. Commonly, the emergency episode occurs in the middle of the night after the child has gone to bed. On EMS arrival, a patient with severe croup may exhibit all the classic signs of respiratory distress. The child may be sitting upright and leaning forward to facilitate breathing (variable); nasal flaring, intercostal retraction, and cyanosis (a late sign of respiratory insufficiency in children) may be present.

Like patients with epiglottitis, children with severe croup are at risk of serious airway obstruction from the narrowed diameter of the trachea. Differentiation of the two syndromes in the prehospital setting may be difficult. Table 27-3 lists different characteristics of croup and epiglottitis.

The prehospital treatments for croup and epiglottitis are essentially the same: airway maintenance, oxygen administration, and transportation in a position of comfort. Medical control may recommend administration of racemic *epinephrine* via a nebulizer. Symptoms may improve dramatically in patients with croup after the child is exposed to cool, humidified air (for example, after moving the patient from his or her residence to

TABLE 27-3 Croup and Epiglottitis Symptoms

Croup	Epiglottitis
Age: 3 months to 3 years	Age: 3 to 7 years
Slow onset	Rapid onset
Patient may lie or sit upright	Patient prefers to sit upright
Barking cough	No barking cough, possible inspiratory stridor
Lack of drooling	Drooling, pain during swallowing
Temperature less than 104° F	Temperature greater than 104° F

the emergency vehicle). Make all efforts to keep the child comfortable and at ease.

Sudden Infant Death Syndrome

Sudden infant death syndrome (SIDS) is the leading cause of death in American infants aged 1 week to 1 year. The syndrome is defined as the sudden death of an apparently healthy infant that remains unexplained by history and a thorough autopsy. SIDS occurs an average of 2 times for every 1000 live births and is responsible for more than 7000 deaths in the United States each year.[4] The disease has been documented since ancient times and may be the condition described in the Old Testament (I Kings 3:19) as "overlaying." (Overlaying is an infant death attributed to suffocation as a result of an adult rolling over onto the infant. Suffocation was ruled out as a cause of SIDS in the 1940s.)

At present, SIDS cannot be predicted or prevented. There is no known cause and no treatment. SIDS occurs during periods of sleep, usually between midnight and 6 AM. The typical age for SIDS is the first year of life, but the majority of SIDS deaths occur within the first 6 months, with a peak incidence between 2 and 4 months. According to most studies, boys die more frequently than girls by a ratio of three to two. The seasonal distribution for SIDS is October through March. The increased incidence with the onset of cool weather is a worldwide phenomenon for which there is no adequate explanation. It is common for a number of SIDS deaths to occur in the same limited geographical area or community (an unexplained phenomenon known as *clustering*).

The cause of SIDS remains a mystery despite years of research. Well-controlled studies have failed to confirm a number of physiological, environmental, genetic, and social factors as causes. From these studies it has been determined, however, that SIDS is *not* caused by external suffocation, location or position during sleep, regurgitation or aspiration of vomitus, child abuse or neglect, hereditary factors, or allergies.

Various physiological aspects that have been suggested to explain SIDS include immaturity of the central nervous system secondary to an prenatal event, idiopathic apnea, upper airway obstruction, hyperactive upper airway reflexes, cardiac conduction disorders, abnormal responses to hypoxia and hypercarbia, abnormal responses to hyperthermia, and alterations in fat metabolism. Although no cause has been identified, several risk factors have been associated with the syndrome. These include:

- Low maternal or paternal age
- Lower socioeconomic groups
- Rank of second or third in birth order, especially in the case of twins and triplets or subsequent siblings of a SIDS victim
- Premature births
- Infants born small for gestational age

SIDS is confirmed by excluding other causes of death. Autopsy findings that occur in most SIDS deaths include smooth muscle thickening in small pulmonary arteries and right ventricular hypertrophy, both felt to be secondary to hypoxia and pulmonary vasculature constriction. Other findings include astrocyte gliosis of the brain stem (a tumor composed of glial [supporting] cells within the nervous system), which may be associated with respiratory center dysfunction, and neuroepithelial bodies in the tracheobronchial tree along with distal atelectasis. In addition, 87% of SIDS victims have intrathoracic petechiae, especially on the thymus, pleura, and pericardium.

External examination reveals the typical SIDS victim to be in a normal state of nutrition and hydration. Body types seem to represent a full cross section of infancy, the great majority of infants being normally plump. Over half of cases exhibit frothy fluids in the mouth and nostrils, which indicates pulmonary edema. The diapers are usually wet and full of stool. In many cases the baby's hands are found to be clutching fibers of blanket material. Emesis is sometimes present on the face. Frequently, the infant has a history of minor illness, such as a cold, within 2 weeks before death.

Management

EMS providers can do little to help the SIDS infant. The primary role of the paramedic is to provide emotional support for parents or other caregivers and loved ones. If the infant is potentially or questionably viable, resuscitation should proceed as for any other infant in cardiac arrest. Even though resuscitation will probably be unsuccessful, it is important for the parents or other caregivers to see that everything possible is being done for their child. The paramedic should follow pediatric resuscitation protocols and consult with medical control regarding decisions to initiate or continue resuscitation efforts.

The paramedic should expect a variety of grief reactions from those who witness the event (parents, family members, neighbors, babysitters). These reactions may vary from shock and disbelief to anger, rage, and self-blame. Arrangements should be made for a relative or neighbor to stay with the family or accompany them to the hospital so that they are not left alone. Many areas have SIDS resource services that provide immediate counseling and support for the family of a SIDS infant.

Because of the mysterious nature of SIDS deaths and classic signs such as postmortem lividity and frothy fluid in the infant's nose and mouth, SIDS victims may appear to have been abused or neglected. Regardless of the circumstances, the paramedic should avoid comments or questions that may imply a suspicion of inappropriate child care. Determining the cause of death is not the responsibility of the EMS crew (although careful scene observation is crucial). The paramedic should document all findings objectively, accurately, and completely. Medical control should be advised if inappropriate child care is suspected.

The death of an infant has a powerful effect on all involved, and it is common for rescuers to experience a range of emotional reactions after a SIDS death. Some EMS services, in conjunction with medical control and SIDS resource agencies, provide counseling and formal debriefing programs by trained professionals. If these services are not available, the EMS crew should be encouraged to openly discuss the event with others involved in the response (co-workers, law enforcement officers) to help relieve feelings of anxiety and stress.

Child Abuse and Neglect

Child abuse and neglect occur in at least 1% of all American children and account for approximately 4000 childhood deaths each year (second only to SIDS as a cause of death in infants 1 to 6 months of age).[5] This crime against children is reportable under law in all 50 states. Paramedics should follow local protocol in reporting suspected abuse and discuss any suspicions of child abuse or neglect with medical control.

Elements of Child Abuse

Child abuse and neglect is the maltreatment of children by their parents, guardians, or other caregivers. Forms of maltreatment include infliction of physical injury ("battered child syndrome"), sexual exploitation, and infliction of emotional pain and neglect (medical neglect, safety neglect, and nutritional deprivation). A number of factors are implicated in the potential for child abuse. These include a care-giver with the potential to abuse, a child with particular characteristics that place him or her at risk for abuse, and an element of crisis.

Characteristics of Abusers

Child abuse reflects a pattern of maladjusted behavior rather than an isolated act of violence. In the majority of cases, the abuser is a related care-giver (90%), a boyfriend of the child's mother (5%), an unrelated babysitter (4%), or a sibling of the abused child (1%).[6] Most abusers tend to be lonely, unhappy, angry adults under tremendous stress. They are usually isolated and incapable of

using support agencies or an extended family in times of crisis. Often, the abusers experienced physical or emotional abuse themselves as children.

As a rule, mothers are more likely to be involved in abuse than fathers, probably because they spend more time with the child; however, there is no difference in likelihood to abuse if the fathers are unemployed. Abusers come from all ethnic, geographical, religious, educational, occupational, and socioeconomic groups. Other factors characteristic of abusers include impoverishment (low socioeconomic conditions) and alcohol or drug dependence. An increased incidence of physical abuse has also been noted in families who live on military bases.[6]

Characteristics of an Abused Child

Abused children often have certain characteristics that increase their potential risk for abuse. Common traits include demanding and difficult behavior, decreased level of functioning (for example, a handicapped or preterm child requiring extra parenting), hyperactivity, and precociousness with intellectual ability equal to or superior to the parent. Often, the abused child is viewed by the parent as "special" or "different" from other siblings. Other factors that tend to increase the potential for child abuse are age (the child is usually less than 5 years old), gender (boys are involved more often than girls), and illegitimacy.

Crises That May Precipitate Abuse

Physical abuse or neglect can occur constantly during a child's life. More often, however, it is intermittent and unpredictable. The abuse is frequently precipitated by stressors in the adult caregiver' life, particularly in situations when the care-giver expects the child to fill emotional needs created by the stress. Failure of the child to respond in an ideal way to the care-giver's needs may lead to an abusive episode. The most common crises associated with an episode of child abuse are:

- Financial stress
- Loss of employment
- Eviction from housing
- Marital or relationship stress

- Physical illness in a child that leads to intractable crying
- Death of a family member
- Diagnosis of an unwanted pregnancy
- Birth of a sibling

History of Injuries Suspicious for Abuse

Physical abuse or neglect is often difficult to determine. The ultimate diagnosis usually begins with suspicions based on unexplained injuries, discrepant history, delays in seeking medical care, and repeated episodes of suspicious injuries. If at any time an injured child indicates that a particular adult caused him or her physical harm, the paramedic should take this report seriously and consult with medical control. In the majority of cases, these accusations are true.[5] The following are fifteen indicators of possible abuse:

1. Any obvious or suspected fractures in a child under 2 years of age
2. Injuries in various stages of healing, especially burns and bruises
3. More injuries than are usually seen in other children of the same age
4. Injuries scattered on many areas of the body
5. Bruises or burns in patterns that suggest intentional infliction
6. Suspected increased intracranial pressure in an infant
7. Suspected intraabdominal trauma in a young child
8. Any injury that does not fit the description of the cause given
9. An accusation that the child injured himself or herself intentionally
10. Long-standing skin infections
11. Extreme malnutrition
12. Extreme lack of cleanliness
13. Inappropriate clothing for the situation
14. Child who withdraws from parent
15. Child who responds inappropriately to the situation (for example, quiet, distant, withdrawn)

Physical Findings Suggestive of Abuse

Some physical findings such as multiple, widely dispersed bruises; welts; and burns are suggestive of nonaccidental trauma. Such physical findings, in conjunction with a vague history or delays in seeking medical care for the child, should alert the paramedic to the possibility of abuse or neglect (Fig. 27-1).

Bruises (Table 27-4)
- Bruises that predominate on the buttocks or lower back are almost always related to punishment.
- Genital area or inner thigh bruises are usually inflicted for toileting mishaps.
- Facial bruises or numerous petechiae on the ear lobe are usually caused by slapping.
- Bruises of the upper lip and labial frenulum are usually caused by forced feedings or from jamming a pacifier into the mouth of a screaming infant.
- Human hand marks resulting from squeezing are pressure bruises in shapes resembling fingertips, fingers, or the entire hand of the abuser.
- Human bite marks result in paired, crescent-shaped bruises that often contain individual teeth marks. The size of the arc distinguishes adult bites from child bites.

Welts
- Strap marks 1 to 2 inches wide are almost always caused by a belt.
- Bizarre-shaped welts or bruises are usually inflicted by a blunt object that resembles its shape (for example, a toy or shoe).
- Choke marks may be seen on the neck.
- Circumferential bruising or abrasions on the ankles or wrist may be caused by rope, cord, or a dog leash.

TABLE 27-4 Dating of Bruises by Color	
Color of Bruise	**Age of Bruise**
Reddish blue or purple	Less than 24 hours
Dark blue to purple	1 to 5 days
Green	5 to 7 days
Yellow	7 to 10 days
Brown	10 to 14 days or longer
Resolution	2 to 4 weeks

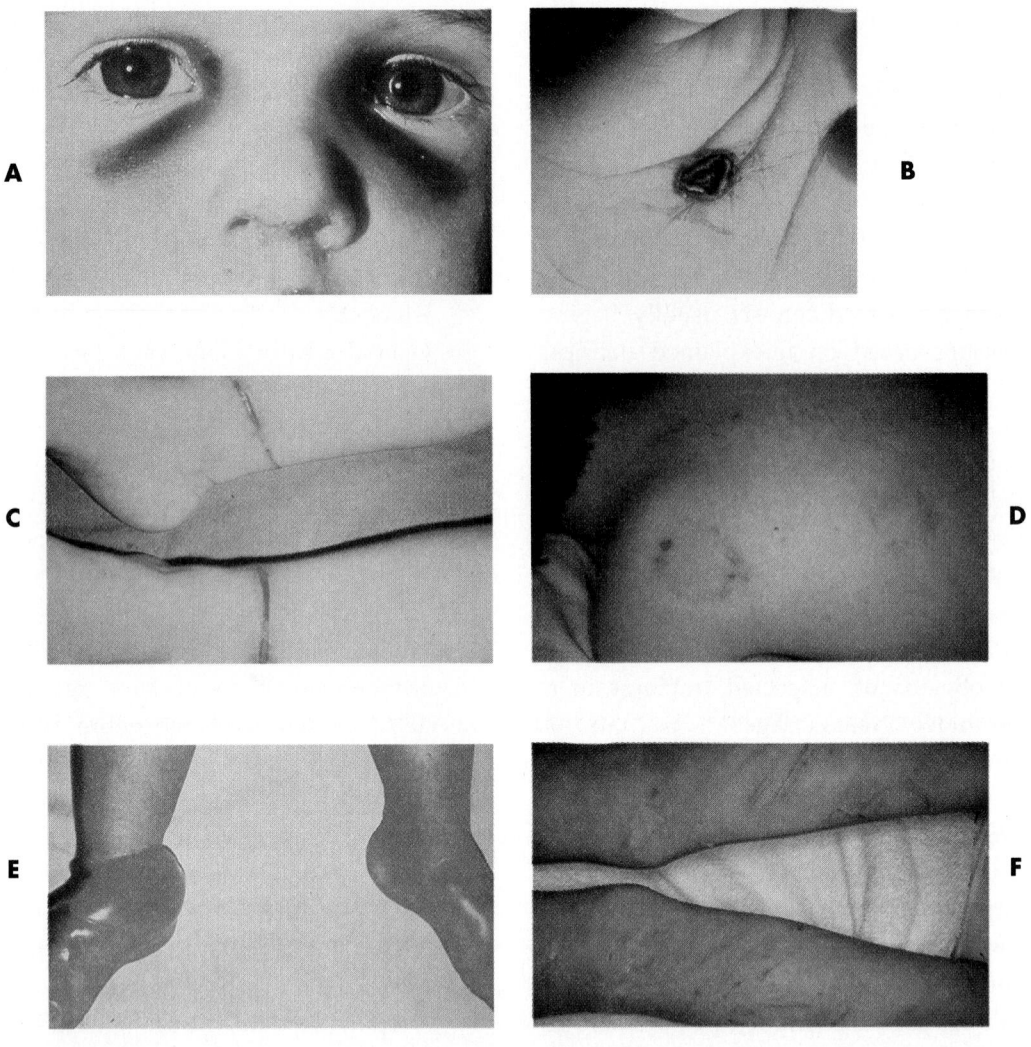

Fig. 27-1 Cutaneous manifestations of child abuse. **A,** "Raccoon eyes," or periorbital bruising, possible indication of anterior fossa skull fracture. **B,** Fresh cigarette burn to palm. **C,** Fresh abrasions of restraint injury. **D,** Human bites. **E,** "Dunking" burns of the feet. **F,** Welts and abrasions to legs as a result of an electrical cord.

Burns

- Cigarette burns are often found on the palms, soles, or abdomen.
- A lighted cigarette, a hot match, or burning incense is sometimes applied to the hand to stop the child from sucking the thumb or to the genital area to discourage masturbation.
- Burns may be inflicted with lighters or other sources of open flame (for example, a gas stove) to teach a child not to play with fire.
- Dry contact burns may result from forcibly holding a child against a heating device (for example, a radiator, hot iron, or electric hot plate).

- The most common hot-water burns or scalds occur from forcible immersion of the hands, feet, or buttocks in scalding water. These injuries often involve both arms or both legs, or they may be circular burns restricted to the buttocks; such burns are incompatible with falling or stepping into a tub of hot water.

Other less visible injuries that may indicate child abuse include brain injury, abdominal visceral injury, and bone fractures.

Subdural Hematoma

Brain injury is the leading cause of death in battered children. The various pathological lesions include cerebral contusions, intraparenchymal hemorrhage, and subdural or even epidural hematomas. Subdural hematomas are among the most common pathological abnormalities associated with intentionally inflicted head injury in children. They should be suspected in any young child who is in a coma or having convulsions, particularly if there is no history of seizure disorder. In many cases, intracranial bleeding is associated with skull fractures or scalp bruises caused by a direct blow from a care-giver's hand or by the child being hit against a wall or door.

Subdural hematomas can also result from vigorous shaking of the child ("shaken baby syndrome"). The acceleration and deceleration forces on the brain associated with shaking cause tearing of the bridging cerebral veins with bleeding into the subdural space. Signs and symptoms of the shaken baby syndrome include retinal hemorrhages, irritability, altered level of consciousness, vomiting, and a full fontanelle.

Abdominal Visceral Injury

Intraabdominal injuries are the second most common cause of death in battered children. These injuries are usually produced by a blunt force such as a punch or blow to the abdomen. Children with abdominal injury often have recurrent vomiting, abdominal distention, absent bowel sounds, and localized tenderness with or without abdominal bruising. Care-givers routinely deny a history of trauma to the child's abdomen in these cases.

Bone Injury

More than 20% of physically abused children have a positive radiological bone survey from previous abusive episodes. Injuries that may only be obvious through radiography include fractures of the ribs, lateral portion of the clavicle, scapula, sternum, and extremities. Multiple fractures in various stages of healing are highly suspicious for physical abuse.

Injuries from Sexual Abuse

Sexual abuse of a child is a symptom of a seriously disturbed family relationship usually associated with physical or emotional neglect or abuse. Often, the sexually abusive adult experienced similar abuse as a child and justifies this maladaptive behavior subconsciously. Family relationships are complex, and silent complicity by at least one parent is usually involved.

Injuries from sexual abuse may be physical and psychological. Sexual abuse may include vaginal intercourse, sodomy (anal intercourse), oral-genital contact, or molestation (fondling, masturbation, or exposure). In most cases, the victimized child is female. Over half of the victims are less than 12 years of age at the time of the first offense. Since many of these incidents are chronic and occur without force (only 35% of cases have positive physical findings), an EMS response is seldom initiated. If, however, a physical injury results from the abuse, emergency care may be summoned. Physical findings suggestive of sexual abuse include pregnancy or veneral disease in a child 12 years of age or younger, painful urination or defecation, tenderness or lacerations to the perineal area, bleeding from the rectum or vagina, and the presence of dried blood, semen, or pubic hair in the genital area of a child.

Emergency care for child victims of sexual abuse should be limited to managing life-threatening injury and providing emotional support during transport to the receiving hospital. These children undergo extensive interviews and examination by the emergency department physician and others. The paramedic should carefully document any statements made by the patient, family member, or care-giver, and any findings should be reported to medical control. These children require compassionate support. In addition, a sexually abused child should not receive the impression that she or he is responsible for any of the abuse or that discussion of the event is inappropriate.

● SPECIAL CONSIDERATIONS FOR THE SERIOUSLY ILL OR INJURED CHILD

Because children vary in size and and differ physiologically from adults, special approaches are used by paramedics in evaluating, managing, and resuscitating children who are seriously ill or injured.

Circulating Blood Volume

Adult blood volumes account for 5% to 6% of total body weight or 70 ml/kg/body weight, whereas pediatric blood volumes account for 7% to 8% of total body weight or 88 ml/kg/body weight. Although pediatric percentages of circulating blood volumes are greater than those of the adult, the absolute blood volume in the child is considerably lower than that of adults. Therefore a relatively small loss of blood may be devastating. For example, a blood loss of 100 ml in an adult is a 2% loss; a similar loss in an infant may be a 15% to 20% loss, resulting in shock. Table 27-5 shows classifications of hemorrhagic shock based on systemic signs.

A child with a volume deficit will maintain stable hemodynamics until all compensatory mechanisms fail. At that point, pediatric shock progresses rapidly, with catastrophic deterioration. Because these efficient compensatory mechanisms can mask a potentially life-threatening condition, the paramedic must maintain a high degree of suspicion. Early recognition, stabilization (airway control, fluid replacement), and rapid patient transport to an appropriate medical facility are especially important when caring for pediatric patients.

Body Surface Area and Hypothermia

Children have a relatively large body surface area in proportion to body weight, and their compensatory mechanisms (for example, shivering) are not well developed. Children in shock can quickly develop hypothermia from exposure and concurrent metabolic acidosis, increased vascular resistance, respiratory depression, and myocardial dysfunction. Because hypothermic states can make resuscitation and medication therapy less effective, every effort must be made by the paramedic to maintain the patient's body temperature through the use of towels and blankets for warming the patient and through warming devices for IV fluids.

TABLE 27-5 Classification of Hemorrhagic Shock in Pediatric Trauma Patients Based on Systemic Signs

System	Very Mild Hemorrhage*	Mild Hemorrhage†	Moderate Hemorrhage‡	Severe Hemorrhage§
Cardiovascular	Normal or mildly increased heart rate	Tachycardia	Significant tachycardia	Severe tachycardia
	Normal pulse rate	Peripheral pulses that may be diminished	Thready peripheral pulses	Thready central pulses
	Normal blood pressure	Normal blood pressure	Hypotension	Significant hypotension
	Normal pH	Normal pH	Metabolic acidosis	Significant acidosis
Respiratory	Normal rate	Tachypnea	Moderate tachypnea	Severe tachypnea
Central nervous system	Slight anxiousness	Irritability, confusion	Irritability or lethargy	Lethargy
		Combative affect	Diminished pain response	Coma
Skin	Warm, pink color	Cool extremities, mottling	Cool extremities, mottling or pallor	Cold extremities, pallor or cyanosis
	Brisk capillary refill	Delayed capillary refill	Prolonged capillary refill	Prolonged capillary refill
Kidneys	Normal urine output	Oliguria, increased specific gravity	Oliguria, increased blood urea nitrogen levels	Anuria

*< 15% blood volume loss.
†15% to 25% blood volume loss.
‡25% blood volume loss.
§40% blood volume loss.

Cardiac Reserve

Because of their already high metabolic needs, infants and children have less cardiac reserve than adults for stressful situations such as shock. It is important to reduce the energy and oxygen requirements of the pediatric patient in shock as much as possible. This can be accomplished by providing ventilatory support, decreasing anxiety, and maintaining moderate ambient temperatures.

Respiratory Fatigue

Respiratory muscle fatigue tends to occur more frequently in infants and children, leading to hypoventilation, hypoxemia, and respiratory failure or arrest. Like other compensatory mechanisms of the child, respiratory compensation in shock syndrome is generally at a maximum until it is depleted, at which time deterioration can be sudden. For this reason, airway control and supplemental oxygen are essential in all pediatric patients who are seriously ill or injured.

Vital Signs and Assessment

Many variables must be considered when evaluating pediatric vital signs. For example, blood pressure and pulse rate vary greatly with age, body temperature, and degree of agitation. Therefore although these parameters should be measured as baseline assessments, they may be of limited value in assessing circulation of the child in shock. The most effective assessment is constant monitoring of the child's physical status and assessing the response to therapy. The following nine evaluation components should be noted when assessing the pediatric patient:

1. Level of consciousness
   a. Anxiety
   b. Agitation
   c. Ability to make eye contact
   d. Ability to recognize family members
2. Skin
   a. Temperature
   b. Moisture
   c. Color
   d. Turgor
   e. Capillary refill
3. Mucous membranes
   a. Color
   b. Moisture
4. Nail beds
   a. Color
   b. Capillary refill
5. Peripheral veins
   a. Collapse
   b. Distention
6. Pulse
   a. Electrocardiogram findings
   b. Rate
   c. Rhythm
   d. Quality
7. Respiration
   a. Rate
   b. Depth
8. Blood pressure
9. Body temperature

● PEDIATRIC RESUSCITATION

Resuscitation of the pediatric patient is similar to that of the adult. The differences in therapeutics and drug modalities reflect the patient's size and weight. Figs. 27-2 and 27-3 are the treatment algorithms recommended by the American Heart Association. These include the bradycardia decision tree and asystole and pulseless arrest decision tree. Drugs used in pediatric advanced life support are listed in Tables 27-6 and 27-7.

Volume Replacement

If necessary, volume replacement should be initiated using isotonic crystalloid solutions such as normal saline or lactated Ringer's solution. The first infusion should be 20 ml/kg administered rapidly (over 5 minutes or less). If the volume loss is in the 20% range, physiological measurements should improve after this infusion. If they do, IV therapy should be continued for maintenance during patient transport.

If there is little response to the first infusion (slight improvement in color and capillary refill and decreased heart rate) or if the patient does not respond to the initial infusion, a second infusion

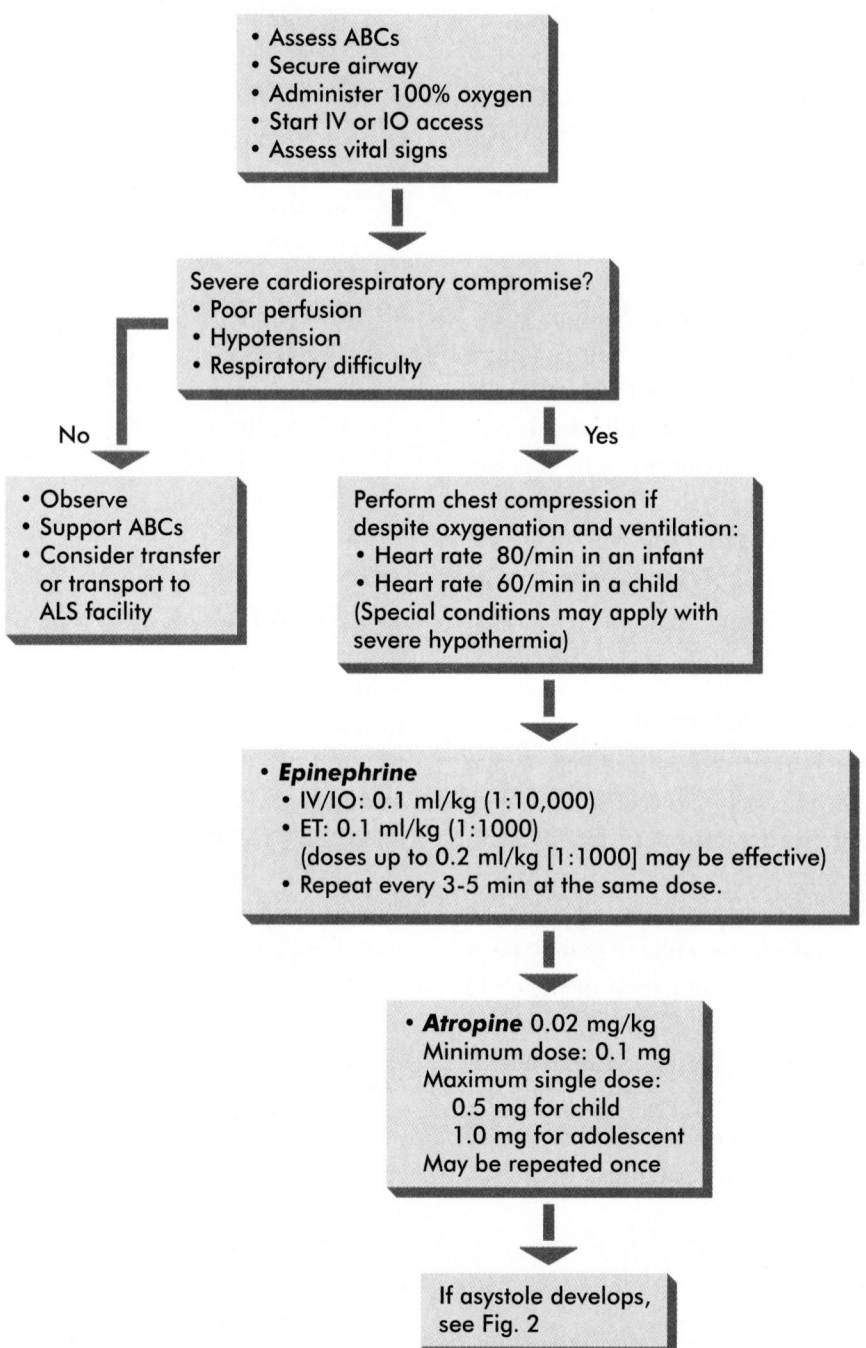

Fig. 27-2 Bradycardia decision tree. (Reproduced with permission. CPR Issue of *JAMA*, Oct 28, 1992. Copyright © American Medical Association.)

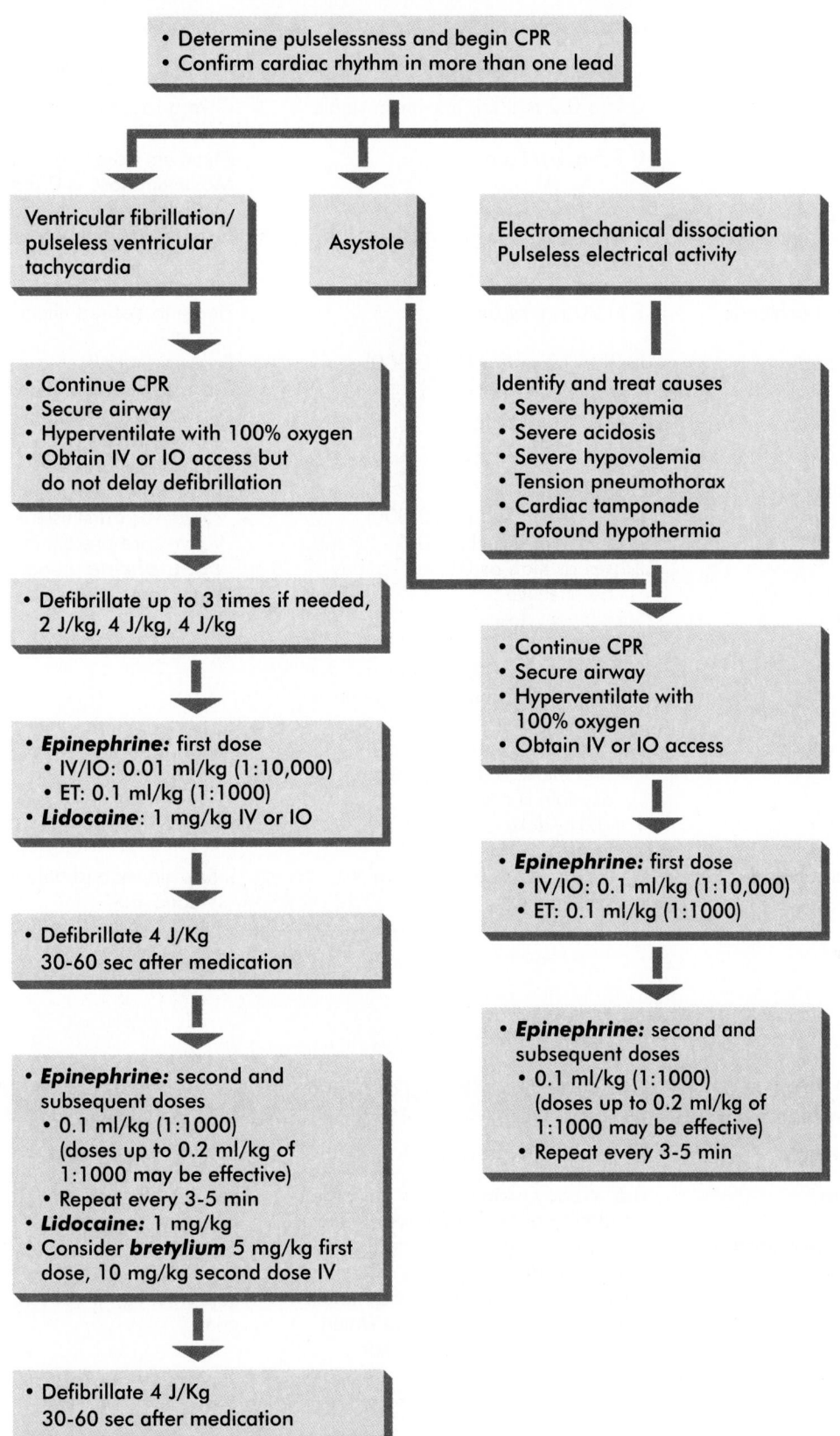

Fig. 27-3 Asystole and pulseless arrest decision tree. (Reproduced with permission. CPR Issue of *JAMA*, Oct 28, 1992. Copyright © American Medical Association.)

TABLE 27-6 Drugs Used in Pediatric Advanced Life Support

Drug	Dose	Remarks
Adenoside	0.1 to 0.2 mg/kg; maximum single dose: 12 mg	Give a rapid IV bolus.
Atropine sulfate	0.2 mg/kg/dose	Minimum dose is 0.1 mg. Maximum dose is 0.5 mg in a child and 1.0 mg in an adolescent.
Bretylium	5 mg/kg; may be increased to 10 mg/kg	Give rapidly through an IV line.
Calcium chloride 10%	20 mg/kg/dose	Give slowly.
Dopamine hydrochloride	2 to 20 μg/kg/min	Titrate to desired effect.
Epinephrine		
For bradycardia	IV/IO: 0.1 ml/kg (1:10,000) ET: 0.1 ml/kg (1:1000)	Be aware of effective dose of preservatives administered (if preservatives are present in **epinephrine** preparation) when high doses are used.
For asystolic or pulseless arrest	First dose: IV/IO: 0.1 ml/kg (1:10,000) ET: 0.1 ml/kg (1:1000) (Doses as high as 0.2 ml/kg may be effective.) Subsequent doses: IV/IO/ET: 0.1 ml/kg (1:1000) (Doses as high as 0.2 ml/kg may be effective.)	Be aware of effective dose of preservatives administered (if preservatives are present in **epinephrine** preparation) when high doses are used.
Epinephrine infusion	Initial dose: 0.1 μg/kg/min (Higher infusion dose is used if asystole is present.)	Titrate to desired effect (0.1 to 1.0 μg/kg/min).
Lidocaine	1 mg/kg/dose	—
Lidocaine infusion	20 to 50 μg/kg/min	—
Sodium bicarbonate	1 mEq/kg/dose or 0.3 × kg × base deficit	Infuse slowly and only if ventilation is adequate.

ET, Endotracheal.

TABLE 27-7 Preparation of Infusions

Drug	Preparation*	Dose
Epinephrine	0.6 × body weight (kg) = milligrams added to diluent† to make 100 ml	Then 1 ml/hr delivers 0.1 μg/kg/min; titrate to effect
Dopamine, dobutamine	6 × body weight (kg) = milligrams added to diluent to make 100 ml	Then 1 ml/hr delivers 1.0 μg/kg/min; titrate to effect
Lidocaine	120 mg of 40 mg/ml solution added to 97 ml of 5% dextrose in water, yielding 1200 μg/ml solution	Then 1 ml/kg/hr delivers 20 μg/kg/min

*Standard concentration may be used to provide more dilute or more concentrated drug solution, but then individual dose must be calculated for each patient and each infusion rate:

$$\text{Infusion rate (ml/hr)} = \frac{\text{Weight (kg)} \times \text{Dose (}\mu\text{g/kg/min)} \times 60 \text{ min/hr}}{\text{Concentration (}\mu\text{g/ml)}}$$

†Diluent may be 5% dextrose in water, 5% dextrose in half-normal saline, normal saline, or lactated Ringer's.

of 20 ml/kg should follow immediately. It is uncommon for children with nonhemorrhagic hypovolemia to be unresponsive to a 40-ml/kg infusion. If there is no response after the second fluid challenge, the patient is probably suffering from hypovolemia caused by hemorrhage. Other possible causes include pneumothorax, sepsis, and myocardial dysfunction.

IV Therapy

Establishing an IV line in children is difficult in the most controlled settings. Accordingly, medical control may recommend that the pediatric patient in shock be stabilized and rapidly transported to an appropriate medical facility. If vascular access is to be attempted in the prehospital setting, the paramedic should consider the following points:

- Use the largest accessible vein.
- If an upper or lower extremity is chosen, secure the site with an armboard or other immobilization device.
- Limit the use of external jugular veins to life-threatening situations.

Peripheral vascular access is described in Chapter 13. Other methods of vascular access in pediatric patients include scalp veins and IO infusion. These procedures require special training and authorization from medical control.

Scalp Vein Cannulation

Veins of the forehead and temporal areas may be used in infants less than 1 year old (Fig. 27-4). To gain access to a scalp vein in an infant, it may be necessary to shave the overlying skin to expose the vein and to provide an adherent surface for tape. A rubber band applied around the level of the forehead may be used as a circumferential tourniquet.

Necessary Equipment

- Alcohol wipes
- Povidone-iodine (betadine wipes)
- Antibiotic ointment
- Tape
- Scalp vein needles: 21 or 23 gauge
- Over-the-needle catheters: 22 gauge

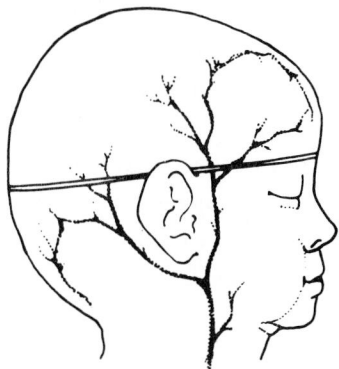

Fig. 27-4 Location of scalp veins. Rubber band used for tourniquet.

- IV tubing: microdrip or pediatric infusion set
- IV fluids (specified by medical control): normal saline, lactated Ringer's solution, special pediatric fluids

Method of Insertion

1. Apply gloves for personal and patient protection.
2. Cleanse the area as for peripheral and central cannulation.
3. Secure the patient and the vein.
4. Insert the scalp vein needle or over-the-needle catheter into the most cephalad portion of the vein and advance caudally.
5. Remove the tourniquet and infuse IV fluid as prescribed by medical control.
6. Secure the IV line with tape and apply bulky dressing to prevent removal by the infant.
7. Document procedure.

Potential Complications

- Inadvertent arterial puncture
- Hematoma
- Residual ecchymosis

IO Infusion

Bone marrow has been used for fluid and drug administration since the early 1920s. With the advent of disposable IV catheters, IO infusion fell into disuse in the 1950s. Studies have shown that this infusion technique is relatively safe and effective when initiated in children under 6 years of age. These studies and the potential requirement for vascular access when peripheral cannulation is unavailable have led to new interest in this technique. The procedure is currently being used by EMS services in many areas of the United States.

Fluids and drugs infused through IO access pass from the marrow cavities into the sinusoids, to large venous channels and emissary veins, and then to the systemic circulation. Normal saline, lactated Ringer's solution, D_5W, plasma, blood, and most ALS medications may be infused quickly through this route (Figs. 27-5 and 27-6).

IO infusion should be considered only in unconscious children under 6 years of age and *only when peripheral cannulation is unobtainable*. Example scenarios include cardiopulmonary arrest and peripheral vascular collapse (as in shock, major trauma, or burns). In addition, IO infusion is rec-

ommended in critically ill children in whom vascular access is impaired by obesity or edema, in small newborns, and in children with life-threatening status asthmaticus. Special training and authorization must be provided by medical control.

The site of choice for initiating this procedure is the tibia, one to two fingerbreadths below the tubercle on the anteromedial surface. An alternative choice would be the femur, two to three fingerbreadths above the lateral condyles in the midline.

Necessary Equipment

- Alcohol wipes
- Povidone-iodine (Betadine) wipes
- Antibiotic ointment
- Tape
- Bone marrow needle or 16-gauge spinal needle
- IV tubing: microdrip or pediatric infusion set
- IV fluids (specified by medical control): normal saline, lactated Ringer's solution, or special pediatric fluids

Method of Insertion

1. Apply gloves for personal and patient protection.
2. Cleanse the site as previously described for peripheral and central cannulation.
3. Prepare bone marrow needle or 16-gauge spinal needle for proper depth during inser-

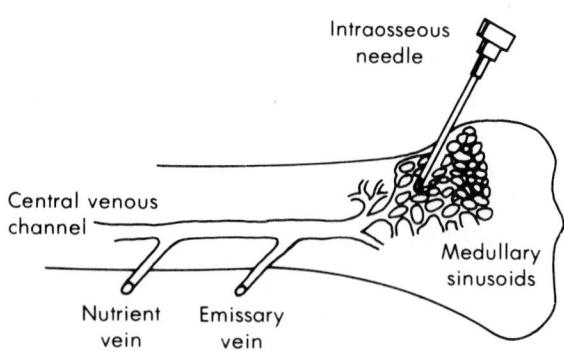

Fig. 27-5 Venous drainage from marrow of long bone with intramedullary needle in place.

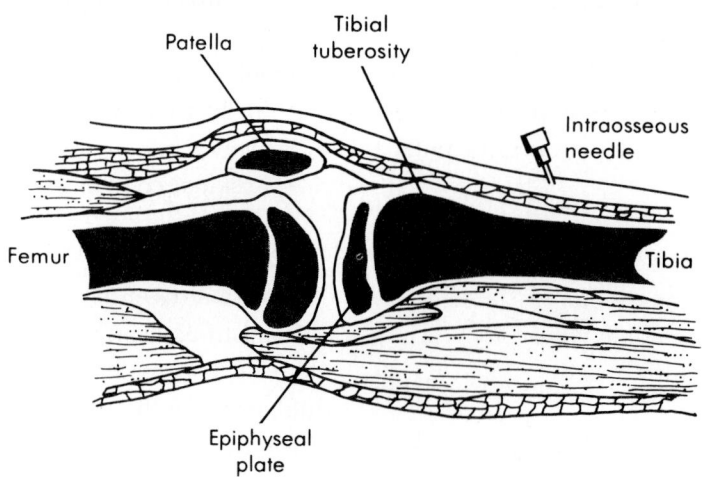

Fig. 27-6 IO insertion of needle.

tion. Insert needle pointing away from epiphyseal plate, advancing to periosteum.

4. Using a boring or screwing motion, advance the needle until it penetrates bone marrow (usually noted by decreased resistance).
5. Remove stylet.
6. Aspirate bone marrow into saline-filled syringe. (Bone marrow will not always be aspirated.)
7. Infuse saline by syringe to ensure placement and to clear clots.
8. Secure needle with tape (although needle is usually well stabilized by the bone).
9. Attach standard IV tubing and fluids to infuse under gravity or pressure as prescribed by medical control.
10. Document procedure.

Contraindications

- Fracture of the site or proximal to the site
- Traumatized extremity
- Cellulitis
- Burns that may be infected by the technique
- Congenital bone disease

Potential Complications

- Technical
  - Subperiosteal infusion from improper placement
  - Penetration of posterior wall of medullary cavity, resulting in soft tissue infusion
  - Slow infusion from clotting of marrow
- Systemic
  - Osteomyelitis (less than 0.6%, usually with prolonged infusion)
  - Fat embolism (not yet reported in children)
  - Slight periostitis at the injection site (usually clearing in 2 to 3 weeks)
  - Infection (acceptably low rate comparable with that of other infusion techniques)
  - Fracture

REFERENCES

1. Ramenofsky M: The need for knowledge, *Emerg Mag* 21(8):8, 1989.
2. National Center for Education in Maternal and Child Health: *Emergency medical services for children: a report to the nation*, Washington, DC, 1991, The Center.
3. *SIDS update*, St Louis, 1991, SIDS Resources.
4. Hazinski M: *Nursing care of the critically ill child*, ed 2, St Louis, 1992, Mosby.
5. Touloukian R: *Pediatric trauma*, ed 2, St Louis, 1990, Mosby.
6. Fuchs S: Managing seizures in children, *Emerg Mag* 22(12):47, 1990.

Summary

Many individuals and agencies focus on identifying specific assessment and management strategies for prehospital pediatric care. To provide optimal medical care to pediatric patients, an EMS system approach must be in place to ensure rapid access and the delivery of advanced emergency care when needed. Children have unique anatomical, physiological, and psychological characteristics that increase their risk for a number of diseases and illnesses. An understanding of these characteristics helps promote confidence in managing the critically ill or injured child.

OB/GYN AND NEONATAL

DIVISION FIVE

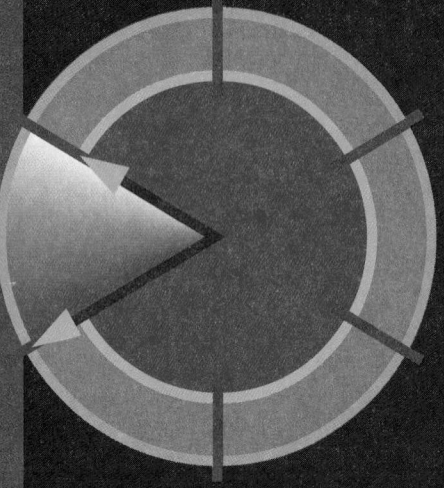

IN THIS DIVISION
28 OBSTETRICAL EMERGENCIES AND NEONATAL RESUSCITATION
29 GYNECOLOGICAL EMERGENCIES

The pinnacle of my career was the day I delivered two babies from two mothers, approximately 15 minutes apart while en route to the hospital. We deal with tragedy every day in this profession. But delivering a precious new life into the world—and doing it twice in one day—well, it made everything seem all right again.

Patricia Dukes, MICT
City and County of Honolulu
Honolulu, Hawaii

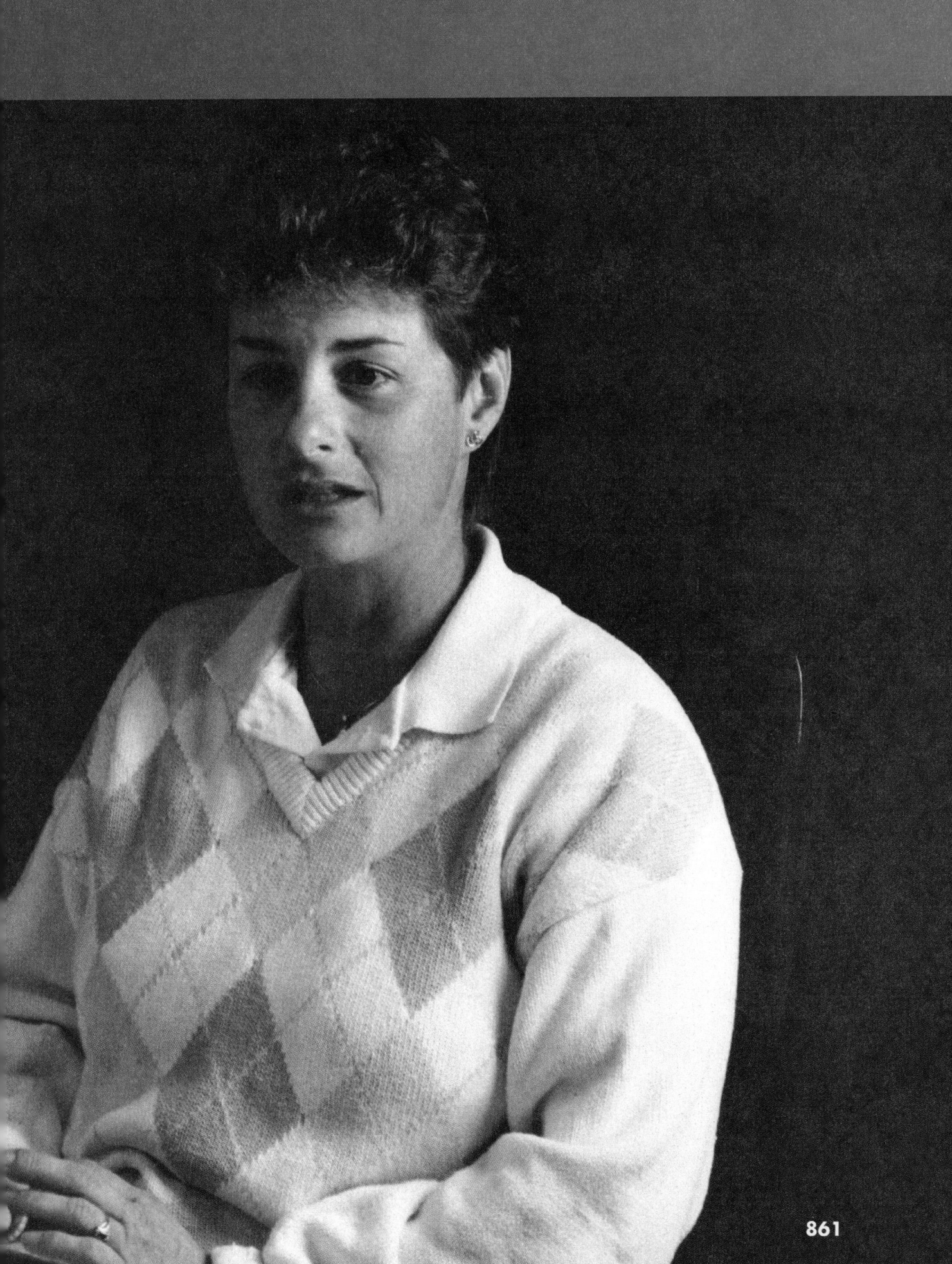

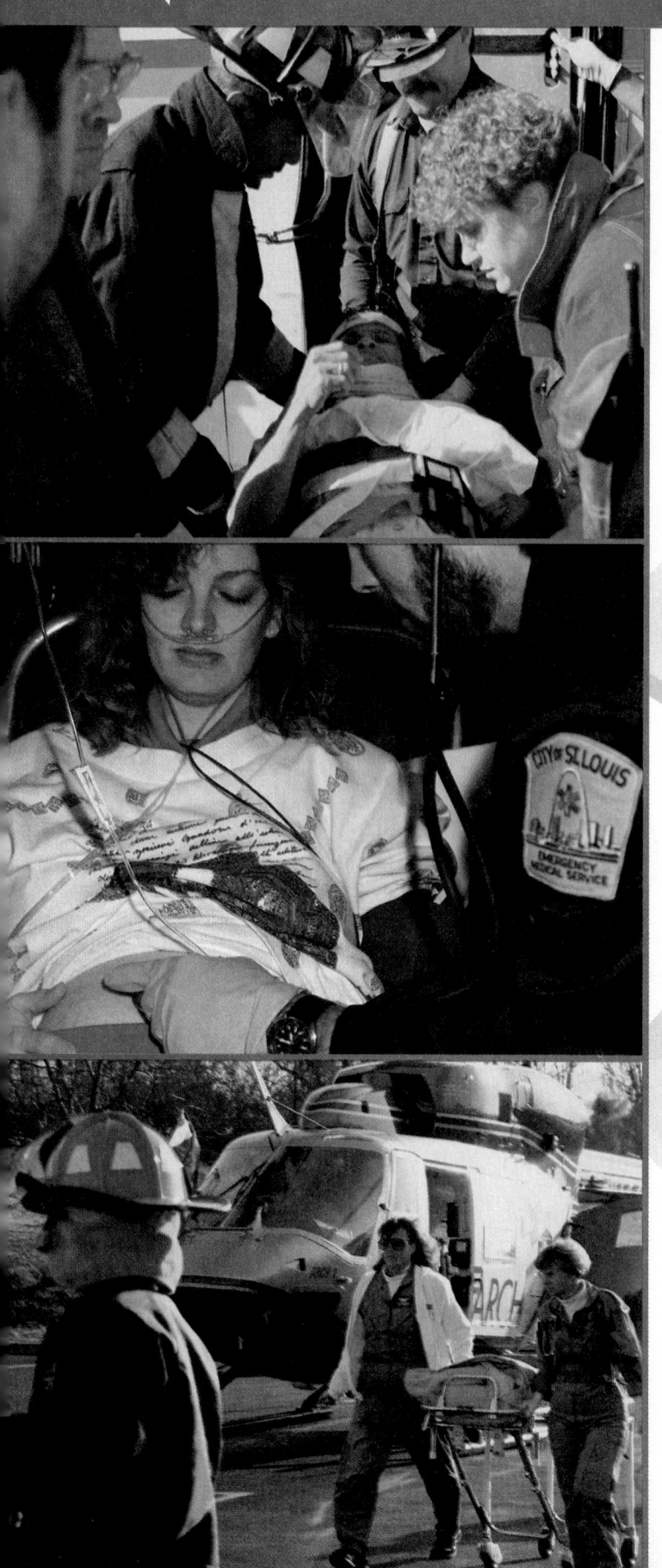

Childbirth is common in the prehospital setting. Most often, EMS personnel only assist in this natural process and provide appropriate care for the mother and newborn. However, obstetrical emergencies can develop suddenly and be life threatening. Therefore paramedics must be prepared to recognize and manage these events and sometimes assist in abnormal deliveries. This chapter presents the etiology and treatment of obstetrical emergencies, the normal and abnormal events associated with pregnancy and childbirth, and initial care and resuscitation of the neonate.

OBJECTIVES

As a paramedic, you should be able to:

1. Label an anatomical diagram of the female reproductive system.
2. Outline the events in the normal menstrual cycle.
3. Outline fetal development from ovulation through birth.
4. Explain normal maternal physiological changes during pregnancy and how they influence prehospital patient care and transport.
5. Describe appropriate information to be elicited during the obstetric patient history.
6. Describe specific techniques for assessing pregnant patients.
7. Discuss the implications of prehospital care based on the effects of trauma on the fetus and mother.
8. Describe the assessment and management of patients with preeclampsia and eclampsia.
9. Explain the pathophysiology, signs and symptoms, and management of the processes that cause vaginal bleeding in pregnancy.
10. Outline the role of the paramedic during normal labor and delivery.
11. Compute an Apgar score for a newborn.
12. Discuss the identification, implications, and prehospital management of complicated deliveries.
13. Describe the pathophysiology, assessment, and prehospital management of maternal pulmonary embolism.
14. Describe prehospital care of the normal neonate.
15. Outline steps in resuscitating a distressed neonate.

Section One
Female Reproductive System

The female reproductive organs are the ovaries, uterine tubes, uterus, vagina, external genital organs, and mammary glands. These structures are explained and illustrated in Chapter 10.

KEY TERMS

Apgar score: The evaluation of an infant's physical condition, usually performed at 1 and 5 minutes after birth, including heart rate, respiratory effort, muscle tone, reflex irritability, and color.

gestation: The period from fertilization of the ovum until birth.

gravida: The number of all current and past pregnancies.

meconium aspiration syndrome: The inhalation of meconium by the fetus or newborn, which can block air passages and result in failure of the lungs to expand or cause other pulmonary dysfunction.

menarche: The first menstruation and the commencement of the cyclic menstrual function.

ovulation: Release of an ovum or secondary oocyte from the vesicular follicle.

para: The number of past pregnancies that have remained viable to delivery.

placenta: A highly vascular fetal-maternal organ through which the fetus absorbs oxygen, nutrients, and other substances and excretes carbon dioxide and other wastes.

trimester: One of three periods of approximately 3 months into which pregnancy is divided.

● MENSTRUATION AND OVULATION

Menstruation is the normal, periodic discharge of blood, mucus, and cellular debris from the uterine mucosa. The normal menstrual cycle is approximately 28 days and occurs at more or less regular intervals from puberty to menopause (except during pregnancy and lactation). The average menstrual flow of 25 to 60 ml usually lasts 4 to 6 days and is fairly constant for each individual from cycle to cycle. The onset of menses (**menarche**) generally begins between ages 12 and 13 and ends permanently (menopause) at an average age of 47 years, with wide variation. Depending on the individual, normal menopause may occur from ages 35 to 60.

Follicle and Oocyte Development

By the fourth month of prenatal life, the ovaries contain approximately 5 million cells from which oocytes (immature ova) develop. At birth, there are approximately 2 million primary oocytes, which decline in number to 300,000 to 400,000 at puberty. Of these primary oocytes, only approximately 400 are eventually released from the ovary. Oocytes are surrounded by a layer of cells (granulosa cells), and the entire structure is known as a *primary follicle* (Fig. 28-1).

The menstrual cycle is associated with hormonal changes that stimulate some of the primary follicles to continue development and become secondary follicles. The secondary follicle continues to enlarge, forming a lump on the surface of the ovary. The fully mature follicle is known as the *vesicular* or *graafian follicle*.

Ovulation

Cellular secretions of the graafian follicle cause it to swell more rapidly than can be accommodated by follicular growth. The follicle expands and ruptures, forcing a small amount of blood and

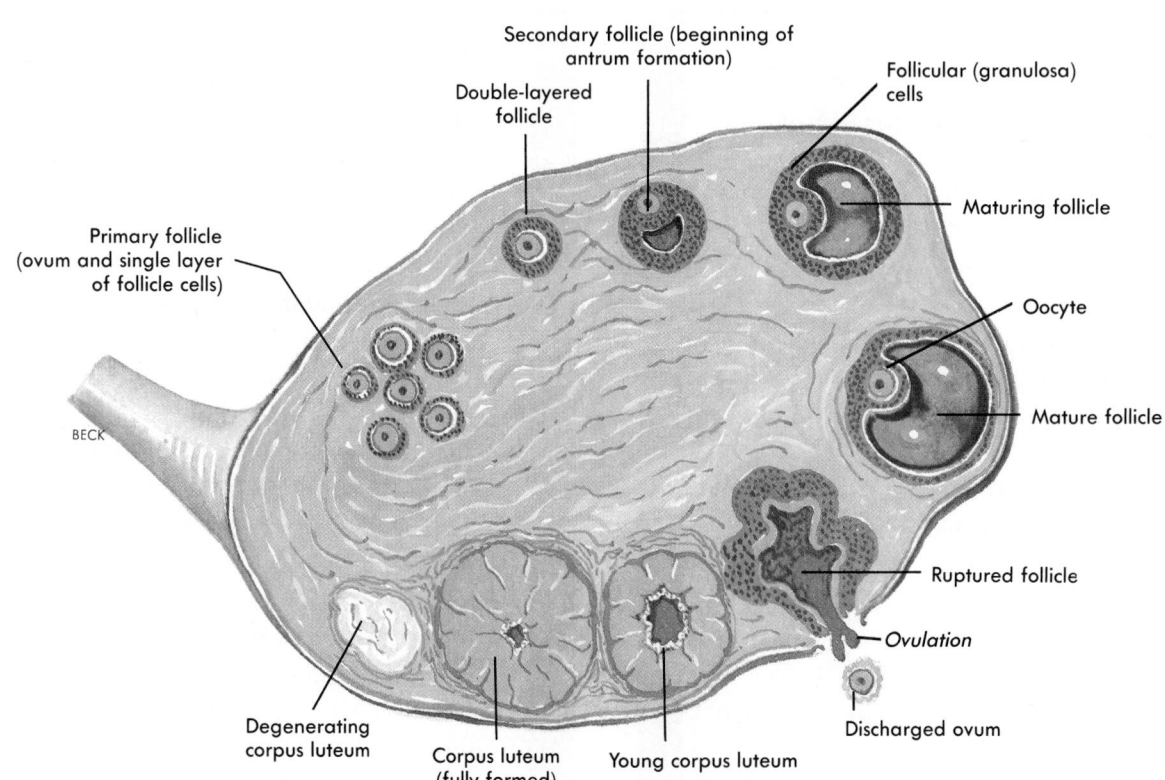

Fig. 28-1 Diagram of ovary and oogenesis. Cross section of mammalian ovary shows successive stages of ovarian (graafian) follicle and ovum development. Begin with the first stage (primary follicle) and follow around clockwise to the final stage (degenerating corpus luteum).

follicular fluid out of the vesicle. Shortly after this initial burst of fluid, an oocyte escapes from the follicle. The release of this secondary oocyte is termed **ovulation.**

After ovulation, the follicle is transformed into a yellow glandular structure called the *corpus luteum,* whose cells secrete large amounts of progesterone and some estrogen. If pregnancy occurs, the fertilized oocyte (zygote) begins releasing a hormonelike substance (chorionic gonadotropin) that keeps the corpus luteum from degenerating. As a result, blood levels of estrogen and progesterone do not decrease, and the menstrual period does not occur. In the absence of pregnancy, the corpus luteum degenerates, and the secondary oocyte passes out of the system with the menstrual flow.

Hormonal Control of Ovulation and Menses

Ovulation and menses are controlled by hormones released from the hypothalamus and anterior pituitary (adenohypophysis). Follicle-stimulating hormone (FSH) stimulates development of the follicle, including cells that produce estrogen. Before ovulation, these cells release estrogen and cause a surge in the pituitary production of luteinizing hormone (LH), which initiates the ovarian cycle (leading to ovulation), which in turn regulates the uterine cycle (Fig. 28-2). Under the influence of the ovarian hormones, the lining of the uterus (endometrium) goes through two phases of development: the proliferative and secretory phases.

The proliferative phase is initiated and maintained by the increasing amounts of estrogen produced by the maturing follicle. The estrogen stimulates the endometrium to grow and increase in thickness, preparing the uterus for implantation of a fertilized ovum. The secretory phase begins after ovulation and is under the combined influence of estrogen and progesterone. During this phase, tortuous secretory glands and spiral vessels develop to prepare the endometrium for implantation of the fertilized ovum. Within 7 days after ovulation (approximately day 21 of the menstrual cycle), the endometrium is ready to receive the developing embryo if fertilization has occurred.

In the absence of fertilization, the ovum can survive only 6 to 24 hours, after which the hormone levels drop and the endometrium is shed as menstrual flow. This process normally occurs on day 28 of the menstrual cycle (approximately 14 days after ovulation).

Fertilization and Implantation

Within several hours after ovulation, the ovum is transported to the ampulla by hair-covered cells (fimbria) of the fallopian tube. The oocyte is capable of being fertilized for up to 24 hours after ovulation, and some spermatozoa remain viable in the female reproductive tract for up to 72 hours. After fertilization, cell division begins rapidly. The developing cells (blastocyst) pass through the fallopian tube and begin to travel toward the uterus, a process that usually takes 3 to 5 days (Fig. 28-3).

Implantation begins within 7 days after fertilization and is completed when the fertilized egg makes contact with maternal circulation (approximately day 12). The process of implantation is assisted by the secretion of proteolytic enzymes by the outer layer of the developing embryonic mass (the trophoblast), which digests the cells of the thickened endometrium and allows invasion of the uterine wall.

● SPECIALIZED STRUCTURES OF PREGNANCY

Specialized structures of pregnancy include the placenta, the umbilical cord, and the amniotic sac and its fluid. These structures transport metabolic fuel and raw materials for the developing embryo and are part of fetal circulation.

Placenta

For approximately 14 days after ovulation, the trophoblast cells continue to develop and form the placenta. The **placenta** is a disklike organ composed of interlocking fetal and maternal tissues. The placenta serves as the organ of exchange between the mother and fetus and is responsible for the following five functions:

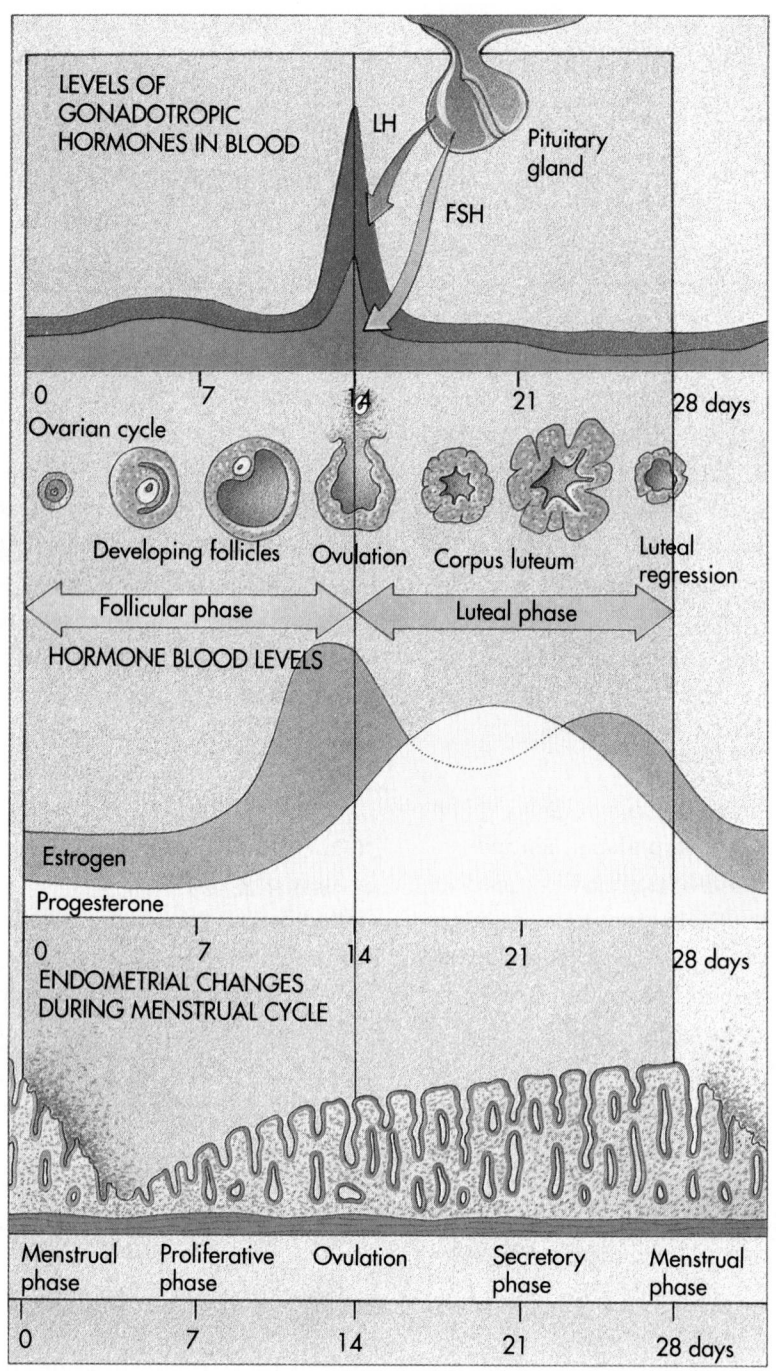

Fig. 28-2 Human menstrual cycle. The interrelationship of pituitary, ovarian, and uterine functions throughout the usual 28-day cycle. A sharp increase in LH levels causes ovulation, whereas menstruation (sloughing of the endometrial lining) is initiated by lower levels of progesterone.

1. Transfer of gases. The diffusion of oxygen and carbon dioxide through the placental membrane is similar to the diffusion that occurs through the pulmonary membranes. Dissolved oxygen in maternal blood passes through the placenta into fetal blood as a result of the pressure gradient between the blood of the mother and fetus. Conversely, as fetal carbon dioxide pressure (P_{CO_2}) accumulates, a low pressure gradient of carbon di-

Uterine (Fallopian) tube

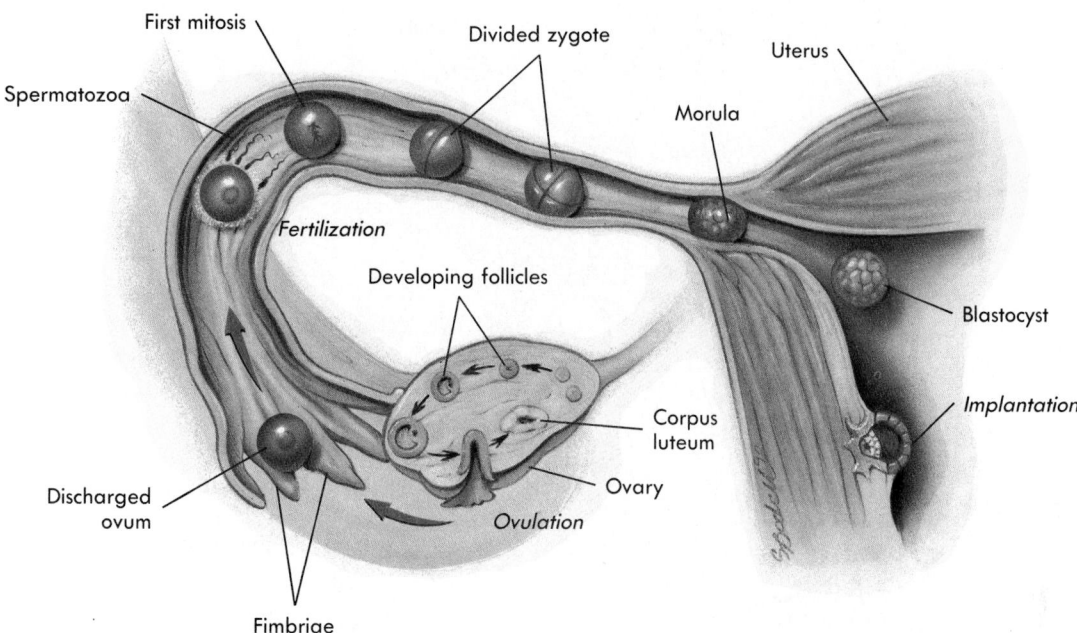

Fig. 28-3 Fertilization and implantation. At ovulation, an ovum is released from the ovary and begins its journey through the uterine tube. While in the tube, the ovum is fertilized by sperm to form the single-celled zygote. After a few days of rapid cell division, a ball of cells called a *morula* is formed. After the morula develops into a hollow ball (blastocyst), implantation occurs.

oxide develops across the placental membrane, and carbon dioxide diffuses from fetal blood to maternal blood.

2. Transport of nutrients. Other metabolic substrates needed by the fetus diffuse into fetal blood in the same manner as oxygen. For example, glucose levels in fetal blood are approximately 20% to 30% lower than levels of glucose in maternal blood, which results in a rapid diffusion of glucose to the fetus. Other substrates transported by way of diffusion include fatty acids, potassium, sodium, and chloride. Some nutrients are also actively absorbed by the placenta from maternal blood.

3. Excretion of wastes. Waste products such as urea, uric acid, and creatinine diffuse from fetal blood into maternal blood, where they are excreted with the waste products of the mother. Wastes transfer from fetus to mother in the same manner as carbon dioxide does.

4. Hormone production. The placenta becomes a temporary endocrine gland, secreting sufficient quantities of estrogen and progesterone so that by the third month of fetal development, the corpus luteum is no longer needed to sustain the pregnancy. Estrogen, progesterone, and other hormones maintain the uterine lining, prevent the occurrence of menses, and stimulate changes in the pregnant woman's breasts, vagina, and cervix that prepare her body for delivery and lactation.

5. Formation of a barrier. The placenta provides a barrier against some harmful substances and chemicals in the mother's circulation. The placental barrier is incomplete and nonselective and therefore does not totally protect the fetus. Among the medications easily transported across the placenta are steroids, narcotics, anesthetics, and some antibiotics.

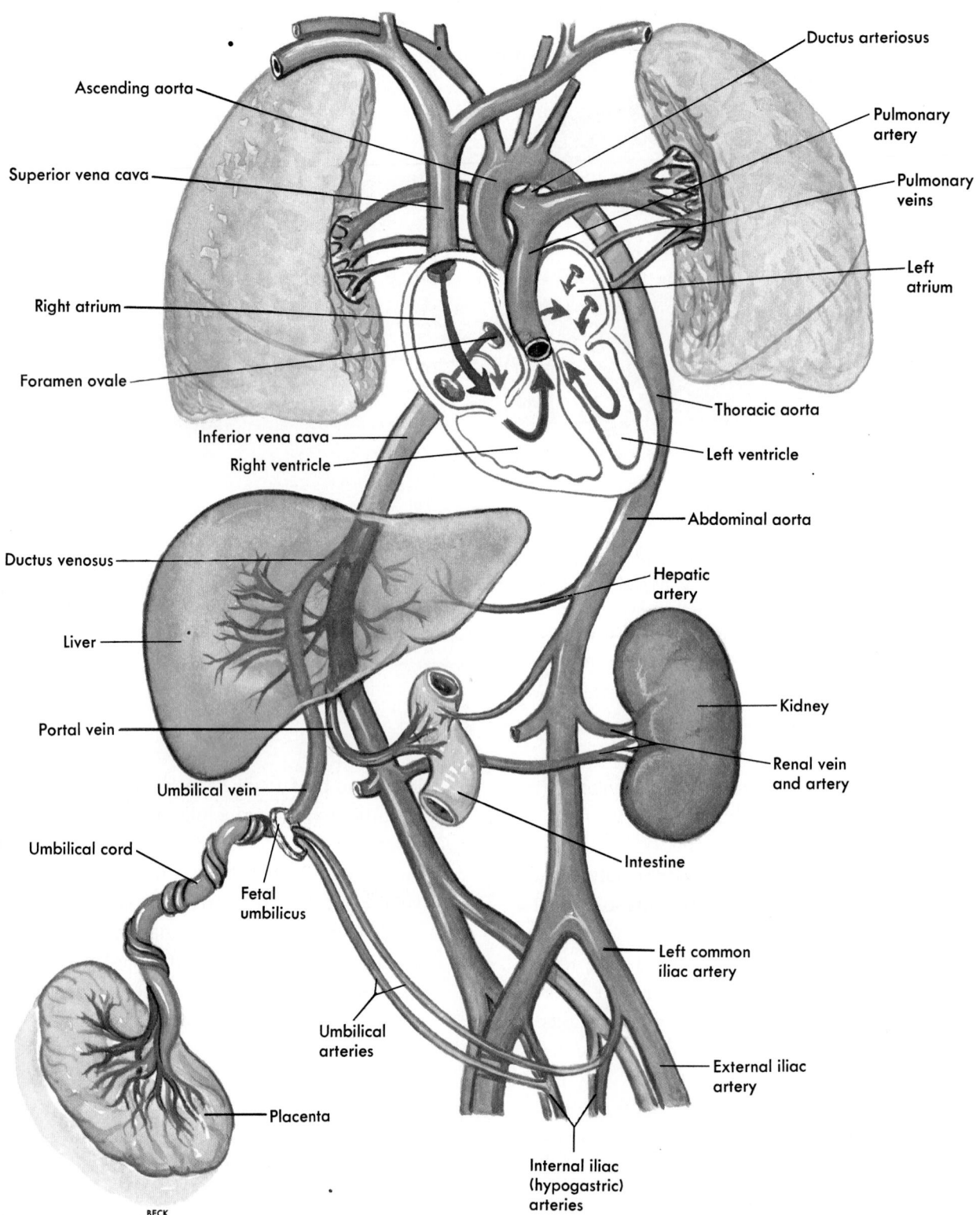

Fig. 28-4 Fetal circulation.

Umbilical Cord

Blood flows from the fetus to the placenta by way of two umbilical arteries carrying deoxygenated blood; oxygenated blood returns to the fetus by an umbilical vein (Fig. 28-4). The blood remains in a closed system independent of and separated from the maternal circulation. Other structures unique to fetal circulation are the ductus venosus, the foramen ovale, and the ductus arteriosus. The ductus venosus is a continuation of the umbilical cord that serves as a shunt to allow most blood returning from the placenta to bypass the immature liver of the embryo and empty directly into the inferior vena cava. The foramen ovale and the ductus arteriosus allow blood to bypass the nonfunctional lungs, which remain collapsed until birth.

The foramen ovale shunts blood from the right atrium directly into the left atrium, and the ductus arteriosus connects the aorta and the pulmonary artery. Thus the well-oxygenated blood from the placenta enters the left side of the heart rather than the right side and is pumped by the left ventricle mainly into vessels of the head and forelimbs. The blood entering the right atrium from the superior vena cava is directed downward through the tricuspid valve into the right ventricle. Most of this blood is deoxygenated blood from the head region of the fetus and is pumped by the right ventricle into the pulmonary artery. From there it passes through the ductus arteriosus into the descending aorta and through the two umbilical arteries into the placenta for oxygenation. At birth, the various arteriovenous shunts close.

Amniotic Sac and Amniotic Fluid

The amniotic sac is a fluid-filled cavity that completely surrounds and protects the embryo. Amniotic fluid originates from several fetal sources, including fetal urine and secretions from the respiratory tract, skin, and amniotic membranes. The fluid accumulates rapidly and amounts to approximately 175 to 225 ml by the fifteenth week of pregnancy and approximately 1 L at birth. The rupture of the amniotic membranes produces the watery discharge at the time of delivery.

● FETAL DEVELOPMENT

During the first 8 weeks of pregnancy, the developing ovum is known as an *embryo,* and thereafter until birth, it is called a *fetus.* The period during which intrauterine fetal development takes place, known as **gestation,** usually averages 40 weeks from time of fertilization to delivery of the newborn. The progress of gestation is usually considered in terms of 90-day periods or **trimesters.** Since conception occurs approximately 14 days after the first day of the last menstrual period, fetal development and the estimated date of confinement (delivery date) can be calculated with reasonable reliability. Rapid fetal growth and development characterize the period of gestation (Fig. 28-5 and Box 28-1).

Adjustments of the Infant to Extrauterine Life

Birth results in the infant's loss of the placental connection with the mother and therefore loss of metabolic support. Especially important are the infant's need to obtain oxygen and excrete carbon dioxide. This requires circulatory adjustments that permit adequate blood flow through the lungs.

After a normal delivery by a mother who has not been depressed with anesthetics, an infant ordinarily begins to breathe with a normal respiratory rhythm immediately or with minimal stimulation. At birth the walls of the alveoli are held together by the surface tension of the viscid fluid that fills them. More than 25 mm Hg of negative pressure is required to oppose the effects of this surface tension, allowing the alveoli to open for the first time. The initial inspirations of the newborn can create as much as 50 mm Hg of negative pressure in the intrapleural space. These powerful first breaths open the alveoli and allow further respirations to occur with much less effort.

The immature liver and nonfunctional lungs of the developing fetus are bypassed by the ductus

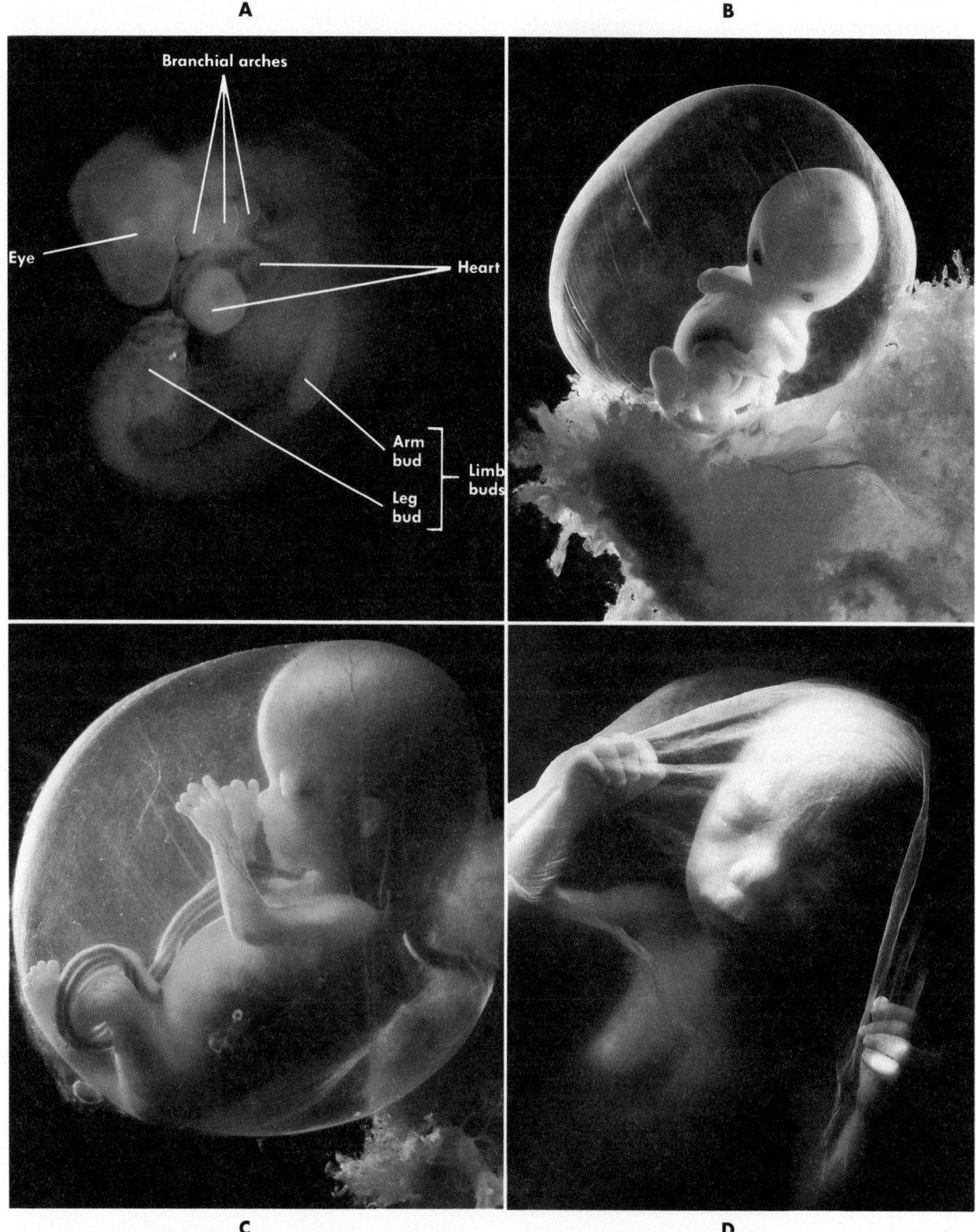

Fig. 28-5 Human embryos and fetuses. **A,** At 35 days. **B,** At 49 days. **C,** At the end of the first trimester. **D,** At 4 months.

BOX 28-1

Embryo and Fetal Development in Utero for Each Lunar Month (28 days)

First Lunar Month
- Foundations are formed for the nervous system, genitourinary system, skin, bones, and lungs.
- Buds of arms and legs begin to form.
- Rudiments of eyes, ears, and nose appear.

Second Lunar Month
- The head is disproportionately large because of brain development.
- Gender differentiation begins.
- The centers of bones begin to ossify.

Third Lunar Month
- Fingers and toes are distinct.
- The placenta is complete.
- Fetal circulation is complete.

Fourth Lunar Month
- Gender is differentiated.
- Rudimentary kidneys secrete urine.
- Heartbeat is present.
- Nasal septum and palate close.

Fifth Lunar Month
- Fetal movements are felt by the mother.
- Heart sounds are perceptible with a fetoscope.

Sixth Lunar Month
- The skin appears wrinkled.
- Eyebrows and fingernails develop.

Seventh Lunar Month
- The skin is red.
- The pupillary membrane disappears from the eyes.
- If born, the infant cries and breathes but frequently dies.

Eighth Lunar Month
- The fetus is viable if born.
- The eyelids open.
- Fingerprints are set.
- Vigorous fetal movement occurs.

Ninth Lunar Month
- The face and body have a loose, wrinkled appearance because of subcutaneous fat deposits.
- Amniotic fluid decreases somewhat.

Tenth Lunar Month
- Skin is smooth.
- Eyes are uniformly slate colored.
- The bones of the skull are ossified and nearly together at sutures.

venous, ductus arteriosus, and foramen ovale. When blood flow through the placenta ceases at birth, there is a resultant increase in systemic vascular resistance and in aortic, left ventricular, and left atrial pressures. In addition, pulmonary vascular resistance decreases greatly because of expansion of the lungs, which reduces the pulmonary arterial, right ventricular, and right atrial pressures. As a result of these changes in pressure gradients, the arteriovenous shunts close normally within a few hours after birth and are eventually occluded by growth of fibrous tissue, a change triggered by certain chemical mediators.

Section Two
Assessment of the Patient

It helps for the paramedic to be familiar with obstetrical terminology and the physiological changes that occur in the pregnant woman.

● OBSTETRICAL TERMINOLOGY

Pregnant patients are described by their gravida and para states. The term **gravida** refers to the

---

BOX 28-2

Obstetrical Terminology

Antepartum: the maternal period before delivery

Grand multipara: a woman who has had seven deliveries or more

Multigravida: a woman who has had two or more pregnancies

Multipara: a woman who has had two or more deliveries

Nullipara: a woman who has never delivered

Perinatal: occurring at or near the time of birth

Postpartum: the maternal period after delivery

Prenatal: existing or occurring before birth

Primigravida: a woman who is pregnant for the first time

Primipara: a woman who has given birth only once

Term: a pregnancy that has reached 40 weeks' gestation

---

number of all of the woman's current and past pregnancies; **para** refers only to the number of the woman's past pregnancies that have remained viable to delivery. For example, a woman who is pregnant for the first time is gravida 1, para 0 (Box 28-2).

● MATERNAL CHANGES DURING PREGNANCY

In addition to cessation of menstruation and the obvious enlargement of the uterus, the pregnant woman undergoes many other physiological changes. These changes affect the genital tract, the breasts, the gastrointestinal system, the cardiovascular system, the respiratory system, and metabolism.

Genital Tract

Uterus
- Uterine size increases from 70 g (nongravid) to 1000 g by term.
- By the second month, the uterus triples in size and weight.
- By the third month, the uterus occupies the entire pelvic cavity and may be palpated suprapubically.
- By the fourth month, the uterus becomes an abdominal organ, and the top of the uterus (fundus) reaches the level of the umbilicus.
- In the last trimester, the uterus recedes a little when the fetus descends into the pelvis.

Cervix
- Increased uterine blood and lymphatic flow cause pelvic congestion and edema. This results in softening and bluish discoloration of the cervix (Chadwick's sign).

Vagina
- The vagina develops a characteristic violet color from increased vascularity.
- The vaginal walls prepare for labor, and the vaginal mucosa increases in thickness.
- Vaginal secretions increase, and the pH decreases to approximately 3.5 because of increased production of lactic acid from glycogen in the vaginal epithelium. (Acidic pH is thought to help keep the vaginal area relatively free of pathogens.)

Bladder
- Frequency of urination occurs from pressure of the expanding uterus on the bladder. (Frequency disappears when the uterus rises out of the pelvis and returns when the fetal head engages in the pelvis near term.)

Breasts
- The breasts become tender in the early weeks of pregnancy.
- By the second month, the breasts increase in size from hypertrophy of the mammary alveoli.

- The nipples become larger, more deeply pigmented, and more erectile early in pregnancy.
- As breast glands proliferate, they begin to secrete a clear fluid by the tenth week after conception.

Gastrointestinal System

- Morning sickness and nausea may occur at any time (usually beginning by the sixth and abating by the fourteenth week). The cause is thought to be related to the high serum levels of chorionic gonadotropin in early pregnancy.
- The patient's stomach and intestines are displaced upward and laterally by the enlarging uterus.
- The liver is displaced backward, upward, and to the right.
- The tone and motility of the gastrointestinal tract decrease, leading to prolonged gastric emptying and relaxation of the pyloric sphincter; heartburn is common.

Cardiovascular System

Heart

- The heart is displaced to the left and upward by elevation of the diaphragm. (Flat or negative T waves may be present in lead III on the electrocardiogram [ECG].)
- Cardiac output rises 30% by the thirty-fourth week.
- The pulse rate may increase 15 to 20 beats/ min above baseline late in the third trimester (variable).
- Pulmonic systolic and apical systolic murmurs are common because lowered blood viscosity and increased flow lead to turbulence in the great vessels.

Circulation

- Total blood volume is increased by 30%, and plasma volume is increased by 50%.
- Blood pressure decreases 10 to 15 mm Hg during the second trimester because of the reduction in peripheral resistance but gradually increases to prepregnancy levels toward term.
- The enlarged uterus interferes with venous return from the legs.
- Hemorrhoids, slight edema of the ankles, and varicose veins may be present.
- The supine position may cause the uterus to compress the inferior vena cava, producing decreased cardiac filling and decreased cardiac output (supine hypotension syndrome). The patient may become faint and hypotensive while lying on her back.

Hematology

- Increased plasma volume results in a drop in hemoglobin and hematocrit concentrations.
- The leukocyte count is elevated.
- Fibrinogen levels increase 50% because of the influence of estrogen and progesterone.

Respiratory System

- Tidal volume and minute ventilation increase by 30% to 40% in late pregnancy.
- Functional residual capacity decreases approximately 25%.
- The respiratory rate may be normal or increased because of elevation of the diaphragm by the uterus.
- P_{CO_2} is normally decreased because of the increased respiratory rate (30 torr versus 40 torr, which provides a gradient for fetal carbon dioxide). This may cause dizziness and a sensation of shortness of breath.

Metabolism

- The mother experiences a normal weight gain of 0.5 kg per week (a total of 9.1 kg [20 pounds]).
- Increased water retention produces increased intracapillary hydrostatic pressure, which favors filtration from the vascular bed and resultant edema.
- The metabolic rate increases, as does caloric demand (especially for protein).

- Glucose escapes into urine as a result of increased glomerular filtration.
- Maternal gestational diabetes mellitus (GDM) may result from an impaired ability to metabolize carbohydrates, which is usually caused by a deficiency of insulin. Generally GDM disappears after delivery, but in some cases it returns years later.
- Fetal demands for calcium and iron may deplete maternal stores if not supplemented through diet.

● HISTORY

When obtaining a history from an obstetrical patient, the paramedic should first gather information on the chief complaint, which may not be related to the pregnancy. Information regarding the onset of signs and symptoms should be solicited in confidence, and privacy should be afforded for all aspects of the physical examination. After ruling out any life-threatening illness or injury, the patient should be interviewed to obtain relevant data, including the following eight points:

1. Obstetric history
   a. Length of gestation
   b. Parity and gravidity
   c. Previous cesarean delivery (removal of the fetus from the uterus through an incision in the mother's abdominal wall and uterus)
   d. Maternal lifestyle (drug or alcohol use, smoking history)
   e. Recent infectious diseases
   f. History of previous gynecological or obstetrical complications (eclampsia, GDM, premature labor, ectopic pregnancy)
2. Presence of pain
   a. Onset (gradual or sudden)
   b. Character
   c. Duration and evolution over time
   d. Location and radiation
3. Presence, quantity, and character of vaginal bleeding
4. Presence of abnormal vaginal discharge
5. Presence of "show" (expulsion of the mucous plug in early labor) or rupture of membranes

6. Current general health and prenatal care
7. Allergies, medications taken
8. Maternal urge to bear down or sensation of imminent bowel movement, indicating imminent delivery

● PHYSICAL EXAMINATION

The patient's chief complaint determines the extent of the physical examination. The prehospital objective in examining an obstetrical patient is to rapidly identify acute surgical or life-threatening conditions or imminent delivery and take appropriate management steps.

The patient's general appearance should be evaluated for skin color. If she is markedly pale, hemorrhage should be suspected. Sunken cheeks, cracked lips, or hollow eyes with a history of vomiting should lead the paramedic to suspect dehydration. Initial vital signs should be assessed and frequently monitored throughout the patient encounter. In addition, orthostatic vital signs may be useful in eliciting the early presence of significant bleeding or fluid loss. The paramedic should recall that normal physiological changes in the pregnant patient can produce variations in vital signs, such as mild tachycardia, a slight fall in systolic and diastolic blood pressures, and an increase in respiratory rate.

The abdomen should be examined for previous scars and any gross deformity, such as that caused by a hernia or marked abdominal distention. Gentle palpation may reveal the presence of masses, enlarged organs, intestinal distention, or a distended bladder, but in late pregnancy, it may be difficult to appreciate these abnormalities. Peritoneal irritation may be discernible during the physical examination and is diagnosed by the presence of tenderness, guarding, or rebound tenderness. If the patient is obviously pregnant, evaluation of uterine size and fetal monitoring may be indicated.

Evaluation of Uterine Size

The uterine contour is usually irregular between weeks 8 and 10. Therefore early uterine enlarge-

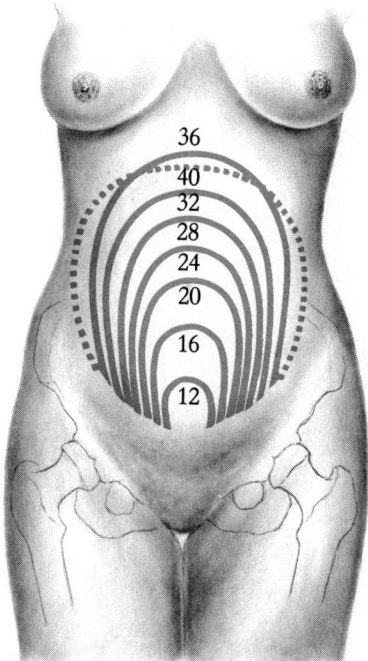

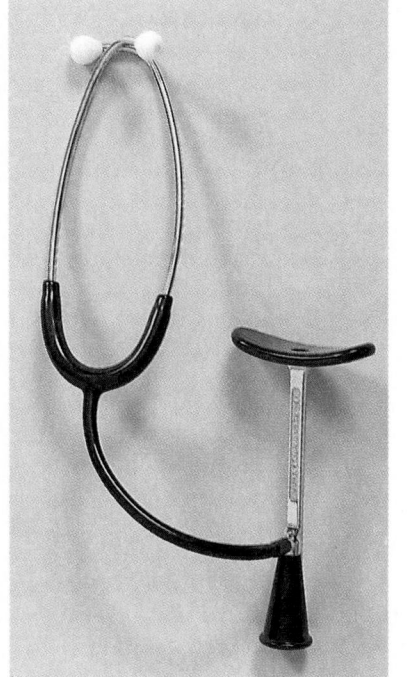

A

Fig. 28-6 Changes in fundal height in pregnancy. Weeks 10 to 12: The uterus is within the pelvis; a fetal heartbeat can be detected with Doppler. Week 12: The uterus is palpable just above the symphysis pubis. Week 16: The uterus is palpable just between the symphysis pubis and umbilicus. Week 20: The uterine fundus is at the lower border of the umbilicus. A fetal heartbeat can be auscultated with a fetoscope. Weeks 24 to 26: The uterus becomes ovoid in shape; the fetus is palpable. Week 28: The uterus is approximately halfway between the umbilicus and xiphoid process; the fetus is easily palpable. Week 34: The uterus fundus is just below the xiphoid. Week 40: Fundal height drops as the fetus begins to engage in the pelvis.

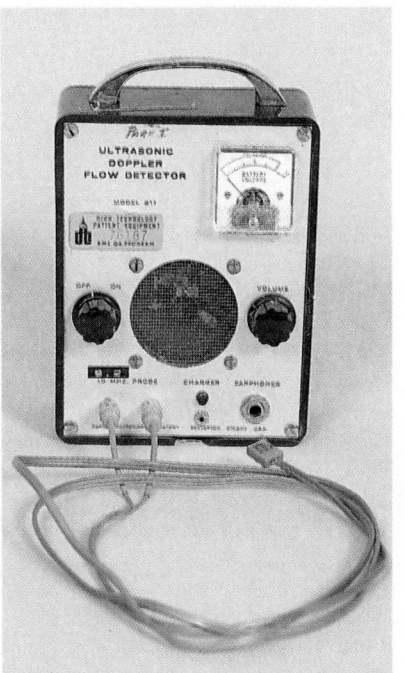

B

ment may not be symmetric, and the uterus may be deviated to one side. At 12 to 16 weeks gestation, the uterus is above the symphysis pubis; at 24 weeks, at the level of the umbilicus; and at term, near the xiphoid process. Changes in fundal height at the various weeks of gestation are shown in Fig. 28-6.

Fig. 28-7 A, Fetoscope. **B,** Doppler.

Fetal Monitoring

Fetal heart sounds may be auscultated between 16 and 40 weeks by use of a stethoscope, fetoscope, or Doppler (Fig. 28-7). The benefits of fetal monitoring include ascertaining the presence or absence of fetal circulation and providing baseline measurements for use in evaluating fetal or maternal distress. Fetal heart rate and maternal vital signs should be evaluated every 5 to 10 minutes.

When auscultating the fetal heart rate, the paramedic should position the high-intensity dia-

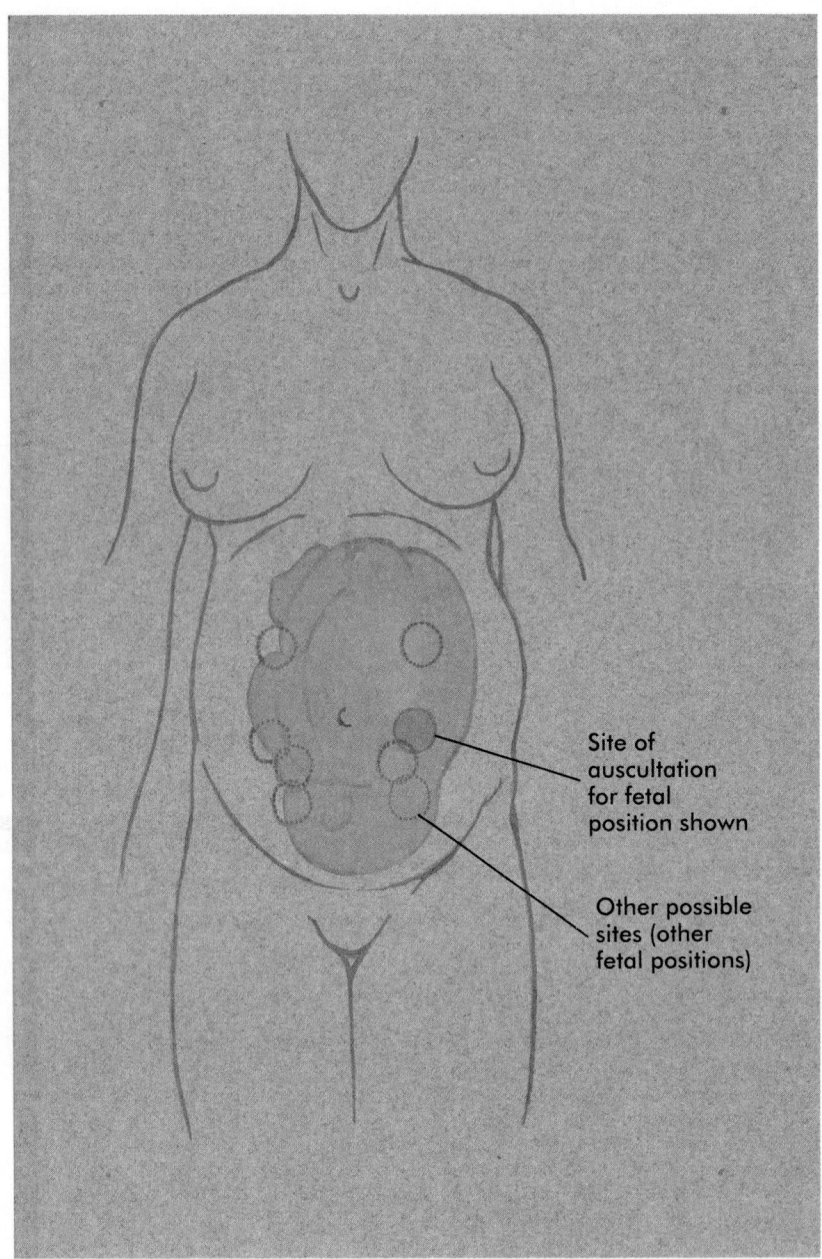

Fig. 28-8 Sites for auscultation of fetal heart tones.

phragm of the stethoscope (the bell of the fetoscope or the microphone of the Doppler) firmly on the mother's abdominal wall. The diaphragm should then be moved in a circular pattern approximately 6 to 8 inches in diameter around the woman's umbilicus until the fetal heart tones can be heard (Fig. 28-8). Once it is located, the fetal heart rate should be measured in beats per minute in the usual fashion.

The normal fetal heart rate is 120 to 160 beats/min. A persistent fetal heart rate above 160 (fetal tachycardia) or below 120 beats/min (fetal bradycardia) is an early sign of fetal distress and fetal or maternal hypoxia. Intermittent, short-term acceleration or deceleration of the fetal heart rate is usually normal and can occur at any time. Short-term periodic changes in fetal heart rate are common during fetal sleep, fetal movement, and contractions associated with labor and delivery.

Section Three
Complications of Pregnancy

Complications associated with pregnancy can result from trauma, medical conditions or prior disease processes that can be aggravated or masked by the pregnancy, the pregnancy itself (vaginal or intraperitoneal hemorrhage), intrauterine abortion, or problems associated with labor and delivery. Often, the patient with gynecological or obstetrical complaints is embarrassed, apprehensive, and if pregnant, concerned about the unborn child. Tact, understanding, and a caring and supportive attitude from the paramedic are important in managing these patients.

● TRAUMA IN PREGNANCY

According to the Committee on Trauma of the American College of Surgeons, accidental injury occurs in 6% to 7% of all pregnancies and is the most common cause of death in the gravid patient.[1] Anatomical and physiological changes associated with pregnancy can alter the patient's response to injury, requiring modified assessment, treatment, and transportation strategies.

Maternal Injury

The causes of maternal injury in decreasing order of frequency are vehicular crashes, falls, and penetrating objects. These injuries can result in trauma to the gravid uterus and to the maternal bladder, liver, and spleen. In addition, an injury that results in a pelvic fracture can produce massive hemorrhage and damage to the fetal skull. As described in Chapter 15, the severity of any injury depends on many factors, and as in a nongravid patient, severe maternal injury often involves multiple organ systems.

During pregnancy, the fetus is well protected within the uterus; amniotic fluid surrounds the fetus and serves as an excellent shock absorber. Because of this protection, it is extremely rare for a fetus to experience physical trauma except as a re-sult of direct penetrating wounds or extensive blunt trauma to the maternal abdomen. The greatest risk of fetal death is from fetal distress and intrauterine demise caused by trauma to the mother or her death. Therefore when dealing with a pregnant trauma patient, the paramedic should promptly assess and intervene on behalf of the mother. Severe abdominal injury may result in premature separation of the placenta, premature labor or abortion, rupture of the uterus, and fetal death. Causes of fetal death from maternal trauma include death of the mother, separation of the placenta, maternal shock, uterine rupture, and fetal head injury.

Assessment and Management

Priorities in assessing and managing a pregnant trauma patient are the same as for a nongravid patient: adequate airway, ventilatory, and circulatory support with spinal precautions; hemorrhage control; and rapid assessment, stabilization, and transport to a medical facility. Resuscitating the mother is the key to survival of both mother and fetus. Therefore during the initial stages of assessment and management, efforts should be directed toward the mother's status. Regardless of the severity of injury, all pregnant trauma patients should be transported for physician evaluation.

The secondary assessment should be thorough. Injuries that would contribute to hypovolemia or hypoxia must be detected, identified, and treated early. With the normal increase in maternal blood volume, the mother can tolerate more blood loss. A 30% to 35% reduction in blood volume can produce minimal changes in blood pressure but will reduce uterine blood flow by 10% to 20%. Thus the mother may achieve homeostasis at the expense of the fetus, and the true magnitude of blood loss may be difficult to discern. Fetal monitoring is the best available indicator of fetal well-being after trauma. However, assessment of fetal heart rate should never delay patient transport.

Accelerations of fetal heart rate above baseline are associated with fetal movement and contractions but may also be an early sign of fetal distress. Decreased fetal movement and increased fetal heart rate can indicate maternal shock.

Decelerations of fetal heart rate below the baseline are associated with a decrease in cardiac output and the presence of hypoxia. A hypoxic fetus in metabolic acidosis cannot accelerate his or her heart rate and thus becomes bradycardic (a heart rate of less than 120 beats/min). Sustained fetal bradycardia (lasting 10 minutes or more) may be a response to increased parasympathetic tone and can only be tolerated for a short time before the fetus becomes acidotic. Fetal bradycardia is usually a late occurrence from maternal hypoxia and decreased maternal circulating volume.

Special Management Considerations

Special considerations in managing the pregnant trauma patient include oxygenation, volume replacement, and hemorrhage control. Labor is also a complication of trauma in pregnancy, so the EMS crew should be prepared to manage imminent delivery or spontaneous abortion.

If cardiac arrest occurs, cardiopulmonary resuscitation (CPR) should be instituted in the usual fashion. An aggressive resuscitation effort is justified in patients near term to allow for emergency cesarean delivery at the emergency department. Fetal survival is good if the interval between maternal death and delivery is less than 5 minutes and poor if longer than 20 to 25 minutes. Advance notice to the receiving emergency department of impending emergency cesarean delivery is paramount.

Oxygenation
- Adequate airway maintenance and oxygenation are essential to prevent fetal hypoxemia.
- Oxygen requirements are 10% to 20% greater than in the nongravid patient. Fetal hypoxia may occur with even small changes in maternal oxygenation.
- If available, pulse oximetry should be used to monitor oxygen saturation.

Volume Replacement
- Signs and symptoms of hypovolemia may not be present until a blood loss is large.
- Blood is preferentially shunted from the uterus to preserve maternal blood pressure.

- Bleeding may also occur inside the patient's uterus.
  - The pregnant uterus can sequester up to 2000 ml of blood after separation of the placenta with little or no evidence of vaginal bleeding.
- Crystalloid fluid replacement is initiated, even in normotensive patients.
- Pneumatic antishock garments are applied (controversial).
  - Only the leg compartments are inflated because they may increase blood loss from disrupted vasculature of the pelvis.
  - Abdominal compartment inflation may be indicated when maternal and fetal death are imminent (by order of medical control).
- Vasopressors are generally not recommended because they decrease uterine blood flow and fetal oxygen delivery.

Hemorrhage Control
- External hemorrhage is controlled.
- Vaginal bleeding may indicate placental separation or uterine rupture
- A vaginal examination should be avoided. It may increase bleeding and precipitate delivery, especially if unsuspected placenta previa presents.
- The amount and color of vaginal bleeding should be documented.
- Any expelled tissue should be collected and transported with the patient to the hospital.

Transportation Strategies

After 3 to 4 months gestation, pregnant patients should not be transported in a supine position because of the potential for supine hypotension. If spinal injury is not suspected, the patient should be transported in a left lateral recumbent position. If spinal injury is suspected, the paramedic should prepare the patient for transport in the following manner:

1. Fully immobilize the patient on a long spine board.
2. After immobilization, carefully tilt the board on its left side by log-rolling the secured patient 10 to 15 degrees.

3. Place a blanket, pillow, or towel under the right side of the board to move the uterus to the left side.

● MEDICAL CONDITIONS AND DISEASE PROCESSES

Medical conditions and disease processes that may be masked or aggravated by pregnancy include acute appendicitis, acute cholecystitis, hypertension, diabetes, infection, neuromuscular disorders, and cardiovascular disease. Two hypertensive disorders, preeclampsia and eclampsia, are specific to pregnancy. Preeclampsia occurs in 5% to 8% of all pregnancies in the United States and is responsible for approximately 25% of maternal deaths and approximately 25% of preterm births.

Preeclampsia and Eclampsia

Preeclampsia is a disease of unknown origin that primarily affects previously healthy, normotensive primigravidae. The disease occurs after the twentieth week of gestation, often near term. The pathophysiology of preeclampsia (which is not reversed until after delivery) is characterized by vasospasm, endothelial cell injury, increased capillary permeability, and activation of the clotting cascade. The signs and symptoms of preeclampsia result from hypoperfusion to the tissue or organs involved (Box 28-3). Eclampsia is characterized by the same signs and symptoms plus seizures or coma.

The criteria for diagnosis of preeclampsia are based on the presence of the "classic triad," which includes hypertension (blood pressure greater than 140/90 mm Hg, a rise of 30 mm Hg in systolic pressure, or a rise of 15 mm Hg in diastolic pressure over prepregnancy levels), proteinuria, and edema. Besides nulliparity, factors predisposing to preeclampsia include advanced maternal age, chronic hypertension, chronic renal disease, vascular disease such as diabetes mellitus and systemic lupus erythematosus, and multiple gestation. Preeclampsia is a clinical diagnosis that may be confirmed by postpartum renal biopsy. When the disease is suspected, most patients are hospitalized or confined to bed rest at home until delivery.

BOX 28-3

Signs and Symptoms of Preeclampsia

Cerebrum
Headache
Hyperreflexia
Dizziness
Confusion
Seizures
Coma

Retina
Blurred vision
Diplopia

Gastrointestinal System
Nausea
Vomiting
Right upper quadrant or epigastric pain and tenderness

Renal System
Proteinuria
Azotemia
Oliguria
Anuria
Hematuria
Hemoglobinuria

Vasculature or Endothelium
Hypertension
Edema
Activation of the clotting cascade

Placenta
Abruptio placentae
Fetal distress

Management

Not all hypertensive patients have preeclampsia, and not all preeclamptic patients have hypertension. Because of the potentially devastating course of the illness, the disease should always be considered when hypertension is present in late pregnancy. If preeclampsia or eclampsia is suspected, prehospital care is directed at preventing or controlling seizures and treating hypertension.

Seizure activity in eclampsia is similar to generalized grand mal seizures of other etiologies and is characterized by tonic-clonic activity. The seizure often begins around the mouth in the form of facial twitching. Eclampsia may be associated with apnea during the seizure. Labor can begin spontaneously and progress rapidly. The regimen for managing severe preeclampsia is:

1. Place the patient in a left lateral recumbent position to maintain or improve uteroplacental blood flow and to minimize risk of insult to the fetus.
2. Handle the patient gently and minimize sensory stimulation to avoid precipitating seizures.
3. Administer high-concentration oxygen and assist respirations as needed.
4. Initiate intravenous therapy per local protocol.
5. Anticipate seizures at any moment and be prepared to provide airway, ventilatory, and circulatory support.
6. Be prepared to administer the following medications per medical control and local protocol:
   a. *Magnesium sulfate* 10% (2-4 g slow intravenous administration)
      i. The paramedic should have an antidote (*calcium gluconate*) close at hand to treat respiratory depression.
   b. *Diazepam* (5-10 mg, slow intravenous or rectal administration)
   c. *Hydralazine* (5 mg, slow intravenous administration) to treat hypertension
      i. It may precipitate a fall in blood pressure.
      ii. It may jeopardize fetal circulation.
      iii. The paramedic should closely monitor vital signs.
7. Gently transport patient to appropriate medical facility.

Vaginal Bleeding

Vaginal bleeding during pregnancy may result from abortion (miscarriage), ectopic pregnancy, abruptio placentae, placenta previa, uterine rupture, or postpartum hemorrhage. Patients who have vaginal bleeding develop varying degrees of blood loss; some require aggressive resuscitation.

Abortion

Abortion is the termination of pregnancy from any cause before the twentieth week of gestation (after which it is known as a *preterm birth*). It is the most frequent cause of vaginal bleeding in pregnant women and occurs in approximately 1 in 10 pregnancies. Common classifications of abortion are listed in the Box 28-4.

Most abortions occur in the first trimester, usually before the tenth week. The patient is often anxious and apprehensive and complains of vaginal bleeding, which may be slight or profuse. In addition, the patient may have suprapubic pain referred to the lower back and described as "cramplike" and similar to the pain of labor or menstruation. When obtaining a history, the paramedic should ascertain the time of onset of pain and bleeding, amount of blood loss (a soaked sanitary pad suggests 20 to 30 ml of blood loss), and whether the patient passed any tissue with the blood. If tissue was passed during bleeding episodes, it should be collected and transported with the patient for analysis.

Management

The assessment of all first-trimester emergencies should include close observation for signs of significant blood loss and hypovolemia. Vital signs (including orthostatic vital signs) should be measured and frequently monitored during transport. Depending on the patient's hemodynamic status, intravenous fluid therapy may be indicated. All patients with suspected abortion should receive oxygen, emotional support, and transport for physician evaluation.

Ectopic Pregnancy

An ectopic pregnancy occurs when a fertilized ovum implants anywhere other than the endometrium of the uterine cavity. More than 90% of ectopic gestations occur within the fallopian tubes; 6% are abdominal pregnancies, and 1% are ovarian and cervical pregnancies. Ectopic gestation occurs in 1 of every 200 pregnancies; it is the lead-

BOX 28-4

Classifications of Abortion

Complete abortion: an abortion in which the patient has passed all of the products of conception.

Incomplete abortion: an abortion in which the patient has passed some but not all of the products of conception.

Induced abortion: an abortion in which the pregnancy is intentionally terminated.

Missed abortion: the retention of the fetus in utero for 4 or more weeks after fetal death.

Spontaneous abortion: an abortion that usually occurs before the twelfth week of gestation (the lay term is *miscarriage*). (Predisposing factors include acute or chronic illness in the mother, abnormalities in the fetus, and abnormal attachment of the placenta. Often, the cause is unknown.)

Therapeutic abortion: a pregnancy legally terminated for reasons of maternal well-being.

Threatened abortion: an abortion in which a patient has some uterine bleeding with an intrauterine pregnancy in which the internal cervical os is closed. A threatened abortion may stabilize and end in normal delivery or progress to an incomplete or complete abortion.

The signs and symptoms of ectopic pregnancy are often difficult to distinguish from those of a ruptured ovarian cyst, pelvic inflammatory disease, appendicitis, or abortion (thus the name the *great imitator*). The classic triad of symptoms includes abdominal pain, vaginal bleeding, and amenorrhea; however, vaginal bleeding may be absent, spotty, or minimal, and amenorrhea may be replaced by oligomenorrhea (scanty flow). The variable presentation of ectopic pregnancy is one reason for its high-risk profile. Other symptoms of ectopic pregnancy include signs of early pregnancy, referred pain to the shoulder, nausea, vomiting, syncope, and the classic signs of shock.

Management

A ruptured ectopic pregnancy is a true emergency that requires initial resuscitation measures and rapid transport for surgical intervention. The patient may deteriorate rapidly and become hemodynamically unstable. If an ectopic pregnancy is suspected, the patient should be managed like any victim of hemorrhagic shock—with airway, ventilatory, and circulatory support and aggressive intravenous fluid resuscitation.

Third-Trimester Bleeding

Third-trimester bleeding occurs in 3% of all pregnancies and is never normal. The majority of bleeding episodes are a result of abruptio placentae, placenta previa, or uterine rupture. Table 28-1 differentiates abruptio placentae, placenta previa, and uterine rupture.

Abruptio Placentae

Abruptio placentae is partial or complete detachment of a normally implanted placenta at more than 20 weeks gestation. It occurs in 0.5% to 2% of all pregnancies and is severe enough to result in fetal death in 1 out of 400 cases of abruption. Predisposing factors to abruptio placentae include maternal hypertension, preeclampsia, multiparity, trauma, and previous abruption.

The common presentation of abruptio placentae is sudden, third-trimester vaginal bleeding and pain. The vaginal bleeding may be minimal and is often out of proportion to the degree of shock, since much of the hemorrhage may be concealed. The more extensive the abruption, the greater the

ing cause of first-trimester death and accounts for more than 11% of all maternal deaths in the United States.[2] Death from ectopic pregnancy is usually the result of hemorrhage.

Though ectopic pregnancy has numerous causes, most involve factors that delay or prevent passage of the fertilized ovum to its normal site of implantation. Predisposing factors include pelvic inflammatory disease, adhesions from previous surgery, tubal ligation, previous ectopic pregnancy, and possibly the presence of intrauterine contraceptive devices (IUDs). Thus obtaining a thorough gynecological history is very important. Although the time from fertilization varies, most ruptures occur by 2 to 12 weeks' gestation.

	TABLE 28-1 Differention of Abruptio Placentae, Placentia Previa,and Uterine Rupture			
History	**Bleeding**	**Abnormal Pain**	**Abdominal Examination**
Abruptio Placentae			
Association with toxemia of pregnancy and hypertension of any cause	Single attack of scant, dark vaginal bleeding (often concealed) that continues until delivery	Present	Localized uterine tenderness Labor Absent fetal heart tones (often)
Placenta Previa			
Lack of association with toxemia of pregnancy	Repeated "warning" hemorrhages over days to weeks	Usually absent	Lack of uterine tenderness (usually) Labor (rare) Fetal heart tones (usually)
Uterine Rupture			
Previous cesarean section	Possible bleeding	Usually present and associated with sudden onset of nausea and vomiting	Diffuse abdominal tenderness Sudden cessation of labor Possible fetal heart tones

uterine irritability, resulting in a tender abdomen and rigid uterus. Contractions may be present. In its severe form, fetal heart sounds are absent because fetal death is likely.

Placenta Previa

Placenta previa is placental implantation in the lower uterine segment encroaching on or covering the cervical os. It occurs in approximately 1 in 200 to 1 in 400 deliveries; the incidence is higher in preterm births. The condition is characterized by painless, bright red bleeding without uterine contraction. The bleeding may occur in repetitive episodes and be slight to moderate, becoming more profuse if active labor ensues. Fetal heart rate is often diminished because of placental insufficiency and hypoxia.

Placenta previa is associated with increasing maternal age, multiparity, previous cesarean section, and previous placenta previa episodes. The bleeding is also frequently precipitated by recent sexual intercourse.

Uterine Rupture

Uterine rupture is a spontaneous or traumatic rupture of the uterine wall; it may result from reopening of a previous uterine scar (for example, a previous cesarean section), a prolonged or obstructed labor, or direct trauma. It occurs in approximately 1 in 1400 deliveries and has a 5% to 15% maternal mortality rate and a 50% fetal mortality rate.

Uterine rupture is characterized by sudden abdominal pain described as steady and "tearing," active labor, early signs of shock (complaints of weakness, dizziness, anxiety), and vaginal bleeding, which may not be visible. On examination, the abdomen is usually rigid with diffuse pain, and fetal parts may be easily palpated through the abdominal wall. A previous cesarean scar may be a good indication of the rupture.

Management

Prehospital management of a patient with third-trimester bleeding is aimed at preventing shock. No attempt should be made to examine the patient vaginally; doing so may increase hemorrhage and precipitate labor. Emergency care measures should include the following:

1. Provide adequate airway, ventilatory, and circulatory support as needed (with spinal precautions if indicated).

2. Place patient in left lateral recumbent position.
3. Begin transport immediately.
4. Initiate intravenous therapy with volume-expanding fluid.
5. Apply a fresh perineal pad and note the time of application to assess bleeding during transport.
6. Check fundal height and document it for baseline measurement.
7. Closely monitor the patient's vital signs en route to the hospital.

Labor and Delivery

Parturition is the process by which the infant is born. Near the end of pregnancy the uterus becomes progressively more irritable and exhibits occasional contractions, which become stronger and more frequent until parturition is initiated. During and as a result of these contractions, the cervix begins to dilate. As uterine contractions increase, complete cervical dilation occurs to approximately 10 cm; the amniotic sac ruptures, and the fetus and shortly thereafter the placenta are expelled from the uterus through the vaginal canal (Fig. 28-9).

Stages of Labor

Labor follows several distinct stages. The length of these stages varies, depending on whether the mother is nullipara or multipara. Therefore the stages of labor should only be used as a guideline in estimating labor progression in the average pregnancy. Approximately 2 to 3 weeks before the onset of active labor, while the cervix undergoes the process of softening, effacement (thinning), and dilation, the uterus begins to become a contractile organ. Contractions, which before 30 weeks' gestation were uncoordinated and of low intensity, begin to steadily increase in intensity and duration; these are termed *Braxton-Hicks contractions*. The patient may not notice the contractions or perceive them as a slight uterine hardening. The contractions eventually strengthen and increase in frequency and duration, heralding the onset of clinical labor.

> **NOTE:**
> There is a great deal of individual variation in the perception and tolerance of uterine contractions. Some mothers experience relatively painless contractions even with the onset of labor, whereas others are quite uncomfortable from the earlier and less intense Braxton-Hicks contractions. In the former group, delivery may be more imminent than anticipated; members of the latter group may develop "false labor" several days to weeks before term.

Labor begins with a prodromal stage that marks the infant's descent into the birth canal. The fetal descent is characterized by a relief of pressure in the upper abdomen and a simultaneous increase in pressure in the pelvis. During this stage a mucous plug (sometimes mixed with blood, thus the name *bloody show*) is expelled from the dilating cervix and discharged from the vagina. The prodromal stage may go unnoticed by the mother.

The first stage of labor begins with the onset of regular contractions and ends with complete dilation of the cervix. The uterine contractions generally occur at 5- to 15-minute intervals and are characterized by cramplike abdominal pains that radiate to the small of the back. As the uterus contracts, the cervix becomes soft and thinned (effaced), and the less muscular segment of the uterus is pulled upward over the presenting part. The first stage usually lasts 8 to 12 hours in the nulliparous mother and approximately 6 to 8 hours in the multiparous mother. In most pregnancies, the amniotic sac ruptures (rupture of membranes) toward the end of the first stage of labor.

The second stage of labor is measured from full dilation of the cervix to delivery of the infant. During the second stage the fetal head enters the birth canal, and the mother's pain and contractions become more intense and frequent (usually 2 to 3 minutes apart). Often, the mother becomes diaphoretic and tachycardiac during this stage. In addition, she generally experiences an urge to bear down with each contraction, and she may express

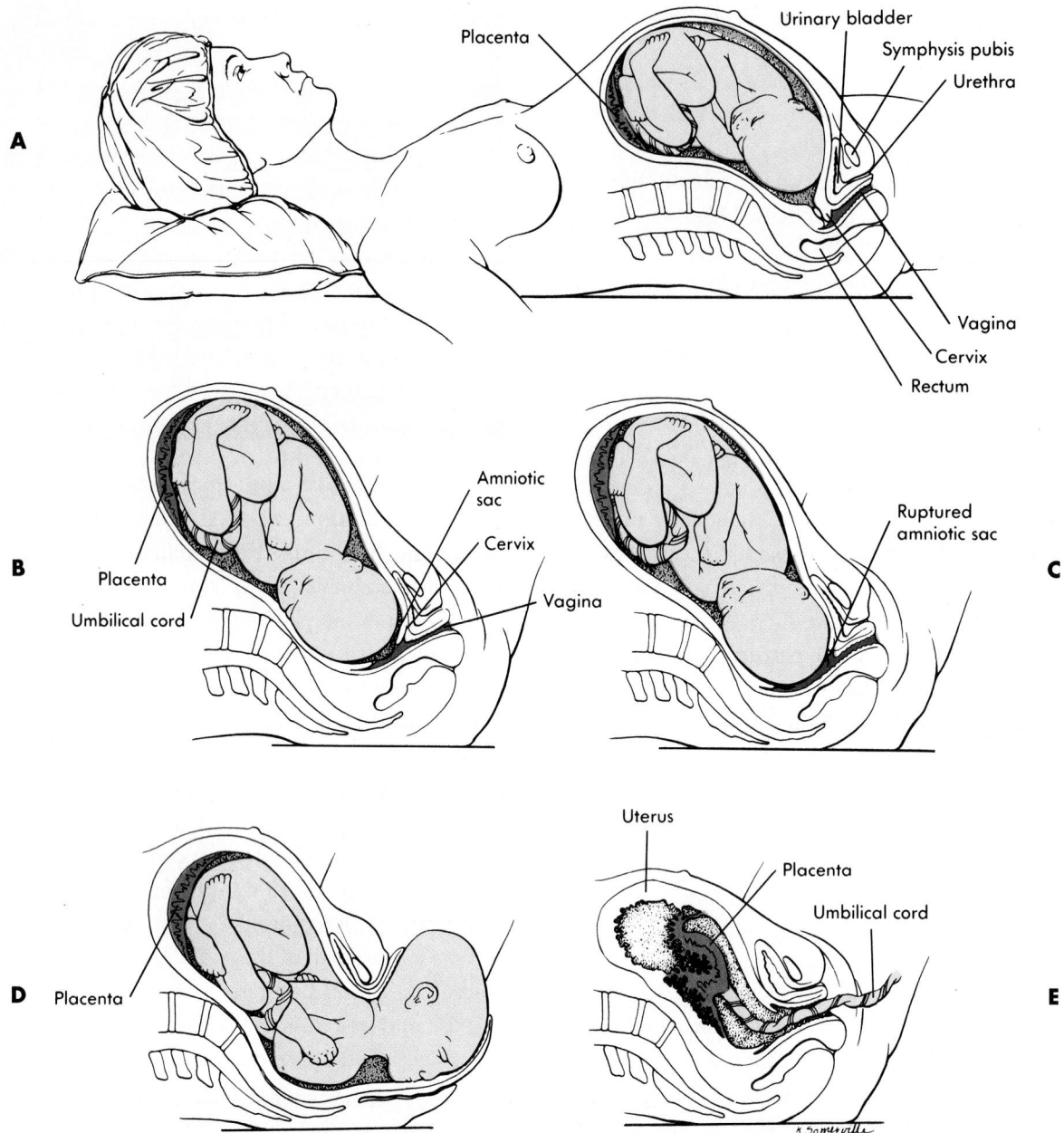

Fig. 28-9 Parturition. **A,** The relation of the fetus to the mother. **B,** The fetus moves into the birth canal. **C,** Dilation of the cervix is complete. **D,** The fetus is expelled from the uterus. **E,** The placenta is expelled.

the need to have a bowel movement (a normal sensation caused by pressure of the fetal head against the mother's rectum). In the second stage of labor, the presenting part of the fetus (usually the head) emerges from the vaginal opening. This process, known as *crowning*, indicates that delivery is imminent. The second stage of labor usu-

ally lasts 1 to 2 hours in the nullipara mother and 30 minutes or less in a woman who is multipara.

The third stage of labor begins with delivery of the infant and ends when the placenta has been expelled and the uterus has contracted. The length of this stage varies from 5 to 60 minutes, regardless of parity.

Signs and Symptoms of Imminent Delivery

The following signs and symptoms indicate that delivery is imminent and that preparations for childbirth should be made at the scene.

- Regular contractions lasting 45 to 60 seconds at 1- to 2-minute intervals. Intervals are measured from the beginning of one contraction to the beginning of the next. If contractions are more than 5 minutes apart, there is generally time to transport the mother to a receiving hospital.
- The mother has an urge to bear down or has a sensation of a bowel movement.
- There is a large amount of bloody show.
- Crowning occurs.
- The mother believes delivery is imminent.

If any of these signs and symptoms are present, the EMS crew should prepare for delivery. Delay or restraint of delivery should never be attempted in any fashion. If complications are anticipated or an abnormal delivery occurs, medical control may recommend expedited transport of the patient to a medical facility.

Preparing for Delivery

When preparing for delivery in the prehospital setting, the paramedic should attempt to provide an area of privacy. The mother should be positioned on a bed, stretcher, or table that has a surface long enough to project beyond the mother's vagina. The delivery area should be as clean as possible and covered with absorbent material to guard against staining and contamination by blood and fecal material.

The mother should be placed on her back with her knees flexed and widely separated (or in another position preferred by the mother), and the vaginal area should be draped appropriately. If delivery occurs in an automobile, the mother should be instructed to lie on her back across the seat with one leg flexed on the seat and the other leg resting on the floorboard. If available, a pillow or blanket should be placed beneath the mother's buttocks to facilitate delivery of the infant's head. The mother's vital signs should be evaluated for baseline measurements, and fetal heart rate should be monitored for signs of fetal distress. Per local protocol and medical control, the paramedic should consider maternal oxygen administration and intravenous access for volume expansion or administration of *oxytocin* if needed.

The paramedic should coach the mother to bear down and push during contractions and to rest between contractions to conserve strength. If the mother finds it difficult to refrain from pushing, she should be encouraged to breathe deeply or "pant" through her mouth between contractions to prevent glottic closure. Deep breathing and panting help decrease the force in bearing down and promote rest.

Delivery Equipment

Prehospital delivery equipment ("OB kit") generally includes the following components (Fig. 28-10):

- Surgical scissors
- Cord clamps or umbilical tape
- Towels
- Surgical masks
- 4 × 4 gauze sponges
- Sanitary napkins
- Bulb syringe/DeLee suction kit
- Baby blanket
- Plastic bag (for placental transport)
- Neonatal resuscitation equipment
- Intravenous fluid supplies

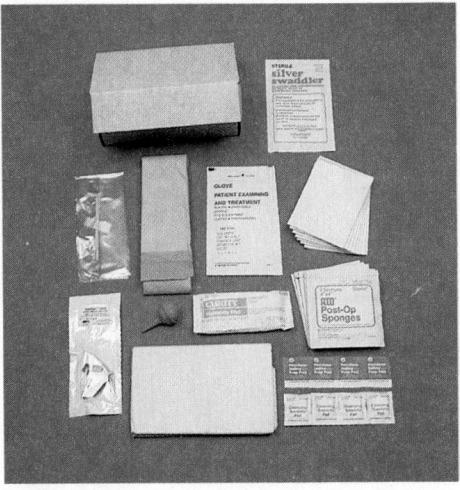

Fig. 28-10 Prehospital delivery equipment.

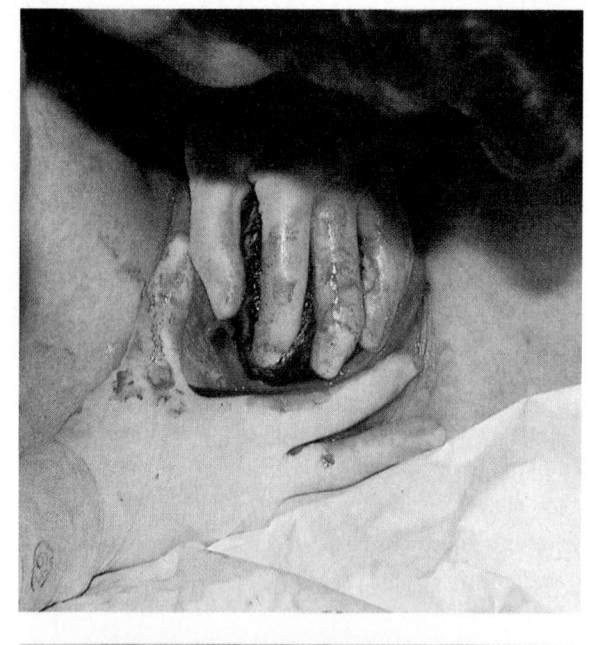
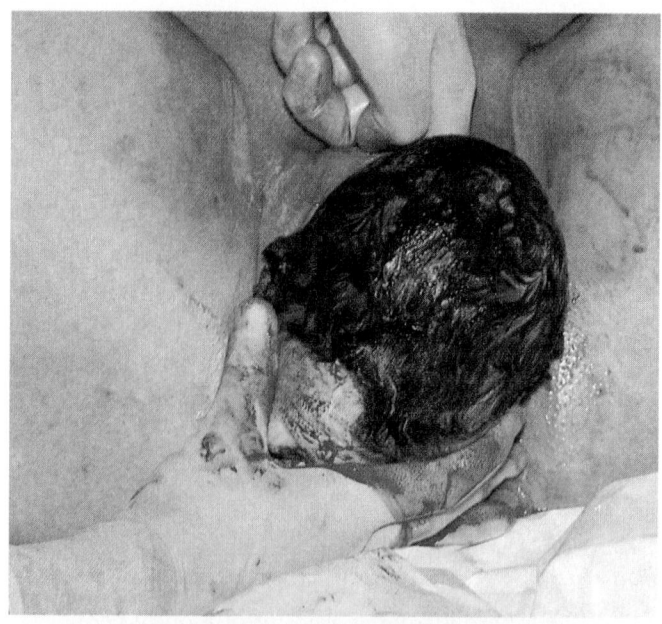
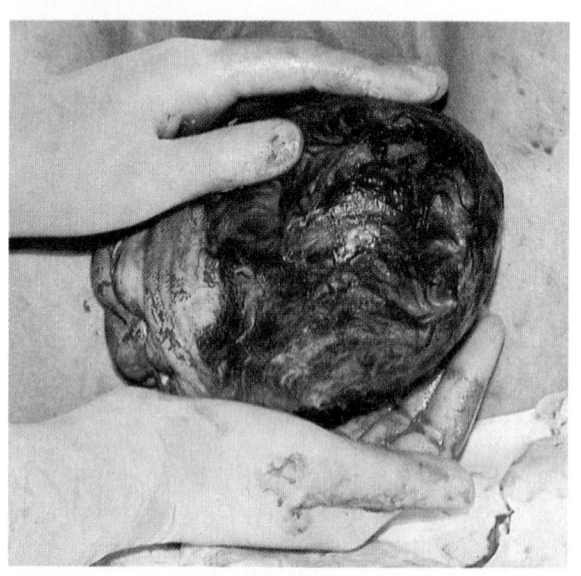
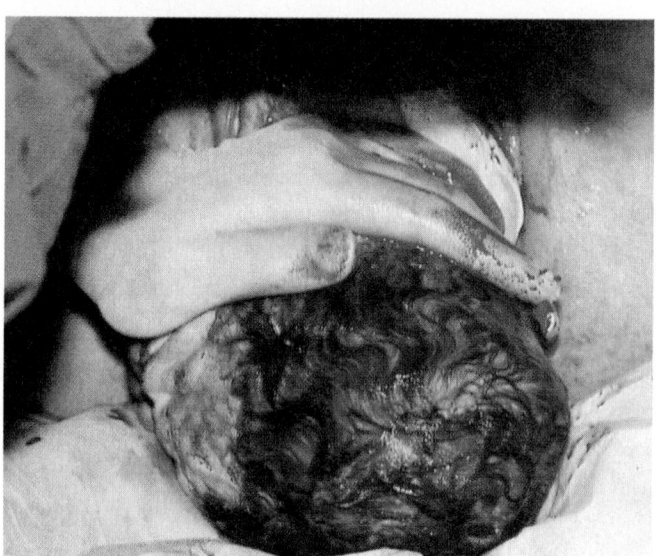
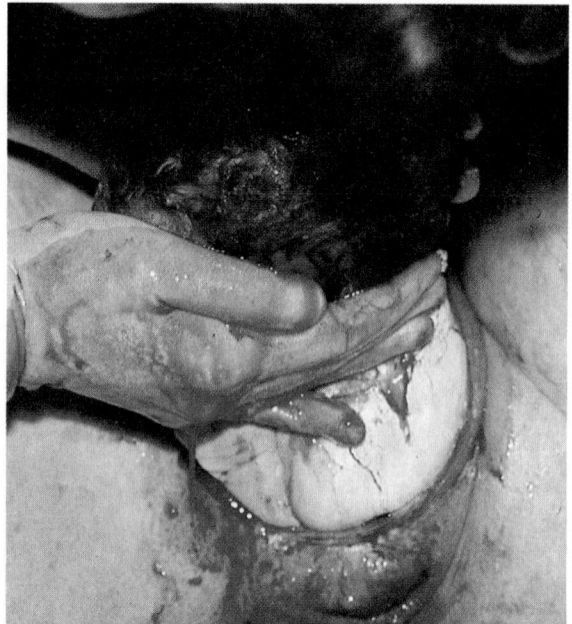

Fig. 28-11 Normal delivery. **A,** When crowning occurs, apply gentle palm pressure to the infant's head. **B,** Examine the neck for the presence of a looped umbilical cord. **C,** Support the infant's head as it rotates for shoulder presentation. **D,** Guide the infant's head downward to deliver the anterior shoulder. **E,** Guide the infant's head upward to release the posterior shoulder.

Before handling this equipment, take personal protective measures and use sterile technique.

Assisting with Delivery

In most cases, the paramedic only assists in the natural events of childbirth. The primary responsibilities of the EMS crew are to prevent an uncontrolled delivery and to protect the infant from cold and stress after the birth. Listed below are the steps in assisting the mother with a normal delivery (Fig. 28-11):

1. Don sterile gloves and other personal protective equipment.
2. When crowning occurs, apply gentle palm pressure to the infant's head to prevent an explosive delivery and tearing of the perineum. If membranes are still intact, tear the sac with finger pressure to allow escape of amniotic fluid.
3. After delivery of the head, examine the infant's neck for a looped umbilical cord. If the cord is looped around the neck, gently slip it over the infant's head or clamp it in two places and cut it between the clamps to release the cord.
4. Suction the infant's mouth and nose with a bulb syringe to clear the airway. Perform suction after the head appears but before the next contraction, which delivers the shoulders and chest. (The birth canal prevents chest expansion and minimizes the risk of aspiration if suction is performed well before the first breath, which usually occurs on delivery of the chest and shoulders.)
5. Support the infant's head as it rotates for shoulder presentation. (Most infants present face down, after which the baby rotates to the left so that the shoulders present in an anterior-posterior position.)
6. With gentle pressure, guide the infant's head downward to deliver the anterior shoulder and then upward to release the posterior shoulder. (The remainder of the infant is delivered quickly by smooth uterine contraction.)
7. Be careful to grasp and support the infant as it emerges. Use care because the baby is very slippery. Hold the infant firmly with its head dependent to facilitate drainage of secretions. Maintain the infant's position at or slightly above the level of the mother's vagina to prevent overtransfusion or undertransfusion of blood from the umbilical cord.
8. Clear the infant's airway of any secretions with sterile gauze and repeat suction of the infant's nose and mouth.
9. Dry the infant with sterile towels and cover the infant (especially the head) to reduce heat loss.
10. Note and record the baby's gender and time of birth.

Evaluating the Infant

After delivery, dry and cover the infant to prevent heat loss, position and clear the airway, and provide tactile stimulation to initiate respirations. If there is no need for resuscitation, use the **Apgar score** at 1 minute and 5 minutes (Table 28-2) to evaluate in the infant. Criteria for computing the Apgar score include appearance (color), pulse (heart rate), grimace (reflex irritability to stimulation), activity (muscle tone), and respiratory effort. Each criterion is rated on a basis of 0 to 2, and the numbers are then added for a total Apgar score.

TABLE 28-2 Evaluation at Birth: Apgar Scoring System			
Evaluation Factor	**0**	**1**	**2**
Heart rate	Absent	Slow (below 100 beats/min)	Over 100 beats/min
Respiratory effort	Absent	Slow or irregular	Good crying
Muscle tone	Limp	Some flexion of extremities	Active motion
Response to catheter in nostril (tested after oropharynx is clear)	No response	Grimace	Cough or sneeze
Color	Blue or pale	Body pink, extremities blue	Completely pink

A score of 10 indicates that the infant is in the best possible condition, 7 to 9 indicates the infant is slightly depressed (near normal), 4 to 6 indicates the infant is moderately depressed, and 0 to 3 indicates the infant is severely depressed. Most newborns have an APGAR score of 8 to 10 at 1 minute after birth. An APGAR score of less than 6 requires neonatal resuscitation.

> **NOTE:**
> **Resuscitation efforts should never be delayed or interrupted to assign an Apgar score.**

Cutting the Umbilical Cord

After delivery and evaluation of the infant, the umbilical cord should be clamped (or tied with umbilical tape) and cut (Fig. 28-12):

1. Clamp the cord approximately 6 to 9 inches away from the infant in two places. Do not strip or milk the cord; doing so may lead to red blood cell destruction, polycythemia, and hyperbilirubinemia.
2. Cut between the two clamps with sterile scissors or a scalpel.
3. Examine the cut ends of the cord to ensure there is no bleeding. If the cut end attached

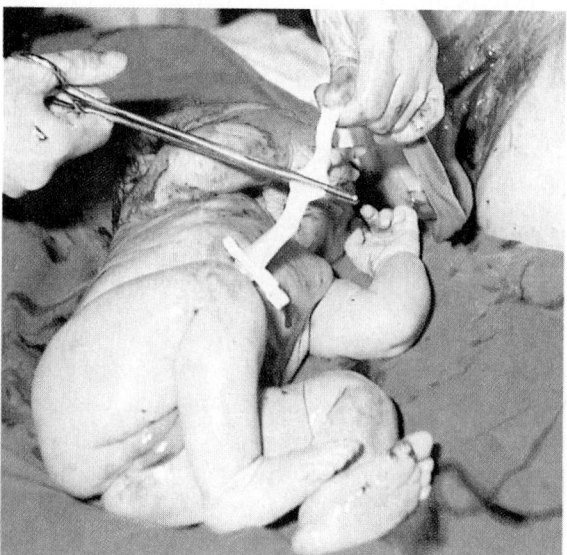

Fig. 28-12 After delivery and evaluation of the infant, the cord is clamped and cut.

to the infant is bleeding, clamp the cord proximal to the previous clamp and reassess for bleeding. Do not remove the first clamp.
4. Handle the cord carefully at all times; it tears easily.

Delivery of the Placenta

The placenta normally delivers within 20 minutes of the infant. Therefore there is no need to delay transport for placental delivery. Sometimes referred to as the *fourth stage of labor*, placental delivery is characterized by episodes of contractions, a palpable rise of the uterus within the abdomen, lengthening of the umbilical cord protruding from the vagina, and a sudden gush of vaginal blood.

As the placenta delivers, the mother should be advised to bear down with contractions. The paramedic should hold the placenta with both hands and gently twist it as it delivers to facilitate complete separation from the uterine wall. (Never pull on the umbilical cord to assist with placental delivery.) When expelled, the placenta should be placed in a plastic bag or other container and transported with the mother and infant to the receiving hospital, where it will be examined for abnormality and completeness. Pieces of placenta retained in the uterus can cause persistent hemorrhage and infection.

After placental delivery, the perineum should be evaluated for tears. If present, the tears should be managed by applying sanitary napkins to the area and maintaining direct pressure. The mother should be closely monitored during transport for signs of hemorrhage or shock. Fundal massage should be initiated to promote uterine contraction. In addition, the administration of *oxytocin* may be prescribed by medical control to manage postpartum hemorrhage.

Postpartum Hemorrhage

Postpartum hemorrhage is more than 500 ml of blood loss after delivery of the newborn. It frequently occurs within the first few hours after delivery but can be delayed up to 24 hours. Postpartum hemorrhage occurs in approximately 5% of all deliveries and often results from ineffective or incomplete contraction of the interlacing uterine muscle fibers. Other causes of postpartum hemorrhage include retained pieces of placenta or membranes in the uterus and vaginal or cervical tears incurred during delivery (rare). Risk factors associated with this condition include uterine atony (lack of tone) from prolonged or tumultuous labor, grand multiparity, twin pregnancy, placenta previa, and a full bladder.

Management

Postpartum hemorrhage can be encountered in the prehospital setting after a field delivery, home delivery, or delivery at an independent birthing center. Assessment and management are similar to those previously described for third-trimester bleeding. In addition, six measures should be taken to encourage uterine contraction:

1. Control external hemorrhage. Manage external bleeding from perineal tears with firm pressure.
2. Uterine massage. Palpate the uterus for firmness or loss of tone. If the uterus does not feel firm, apply fundal pressure by supporting the lower uterine segment with the edge of one hand just above the symphysis and massaging the fundus with the other hand. Continue massaging until the uterus feels firm. The patient should be re-evaluated every 10 minutes; note the location of the fundus in relation to the level of the umbilicus, the degree of firmness, and vaginal flow.
3. Encourage the infant to breastfeed. If the mother is stable, place the newborn to her breast and encourage the infant to breastfeed. Stimulation of the breasts may promote uterine contraction.
4. *Administer oxytocin.* Per medical control and after ensuring that a second fetus is not present in the uterus, add 10 units of *oxytocin* to 1000 ml lactated Ringer's solution and infuse at 20 to 30 drops/min via microdrip tubing (titrated to the severity of hemorrhage and uterine response). Continue with fluid resuscitation as indicated by the patient's hemodynamic status.
5. Do not attempt a vaginal examination or vaginal packing to control hemorrhage.
6. Rapidly transport the patient for physician evaluation.

Section Four
Delivery Complications

As previously stated, most women have routine pregnancies. Prehospital deliveries seldom present any significant problems for the mother, newborn, or emergency crew. The delivery complications discussed in this chapter include cephalopelvic disproportion, abnormal presentation, premature birth, multiple gestation, precipitous delivery, uterine inversion, pulmonary embolus, and fetal membrane disorders. Box 28-5 lists factors that should alert the paramedic to anticipate an abnormal delivery.

● CEPHALOPELVIC DISPROPORTION

Cephalopelvic disproportion produces a difficult labor because of the presence of a small pelvis, an oversized fetus, or fetal abnormalities (hydrocephalus, conjoined twins, fetal tumors). The mother is often primigravida and experiencing strong, frequent contractions for a prolonged period. Definitive care is cesarean delivery because uterine rupture and fetal demise are possible. Prehospital care is limited to maternal oxygen administration, intravenous access for fluid resuscitation if needed, and rapid transport to the receiving hospital.

● ABNORMAL PRESENTATION

Most infants are born head first (cephalic or vertex presentation). However, on rare occasions, a presentation is abnormal, as in a breech presentation, shoulder dystocia, shoulder presentation, and a cord presentation (prolapsed umbilical cord).

Breech Presentation

In breech presentations, the largest part of the fetus (the head) is delivered last. Breech presenta-

---

BOX 28-5

Factors Associated with High Risk of Abnormal Delivery

Maternal Factors
- Maternal age: very young or very old
- Absence of prenatal care
- Maternal lifestyle: alcohol, tobacco, or drug usage
- Preexisting maternal illness, including diabetes, chronic hypertension, or Rh sensitization
- Previous obstetrical history
  Premature delivery or miscarriage
  Perinatal loss
  Previous malformed neonate
  Previous multiple births
  Previous cesarean delivery
- Intrapartum disorders
  Preeclampsia
  Prolonged rupture of membranes
  Prolonged labor
  Abnormal presentation
  Abruptio placentae
  Placenta previa

Fetal Factors
- Lack of fetal well-being
  History of decreased fetal movement
  History of heart rate abnormalities
  Evidence of fetal distress
- Fetal immaturity: prematurity as established by dates, ultrasound, uterine size, amniocentesis
- Fetal growth: history of poor intrauterine growth or postdate delivery
- Specific fetal malformation detected by ultrasound: diaphragmatic hernia or omphalocele

---

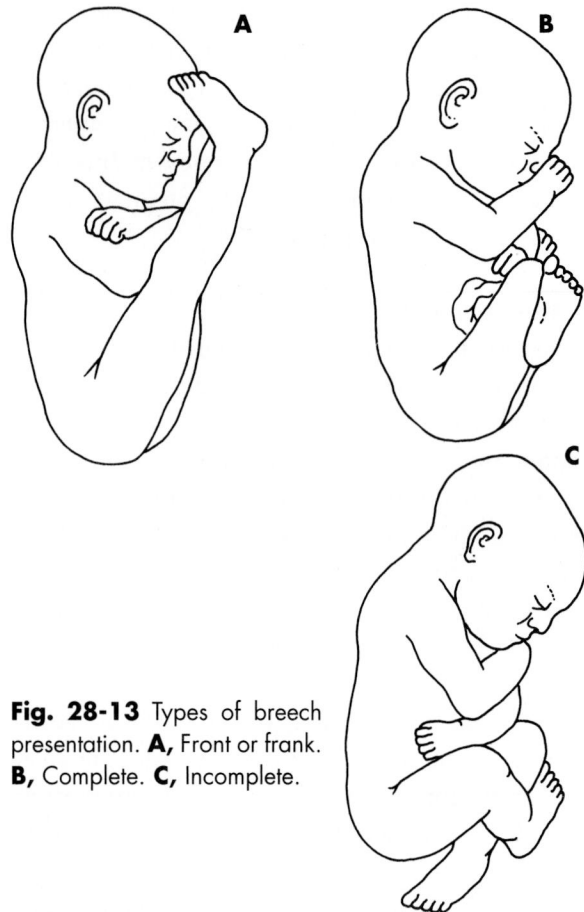

Fig. 28-13 Types of breech presentation. **A,** Front or frank. **B,** Complete. **C,** Incomplete.

Management

An infant in a breech presentation is best delivered in a hospital where emergency cesarean section is a possible alternative to vaginal delivery. However, it is sometimes necessary to assist in a breech delivery in the prehospital setting. If delivery is imminent, the EMS crew should proceed as follows:

1. Prepare the mother for delivery as previously described.
2. Provide supplemental oxygen and intravenous access and continuously monitor the fetal heart rate.
3. Allow the fetus to deliver spontaneously up to the level of the umbilicus. If the fetus is in a front presentation, gently extract the legs downward after the buttocks are delivered.
4. After the infant's legs are clear, support the baby's body with the palm of the hand and volar surface of the arm.
5. After the umbilicus is visualized, gently extract a 4- to 6-inch loop of umbilical cord to

tion occurs in 3% to 4% of deliveries at term and is more frequent with multiple births and when labor occurs before 32 weeks' gestation. Fig. 28-13 illustrates three types of breech presentation (Box 28-6).

BOX 28-6

Categories of Breech Presentation

- Front or frank breech: The fetal hips are flexed and the legs extend in front of the fetus. The buttocks are the presenting part. Frank breech accounts for approximately 60% of breech presentations.
- Complete breech: The fetus has both knees and hips flexed. The buttocks are the presenting part. Complete breech accounts for approximately 5% of breech presentations.
- Incomplete breech: The fetus has one or both hips incompletely flexed, resulting in presentation of one or both lower extremities (often a foot). Incomplete breech accounts for approximately 30% of breech presentations.

allow delivery without excessive traction on the cord. Gently rotate the fetus to align the shoulders in an anterior-posterior position. Continue with gentle traction until the axilla is visible.

6. Gently guide the infant upward to allow delivery of the posterior shoulder.
7. Gently guide the infant downward to deliver the anterior shoulder.
8. During a breech delivery, avoid having the fetal face or abdomen toward the maternal symphysis.
9. Be aware that after shoulder delivery, the head is often delivered without difficulty. Be careful to avoid excessive head and spine manipulation or traction.

If the head does not deliver immediately, action must be taken to prevent suffocation of the infant. The paramedic should place a gloved hand in the vagina with the palm toward the baby's face. With index and middle fingers, a V should be formed on either side of the baby's nose. The vaginal wall should then be gently pushed away from the baby's face until the head is delivered. If the head

does not deliver within 3 minutes, the baby's airway should be maintained with the V formation, and the mother should be rapidly transported to the receiving hospital.

Shoulder Dystocia

Shoulder dystocia occurs when the fetal shoulders impact against the maternal symphysis pubis, blocking shoulder delivery. In this presentation, the head delivers normally but then pulls back tightly against the maternal perineum. The incidence of shoulder dystocia is small but increases significantly with increasing birth weight (up to 10% incidence with birth weights of 10 or more pounds). Complications include brachial plexus damage, fractured clavicle, and fetal anoxia from cord compression.

Management

Shoulder dystocia delivery entails dislodging one shoulder and rotating the fetal shoulder girdle into the wider oblique pelvic diameter. Because of the potential for cord compression, the anterior shoulder should be delivered immediately after the head (before suctioning of the nares and mouth). A number of maneuvers can help successfully deliver an infant when this complication arises. The following steps constitute a reasonable field approach to this problem:

1. Position the mother on her left side in a dorsal-knee-chest position to increase the diameter of the pelvis.
2. Attempt to guide the infant's head downward to allow the anterior shoulder to slip under the symphysis pubis. Avoid excessive force or manipulation.
3. Gently rotate the fetal shoulder girdle into the wider oblique pelvic diameter. The posterior shoulder usually delivers without resistance. Medical control may recommend attempting delivery of the posterior shoulder first. This may be accomplished by rotating the posterior shoulder downward and into the left posterior quadrant. The anterior shoulder usually follows.
4. After delivery, continue with resuscitative measures as needed.

Shoulder Presentation

Shoulder presentation (transverse presentation) results when the long axis of the fetus lies perpendicular to that of the mother. This position usually results in the fetal shoulder lying over the pelvic inlet, thus the name. The fetal arm or hand may be the presenting part. This abnormal delivery occurs in only 0.3% of deliveries but may occur in 10% of second twins.

Management

Spontaneous delivery of a shoulder presentation is not possible. The mother should be provided with adequate oxygen, ventilatory and circulatory support, and rapid transport to the receiving hospital. Cesarean section is required whether the fetus is viable or nonviable.

Cord Presentation

Cord presentation occurs when the cord slips down into the vagina or presents externally after the amniotic membranes have ruptured. The umbilical cord is compressed against the presenting part, diminishing fetal oxygenation from the placenta. Prolapsed cord occurs in approximately 1 in every 200 pregnancies and should be suspected when fetal distress is present. Predisposing factors include breech presentation, premature rupture of membranes, a large fetus, multiple gestation, a long cord, and preterm labor.

Management

Fetal asphyxia may rapidly ensue if circulation through the cord is not re-established and maintained until delivery. If the umbilical cord can be seen or felt in the vagina, the paramedic should take the following steps:

1. Position the mother with hips elevated as much as possible. The Trendelenburg or knee-chest position may relieve pressure on the cord.
2. Administer oxygen to the mother.
3. Instruct the mother to "pant" with each contraction to prevent bearing down.
4. If assistance is available, apply moist sterile dressings to the exposed cord to minimize temperature changes that may cause umbilical artery spasm.

5. With a gloved hand, gently push the baby back into the vagina and elevate the presenting part to relieve pressure on the cord. The cord may spontaneously retract, but no attempt should be made to reposition the cord.
6. Maintain this hand position during rapid transport to the receiving hospital. The definitive treatment is cesarean section.

Other Abnormal Presentations

Other abnormal presentations include occiput posterior presentation, in which the infant's head is delivered face up instead of face down, and face or brow presentation. Nonvertex presentations result in increased perinatal morbidity and mortality as a result of difficult labor and delivery and associated abnormalities. These presentations may require cesarean section. Therefore early recognition of potential complications, maternal support and reassurance, and rapid transport for definitive care are the goals of prehospital management.

● PREMATURE BIRTH

A premature infant is one born before 37 weeks of gestation. Low birth weight (less than 2.5 kg [5.5 pounds]) has also been used to determine prematurity, although the conditions are not synonymous. Premature deliveries occur in 6% to 9% of all pregnancies. After a preterm labor, the newborn is at increased risk for hypothermia because of a large surface-mass ratio and for cardiorespiratory distress because the cardiovascular system is premature. Therefore these infants require special care and observation. After delivery, prehospital management for a premature infant includes the following:

- Keep the infant warm. Dry the infant, wrap it in a warm blanket, place it on the mother's abdomen, and cover both mother and infant.
- Frequently suction the infant's mouth and nares.
- Carefully monitor the cut end of the umbilical cord for oozing. If bleeding is present, manage as previously described.
- Administer humidified free-flow oxygen through a makeshift oxygen tent. Aim oxygen

flow toward the top of tent; do not allow it to flow directly into the baby's face.

- Protect the infant from contamination. Don mask and gown and minimize family member and bystander contact with the baby.
- Gently transport the mother and infant to the receiving hospital.

● MULTIPLE GESTATION

A multiple gestation is a pregnancy with more than one fetus. Twins occur in 1 of every 80 to 90 births, and triplets occur in 1 out of 8000 births (Box 28-7). Multiple gestation places additional stress on the maternal system and is accompanied by an increased complication rate. Associated complications include premature labor and delivery (30% to 50% of twin deliveries are premature), premature rupture of membranes, abruptio placentae, postpartum hemorrhage, and abnormal presentation. A mother who has not had any prenatal care is often unaware of her multiple pregnancy.

Delivery Procedure

First-twin delivery is identical to single delivery with the same presentation. However, up to 50% of second-twin deliveries are in nonvertex presentation. Because fetuses are smaller in multiple births, the breech presentation of the second twin does not usually pose significant delivery problems.

After delivery of the first twin, clamp (or tie) and cut and clamp the umbilical cord in the usual fashion, as previously described. Within 5 to 10 minutes after delivery of the first twin, uterine contractions begin again. Delivery of the second twin usually occurs within 30 to 45 minutes. (Medical control may recommend transport before delivery of the second twin.) As a rule, both twins are born before placental delivery.

Infants in multiple births are often smaller than infants of term births. Special attention should be given to keeping these infants warm, well oxygenated, and free from unnecessary contamination as described for premature infants. Postpartum hemorrhage may be more severe after multiple births,

---

> ### BOX 28-7
>
> ## Twin Terminology
>
> **Fraternal twins** result from the fertilization of two ova by two spermatozoa. Each fraternal twin has a separate placenta and is separated by individual amniotic membranes. Fraternal twins are not identical in appearance and are often of different gender.
>
> **Identical twins** result from the fertilization of a single ovum; they may share a common placenta and amniotic sac or have separate placental structures. Identical twins are less common than fraternal twins (occurring in one out of three twin conceptions). Unlike fraternal twins, they look alike, are of the same gender, and are genetically identical.

---

requiring fluid resuscitation, uterine massage, and even *oxytocin* infusion.

● PRECIPITOUS DELIVERY

A precipitous delivery is a rapid spontaneous delivery, with less than 3 hours from onset of labor to birth. It results from overactive uterine contractions and little maternal soft tissue or bony resistance. A precipitous delivery occurs most frequently in a mother who is grand multipara. It can be associated with soft tissue injury and uterine rupture (rare) and has an increased perinatal mortality rate secondary to trauma and hypoxia. The primary danger to the fetus is from cerebral trauma or tearing of the umbilical cord.

If a precipitous delivery is anticipated, the paramedic should attempt to prevent an explosive delivery by providing gentle counterpressure to the infant's head. (No attempt should be made to detain fetal head descent.) After the delivery, the infant should be kept dry and warm to prevent any heat loss, and the mother should be examined for the perineal tears that often accompany a rapid birth.

● UTERINE INVERSION

Uterine inversion is an infrequent but serious complication of childbirth, occurring in approximately 1 in 2100 deliveries. It is essentially a turning "inside out" of the uterus. It may occur spontaneously after a contraction or with increased abdominal pressure caused by coughing or sneezing. It is thought, however, to be more often iatrogenic (caused by medical personnel or a medical procedure) secondary to excessive cord traction and fundal pressure, particularly when fundal implantation of the placenta has occurred. Uterine inversion is considered incomplete if the uterine fundus does not extend beyond the cervix and complete if the entire uterus protrudes through the cervical ring. Signs and symptoms of uterine inversion include postpartum hemorrhage, which may be profuse, and sudden and severe lower abdominal pain. Hypovolemic shock may develop quickly.

Management

Prehospital care for uterine inversion includes airway, ventilatory, and circulatory support and rapid transport. In addition, medical control may recommend that manual replacement of the uterus be attempted, provided that the cervix has not yet constricted.

> **NOTE:**
> Manual replacement may be very painful to the patient. The use of analgesics may be indicated per medical control, and the need for the procedure should be explained.

The technique for manual replacement is listed below:

1. Place the patient supine.
2. Make no attempt to remove the placenta, which will increase hemorrhage.
3. Apply pressure with the fingertips and palm of a gloved hand and push the fundus upward and through the cervical canal. If this is ineffective, cover all protruding tissues with moist sterile dressings and rapidly transport the patient.

● PULMONARY EMBOLISM

The development of pulmonary embolism during pregnancy, labor, or the postpartum period is one of the most common causes of maternal death. The embolus is frequently the result of a blood clot in the pelvic circulation (venous thromboembolism); it is more commonly associated with cesarean section than vaginal delivery. The patient often has classic signs and symptoms, including sudden dyspnea; sharp, focal chest pains; tachycardia; tachypnea; and occasionally hypotension. If the embolism occurs in the prehospital setting, emergency care for the patient is directed at airway, ventilatory, and circulatory support; ECG monitoring; and rapid transport for physician evaluation.

● FETAL MEMBRANE DISORDERS

The fetal membrane disorders to be discussed in this chapter include premature rupture of membranes, amniotic fluid embolism, and meconium staining.

Premature Rupture of Membranes

Premature rupture of the membranes is a rupture of the amniotic sac before the onset of labor, regardless of gestational age. Premature rupture occurs in approximately 1 of 10 pregnancies. At term, 70% of patients are in labor within 12 hours of premature rupture of membranes, and 85% are in labor within 24 hours. Signs and symptoms include a history of a "trickle" or sudden gush of fluid from the vagina. Patients should be transported for physician evaluation. In-hospital delivery preparations will be made if the patient enters the advanced stages of labor or if an infection of fetal membranes (chorioamnionitis) is diagnosed.

Chorioamnionitis is associated with premature rupture of membranes of greater than 24 hours duration or with prolonged labor. The infection is generally accompanied by maternal fever, chills, and uterine pain and is treated with antibiotic therapy. The definitive treatment for the maternal infection is delivery of the fetus.

Amniotic Fluid Embolism

An amniotic fluid embolism may occur when amniotic fluid gains access to maternal circulation during labor or delivery or immediately after delivery. Probable routes of entry include lacerations of the endocervical veins during cervical dilation, of the lower uterine segment or placental site, and of uterine veins at sites of uterine trauma. Particulate matter in the amniotic fluid (meconium, lanugo hairs, fetal squamous cells) forms an embolus and obstructs the pulmonary vasculature. Amniotic fluid embolism is rare, occurring in 1 of 20,000 to 30,000 deliveries. The condition is most commonly seen in multiparous women late in the first stage of labor. Other conditions that can increase the incidence of this severe complication are placenta previa, abruptio placentae, and intrauterine fetal death. The maternal mortality rate is near 90%.

Signs and symptoms of amniotic fluid embolism are the same as those described for pulmonary embolism and may include cardiopulmonary arrest. The patient should be managed with airway, ventilatory, and circulatory support; fluid resuscitation; and rapid transport.

Meconium Staining

Meconium staining is the presence of fetal stool in amniotic fluid. The condition occurs in from 8% to over 30% of all deliveries, becoming more common in relation to gestational age. The cause of meconium staining is not clear. Some believe it results from asphyxia of the fetus or cord compression. Others believe it results from fetal maturity. Regardless of the underlying cause, meconium staining is associated with increased perinatal mortality. Depending on the amount of meconium particles and the amount of amniotic fluid, the staining may range from a slight yellow or light green to a thick meconium that has a "pea-soup" appearance. When thick meconium is present in amniotic fluid, there is a chance the particles will be aspirated into the infant's mouth and potentially into the trachea and lungs **(meconium aspiration syndrome).**

After meconium is observed in the amniotic fluid, intervention is aimed at preventing or minimizing the risk of aspiration by the newborn. Because the presence of meconium can only be determined after the membranes have ruptured, it is important that the proper equipment be readily available and that the EMS crew be organized to act instantly. Emergency care includes the following:

1. Prepare the necessary equipment (intubation equipment, DeLee suction or bulb syringe, 10-French or larger suction catheter, portable suction, gauze pads, pediatric bag-valve device).

2. As the baby's head is delivered (and before shoulder delivery), clear the infant's airway and thoroughly suction the mouth, pharynx, and nose in that order.

3. After delivery of the infant, remove residual meconium in the hypopharynx by suction under direct visualization.

4. If the neonate is depressed or the meconium is thick or particulate, perform direct endotracheal suctioning using the endotracheal tube as a suction catheter. Quickly intubate the trachea (preferably before the baby has taken its first breath). Apply suction to the proximal end of the endotracheal tube while withdrawing the tube. During intubation and suction, aim 100% oxygen toward the infant's face, and monitor the fetal heart rate for bradycardia. If bradycardia develops, ventilate the infant's lungs using a bag-valve device after suctioning to prevent persistent bradycardia and hypoxia.

5. Repeat the intubation-suction-extubation cycle until no further meconium is obtained. Do not ventilate between intubations.

6. After tracheal suction is complete, continue resuscitative measures as needed. If respirations are adequate, manage the infant's airway in the normal fashion.

Section Five
Neonatal Resuscitation

According to the American Heart Association and the American Academy of Pediatrics, the initial steps of neonatal resuscitation (with the excep-

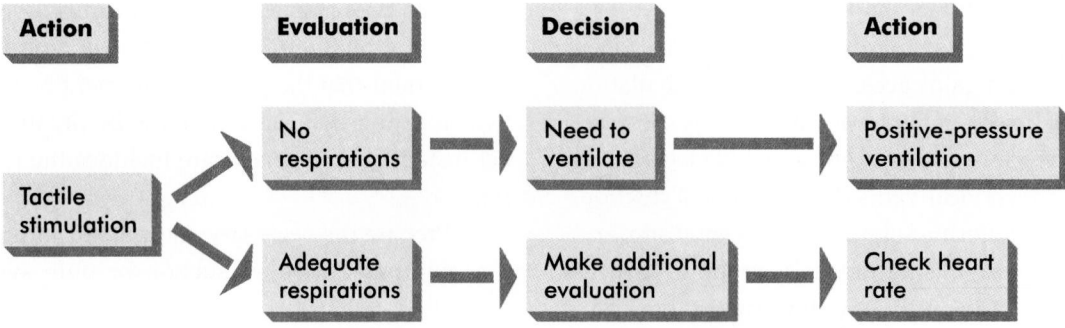

Fig. 28-14 Action-evaluation-decision cycle.

tion of infants born through meconium) are (1) prevent heat loss, (2) clear the airway by positioning and suctioning, (3) provide tactile stimulation and initiate breathing if necessary, and (4) further evaluate the infant (Fig. 28-14).[3] These steps enable the paramedic to immediately recognize an infant in need of resuscitation and leads to efficient and effective emergency care delivery.

● PREVENTION OF HEAT LOSS

Even healthy term infants are limited in their ability to conserve heat when exposed to a cold environment. Therefore immediately after delivery, the infant's body and head should be dried to prevent evaporative heat loss and metabolic problems that may be brought on by cold stress. The act of drying also provides gentle stimulation, which may initiate or help maintain respirations. Care should be taken to remove the wet towel or blanket from the infant, or evaporative heat loss will continue. Cover the infant again with dry wrappings. The majority of heat loss can be prevented by covering the newborn's head.

● OPENING OF THE AIRWAY

After the infant has been dried and covered, the next step is to establish an open airway by correctly positioning the infant and suctioning the mouth and nose. The neonate should be placed on the back or side with the neck slightly extended

(sniffing position). As described in Chapter 12, care should be taken to prevent hyperextension or underextension, which may compromise the airway. Placing a blanket or towel under the infant's shoulders can help maintain the correct position.

After the infant has been positioned, the mouth and nose should be suctioned with a bulb syringe or mechanical suction. It is preferable to suction the mouth first to prevent aspiration in case the infant gasps when the nose is cleared of secretions. Each application of suction should last no more than 5 seconds to prevent hypoxia. In addition (except in meconium-stained newborns), the paramedic should be careful to avoid deep or vigorous suction because stimulation of the posterior pharynx can produce a vagal response with resulting bradycardia, apnea, or both. Suctioning also provides a degree of tactile stimulation that may initiate respirations.

● PROVISION OF TACTILE STIMULATION

If drying and suctioning do not induce respirations in the infant, additional tactile stimulation should be provided. The two safe and appropriate methods of tactile stimulation are slapping or flicking the soles of the feet and rubbing the infant's back. If the infant remain apneic after two attempts at stimulation, positive-pressure ventilation should be initiated immediately with a pediatric bag-valve device and supplemental oxygen (40 to 60 ventilations/min).

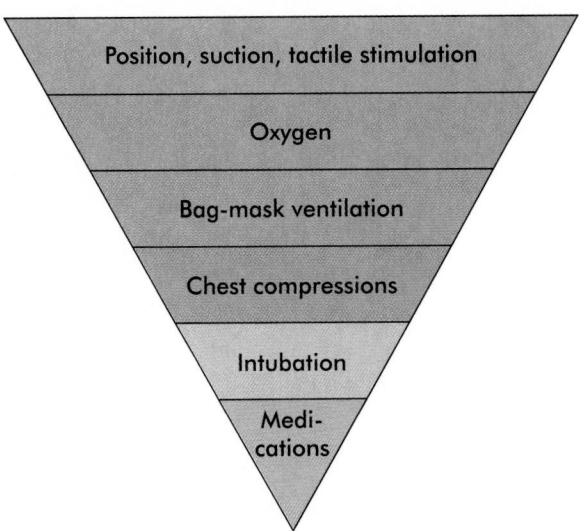

Fig. 28-15 Inverted pyramid reflecting the approximate relative frequency of neonatal resuscitative efforts. Note that a majority of infants respond to simple measures.

(Pyramid labels, top to bottom:)
Position, suction, tactile stimulation
Oxygen
Bag-mask ventilation
Chest compressions
Intubation
Medi-cations

● EVALUATION OF THE INFANT

Positioning, suctioning, and stimulating are necessary in every infant at birth and are used to clear the airway and to initiate respirations. The next step in the resuscitation process depends on evaluation of the infant's respiratory effort, heart rate, and color. The following steps are suggested for monitoring and evaluating the newborn (Fig. 28-15):

1. Observe and evaluate the infant's respirations. If they are normal (crying), continue the evaluation. If the respiratory response is inappropriate (slow, shallow, or absent), begin positive-pressure ventilation.
2. Evaluate the infant's heart rate by stethoscope or by palpating the pulse in the umbilical cord or brachial artery. If it is above 100 beats/min, continue the evaluation. If it is less than 100 beats/min, initiate positive-pressure ventilation. If the heart rate is less than 80 beats/min and does not increase despite 30 seconds of positive-pressure ventilation, initiate chest compressions (½ to ¾ inch in depth) at a rate of 120/min.
3. Evaluate the infant's color. If central cyanosis is present in an infant with spontaneous

respirations and an adequate heart rate, administer free-flow oxygen at 5 L/min. A maximum oxygen concentration of approximately 80% can be achieved when the tube is ½ inch from the infant's nose. The tubing should be held steady and aimed at the nares. Waving the end of the tubing back and forth or withdrawing the tube 1 or 2 inches from the infant's face decreases oxygen concentration considerably.

● RESUSCITATION OF THE DISTRESSED NEONATE

Approximately 6% of infants born in U.S. hospitals require resuscitation immediately after birth, and this figure is thought to be much higher for prehospital deliveries. Risk factors associated with the need for resuscitation include premature delivery, maternal health problems, complicated pregnancies, and delivery complications. If, with continued assisted ventilations, the infant's condition continues to deteriorate or fails to improve, the infant may require endotracheal intubation (see Chapter 12) and the administration of drugs. Before the paramedic considers intubation or pharmacological therapy, the following two components of the resuscitation process should be reevaluated:

1. Is chest movement adequate? Check for adequacy of chest expansion and auscultate for bilateral breath sounds.
   a. Is the face-mask seal tight? A relatively large mask should be turned upside down for a better fit.
   b. Is the airway blocked from improper head position or secretions in the nose, mouth, or pharynx?
   c. Is adequate ventilatory pressure being used? A bag-valve mask pop-off valve may need to be disabled, especially for premature or meconium-aspiration delivery.
   d. Is air in the stomach interfering with chest expansion? Consider nasogastric or orogastric decompression per protocol.

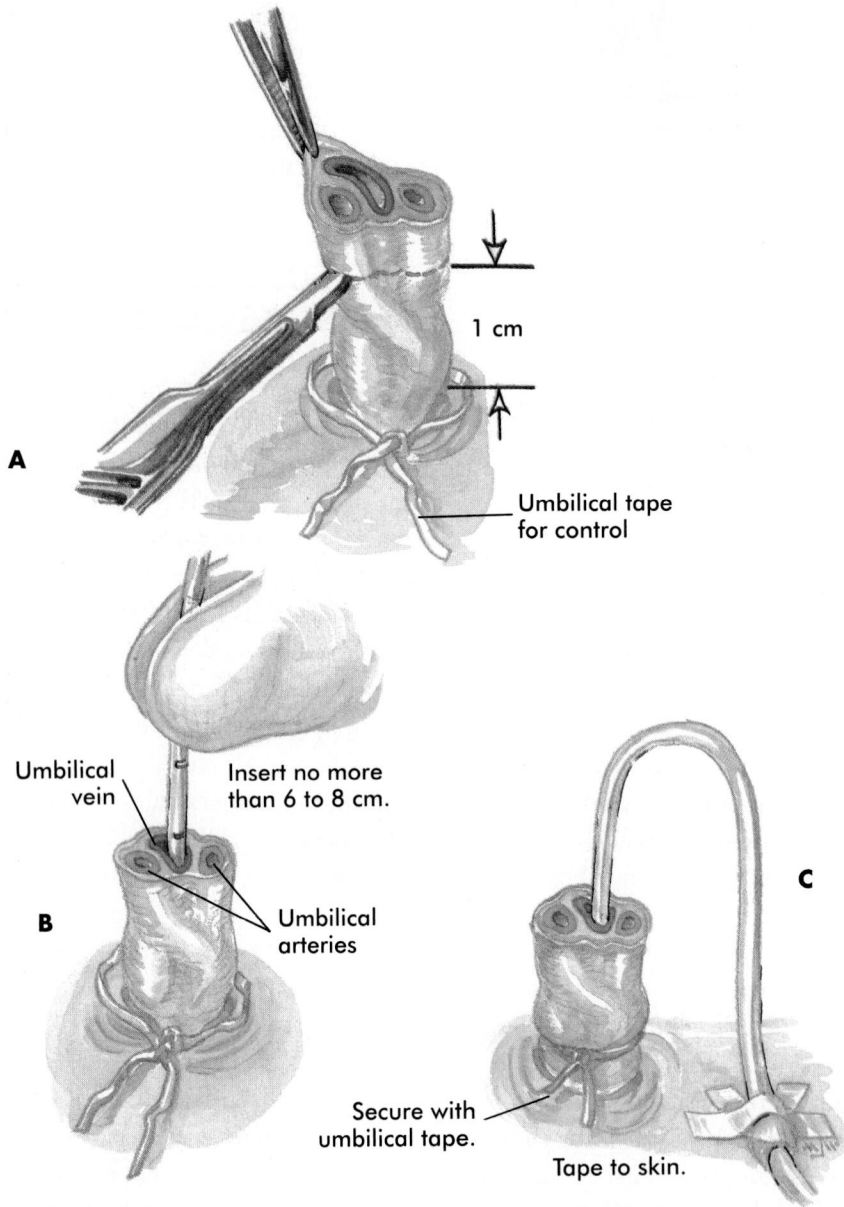

Fig. 28-16 Umbilical vein cannulation procedure. **A,** Identify the umbilical vein after trimming the cord. **B,** Insert the umbilical catheter or angiocatheter into the vein. **C,** Secure the base of the cord to hold the catheter in place and stabilize the catheter with tape.

TABLE 28-3 Medications for Neonatal Resuscitation

Indications and Use	Concentration	Preparation	Dosage and Route	Total Dose for Infant		Rate and Precautions
				Weight	Total Dose	
Epinephrine Asystole, spontaneous heart rate of less than 80 beats/min despite adequate ventilation with 100% oxygen and chest compression	1:10,000	10 ml	0.1-0.2 ml/kg IV, ET, IO	1 kg 2 kg 3 kg 4 kg	0.1-0.2 ml 0.2-0.4 ml 0.3-0.6 ml 0.4-0.8 ml	Give rapidly.
Volume Expanders Resuscitation of a newborn who is hypovolemic	Normal saline, lactated Ringer's solution	40 ml	10 ml/kg IV, IO	1 kg 2 kg 3 kg 4 kg	10 ml 20 ml 30 ml 40 ml	Give over 5-10 minutes.
Naloxone Reversal of respiratory depression induced by narcotics given to the mother within 4 hours of delivery	0.4 mg/ml	1 ml	0.1 mg/kg (0.25 ml/kg) IV, IM, IO, ET, SQ	1 kg 2 kg 3 kg 4 kg	0.1 mg 0.25 ml 0.2 mg 0.50 ml 0.3 mg 0.75 ml 0.4 mg 1.00 ml	Give rapidly. Use IV, IO, and ET routes (preferred).
	1.0 mg/ml	1 ml	0.1 mg/ml (0.1 ml/kg) IV, IM, IO, ET, SQ	1 kg 2 kg 3 kg 4 kg	0.1 mg 0.1 ml 0.2 mg 0.2 ml 0.3 mg 0.3 ml 0.4 mg 0.4 ml	Use IM and SQ routes (acceptable).

IV, Intravenous; *ET*, endotracheal; *IO*, intraosseous; *IM*, intramuscular; *SQ*, subcutaneous.

2. Is 100% oxygen being administered?
   a. Is the oxygen tubing attached to the bag and to the flowmeter?
   b. If using a self-inflating bag, is the oxygen reservoir attached?

Routes of Drug Administration

Drugs and fluids may be administered to the neonate via peripheral cannulation or intraosseous infusion (see Chapter 27), and some drugs may be given through the endotracheal tube (see Chapter 14). Another common site for vascular access in the neonate is the umbilical vein; this pro-

cedure requires special training and authorization from medical control (Fig. 28-16).

To review, the umbilical cord contains three vessels: two arteries and one vein. The vein in the umbilical cord has a thin wall and is larger than the arteries, which are thick walled and usually paired. To gain access to the umbilical vein, the paramedic should perform the following steps:

1. Set up intravenous fluid (per protocol) and tubing with a three-way stopcock.
2. Select a 3.5-French or 5.0-French umbilical catheter.
3. Connect the catheter to the stopcock and purge the air from the catheter.

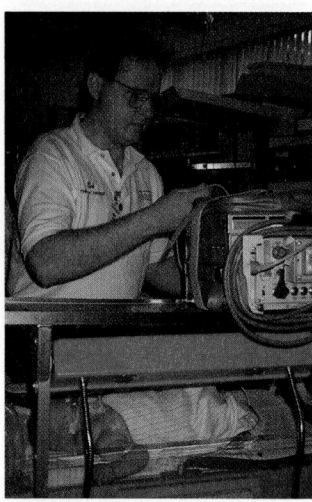

Fig. 28-17 Neonatal transport team.

4. Cleanse the umbilical stump and surrounding skin with antibacterial solution.
5. Loosely tie umbilical tape around the cord so that pressure can be applied to control bleeding.
6. Hold the umbilical stump firmly, and with a scalpel, trim the cord 1 cm above the abdomen.
7. Locate the umbilical vein and insert the catheter until blood is freely obtained. Do not insert the catheter more than 6 to 8 cm. (If the catheter is inserted farther, there is a risk of infusing solutions directly into the liver rather than into the systemic circulation.)

8. Draw blood for a sample if needed.
9. Start the infusion and regulate the fluid flow per medical control.
10. Secure the catheter in place with tape and cover with a sterile dressing.
11. Document the procedure.

The umbilical cord may also be cannulated by using a typical intravenous catheter. Insert the catheter-over-needle through the side of the proximal end of the cord into the vein and advance it upward through the translucent wall. Start the infusion, adjust the fluid flow per medical control, and secure the catheter in place with tape.

Medications Used in Neonatal Resuscitation

Medications most frequently used during neonatal resuscitation are *epinephrine*, volume expanders, and *naloxone*. Table 28-3 lists the medications recommended by the American Heart Association and the American Academy of Pediatrics.

● NEONATAL TRANSPORT

During transport of the neonate, it is important to maintain body temperature, oxygen administration, and ventilatory support. In the initial prehospital phase of care, transport strategies are usually limited to providing a warm ambulance, free-flow oxygen administration, and warm blankets. Specialized transport equipment such as isolettes and radiant heating units are often used for interhospital transfers and require special training. Highly trained neonatal transport teams consisting of paramedics, nurses, respiratory therapists, and physicians are part of several well-organized regional referral systems throughout the United States (Fig. 28-17).

REFERENCES

1. Moore E et al: *Early care of the injured patient*, ed 4, Philadelphia, 1990, BC Decker.
2. Shaffer M, Franaszek J, editors: OB/GYN emergencies, *Top Emerg Med* 7(2):27, 1985.
3. American Heart Association. *Textbook of neonatal resuscitation*, Dallas, 1990, The Association.

Summary

Participating in childbirth is an exciting and rewarding experience. In most cases, paramedic involvement is limited to providing minimal delivery assistance to the mother and initial care to the mother and newborn. However, if an obstetrical emergency arises, care of the mother and infant requires special knowledge and skills in physical assessment, patient management, and neonatal resuscitation. These talents can greatly reduce maternal and infant morbidity and mortality.

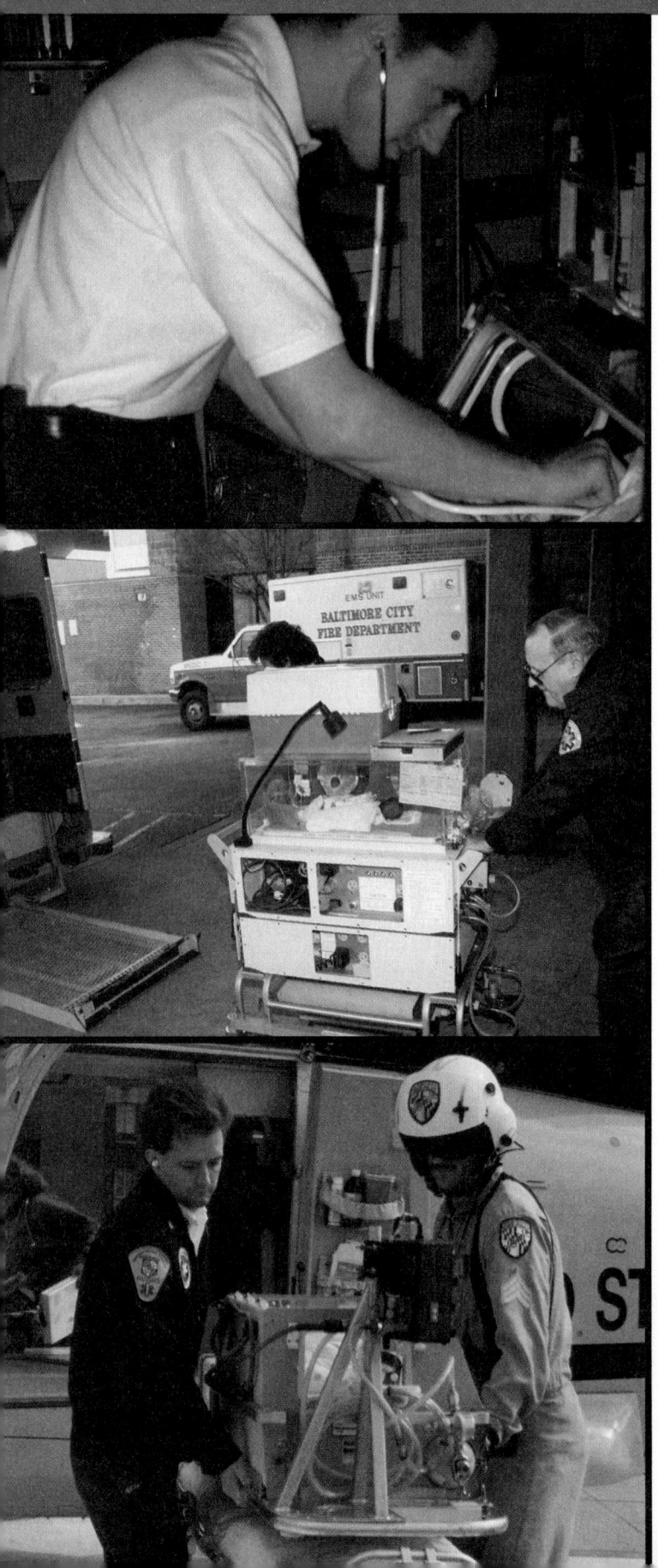

A number of disorders can occur in the female reproductive system, some of which lead to gynecological emergencies. This chapter explains the etiology and emergency care measures for common problems associated with the female reproductive system.

As a paramedic, you should be able to:

1. Describe the pathophysiology, assessment, and management of the following causes of abdominal pain in females: dysmenorrhea, mittelschmerz, pelvic inflammatory disease, and ruptured ovarian cyst.
2. Outline the assessment and physical and psychological management of the sexual assault victim.
3. Describe specific prehospital measures to preserve evidence in sexual assault cases.

● ABDOMINAL PAIN

In addition to the gastrointestinal causes of abdominal pain described in Chapter 21, acute or chronic infection involving the patient's uterus, ovaries, fallopian tubes, and adjacent structures may be a source of severe abdominal pain. The scope of abdominal pain associated with the female reproductive system may range from benign episodes of difficult menstruation to a potentially life-threatening hemorrhage from a ruptured ovarian cyst or ectopic pregnancy. Common causes of abdominal pain in women in their reproductive or childbearing years include dysmenorrhea and mittelschmerz, endometriosis, pelvic inflammatory disease (PID), ectopic pregnancy (see Chapter 28), and ruptured ovarian cyst (Table 29-1).

Dysmenorrhea and Mittelschmerz

Many women experience dysmenorrhea during menstruation. **Dysmenorrhea** is characterized by painful menses but may also be associated with headache, faintness, dizziness, nausea, diarrhea, backache, and leg pain. In severe cases, chills, headache, diarrhea, nausea, vomiting, and syncope can occur. Occurrence is more common in unmarried women and in women who have not borne children. The lower abdominal pains associated with dysmenorrhea are thought to be related to muscular contraction of the myometrium (the muscular layer of the uterus), mediated by local prostaglandins. Other factors associated with dysmenorrhea include infection, inflammation, and the presence of an intrauterine contraceptive device (IUCD).

Mittelschmerz (German for "middle pain") is another cause of pain from the rupture of the graafian follicle and bleeding from the ovary during the menstrual cycle. Mittelschmerz is characterized by right or left lower quadrant abdominal pain that occurs in the normal midcycle of a menstrual period (after ovulation). The hormones produced by the ovary may also produce slight endometrial bleeding and low-grade fever. Dysmenorrhea and mittelschmerz are not life-threatening conditions, but physician evaluation is required to rule out more serious causes of menstrual pain.

Endometriosis

Endometriosis is an abnormal gynecological condition characterized by ectopic growth and functioning of endometrial tissue. The disease is thought to result from fragments of endometrium

---

KEY TERMS

dysmenorrhea: Pain associated with menstruation.

pelvic inflammatory disease: Any inflammatory condition of the female pelvic organs.

sexual assault: A forcible act of sexual contact with the body of another person, male or female, without his or her consent.

TABLE 29-1 Characteristics of Abdominal Pain in Gynecological Emergencies

Onset	Location	Quality	Radiation	Vaginal Discharge	Menstrual History
Ruptured Ectopic Pregnancy					
Rapid (can become generalized)	Unilateral (can generalize)	Cramplike, then steady	Shoulder (may indicate intraperitoneal bleeding)	Vaginal bleeding (75% of cases)	Amenorrhea, 6 weeks or more since last period
Ruptured Ovarian Cyst					
Sudden	Unilateral (can generalize)	Steady	Shoulder (may indicate intraperitoneal bleeding)	Possible vaginal bleeding	Usually 1 week before period
PID					
Gradual (can become generalized)	Diffuse, bilateral	Steady ache	Right upper quadrant	Watery, foul-smelling discharge	Usually within 1 week after period

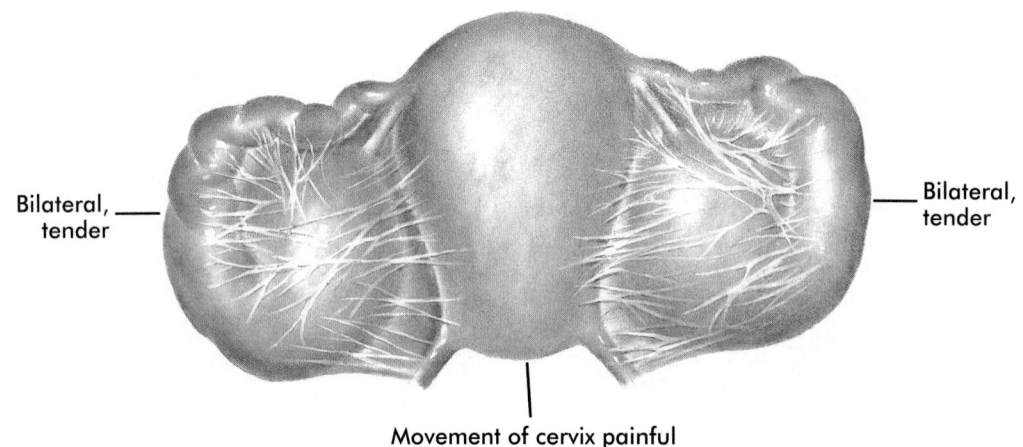

Bilateral, tender

Bilateral, tender

Movement of cervix painful

Fig. 29-1 Pelvic inflammatory disease.

from the lining of the uterus regurgitated backward during menstruation through the fallopian tubes into the peritoneal cavity, where they attach and grow as small cystic structures. The endometrial tissue of endometriosis functions cyclically and undergoes periodic menstrual breakdown that results in bleeding within cysts, stretching of the cyst wall, and pain.

Endometriosis is more common in women who defer pregnancy. The average age of women found to have endometriosis is 37 years. Characteristic symptoms of endometriosis are pain (particularly dysmenorrhea), painful defecation, and suprapubic soreness. Other common symptoms

include premenstrual vaginal staining of blood and infertility. After physician evaluation, treatment may consist of medication with analgesics or hormones and sometimes surgery.

PID

Pelvic inflammatory disease affects about 1 million women annually and is responsible for more than 250,000 hospitalizations each year. The disease results from infection of the cervix, uterus, fallopian tubes, and ovaries and their supporting structures (Fig. 29-1). It is usually caused by sexually transmitted bacteria, most commonly

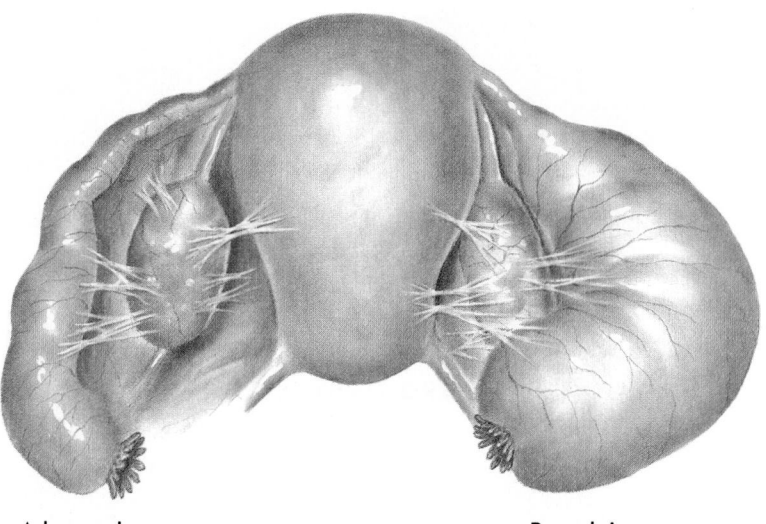

Advanced   Pyosalpinx

Fig. 29-2 Salpingitis.

Neisseria gonorrheae, chlamydia, or both. Staphylococci, streptococci, and other pathogens may also cause infection, but these organisms are usually transmitted by doctor's instruments.

Ascending infection from the vaginal area infects the cervix (cervicitis) initially, followed by the uterus proper (endometritis) and the fallopian tubes (salpingitis) (Fig. 29-2) and finally the associated contiguous supporting structures around the uterus and fallopian tubes (parametritis). The infection is polymicrobial in etiology, producing diffuse lower abdominal pain associated with low-grade fever (variable), vaginal discharge, and dyspareunia (pain with sexual intercourse). The inflammation frequently follows the onset of menstrual bleeding by 7 to 10 days, when reproductive organs are especially vulnerable to bacterial infection from the presence of relatively avascular endometrial tissue that sloughs during menstruation. In many cases, the presence of PID is accompanied by pain on ambulation, with the patient bent forward; taking short, slow steps; and often guarding the abdomen (the "PID shuffle"). Consequences include secondary infertility, ectopic pregnancies, and tuboovarian abscesses; in severe cases, reproductive organs may require surgical removal. Definitive treatment usually consists of antibiotic therapy to eradicate the infection and to preserve fallopian tube structure and function.

Ruptured Ovarian Cyst

A ruptured ovarian cyst is a gynecological emergency that can result in significant internal hemorrhage. An ovarian cyst is a thin-walled, fluid-filled sac located on the surface of the ovary (Fig. 29-3). The abdominal pain caused by an ovarian cyst may result from rapid expansion, torsion that produces ischemia, or acute rupture. The type of cyst most prone to rupture is the corpus luteum cyst, which forms as a result of hemorrhage in a mature corpus luteum. Since the corpus luteum develops after ovulation (day 14 of the 28-day cycle), most ruptures occur approximately 1 week before menstrual bleeding is due to begin. However, some patients with a ruptured ovarian cyst have vaginal bleeding or report a late or missed period at the time of rupture.

A ruptured ovarian cyst, like a ruptured ectopic pregnancy, can result in localized, unilateral lower abdominal pain or in generalized signs of peritonitis if massive hemorrhage has occurred. The onset of pain is frequently associated with minimal abdominal trauma, sexual intercourse, or exercise.

Management

Precise diagnosis of lower abdominal pain in the female is difficult because many gynecological conditions produce common clinical character-

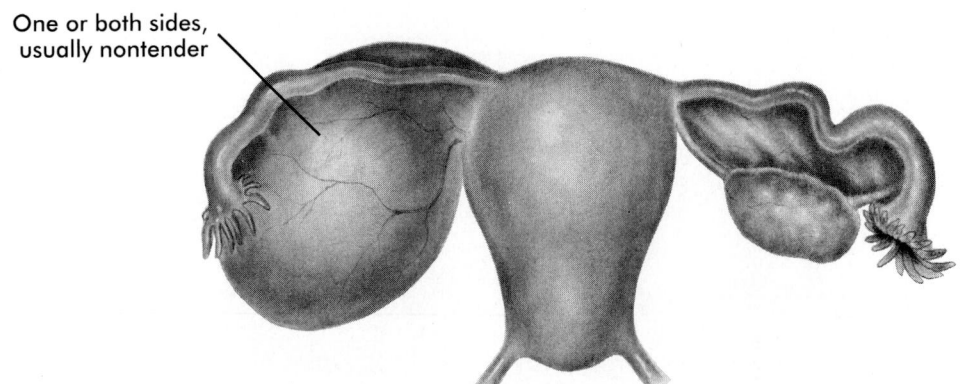

One or both sides,
usually nontender

Fig. 29-3 Ovarian cyst.

istics. For example, ectopic pregnancy, ruptured ovarian cyst, PID, and appendicitis can have identical presentations. The goal of prehospital management is quick identification of conditions that require aggressive therapy and rapid transport for surgical intervention. Prehospital care includes obtaining a thorough gynecological history; providing airway, ventilatory, and circulatory support as needed; and transporting the patient for physician evaluation.

● SEXUAL ASSAULT

Sexual assault is a crime of violence with serious physical and psychological implications. Anyone of either gender at any age can be sexually assaulted. However, women and girls are most often the victims. It is estimated that one in three women will be raped during their lifetimes and that only 10% to 30% of these crimes will be reported.[1] Often, the paramedic is first to encounter

these patients. Tact, kindness, and sensitivity during the patient care episode are essential.

The victim of sexual assault should be initially cared for like any other injured patient. However, after the management of life-threatening injury, the paramedic's approach to the patient should be somewhat modified with reference to history taking and the physical examination. Before gathering a history or performing a physical examination, the patient should be moved to a private area. If possible, the patient should be given the opportunity to be interviewed and examined by a paramedic of the same gender.

History Taking

As a rule, victims of sexual assault should not be questioned in detail about the incident in the prehospital setting. The history should be limited to elements that are necessary to provide emergency medical care. For example, questions regarding penetration or inquiries about the patient's sexual history or practices are irrelevant to prehospital care and only add to the patient's emotional stress. Allow the patient to speak openly if he or she wishes, and record all information accurately and thoroughly.

Assessment

The purpose of the physical examination is to identify any physical trauma outside of the pelvic area for which the patient needs immediate attention. It is not uncommon to find facial fractures, human bites of the hands and breasts, long bone fractures, broken ribs, or trauma to the abdomen. The paramedic should examine the genitalia only if severe injury is present or suspected. When possible, all procedures should be explained to the patient before the examination takes place. All observations of the physical examination should be documented, including the patient's emotional state, the condition of the victim's clothing, obvious injuries, and any patient care rendered.

Management

After managing life-threatening injury, emotional support is the most important patient care procedure that can be offered to a victim of sexual abuse. The paramedic should provide a safe environment for the patient and respond appropriately to the victim's physical and emotional needs. Paramedics should also be aware of the need to preserve evidence from the crime scene. Special considerations include the following:

- Handle clothing as little as possible.
- Do not clean wounds.
- Do not use plastic bags for blood-stained articles.
- Bag each clothing item separately.
- Ask the victim not to change clothes or bathe.
- Disturb the crime scene as little as possible.

REFERENCE

1. Williams D: Sensitive emergency management of rape victims, *Rep Emerg Nurs* 1(11):14, 1990.

Summary

Gynecological emergencies are common in the prehospital setting. The paramedic should approach these patients with a high index of suspicion for serious illness or injury that may require rapid intervention and maintain a sensitive and professional rapport during the patient care encounter.

BEHAVIORAL

DIVISION SIX

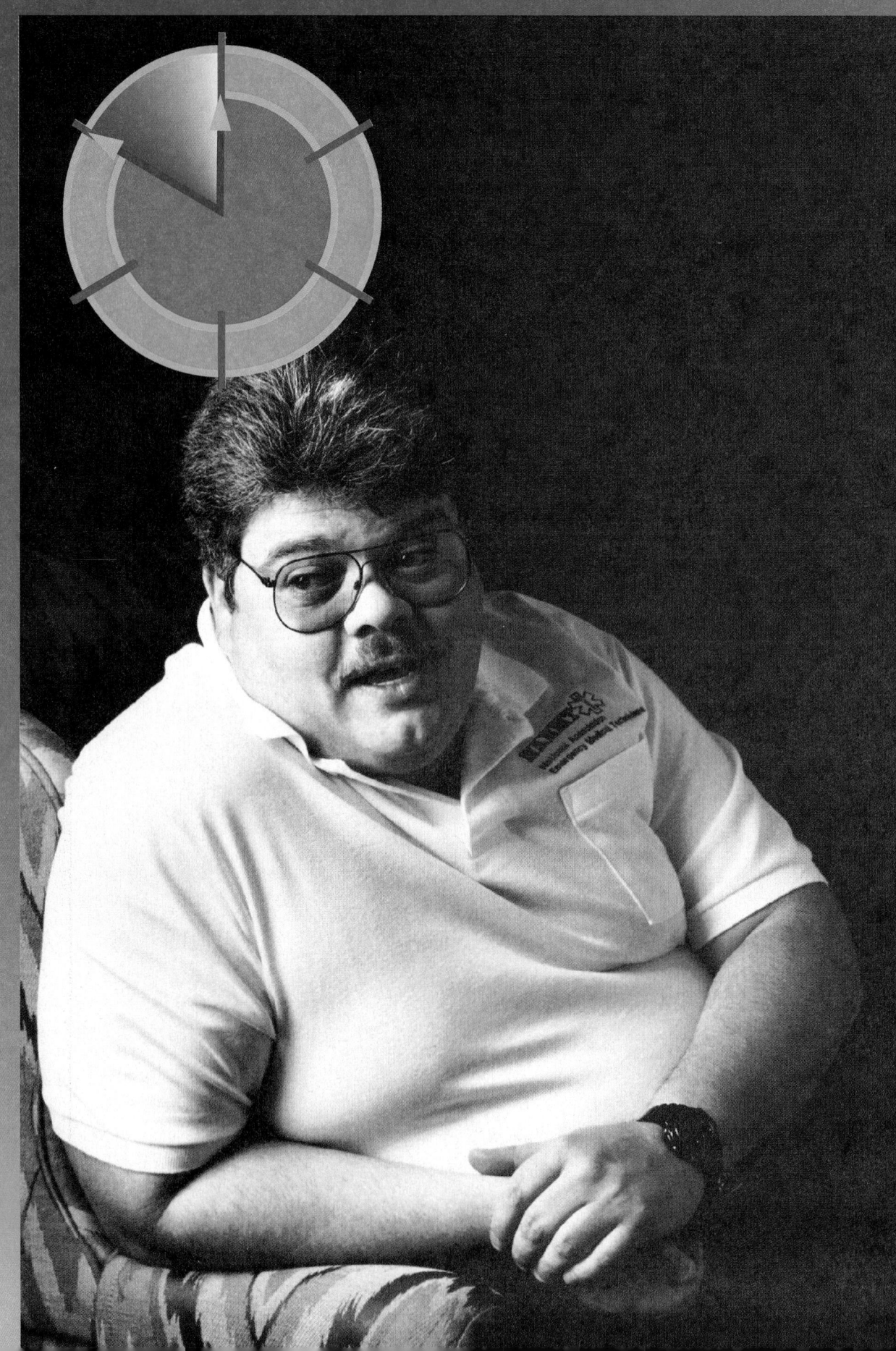

Violent or disturbed patients can be the most challenging and frustrating. Just remember your people skills and your ability to build rapport with patients. Take control of the situation, so you don't become part of the problem.

Kevin Agard, EMT-P
New York City EMS
New York, New York

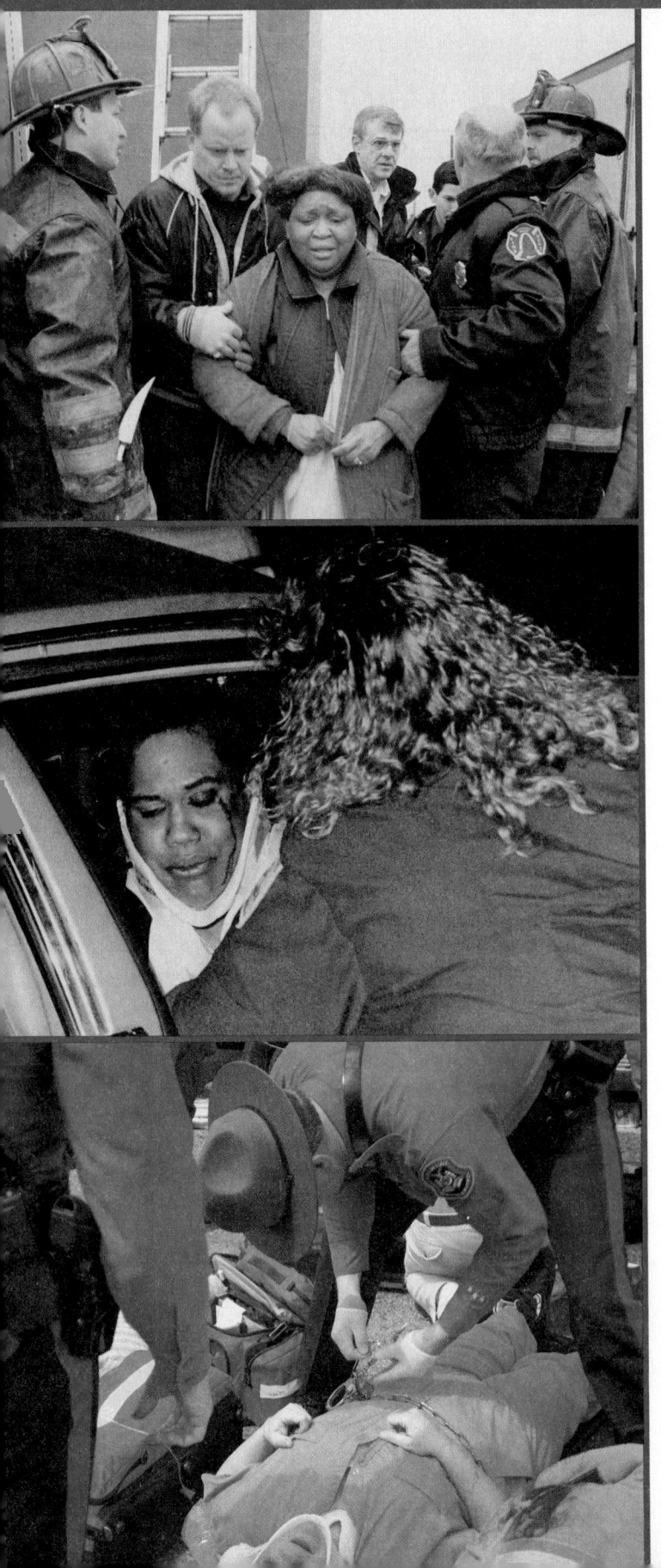

Behavioral emergencies require a different approach than medical or trauma-related calls. There are no scientific tools with which to assess the situation and no firm protocols to ensure a positive outcome. Therefore it is common for EMS personnel to feel uncertain and lack confidence in their ability to deal with patients experiencing behavioral emergencies. This chapter stresses that intervention in such emergencies is essential to prevent the escalation of a crisis, that paramedics can make a significant difference in patient outcome, and that these emergencies can be approached and evaluated in an organized manner.

As a paramedic, you should be able to:

1. List examples of interpersonal, situational, organic, and intrapsychic causes of behavioral emergencies.
2. List three critical principles in dealing with a patient having a behavioral emergency.
3. Describe effective interviewing techniques.
4. Distinguish among key symptoms and management techniques for selected behavioral (psychiatric) illnesses.
5. Identify factors that must be considered when assessing suicide risk.
6. Formulate appropriate interview questions to determine suicidal intent.
7. Explain management techniques for the patient who has attempted suicide.
8. Describe assessment of the potentially violent patient.
9. List situations when patient restraint can be used.
10. Outline steps in patient restraint.
11. Describe general safety measures to be taken when patient violence is anticipated.
12. Describe steps for self-protection when confronted with a violent patient.

● UNDERSTANDING BEHAVIORAL EMERGENCIES

A *behavioral emergency* can be defined as a change in mood or behavior that cannot be tolerated by the involved person or others and that requires immediate attention. Behavioral emergencies may range from disordered and disturbed patients who are dangerous to themselves and others to less intense situations in which the patient has a transient inability to cope with stress or anxiety. Most behavioral emergencies result from interpersonal, situational, organic, or intrapsychic causes.

Interpersonal and Situational Causes

Most people maintain a delicate balance among emotions, thoughts, and actions. When this equilibrium shifts rapidly, the person may experience emotional turmoil that results in crisis. Changes in behavior caused by interpersonal or situational stress are frequently linked to specific incidents or series of incidents. Examples include death of a loved one, rape, and natural or manmade disasters.

Organic Causes

Physical or biochemical disturbances can also result in significant changes in behavior. Examples

KEY TERMS

mania: A phase of bipolar disorder characterized by elation, agitation, hyperexcitability, hyperactivity, and increased speed of thought or speech.

neurosis: Any faulty or inefficient way of coping with anxiety or inner conflict that may lead to a neurotic disorder.

psychosis: Any major mental disorder of organic or emotional origin that is characterized by extreme derangement or disorganization of the personality, often accompanied by severe depression, agitation, regressive behavior, illusions, delusions, and hallucinations and in which the individual loses touch with reality and is incapable of functioning normally in society.

BOX 30-1

Common Medical Conditions Presenting as Behavioral Disorders

Metabolic Disorders
Glucose, sodium, calcium, or magnesium imbalance
Acid-base imbalance
Acute hypoxia
Renal failure
Hepatic failure

Endocrine Disorders
Thyroid disease
Parathyroid disease
Adrenal hormone imbalance

Infectious Diseases
Encephalitis
Meningitis
Brain abscess
Severe systemic infection

Trauma
Concussion
Intracranial hematoma (especially subdural hematoma)

Cardiovascular Disorders
Cardiac dysrhythmia
Hypotension
Transient ischemic attack
Cardiovascular accident
Hypertensive encephalopathy

Neoplastic Diseases
Central nervous system tumors or metastases

Degenerative Diseases
Dementia of the Alzheimer's type
Other dementias

Drug Abuse
Alcohol
Barbiturates
Sedative hypnotics
Amphetamines and other stimulants
Hallucinogens

Drug Reactions
Beta-adrenergic blockers
Antihypertensives
Cardiac drugs
Bronchodilators
Beta-adrenergic agonists
Anticonvulsants

---

of organic causes of behavioral emergencies have been discussed throughout this text and include substance abuse, trauma, illness such as diabetes and electrolyte imbalance, and dementia. It is important to consider the possibility of organic causes in all behavioral emergencies (Box 30-1).

Intrapsychic Causes

Acute or chronic episodes of an underlying psychiatric condition may result in a behavioral emergency that requires EMS assistance. Most intra-

psychic illnesses are of unknown etiology and are characterized by **neurosis** (a restricted ability to achieve optimal functioning in social life) or **psychosis** (maladaptive behavior that involves major distortions of reality). The behavioral changes associated with psychiatric illness manifest in a wide range of psychological and physiological responses, including:

- Depression
- Withdrawal
- Catatonic state
- Violence

- Suicidal acts
- Paranoid reactions
- Phobia
- Disorientation or disorganization

● DOMESTIC VIOLENCE

Domestic violence can be defined as behavior among family or household members that threatens to cause or does cause serious physical harm. Examples of domestic violence include battered spouses and child and elder abuse and neglect. The paramedic should be aware that in these situations the danger of violence is very real and that volatile hostility may be directed toward the EMS crew. As in any emergency response, personal safety is of prime importance. In most situations, police should be summoned for assistance in containing the crisis.

● ASSESSMENT OF BEHAVIORAL EMERGENCIES

The first step in assessing a behavioral emergency is to protect the EMS crew. Because of the nature of these responses, injury to an emergency medical provider is always a possibility. Therefore evaluating the scene for possible danger must be the highest priority. Most EMS services operate under protocol that includes a police response for any behavioral emergency. If a dangerous situation is suspected, the EMS crew should not approach the patient until police are present and the potential for danger is controlled. Three general principles must be remembered when dealing with behavioral emergencies:
1. Contain the crisis.
2. Render appropriate emergency medical care.
3. Transport the patient to an appropriate health care facility.

Assessment

Patient assessment should begin by gathering the information necessary for immediate management of life-threatening conditions. On arrival, the scene should be surveyed for patient care information such as evidence of violence, substance abuse, or a suicide attempt. Other information can be volunteered by the patient, obtained from the patient interview, or provided by family, bystanders, and first responders. During the patient assessment, an attempt should be made to gather the following data:
- The patient's mental state (alertness, orientation, and ability to communicate)
- Patient's name and age
- Past medical history
- Past psychiatric problems
- Precipitating situation or problem

Interview Techniques

After any life-threatening illness or injury has been managed, alert and communicative patients should be interviewed. The paramedic should not ask for more information than is necessary, but a limited and supportive interview helps strengthen the paramedic's rapport with the patient and can help establish and maintain a relationship during the patient encounter. Ten useful interviewing skills are listed in the sidebar on p. 914.[1]

Other Patient Care Measures

After the primary survey and history taking, the remainder of the examination is determined by the patient's overall condition and the nature of the psychiatric problem. The benefits of a thorough secondary assessment must be weighed against the risks involved in an encounter that the patient may construe as a physical violation. If there is reason to suspect an organic cause that might be further elucidated by a secondary survey and the patient demonstrates no apprehension or disapproval, the secondary survey should be performed. Otherwise, prehospital management may be limited to maintaining an effective rapport with the patient during transfer to the hospital.

Elements of the secondary survey that may be associated with a behavioral emergency include abnormal pupillary size and reactivity (indicating toxic ingestion or an intracranial process), a breath

Ten Useful Interviewing Skills for Behavioral Emergencies

1. Listen to the patient in a caring, concerned, and receptive manner. Be aware of nonverbal communications such as eye contact, facial expression, and posture, which can reassure the patient that you are responding with empathy.

2. Elicit feelings as well as facts to help develop a more accurate impression of the patient. If the patient is anxious, encourage him or her to share information relevant to that feeling.

3. Respond to the patient's feelings by acknowledging and labeling them (for example, "You seem angry"). This may help validate and legitimize the patient's intense and sometime overwhelming feelings.

4. Correct cognitive misconceptions or distortions. If a distorted sense of reality is producing fear or anxiety, offer a simple and correct explanation.

5. Provide information on the nature of the intervention or the care the patient can expect after arrival at the hospital.

6. Offer honest and realistic reassurance and support. Providing this support helps calm the patient and establishes rapport.

7. Ask effective questions. When seeking immediate information, ask closed-ended questions such as "Are you thinking of hurting yourself?" and "What medicines did you take?" More open-ended questions are appropriate after identifying problems that require immediate attention; such questions permit the individual to develop answers that usually help the paramedic completely understand the problem.

8. Avoid questions that may lead the person to say things he or she did not intend.

9. Structure the interview to develop a pattern rather than permitting a natural flow of information. Chronologically reported histories or sequences of events usually permit more complete understanding of the patient's problem (particularly causal relationships) and help the patient to organize thoughts. Keep the patient's responses focused by comments such as "What happened next?" and "Was that before or after what you were just telling me about?"

10. Conclude the interview. After obtaining relevant information, encourage the patient to describe other important events or feelings.

---

odor of alcohol, needle tracks on the extremities, and unilateral weakness or loss of sensation.

● SPECIFIC PSYCHIATRIC DISORDERS

More than 250 psychiatric conditions have been identified by mental health workers. Common classifications of psychiatric illness include anxiety disorders, phobia, conversion hysteria, depression, manic disorders, suicide and suicide threats, and paranoia.

Anxiety Disorders

As discussed in Chapter 8, a certain amount of anxiety is useful and necessary in adapting constructively to stress. However, a patient who suffers from an anxiety disorder displays a persistent, fearful feeling that cannot be consciously related to reality. This type of illness may be disabling as the patient withdraws from daily activities in a usually unsuccessful attempt to avoid the episodes of intense activity. Severe anxiety disorders may manifest in a "panic attack" with the following signs and symptoms:

- Hyperventilation
- Fear of losing control
- Fear of dying
- Somatic complaints
  - Chest discomfort
  - Palpitations or tachycardia
  - Dyspnea
  - Choking
  - Faintness

- ◦ Syncope
- ◦ Vertigo
- Trembling and sweating
- Urinary frequency and diarrhea

Patient management is primarily supportive. The paramedic should assure these patients that, although they may feel like they are dying, they are not and that effective treatment is available. Panic attacks may mimic a number of medical emergencies. Therefore any patient who exhibits the signs and symptoms previously described should be thoroughly assessed at the scene and transported for physician evaluation. Patients with anxiety disorders should not be left alone.

Phobia

A phobic patient is one who has transferred anxiety onto a situation or object in the form of an irrational, intense fear (for example, fear of heights, water, other people). As the object or situation comes closer to the person, the anxiety increases. If the crisis is allowed to continue, the patient's anxiety may escalate into a panic attack. These patients generally recognize that their fear is unreasonable, but they cannot prevent the phobia. In some cases, the phobia did not initiate the EMS response but becomes a secondary complication in emergency care. An example is a submerged motor vehicle crash in which a patient who is phobic of water is trapped in the automobile.

In caring for these patients, the paramedic should be careful to explain each step involved in an emergency or rescue procedure. A careful rehearsal with the patient, explaining exactly what and how care will be accomplished, is important. In addition, the EMS crew should show patience and understanding of the phobia and assure the patient that no forceful steps will be taken to make him or her do anything he or she does not want to do.

Conversion Hysteria

In conversion hysteria there is a loss of sensory, motor, or special sense function without organic pathology. The individual suddenly cannot hear or see or feel, an arm or leg is paralyzed, or he or she is unable to speak. In many cases, the areas of the body affected do not correspond to the actual arrangement of neural pathways. The hysterical symptoms may also come and go or appear at different times and in different areas of the body.

The paramedic should treat the symptoms as if they are real, since it may be difficult to differentiate an organic ailment from a hysterical one. It is important to recognize that these patients are not "faking"; they believe their loss of function to be real and often will actually sustain bodily harm (such as burns) in the area affected. These patients require physician evaluation.

Depression

The depressed patient may show feelings of hopelessness, extreme isolation, tenseness, and irritability. In severe cases, the depression may be followed by sleeplessness, loss of appetite, decreased libido, and deep feelings of worthlessness and guilt. Care in this situation is directed at quietly talking to the patient about things that appear to be of interest to him or her and at attempting to gain responsiveness.

Manic Disorders

Mania is characterized by excessive elation, talkativeness, flight of ideas, motor activity, irritability, accelerated speech, and frequently, delusions that center around personal grandeur. Patients with mania are often suffering from bipolar disorder (manic-depressive illness), in which depressive and manic episodes alternate with one another.

Manic states sometimes begin gradually, but they may occur abruptly and be precipitated by a single event. The manic phase can last weeks or months. Compared with depression, mania is rare. The most frequent age for initial episodes is between 20 and 35 years, with initial attacks of depression occurring approximately 10 years later.

Prehospital care should consist of calm, firm emotional support and transport for physician evaluation. If this is the patient's first manic episode, the paramedic should consider the possibility of drug abuse. It is generally recommended to keep sensory stimulation to a minimum, so if the

Mythology of Suicide[2]

MYTH: People who talk about killing themselves rarely commit suicide.

FACT: Most people who commit suicide have given some clue or warning of their intent; therefore suicidal threats and attempts should always be treated seriously.

MYTH: The tendency toward suicide is inherited and passed from generation to generation.

FACT: Although suicide does tend to "run in families," it appears that it is not transmitted genetically.

MYTH: All suicidal people are deeply depressed.

FACT: Although depression is often associated with suicidal feelings, not all people who kill themselves are obviously depressed. In fact, some suicidal people appear to be happier than they have been in quite a while because they have decided to "resolve" all of their problems at the same time.

MYTH: There is a very low correlation between alcoholism and suicide.

FACT: Alcoholism and suicide often go hand in hand. Alcoholics are prone to suicide, and even people who do not normally drink often ingest alcohol shortly before killing themselves.

MYTH: Suicidal people are mentally ill.

FACT: Although many suicidal people are depressed and distraught, most of them would not be diagnosed as mentally ill.

MYTH: If someone attempts suicide, he or she will always entertain thoughts of suicide.

FACT: Most people who are suicidal are that way for only a brief period in their lives. If the attempter receives the proper assistance and support, he or she will probably never be suicidal again. Only about 10% of attempters later complete the act.

MYTH: If you ask the person about his or her suicidal intentions, you will encourage the person to kill himself or herself.

FACT: Actually, the opposite is true. Asking someone directly about suicidal intent often lowers the anxiety level and acts as a deterrent to suicidal emotions.

MYTH: Suicide is more common among the lower classes.

FACT: Suicide crosses all socioeconomic groups, and no one class is more susceptible to it than another.

MYTH: Suicidal people rarely seek medical attention.

FACT: Research has consistently shown that about 75% of suicidal people visit a physician within 3 months before they kill themselves.

MYTH: Suicide is basically a problem limited to young people.

FACT: The suicide rate rises with age and reaches a peak among older white men.

MYTH: Professional people do not kill themselves.

FACT: Physicians, lawyers, dentists, and pharmacists may have high suicide rates.

MYTH: When a person's depression lifts, there is no longer any danger of suicide.

FACT: The greatest danger of suicide exists during the first 3 months after a person recovers from a deep depression.

MYTH: Suicide is a spontaneous activity that occurs without warning.

FACT: Most people plan their self-destruction and then present clues indicating that they have become suicidal.

MYTH: Because it includes the Christmas season, December has a high suicide rate.

FACT: There is not a rash of suicides at Christmas, and December has the lowest rate of any month.

patient's condition permits, EMS transport should proceed without lights or sirens.

Suicide and Suicide Threats

A threat of suicide is an indication that a patient has a serious crisis that requires immediate intervention. In many cases, suicide attempts are a cry for help or a form of direct or indirect communication, such as "I don't want to live" or "I am angry with you." Other suicide attempts are an effort to manipulate relationships such that the suicidal patient will be surrounded by individuals ready and willing to provide advice and support. In assessing the risk of suicide, consider these seven facts:

1. Suicide is the third leading cause of death in people 15 to 25 years of age and the fourth leading cause of death in people between the ages of 25 and 45.
2. Women *attempt* suicide more often than men.
3. Men *commit* suicide more often than women.
4. An older man (55 years or more) presents the greatest threat of actual suicide and a younger woman the least.
5. Men use more violent means (guns, knives) than women (pills, razors).
6. Approximately 60% of successful suicides have a history of a previous attempt.
7. The more specific and detailed the suicide plan, the greater the suicide potential.

Other factors associated with suicide threats include recent loss of a spouse or a significant relationship, financial setback or job loss, chronic or debilitating illness, social isolation, drug or alcohol abuse, and schizophrenia. If a suicide attempt is suspected, it is generally recommended that these suspicions be discussed with the patient. Questions such as "Do you have thoughts about killing yourself?" or "Have you ever tried to kill yourself?" are appropriate; many depressed patients are willing to discuss their suicidal thoughts.

When responding to a suicide attempt, the paramedic should request police protection before approaching the scene. After scene safety is ensured and access to the patient is gained, the scene should be evaluated for the presence of dangerous objects. Armed patients must be considered homicidal as well as suicidal.

The first priority in patient management is medical care. Unconscious patients should be managed with airway, ventilatory, and circulatory support and rapid transport. If the patient is conscious, it is important to develop a rapport within a relatively short period. The paramedic should conduct a brief interview to assess the situation and to determine the need and direction for further action. The following five steps should reduce the potential for suicide in most situations:

1. Provide support and honest assurance about the patient's well-being if possible.
2. Provide for physical safety as well as emotional security. Establish protective limits and measures to prevent the person from injuring himself or herself or others. This conveys to patients that you will help them control their behavior until they can gain self-control.
3. Listen to the person, even if his or her talk seems bizarre, inappropriate, or unrealistic. Do not feel that you must answer every statement or give advice or opinions. During the interview, acknowledge the patient's feelings, and do not argue with his or her wish to die. Explain alternatives to suicide that the patient may not have considered.
4. Determine the patient's support system or significant others when possible. Others may be better able to communicate with and calm the patient and direct him or her to appropriate activity.
5. Encourage the patient to discuss feelings and reassure the patient that he or she can be helped through this crisis.

Paranoia

Paranoia is a rare psychosis characterized by logical and highly developed delusional systems with little or no indication of other psychotic symptoms. Transient, nonrecurring episodes of paranoia do occur in some individuals. The more common chronic or recurrent paranoia generally indicates an underlying diagnosis of schizophrenia.

Schizophrenia

Schizophrenia is a group of disorders characterized by recurrent episodes of psychotic behavior, which may include abnormalities of thought process, thought content (delusions), perception (auditory hallucinations are particularly common), and judgment. There is often a family history of schizophrenia, and the disorder usually becomes apparent during adolescence or early adulthood. Most schizophrenics function poorly between frank psychotic episodes. Management of paranoid reactions should include:

1. Clearly identifying yourself as a paramedic and expressing your intent to provide help.
2. Exhibiting an attitude that is friendly, yet somewhat distant and neutral. Kindness and warmth may be interpreted by the patient as an attempt to gain his or her confidence for ulterior motives.
3. Never responding to the patient's anger.
4. Not speaking with family members or bystanders in hushed or secretive tones.
5. Using tact and firmness in persuading the patient to be transported to the hospital.
6. Remembering that paranoid reactions can lead to violent behavior; precautions regarding personal safety must be a priority.

● ASSESSING THE POTENTIALLY VIOLENT PATIENT

Only a small proportion of persons with mental health problems are potentially violent. Nonetheless, assessment and management of the potentially violent patient should be part of an EMS protocol. The following four factors may help determine the potential for a violent episode[3]:

1. Past history: Has the patient exhibited hostile, aggressive, or violent behavior?
2. Posture: Is the patient sitting or standing? Does the patient appear to be tense or rigid?
3. Vocal activity: Loud, obscene, and erratic speech indicates emotional distress.
4. Physical activity: Is the patient pacing or agitated or displaying protection of physical boundaries?

If any of these signs of potentially violent behavior are present, the paramedic should attempt to reduce the impact of the stress but avoid confrontation and prepare a way to cope with the crisis that reduces the potential for a life-threatening incident or psychologically damaging consequences.

Controlling Violent Situations

Severely disturbed patients who pose a threat to themselves or others may need to be restrained, transported, and hospitalized against their will. Each state has a statute covering the criteria for involuntary commitment, and the paramedic should be familiar with all applicable laws. The premise on which most state laws are based suggests that one person may restrain another to protect life or prevent injury.

When a psychiatric patient refuses care in the prehospital setting, EMS personnel should consult with medical control. The decision to restrain, treat, or release the patient is a medical control decision. If violent behavior must be contained, "reasonable force" to restrain the patient should be used as humanely as possible. In most cases, the restraint duty (if necessary) should be given to law enforcement personnel. As in all other aspects of health care, details of the incident should be carefully recorded for future reference.

Restraint Guidelines

- If the patient is homicidal, do not attempt restraint. If the patient is armed, move everyone out of range and wait for law enforcement personnel.
- Remember that the patient may not be responsible for his or her actions.
- Plan your restraining action to include a back-up plan in case the initial action fails.
- Be sure that adequate man power is available. Make sure that a minimum of four capable individuals are available to help restrain an adult patient.
- Remember that the potential for personal injury and legal liability is always present.

Restraint Methods

A number of restraint methods can be used to manage a violent patient. The techniques used to contain violent behavior should begin with a gentle, nonthreatening, low-profile approach and progress to more direct intervention as needed. Always explain the options of physical restraint to the patient before applying force. If the patient is still unwilling to cooperate, advise him or her that restraint is necessary to protect himself or herself and others from injury. Tell the patient that he or she will be assisted in maintaining self-control by restraint and need not fear actual or possible loss of self-control.

Before approaching the violent patient, the paramedic should be aware of the patient's surroundings. Note seemingly harmless items including ashtrays, lighted cigarettes, hot coffee, letter openers, soda bottles, cans, and furniture. The paramedic should make no attempt to enter the patient's physical space (usually considered to be one arm's length) until the other members involved in the restraint action are ready to proceed.

The paramedic should consider the patient's muscle groups and potential range of motion before initiating restraint procedures. Plan to position the patient in a way that limits the effectiveness of his or her strength and range of motion. Each member of the restraint team should be assigned a specific body part or responsibility before actual restraint activity.

The paramedic must be familiar with the restraint devices available and should be able to improvise if the need arises. The preferred method is to use commercially manufactured leather restraints with padded bracelets for wrists and ankles, a waist belt, and straps (Fig. 30-1). Effective restraints may also be improvised using common materials such as:

- Small towels that can be wrapped around the patient's wrists and ankles and secured with tape to the stretcher
- Cravats
- Webbed straps ordinarily used to secure patients to spine boards
- Roll bandage
- Blanket roll

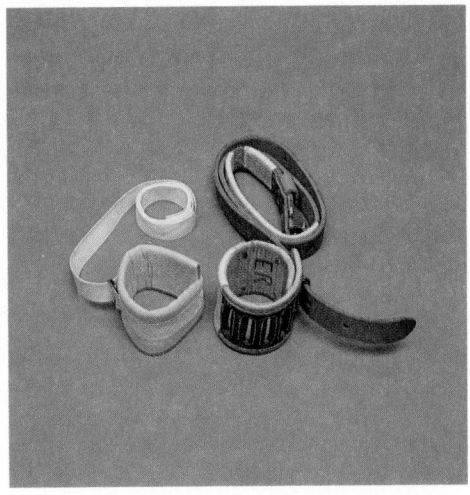

Fig. 30-1 Restraint devices.

Regardless of the types of restraint used, they should be strong enough to produce the desired effect without compromising circulatory or respiratory status.

Sequence of Restraint Actions

Many restraint techniques can be used by trained personnel. The following sequence is an example of a restraint action that may be used to contain violent behavior:

1. The paramedic offers the patient one final opportunity to cooperate.
2. If there is no response, a minimum of two rescuers should move swiftly toward the patient and position themselves close to and slightly behind the patient. Each rescuer should then position an inside leg in front of the patient's leg to force the patient into a prone position if needed (Fig. 30-2). Swift movement by two or more rescuers minimizes the patient's ability to focus on restraint actions and decreases the accuracy of kicks or blows. During the restraint procedure, the patient should be continually reassured by a rescuer not involved in the physical maneuver.
3. If the patient calms and agrees to be transported without restraints, the paramedic po-

sitions the patient face down on a stretcher (if not contraindicated by mechanism of injury or medical condition) and secures him or her with straps to limit range of motion. If the patient becomes dangerous to himself or herself or others, the paramedic restrains him or her en route.

4. If the patient continues to resist, the rescuers should force the patient into a prone position. The prone position prevents the patient from using strong abdominal muscles to sit up and

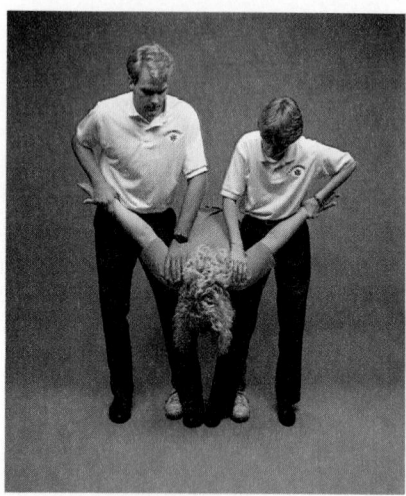

Fig. 30-2 Control position. Rescuers face the same direction. Inside legs are placed in front of patient. Rescuers' outside hands hold patient's wrists. Rescuers' inside hands form a C on the patient's shoulders.

allows the arms to be easily restrained. In addition, a face-down position makes kicking less effective and helps to control biting and spitting.

5. Once the patient is positioned face down on the stretcher, restraint must be continued to maintain control (Fig. 30-3). One arm should be secured to the stretcher at the patient's side and the other arm secured above his or her head to prevent large muscle groups from working together. Webbed straps should be placed across the patient's shoulder region, lumbar region, and legs. After applying straps, the patient's ankles should be secured to the stretcher and to one another.

6. Once applied, restraints should not be removed until the patient is delivered to the emergency department or until there are adequate resources to control the situation. Restrained limbs should be checked periodically for adequacy of circulation and the presence of soft tissue injury. If a change in the restraints is required, adequate assistance must be available and only one limb should be repositioned at a time.

Restraint procedures should be thoroughly documented on the prehospital care report. Attempts at negotiations and the sequence of patient behavior that led to the need for restraint should be clearly described. Documentation

A 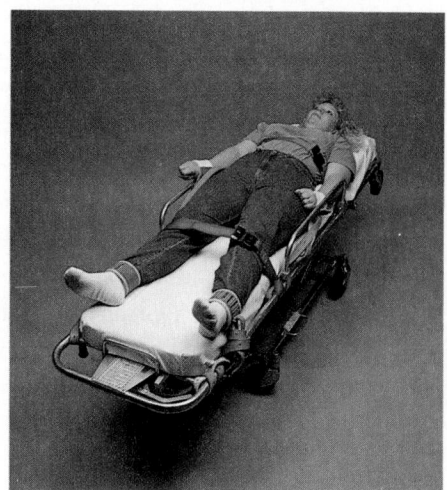 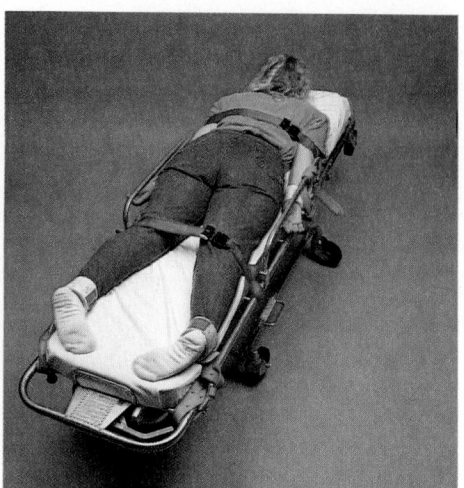 B

Fig. 30-3 Patient restraint in supine **(A)** and prone **(B)** positions.

should also verify that circulatory evaluation and continued monitoring of the patient were performed after restraint. Again, physical restraint is only recommended when all verbal and nonverbal techniques have been exhausted and only when an individual presents a danger to self or others.

● PERSONAL SAFETY

Although personal safety should be considered in any emergency response, behavioral emergencies are more likely to require that the paramedic protect himself or herself and the crew from hostile injury. The following methods to avoid personal injury should be considered:

- When possible, remain a safe distance from the patient.
- Do not allow the patient to block your exit.
- Keep large furniture between you and the patient.

- Do not allow a single paramedic to remain alone with the patient.
- Avoid threatening statements.
- Use folded blankets or cushions to absorb the impact of thrown objects.

Various training programs have been developed to provide safety and security to the rescuer and to the violent patient. Nonviolent personal protection maneuvers should be learned and practiced under the supervision of someone trained in these procedures.

REFERENCES

1. Bassuk E et al: *Behavioral emergencies: a field guide for EMTs and paramedics,* Boston, 1983, Little, Brown.
2. *The mythology of suicide,* Denver, 1987, Suicide Prevention Allied Regional Effort (SPARE).
3. Judd R, Peszke M: Psychological and behavioral emergencies, *Top Emerg Med* 4(4):7, 1983.

Summary

Most behavioral emergencies require only supportive measures to prevent the escalation of a crisis. In many cases, the paramedic's primary role is to provide understanding, compassion, and direction to someone with temporary emotional turmoil. In some instances, however, it is necessary to use direct verbal or physical intervention skills to prevent injury to the patient, bystanders, or members of the paramedic crew. EMS personnel must be oriented to helping and protecting these patients in a humane manner until they are able to gain control of themselves or until other therapeutic skills can be applied.

EMERGENCY DRUG INDEX

The Emergency Drug Index is a list of commonly prescribed medications used in prehospital care; it is not a complete guide to all emergency medications. For additional drug information, the consult other standard references or pharmacology textbooks. Drugs are listed alphabetically by generic name. Trade names are shown in parenthesis after the generic listing.

● ACTIVATED CHARCOAL
(CHARCOAIDE)

Class
Adsorbent

Description
Activated charcoal is a fine black powder that binds and adsorbs ingested toxins. Once bound to the activated charcoal, the combined complex is excreted from the body.

Onset and Duration
Onset: Immediate
Duration: Continual while in GI tract

Indications
Many oral poisonings, medication overdoses, and IV poisons

Contraindications
Corrosives, caustics, or petroleum distillates (relatively ineffective and may induce vomiting)

Adverse Reactions
May indirectly induce nausea and vomiting
May cause constipation

Drug Interactions
Syrup of ipecac is adsorbed by activated charcoal.

How Supplied
25 g (black powder)/125-ml bottle (200 mg/ml)
50 g (black powder)/250-ml bottle (200 mg/ml)

Dosage and Administration
Approximately 5-10 times the amount of the poison (larger amounts if food is also present)

Adult: 0.5-1.0 g/kg diluted to a
               500-ml aqueous slurry
               Administered PO or slowly
               by nasogastric tube
Pediatric: 0.6-2.0 g/kg diluted with
               8 oz water in a slurry
               solution
               Administered PO or slowly
               by nasogastric tube

Special Considerations
Pregnancy safety: Not established.
Activated charcoal may also be known as *AC.*
Is relatively insoluble in water.
May blacken feces.
Must be stored in a closed container.
Different charcoal preparations may have varying rates of adsorption.
Does not adsorb all drugs and toxic substances (for example, cyanide, lithium, iron, lead, and arsenic).

● ADENOSINE (ADENOCARD)

Class
Endogenous nucleotide

Description
Adenosine is primarily formed from the breakdown product of adenosine triphosphate (ATP). Both compounds are found in every cell of the human body and have a wide range of metabolic roles. Adenosine slows tachycardias associated with the AV node via modulation of the autonomic nervous system without causing negative inotropic effects. It acts directly on sinus pacemaker cells and vagal nerve terminals to decrease chronotropic and dromotropic activity. Adenosine is the drug of choice for paroxysmal supraventricular tachycardia (PSVT) and can be used diagnostically for stable, wide-complex tachycardias of unknown type after two doses of *lidocaine.*

Onset and Duration
Onset: 30 sec
Duration: 10 sec

Indications
Conversion of PSVT to sinus rhythm

Contraindications
Second- or third-degree AV block, or sick-sinus syndrome
Atrial flutter
Atrial fibrillation
Ventricular tachycardia
Hypersensitivity to adenosine

Adverse Reactions
Facial flushing
Lightheadedness
Paresthesia
Headache
Diaphoresis
Palpitations
Chest pain
Hypotension
Shortness of breath
Nausea
Metallic taste

Drug Interactions

Methylxanthines (for example, caffeine and theophylline) antagonize the action of adenosine.

Dipyridamole potentiates the effect of adenosine; reduction of adenosine dose may be required.

Carbamazepine may potentiate the AV-nodal blocking effect of adenosine.

How Supplied

Parenteral for IV injection
3 mg/ml in 2-ml flip-top vials

Dosage and Administration

Adult:

Initial dose:	6 mg over 1-3 sec
Repeat dose:	If no response is observed after 1-2 min, administer 12 mg over 1-3 sec.
	The second 12-mg dose may be repeated once if needed (maximum 30-mg dose).
Pediatric:	0.1-0.2 mg/kg rapid IV; maximum single dose; 12 mg

Special Considerations

Pregnancy safety: Category C.

May produce bronchoconstriction in patients with asthma or bronchopulmonary disease.

● ALBUTEROL (PROVENTIL, VENTOLIN)

Class

Sympathomimetic, bronchodilator

Description

Albuterol is a sympathomimetic that is selective for beta$_2$-adrenergic receptors. It relaxes smooth muscles of the bronchial tree and peripheral vasculature by stimulating adrenergic receptors of the sympathetic nervous system.

Onset and Duration

Onset:	5-15 min after inhalation; 30 min PO
Duration:	3-4 hr after inhalation; 4-6 hr PO

Indications

Relief of bronchospasm in patients with reversible obstructive airway disease

Prevention of exercise-induced bronchospasm

Contraindications

Prior hypersensitivity reaction to albuterol

Cardiac dysrhythmias associated with tachycardia

Tachycardia caused by digitalis intoxication

Pregnancy Category Ratings for Drugs

Drugs have been categorized by the Food and Drug Administration (FDA) according to the level of risk to the fetus. These categories are listed for each herein under "Pregnancy Safety" and are interpreted as follows[1]:

Category A: Controlled studies in women fail to demonstrate a risk to the fetus in the first trimester, and there is no evidence of risk in later trimesters; the possibility of fetal harm appears to be remote.

Category B: Either (1) animal reproductive studies have not demonstrated a fetal risk but there are no controlled studies in pregnant women or (2) animal reproductive studies have shown an adverse effect (other than decreased fertility) that was not confirmed in controlled studies on women in the first trimester and there is no evidence of risk in later trimesters.

Category C: Either (1) studies in animals have revealed adverse effects on the fetus and there are no controlled studies in women or (2) studies in women and animals are not available. Drugs in this category should be given only if the potential benefit justifies the risk to the fetus.

Category D: There is positive evidence of human fetal risk, but the benefits for pregnant women may be acceptable despite the risk, as in life-threatening diseases for which safer drugs cannot be used or are ineffective. An appropriate statement must appear in the "Warnings" section of the labeling of drugs in this category.

Category X: Studies in animals or humans have demonstrated fetal abnormalities, there is evidence of fetal risk based on human experience, or both; the risk of using the drug in pregnant women clearly outweighs any possible benefit. The drug is contraindicated in women who are or may become pregnant. An appropriate statement must appear in the "Contraindications" section of the labeling of drugs in this category.

Adverse Reactions

Usually dose related
Restlessness, apprehension
Dizziness
Palpitations
Increase in blood pressure
Dysrhythmias
Increased hypoxemia

Drug Interactions

Sympathomimetics may exacerbate adverse cardiovascular effects.
Antidepressants may potentiate the effects on the vasculature.
Beta blockers may antagonize albuterol.
Albuterol may potentiate diuretic-induced hypokalemia.

How Supplied

Syrup (as sulfate): 2 mg/5 ml
Tablet (as sulfate): 2 and 4 mg
Tablet/extended release (as sulfate): 4 mg
MDI: 90 mcg/metered spray (17-g canister with 200 inhalations)
Solution for aerosolization: 0.5% (5 mg/ml)

Dosage and Administration

Bronchial asthma
  Adult:
    Tablet: 2-4 mg tid-qid as tab (maximum dose 8 mg qid) or 4-8 mg q 12 hr extended release (maximum dose 16 mg bid)
    MDI: 1-2 inhalations (90-180 mcg) q 4-6 hr (wait 5 min between inhalations)
    Solution: 2.5 mg (0.5 ml of 0.5% solution) diluted to 3 ml with 0.9% NaCl (0.083% solution). Administer over 5-15 min
  Pediatric:
    Syrup: 6-14 years—2 mg, three to four times daily (maximum dose 24 mg/day)
        2-6 years—0.1 mg/kg, three times daily (maximum dose 4 mg, three times a day)
    Solution: 0.01-0.03 ml (0.05-0.15 mg)/kg/dose to maximum of 0.50 ml/dose diluted in 2 ml of 0.9 NS; may be repeated q 20 min three times
Exercise-induced bronchospasm
  Adult:
    MDI: Two inhalations 15 minutes before exercise
    Pediatric: Safety not documented

Special Considerations

Pregnancy safety: Category C.
May precipitate angina pectoris and dysrhythmias.
Should be used with caution in patients with diabetes mellitus, hyperthyroidism, prostatic hypertrophy, or seizure disorder.
In prehospital emergency care, albuterol should only be administered via inhalation.

● AMINOPHYLLINE (AMOLINE, SOMOPHYLLIN, AMINOPHYLLIN)

Class

Xanthine bronchodilator (theophylline derivative)

Description

Aminophylline achieves bronchodilation via different mechanisms than sympathomimetics and may be effective when sympathomimetics are not. Aminophylline is a respiratory stimulant as well as a bronchodilator; it has mild diuretic properties and positive chronotropic and inotropic effects (in large doses). In emergency care, aminophylline is usually administered by slow intravenous infusion. It has been reduced to a second-line drug in the emergency setting with the advent of more efficacious agents and controversy over its usefulness; it is used in life-threatening conditions after other agents have proven ineffective.

Onset and Duration

  Onset: Less than 15 min IV
  Duration: 4½ hr

Indications

Bronchospasm (associated with asthma, chronic bronchitis, emphysema)
Bronchospasm associated with pulmonary edema
May be effective when sympathomimetics have been ineffective
Congestive heart failure

Contraindications

Allergy to xanthine compounds (for example, caffeine)
Hypersensitivity to the drug
Cardiac dysrhythmias

Adverse Reactions

Tachycardia
Palpitations
PVCs
Angina pectoris
Dizziness
Anxiety
Headache
Seizure
Nausea and vomiting
Abdominal cramps

Drug Interactions

Beta blockers may oppose effects.

Barbiturates, *phenytoin*, and smoking may decrease theophylline levels.

How Supplied

500 mg/10-ml ampule (50 mg/ml)

500 mg/20-ml ampule, preload (25 mg/ml)

250 mg/10-ml ampule, preload (25 mg/ml)

Dosage and Administration

Loading Dose

Adult:	5-6 mg/kg in 50-100 ml of diluent over 30 min (not to exceed 20 mg/min); loading dose should be lower in patients who have been receiving the-ophylline preparations
Pediatric:	5-6 mg/kg in 50-100 ml IV infusion (not to exceed 20 mg/min)

Maintenance infusion (mg/kg/hr):

Patient category	First 12 hours	Subsequently (based on serum aminophylline levels)
Children	1	0.8
Young adults (smokers)	1	0.8
Young adults (non-smokers)	0.7	0.5
Elderly patients	0.6	0.3
Patients with heart failure or liver disease	0.5	0.1-0.2

Special Considerations

Pregnancy safety: Category C.

Aminophylline should be used with caution in patients with cardiovascular disease, hypertension, or hepatic or renal insufficiency.

Doses should be reduced by half in patients who have had a theophylline preparation within the past 6-24 hours.

Hypotension may occur after rapid administration.

Therapeutic-to-toxic ratio is narrow.

● AMRINONE LACTATE (INOCOR LACTATE)

Class

Inotropic agent

Description

Amrinone is a rapid-acting inotropic agent that increases cardiac output after IV administration. It is a phosphodiesterase (class III) inhibitor that increases myocardial contractility and produces systemic vasodilation without stimulating either alpha- or beta-adrenergic receptors. Amrinone's net hemodynamic effects are similar to those of *dobutamine*, but because the drug does not stimulate beta-adrenergic receptors, it may be effective in patients with congestive heart failure who do not respond to *dobutamine* or other inotropic agents.

Onset and Duration

Onset:	10-15 min after loading dose
Duration:	Dose dependent; approximately 0.5 hr after 0.75 mg/kg and 2 hr after 3 mg/kg

Indications

Short-term management of refractory congestive heart failure that is not associated with myocardial infarction

Contraindications

Hypersensitivity to amrinone or bisulfite

Idiopathic hypertrophic subaortic stenosis (IHSS)

Hypotension

Adverse Reactions

Tachydysrhythmias (dose related)

Nausea and vomiting

Thrombocytopenia (dose related)

Fever, flulike symptoms

Increase in liver enzyme levels

Drug Interactions

Hypotension may develop when amrinone is used with disopyramide or other agents with negative inotropic effects or vasodilatory activity.

Potentiates inotropic, chronotropic, and arrhythmogenic response to catecholamine and theophylline.

Incompatible with *furosemide*.

How Supplied

IV injection: 5 mg/ml (20-ml ampule)

Dosage and Administration

Adult:

Loading dose:	0.75 mg/kg IV administered slowly over 2-3 min.
Maintenance dose:	5-15 mcg/kg/min, titrated to hemodynamic effect. May be prepared by placing 100 mg (one ampule) in 500 ml of 0.9% NaCl to achieve a concentration of 0.2 mg/ml (200 mcg/ml).

> **NOTE:** Amrinone is incompatible with dextrose solutions.

Pediatric dose:	Safety not documented

Special Considerations
Pregnancy safety: Category C.
Can induce or worsen myocardial ischemia.

● AMYL NITRITE

Class
Coronary vasodilator

Description
Amyl nitrite is chemically related to **nitroglycerin** and has been used for many years to treat angina pectoris. It is also effective in the emergency management of cyanide poisoning by causing the oxidation of hemoglobin to the compound methemoglobin. Methemoglobin reacts with the cyanide ion to form cyanomethemoglobin, which has less affinity for oxygen, thus freeing hemoglobin to react with oxygen.

Onset and Duration
Onset:	30 sec inhaled
Duration:	3-20 min

Indications
Cyanide poisoning
May be used in the treatment of symptomatic angina pectoris

Contraindications
None when used for cyanide poisoning

Adverse Reactions
Hypotension	Syncope
Tachycardia	Headache
Palpitations	Nausea

Drug Interactions
There are no significant drug interactions with other emergency medications.

How Supplied
0.3 ml/glass ampule (capsule covered with woven gauze)

Dosage and Administration
Adult:	Glass ampule should be broken and inhaled for 30-60 sec. May be repeated as necessary.
Pediatric:	Same as adult.

Special Considerations
Pregnancy safety: Category C.
Frequently abused (claimed to be an aphrodisiac).
Also known as *amy*.
Cyanide poisoning often produces a bitter-almond breath odor (not all persons can detect the odor).

● ANISOYLATED PLASMINOGEN STREPTOKINASE ACTIVATOR (EMINASE)

Class
Thrombolytic agent

Description
Anisoylated plasminogen streptokinase activator is a complex that converts plasminogen to the proteolytic enzyme plasmin. Plasmin degrades fibrin clots as well as fibrinogen and certain other plasma proteins. After administration, plasma fibrinogen levels are decreased for 24-36 hours, and thrombin time may remain prolonged for 24 hours.

Onset and Duration
Onset:	10-20 min
Duration:	12-24 hr

Indications
Acute evolving transmural myocardial infarction

Contraindications
Active bleeding
Recent CVA
Intracranial or intraspinal surgery
Intracranial neoplasm
Uncontrolled hypertension
Severe allergy to the product
Prolonged CPR
Trauma
Recent surgery (within 2-3 weeks)
Peptic ulcer disease

Adverse Reactions
Bleeding
Dysrhythmias (idioventricular, sinus bradycardia, second- and third-degree heart blocks)
Allergic reactions

Drug Interactions
Aspirin and **heparin** may increase risk of bleeding (both agents may be given concurrently to improve overall efficacy).

How Supplied
Injection:	30 units (1 unit equals 1 mg, which contains 36,000 IU of **streptokinase**) Store at 5° C

Dosage and Administration
Adults: 30 units reconstituted in water or NS for injection, administered over 4-5 min. Medication must be used within 30 min after reconstitution.

Pediatric: Safety has not been established.

Special Considerations
Pregnancy safety: Contraindicated.

● ATROPINE SULFATE (ATROPINE AND OTHERS)

Class
Anticholinergic agent

Description
Atropine sulfate, a potent parasympatholytic, inhibits actions of acetylcholine at postganglionic parasympathetic neuroeffector sites. Small doses inhibit salivary and bronchial secretions; moderate doses dilate pupils and increase heart rate. Large doses decrease GI motility, inhibit gastric acid secretion, and may block nicotinic receptor sites at the autonomic ganglia and at the neuromuscular junction. Blocked vagal effects result in positive chronotropy and positive dromotropy (limited or no inotropic effect). In emergency care, it is primarily used to increase the heart rate in life-threatening bradycardias.

Onset and Duration
Onset: Rapid
Duration: 2-6 hr

Indications
Hemodynamically significant bradycardia
Asystole
Organophosphate poisoning (drug of choice)
Bronchospastic pulmonary disorders

Contraindications
Tachycardia
Hypersensitivity
Unstable cardiovascular status in acute hemorrhage and myocardial ischemia
Narrow-angle glaucoma

Adverse Reactions
Tachycardia
Paradoxical bradycardia when pushed slowly or when used at doses less than 0.5 mg
Palpitations
Dysrhythmias
Headache
Dizziness
Anticholinergic effects (dry mouth or nose, photophobia, blurred vision, urine retention)
Nausea and vomiting
Flushed, hot, dry skin
Allergic reactions

Drug Interactions
Anticholinergics may increase vagal blockade. Potential adverse effects when administered in conjunction with digitalis, cholinergics, neostigmine. The effects of atropine may be enhanced by antihistamines, *procainamide*, quinidine, antipsychotics, antidepressants, and benzodiazepines.

How Supplied
Tablet: 0.4, 0.6 mg
Parenteral: There are various injection preparations. In emergency care, atropine is usually supplied in prefilled syringes containing 1.0 mg in 10 ml of solution.
Nebulizer: 0.2% (1 mg in 0.5 ml UD), 0.5% (2.5 mg in 0.5 ml UD)

Dosage and Administration
Bradydysrhythmias
Adult: 0.5-1.0 mg IV q 3-5 min as needed
Pediatric: 0.02 mg/kg IV (minimum dose of 0.1 mg; maximum single dose of 0.5 mg for a child and 1.0 mg for an adolescent)
Asystole
Adult: 1.0 mg IV (maximum of 0.04 mg/kg)
Pediatric: Same as for dysrhythmias

Special Considerations
Pregnancy safety: Category C.

● BRETYLIUM TOSYLATE (BRETYLOL)

Class
Antidysrhythmic (class III)

Description
Bretylium is an adrenergic neuronal blocking agent that has both adrenergic and direct myocardial effects. Although the antidysrhythmic action of bretylium is poorly understood, like *lidocaine* it has been found to be effective in treating ventricular fibrillation and ventricular tachycardia. Bretylium produces a prompt increase in ventricular fibrillation threshold, perhaps through postganglionic adrenergic blockade. At present, its use is reserved for patients who fail to respond to *lidocaine* or other first-line antidysrhythmics.

Onset and Duration
Onset: Antifibrillatory effects are seen 2-15 min after IV administration. The suppression of ventricular tachycardia and other ventricular dysrhythmias occurs in 20 min or longer after IV administration.

Duration: 2-6 hr (ventricular fibrillation). Up to 24 hr (ventricular tachycardia)

Indications
Treatment of VF and VT refractory to *lidocaine*

Contraindications
None in the treatment of life-threatening dysrhythmias

Adverse Reactions
Vertigo
Dizziness
Syncope
Hypotension
Bradycardia
Increase in PVCs
Angina pectoris

Drug Interactions
Digoxin toxicity may be aggravated by the initial release of *norepinephrine* from bretylium.

How Supplied
Parenteral: 50 mg/ml in 10-ml vials

Dosage and Administration
Ventricular fibrillation
    5 mg/kg rapid IV bolus. Repeated at a dose of 10 mg/kg (maximum dose of 30-35 mg/kg).
Refractory or recurrent ventricular tachycardia
    Dilute 500 mg (10 ml) to 50 ml, and administer 5-10 mg/kg IV over 8-10 min.
    May be repeated in 1-2 hr, and if needed, q 6-8 hr thereafter.
    Bretylium may be administered as an IV infusion at a rate of 1-2 mg/min.
Pediatric: 5 mg/kg rapid IV; may be increased to 10 mg/kg

Special Considerations
Pregnancy safety: Safety has not been established.
Postural hypotension occurs in 50% of patients receiving bretylium (patient should be kept in supine position).
In ventricular fibrillation, bretylium is usually only effective if followed by defibrillation.
Ventricular tachycardia does not respond to bretylium as rapidly as ventricular fibrillation.

● BUTORPHANOL TARTRATE
(STADOL)

Class
Opioid agonist-antagonist analgesic

Description
Butorphanol is a synthetic analgesic with effects similar to those of *morphine* (2 mg of butorphanol is equivalent to 10 mg MS or 80 mg *meperidine*). It has narcotic agonist and antagonist properties and should be used with caution in patients who are narcotic-dependent. At present, butorphanol is not restricted under the Controlled Substance Act.

Onset and Duration
Onset: 10 min IM, 1-5 min IV
Duration: 3-4 hr

Indications
Relief of moderate to severe pain
Preoperative or preanesthetic medication
Used to relieve prepartum pain

Contraindications
Hypersensitivity
Head injury
Use with caution in patients with respiratory depression

Adverse Reactions
Sedation
Headache
Vertigo
Hallucinations
Palpitation
Increase or decrease in blood pressure
Respiratory depression (naloxone [Narcan] should be available)
Possible withdrawal symptoms

Drug Interactions
Phenothiazines, droperidol, tranquilizers, and barbiturates may potentiate the actions of butorphanol.

How Supplied
Parenteral: 1 mg/ml in 1-ml vials
    2 mg/ml in 1-, 2-, 10-ml vials

Dosage and Administration
IM: 2 mg q 3-4 hr as needed (range of 1-4 mg)
IV: 1 mg q 3-4 hr as needed (range of 0.5-2 mg q 3-4 hr)
Pediatric: Safety and efficacy in children less than 18 have not been established

Special Considerations
Pregnancy safety: Has not been established.
May increase cardiac work load in patients with congestive heart failure, acute myocardial infarction, ventricular dysfunction, or coronary insufficiency.
Use with caution in patients with end-stage liver disease.
Has potential for abuse.

● CALCIUM CHLORIDE

Class
Electrolyte

Description
Calcium is an essential component for functional integrity of the nervous and muscular systems, normal cardiac contractility, and the coagulation of blood. Calcium chloride contains 27.2% elemental calcium. Calcium chloride should only be administered intravenously (slowly, not exceeding 1 ml/min).

Onset and Duration
Onset: 5-15 min
Duration: Dose dependent (effects may persist for 4 hr after IV administration)

Indications
Hypocalcemia (prompt increase in serum calcium levels)
Adjunctive therapy in the treatment of insect bites and stings (especially black widow spider and scorpion)
Magnesium sulfate overdose
Hyperkalemia
Cardiac resuscitation (questionable value)
Calcium channel blocker toxicity

Contraindications
VF during cardiac resuscitation
In patients with digitalis toxicity
Hypercalcemia

Adverse Reactions
Decrease in heart rate (may cause asystole)
Decrease in blood pressure
Peripheral vasodilation
Metallic taste
Severe local necrosis and sloughing after IM use or IV infiltration

Drug Interactions
Calcium may worsen dysrhythmias secondary to digitalis.
May antagonize effects of *verapamil.*

NOTE: It is important to flush IV line between administration of *calcium chloride* and *sodium bicarbonate* to avoid precipitation.

How Supplied
10% solution in 10 ml ampules, vials, and prefilled syringes (100 mg/ml)

Dosage and Administration
Adult: 2-4 mEq/kg of 10% solution IV. Repeat as necessary at 10-min intervals.
Pediatric: 20 mg/kg/dose of 10% solution slow IV (maximum 1 g dose); may be repeated once in 10 min.

Special Considerations
Pregnancy safety: Category C.
Calcium may produce vasospasm in coronary and cerebral arteries.

● DEXAMETHASONE
(DECADRON, HEXADROL, AND OTHERS)

Class
Glucocorticoid

Description
Dexamethasone is a synthetic steroid chemically related to the natural hormones secreted by the adrenal cortex. The drug suppresses acute and chronic inflammation, potentiates the relaxation of vascular smooth muscle by beta-adrenergic agonists, and possibly alters airway hyperreactivity. In emergency care, dexamethasone is generally used to treat allergic reactions, asthma, and spinal cord injury and occasionally in the management of shock.

Onset and Duration
Onset: 4-8 hr
Duration: 24-72 hr

Indications
Cerebral edema (controversial)
Endocrine, rheumatic, hematological disorders
Allergic states

Contraindications
Hypersensitivity to the product

Adverse Reactions
Hypertension
Sodium and water retention
GI bleeding

Prolonged wound healing
Suppression of adrenocortical steroid production

Drug Interactions

There are no significant drug interactions with other emergency medications.

How Supplied

Dexamethasone is available in many forms, including tablet, elixir, gel, and ointment. The preparations most commonly used in emergency care are for intravenous administration and are listed below:
4 mg/ml in 1-, 5-, 10-, 25-, 30-ml vials
10 mg/ml in 10-ml vials, 1-ml syringe, 1-ml ampule
20 mg/ml in 5-ml vials (IV or IM), 5-ml syringe (IV)
24 mg/ml (IV only) in 5-, 10-ml vials

Dosage and Administration

Adult: There is considerable variance in recommended dexamethasone doses. The usual range in emergency care is 4-24 mg IV. Some physicians prefer significantly higher doses (up to 100 mg) for unusual indications.

Pediatric: 0.25-0.5 mg/kg/dose IV q 6 hr

Special Considerations

Pregnancy safety: Not established.
          Crosses the placenta and may cause fetal damage.
Medication should be protected from heat.
Because the onset of action is 4-8 hr, dexamethasone should not be considered a first-line medication for allergic reactions.

● DEXTROSE 50%

Class

Carbohydrate, hypertonic solution

Description

The term *dextrose* is used to describe the six-carbon sugar d-glucose, the principal form of carbohydrate used by the body. D_{50} is used in emergency care to treat hypoglycemia and to manage coma of unknown origin.

Onset and Duration

Onset: ≤1 min
Duration: Depends on the degree of hypoglycemia

Indications

Hypoglycemia
Altered level of consciousness
Coma of unknown etiology

Seizure of unknown etiology
Refractory cardiac arrest (controversial)

Contraindications

There are no significant contraindications for IV administration of 50% dextrose in emergency care.

Adverse Reactions

Warmth, pain, burning from medication infusion, thrombophlebitis, rhabdomyositis

Drug Interactions

There are no significant drug interactions with other emergency medications.

How Supplied

25 g/50 ml prefilled syringe (500 mg/ml)

Dosage and Administration

Adult: 12.5-25 g slow IV
              May be repeated once
Pediatric: 0.5-1 g/kg/dose slow IV
              May be repeated once

Special Considerations

Pregnancy safety: NA.
Draw blood sample before administration if possible.
Use blood-glucose reagent strips (Dextrostix) or glucometer before administration if possible.
Extravasation may cause tissue necrosis; use a large vein and aspirate occasionally to ensure route patency.
D_{50} sometimes precipitates severe neurological symptoms (Wernicke's encephalopathy) in *thiamine*-deficient patients such as alcoholics. (This can be prevented by administering 100 mg of *thiamine*, IV.)

● DIAZEPAM (VALIUM AND OTHERS)

Class

Benzodiazepine sedative-hypnotic, anticonvulsant

Description

Diazepam is frequently prescribed to treat anxiety and stress. In emergency care, it is used to treat alcohol withdrawal and grand mal seizure activity. Diazepam acts on the limbic, thalamic, and hypothalamic regions of the CNS to potentiate the effects of inhibitory neurotransmitters, raising the seizure threshold in the motor cortex. It may also be used in conscious patients during cardioversion to induce amnesia and sedation. Though the drug is still widely used as an anticonvulsant, it is relatively weak and of short duration. Rapid IV administration may be followed by respiratory depression and excessive sedation.

Onset and Duration
Onset: (IV) 1-5 min
            (IM) 15-30 min
Duration: (IV) 15 min-1 hr
            (IM) 15 min-1 hr

Indications
Acute anxiety states
Acute alcohol withdrawal
Muscle relaxant
Seizure activity
Preoperative sedation

Contraindications
Hypersensitivity to the drug
Substance abuse
Coma
Shock

Adverse Reactions
Hypotension
Reflex tachycardia
Respiratory depression
Ataxia
Psychomotor impairment
Confusion
Nausea

Drug Interactions
Diazepam may precipitate CNS depression and psychomotor impairment when the patient is taking CNS depressant medications.
Should not be administered with other drugs because of possible precipitation (incompatible with most fluids; should be administered into an IV of normal saline solution).

How Supplied
Tablet: 2, 5, 10 mg
Parenteral: 5 mg/ml vials, ampules, Tubex

Dosage and Administration
Seizure activity
Adult: 5-10 mg IV q 10-15 min prn (maximum dose 30 mg)
Pediatric: 0.2-0.3 mg/kg/dose IV (≤1 mg/min) q 2-5 min prn (maximum total dose 10 mg)
Amnesia for cardioversion
Adult: 5-15 mg IV, 5-10 min before procedure

Special Considerations
Pregnancy safety: Category D.
May cause local venous irritation.
Has short duration of anticonvulsant effect.
Reduce dose by 50% in elderly patients.
Resuscitation equipment should be readily available.

● DIGOXIN (LANOXIN)

Class
Inotropic agent

Description
Digoxin is a rapid-acting cardiac glycoside that has both direct and indirect effects. The direct effects include increased force and velocity of myocardial systolic contraction, increased refractory period of the AV node, and increased total peripheral resistance. An indirect vagomimetic action depresses the SA node and prolongs AV-node conduction. High doses of digoxin may enhance automaticity.

Onset and Duration
Onset: (PO) 30-120 min
           (IV) 5-30 min
Duration: Several days

Indications
Congestive heart failure
Supraventricular tachycardias, especially atrial flutter and atrial fibrillation

Contraindications
Ventricular fibrillation
Ventricular tachycardia
Digitalis toxicity
Hypersensitivity to digoxin

Adverse Reactions (mostly related to digitalis toxicity)
Headache
Weakness
Visual disturbances (blurred yellow or green vision, halo effect)
Confusion
Seizures
ECG abnormalities
Dysrhythmias
Nausea and vomiting
Skin rash

Drug Interactions
Amiodarone, *verapamil*, and quinidine may increase serum digoxin concentrations by 50%-70%.
Concurrent administration of IV digoxin and IV *verapamil* may lead to severe heart block.
Erythromycin and tetracycline can increase serum concentrations by reducing hepatic breakdown.
Diuretics may potentiate digoxin cardiotoxicity.
Sympathomimetics may augment the inotropic and cardiotoxic effects of digoxin.
Kaolin, pectin, and antacids may reduce digoxin absorption.

How Supplied
Digoxin is available in a number of preparations, including tablets, capsules, and elixirs. In emergency care, the common form of digoxin is supplied in 2-ml ampules containing 0.5 mg of the drug.

Dosage and Administration

Adult: 0.25-0.5 mg slow IV push
Pediatric: 25-40 mcg/kg slow IV push

Special Considerations

Pregnancy safety: Category A.

Patient should be constantly monitored for signs of digitalis toxicity.

Patients with myocardial infarction or renal failure are prone to develop digitalis toxicity.

Digitalis toxicity is potentiated in patients with hypokalemia, hypomagnesemia, and hypercalcemia.

Use only if necessary in patients with Wolff-Parkinson-White (WPW) syndrome because of possible ventricular dysrhythmias.

● DILTIAZEM (CARDIZEM) INJECTABLE

Class

Slow channel blocker or calcium channel antagonist

Description

Diltiazem is a calcium-channel-blocking agent that slows conduction and increases refractoriness in the AV node. The drug is used to control ventricular response rates in patients with atrial fibrillation, flutter, or multifocal atrial tachycardias.

Onset and Duration

Onset: 2-5 min
Duration: 1-3 hr

Indications

Atrial fibrillation
Atrial flutter
PSVT

Contraindications

Sick sinus syndrome
Second- or third-degree AV block
Severe hypotension
Cardiogenic shock
Hypersensitivity to diltiazem
Atrial fibrillation or atrial flutter associated with WPW syndrome or a short PR syndrome

Adverse Reactions

Atrial flutter
First- and second-degree AV block
Bradycardia
Chest pain
Congestive heart failure
Syncope
Ventricular dysrhythmia
Ventricular fibrillation
Ventricular tachycardia
Sweating
Nausea and vomiting
Dizziness
Dry mouth

Dyspnea
Headache

Drug Interactions

Caution is warranted in patients receiving medications that affect cardiac contractility or SA or AV node conduction.

How Supplied

25 mg (5-ml vial); 50 mg (10-ml vial)

Dosage and Administration

Bolus Injection: 0.25 mg/kg over 2 min; may be repeated in 15 min (0.35 mg/kg over 2 min) if response is inadequate

Infusion: Dilute 125 mg (25 ml) in 100 ml of NS, D_5W, or D_5W/0.45% NaCl for a final concentration of 1.0 mg/ml; infuse 5-10 mg/hr (5-15 ml/hr)

Pediatric: Not recommended

Special Considerations

Pregnancy safety: Category C.

Use with caution in patients with impaired renal or hepatic function.

Hypotension may occasionally result (carefully monitor vital signs).

PVCs may be present on conversion of PSVT to sinus rhythm.

● DIPHENHYDRAMINE (BENADRYL)

Class

Antihistamine

Description

Antihistamines prevent the physiological actions of histamine by preventing histamines from reaching H_1- and H_2-receptor sites. Antihistamines provide short-lived benefits and provide only symptomatic relief. Antihistamine is specific for conditions in which histamine excess is present (for example, acute urticaria) but is adjunctive therapy in the treatment of anaphylactic shock because *epinephrine* is more effective. Antihistamines are quite specific for reversing extrapyramidal reactions and are probably efficacious as drying agents in upper respiratory and sinus conditions.

Onset and Duration

Onset: Maximal effects 1-3 hr
Duration: 6-12 hr

Indications

Symptomatic relief of allergies
Allergic reactions
Anaphylaxis
Acute dystonic reactions

Contraindications

Lower respiratory diseases such as asthma attacks
Patients taking MAOIs
Hypersensitivity
Narrow-angle glaucoma

Adverse Reactions

Dose-related drowsiness
Sedation
Disturbed coordination
Hypotension
Palpitations
Tachycardia, bradycardia
Thickening of bronchial secretions
Dry mouth and throat

Drug Interactions

CNS depressants may increase depressant effects.
MAOIs may prolong and intensify anticholinergic effects of antihistamines.

How Supplied

Tablet: 25, 50 mg
Capsule: 25, 50 mg
Elixir: 12.5 mg/5 ml
Parenteral: 10, 50 mg/ml vials, prefilled syringe

Dosage and Administration

Adult: The standard dose of diphenhydramine is 25-50 mg, either IM or IV.
Pediatric: 5 mg/kg/24 hr q 6 hr PO. 2-5 mg/kg IV or IM.

Special Considerations

Pregnancy safety: Category B.

● DOBUTAMINE (DOBUTREX)

Class

Sympathomimetic

Description

Dobutamine is a synthetic catecholamine that stimulates alpha-, beta$_1$- and beta$_2$-adrenergic receptors. The effects of this drug include positive inotropic effects with minimal changes in chronotropic activities or systemic vascular resistance. For these reasons, dobutamine is useful in managing congestive heart failure when an increase in heart rate is not desired.

Onset and Duration

Onset: 1-2 min; peak after 10 min
Duration: 10-15 min

Indications

Inotropic support for patients with left ventricular dysfunction

Contraindications

Tachydysrhythmias
Severe hypotension

Adverse Reactions

Headache
Dose-related tachydysrhythmias
Hypertension
PVCs

Drug Interactions

Beta-adrenergic antagonists may blunt inotropic responses.
Sympathomimetics and phosphodiesterase inhibitors may exacerbate dysrhythmia responses.
Incompatible with *sodium bicarbonate* and *furosemide.*

How Supplied

250 mg/20 ml vials

Dosage and Administration

Adult: The drug is infused at 2-20 mcg/kg/min (instead of 2.5-20).
Pediatric: 2-20 mcg/kg/min (titrated to desired effect).

Special Considerations

Pregnancy safety: Not well established.
May be administered through a Y-site with concurrent *dopamine, lidocaine,* nitroprusside, and potassium chloride infusions.
Blood pressure should be closely monitored.
Increases in heart rate of more than 10% may induce or exacerbate myocardial ischemia.
Lidocaine should be readily available.

● DOPAMINE (INTROPIN)

Class

Sympathomimetic

Description

Dopamine is chemically related to *epinephrine* and *norepinephrine.* It acts primarily on alpha$_1$- and beta$_1$-adrenergic receptors, increasing systemic vascular resistance and exerting a positive inotropic effect on the heart. In addition, the actions of this drug on dopaminergic receptors dilate renal and splanchnic vasculature, maintaining blood flow. Dopamine is commonly used to treat hypotension associated with cardiogenic shock.

Onset and Duration

Onset: 2-4 min
Duration: 10-15 min

Indications

Hypotension
Low cardiac output states

Contraindications

Tachydysrhythmias
Ventricular fibrillation
Patients with pheochromocytoma

Adverse Reactions

Dose-related tachydysrhythmias
Hypertension
Increased myocardial oxygen demand

Drug Interactions

May be deactivated by alkaline solutions (*sodium bicarbonate* and *furosemide*).
MAOIs and *bretylium* may potentiate the effect of dopamine.
Sympathomimetics and phosphodiesterase inhibitors exacerbate dysrhythmia response.
Beta-adrenergic antagonists may blunt inotropic response.
When administered with *phenytoin,* hypotension, bradycardia, and seizures may develop.

How Supplied

200 mg/5 ml, 400 mg/5 ml prefilled syringe and ampule for IV infusion (IV piggyback)

Dosage and Administration

Adult:	Usually prepared by placing 800 mg in 500 ml D_5W or 200 mg in 250 ml D_5W to achieve a concentration of 1600 mcg/ml; infuse at 2.5-20 mcg/kg/min (titrated to patient response)
	Dopaminergic response: 2-4 mcg/kg/min
	Beta-adrenergic response: 5-10 mcg/kg/min
	Adrenergic response: 10-20 mcg/kg/min
Pediatric:	2-20 mcg/kg/min (titrated to patient response)

Special Considerations

Pregnancy safety: Not well established.
Infuse through a large, stable vein to avoid the possibility of extravasation injury.
Monitor patient for signs of compromised circulation.

● EPINEPHRINE (ADRENALIN)

Class

Sympathomimetic

Description

Epinephrine stimulates alpha-, $beta_1$-, and $beta_2$-adrenergic receptors in dose-related fashion. It is the initial drug of choice for treating bronchoconstriction and hypotension resulting from anaphylaxis as well as all forms of cardiac arrest. It is useful in managing reactive airway disease, but beta-adrenergic agents are often used initially because of their convenience and oral inhalation route. Rapid injection produces a rapid increase in systolic pressure, ventricular contractility, and heart rate. In addition, epinephrine causes vasoconstriction in the arterioles of the skin, mucosa, and splanchnic areas and antagonizes the effects of histamine.

Onset and Duration

Onset:	(SQ) 5-10 min
	(IV) 1-2 min
Duration:	5-10 min

Indications

Bronchial asthma
Acute allergic reaction
Cardiac arrest
    Asystole
    Electromechanical dissociation
    Ventricular fibrillation unresponsive to initial defibrillatory attempts

Contraindications

Hypersensitivity
Hypovolemic shock
Coronary insufficiency
Hypertension

Adverse Reactions

Headache
Nausea
Restlessness
Weakness
Dysrhythmias
Hypertension
Precipitation of angina pectoris

Drug Interactions

MAOIs and *bretylium* may potentiate the effect of epinephrine.
Beta-adrenergic antagonists may blunt inotropic response.
Sympathomimetics and phosphodiesterase inhibitors may exacerbate dysrhythmia response.
May be deactivated by alkaline solutions (*sodium bicarbonate, furosemide*).

How Supplied

Parenteral:	1 mg/ml (1:1000), 0.1 mg/ml (1:10,000) ampule and prefilled syringe Autoinjector (EpiPen) 0.5 mg/ml (1:2000) 0.01 mg/ml (1:100,000) pediatric

Dosage and Administration

Asystole, pulseless electrical activity, or ventricular fibrillation

Adult:

Initial:	1 mg IV push, repeat q 3-5 min
Intermediate:	2-5 mg IV push q 3-5 min
Escalating:	1 mg–3 mg–5 mg IV (3 min apart)
High:	0.1 mg/kg IV push, q 3-5 min

Pediatric:

First dose:	Standard (0.1 ml/kg 1:10,000) IV/IO
	High (0.1 ml/kg 1:1000) ET
Second and subsequent doses:	High (0.1 ml/kg 1:1000) IV/IO
	High (0.1 ml/kg 1:1000) ET

Bradycardia refractory to other interventions

Adult:	2-10 mcg/min (1 mg 1:1,000 in 500 ml of normal saline or D_5W)

Pediatric:

Standard:	0.1 ml/kg 1:10,000 IV/IO
High:	0.1 ml/kg 1:1000 ET

Special Considerations

Pregnancy safety: Category C.

Syncope has occurred after epinephrine administration to asthmatic children.

May increase myocardial oxygen demand.

● EPINEPHRINE RACEMIC
(MICRONEFRIN, VAPONEFRIN)

Class

Sympathomimetic

Description

Like other forms of epinephrine, racemic epinephrine acts as a bronchodilator that stimulates $beta_2$ receptors in the lungs, resulting in relaxation of bronchial smooth muscle. This alleviates bronchospasm, increases vital capacity, and reduces airway resistance. It is also useful in treating laryngeal edema. Racemic epinephrine also inhibits the release of histamine.

Onset and Duration

Onset:	Within 5 min
Duration:	1-3 hr

Indications

Bronchial asthma

Prevention of bronchospasm

Croup (laryngotracheobronchitis)

Laryngeal edema

Contraindications

Hypertension

Underlying cardiovascular disease

Epiglottis

Adverse Reactions

Tachycardia

Dysrhythmias

Drug Interactions

MAOIs and *bretylium* may potentiate the effect of epinephrine.

Beta-adrenergic antagonists may blunt the bronchodilating response.

Sympathomimetics and phosphodiesterase inhibitors may exacerbate dysrhythmia response.

How Supplied

MDI: 0.16-0.25 mg/spray

Solution: 7.5, 15, 30 ml in 1%, 2.25% solution

Dosage and Administration

MDI

Adult:	2-3 inhalations, repeated once in 5 min prn

Solution

Adult:	Dilute 5 ml (1%) in 5-ml saline, administer over 15 minutes
Pediatric:	Dilute 0.25 ml (0.1%) in 2.5 ml saline (if less than 20 kg); 0.5 ml in 2.5 ml saline (if 20-40 kg); 0.75 ml in 2.5 ml saline (if greater than 40 kg); administer by aerosolization

Special Considerations

May produce tachycardia and other dysrhythmias.

Monitor vital signs closely.

Excessive use may cause bronchospasm.

● FLUMAZENIL (MAZICON)

Class

Benzodiazepine receptor antagonist

Description

Flumazenil antagonizes the actions of benzodiazepines on the central nervous system. It has been shown to antagonize the sedation, impairment of recall, and psychomotor impairment produced by benzodiazepines. Flumazenil does not antagonize the CNS effects of ethanol, barbiturates, or opioids.

Onset and Duration

Onset:	1-2 min
Duration:	Related to plasma concentration of benzodiazepine

Indications

Reversal of benzodiazepine sedation

Contraindications

Hypersensitivity to flumazenil or to benzodiazepines
Cyclic antidepressant overdose

Adverse Reactions

Nausea and vomiting
Dizziness
Agitation
Injection-site pain
Cutaneous vasodilation
Abnormal vision
Seizures

Drug Interactions

Toxic effects of mixed drug overdose (especially cyclic antidepressants) may emerge with the reversal of the benzodiazepine effects.

How Supplied

5- and 10-ml vials (0.1 mg/ml)

Dosage and Administration

For suspected benzodiazepine overdose:

Adult: 0.2 mg (2 ml) IV over 30 seconds; an additional dose of 0.3 mg (3 ml) may be given in 30 seconds, followed by 0.5 mg (5 ml) at 1- min intervals (maximum dose of 3 mg)

Pediatric: Not recommended

Special Considerations

Pregnancy safety: Category C.

To minimize the likelihood of injection-site pain, administer through an intravenous infusion established in a large vein.

Be prepared to manage seizures in patients who are physically dependent on benzodiazepines to control seizures or who have ingested large doses of other drugs.

Flumazenil may precipitate withdrawal syndromes in patients dependent on benzodiazepines.

Patients should be monitored for possible resedation, respiratory depression, or other residual benzodiazepine effects.

Be prepared to establish and assist ventilation.

● FUROSEMIDE (LASIX)

Class

Diuretic

Description

Furosemide is a potent diuretic that inhibits the reabsorption of sodium and chloride in the proximal tubule and loop of Henle.

Onset and Duration

Onset: (PO) 30-60 min
(IV) Within 15-20 min
Duration: 4-6 hr

Indications

Pulmonary edema
Congestive heart failure

Contraindications

Anuria
Hypersensitivity
States of severe electrolyte depletion

Adverse Reactions

Hypotension
ECG changes
Chest pain
Dry mouth
Hypochloremia
Hypokalemia
Hyponatremia
Hyperglycemia

Drug Interactions

Digitalis toxicity may be potentiated by the potassium depletion that can result from furosemide administration.

Lithium toxicity may be potentiated by sodium depletion.

Compatible with D_5W, NS, LR solutions.

How Supplied

Tablet: 20, 40, 80 mg
Parenteral: 10 mg/ml in 2-ml ampule, 100 mg/ml in 10-ml vial

Dosage and Administration

Adult: 0.5-1.0 mg/kg IV injected slowly
Pediatric: 1 mg/kg/dose q 12 hr

Special Considerations

Pregnancy safety: Category C.

Furosemide has been known to cause fetal abnormalities.

Should be protected from light.

● GLUCAGON

Class

Pancreatic hormone, insulin antagonist

Description

Glucagon is a protein secreted by the alpha cells of the pancreas. When released, it elevates blood glucose levels by increasing the breakdown of glycogen to glucose and inhibiting glycogen synthesis. In addition, glucagon exerts positive inotropic action on the heart and decreases renal vascular resistance. The drug is only effective in treating hypoglycemia if liver glycogen is available. Therefore it may be ineffective in chronic hypoglycemia, starvation, and adrenal insufficiency.

Onset and Duration

Onset: Within 1 min
Duration: 9-17 min

Indications

Altered level of consciousness where hypoglycemia is suspected.
May be used as an inotropic agent in beta-blocker overdose.

Contraindications

Hypersensitivity (allergy to proteins)

Adverse Reactions

Tachycardia
Hypertension
Nausea and vomiting

Drug Interactions

There are no significant drug interactions with other emergency medications.

How Supplied

Glucagon must be reconstituted (with provided diluent) before administration. Dilute 1 unit (1 mg) white powder in 1 ml of diluting solution (1 mg/ml).

Dosage and Administration

Adult: 0.5-1 mg IM, SQ, or slow IV; repeat in 20 min prn
Pediatric: 0.03-0.1 mg/kg/dose (not to exceed 1 mg) q 20 min IM, SQ, IV, prn

Special Considerations

Pregnancy safety: Category B.
Should not be considered a first-line choice for hypoglycemia.
Intravenous glucose must be administered if the patient does not respond to a second dose of glucagon.

● HALOPERIDOL (HALDOL)

Class

Tranquilizer

Description

Haloperidol has pharmacological properties similar to those of the phenothiazines. The exact mechanism of action has not yet been determined, but the drug is thought to block dopamine receptors in the brain, altering mood and behavior. In emergency care, haloperidol is usually administered IM but may also be given IV.

Onset and Duration

Onset: (IV) 10-20 min
            (IM) 30-60 min
            (PO) 1-2 hr
Duration: 12-24 hr

Indications

Acute psychotic episodes

Contraindications

CNS depression
Coma
Hypersensitivity
Pregnancy

Adverse Reactions

Dose-related:
    Pseudoparkinsonism
    Akathisia
    Dystonias
Hypotension
Orthostatic hypotension
Nausea, vomiting
Allergic reactions
Blurred vision

Drug Interactions

Other CNS depressants may potentiate effects.
May inhibit vasoconstrictor effects of *epinephrine.*

How Supplied

5 mg/ml ampule

Dosage and Administration

Adult: 2-5 mg IM
Pediatric: Not recommended

Special Considerations

Pregnancy safety: Not established.

● HEPARIN (HEPARIN-LOCK FLUSH SOLUTIONS)

Class

Anticoagulant

Description

Heparin inhibits the clotting cascade by activating specific plasma proteins. The drug is used to prevent and treat all types of thromboses and emboli, DIC, arterial occlusion, and thrombophlebitis and prophylactically to prevent clotting before and after surgery. In emergency care, heparin is used to prevent coagulation of laboratory samples and to maintain patency of indwelling catheters. (This discussion is limited to heparin-lock flush solutions.)

Onset and Duration
Onset: Immediate
Duration: 4-8 hr

Indications
To maintain patency of IV injection devices and indwelling catheters

Contraindications
Hypersensitivity

Adverse Reactions
Allergic reaction (chills, fever, back pain)

Drug Interactions
Salicylates, some antibiotics, and quinidine may increase risk of bleeding.

How Supplied
Heparin-lock flush solutions are available in 10-and 100-unit/ml ampules and prefilled syringes.

Dosage and Administration
Lock flush solution:
Inject 1 ml of heparin-lock flush solution into the indwelling vein puncture device. If the device is being used to administer a drug that is incompatible with heparin, the device should be flushed with sterile water or 0.9% sodium chloride for injection before and after the drug is given. Inject the heparin-lock flush solution after the second flush of sterile water or sodium chloride. If the device is being used to obtain blood samples for laboratory analysis, the heparin solution should be cleared from the device by aspirating and discarding 1 ml of solution from the device before the blood sample is taken. After the blood sample is drawn, the device is again filled with 1 ml of heparin-lock flush solution.

Special Considerations
Pregnancy safety: NA for heparin-lock flush solution.
The recommended dose of heparin-lock flush solutions varies by medical control agency and hospital policy.
NS may be preferred instead of heparin to irrigate and maintain catheter patency.

● HYDRALAZINE (APRESOLINE)

Class
Antihypertensive

Description
Hydralazine is an arteriolar vasodilating agent used to manage hypertensive crisis. The effects of the drug

include a decrease in arterial pressure, a decrease in peripheral resistance, and an increase in cardiac output (as a result of the baroreceptor reflex).

Onset and Duration
Onset: (IV) 5-30 min
(IM) 10-40 min
Duration: 2-6 hr

Indications
Hypertensive crisis
Hypertension associated with renal failure, preeclampsia, and eclampsia

Contraindications
Compensatory hypertension
Coronary artery disease
Dissecting aneurysm
Hypersensitivity

Adverse Reactions
Reflex tachycardia
Hypotension
Facial flushing
Headache
Diaphoresis
Anxiety
Nausea and vomiting

Drug Interactions
Concurrent use of diazoxide may result in severe hypotension.
Color changes may occur when given with glucose solutions.

How Supplied
20 mg in 1-ml ampule (20 mg/ml)

Dosage and Administration
Adult: 10-40 mg IM or IV; may be repeated in 10-min prn
Infusion: 20 mg in 250 ml NS or LR at 5-20 mg/hr
Pediatric: 0.1-0.2 mg/kg/dose q 4-6 hr IM, IV; may be repeated prn
Infusion: 0.75-3 mg/kg q 6-12 hr

Special Considerations
Pregnancy safety: Category C.
Blood pressure and ECG should be continuously monitored.

● HYDROXYZINE (ATARAX, VISTARIL)

Class
Antihistamine, antiemetic, antianxiety

Description

Hydroxyzine is clinically effective in managing neuroses and emotional disturbances manifested by anxiety and tension. The drug has a calming effect without impairing mental alertness; antiemetic and antihistaminic effects have also been demonstrated with hydroxyzine. When administered concurrently with analgesics, it tends to potentiate their effects.

Onset and Duration

Onset: (IM) 15-30 min
               (IV) Immediate
Duration: 4-6 hr

Indications

To potentiate the effects of analgesics
Nausea and vomiting
Anxiety reactions
Preoperative and postoperative sedation
Motion sickness

Contraindications

Hypersensitivity

Adverse Reactions

Dry mouth
Drowsiness

Drug Interactions

The potentiating action of hydroxyzine must be considered when the drug is used in conjunction with CNS depressants such as narcotics, barbiturates, and alcohol.

How Supplied

25, 50 mg/ml in 1-ml vials

Dosage and Administration

Adult: 25-100 mg IM
Pediatric: 0.5-1 mg/kg/dose IM

Special Considerations

Hydroxyzine should be administered by IM injection only.
Localized burning at the injection site is a common complaint.

● INSULIN (REGULAR, NPH, ULTRALENTE, AND OTHERS)

Class

Hormone

Description

Insulin is secreted by the beta cells (islets of Langerhans) of the pancreas and is required for proper glucose use by the body. If insulin secretion is diminished (as in diabetes mellitus), supplemental insulin must be obtained by injection. Insulin preparations are classified as rapid acting (Regular), intermediate acting (NPH), and long acting (Ultralente). Insulin is seldom administered in the prehospital setting and then only when ketoacidosis is confirmed.

Onset and Duration

Onset: 0.5-1 hr (rapid-acting)
            1-1.5 hr (intermediate-acting)
            4-6 hr (long-acting)
Duration: 6-8 hr (rapid-acting)
            24 hr (intermediate-acting)
            36 hr (long-acting)

Indications

Type I diabetes mellitus
Type II diabetes mellitus if oral hypoglycemic agents do not adequately control plasma glucose
Diabetic ketoacidosis
Nonketotic hyperosmolar coma
Insulin and *dextrose 50%* administration are given together to lower potassium levels in hyperkalemia

Contraindications

Hypoglycemia

Adverse Reactions

Hypoglycemia
Fatigue
Weakness
Confusion
Headache
Tachycardia
Rapid, shallow breathing
Nausea
Diaphoresis
Allergic reaction

Drug Interactions

Corticosteroids, *dobutamine, epinephrine,* and thiazide diuretics may antagonize (decrease) the hypoglycemic effects of insulin.
Alcohol, beta-adrenergic blockers, MAOIs, and salicylates may potentiate the hypoglycemic effects of insulin.

How Supplied

100 units/ml in 10-ml vials

Dosage and Administration

Insulin may be administered SQ, IM, or IV, and dosage is governed by the clinical presentation of the patient. A standard dose of insulin administration in diabetic coma is listed below:

Adult: 10-25 units regular insulin IV, followed by an infusion of 0.1 units/kg/hr
Pediatric: 0.1-0.2 units/kg/hr IM
            Infusion: 50 units of regular insulin mixed in 250 ml of NS (0.2 units/ml), infused at a rate of 0.1-0.2 units/kg/hr

Special Considerations

Pregnancy safety: Not established.

Insulin is the drug of choice for control of diabetes in pregnancy.

Regular insulins are clear; modified insulins are cloudy.

Insulin injected into the abdominal wall is absorbed most rapidly, insulin in the arm is absorbed more slowly, and insulin injected into the thigh is absorbed slowest.

● ISOPROTERENOL (ISUPREL)

Class

Sympathomimetic

Description

Isoproterenol is a synthetic catecholamine that stimulates both beta$_1$- and beta$_2$-adrenergic receptors (no alpha-receptor capabilities). The drug affects the heart by increasing inotropic and chronotropic activity. In addition, isoproterenol causes arterial and bronchial dilation and is sometimes administered via aerosolization as a bronchodilator to treat bronchial asthma and bronchospasm. (Because of the undesirable beta$_2$ cardiac effects, the use of this drug as a bronchodilator is uncommon in the prehospital setting.)

Onset and Duration

Onset: 1-5 min
Duration: 15-30 min

Indications

Hemodynamically stable bradycardias that are resistant to *atropine*

Heart blocks with palpable pulse

Management of torsades de pointes

Contraindications

Ventricular tachycardia

Ventricular fibrillation

Hypotension

Pulseless idioventricular rhythm

Ischemic heart disease

Cardiac arrest

Adverse Reactions

Dysrhythmias

Hypotension

Precipitation of angina pectoris

Facial flushing

Drug Interactions

MAOIs and *bretylium* potentiate the effects of catecholamines.

Beta-adrenergic antagonists may blunt inotropic response.

Sympathomimetics and phosphodiesterase inhibitors may exacerbate dysrhythmia response.

How Supplied

1 mg in 1-ml or 5-ml ampule and prefilled syringe

Dosage and Administration

Adult: Dilute 1 mg in 500 ml of D$_5$W (2 mcg/ml); infuse at 2-10 mcg/min or until the desired heart rate is obtained.

Pediatric: 0.05-1.5 mcg/kg/min IV infusion, titrated to patient response.

Special Considerations

Pregnancy safety: Category C.

Isoproterenol increases myocardial oxygen demand and can induce serious dysrhythmias (including ventricular tachycardia and ventricular fibrillation).

May exacerbate tachydysrhythmias because of digitalis toxicity or hypokalemia.

Newer inotropic agents have replaced isoproterenol in most clinical settings.

If electronic pacing is available, it should be used instead of isoproterenol or as soon as possible after the drug has been initiated.

● KETOROLAC TROMETHAMINE (TORADOL IM)

Class

Nonsteroidal antiinflammatory

Description

Ketorolac tromethamine is an antiinflammatory drug that also exhibits peripherally acting nonnarcotic analgesic activity by inhibiting prostaglandin synthesis.

Onset and Duration

Onset: Within 10 min
Duration: 2-6 hr

Indications

Short-term management of moderate to severe pain

Contraindications

Hypersensitivity to the drug

Patients with history of asthma

Patients with allergies to aspirin or other nonsteroidal antiinflammatory drugs

Bleeding disorders

Renal failure

Hypotension

Adverse Reactions

Anaphylaxis from hypersensitivity

Edema

Sedation

Hypertension or hypotension

Bleeding disorders
Rash
Nausea
Headache

Drug Interactions
Ketorolac tromethamine may increase bleeding time when administered to patients taking anticoagulants.

How Supplied
15 mg or 30 mg in 1 ml or 60 mg in 2 ml

Dosage and Administration
Adult: 30-60 mg IM
Pediatric: Not recommended

Special Considerations
Pregnancy Safety: Category C
Solution is clear and slightly yellow in color.
Use with caution and reduced doses when administering to older patients.
Is also being evaluated for IV use (10-30 mg over 5 min) by the FDA.

● LABETALOL (NORMODYNE, TRANDATE)

Class
Alpha- and beta-adrenergic blocker

Description
Labetalol is a competitive alpha$_1$-receptor blocker as well as a nonselective beta-receptor blocker used to lower blood pressure in a hypertensive crisis. Because of alpha- and beta-blocking properties, blood pressure is reduced without reflex tachycardia, and total peripheral resistance is decreased without a significant alteration in cardiac output. In emergency care, labetalol is administered intravenously.

Onset and Duration
Onset: Within 5 min
Duration: 3-6 hr

Indications
Hypertension

Contraindications
Bronchial asthma
Congestive heart failure
Second- and third-degree heart block
Bradycardia
Cardiogenic shock

Adverse Reactions
Headache
Dizziness
Ventricular dysrhythmias

Hypotension
Dyspnea
Allergic reaction
Facial flushing
Diaphoresis
Postural hypotension

Drug Interactions
Bronchodilator effects of beta-adrenergic agonists may be blunted by labetalol.
Nitroglycerin may augment hypotensive effects.

How Supplied
100 mg in 20 ml of solvent ampule (5 mg/ml)

Dosage and Administration
Adult: 5-20 mg slow IV over 2 min; additional injections of 10-40 mg can be given at 10-min intervals prn
Infusion: Mix 200 mg in 250 ml D$_5$W (0.8 mg/ml); infuse at a rate of 2 mg/min, titrated to supine blood pressure.
Pediatric: Safety has not been established.

Special Considerations
Pregnancy safety: Category C.
Blood pressure, pulse rate, ECG should be continuously monitored.
Observe for signs of congestive heart failure, bradycardia, bronchospasm.
Labetalol should only be administered with the patient in a supine position.

● LIDOCAINE (XYLOCAINE)

Class
Antidysrhythmic (class Ib)

Description
Lidocaine decreases phase-4 diastolic depolarization and suppresses premature ventricular contractions. In addition, it is used to treat ventricular tachycardia and some cases of ventricular fibrillation. Lidocaine also raises the ventricular fibrillation threshold.

Onset and Duration
Onset: 30-90 sec
Duration: 2-4 hr

Indications
Acute ventricular dysrhythmias

Contraindications
Hypersensitivity
Stokes-Adams syndrome
Second- or third-degree heart block in the absence of an artificial pacemaker

Adverse Reactions

Lightheadedness
Confusion
Blurred vision
Hypotension
Cardiovascular collapse
Bradycardia
CNS depression (altered level of consciousness, irritability, muscle twitching, seizures) with high doses

Drug Interactions

Metabolic clearance of lidocaine may be decreased in patients taking beta-adrenergic blockers or in patients with liver dysfunction.

Apnea induced with *succinylcholine* may be prolonged with large doses of lidocaine.

Cardiac depression may occur if lidocaine is given concomitantly with IV *phenytoin.*

Additive neurological effects may occur with *procainamide.*

How Supplied

Prefilled syringes:	100 mg in 5 ml of solution
	1 and 2 g additive syringes
Ampules:	100 mg in 5 ml of solution
	1- and 2-g vials in 30 ml of solution
	5 ml containing 100 mg/ml

Dosage and Administration

Ventricular fibrillation or pulseless ventricular tachycardia

Adult:	1.5 mg/kg Repeat once in 3-5 min (maximum dose 3 mg/kg)
Pediatric:	1 mg/kg IV/IO per dose; Infusion: 20-50 mcg/kg/minute

Ventricular ectopy with a pulse

Adult:	1-1.5 mg/kg IV push. Additional boluses of 0.5-0.75 mg/kg can be given every 5-10 min (maximum dose 3 mg/kg). With resolution of ventricular ectopy, continuous infusion should be inititated at 2-4 mg/min.
Pediatric:	1 mg/kg IV/IO per dose; Infusion: 20-50 mcg/kg/min

Special Considerations

Pregnancy safety: Category B.

Therapeutic plasma levels of lidocaine between 2-6 mcg/ml suppress ventricular dysrhythmias.

A 75- to 100-mg bolus maintains adequate blood levels for only 20 min.

If bradycardia occurs in conjunction with PVCs, always treat the bradycardia first with *atropine, isoproterenol,* or both.

Exceedingly high doses of lidocaine can result in coma or death.

Avoid lidocaine for reperfusion dysrhythmias after thrombolytic therapy.

● LORAZEPAM (ATIVAN INJECTION)

Class

Benzodiazepine

Description

Lorazepam is a benzodiazepine with antianxiety and sedative effects. When given by injection, it appears to suppress the propagation of seizure activity produced by foci in the cortex, thalamus, and limbic areas.

Onset and Duration

Onset:	1-5 min
Duration:	6-8 hr

Indications

Initial control of status epilepticus or severe recurrent seizures

Contraindications

Hypersensitivity to the drug
Substance abuse
Coma
Shock

Adverse Reactions

Respiratory depression
Bradycardia
Hypotension
Sedation
Ataxia
Psychomotor impairment
Confusion

Drug Interactions

Lorazepam may precipitate CNS depression and psychomotor impairment when the patient is taking CNS depressant medications.

How Supplied

2- and 4-mg/ml concentrations in 1-ml vials

Dosage and Administration

Before IV administration, lorazepam must be diluted with an equal volume of sterile water or sterile saline. When given IM, lorazepam is not to be diluted.

Adult:	2-4 mg slow IV at 2 mg/min; may be repeated in 15-20 min to a maximum dose of 8 mg.
Pediatric:	0.05 to 0.15 mg/kg slow IV over 2 min; may be repeated in 15-20 min to a maximum dose of 0.2 mg/kg.

Special Considerations

Pregnancy safety: Category D.

Monitor respiratory rate and blood pressure during administration.

Have suction and intubation equipment available.

Inadvertent intraarterial injection may produce arteriospasm resulting in gangrene that may require amputation.

Lorazepam expires in 6 weeks when not refrigerated.

● MAGNESIUM SULFATE

Class
CNS depressant

Description
Magnesium sulfate reduces striated muscle contractions and blocks peripheral neuromuscular transmission by reducing acetylcholine release at the myoneural junction. In emergency care, magnesium sulfate is used to manage seizures associated with toxemia of pregnancy. Other uses include uterine relaxation (to inhibit contractions of premature labor), as a bronchodilator after beta-agonist and anticholinergic agents have been used, replacement therapy for magnesium deficiency, as a cathartic to reduce the absorption of poisons from the GI tract, and in the initial therapy for convulsions. Magnesium sulfate is gaining popularity as an initial treatment in the management of various dysrhythmias, particularly torsades de pointes, and dysrhythmias secondary to a tricyclic antidepressant overdose or digitalis toxicity. The drug is also considered as a class IIa agent (probably helpful) for refractory ventricular fibrillation and ventricular tachycardia after administration of *lidocaine* or *bretylium* doses.

Onset and Duration
Onset: Immediate
Duration: 3-4 hr

Indications
Seizures of eclampsia (toxemia of pregnancy)
Torsades de pointes

Contraindications
Heart block

Adverse Reactions
Diaphoresis
Facial flushing
Hypotension
Depressed reflexes
Hypothermia
Reduced heart rate
Circulatory collapse
Respiratory depression

Drug Interactions
CNS depressant effects may be enhanced if the patient is taking other CNS depressants.
Serious changes in cardiac function may occur with cardiac glycosides.

How Supplied
5 and 10 ml of a 10% solution in prefilled syringe

Dosage and Administration
Seizure activity associated with pregnancy
Adult: 1-4 g (8-32 mEq); maximum
              dose of 1.5 ml/min
Pediatric: NA
For magnesium deficiency related to cardiac dysrhythmias, torsades de pointes, or refractory ventricular fibrillation:
Adult: 1-2 g diluted in 100 ml of D_5W
              administered over 1-2 minutes
Pediatric: Not recommended

Special Considerations
Pregnancy safety: Magnesium sulfate is administered to treat toxemia of pregnancy. It is recommended that the drug not be administered in the 2 hours before delivery, if possible.
IV calcium gluconate or *calcium chloride* should be available as an antagonist to magnesium if needed.
Convulsions may occur up to 48 hr after delivery, necessitating continued therapy.
The "cure" for toxemia is delivery of the baby.
Magnesium must be used with caution in patients with renal failure, since it is cleared by the kidneys and can reach toxic levels easily in those patients.
Prophylactic administration of magnesium sulfate for patients with acute myocardial infarction should be considered.

● MANNITOL (OSMITROL)

Class
Osmotic diuretic

Description
Because of mannitol's osmotic properties, it promotes the movement of fluid from the intracellular into the extracellular space. In emergency care, mannitol is used to treat head injury to decrease cerebral edema and intracranial pressure and in the promotion of urinary excretion of toxic substances.

Onset and Duration
Onset: 1-3 hr (for diuretic effect)
             15 min (for reduction of intracranial pressure)
Duration: 4-6 hr (for diuretic effect)
             3-8 hr (for reduction of intracranial pressure)

Indications
Cerebral edema
Other causes of increased intracranial pressure (space-occupying lesions)
Rhabdomyolysis (myoglobinuria)
Blood transfusion reactions

Contraindications
Severe hypotension
Profound hypovolemia

Dehydration
Hyponatremia
Pulmonary edema
Congestive heart failure

Adverse Reactions

Transient volume overload
Pulmonary edema
Renal failure
Congestive heart failure
Hypotension (from excessive diuresis)
Sodium depletion

Drug Interactions

When given concurrently with digitalis glycosides, an increase in digitalis toxicity may develop.

How Supplied

250 and 500 ml of a 20% solution for IV infusion (200 mg/ml)
25% solution in 50 ml for slow IV push

Dosage and Administration

Adult:	0.25-2 g/kg IV infusion over 15 min; may be repeated after 5 min if no effect
Pediatric:	0.2-0.5 g/kg/dose IV infusion over 30-60 min; may be repeated after 30 min if no effect

Special Considerations

Pregnancy safety: Category C.
Mannitol may crystalize at low temperatures (approximately 7.8° C or colder) and may need to be warmed in boiling water until clear (cool to body temperature before use).
In-line filter should always be used.
Effectiveness depends on large doses and an intact blood-brain barrier.
The use of mannitol and its dosages in emergency care are controversial.

● MEPERIDINE (DEMEROL)

Class

Opioid analgesic

Description

Meperidine is a synthetic opioid agonist that works on opioid receptors to produce analgesia, euphoria, and respiratory and physical depression. It has a tendency for physical dependence and abuse and is classified as a schedule II drug.

Onset and Duration

Onset:	(IM) 10-45 min
	(IV) Less than 1 min
Duration:	2-4 hr

Indications

Moderate to severe pain
Preoperative medication
OB analgesia

Contraindications

Hypersensitivity to narcotics
Diarrhea caused by poisoning
Patients taking MAOIs
During labor or delivery of a premature infant
Undiagnosed abdominal pain or head injury

Adverse Reactions

Respiratory depression
Euphoria
Delirium
Agitation
Hallucination
Seizures
Headache
Visual disturbances
Coma
Facial flushing
Circulatory collapse
Dysrhythmias
Allergic reaction

Drug Interactions

Respiratory depression, hypotension, or sedation may be potentiated by CNS depressants.
Therapeutic doses of meperidine have caused fatal reactions in patients taking MAOIs within the previous 14 days.

How Supplied

Tablet:	50, 100 mg
Parenteral:	50 mg/ml in 1-ml prefilled syringe and Tubex

Dosage and Administration

Adult:	50-100 mg IM
	10-25 mg IV
Pediatric:	1-2 mg/kg/dose IM or IV

Special Considerations

Pregnancy safety: Category C.
Use with caution in patients with asthma and chronic obstructive pulmonary disease.
May aggravate seizures in those with convulsive disorders.
Use with caution in those susceptible to CNS depression.
Naloxone should be readily available.

● METAPROTERENOL (ALUPENT)

Class

Sympathomimetic, bronchodilator

Description

Metaproterenol relaxes the smooth muscles of the bronchial tree and peripheral vasculature by stimulating beta$_2$-adrenergic receptors of the sympathetic nervous system.

Onset and Duration
Onset: 1 min after inhalation
Duration: 3-6 hr

Indications

Bronchial asthma
Reversible bronchospasm (bronchitis, emphysema)

Contraindications

Hypersensitivity
Cardiac dysrhythmias
Tachycardia caused by digitalis toxicity

Adverse Reactions

Restlessness, apprehension
Palpitations
Tachycardia
Dysrhythmias
Decreased blood pressure
Coughing
Facial flushing
Diaphoresis

Drug Interactions

Other sympathomimetics may exacerbate adverse cardiovascular effects.
MAOIs may potentiate hypotensive effects.
Beta blockers may antagonize metaproterenol.

How Supplied
MDI: 0.65/mg/spray (15- ml inhaler)
Solution: 0.6% (2.5 ml dose); 5% (0.3 ml dose)

Dosage and Administration
MDI
Adult: 2-3 inhalations q 3-4 hr (2 min
            between inhalations); maximum
            dose of 12 inhalations/day
Pediatric: Not recommended
Solution
Adult: 5-15 inhalations of 5% solution
Pediatric: Not recommended

Special Considerations

Pregnancy safety: Category C.
Monitor vital signs for hypotension and tachycardia.
Use with caution in patients with coronary artery disease and diabetes mellitus.

● METHYLPREDNISOLONE (SOLU-MEDROL)

Class

Glucocorticoid

Description

Methylprednisolone is a synthetic steroid that suppresses acute and chronic inflammation. In addition, it potentiates vascular smooth muscle relaxation by beta-adrenergic agonists and may alter airway hyperactivity. A newer usage is for reduction of posttraumatic spinal cord edema.

Onset and Duration
Onset: 1-2 hrs
Duration: 8-24 hr

Indications

Anaphylaxis
Bronchodilator for unresponsive asthma
Shock (controversial)
Acute spinal cord injury

Contraindications

Use with caution in patients with GI bleeding and diabetes mellitus.

Adverse Reactions

Headache
Hypertension
Sodium and water retention
Hypokalemia
Alkalosis

Drug Interactions

Hypoglycemic responses to *insulin* and oral hypoglycemic agents may be blunted.
Potassium-depleting agents may potentiate hypokalemia induced by corticosteroids.

How Supplied

40-, 125-, 500-, 1000-mg vials

Dosage and Administration
Adult: Variable; usually within the
            range of 40-125 mg IV, ex-
            cept for spinal cord injury
            where the initial dose is 30
            mg/kg IV bolus followed by
            an IV infusion of 5.4 mg/kg/hr
Pediatric: 1-2 mg/kg/dose IV

Special Considerations

Pregnancy safety: Not established.
Crosses the placenta and may cause fetal harm.

● MIDAZOLAM HYDROCHLORIDE (VERSED)

Class

Short-acting benzodiazepine CNS depressant

Description

Midazolam HCl is a water-soluble benzodiazepine that may be administered for conscious sedation to relieve apprehension or impair memory before endotracheal or nasotracheal intubation.

Onset and Duration
Onset: 1-3 min (IV); dose dependent
Duration: 2-6 hr; dose dependent

Indication
Premedication for tracheal intubation

Contraindications
Hypersensitivity to midazolam
Glaucoma
Shock
Coma
Alcohol intoxication
Overdose
Depressed vital signs
Concomitant use of barbiturates, alcohol, narcotics, or other CNS depressants

Adverse Reactions
Hiccough
Cough
Oversedation
Pain at the injection site
Nausea and vomiting
Headache
Blurred vision
Fluctuations in vital signs
Hypotension
Respiratory depression
Respiratory arrest

Drug Interactions
Sedative effect of midazolam may be accentuated by concomitant use of barbiturates, alcohol, or narcotics (it should therefore not be used in patients who have taken CNS depressants).

How Supplied
2-, 5-, 10-ml vials (1 mg/ml)
1-, 2-, 5-, 10-ml vials (5 mg/ml)

Dosage and Administration
Adult: 2-2.5 mg slow IV (over 2-3 min); may be repeated if necessary in small increments (total maximum dose not to exceed 0.1 mg/kg)
Pediatric: Not recommended

Special Considerations
Pregnancy safety: Category D.
Administer immediately before the intubation procedure.
Provide continuous monitoring of respiratory and cardiac function.
Have resuscitation equipment and medication readily at hand.
Never administer medication as IV bolus.

● MORPHINE SULFATE
(ASTRAMORPH/PF, AND OTHERS)

Class
Opioid analgesic

Description
Morphine sulfate is a natural opium alkaloid that increases peripheral venous capacitance and decreases venous return ("chemical phlebotomy"). It promotes analgesia, euphoria, and respiratory and physical depression. Secondary pharmacological effects of morphine include depressed responsiveness of alpha-adrenergic receptors (producing peripheral vasodilation) and baroreceptor inhibition. In addition, because morphine decreases both preload and afterload, it may decrease myocardial oxygen demand. The properties of this medication make it extremely useful in emergency care. Morphine sulfate is a schedule II drug.

Onset and Duration
Onset: Immediate
Duration: 2-7 hr

Indications
Chest pain associated with myocardial infarction
Moderate to severe acute and chronic pain
Should be used with caution in chronic pain syndromes
Pulmonary edema, with or without associated pain

Contraindications
Hypersensitivity to narcotics
Diarrhea caused by poisoning
Hypovolemia
Hypotension
Head injury or undiagnosed abdominal pain
Patients who have taken MAOIs within 14 days

Adverse Reactions
Hypotension
Tachycardia or bradycardia
Palpitations
Syncope
Facial flushing
Respiratory depression
Euphoria
Bronchospasm
Dry mouth
Allergic reaction

Drug Interactions
CNS depressants may potentiate effects of morphine (respiratory depression, hypotension, sedation).
Chlorpromazine may potentiate analgesia.
MAOIs may cause paradoxical excitation.

How Supplied
Morphine is supplied in tablets, suppositories, and solution. In emergency care, morphine sulfate is usu-

ally administered IV. Parenteral preparations are available in many strengths. A common preparation is 10 mg in 1 ml of solution, ampules, and Tubex syringes.

Dosage and Administration
Adult: 1-3 mg IV q 5 min (titrated to relief of pain)
Pediatric: 0.1-0.2 mg/kg/dose IV (maximum 15-mg dose)

Special Considerations
Pregnancy safety: Category C.
Narcotics rapidly cross the placenta.
Safety in neonates has not been established.
Use with caution in older adults, those with asthma, and those susceptible to CNS depression.
May worsen bradycardia or heart block in inferior myocardial infarction (vagotonic effect).
Naloxone should be readily available.

● NALBUPHINE (NUBAIN)

Class
Opioid analgesic

Description
Nalbuphine is a synthetic analgesic with a potency equivalent to that of morphine sulfate on a milligram-to-milligram basis. It has both agonist and antagonist properties. Nalbuphine may be preferred for treating chest pain associated with myocardial infarction because it reduces the oxygen needs of the heart without reducing blood pressure. Nalbuphine is not presently regulated under the Controlled Substance Act.

Onset and Duration
Onset: 2-3 min
Duration: 3-6 hr

Indications
Chest pain associated with myocardial infarction
Moderate to severe acute pain
May be necessary in some chronic pain syndromes
Pulmonary edema, with or without associated pain (*morphine* is a first-line medication in this class)

Contraindications
Hypersensitivity to narcotics
Diarrhea caused by poisoning
Hypovolemia
Hypotension
Head injury or undiagnosed abdominal pain

Adverse Reactions
Hypotension
Bradycardia
Facial flushing
Respiratory depression
CNS depression
Euphoria

Paradoxical CNS stimulation
Blurred vision

Drug Interactions
CNS depressants may potentiate effects.

How Supplied
10 mg in 1-ml ampule (10 mg/ml)
20 mg in 1-ml ampule

Dosage and Administration
Adult: 2-5-mg slow IV; may be augmented with 2-mg doses prn
Pediatric: Not recommended

Special Considerations
Pregnancy safety: Category B.
Use with caution in patients with impaired respiratory function.
Has a weak narcotic antagonist effect and may precipitate withdrawal syndrome in narcotic-dependent patients.
Naloxone should be readily available.

● NALOXONE (NARCAN)

Class
Synthetic opioid antagonist

Description
Naloxone is a competitive narcotic antagonist used in the management and reversal of overdoses caused by narcotics and synthetic narcotic agents. Unlike other narcotic antagonists, which do not completely inhibit the analgesic properties of opiates, naloxone antagonizes all actions of **morphine.**

Onset and Duration
Onset: Within 2 min
Duration: 30-60 min

Indications
For the complete or partial reversal of CNS and respiratory depression induced by opioids:
Narcotic agonist
  Morphine sulfate
  Heroin
  Hydromorphone (Dilaudid)
  Methadone
  Meperidine (Demerol)
  Paregoric
  Fentanyl citrate (Sublimaze)
  Oxycodone (Percodan)
  Codeine
  Propoxyphene (Darvon)
Narcotic agonist and antagonist
  Butorphanol tartrate (Stadol)
  Pentazocine (Talwin)
  Nalbuphine (Nubain)
Decreased level of consciousness

Coma of unknown origin

Circulatory support in refractory shock (investigational)

Contraindications

Hypersensitivity

Use with caution in narcotic-dependent patients who may experience withdrawal syndrome (including neonates of narcotic-dependent mothers)

Adverse Reactions

Tachycardia

Hypertension

Dysrhythmias

Nausea and vomiting

Diaphoresis

Drug Interactions

Is incompatible with bisulfite and with alkaline solutions.

How Supplied

0.02 mg/ml (neonate), 0.4 mg/ml, 1 mg/ml

Dosage and Administration

Adult: 0.4-2 mg IV, IM, SQ (or ET diluted); minimum recommended dosage is 2 mg; may be repeated at 5-min intervals to a maximum of 10 mg

Infusion: 2 mg in 500 ml of D_5W (4 mcg/ml), infuse at 0.4 mg/hr (100 ml/hr)

Pediatric: 0.1 mg/kg/dose IV, IM, SQ (or ET diluted); maximum dose of 0.8 mg; if no response in 10 min, administer an additional 0.1 mg/kg/dose

Special Considerations

Pregnancy safety: Category B.

Seizures have been reported (no causal relationship established).

May not reverse hypotension.

Caution should be exercised when administering *naloxone* to narcotic addicts (may precipitate withdrawal with hypertension, tachycardia, and violent behavior).

● NIFEDIPINE (PROCARDIA)

Class

Calcium-channel blocker

Description

Nifedipine inhibits the movement of calcium ions across cell membranes. By blocking the entry of calcium into cells, it depresses smooth muscle contraction. Nifedipine dilates coronary arteries and arterioles in normal and ischemic tissue, prevents coronary artery spasm, dilates peripheral vessels, and decreases total peripheral resistance (reducing myocardial oxygen demand). When arterial pressure is reduced, a reflex is stimulated, causing a small increase in heart rate and a mild elevation in the force of myocardial contraction. Nifedipine does not slow SA nodal activity or prolong AV nodal conduction.

Onset and Duration

Onset: 15-30 min

Duration: 6-8 hr

Indications

Angina pectoris

Hypertensive urgencies (investigational)

Pulmonary edema (investigational)

Contraindications

Hypersensitivity

Compensatory hypertension

Hypotension

Adverse Reactions (in order of prevalence)

Dizziness, lightheadedness

Flushing, heat sensation

Headache

Weakness

Nausea

Muscle cramps

Peripheral edema

Mood changes

Palpitations

Hypotension

Myocardial infarction

Allergic reaction

Facial flushing

Drug Interactions

Beta blockers may potentiate effects.

Antihypertensives may potentiate hypotensive effects.

Effects of theophylline may be increased.

How Supplied

Soft gelatin capsules: 10, 20 mg (Puncture end of capsule with needle and squeeze; may administer sublingually or buccally or have patient bite and swallow; both methods allow for rapid absorption.)

Extended-release tablets: 30, 60, 90 mg

Dosage and Administration

Adult: 10 mg SL or buccal; repeat in 30 min prn

Pediatric: Not recommended

Special Considerations

Pregnancy safety: Category C.

A beta blocker should be available for management of reflex tachycardia.

May produce hypotension and precipitate angina pectoris in older patients.

● NITROGLYCERIN (NITROSTAT AND OTHERS)

Class
Vasodilator

Description
It was originally believed that nitrates and nitrites dilated coronary blood vessels, thereby increasing blood flow to the heart. It is now believed that atherosclerosis limits coronary dilation and that the benefits of nitrates and nitrites result from dilation of arterioles and veins in the periphery. The resulting reduction in preload and to a lesser extent in afterload decreases the work load of the heart and lowers myocardial oxygen demand. Nitroglycerin is very lipid soluble and is thought to enter the body from the GI tract through the lymphatics rather than the portal blood.

Onset and Duration
Onset: 1-3 min
Duration: 20-30 min

Indications
Ischemic chest pain
Hypertension
Congestive heart failure

Contraindications
Hypersensitivity
Hypotension
Head injury
Cerebral hemorrhage

Adverse Reactions
Transient headache
Postural syncope
Reflex tachycardia
Hypotension
Nausea and vomiting
Allergic reaction
Muscle twitching
Diaphoresis

Drug Interactions
Other vasodilators may have additive hypotensive effects.

How Supplied
Tablets: 0.15 mg (1/400 gr), 0.3 mg (1/200 gr), 0.4 mg (1/150 gr), 0.6 (1/100 gr)
MDI: 0.4-mg metered dose
Parenteral: 0.8, 5 mg/ml

Dosage and Administration
Adult: Tablet: 0.3-0.4 mg SL; may be repeated in 3-5 min three times
Pediatric: Not recommended

Special Considerations
Pregnancy safety: Category C.
Susceptibility to hypotension in older adults increases.
Nitroglycerin decomposes when exposed to light or heat.
Must be kept in airtight containers.
Active ingredient of nitroglycerin "stings" when administered SL.

● NITROPASTE (NITRO-BID OINTMENT)

Class
Vasodilator

Description
Nitropaste contains a 2% solution of nitroglycerin in an absorbent paste. It is applied to the skin (usually the chest wall), where it is absorbed transdermally over 24 hours. The paste or polymer-bonded adhesive bandage should be applied to a site that is free of hair; it should be placed at a new site each time to avoid irritation.

Onset and Duration
Onset: 30 min
Duration: 18-24 hr

Indications
Angina pectoris
Chest pain associated with AMI (less easily titratable than IV nitroglycerin)

Contraindications
Hypersensitivity
Hypotension
Head injury
Cerebral hemorrhage

Adverse Reactions
Transient headache
Postural syncope
Reflex tachycardia
Hypotension
Nausea and vomiting
Allergic reaction
Muscle twitching
Diaphoresis

Drug Interactions
Other vasodilators may have additive hypotensive effects.

How Supplied
20-, 60-g tubes of paste (measuring applicators are supplied)
Transdermal units of varying dosages

Dosage and Administration

Adult

Paste: Apply ½ to ¾ inch (1-2 centimeters), 15-30 mg, cover with transparent wrap and secure with tape; maximum of 5 inches (75 mg) per application

Transdermal: Apply unit to intact skin Dosage adjustments made by changing the dose to the next larger dose or by using a combination of nitroglycerin preparations

Pediatric: Not recommended

Special Considerations

Pregnancy safety: Category C.

Avoid using fingers to spread paste.

Do not massage or rub paste (rapid absorption interferes with the drug's sustained action).

Store paste in a cool place with the tube tightly capped.

Although the adverse effects for nitropaste are the same as for SL nitroglycerin, their frequency and severity are usually considerably less with the sustained-release preparations because of the slower absorption and a less erratic change in serum levels.

● NITROUS OXIDE:OXYGEN (50:50) (NITRONOX)

Class

Gaseous analgesic and anesthetic

Description

Nitrous oxide:oxygen is a blended mixture of 50% nitrous oxide and 50% oxygen. When inhaled, nitrous oxide and oxygen depresses the CNS, causing anesthesia. In addition, the high concentration of oxygen delivered along with the nitrous oxide increases oxygen tension in the blood, thereby reducing hypoxia. Nitrous oxide:oxygen is self-administered.

Onset and Duration

Onset: 2-5 min
Duration: 2-5 min

Indications

Moderate to severe pain
Anxiety
Apprehension

Contraindications

Impaired LOC
Head injury
Chest trauma (pneumothorax)
Inability to comply with instructions
Decompression sickness (nitrogen narcosis, air embolus, air transport)
Undiagnosed abdominal pain or marked distention
Bowel obstruction
Hypotension
Shock
COPD (with history or suspicion of CO_2 retention)

Adverse Reactions

Dizziness
Apnea
Expansion of gas-filled pockets
Cyanosis
Nausea and vomiting
Malignant hyperthermia (rare but dangerous)

Drug Interactions

There are no significant drug interactions with other emergency medications.

How Supplied

D and E cylinders (blue and white in Canada, blue and green in United States) of 50% nitrous oxide and 50% oxygen compressed gas

Dosage and Administration

Adult: Invert cylinder several times before use; instruct the patient to inhale deeply through demand valve and mask or mouthpiece

Pediatric: Same as adult

Special Considerations

Pregnancy safety: Nitrous oxide has been shown to increase the incidence of spontaneous abortion.

Nitrous oxide is 34 times as soluble as nitrogen and diffuses into pockets of trapped gas in the patient (intestinal obstruction, pneumothorax, blocked middle ear). As the nitrogen leaves and is replaced by larger amounts of nitrous oxide, increased pressures or volumes may cause serious damage, for example, intestinal rupture.

Nitrous oxide is a nonexplosive gas.

NOTE: When delivering nitrous oxide and oxygen from a single tank, it is important to ensure that enough oxygen remains in the tank to provide adequate oxygenation. Inverting the cylinder several times to mix the gases is important for this reason. It is also reasonable to monitor oximetry during administration of nitrous oxide.

● NOREPINEPHRINE (LEVOPHED)

Class
Sympathomimetic

Description
Norepinephrine is an alpha- and beta$_1$-adrenergic agonist. It is a potent vasoconstrictor that increases myocardial contractility and peripheral vascular resistance. Because norepinephrine tends to constrict the renal and mesenteric blood vessels, it is rarely used in the prehospital setting.

Onset and Duration
Onset: 1-3 min
Duration: 5-10 min

Indications
Cardiogenic shock
Neurogenic shock
Inotropic support

Contraindications
Hypotensive patients with hypovolemia

Adverse Reactions
Headache
Dysrhythmias
Tachycardia
Reflex bradycardia
Angina pectoris
Hypertension

Drug Interactions
Can be deactivated by alkaline solutions.
MAOIs and *bretylium* may potentiate the effects of catecholamines.
Beta-adrenergic antagonists may blunt inotropic response.
Sympathomimetics and phosphodiesterase inhibitors may exacerbate dysrhythmia response.

How Supplied
1 mg/ml, 4-ml ampule

Dosage and Administration
Adult: Dilute 8 mg in 500 ml of D$_5$W or 4 mg in 250 ml of D$_5$W (16 mcg/ml); infuse by IV piggyback at 0.5-1.0 mcg/min, titrated to patient response
Pediatric: 0.1-1 mcg/min IV infusion, titrated to patient response

Special Considerations
Pregnancy safety: Not established.
May cause fetal anoxia when used in pregnancy.
Infuse norepinephrine through a large stable vein to avoid tissue necrosis.

● OXYGEN

Class
Naturally occurring atmospheric gas

Description
Oxygen is an odorless, tasteless, colorless gas present in room air at a concentration of approximately 21%. It is an important emergency drug used to reverse hypoxemia; in doing so it helps oxidize glucose to produce ATP (aerobic metabolism) and helps reduce the area of infarcted tissue during an acute myocardial infarction (in patients who are hypoxemic on room air).

Onset and Duration
Onset: Immediate
Duration: Less than 2 min

Indications
Confirmed or suspected hypoxia
Ischemic chest pain
Respiratory insufficiency
Prophylactically during air transport
Confirmed or suspected carbon monoxide poisoning and other causes of decreased tissue oxygenation (cardiac arrest)

Contraindications
Oxygen should never be withheld in any critical patient

Adverse Reactions
High-concentration oxygen may cause decreased LOC and respiratory depression in patients with chronic carbon dioxide retention.
High concentrations of oxygen administered to premature infants may result in retrolental fibroplasia (maintain between 30% and 40%).

Drug Interactions
There are no significant drug interactions with other emergency medications.

How Supplied
Oxygen cylinders (usually green and white) of 100% compressed oxygen gas

Dosage and Administration
Adult:
   Cardiac arrest or carbon monoxide poisoning: As near to 100% as possible
   Hypoxia: 10-15 L/min (via nonrebreather)
   COPD: 0-2 L/min (via nasal cannula or 28%-35% venturi mask); if additional oxygen therapy is needed, be prepared to provide ventilatory support
Pediatric: Same as for adult (with the exceptions noted above)

Special Considerations
Pregnancy safety: NA.
Oxygen vigorously supports combustion.

● OXYTOCIN (PITOCIN)

Class
Hormone

Description
Oxytocin means "rapid birth." It is a synthetic hormone named for the natural posterior pituitary hormone. It stimulates uterine smooth muscle contractions indirectly and helps expedite the normal contractions of spontaneous labor. As in all significant uterine contractions, there is a transient reduction in uterine blood flow. Oxytocin also stimulates the mammary glands to increase lactation without increasing the production of milk. The drug is administered in the prehospital setting to control postpartum bleeding.

Onset and Duration
Onset: (IV) Immediate
(IM) Within 3-5 min
Duration: (IV) 20 minutes after the infusion is stopped
(IM) 30-60 min

Indications
Postpartum hemorrhage after infant and placental delivery

Contraindications
Presence of a second fetus

Adverse Reactions
Hypotension or hypertension
Tachycardia
Dysrhythmias
Angina pectoris
Anxiety
Seizure
Nausea and vomiting
Allergic reaction
Uterine rupture (from excessive administration)

Drug Interactions
Other vasopressors may potentiate hypertension.

How Supplied
10 USP units/1-ml ampule (10 U/ml) and prefilled syringe
5 USP units/1-ml ampule (5 U/ml) and prefilled syringe

Dosage and Administration
IM: 3-10 units IM after delivery of placenta
IV: Mix 5-20 units in 500 ml of D$_5$W, NS, or LR; infuse at 20-40 milliunits/min, titrated to severity of bleeding and uterine response

Special Considerations
Pregnancy safety: NA.
Vital signs (including fetal heart rate) and uterine tone should be closely monitored.

● PANCURONIUM (PAVULON)

Class
Neuromuscular blocker (nondepolarizing)

Description
Pancuronium produces complete muscular relaxation by binding to the receptor for acetylcholine at the neuromuscular junction, without initiating depolarization of the muscle membrane. As the concentration of acetylcholine rises in the neuromuscular junction, pancuronium is displaced and muscle tone is regained. Neuromuscular blocking agents are used to provide muscle relaxation during surgery (particularly relaxation of the abdominal muscles) without general anesthesia and to prevent convulsive muscle spasms during electroconvulsive therapy. In emergency care, pancuronium is used to optimize conditions for endotracheal intubation and assisted ventilations.

Onset and Duration
Onset: Paralysis in 3-5 min
Duration: 45-60 min

Indications
Induction or maintenance of paralysis after intubation to assist ventilations

Contraindications
Known hypersensitivity to the drug
Inability to control airway and support ventilations with *oxygen* and positive pressure
Neuromuscular disease (e.g., myasthenia gravis)

Adverse Reactions
Transient hypotension
Tachycardia
Dysrhythmias
Increased blood pressure
Excessive salivation
Pain, burning at IV injection site

Drug Interactions
Positive chronotropic drugs may potentiate tachycardia.

How Supplied
4 mg/2-ml ampule

Dosage and Administration
Adult: 0.1 mg/kg slow IV; repeat q 30-60 min prn
Pediatric: Same as adult

NOTE: If the patient is conscious, explain the effects of the medication before administration, and always sedate the patient before using a neuromuscular blocking agent.

Special Considerations
Pregnancy safety: Not established.

NOTE: Neuromuscular blocking agents produce respiratory paralysis. Therefore intubation and ventilatory support must be readily available.

Carefully monitor the patient and be prepared to resuscitate.

The effects of pancuronium may be reversed with neostigmine (Prostigmin) 0.05 mg/kg and should be accompanied by *atropine* (0.6-1.2 mg IV).

Pancuronium has no effect on consciousness or pain.

Will not stop neuronal seizure activity or decrease CNS damage secondary to seizures.

Heart rate, cardiac output, and atrial pressure are increased.

Pancuronium is excreted in the urine; doses should be decreased for patients with renal disease.

● PHENOBARBITAL (LUMINAL)

Class
Barbiturate, anticonvulsant

Description
Phenobarbital is a drug of choice in treating grand mal and focal motor epilepsy. In addition, it is used prophylactically for febrile seizures in children. The exact mode and site of action of phenobarbital (and other barbiturates) in suppression of seizure activity are unknown. It is thought that the drugs work by reducing neuronal excitability and by increasing the motor cortex threshold to electrical stimulation.

Onset and Duration
Onset: 3-30 min
Duration: 4-6 hr

Indications
Prevention and treatment of seizure activity
Prophylaxis for febrile seizures
Anxiety
Apprehension

Contraindications
Hypersensitivity
Patients with porphyria
Severe liver or respiratory disease

Adverse Reactions
Hypotension
Bradycardia
Respiratory depression
CNS depression
Ataxia
Nystagmus
Nausea and vomiting
Pupil constriction
Burning at injection site

Drug Interactions
Other anticonvulsants, CNS depressants, and MAOIs may potentiate effects.

How Supplied
Elixir: 20 mg/5 ml
Tablets: 8, 15, 30, 60, 90, 100 mg
Parenteral: 65-, 130-mg/ml ampule; dose may be diluted with 9 ml of D_5W (6.5, 13 mg/ml)

Dosage and Administration
Seizure activity
Adult: 100-250 mg slow IV; repeat as needed in 20-30 min
Pediatric: 10-15 mg/kg IV (less than 1 mg/kg/min); repeat as needed in 20-30 min

Special Considerations
Pregnancy safety: Category B.

Has potential for abuse.

Carefully monitor vital signs.

Phenobarbital may be substituted for other barbiturates to decrease the incidence of withdrawal symptoms while weaning patients off barbiturates.

Use with caution in patients with pulmonary, cardiovascular, hepatic, or renal insufficiency.

Hypoglycemic seizures should be treated with glucose, not phenobarbital, which does not resolve the hypoglycemic state or prevent CNS injury.

Use a large, stable vein for injection (extravasation may cause tissue necrosis).

● PHENYTOIN (DILANTIN)

Class
Anticonvulsant, antidysrhythmic (class 1b)

Description
Phenytoin (a hydantoin) is a drug of choice in controlling grand mal and focal motor seizure activity. It was developed as an alternative anticonvulsant that would cause less sedation than barbiturates. Phenytoin

appears to inhibit the spread of seizure activity by promoting sodium efflux from neurons, thereby stabilizing the neuron's threshold against excitability caused by excess stimulation. Phenytoin has also been used to treat digitalis-induced atrial and ventricular dysrhythmias by stabilizing the sodium influx in Purkinje fibers of the heart, decreasing abnormal ventricular automaticity, and decreasing the refractory period.

Onset and Duration
Onset: 20-30 min for seizure disorder
Duration: As long as 15 days

Indications
Major motor seizures
Digitalis-induced dysrhythmias

Contraindications
Hypersensitivity
Bradycardia
Second- and third-degree heart block

Adverse Reactions
Hypotension with rapid IV push (greater than 50 mg/min)
Heart block
Cardiovascular collapse
Dysrhythmias
Respiratory depression
CNS depression
Ataxia
Nystagmus
Nausea and vomiting
Pain from injection site

Drug Interactions
Anticoagulants, *cimetidine*, sulfonamides, and salicylates may increase serum phenytoin levels.
Chronic alcohol speeds metabolism of the drug.
Lidocaine, propranolol, and other beta-blocking agents may increase cardiac depressant effects.
Xanthines may result in decreased phenytoin absorption.
Precipitation may occur when mixed with D_5W.
Incompatible with many solutions and medications.

How Supplied
50 mg/ml in 2- and 5-ml ampules, 2-ml prefilled syringe.
May be diluted in NS (1-10 mg/ml, per protocol); use in-line filter.
IV line should be flushed with 0.9% NS before and after the drug is administered.

Dosage and Administration
Seizures
Adult: 10-20 mg/kg slow IV (not to exceed 1 g or rate of 50 mg/min)
Pediatric: 10-20 mg/kg slow IV (1-3 mg/kg/min)

Dysrhythmias
Adult: 50-100 mg (diluted) slow IV q 5-15 min prn; maximum dose 1 g
Pediatric: 5 mg/kg slow IV

Special Considerations
Pregnancy safety: Not established.
Phenytoin may normally have slight yellow color.
Carefully monitor vital signs.
Venous irritation can result from the alkalinity of the solution.
Use with caution in patients with pulmonary, cardiovascular, hepatic, or renal insufficiency.
Use large, stable vein for injection (extravasation may cause tissue necrosis).

● PROCAINAMIDE (PRONESTYL)

Class
Antidysrhythmic (class Ia)

Description
Procainamide suppresses phase-4 depolarization in normal ventricular muscle and Purkinje fibers, reducing the automaticity of ectopic pacemakers. It also suppresses reentry dysrhythmias by slowing intraventricular conduction. Procainamide may be effective in treating PVCs and recurrent ventricular tachycardia that cannot be controlled with *lidocaine.*

Onset and Duration
Onset: 10-30 min
Duration: 3-6 hr

Indications
Suppressing PVCs refractory to *lidocaine*
Suppressing ventricular tachycardia (with a pulse) refractory to *lidocaine*
Suppressing ventricular fibrillation refractory to *lidocaine* when *bretylium tosylate* is not readily available
PSVTs with wide-complex tachycardia of unknown origin (drug of choice when associated with WPW)

Contraindications
Second- and third-degree AV block
Digitalis toxicity
Torsades de pointes

Adverse Reactions
Hypotension
Bradycardia
Reflex tachycardia
AV block
Widened QRS
Prolonged PR or QT interval
PVCs
Ventricular tachycardia, ventricular fibrillation, asystole

CNS depression
Confusion
Seizure

Drug Interactions

There are no significant drug interactions with other emergency medications.

How Supplied

1 g in 10-ml vial (100 mg/ml)
1 g in 2-ml vials (500 mg/ml) for infusion

Dosage and Administration

Adult:	20 mg/min (30 mg/min for refractory VF): maximum dose is 17 mg/kg
	Maintenance infusion (after resuscitation from cardiac arrest; is 1-4 mg/min
Pediatric:	3-5 mg/kg q 15 min; maximum dose is 17 mg/kg

NOTE: Discontinue if the dysrhythmia is suppressed, hypotension develops, the QRS complex is widened by 50% of its original width, or a total of 1 g has been administered.

Special Considerations

Pregnancy safety: Category C.
Procainamide has potent vasodilating and inotropic effects.
Rapid injection may cause procainamide-induced hypotension.
Carefully monitor vital signs and ECG.
Administer cautiously to patients with asthma, digitalis-induced dysrhythmias, acute myocardial infarction, or cardiac, hepatic, or renal insufficiency.

● PROMETHAZINE (PHENERGAN)

Class

Antihistamine

Description

Promethazine is an H_1-receptor antagonist that blocks the actions of histamine by competitive antagonism at the H_1 receptor. In addition to antihistaminic effects, promethazine possesses sedative, antimotion, antiemetic, and considerable anticholinergic activity. It is often administered with analgesics, particularly narcotics, to potentiate their effects, though the occurrence of potentiation is controversial.

Onset and Duration

Onset:	IV (rapid)
	PO (20 min)
Duration:	4-6 hr

Indications

Nausea and vomiting
Motion sickness
Preoperative and postoperative, obstetric (during labor) sedation
To potentiate the effects of analgesics

Contraindications

Hypersensitivity
Comatose states
Patients who are CNS depressed (alcohol, barbiturates, narcotics)
When signs of Reye's syndrome are present

Adverse Reactions

Sedation
Dizziness
May impair mental and physical ability
Allergic reactions
Dysrhythmias
Nausea and vomiting
Hyperexcitability
Use in children may cause hallucinations, convulsions, and sudden death

Drug Interactions

Concomitant use of CNS depressants may have an additive sedative effect.
The incidence of extrapyramidal effects increases when given with some MAOIs.

How Supplied

25, 50 mg/ml in 1-ml ampules and Tubex syringes

Dosage and Administration

Adult:	12.5-25 mg IV, deep IM
Pediatric:	0.5-1 mg/kg/dose IM

Special Considerations

Pregnancy safety: Category C (generally considered safe for use during labor).
Use caution in patients with asthma, peptic ulcer, and bone marrow depression.
Antiemetics should not be used in children with vomiting of unknown etiology.
Care must be taken to avoid accidental intraarterial injection.
IM injections are the preferred route of administration.

● PROPRANOLOL (INDERAL)

Class
Beta-adrenergic blocker, antidysrhythmic (class II)

Description
Propranolol is a nonselective beta-adrenergic blocker that inhibits chronotropic, inotropic, and vasodilator response to beta-adrenergic stimulation. It slows the sinus rate, depresses AV conduction, decreases cardiac output, and reduces blood pressure. In addition, propranolol decreases myocardial oxygen demand and reduces the risk of sudden death in patients with AMI.

Onset and Duration
Onset:	15-60 min
Duration:	6-12 hr

Indications
Hypertension
Angina pectoris
Ventricular tachycardia and ventricular fibrillation refractory to *lidocaine* and *bretylium*
Selected supraventricular tachycardias

Contraindications
Sinus bradycardia
Second- or third-degree AV block
Asthma
Congestive heart failure
COPD

Adverse Reactions
Bradycardia	Dizziness
Heart blocks	Angina pectoris
Bronchospasm	Palpitations
Dyspnea	Syncope
Anxiety	Nausea and vomiting
Hallucinations	Visual disturbances

Drug Interactions
Catecholamine-depleting drugs may potentiate hypotension.
Sympathomimetic effects may be antagonized.
Verapamil may worsen AV conduction abnormalities.
Succinylcholine effects may be enhanced.
Isoproterenol, norepinephrine, dopamine, and *dobutamine* may reverse effects of propranolol.
Epinephrine may cause a rise in blood pressure, a decrease in heart rate, and severe vasoconstriction.
Hypoglycemic effects of *insulin* may be prolonged.

How Supplied
Propranolol is available in tablet, capsule, and solution (1 mg/ml vial). It is administered intravenously in the treatment of life-threatening tachydysrhythmias (although newer beta blockers may be preferable).

Dosage and Administration
Adult: Dilute 1-3 mg in 10-30 ml of D_5W; administer slow IV (less than 1 mg/min); repeat in 5-10 min prn (maximum dose 5 mg)

Pediatric: 0.01-0.05 mg/kg/dose (diluted) slow IV over 10 min; repeat q 5 min prn (maximum 3 mg)

Special Considerations
Pregnancy safety: Category C.
Propranolol may produce life-threatening side effects; closely monitor patient during administration.
Use with caution in older patients.
Use with caution in patients with impaired hepatic or renal function.
Atropine should be readily available.

> **NOTE:** Beta₁-selective drugs now available are more commonly used for cardiac emergencies.

● SODIUM BICARBONATE

Class
Buffer

Description
Sodium bicarbonate reacts with hydrogen ions to form water and carbon dioxide and thereby can act to buffer metabolic acidosis. Increasing the plasma concentration of bicarbonate causes blood pH to rise.

Onset and Duration
Onset:	2-10 min
Duration:	30-60 min

Indications
Known preexisting bicarbonate-responsive acidosis
Intubated patient with continued long arrest interval
Upon return of spontaneous circulation after long arrest interval
Tricyclic antidepressant overdose
Alkalinization for treatment of specific intoxications

Contraindications
In patients with chloride loss from vomiting and GI suction
Metabolic and respiratory alkalosis
Hypocalcemia
Hypokalemia

Adverse Reactions
Metabolic alkalosis
Hypoxia
Rise in intracellular P_{CO_2} and increased tissue acidosis

Electrolyte imbalance (tetany)
Seizures
Tissue sloughing at injection site

Drug Interactions

May precipitate in calcium solutions.
Alkalinization of urine may increase half-lives of certain drugs.
Vasopressors may be deactivated.

How Supplied

50 mEq in 50 ml of solvent

Dosage and Administration

Urgent forms of metabolic acidosis
    Adult: 1 mEq/kg IV; repeat with 0.5
                 mEq/kg q 10 min
    Pediatric: Same as adult

Special Considerations

Pregnancy safety: Category C.
When possible, blood gas analysis should guide bicarbonate administration.
Bicarbonate administration produces carbon dioxide, which crosses cell membranes more rapidly than bicarbonate, potentially worsening intracellular acidosis.
May increase edematous or sodium-retaining states.
May worsen congestive heart failure.

● STREPTOKINASE (STREPTASE)

Class

Thrombolytic agent

Description

Streptokinase combines with plasminogen to produce an activator complex that converts free plasminogen to the proteolytic enzyme plasmin. The plasmin in turn functions as an enzyme that degrades fibrin threads as well as fibrinogen, causing lysis of the blood clot. In the prehospital setting, streptokinase is administered to selected patients with acute evolving myocardial infarctions.

Onset and Duration

    Onset: 10-20 min (fibrinolysis, 10-20
                min; clot lysis, 60-90 min)
    Duration: 3-4 hr (prolonged bleeding
                times up to 24 hr)

Indications

Acute evolving myocardial infarction
Massive pulmonary emboli
Arterial thrombosis and embolism
To clear arteriovenous cannulas

Contraindications

Hypersensitivity
Active bleeding

Recent surgery (within 2-3 weeks)
Recent cerebrovascular accident
Prolonged CPR
Intracranial or intraspinal surgery
Recent significant trauma (particularly head trauma)
Uncontrolled hypertension

Adverse Reactions

Bleeding (GI, GU, intracranial, other sites)
Allergic reactions
Hypotension
Chest pain
Reperfusion dysrhythmias
Abdominal pain

Drug Interactions

Acetylsalicylic acid may increase risk of bleeding (may also be beneficial in improving overall effectiveness).
Heparin and other anticoagulants may increase risk of bleeding as well as improve overall outcome.

How Supplied

250,000-, 600,000-, 750,000-, 1,500,000-IU vials
Reconstitute by slowly adding 5 ml of sodium chloride or D_5W, directing the stream toward the side of the vial rather than into the powder. Do not shake the vial, but gently roll and tilt it for reconstitution. Slowly dilute the entire contents of the vial to total of 45 ml.

Dosage and Administration

Evolving acute myocardial infarction
    Adult: 500,000-1,500,000 IU di-
                luted to 45 ml (IV) over 1 hr
    Children: Safety not established

Special Considerations

Pregnancy safety: Category A.
Do not administer IM injections to patients receiving thrombolytic drugs.
Obtain blood sample for coagulation studies before administration.
Carefully monitor vital signs.
Observe the patient for bleeding.
Use caution when moving patient to avoid bruising or bleeding.
Do not draw arterial blood gas specimens in thrombolytic therapy candidates.

● SUCCINYLCHOLINE (ANECTINE)

Class

Neuromuscular blocker (depolarizing)

Description

Succinylcholine has the briefest duration of action of all neuromuscular blocking drugs, making it a drug of choice for such procedures as terminating laryngospasm, endotracheal intubation, and electroconvulsive shock therapy. Like nondepolarizing blockers, depolarizing drugs also bind to the receptors for acetylcholine. However, because they cause depolarization of the muscle membrane, they often lead to fasciculations and some muscular contractions.

Onset and Duration
Onset: Less than 1 min
Duration: 5 min

Indications
To facilitate intubation
To terminate laryngospasm
For muscle relaxation

Contraindications
Penetrating eye injury (succinylcholine increases intraocular pressure)
Inability to control airway or support ventilations with oxygen and positive pressure

Adverse Reactions
Hypotension
Bradycardias
Dysrhythmias
Initial muscle fasciculation
Excessive salivation
Malignant hyperthermia
Allergic reaction
Can exacerbate hyperkalemia in trauma patients (hours posttrauma)

Drug Interactions
Oxytocin, beta blockers, and organophosphates may potentiate effects.
Diazepam may reduce duration of action.
Cardiac glycosides may induce dysrhythmias.

How Supplied
40 mg in 2-ml ampule (20 mg/ml)
100 mg in 5-ml ampule (20 mg/ml)
Multidose vial

Dosage and Administration

NOTE: If the patient is conscious, explain the effects of the medication before administration. Premedication with *atropine* should be strongly considered, particularly in the pediatric age group. Premedicating with *lidocaine* may blunt any increase in intracranial pressure associated with intubation. Finally, *diazepam* or another sedative should be used in any conscious patient undergoing neuromuscular blockade.

Adult: 1.5 mg/kg rapid IV; repeat once if needed

Pediatric: 1 mg/kg dose rapid IV; repeat once if needed

Special Considerations
Pregnancy safety: Category C.

NOTE: Neuromuscular blocking agents will produce respiratory paralysis. Therefore intubation and ventilatory support must be readily available.

Carefully monitor the patient and be prepared to resuscitate.
Administer with caution to patients with severe trauma, burns, and electrolyte imbalances (high potassium levels).
Brain or spinal cord injury may prolong effects.
Children are not as sensitive to succinylcholine on a weight basis as adults and may require higher doses.
Succinylcholine has no effect on consciousness or pain.
Will not stop neuronal seizure activity.

● SYRUP OF IPECAC

Class
Emetic

Description
Syrup of ipecac acts as a local irritant on the gastric mucosa and on emetic centers of the brain. Vomiting induced by syrup of ipecac occurs in 80%-99% of patients. The drug is available over the counter, but medical control, a poison control center, or both should be consulted before administration.

Onset and Duration
Onset: Generally 15-20 min
Duration: 80 min

Indications
Acute oral drug or toxin overdose in alert patients

Contraindications
Caustics, corrosives, petroleum distillates
Unprotected airways
Absent gag reflex
Unknown ingestion
Children less than 6 months of age
Rapidly acting CNS depressants (causing decreased level of consciousness faster than ipecac can work)

Adverse Reactions
Prolonged vomiting
Muscle aching, weakness

Cardiac conduction disturbances or dysrhythmias
Chest pain
Hypotension

Drug Interactions
Activated charcoal adsorbs ipecac.

How Supplied
15-, 30-ml vials

Dosage and Administration
Adult:	30 ml PO followed by 1-2 glasses of water; may repeat once in 25-30 min if ineffective
Pediatric (1-12 years):	15 ml PO followed by water (4 ml/kg)
(6-12 months):	5-10 ml PO followed by a couple of swallows of water; may repeat once if ineffective

Special Considerations
Pregnancy safety: Not established.
Carefully monitor patient's airway.
Within ½ hour of administration, 90% of patients vomit (average time is 20 min).
Activated charcoal should be administered only after complete gastric emptying.
Use of syrup of ipecac is that persistent vomiting may preclude use of activated charcoal.
Save emesis sample for evaluation.
Patients usually vomit two or three times per dose over one or two periods. Keep patient awake.
Administer with caution in TCA overdose as TCA rapidly progresses to seizures and unconsciousness (within 30 min); ipecac should not be given unless overdose was witnessed, such as when acetaminophen ingestion was witnessed by a parent.

NOTE: Several studies show ipecac to be less effective than charcoal in decreasing toxin absorption. Consequently, enthusiasm for the use of ipecac has waned. It may continue to be useful in poisonings where charcoal is ineffective and when there is a considerable delay in transportation for definitive care.

● TERBUTALINE (BRETHINE)

Class
Sympathomimetic, bronchodilator

Description
Terbutaline is selective for beta$_2$-adrenergic receptors, resulting in relaxation of smooth muscles of the bronchial tree and peripheral vasculature. It is effective in producing immediate bronchodilation with minimal cardiac effects.

Onset and Duration
Onset:	(SQ) 15-30 min
	(MDI) 5-30 min
Duration:	(SQ) 1.5-4 hr
	(MDI) 3-6 hr

Indications
Bronchial asthma
Reversible bronchospasm associated with exercise, chronic bronchitis, and emphysema

Contraindications
Hypersensitivity
Tachydysrhythmias
Digitalis-induced tachycardia

Adverse Reactions
Usually transient and dose related
Restlessness, apprehension
Palpitations
Tachycardia
Chest pain
Coughing
Bronchospasm
Nausea
Facial flushing

Drug Interactions
Other sympathomimetics may exacerbate adverse cardiovascular effects.
MAOIs may potentiate tachydysrhythmias.
Beta blockers may antagonize terbutaline.

How Supplied
Tablet:	2.5, 5 mg
MDI:	200 mcg/metered spray
Parenteral:	1 mg/ml ampule

Dosage and Administration
Adult:	0.25 mg SQ; may repeat in 15-30 min (maximum dose 0.5 mg/4 hr)
	400 mcg (two inhalations by MDI) q 4-6 hr; allow 1-2 min between inhalations
Pediatric:	Not recommended for children under 12
	0.01 mg/kg/dose SQ q 15-20 min prn (maximum 0.25 mg dose)
	0.03-0.05 mg/kg in 1.25 ml saline for aerosolization q 4 hr

Special Consideration
Pregnancy safety: Category B.
Carefully monitor vital signs.
Use with caution in patients with cardiovascular disease or hypertension.

> **NOTE:** Bronchodilators may initially worsen hypoxemia by increasing ventilation-perfusion mismatching. Thus these patients should receive *oxygen* before and during bronchodilator administration.

● THIAMINE (BETAXIN)

Class
Vitamin (B_1)

Description
Thiamine combines with ATP to form thiamine pyrophosphate coenzyme, a necessary component for carbohydrate metabolism. Most vitamins required by the body are obtained through diet, but certain states, such as alcoholism and malnourishment, may affect the intake, absorption, and use of thiamine. The brain is extremely sensitive to thiamine deficiency.

Onset and Duration
Onset: Rapid
Duration: Depends on the degree of
                  deficiency

Indications
Coma of unknown origin (before the administration
    of *dextrose 50%* or *naloxone*)
Delirium tremens
Beriberi (rare)
Wernicke's encephalopathy

Contraindications
There are no significant drug interactions with other
    emergency medications.

Adverse Reactions
Hypotension (from rapid injection or large dose)
Anxiety
Diaphoresis
Nausea and vomiting
Allergic reaction (usually from IV injection; very rare)

Drug Interactions
There are no significant drug interactions with other
    emergency medications.

How Supplied
1000 mg in 10-ml vial (100 mg/ml)

Dosage and Administration
Adult: 100 mg slow IV or IM
Pediatric: 10-25 mg slow IV or IM

Special Considerations
Pregnancy safety: Category A.
Large IV doses may cause respiratory difficulties.
Anaphylactic reactions have been reported.

● TISSUE PLASMINOGEN ACTIVATOR (T-PA, RECOMBINANT ALTEPLASE)

Class
Thrombolytic agent

Description
Tissue plasminogen activator is a naturally occurring enzyme derived from DNA technology. The enzyme binds to fibrin-bound plasminogen at the site of an arterial clot, thus converting plasminogen to plasmin. Plasmin digests the fibrin strands of the clot and restores perfusion to the occluded artery. In emergency care, thrombolytic agents are used to treat selected patients with acute evolving myocardial infarction.

Onset and Duration
Onset: Clot lysis often occurs within
                  60-90 min
Duration: ½ hr (80% cleared in 10 min)

Indications (same as other thrombolytic agents)
Acute evolving myocardial infarction
Massive pulmonary emboli
Arterial thrombosis and embolism
To clear arteriovenous cannulas

Contraindications
Active bleeding
Recent surgery (within 2-3 weeks)
Recent CVA
Prolonged CPR
Intracranial or intraspinal surgery
Recent significant trauma (particularly head trauma)
Uncontrolled hypertension

Adverse Reactions
Bleeding (GI, GU, intracranial, other sites)
Allergic reactions
Hypotension
Chest pain
Reperfusion dysrhythmias
Abdominal pain
Active bleeding
Recent CVA
Prolonged CPR
Recent surgery (within 2-3 weeks)
Peptic ulcer disease
Recent intracranial or intraspinal surgery or trauma
Uncontrolled hypertension

Drug Interactions
Acetylsalicylic acid may increase risk of bleeding
    (may also be beneficial in improving overall effec-
    tiveness).
Heparin and other anticoagulants may also increase
    risk of bleeding and improve overall effectiveness.

How Supplied

20 mg (with 20 ml of diluent)
50 mg (with 50 ml of diluent)
May further dilute with equal amounts of 0.9% sodium chloride or D_5W

Dosage and Administration

Adult:	10-mg bolus (IV) over 2 min, then 50 mg over 1 hr, then 20 mg over the second hr, and 20 mg over the third hour for a total dose of 100 mg (other doses may be prescribed by medical control)
Pediatric:	Safety not established

Special Considerations

Pregnancy safety: Contraindicated.
Closely monitor vital signs.
Observe for bleeding.
Obtain blood sample for coagulation studies before administration.
Do not administer IM injections to patients receiving thrombolytic drugs.
No arterial blood gas specimens should be drawn on potential thrombolytic therapy candidates because of bleeding tendency.
Use caution when moving patient to avoid bleeding or bruising.

● VERAPAMIL (ISOPTIN)

Class

Calcium channel blocker (class IV antidysrhythmic)

Description

Verapamil is used as an antidysrhythmic and antianginal agent. It works by inhibiting the movement of calcium ions across cell membranes. The slow calcium ion current blocked by verapamil is more important for the activity of the SA and AV nodes than for many other tissues in the heart. By interfering with this current, calcium channel blockers achieve some selectivity of action. Verapamil decreases atrial automaticity, reduces AV conduction velocity, and prolongs the AV nodal refractory period. In addition, verapamil depresses myocardial contractility, reduces vascular smooth muscle tone, and dilates coronary arteries and arterioles in normal and ischemic tissues.

Onset and Duration

Onset:	2-5 min
Duration:	30-60 min

Indications

PSVTs
Atrial flutter with a rapid ventricular response
Atrial fibrillation with a rapid ventricular response

Contraindications

Hypersensitivity
Sick-sinus syndrome (unless the patient has a functioning pacemaker)
Second- or third-degree heart block
Hypotension
Cardiogenic shock
Severe congestive heart failure
WPW with atrial fibrillation or flutter
Patients receiving intravenous beta blockers
Wide-complex tachycardias (ventricular tachycardia can deteriorate into ventricular fibrillation when calcium channel blockers are given)

Adverse Reactions

Dizziness
Headache
Nausea and vomiting
Hypotension
Bradycardia
Complete AV block
Peripheral edema

Drug Interactions

Verapamil increases serum concentration of *digoxin.*
Beta-adrenergic blockers may have additive negative inotropic and chronotropic effects.
Antihypertensives may potentiate hypotensive effects.

How Supplied

Tablet: 40, 80, 120 mg
Parenteral: 5 mg/2 ml in 2-, 4-, 5-ml vials or 2-, 4-ml ampules

Dosage and Administration

> **NOTE: Many physicians recommend slow IV administration of 500 mg *calcium chloride* before dose of verapamil to minimize the untoward results of hypotension and bradycardia.**

Adult:	2.5-5.0 mg IV bolus over 2 min; repeat doses of 5-10 mg may be given every 15-30 min (maximum of 20 mg)
Pediatric:	0.1-0.2 mg/kg/dose IV over 2 min; repeat in 30 min if not effective

Special Considerations

Pregnancy safety: Category C.
Closely monitor patient's vital signs.
Be prepared to resuscitate.
AV block or asystole may occur as a result of slowed AV conduction.

BIBLIOGRAPHY

CHAPTER 1

Ampolsk A: National perspective, *Emerg Mag* May, 1989.

Damus A: Emergency medicine: historical perspectives, *Mercy Med* 8(2,3):1989.

Dorsey J: *Psychology of ethics*, Detroit, 1974, Center for Health Education.

E.M.T. paramedic national standard curriculum instructor's lesson plan, Washington, DC, 1985, US Government Printing Office.

Emergency medical services transportation systems and available facilities, Lexington, Mass, 1988, National EMS Clearinghouse.

Federal Emergency Management Agency: *Introduction to emergency medical services*, Emmitsburg, 1984, The Agency.

Fenichel D: Growing pains, *Emerg Mag* March, 1989.

Fitch J: *Beyond the street*, Solana Beach, 1988, JEMS Publications.

Gonsalves D: Historical background of emergency medical services in the United States, *Emerg Care Q* November, 1988.

Haller J: The beginnings of urban ambulance service in the United States and England, *J Emerg Med* 8: 1990.

Hinman A: 1889 to 1989: a century of health and disease, *Pub Health Rep* July-August, 1990.

Kuehl A: *EMS medical director's handbook*, National Association of EMS Physicians, St Louis, 1989, Mosby.

McKay J: Historical review of emergency medical services: EMT roles, and EMT utilization in emergency departments, *Emerg Nurs* 11(1):1985.

McKechnie J, editor: *Webster's new universal unabridged dictionary*, ed 2, New York, 1988, Simon & Schuster.

Page J: A brief history of EMS, *JEMS* August, 1989.

Page J: *The paramedics*, Morristown, 1976, Backdraft Publications.

Rockwood C et al: History of emergency medical services in the United States, *J Trauma* 16(4):1986.

Roush W, editor: *Principles of EMS systems*, Dallas, 1989, American College of Emergency Physicians.

Salomone J: Ethics in EMS, *JEMS* May, 1989.

Training and certification of EMS personnel, Lexington, Mass, 1990, National EMS Clearinghouse.

US Department of Transportation National Highway Traffic Safety Administration: *Emergency medical services: 1990 and beyond*, Washington, DC, 1990, The Administration.

US emergency medicine statistical/historical profile, *ACEP News* April, 1990.

CHAPTER 2

American Heart Association: *Textbook of advanced cardiac life support*, ed 2, Dallas, 1990, The Association.

Association of Air Medical Services: *Standards, minimum quality standards and safety guidelines*, Pasadena, Calif, 1988, The Association.

Burney R: Ground versus air transport of trauma victims: medical and logistical considerations, *Ann Emerg Med* December, 1986.

Committee on Trauma, American College of Surgeons. *Resources for optimal care of the injured patient*, Chicago, 1990, The College.

E.M.T. paramedic national standard curriculum instructor's lesson plan, Washington, DC, 1985, US Government Printing Office.

Federal Emergency Management Agency: *Introduction to emergency medical services*, Emmitsburg, Md, 1984, The Agency.

Federal Emergency Management Agency, US Fire Administration. *Rockville report*, Washington, DC, 1980, The Administration.

Fitch J: *Beyond the street*, Solana Beach, 1988, JEMS Publications.

Kuehl A, editor: *EMS medical director's handbook*, St Louis, 1989, Mosby.

McNeil E: *Airborne care of the ill and injured*, New York, 1983, Springer-Verlag.

Page J: A brief history of EMS, *JEMS* August, 1989.

Rockwood C et al: History of emergency medical services in the United States, *J Trauma* 16(4):1986.

Roush W, editor: *Principles of EMS systems*, Dallas, 1989, American College of Emergency Physicians.

Sargent K, editor: Helicopter EMS, *Emerg Care Q* 2(3):1986.

Standard specification for minimum performance requirements for emergency medical services ground vehicles (F1230-89), *ASTM* November, 1989.

Stanford T: Thirty years too late, *Emerg Mag* April, 1988.

US Department of Transportation, National Highway Safety Administration: *Air medical crew national standard curriculum*, Washington, DC, 1988, The Department.

CHAPTER 3

Ayres J: Current controversies in prehospital resuscitation of the terminally ill patient, *Prehosp Dis Med* January-March, 1990.

Criminal liability for failure to treat: New York's toughest new law, *Emerg Medl Tech Leg Bull* 8(4):1984.

Crimmins T: The need for a prehospital DNR system, *Prehosp Dis Med* January-March, 1990.

EMS negligence? Let the jury decide, *Emerg Med Tech Leg Bull* 10(3):1986.

E.M.T. paramedic national standard curriculum instructor's lesson plan, Washinton, DC, 1985, US Government Printing Office.

Fitch J: *Beyond the street,* Solana Beach, 1988, JEMS Publications.

Foster F: Law of consent: expressed-implied-refused, *Mo Emerg Med Serv* March-April, 1982.

Foster F: Legal precautions, *Mo Emerg Med Serv* November, 1983.

Frew S: *Street law,* Reston, 1983, Reston Publishing.

Goldstein A: *EMS and the law,* Bowie, 1983, Brady Company.

Good samaritan immunity challenged, *Emerg Med Tech Leg Bull* 12(4):1988.

Hall S: New act compels EMS to define new roles, *JEMS* January, 1992.

Interference at the scene, *Emerg Med Tech Leg Bull* 11(3):1987.

Lazar R: *EMS law,* Rockville, Md, 1989, Aspen Publications.

Page J: *EMS legal primer,* Solana Beach, 1985, JEMS Publications.

Shanaberger C: The moment of death, *JEMS* 1988.

Stratton S: Withholding CPR in the prehospital setting, *Prehosp Dis Med* 1990.

CHAPTER 4

Clawson J: Dispatch life support: establishing standards that work, *JEMS* July, 1990.

Cross M, Maniscalco P: Cellular technology: an EMS overview, *Emerg Med Serv* 18(7):1988.

E.M.T. paramedic national standard curriculum, instructor's lesson plan, Washington, DC, 1985, US Government Printing Office.

Emergency medical services dispatcher national standard curriculum, ed 2, Washington, DC, 1983, US Government Printing Office.

Felt H: A primer on radio communications. I. Understanding the language, *JEMS* 5(4):1980.

Felt H: A primer on radio communications. II. Characteristics and considerations, *JEMS* 5(5):1980.

Felt H: A primer on radio communication. III. Configurations, *JEMS* 5(6):1980.

Johnson M et al: Is EMS communicating with the FCC? *JEMS* July, 1989.

Kleindienst R: The wave of the future, *Emerg Mag* January, 1990.

Public safety communications standard operating procedure manual, ed 19 (rev), 1982, Associated Public-Safety Communications Officers.

Roush W, editor: *Principles of EMS systems,* Dallas, 1989, American College of Emergency Physicians.

Rules and regulations, part 90, Washington, DC, 1979, US Government Printing Office.

Stanford T: *EMS report writing: a pocket reference,* Englewood Cliffs, NJ, 1992, Brady Publishing.

Talley D: *Radio engineering and field survey transmission methods for mobile telephone systems,* Institute of Electrical and Electronic Engineers, Inc, VC-14(1):1965.

US Department of Transportation, National Highway Traffic Safety Administration: *Training program for emergency medical technician: dispatcher,* Washington, DC, 1976, US Government Printing Office.

Wilson M, editor: *The 1988 ARRL handbook,* Newington, 1988, American Radio Relay League.

Yamamoto L: Cellular telephone communication between hospitals and ambulances, *Am J Emerg Med* 6(1):1988.

CHAPTER 5

American Academy of Orthopaedic Surgeons: *Basic rescue and emergency care,* Park Ridge, 1990, The Academy.

Cotter M: Firefighting skills for EMTs, *JEMS* June, 1984.

E.M.T. paramedic national standard curriculum, instructor's lesson plan, Washington, DC, 1985, US Government Printing Office.

Essentials of fire fighting, ed 2, Stillwater, International Fire Service Training Association, 1983, Fire Protection Publications.

Moore R: *Vehicle rescue and extrication,* St Louis, 1991, Mosby.

US Department of Labor Occupational Safety and Health Administration: *General industry,* OSHA 2206, Washington, DC, 1981, The Department.

CHAPTER 6

Air medical crew national standard curriculum, Pasadena, 1988, ASHBEAMS, US Department of Transportation/NHTSA.

American Academy of Orthopaedic Surgeons: *Basic rescue and emergency care,* Park Ridge, 1990, The Academy.

Association of Air Medical Services. *Standards, minimum quality standards and safety guidelines,* Pasadena, Calif, 1988, The Association.

Auf Der Heide E: *Disaster response,* St Louis, 1989, Mosby.

Burney R: Ground versus air transport of trauma victims: medical and logistical considerations, *Ann Emerg Med* 1986.

Champion H: Helicopter triage, *Emerg Care Q* 2(3):1986.

Cleary V et al: *Prehospital care administrative and clinical management,* Rockville, Md, 1987, Aspen Publications.

Committee on Trauma, American College of Surgeons. *Resources for optimal care of the injured patient,* Chicago, 1990, The College.

E.M.T. paramedic national standard curriculum instructor's lesson plan, Washington, DC, 1985, US Government Printing Office.

Greater St Louis Area Fire Chiefs Association: *The incident command system,* St Louis, 1988, The Association.

Kuehl A, editor: *EMS medical directors' handbook,* St Louis, 1989, Mosby.

Lee G: *Flight nursing: principles and practice,* St Louis, 1991, Mosby.

McNeil E: *Airborne care of the ill and injured,* New York, 1983, Springer-Verlag.

Moore R: *Vehicle rescue and extrication,* St Louis, 1991, Mosby.

Morris G: Applying the incident command system to mass casualty incidents, *Emerg Care Q* 2(1):1986.

National Fire Protection Association. *NFPA 1500 standard on fire department occupational safety and health program,* Quincy, Mass, 1987, The Association.

Rhodes M: A prospective study of field triage for helicopter transport, *Emerg Care Q* 2(3):1986.

Roush W, editor: *Principles of EMS systems,* Dallas, 1989, American College of Emergency Physicians.

US Environmental Protection Agency: *Title III fact sheet,* Washington, DC, 1988, The Agency.

CHAPTER 7

Adkins J: *Formula for safety,* Washington, DC, 1989, Atlantic Information Services.

Barker S: Hazardous materials emergencies: response and control, *Emerg Care Q* 2(1):1986.

Borak J et al: *Hazardous materials exposure,* Englewood Cliffs, NJ, 1991, Brady Publishing.

Bronstein A, Currance P: *Emergency Care for hazardous materials exposure,* St Louis, 1988, Mosby.

Burton B, Bayer M: Hazardous materials, *Top Emerg Med* 7(1):1985.

Carafano P: Handle with care, *Fire Command* 56(5):1989.

Currance P: EMS crosses hazmat lines, *JEMS* 1989.

E.M.T. paramedic national standard curriculum instructor's lesson plan, Washington, DC, 1985, US Government Printing Office.

Fire Service Training Association: *Hazardous materials for first responders,* ed 1, Stillwater, 1988, International Fire Protection Publications.

Manning R: Expose yourself to radiation (accident management), *JEMS* 1988.

Noll G et al: *Hazardous materials: managing the incident,* Stillwater, 1988, Fire Protection Publications.

Office of the Federal Register, National Archives and Records Service, General Services Administration: *Code of federal regulations,* 49 CFR, 173.500, Parts 100-177, Washington, DC, 1981.

Ricks R: *Prehospital management of radiation accidents,* Oak Ridge, 1984, Oak Ridge Associated Universities.

Stutz D, Janusz S: *Hazardous materials injuries: a handbook for pre-hospital care,* ed 2, Beltsville, Md, 1988, Bradford Communications.

Title III list of lists, Washington, DC, 1990, Environmental Protection Agency, EPA 560/4-90-011.

US Department of Transportation: *Emergency response guidebook,* DOT P 5800.5, Washington, DC, 1990, The Department.

Verdile V, Full R: EMS and the hazmat response, *Emerg Mag* 1990.

CHAPTER 8

Aguilera D, Messick J: *Crisis intervention,* ed 6, St Louis, 1990, Mosby.

Bassuk E et al: *Behavioral emergencies,* Boston, 1983, Little, Brown.

Edwards D: *General psychology,* London, 1968, Macmillan.

E.M.T. paramedic national standard curriculum, instructor's lesson plan, Washington, DC, 1985, US Government Printing Office.

Everly G: *A clinical guide to the treatment of the human stress response,* New York, 1989, Plenum Press.

Freud dictionary of psychoanalysis, Greenwich, 1958, Fawcett Publications.

Haffen B, Frandsen K: *Psychological emergencies and crisis intervention,* Englewood, 1985, Morton Publishing.

Hall C, Gardner L: *Theories of personality,* New York, 1970, Wiley & Sons.

Judd R, editor: Behavioral and psychological crisis in emergency medical services, *Top Emerg Med* 4(4):1983.

Mitchell J, Bray G: Critical incident stress management, *Resp Mag* September/October, 1986.

Mitchell J, Bray G: *Emergency services stress,* Englewood Cliffs, NJ, 1990, Brady Publishing.

Mitchell J, Bray G: When disaster strikes. . . , *JEMS* 1983.

National Institute of Mental Health, Center for Mental Health Studies of Emergencies, U.S. Department of Health and Human Services: *Role stressors and supports for emergency workers,* Rockville, Md, 1985, The Department.

Patterson C: *Theories of counseling and psychotherapy,* ed 2, New York, 1973, Harper & Row.

Sarason I: *Abnormal psychology: the problem of maladaptive behavior,* New York, 1972, Meredith Corporation.

Selye H: *The stress of life,* New York, 1956, McGraw-Hill.

Selye H: *Stress without distress,* Philadelphia, 1974, Lippincott.

Selye H: *Stress in health and diseases,* Boston, 1976, Butterworth.

Spitzer C: Stress: the invisible toll on rescue workers, *Washington Post Health* May 10, 1988.

Windham R: An overview of stress in emergency services, *Calif Fireman* September, 1989.

CHAPTER 9

Cordón M: *Clinical calculations for nurses,* Englewood Cliffs, NJ, 1984, Prentice-Hall.

Dorland's illustrated medical dictionary, ed 25, Philadelphia, 1974, WB Saunders.

E.M.T. paramedic national standard curriculum instructor's lesson plan, Washington, DC, 1985, US Government Printing Office.

Everything you always wanted to know about metrics, Valdese, 1978, R&R Enterprises.

McKenry L, Salerno E: *Mosby's pharmacology in nursing,* ed 18, St Louis, 1992, Mosby.

Seeley R et al: *Anatomy & physiology,* ed 2, St Louis, 1992, Mosby.

CHAPTER 10

Berne R, Levy M: *Physiology,* ed 2, St Louis, 1988, Mosby.

Luciano D et al: *Human function and structure,* New York, 1978, McGraw-Hill.

Seeley R et al: *Anatomy and physiology,* ed 2, St Louis, 1992, Mosby.

Solomon E, Phillips G: *Understanding human anatomy and physiology,* Philadelphia, 1987, WB Sanders.

Thibodeau G: *Structure and function of the body,* ed 9, St Louis, 1992, Mosby.

CHAPTER 11

Assessing your patients, Horsham, 1981, Intermed Communications.

Bassuk E et al: *Behavioral emergencies, a field guide for EMTs and paramedics,* Boston, 1983, Little, Brown.

Burnside J: *Physical diagnosis,* ed 16, Baltimore, 1981, Williams & Wilkins.

Campbell J, editor: *BTLS basic prehospital trauma care,* ed 2, Englewood Cliffs, NJ, 1988, Brady Publishing.

Cosgriff J, Anderson D: *The practice of emergency care,* ed 2, Philadelphia, 1984, Lippincott.

Cugell D: Lung sound nomenclature, *Am Rev Respir Dis* 136:1987.

Curriculum guide for public-safety and emergency-response workers: prevention of transmission of human immunodeficiency virus and hepatitis B virus, Atlanta, 1989, US Government Printing Office.

Dierking B: The stress of trauma, psychological response of the pediatric patient, *JEMS* 1988.

Dierking B et al: Initial prehospital assessment of the pediatric patient, *JEMS* April, 1988.

E.M.T. paramedic national standard curriculum instructor's lesson plan, Washington, DC, 1985, US Government Printing Office.

Erickson B: *Heart sounds and murmurs,* St Louis, 1987, Mosby.

Luciano D et al: *Human function and structure,* New York, 1978, McGraw-Hill.

McSwain N et al, editors: *PHTLS basic and advanced prehospital trauma life support,* ed 2, Akron, Ohio, 1990, Emergency Training.

Mikami R et al: International symposium on lung sounds, *Chest* 92(2):1987.

Moore P: When you have to think small for a neurological exam, *RN Mag* 1988.

Rey R, editor: *Emergency nursing core curriculum,* ed 3, Philadelphia, 1987, WB Saunders.

Rothenberg M: *Advanced medical life support: adult medical emergencies,* St Louis, 1987, Mosby.

Seeley R et al: *Anatomy and physiology,* ed 2, St Louis, 1992, Mosby.

Seidel H et al: *Mosby's guide to physical examination,* ed 2, St Louis, 1992, Mosby.

Seidel J, Henderson D, editors: *Prehospital care of pediatric patients,* California EMSC Project, Los Angeles, 1987, American Academy of Pediatrics.

Silverman M: *Examination of the heart,* Dallas, 1978, American Heart Association.

Simon J, Goldberg A: *Prehospital pediatric life support,* St Louis, 1989, Mosby.

Solomon E, Phillips G: *Understanding human anatomy and physiology,* Philadelphia, 1987, WB Saunders.

Ward J: Lung sounds: easy to hear, hard to describe, *Respir Care* 34(1):1989.

Wilkins R et al: *Lung sounds: a practical guide,* St Louis, 1988, Mosby.

CHAPTER 12

American Heart Association: *Health provider's manual for basic life support,* Dallas, 1988, The Association.

American Heart Association. *Textbook of advanced cardiac life support,* Dallas, 1987, The Association.

American Heart Association. *Textbook of pediatric basic life support,* Dallas, 1988, The Association.

Benjamin G: Aspiration pneumonia, empyema, and lung abscess. In *Emergency medicine,* ed 2, New York, 1988, American College of Emergency Physicians, McGraw-Hill.

Berne R, Levy M: *Physiology,* ed 2, St Louis, 1988, Mosby.

Bosker G et al: *Geriatric emergency medicine,* St Louis, 1990, Mosby.

Burke S: *Human biology in health and disease,* New York, 1975, Wiley & Sons.

Campbell J, editor: *BTLS basic prehospital trauma care,* ed 2, Englewood Cliffs, NJ, 1988, Brady Publishing.

Currents in emergency cardiac care, American Heart Association and the Citizen CPR Foundation 1(1):1990.

E.M.T. paramedic national standard curriculum instructor's lesson plan, Washington, DC, 1985, US Government Printing Office.

Frass M et al: The esophageal tracheal combitube: preliminary results with a new airway for CPR, *Ann Emerg Med* 16:1987.

Frass M et el: Evaluation of esophageal tracheal combitube in cardiopulmonary resuscitation, *Crit Care Med* 15(6):1986.

Fuhrman G et al: Blunt laryngeal trauma: classification and management protocol, *J Emerg Nurs* 1990.

Garnett R et al: End-tidal carbon dioxide monitoring during cardiopulmonary resuscitation, *JAMA* 257(4): 1987.

Giard D, Ross C: The use of pulse oximetry in prehospital treatment and transport, *BOC Health Care* 1989.

Goldberg J et al: Colorimetric end-tidal carbon dioxide monitoring for tracheal intubation, *Anesth Analg* 70:1990.

Gorback M: *Emergency airway management,* Philadelphia, 1990, BC Decker.

Guyton A: *Human physiology and mechanisms of disease,* Philadelphia, 1982, WB Saunders.

Kalish M: Airway management in maxillofacial trauma, *Emerg Med Serv Mag* July, 1989.

Luicano D et al: *Human function and structure,* New York, 1978, McGraw-Hill.

McGuire T, Pointer J: Evaluation of a pulse oximeter in the prehospital setting, *Ann Emerg Med* 17(10):1988.

McSwain N et al, editors: *PHTLS basic and advanced prehospital trauma life support,* ed 2, Akron, Ohio, 1990, Emergency Training.

Miller K: The ABGs of emergency care, *Emerg Mag* 1988.

Morrow J: Simplifying nursing management of pediatric airways and intravenous infusions, *J Emerg Nurs* March/April, 1988.

Mullen R et al: Guidelines for prevention of transmission of human immunodeficiency virus and hepatitis B to health care and public safety workers, *MMWR* 1989.

National Safety Council: *Accident facts,* Chicago, 1991, The Council.

Ornato J: Providing CPR and emergency care during the AIDS epidemic, *Emerg Med Serv* 1989.

Rothstein R, editor: Respiratory emergencies. I and II. *Top Emerg Med* 2(1,2):1980.

Seeley R, et al: *Anatomy and physiology,* ed 2, St Louis, 1992, Mosby.

Sheehy S: *Mosby's manual of emergency care,* ed 3, St Louis, 1990, Mosby.

Simon J, Goldberg A: *Prehospital pediatric life support,* St Louis, 1989, Mosby.

Solomon E, Phillips G: *Understanding human anatomy and physiology,* Philadelphia, 1987, WB Saunders.

Stanford T: ET: a different approach, *Emerg Mag* December, 1988.

Stanford T: A sizeable difference, *Emerg Mag* October, 1987.

US Department of Health and Human Services, Centers for Disease Control. *Curriculum guide for public-safety and emergency-response workers: prevention of transmission of human immunodeficiency virus and hepatitis B virus,* Atlanta, 1989, The Centers.

CHAPTER 13

American Heart Association: *Textbook of advanced cardiac life support,* Dallas, 1987, The Association.

Baxt W: *Trauma: the first hour,* Norwalk, 1985, Appleton-Century-Crofts.

Berk J, Sampliner J, editors: *Handbook of critical care,* Boston, 1990, Little, Brown.

Beren R, Levy M: *Physiology,* ed 2, St Louis, 1988, Mosby.

Bourn S: Cardiogenic shock: a case of body power failure, *JEMS* January, 1989.

Bourn S, Taigman M: Seeking approval for the antishock garment, *JEMS* January, 1989.

Broughton J: *Understanding blood gases,* Akron, Ohio, 1971, Ohio Medical Products.

Campbell J, editor: *BTLS basic prehospital trauma care,* ed 2, Englewood Cliffs, NJ, 1988, Brady Publishing.

Cason D: Anaphylactic shock, *JEMS* February, 1989.

Clark M: *Contemporary biology,* Philadelphia, 1973, WB Saunders.

Dison N: *Simplified drugs and solutions for nurses,* ed 10, St Louis, 1992, Mosby.

Elrich F: *Pediatric trauma, Top Emerg Med* 4(3):1982.

E.M.T. paramedic national standard curriculum instructor's lesson plan, Washington, DC, 1985, US Government Printing Office.

Gorgen A: Shock: the lay-up, the sinker, the bounce, *JEMS* December, 1988.

Gorgen A: An unpleasant surprise: compensated shock, *JEMS* December, 1988.

Guyton A: *Human physiology and mechanisms of disease,* Philadelphia, 1982, WB Saunders.

Hardaway R, editor: *Shock: the reversible stage of dying,* Littleton, 1988, PSG Publishing.

Haynes B et al: Catheter introducers for rapid fluid resuscitation, *Ann Emerg Med* 12(10): 1983.

Ho M, Saunders C, editor: *Current emergency diagnosis and treatment,* Norwalk, Conn, 1990, Appleton & Lange.

Koepke J: *Guide to clinical laboratory diagnosis,* ed 2, New York, 1979, Appleton-Century-Crofts.

Luciano D et al: *Human function and structure,* New York, 1978, McGraw-Hill.

Manual of pediatric advanced cardiac care and trauma support for life, St Louis, 1986, Cardinal Glennon Children's Hospital.

McHugh M: IO infusion in children, *Emerg Mag* January, 1990.

McKenry L, Salerno E: *Mosby's pharmacology in nursing,* ed 18, St Louis, 1992, Mosby.

McSwain N, Kernstein M: *Evaluation and management of trauma,* Norwalk, Conn, 1987, Appleton-Century-Crofts.

McSwain N, Kernstein M: Pneumatic anti-shock garment: state of the art 1988, *Ann Emerg Med* May, 1988.

McSwain N et al, editors: *PHTLS basic and advanced prehospital trauma life support,* ed 2, Akron, Ohio, 1990, Emergency Training.

Morrison M, editor: *Respiratory intensive care nursing,* ed 2, Boston, 1979, Little, Brown.

Needle and cannula techniques, North Chicago, 1977, Abbott Laboratories.

O'Keefe J: The Hickman indwelling catheter in prehospital use, *JEMS* June, 1986.

Pratt J: Intraosseous infusion, *Int Pediatr* 4(1):1989.

Prehospital care of pediatric patients, Los Angelos, 1987, The California EMSC Project, Los Angeles Pediatric Society; Chapter 2, American Academy of Pediatrics.

Seeley R et al: *Anatomy and physiology,* ed 2, St Louis, 1992, Mosby.

Sheehy S: *Mosby's manual of emergency care,* ed 3, St Louis, 1990, Mosby.

Sheeler P, Bianchi D: *Cell biology,* New York, 1980, Wiley & Sons.

Sholtis B et al: The *Lippincott manual of nursing practice,* ed 3, Philadelphia, 1982, JB Lippincott.

Tintinalli J et al, editors: *Emergency medicine: a comprehensive study guide,* ed 2, New York, 1988, McGraw-Hill.

Trauma reference manual, Bowie, 1985, Maryland Institute for Emergency Medical Services Systems, Brady Publishing.

Warren C: Shock: assessment and intervention, *Curr Con Trauma Care* 1980.

CHAPTER 14

American Heart Association: Guidelines for cardiopulmonary resuscitation and emergency cardiac care, *JAMA* 268(16):2172, 1992.

American Heart Association: *Textbook of advanced cardiac life support,* Dallas, 1987, The Association.

Barkin R, Rosen P: *Emergency pediatrics,* ed 3, St Louis, 1990, Mosby.

Bayer M, Rumack B, editors: Poisonings and overdose, *Top Emerg Med* 1(3):1979.

Brunner L, Suddarth D: *Lippincott manual of nursing practice,* ed 3, Philadelphia, 1982, JB Lippincott.

Clark J, Pringle R: Pediatric respiratory drugs, *Emerg Mag* December, 1990.

Clark J et al: *Pharmacologic basis of nursing practice,* ed 4, St Louis, 1993, Mosby.

Collier C: *Recommendations for needle-stick, puncture wounds, and muco-cutaneous blood and body fluid exposure in health care workers,* Jefferson City, Mo, 1992, Missouri Department of Health Bureau of Communicable Disease Control.

Cordón M: *Clinical calculations for nurses,* Englewood Cliffs, NJ, 1984, Prentice-Hall.

DiMarco J et al: *Adenosine for paroxysmal supraventricular tachycardia: dose ranging and comparison with verapamil,* Dallas, 1990, The American College of Physicians.

E.M.T. paramedic national standard curriculum instructor's lesson plan, Washington, DC, 1985, US Government Printing Office.

Fedson D: *Immunizations for health care workers and patients in hospitals. Prevention and control of nosocomial infections,* Baltimore, 1987, Williams & Wilkins.

Glanze W, editor: *Mosby's medical, nursing, and allied health dictionary,* ed 3, St Louis, 1990, Mosby.

Goldberg E: *Treatment of cardiac emergencies,* ed 5, St Louis, 1990, Mosby.

Gonzalez E, Ornato J: Field drug reference for emergency care providers, Hamilton, 1990, Drug Intelligence Publications.

Gorback M: *Emergency airway management,* Philadelphia, 1990, BC Decker.

Harris L, Mistovich J: Prehospital administration of aerosolized bronchodilators, *EMS Mag* October, 1988.

Katzung B: *Basic and clinical pharmacology,* ed 4, Norwalk, Conn, 1989, Appleton & Lange.

Lee G: *Flight nursing: principles and practice,* St Louis, 1991, Mosby.

Levy D: Adenosine: a new drug for PSVT, *Emerg Mag* November, 1990.

Levy D: A benzodiazepine breakthrough, *Emerg Mag* September, 1989.

Levy D: Emergency use of bronchodilators, *Emerg Mag* April, 1988.

Madigan K: *Prehospital emergency drugs,* St Louis, 1990, Mosby.

McKenry L, Salerno E: *Mosby's pharmacology in nursing,* ed 18, St Louis, 1992, Mosby.

National Institute for Occupational Safety and Health,

Centers for Disease Control: *Guidelines for prevention of transmission of human immunodeficiency virus and hepatitis B virus to health-care and public-safety workers,* Atlanta, 1989, The Centers.

Needle and cannula techniques, Chicago, 1977, Abbott Laboratories.

Pratt J: Intraosseous infusion, *Int Pediatr* 4(1):19, 1989.

Protection against occupational exposure to hepatitis B virus (HBV) and human immunodeficiency virus (HIV), *Federal Register,* Washington, DC, 1987, Department of Labor, Department of Health and Human Services.

Rosen P et al: *Essentials of emergency medicine,* St Louis, 1991, Mosby.

Seeley R et al: *Anatomy and physiology,* ed 2, St Louis, 1992, Mosby.

St. Louis Post Dispatch, St Louis, Mo, July 7, 1988. p. 1D

Stein L, Cole R: *Early administration of corticosteroids in emergency room treatment of acute asthma,* Dallas, 1990, American College of Physicians.

Syverud S, et al: Prehospital use of neuromuscular blocking agents in a helicopter ambulance program, *Ann Emerg Med* 17(3):237, 1988.

Thibodeau G: *Structure and function of the body,* ed 9, St Louis, 1992, Mosby.

Wickham R: Advances in venous access devices and nursing management strategies, *Nurs Clin North Am* 25(2):1990.

Wilson S, Thompson J: *Respiratory Disorders,* St Louis, 1990, Mosby.

CHAPTER 15

American College of Surgeons: *A guide to emergency care of eye injuries,* Chicago, 1977, The College.

Campbell J, editor: *BTLS basic prehospital trauma care,* ed 2, Englewood Cliffs, NJ, 1988, Brady Publishing.

Committee on Trauma, American College of Surgeons: *Resources for optimal care of the injured patient,* Chicago, 1990, The College.

Emergency Nurses Association: *Trauma nursing core course (provider) manual,* ed 2, Chicago, 1986, The Association.

Fackler M: Wound ballistics: a review of common misconceptions, *JAMA* 1988.

Goldman R: For your eyes only, *Emerg Med Serv* July, 1989.

Krasner P: Management of avulsed teeth, *Emerg Med Serv* July, 1989.

Lee G: *Flight nursing: principles and practice,* St Louis, 1991, Mosby.

London P: *Color atlas of diagnosis after recent injury,* St Louis, 1990, Mosby.

Managing contact lens removal, *Emerg Mag* October, 1980.

Manson P, Kelly K: Evaluation and management of the patient with facial trauma, *Emerg Med Serv* July, 1989.

McSwain N, Kerstein M: Evaluation and management of trauma, Norwalk, Conn, 1987, Appleton-Century-Crofts.

McSwain N et al, editors: *PHTLS basic and advanced pre-hospital trauma life support,* ed 2, Akron, Ohio, 1990, Emergency Training.

Moore E, editor: *Early care of the injured patient,* ed 4, Philadelphia, 1990, Committee on Trauma, American College of Surgeons, BC Decker.

Ragge N, Easty D: *Immediate eye care,* St Louis, 1991, Mosby.

Sheehy S: *Mosby's manual of emergency care,* ed 3, St Louis, 1990, Mosby.

Shires T: *Care of the trauma patient,* ed 2, New York, 1979, McGraw-Hill.

Tintinalli J et al, editors: *Emergency medicine: a comprehensive study guide,* ed 2, New York, 1988, McGraw-Hill.

Trunkey D, Lewis F: *Current therapy of trauma,* ed 3, St Louis, 1991, Mosby.

US Department of Justice, Federal Bureau of Investigation: *Handbook of forensic science,* Washington, DC, 1981, The Department.

Weigelt J, McCormack A: *Mechanism of injury: trauma nursing from resuscitation through rehabilitation,* Philadelphia, 1988, WB Saunders.

CHAPTER 16

Achauer B: *Management of the burned patient,* Norwalk, Conn, 1987, Appleton & Lange.

American Burn Association: Hospital and prehospital resources for optimal care of patients with burn injury, *J Burn Care Rehab* 1988.

Better O, Stein J: Early management of shock and prophylaxis of acute renal failure in traumatic rhabdomyolysis, *New Engl J Med* March, 1990.

Committee on Trauma, American College of Surgeons: *Resources for optimal care of the injured patient,* Chicago, 1990, The College.

Demling R, LaLonde C: *Burn trauma,* New York, 1989, Thieme Medical Publishers.

Dressler D et al: *Thermal injury,* St Louis, 1988, Mosby.

E.M.T. paramedic national standard curriculum instructor's lesson plan, Washington, DC, 1985, US Government Printing Office.

Epifano P: *Trauma nursing: from resuscitation through rehabilitation,* Philadelphia, 1988, WB Saunders.

Guyton A: *Human physiology and mechanism of disease,* Philadelphia, 1982, WB Saunders.

Kobernick M: Electrical injuries: pathophysiology and emergency management, *Ann Emerg Med* 1982.

Kunkle R: *Medical care of entrapped patients in confined spaces: proceedings of the International Workshop on Earthquake Injury Epidemiology for Mitigation and Response,* Johns Hopkins University, Rockville, Md, July, 1989.

Lavin R: The high-pressure demands of compartment syndrome, *RN* 1989.

Lee G: *Flight nursing: principles and practice,* St Louis, 1991, Mosby.

Martyn J: *Acute management of the burned patient,* Philadelphia, 1990, WB Saunders.

McLaughlin E: *Critical care of the burned patient,* Rockville, Md, 1990, Aspen Publishers.

McSwain N, Kerstein M: *Evaluation and management of trauma,* Norwalk, Conn, 1987, Appleton-Century-Crofts.

McSwain N et al, editors: *PHTLS basic and advanced pre-hospital trauma life support,* ed 2, Akron, Ohio, 1990, Emergency Training.

Nebraska Burn Institute: *Advanced burn life support course provider's manual,* Lincoln, Neb, 1990, The Institute.

Noji E: *Training of search and rescue teams for structural collapse events: a multidisciplinary approach, new aspects of disaster medicine,* Tokyo, Japan, 1989, Hersu Publishing.

Orlando R: Smoke inhalation injury, *Emerg Care Q* 1985.

Proehl J: Compartment syndrome, *J Emerg Nurs* 1988.

Rea R et al: *Emergency nursing core curriculum,* Philadelphia, 1987, Emergency Nurses Association, WB Saunders.

Seward P: Electrical injuries: trauma with a difference, *Emerg Med* 1987.

Stockwell S: Muscle damage acts as a red flag for crush syndrome, *Emerg Med News* May, 1990.

Tintinalli J et al, editors: *Emergency medicine: a comprehensive study guide,* ed 2, New York, 1988, McGraw-Hill.

Trunkey D, Frank L: *Current therapy of trauma,* ed 3, St Louis, 1991, Mosby.

CHAPTER 17

American Heart Association: *Healthcare provider's manual for basic life support,* Dallas, 1988, The Association.

American Heart Association: *Textbook of advanced cardiac life support,* Dallas, 1988, The Association.

American Heart Association: *Textbook of pediatric basic life support,* Dallas, 1988, The Association.

Berk J, Sampliner J, editors: *Handbook of critical care,* ed 3, Boston, 1990, Little, Brown.

Bosker G et al: *Geriatric emergency medicine,* St Louis, 1990, Mosby.

Callaham M: *Current practice of emergency medicine,* ed 2, Philadelphia, 1991, BC Decker.

Cosgriff J et al: *The practice of emergency care,* ed 2, Philadelphia, 1984, Lipincott.

E.M.T. paramedic national standard curriculum instructor's lesson plan, Washington, DC, 1985, US Government Printing Office.

Gorback M: *Emergency airway management,* Philadelphia, 1990, BC Decker.

Grimes D: *Infectious diseases,* St Louis, 1991, Mosby.

Hale D: Asthma deaths on rise in U.S., *New York Times,* August 2, 1990.

Katzung B: *Basic and clinical pharmacology,* Norwalk, Conn, 1989, Appleton & Lange.

Lee G: *Flight nursing: principles and practice,* St Louis, 1991, Mosby.

Lodge D, Grant H: *Handbook of emergency care procedures,* Englewood Cliffs, NJ, 1988, Brady Publishing.

National Safety Council: *Accident facts*, Chicago, 1991, The Council.

O'Doherty D, Fermaglich J: *Handbook of neurologic emergencies*, Flushing, 1977, Medical Examination Publishing.

Rosen P et al: *Essentials of emergency medicine*, St Louis, 1991, Mosby.

Thibodeau G: *Structure and function of the body*, ed 9, St Louis, 1992, Mosby.

Tintinalli J et al, editors: *Emergency medicine: a comprehensive study guide*, ed 2, New York, 1988, McGraw-Hill.

Wilson S, Thompson J: *Respiratory disorders*, St Louis, 1990, Mosby.

CHAPTER 18

American Heart Association: *Health care provider's manual for basic life support*, Dallas, 1988, The Association.

American Heart Association: *Instructor's manual for advanced cardiac life support (early defibrillation)*, Dallas, 1990, The Association.

American Heart Association: *Textbook of advanced cardiac life support*, Dallas, 1987.

Atwood S et al: *Introduction to basic cardiac dysrhythmias*, St Louis, 1990, Mosby.

Balke L et al: *Defibrillation: a manual for the EMT*, Philadelphia, 1985, JB Lippincott.

Brown K, Jacobson S: *Mastering dysrhythmias: a problem-solving guide*, Philadelphia, 1988, FA Davis.

Callaham M: *Current practice of emergency medicine*, ed 2, Philadelphia, 1991, BC Decker.

Cosgriff J, Anderson D: *The practice of emergency care*, ed 2, Philadelphia, 1984, JB Lippincott.

Crockett P, Grose L: *Noninvasive pacing: what you should know*, Redmond, 1988, Physio-Control.

Currents in emergency cardiac care, American Heart Association and the Citizen CPR Foundation 2(2): 1991.

Dubin D: *Rapid interpretation of EKG's*, ed 3, Tampa, Fla, 1974, Cover Publishing.

E.M.T. paramedic national standard curriculum instructor's lesson plan, Washington, DC, 1985, US Government Printing Office.

Friery J, Cahill J: *Cardiac pacing*, *Emerg Mag* July, 1989.

Goldberg E: *Treatment of cardiac emergencies*, St Louis, 1990, Mosby.

Grauer Ken: *A practical guide to ECG interpretation*, St Louis, 1992, Mosby.

Grubbs T: The ultimate emergency: managing aortic aneurysms, *JEMS* 1991.

Higgins S: *Defibrillation: what you should know*, Redmond, 1978, Physio-Control.

Huszar R: *Basic dysrhythmias: interpretation and management*, St Louis, 1988, Mosby.

Little R, Little W: *Physiology of the heart and circulation*, ed 4, St Louis, 1989, Mosby.

Marriott H, Conover M: *Advanced concepts in arrhythmias*, ed 2, St Louis, 1989, Mosby.

Marriott H, Conover M: *Practical electrocardiography*, ed 8, Baltimore, 1988, Williams & Willkins.

Seeley R et al: *Anatomy and physiology*, ed 2, St Louis, 1992, Mosby.

Sheehy S: *Mosby's manual of emergency care*, ed 3, St Louis, 1990, Mosby.

Taigman M, Canan S: Cardiology practicum: precursors to complete heart block, *JEMS* September, 1991.

Taigman M, Canan S: Reading bundle branch blocks, *JEMS* 15(5):41, 1990.

Tintinalli J et al, editors: *Emergency medicine: a comprehensive study guide*, ed 2, New York, 1988, McGraw-Hill.

Weaver D et al: Use of the automatic external defibrillator in the management of out-of-hospital cardiac arrest, *New Engl J Med* 319:1988.

CHAPTER 19

Bourn S: Diabetic ketoacidosis: recognition and management in the field, *JEMS* May, 1988.

Callaham M: *Current practice of emergency medicine*, ed 2, Philadelphia, 1991, BC Decker.

E.M.T. paramedic national standard curriculum instructor's lesson plan, Washington, DC, 1985, US Government Printing Office.

Emergency treatment of the diabetic, New York, 1978, Cambridge Book.

Guyton A: *Human physiology and mechanisms of disease*, ed 3, Philadelphia, 1982, WB Saunders.

Seeley R et al: *Anatomy and physiology*, ed 2, St Louis, 1992, Mosby.

Rosen P et al: *Essentials of emergency medicine*, St Louis, 1991, Mosby.

A team approach to diabetes, *Barnes Health News* 8(4):1989.

Tintinalli J et al, editors: *Emergency medicine: a comprehensive study guide*, ed 2, New York, 1988, McGraw-Hill.

CHAPTER 20

American Heart Association: *1990 heart and stroke facts*, Dallas, 1989, The Association.

Berk J, editor: *Handbook of critical care*, ed 3, Boston, 1990, Little, Brown.

Callaham M: *Current practice of emergency medicine*, ed 2, Philadelphia, 1991, BC Decker.

E.M.T. paramedic national standard curriculum instructor's lesson plan, Washington, 1985, U.S. Government Printing Office.

Gallagher J, editor: Neurological emergencies, *Top Emerg Med* 4(2):1982.

Guidelines for cardiopulmonary resuscitation and emergency cardiac care, *JAMA* 268(16):1992.

Guyton A: *Human physiology and mechanisms of disease*, ed 3, Philadelphia, 1982, WB Sanders.

Lee G: *Flight nursing: principles and practice*, St Louis, 1991, Mosby.

O'Doherty D, Fermaglich J: *Handbook of neurologic emergencies*, Flushing, NY, 1977, Medical Examination Publishing.

Reid D, Fontanarosa P: It's all in your head: treating acute non-traumatic headaches, *JEMS* April, 1991.

Seeley R et al: *Anatomy and physiology*, ed 2, St Louis, 1992, Mosby.

Tintinalli J et al, editors: *Emergency medicine: a comprehensive study guide*, ed 2, New York, 1988, McGraw-Hill.

CHAPTER 21

Berk J, Sampliner J: *Handbook of critical care*, ed 3, Boston, 1990, Little, Brown.

Brunner L, Suddarth D: *The Lippincott manual of nursing practice*, ed 3, Philadelphia, 1982, JB Lippincott.

Callaham M: *Current practice of emergency medicine*, ed 2, Philadelphia, 1992, BC Decker.

Cosgriff J, Anderson D: *The practice of emergency care*, ed 2, Philadelphia, 1984, JB Lippincott.

Costrini N, Thomson W: *Manual of medical therapeutics*, ed 22, Boston, 1977, Little, Brown.

E.M.T. paramedic national standard curriculum instructor's lesson plan, Washington, DC, 1985, U.S. Government Printing Office.

Ho M, Saunders C: *Current emergency diagnosis and treatment*, ed 3, Norwalk, Conn, 1990, Appleton & Lange.

Lee G: *Flight nursing: principles and practices*, St Louis, 1991, Mosby.

Sanders J, Gardner L: *Handbook of medical emergencies*, ed 22, Garden City, 1978, Medical Examination Publishing.

Seeley R et al: *Anatomy and physiology*, ed 2, St Louis, 1992, Mosby.

Sheehy S: *Emergency nursing: principles and practice*, ed 3, St Louis, 1992, Mosby.

Thibodeau G: *Structure and function of the body*, ed 9, St Louis, 1992, Mosby.

Tintinalli J et al, editors: *Emergency medicine: a comprehensive study guide*, ed 2, New York, 1988, McGraw-Hill.

CHAPTER 22

Adamski D: Assessment and treatment of allergic response to stinging insects, *J Emerg Nurs* April, 1990.

Barkin R, Rosen P: *Emergency pediatrics*, ed 3, St Louis, 1990, Mosby.

Callaham M: *Current practice of emergency medicine*, ed 2, Philadelphia, 1991, BC Decker.

Cason D: Anaphylactic shock, *JEMS* February, 1989.

Costa A: Anaphylactic shock, *Postgrad Med* March, 1988.

E.M.T. paramedic national standard curriculum instructor's lesson plan, Washington, DC, 1985, US Government Printing Office.

Grabenstein J, Smith L: Incidence of anaphylactic self-treatment in an outpatient population, *Ann Allergy* September, 1989.

Grimes D: *Infectious diseases*, St Louis, 1991, Mosby.

Hardaway R, editor: *Shock: the reversible stage of dying*, 1988, PSG Publishing.

Muir B: *Pathophysiology: an introduction to mechanisms of disease*, New York, 1990, Wiley & Sons.

O'Keefe J: The Hickman indwelling catheter in prehospital use, *JEMS* 11(6):51, 1986.

Solomon E, Phillips G: *Understanding human anatomy and physiology*, Philadelphia, 1977, WB Saunders.

Soreide E et al: Severe anaphylactic reactions outside hospital: etiology, symptoms, and treatment, *Acta Anaesth Scand* May, 1988.

Stafford C: Life-threatening allergic reaction, *Postgrad Med* July, 1989.

Thibodeau G: *Structure and function of the body*, ed 9, St Louis, 1992, Mosby.

Tintingalli J et al, editors: *Emergency medicine: a comprehensive study guide*, ed 2, New York, 1988, McGraw-Hill.

Yarbrough J et al: Cimetidine in the treatment of refractory anaphylaxis, *Ann Allergy* September, 1989.

CHAPTER 23

Auerbach P, Geehr E, editors: Environmental medical emergencies, *Top Emerg Med* 2(3):1980.

Auerbach P, Geehr E, editors: *Management of wilderness and environmental emergencies*, ed 2, St Louis, 1989, Mosby.

Bayer M, Rumack B, editors: Poisonings and overdose, *Top Emerg Med* 1(3):1979.

Borak J et al: *Hazardous material exposure*, Englewood Cliffs, NJ, 1991, Brady Publishing.

Burton B, Bayer M, editors: Hazardous materials, *Top Emerg Med* 7(1):1985.

Callaham M: *Current practice of emergency medicine*, ed 2, Philadelphia, 1991, BC Decker.

Daniels P, LePard A: Organophosphates: the pervasive poison, *JEMS* November, 1991.

Dillmann J: Designer drugs: an update of street drug names, *JEMS* July, 1988.

E.M.T. paramedic national standard curriculum instructor's lesson plan, Washington, DC, 1985, US Government Printing Office.

Heckman J, editor: *Emergency care and transportation of the sick and injured*, ed 5, Chicago, 1992, American Academy of Orthopaedic Surgeons.

Levy D: Narcotic review, *Emerg Mag* January, 1988.

Litovitz T et al: 1990 annual report of the American Association of Poison Control Centers national data collection system, *Am J Emerg Med* 9:1991.

Maddad L, Winchester J: *Clinical manifestations of poisoning and drug overdose*, ed 2, Philadelphia, 1990, WB Saunders.

Mark J, Jorden R, editors: Alcohol-related emergencies, *Top Emerg Med* 6(2):1984.

McKenry L, Salerno E: *Mosby's pharmacology in nursing*, ed 18, St Louis, 1993, Mosby.

Moore E et al: *Early care of the injured patient*, ed 4, Philadelphia, 1990, BC Decker.

National Safety Council: *Accident facts*, 1991, Chicago, 1990, The Council.

Peppers M: Alcohol withdrawal syndrome, *Emerg Mag* December, 1991.

Tintinalli J et al, editors: *Emergency medicine: a comprehensive study guide*, ed 2, New York, 1988, McGraw-Hill.

CHAPTER 24

Auerbach P, Geehr E, editors: *Management of wilderness and environmental emergencies*, ed 2, St Louis, 1989, Mosby.

Bettoli E: Herpes: facts and fallacies, *Am J Nurs* June, 1982.

Bartlett J: *The Johns Hopkins Hospital Guide to medical care of patients with HIV infection*, ed 3, Baltimore, 1993, Williams & Wilkins.

Curriculum guide for public-safety and emergency-response workers, Atlanta, 1989, US Department of Health and Human Services, Centers for Disease Control.

E.M.T. paramedic national standard curriculum instructor's lesson plan, Washington, DC, 1985, US Government Printing Office.

Geiderman J, Baraff L, editors: Infectious disease emergencies, *Top Emerg Med* 4(1):1982.

Grimes D: *Infectious diseases*, St Louis, 1991, Mosby.

Guidelines for prevention of transmission of human immunodeficiency virus and hepatitis B virus to health-care and public safety workers, Washington, DC, 1989, US Department of Health and Human Services, Centers for Disease Control, National Institute of Occupational Safety and Health, vol 38, Nos. 5-6.

Peppers M, Brown D: Viral vaccines, *Emerg Mag* March, 1992.

Sacks S: *The truth about herpes*, Cloverdale, 1986, Verdant Press.

Sexual transmission of hepatitis C linked to HIV, *Emerg Mag* 24(3):1992.

Tintinalli J et al, editors: *Emergency medicine: a comprehensive study guide*, ed 2, New York, 1988, McGraw-Hill.

Title 29 code of federal regulations (CFR), Part 1910.1030, December 1991.

US Department of Health and Human Services, Centers for Disease Control and Prevention: 1993 revised classification system for HIV infection and expanded surveillance case definition for AIDS among adolescents and adults, *MMWR* 41: RR-17 1993.

US Department of Labor, Occupational Safety and Health Administration: *Occupational exposure to bloodborne pathogens: precautions for emergency responders*, OSHA 3130, Washington, DC, 1992, The Administration.

West K: Assessing the risks, *Emerg Mag* 34(30):1992.

CHAPTER 25

Auerbach P, Geehr E, editors: *Management of wilderness and environmental emergencies*, ed 2, St Louis, 1989, Mosby.

Callaham M: *Current practice of emergency medicine*, ed 2, Philadelphia, 1991, BC Decker.

Colby P: Plunging into water rescue, *JEMS* July, 1990.

DeLapp T: Accidental hypothermia, *Am J Nurs* January, 1983.

E.M.T. paramedic national standard curriculum instructor's lesson plan, Washington, DC, 1985, US Government Printing Office.

Guidelines for cardiopulmonary resuscitation and emergency cardiac, *JAMA* 268(16):1992.

National Safety Council: *Accident facts*, Chicago, 1991, The Council.

Pruessner H et al: Management of the near-drowning victim, *APP* May, 1988.

Schottelius B, Schottelius D: *Textbook of physiology*, ed 17, St Louis, 1973, Mosby.

Smith D: Living death: don't let hypothermia fool you into a fatal mistake, *RN* January, 1983.

Stanford T: Near-drowning, *Emerg Mag* June, 1989.

Tintinalli J et al, editors: *Emergency medicine: a comprehensive study guide*, ed 2, New York, 1988, McGraw-Hill.

Webb J: Cold to the core: treating the hypothermic patient, *JEMS* December, 1989.

CHAPTER 26

Bayer A: Changing presentation of myocardial infarction with increasing old age, *J Am Geriatr Soc* 34:1986.

Bosker G et al: *Geriatric emergency medicine*, St Louis, 1990, Mosby.

Buchner D: Falls and syncope in the elderly, *Audio Dig Emerg Med* 8(10):1991.

E.M.T. paramedic national standard curriculum instructor's lesson plan, Washington, DC, 1985, US Government Printing Office.

Janing J: Reflections on aging: communicating with elderly patients, *JEMS* 1991.

Kaudner D, Schwab W: Trauma in the elderly, *Emerg Mag* February, 1991.

Moore E, editor: *Early care of the injured patient*, ed 4, Philadelphia, 1990, Committee on Trauma, American College of Surgeons, BC Decker.

National Safety Council: *Accident facts*, Chicago, 1991, The Council.

Rose C, editor: Emergency care of the elderly, *Emerg Med Clin North Am* May, 1990.

Westfall L, Pavlis R: Why the elderly are so vulnerable to drug reactions, *RN* November, 1987.

CHAPTER 27

Barkin R, Rosen P: *Emergency pediatrics*, ed 3, St Louis, 1990, Mosby.

Beckwith B: *Sudden infant death syndrome*, Rockville, Md, 1975, US Department of Health, Education, and Welfare.

Callaham M: *Current practice of emergency medicine*, ed 2, Philadelphia, 1991, BC Decker.

Corr C et al: *Sudden infant death syndrome: who can help and how*, New York, 1991, Springer Publishing.

Doughtery J: SIDS: the silent killer, *Emerg Mag* October, 1987.

Emergency medical services for children: a report to the nation, Washington, DC, 1991, National Center for Education in Maternal and Child Health.

E.M.T. paramedic national standard curriculum instructor's lesson plan, Washington, DC, 1985, US Government Printing Office.

Fuchs S: Managing seizures in children, *Emerg Mag* 22(12):47, 1990.

Harris J, Liebert R: *The child: development from birth to adolescence,* ed 2, Englewood Cliffs, NJ, 1984, Prentice-Hall.

Hazinski M: *Nursing care of the critically ill child* ed 2, St Louis, 1992, Mosby.

Pierog J, Pierog L, editors: Pediatric emergencies, *Top Emerg Med* 3(1):1981.

Ramenofsky M: The need for knowledge, *Emerg Mag* 21(8):1989.

Rothstein R, editor: Respiratory emergencies. I. *Top Emerg Med* 2(1):1980.

Touloukian R: *Pediatric trauma,* ed 2, St Louis, 1990, Mosby.

US Department of Health and Human Services. *Sudden infant death syndrome: a review of the medical literature,* Rockville, Md, 1980, The Department.

CHAPTER 28

American Heart Association: *Textbook of advanced cardiac life support,* Dallas, 1987, The Association.

American Heart Association, American Academy of Pediatrics: *Textbook of neonatal resuscitation,* Elk Grove Village, 1990, The Association.

Callaham M: *Current practice of emergency medicine,* ed 2, Philadelphia, 1991, BC Decker.

Cosgriff J, Anderson D: *The practice of emergency care,* ed 2, Philadelphia, 1984, JB Lippincott.

Dolgan D, Roush W: Third trimester bleeding, *JEMS* July, 1986.

E.M.T. paramedic national standard curriculum instructors' lesson plan, Washington, DC, 1985, US Government Printing Office.

Moore E et al: *Early care of the injured patient,* ed 4, Philadelphia, 1990 BC Decker.

PACTS for life, St. Louis, 1986, Cardinal Glennon Children's Hospital, Saint Louis University School of Medicine.

Previte J: *Human physiology,* New York, 1983, McGraw-Hill.

Seeley R et al: *Anatomy and physiology,* ed 2, St Louis, 1992, Mosby.

Shaffer M, Franaszek J, editors: OB/GYN emergencies, *Top Emerg Med* 7(2):1985.

CHAPTER 29

Dickinson E: Life-threatening gynecologic emergencies: when pain calls for quick action, *JEMS* March, 1990.

E.M.T. paramedic national standard curriculum instructor's lesson plan, Washington, DC, 1985, US Government Printing Office.

Sheehy S: *Emergency nursing: principles and practice,* ed 3, St Louis, 1992, Mosby.

Williams D: Sensitive emergency management of rape victims, *Rep Emerg Nurs* 1(11):1990.

CHAPTER 30

Aguilera D: *Crisis intervention: theory and methodology,* St Louis, 1990, Mosby.

Bassuk E et al: *Behavioral emergencies: a field guide for EMTs and paramedics,* Boston, 1983, Little, Brown.

Butler J: Safe transport of the psychiatric patient, *JEMS* March, 1988.

Dernocoeur K: *Streetsense: communication, safety and control,* Bowie, 1985, Brady Publishing.

E.M.T. paramedic national standard curriculum instructor's lesson plan, Washington, DC, 1985, US Government Printing Office.

Hafen B, Frandsen K: *Psychological emergencies: crisis intervention,* Englewood, 1985, Morton Publishing.

Judd R, Peszke M, editors: Psychological and behavioral emergencies, *Top Emerg Med* 4(4):1983.

The mythology of suicide, Denver, 1987, Suicide Prevention Allied Regional Effort (SPARE).

National Crisis Prevention Institute: *Nonviolent crisis intervention,* Brookfield, 1987, The Institute.

Rathus S: *Psychology,* ed 3, New York, 1987, Holt, Rinehart & Winston.

Sarason I: *Abnormal psychology,* New York, 1972, Appleton-Century-Crofts.

EMERGENCY DRUG INDEX

American Heart Association: Guidelines for cardiopulmonary resuscitation and emergency cardiac care, *JAMA* 268(16):1992.

American Heart Association: *Textbook of advanced cardiac life support,* Dallas, 1987, The Association.

Barkin R, Rosen P: *Emergency pediatrics,* ed 3, St Louis, 1990, Mosby.

Beck R: *Pharmacology for prehospital emergency care,* Philadelphia, 1992, FA Davis.

Clark J, Pringle R: Pediatric respiratory drugs, *Emerg Mag* 22(12):1990.

Goldberg E: *Treatment of cardiac emergencies,* ed 5, St Louis, 1990, Mosby.

Gonzalez E, Ornato J: *Field drug reference for emergency care providers,* Hamilton, Ill, 1990, Drug Intelligence Publications.

Katzung B: *Basic and clinical pharmacology,* ed 4, Norwalk, Conn, 1989, Appleton & Lange.

McKenry L, Salerno E: *Mosby's pharmacology in nursing,* ed 18, St Louis, 1992, Mosby.

Rosen P et al: *Essentials of emergency medicine,* St Louis, 1991, Mosby.

Tintinalli J et al, editors: *Emergency medicine: a comprehensive study guide,* ed 2, New York, 1988, McGraw-Hill.

GLOSSARY

abandonment Terminating medical care without legal excuse or turning care over to less qualified personnel, thereby injuring the patient.

abdominal Pertaining to the abdomen.

abduction Movement away from the midline.

abnormal Away from the normal.

abruptio placenta Separation of the placenta implanted in a normal position in a pregnancy of 20 weeks or more, during labor, or during delivery of the fetus.

absolute refractory period The portion of the action potential during which the membrane is insensitive to all stimuli, regardless of strength.

absorption The passage of substances across and into tissues, such as the passage of digested food molecules into intestinal cells or the passage of liquids into kidney tubules.

accelerated AV conduction See *anomalous conduction.*

acclimatization The physical adjustment to a different climate or to changes in altitude or temperature.

acetabulum The large, cup-shaped articular cavity at the juncture of the ilium, the ischium, and the pubis, containing the ball-shaped head of the femur.

acetoacetic acid A colorless, oily ketone body produced by the metabolism of lipids and pyruvates; excreted in trace amounts in normal urine and in elevated levels in diabetes mellitus, especially in ketoacidosis.

acetonemia The presence of acetone in the blood; characterized by the fruity breath odor of ketoacidosis.

acetylcholine (ACh) A neurotransmitter substance widely distributed in body tissues, with the primary function of mediating the synaptic activity of the nervous system.

acetylcholinesterase (AChE) An enzyme found in the synaptic cleft that causes the breakdown of acetylcholine to acetic acid and choline, thus limiting the stimulatory effect of acetylcholine.

acinus A small lobule of a compound gland; the exocrine portion of the pancreas that produces pancreatic juice.

acquired immunodeficiency syndrome (AIDS) Infection with the human immunodeficiency virus (HIV), which affects the immune system and can produce opportunistic infections and malignancies.

acromegaly A chronic metabolic condition characterized by a gradual, marked enlargement and elongation of the bones of the face, jaw, and extremities.

acromion process The lateral extension of the spine of the scapula; gives attachment to the deltoideus and trapezius.

actin A protein found in muscle fibers that acts with myosin to bring about contraction and relaxation.

actinomycosis A chronic systemic disease characterized by deep, lumpy abscesses that extrude a granular pus through multiple sinuses.

action potential A change in membrane potential in an excitable tissue that acts as an electrical signal and is propagated in an all-or-none fashion.

active transport A carrier-mediated process that can move substances against a concentration gradient.

active tubular secretion Secretion that involves the transport of free drug from the blood across the proximal tubular cell and into the tubular urine by an active process, against a concentration gradient.

acute dystonia A sudden impairment of muscle tone; commonly involves the head, neck, or tongue, and often occurs as an adverse effect to medication.

acute mountain sickness (AMS) A common high-altitude illness that results from rapid ascent of an unacclimatized person to altitudes of 8000 feet or more.

acute pain Severe pain, such as may follow trauma or accompany myocardial infraction or other conditions and diseases.

Addison's disease A life-threatening condition caused by partial or complete failure of adrenocortical function.

adduction Movement toward the midline.

adenohypophysis The anterior lobe of the pituitary gland.

adenoma A tumor of glandular epithelium in which the cells of the tumor are arranged in a recognizable glandular structure.

adenosine A compound derived from nucleic acid, composed of adenine and a sugar.

adenosine diphosphate (ADP) A product of the hydrolysis of adenosine triphosphate.

adenosine monophosphate (AMP) A compound that affects energy release in work done by muscles.

adenosine triphosphate (ATP) Adenosine, an organic base, with three phosphate groups attached to it. It serves to store energy in muscles.

adhesion The quality of remaining in close ccontact with or stuck to another entity; also, a structure that joins several parts, sometimes abnormally.

adipose tissue A specialized connective tissue that stores lipids. Also known as *fat tissue.*

adrenal gland Either of two secretory glands perched atop the kidneys. Each gland consists of two parts, the cortex and medulla, that have independent functions.

adrenal medullary mechanism The mechanism by which epinephrine and norepinephrine are released from the adrenal medulla as a result of the same stimuli that increase sympathetic stimulation of the heart and blood vessels.

Adrenalin Proprietary name for *epinephrine.*

adrenergic Of or pertaining to sympathetic nerve fibers of the autonomic nervous system that use epinephrine or epinephrine-like substances as neurotransmitters.

adrenocorticotropic hormone (ACTH) A hormone of the anterior pituitary gland that stimulates growth of the adrenal gland cortex and secretion of corticosteroids.

adsorption A substance's capacity to attract and hold other materials or particles on its surface.

adult respiratory distress syndrome (ARDS) A group of symptoms accompanying fulminant pulmonary edema and resulting in acute respiratory failure. Also known as *noncardiogenic pulmonary edema*.

aerobic Of or pertaining to the presence of air or oxygen.

aerosol Pressurized gas containing a finely nebulized medication for inhalation therapy.

affective disorder Any of a group of psychotic disorders characterized by severe and inappropriate emotional responses, prolonged and persistent disturbances of mood and related thought distortions, and other symptoms associated with depressed or manic states.

afferent division Nerve fibers that send impulses from the periphery to the central nervous system.

affinity The propensity of a drug to bind or attach itself to a given receptor site.

afterdrop phenomenon A sudden return of cold blood and waste products to the body's core as a result of rewarming methods used to treat hypothermia.

afterload See *peripheral vascular resistance.*

agglutination An aggregation clumping together of cells as a result of their interaction with specific antibodies called "agglutinins."

agglutinin A kind of antibody whose interaction with antigens is manifested as agglutination.

agonal rhythm A ventricular escape complex or rhythm that occurs when the electrical impulses from the SA node, atria, or AV junction fail to reach the ventricles because of sinus arrest or high degree AV block; frequently seen as the last rhythm in an unsuccessful resuscitation.

agonist A drug that combines with receptors and initiates a sequence of biochemical and physiologic changes; possesses both affinity and efficacy.

air trapping The result of a prolonged but inefficient expiratory effort. Usually results from chronic obstruction of the pulmonary tree, as is commonly seen in chronic obstructive pulmonary disease (COPD) or asthma.

akathisia An abnormal condition characterized by restlessness and agitation.

albumin A water-soluble protein containing carbon, hydrogen, oxygen, nitrogen, and sulfur.

aldosterone A steroid hormone produced by the adrenal cortex to regulate sodium and potassium balance in the blood.

aliquot A sample that is representative of the whole.

allergen A substance that can produce a hypersensitive reaction in the body; it is not necessarily intrinsically harmful.

all-or-none principle The principle that when a stimulus is applied to a cell, an action potential either is produced or is not.

alpha-adrenergic receptor Any one of the postulated adrenergic components of receptor tissues that responds to norepinephrine and to various blocking agents.

alpha cell A constituent of the islet of Langerhans; secretes insulin.

alveolar duct Part of the respiratory passages beyond a respiratory bronchiole; from it arise alveolar sacs and alveoli.

alveolus A small cavity; the terminal ending of a secretory gland. Alveoli of the lungs are microscopic saclike dilations of terminal bronchioles.

amaurosis fugax Unilateral vision loss as a result of internal carotid artery plaque emboli.

amenorrhea The absence of menstruation.

amino acid An organic chemical compound composed of one or more basic amino groups and one or more acidic carboxyl groups.

ammonia A colorless, aromatic gas consisting of nitrogen and hydrogen.

amniocentesis An obstetric procedure in which a small amount of amniotic fluid is removed for laboratory analysis; aids in diagnosis of fetal abnormalities.

amniotic fluid embolism An embolism that occurs when particulate matter in amniotic fluid forms an embolus and gains access to maternal circulation during labor or delivery or immediately after delivery.

amplitude modulation (AM) A transmitted radio frequency carrier fixed in frequency but increasing or decreasing in amplitude in accordance with the strength of the applied audio.

ampulla A rounded, saclike dilation of the uterine tube.

amylase A starch-splitting enzyme.

anabolic steroid Any of several compounds derived from testosterone or prepared synthetically to promote general body growth, to oppose the effects of endogenous estrogen, or to promote masculinizing effects.

anaerobic metabolism Metabolism that occurs in the absence of oxygen.

anal canal The final portion of the alimentary tract between the rectal ampulla and the anus.

anal triangle The posterior portion of the perianal region through which the anal canal opens.

anaphylactic shock Shock that occurs when the body is exposed to a substance that produces a severe allergic reaction.

anasarca Generalized, massive edema.

anastomosis The joining of two parts.

anatomic dead space The volume of the conducting airways from the external environment down to the terminal bronchioles.

anatomical position A person standing erect with feet and palms facing the examiner.

androgen Any steroid hormone that increases male characteristics.

anemia A decrease in blood hemoglobin.

anesthesia Without sensation.

angioedema An acute, painless dermal, subcutaneous, or submucosal swelling of short duration involving the face, neck, lips, larynx, hands, feet, genitalia, or viscera.

angiogram A study of vessels.

angioplasty Repair of damaged vessels.

angle of Louis See *sternal angle.*

anion An ion with a negative charge.

anisocoria Normal or congenital unequal pupil size.

anomalous conduction A preexcitation syndrome; a clinical condition associated with abnormal conduction pathways between the atria and ventricles that bypass the AV node and bundle of His and allow the electrical impulses to initiate depolarization of the ventricles earlier than usual. Also known as *accelerated AV conduction.*

anorexia Lack or loss of appetite, resulting in the inability to eat.

antagonism The opposition between two or more medications; occurs when the combined (conjoint) effect of two drugs is less than the sum of the drugs acting separately.

antagonist muscle A muscle that works in opposition to another muscle.

antagonist An agent designed to inhibit or counteract effects produced by other drugs or undesired effects caused by normal or hyperactive physiologic mechanisms.

antecubital fossae See *antecubital space.*

antecubital space (AC space) The depressed area in front of the elbow or at the bend of the elbow. Also known as *antecubital fossae.*

antegrade amnesia The loss of memory for events that occurred immediately after recovery of consciousness.

antenatal Occurring or formed before birth.

antepartum The maternal period before delivery.

anterior chamber of eye The chamber of the eye between the cornea and the iris.

anterior communicating artery The artery that connects with the anterior cerebral arteries and completes the circle of Willis.

anterior cord syndrome A spinal cord injury usually seen in flexion injuries; caused by pressure on the anterior aspect of the spinal cord by a ruptured intervertebral disc or fragments of the vertebral body extruded posteriorly into the spinal canal.

anterior superior iliac spine One of two bony segments that form the iliac crest.

antibody A substance produced by the body that destroys or inactivates a specific substance (antigen) that has entered the body.

anticoagulant A substance that prevents or delays coagulation of the blood.

antidiuretic hormone (ADH) A hormone produced in the posterior pituitary gland to regulate the balance of water in the body by accelerating the reabsorption of water.

antidotel A drug or other substance that opposes the action of a poison.

antigen A substance, usually a protein, that causes the formation of an antibody and reacts specifically with that antibody.

antigenic site A site capable of binding to and reacting with an antibody.

antiplatelet A drug that interferes with platelet aggregation.

antipyretic Something that works against fever.

antivenin A suspension of venom-neutralizing antibodies prepared from the serum of immunized horses.

anuria The inability to urinate; the cessation of urine production; a diminished urinary output of less than 100 to 250 ml per day.

anus The distal end or outlet of the rectum.

anxiety A state or feeling of apprehension, uneasiness, agitation, uncertainty, and fear resulting from the anticipation of some threat or danger.

aorta The main and largest artery in the body.

aortic aneurysm A localized dilation of the wall of the aorta.

aortic body Any of the specialized nerve cells located in the arch of the aorta, where they monitor levels of oxygen and hydrogen ions in the cardiovascular system.

aortic semilunar valve A valve that guards the orifice between the left ventricle and the aorta.

apex of the heart The top or tip of the heart opposite the base.

Apgar score The evaluation of an infant's physical condition, usually performed at 1 minute and again at 5 minutes after birth; evaluation components include heart rate, respiratory effort, muscle tone, reflex irritability, and color.

aphasia Loss of speech power.

apical impulse A pulsation of the left ventricle of the heart, palpable and sometimes visible at the fifth intercostal space to the left of the midline.

apnea Without breath.

apneustic center A group of neurons in the pons that has a stimulatory effect on the inspiratory center.

apocrine gland A gland whose cells contribute cytoplasm to its secretion, such as a mammary gland.

apothecary A system of graduated liquid volumes arranged in order of heaviness; based on the "grain."

apparatus A vehicle used for fire suppression or rescue. Does not include staff vehicles.

appendicular region The limbs or extremities.

appendicular skeleton The bones of the upper and lower extremities of the body.

appendix A wormlike blunt process extending from the cecum. Also known as *vermiform appendix.*

aqueous humor The clear, watery fluid circulating in the anterior and posterior chambers of the eye.

arachnida A large class of arthropods that includes spiders, scorpions, mites, and ticks.

arachnoid layer A delicate, weblike middle membrane covering the brain.

areflexia A neurologic condition characterized by absence of the reflexes.

areola The circular pigmented area surrounding the nipple.

areolar connective tissue A loose tissue that consists of delicate webs of fibers and a variety of cells embedded in a matrix of soft, sticky gel.

areolar gland A gland that forms small rounded projections from the surface of the areola of the mamma.

arrector pili Smooth muscles of the skin attached to hair follicles; when contraction occurs, the hair rises, resulting in "gooseflesh."

arterial capillary The ends of capillaries closest to arterioles.

arteriogram A study of arteries.

arteriole A small branch of an artery.

arteriovenous anastomosis A vessel that allows blood to flow from arteries to veins without passing through capillaries. Also known as an **AV shunt.**

artery A vessel that carries blood away from the heart.

arthritis An inflammatory condition of the joints, characterized by pain and swelling.

arthroscopy Inspection of a joint.

artifact A deflection on the ECG display or tracing produced by factors other than the heart's electrical activity.

arytenoid cartilages Small, pyramidal laryngeal cartilages that articulate with the cricoid cartilage.

asbestosis A chronic lung disease caused by the inhalation of asbestos fibers; results in the development of alveolar, interstitial, and pleural fibrosis.

ascending colon The segment of the colon that extends from the cecum in the right lower quadrant of the abdomen to the transverse colon at the hepatic flexure on the right side; usually at the level of the umbilicus.

ascites An abnormal intraperitoneal accumulation of fluid containing large amounts of protein and electrolytes.

aseptic Sterile, without germs.

asphyxiation A state of suffocation caused by severe hypoxia, leading to hypoxemia and hypercapnia, loss of consciousness, and if not corrected, death.

aspiration The inhalation of foreign substances into the pulmonary system.

assault Creating apprehension, or unauthorized handling and treatment of a patient.

asthma A respiratory disorder characterized by recurring episodes of paroxysmal dyspnea, wheezing on expiration due to constriction of the bronchi, coughing, and viscous mucoid bronchial secretions.

astigmatism An abnormal condition of the eye in which the light rays cannot be focused clearly on a point on the retina because the spheric curve of the cornea is not equal in all meridians.

astrocyte gliosis A tumor composed of glial cells within the nervous system; may be associated with respiratory center dysfunction and neuroepithelial bodies in the tracheobronchial tree, along with distal atelectasis.

ataxia Failure of muscle coordination.

ataxic breathing A type of cluster or irregular breathing pattern characterized by a series of inspirations and expirations.

atelectasis An abnormal condition characterized by the collapse of lung tissue, preventing the respiratory exchange of oxygen and carbon dioxide.

atelectatic breathing A modified respiratory effort thought to be a protective reflex to hyperinflate the lungs and reexpand alveoli that might have been collapsed.

atheroma A hard, atherosclerotic plaque.

atherosclerosis A common arterial disorder characterized by yellowish plaques of cholesterol, lipids, and cellular debris in the inner layers of the walls of large and medium-sized arteries.

atlantooccipital joint One of a pair of condyloid joints formed by the articulation of the atlas of the vertebral column with the occipital bone of the skull.

atlas The first cervical vertebra, articulating with the occipital bone and the axis.

atmospheric pressure The pressure exerted by the weight of the atmosphere. At sea level this pressure is 760 mm Hg.

atony Weak muscle tone.

atria A chamber or cavity, such as the atria of the heart.

atrial natriuretic factor A peptide released from the atria when atrial blood pressure is increased; lowers blood pressure by increasing urine production, thus reducing blood volume.

atrial synchronous ventricular pacemaker An artificial pacemaker synchronized with the patient's atrial rhythm, pacing the ventricles only when an AV block occurs.

atrial-ventricular demand pacemaker An artificial pacemaker that paces either the atria or ventricles when the intrinsic rate of the paced chamber drops dangerously low.

atrioventricular canal The path through which the atria open into the ventricles.

atrioventricular node (AV node) An area of specialized cardiac muscle that receives the cardiac impulse from the sinoatrial node and conducts it to the bundle of His.

atrioventricular valve A valve in the heart through which blood flows from the atria to the ventricles.

atrophy Wasting.

auditory Of or pertaining to hearing or the organs of hearing.

auditory ossicles The incus, malleus, and stapes; small bones in the middle ear that articulate with each other and the tympanic membrane.

auditory tube The auditory canal; extends from the middle ear to the nasopharynx. Also known as *eustachian tube.*

auricle The part of the external ear that protrudes from the head. Also known as **pinna.**

autolysis The spontaneous disintegration of tissues or cells by the action of their own autogenous enzymes.

automatic implanted cardiac defibrillator (AICD) A surgically implanted device that monitors a person's heart rate. Designed to deliver defibrillatory shocks as needed.

automatic vehicle location (AVL) A radio communications subsystem that uses one or more electronic methods to periodically determine a land, marine, or air vehicle's position and relay that information via radio to a communications center.

automatism Abnormal repetitive motor behavior such as lip smacking, chewing, or swallowing, during which time the patient is amnestic.

autonomic nervous system (ANS) The part of the nervous system that regulates involuntary vital functions, including the activity of cardiac muscle, smooth muscle, and glands. Subdivided into sympathetic and parasympathetic divisions.

autophagia Nutrition of the body by consumption of its own tissues.

avascular Having blood vessels.

AV dissociation P waves and QRS complexes that occur rhythmically, but without a relationship to each other.

Avogardro's number The number of molecules in 1 gram molecule of a substance.

AV sequential pacemaker An artificial pacemaker that paces the atria first and then the ventricles when spontaneous activity is absent or slowed in both the atria and ventricles.

AV shunt See *arteriovenous anastomosis.*

axial region The head, neck, thorax, abdomen, and pelvis.

axial skeleton The bones of the head, neck, and torso.

axillae Armpits.

axillary node One of the lymph glands of the axillae that help fight infections in the chest, armpit, neck, and arm and drain lymph nodes from those areas.

axis The second cervical vertebra about which the atlas rotates, allowing the head to be turned, extended, or flexed.

axon The main central process of a neuron that normally conducts action potentials away from the neuron cell body.

azotemia Retention in the blood of excess amounts of nitrogenous compounds; caused by failure of the kidneys to remove urea from the blood and characterized by uremia.

Babinski's sign Plantar reflex; a reflex movement in which the great toe bends upward when the outer edge of the sole of the foot is scratched.

bacteriocidal Destructive to bacteria.

bacteriostatic Tending to restrain the development or the reproduction of bacteria.

ball-and-socket joint A joint that consists of a ball (head) at the end of one bone and a socket in an adjacent bone into which a portion of the ball fits.

baroreceptor A sensory nerve ending in the walls of the atria of the heart, venae cavae, aortic arch, and carotid sinuses; sensitive to stretching of the walls caused by increased blood pressure.

barotitis An inflammation of the ear caused by changes in atmospheric pressure.

barotrauma A physical injury sustained as a result of exposure to increased environmental pressure.

Bartholin's gland One of two small, mucus-secreting glands located on the posterior and lateral aspect of the vestibule of the vagina.

Barton's bandage A circumferential head dressing applied to restrict jaw movement and minimize pain.

base of the heart The portion of the heart opposite the apex, directed to the right side of the body.

base station A grouping of radio equipment consisting of at least a transmitter, a receiver, a transmission line, and an antenna located at a specific fixed location.

basilar artery The single arterial trunk formed by the junction of the two vertebral arteries at the base of the skull.

basilar fracture A fracture that may occur when the mandibular condyles perforate into the base of the skull, but more commonly results from extension of a linear fracture into the floor of the anterior and middle fossae.

basophil A white blood cell that promotes inflammation; readily stains with specific dyes.

battery Physical contact with a person without their consent and without legal justification.

Battle's sign Ecchymosis over the mastoid process caused by fracture of the temporal bone.

Beck's triad A combination of three symptoms that characterize pericardial tamponade: elevated venous pressure, decreased arterial pressure, and a small, quiet heartbeat.

beta-adrenergic receptor Any of the postulated adrenergic components of receptor tissues that respond to epinephrine and various blocking agents.

beta cell A constituent of the islet of Langerhans' secretes glucagon.

beta-hydroxybutyric acid One of the ketone bodies, occurring in abnormal amounts in diabetic ketoacidosis as a result of fatty acid oxidation.

bicarbonate buffer system The principal mechanism for stabilizing of acid-base balance.

biceps brachii The biceps muscle of the arm that flexes and supinates the forearm.

bicuspid valve One of the two atrioventricular valves located between the left atrium and ventricle. Also known as *mitral valve.*

bifurcate Divided into two branches.

bilateral Having or occuring on two sides.

bile A bitter, yellow-green secretion of the liver; stored in the gallbladder.

biology The study of life.

biosynthesis A chemical reaction that continually occurs throughout the body in which molecules form more complex molecules.

biotransformation The process whereby a drug is chemically converted to a metabolite.

Biot's respiration A respiratory pattern that consists of irregular respirations varying in depth and interrupted by intervals of apnea.

biphasic complex A QRS complex that is partly positive, partly negative.

bipolar lead A lead composed of two electrodes of opposite polarity.

bipolar disorder See *manic-depressive disorder.*

blastocyst The stage of mammalian embryos in which the embryo consists of the inner cell mass and a thin trophoblast layer.

blood The fluid and its suspended formed elements circulated through the heart, arteries, capillaries, and veins.

blood-brain barrier An anatomic-physiologic feature of the brain thought to consist of walls of capillaries in the central nervous system and surrounding glial membranes; functions in preventing or slowing the passage of chemical compounds from the blood into the central nervous system.

blood clot The end result of the clotting process in blood; normally consists of red cells, white cells, and platelets enmeshed in an insoluble fibrin network.

blood colloid osmotic pressure Osmotic pressure caused by the presence of plasma proteins (mostly albumin) too large to pass through the wall of the capillary. Also known as *oncotic pressure.*

blowout fracture A fracture of the floor of the orbit caused by a blow that suddenly increases the intraocular pressure.

blunt trauma An injury produced by the wounding forces of compression and change of speed, both of which may disrupt tissue.

B lymphocyte A type of lymphocyte responsible for antibody-mediated immunity.

body The largest or main part of any organ or structure.

bone A highly specialized form of hard, connective tissue; consists of living cells and mineralized matrix.

bony labyrinth Part of the inner ear; contains the membranous labyrinth.

botulism An often fatal form of food poisoning caused by an endotoxin produced by the bacillus *Clostridium botulinum.*

Bowman's capsule The expanded beginning of a renal tubule.

boxer's fracture Fracture of the fifth metacarpal bone from direct trauma to a closed fist.

Boyle's law See *general gas law.*

brachial plexus A network of nerves in the neck passing under the clavicle and into the axilla, originating in the fifth, sixth, seventh, and eighth cervical and first two thoracic spinal nerves; innervates the muscles and the skin of the chest, shoulders, and arms.

bradycardia A heart rate of less than 60 beats per minute.

bradypnea A persistent respiratory rate slower than 12 breaths per minute.

brain stem The midbrain, pons, and medulla.

brand name See *trade name.*

Braxton-Hicks contraction Irregular tightening of the pregnant uterus that begins in the first trimester and increases in frequency, duration, and intensity as pregnancy progresses.

breech presentation The intrauterine position of the fetus in which the buttocks or feet present.

broad ligament A folded sheet of peritoneum draped over the uterine tubes, uterus, and ovaries.

bronchiectasis An abnormal condition of the bronchial tree, characterized by irreversible dilation and destruction of the bronchial walls.

bronchiole A small branch of a bronchus.

bronchiolitis An acute viral infection of the lower respiratory tract that occurs primarily in infants under 18 months of age; characterized by expiratory wheezes, respiratory distress, inflammation, and obstruction at the level of the bronchioles.

Brown-Séquard syndrome A hemitransection of the spinal cord; pressure on one half of the spinal cord results in weakness of the upper and lower extremities on the ipsilateral side and loss of pain and temperature sensation on the contralateral side.

brow presentation See *face presentation.*

buccal route A route of medication administration in which the agent is placed between the teeth and mucous membrane of the cheek.

bulbourethral glands Small glands, located just below the prostate gland, that lubricate the terminal portion of the urethra and contribute to seminal fluid. Also known as *Cowper's glands.*

bullet tumble See *bullet yaw.*

bullet yaw The forward rotation of a bullet around its center of mass, which causes an end-over-end motion, producing a greater energy exchange and greater tissue damage. Also known as **bullet tumble.**

bundle of His A band of fibers in the myocardium through which the cardiac impulse is transmitted from the atrioventricular node to the ventricles.

bundle of Kent Fibers that connect atrial muscle to ventricular muscle, bypassing the AV node. Also known as *Kent fibers.*

burette An intravenous device used to deliver a wide range of accurate specific volumes.

bursitis An inflammation of the bursa, the connective tissue structure surrounding a joint.

Caesarean delivery A surgical procedure in which the abdomen and uterus are incised and the newborn is delivered transabdominally.

calcaneus The heel bone, the largest of the tarsal bones.

calipers An instrument with two hinged, adjustable legs used to measure components of the electrocardiogram.

canaliculus A very small tube or channel.

cancellous bone Latticelike tissue normally present in the interior of many bones where spaces are usually filled with marrow. Also known as *spongy bone.*

capillary A tiny vessel that connects an arteriole to a venule.

capillary refill test A test used to evaluate the rate of blood flow through peripheral capillary beds.

capitulum The lateral aspect of the humerus; articulates with the head of the radius.

carbaminohemoglobin A chemical complex formed by carbon dioxide and hemoglobin after the release of oxygen by the hemoglobin to a tissue cell.

carbonic acid An aqueous solution of carbon dioxide.

carbonic anhydrase The enzyme that converts carbon dioxide into carbonic acid.

carcinogenic Cancer-causing.

cardiac cycle The complete round of cardiac systole and diastole.

cardiac muscle A special striated muscle of the myocardium, containing dark, intercalated disks at the junctions of the abutting fibers; characterized by special contractile abilities.

cardiac output The volume of blood pumped by the heart per minute.

cardiac plexus One of several nerve complexes situated close to the arch of the aorta.

cardiac sphincter A ring of muscle fibers at the juncture of the esophagus and stomach.

cardiogenic shock Shock that results when cardiac action is unable to deliver sufficient circulating blood volume for tissue perfusion.

cardiography Recording the movements of the heart.

cardiomyopathy Any disease that affects the myocardium.

cardiopulmonary Of or pertaining to the heart and lungs.

carina of the trachea A downward and backward projection of the lowest tracheal cartilage, forming a ridge between the openings of the right and left primary bronchi.

carotid body A small structure containing neural tissue at the bifurcation of the carotid arteries. It monitors the oxygen content of the blood and helps regulate respiration.

carotid sinus massage See *carotid sinus pressure.*

carotid sinus pressure A technique used to increase vagal tone to convert paroxysmal supraventricular tachycardia to sinus rhythm. Also known as *carotid sinus massage.*

carpal Pertaining to the carpus, or wrist.

carpometacarpal joint The joint of the thumb.

carrier A radio signal of specific frequency generated by a transmitter without audio information imposed on it.

carrier molecule A protein that combines with solutes on one side of a membrane, transporting the solute to the other side; used in mediated transport mechanisms.

cartilage Firm, smooth, nonvascular connective tissue.

cartilaginous joint See **joint.**

catabolic Pertaining to the destruction of complex substances by living cells to form simple compounds.

catecholamine Any of a group of sympathomimetic amines, including *dopamine, epinephrine,* and *norepinephrine.*

cathartic Causing evacuation of the bowel.

cation An ion with a positive charge.

cavitation A temporary or permanent opening produced by a force that pushes body tissues laterally away from the track of a projectile.

cecum A cul-de-sac constituting the first part of the large intestine.

cell body The part of the cell that contains the nucleus and surrounding cytoplasm, exclusive of any projections or processes; concerned more with metabolism of the cell than with a specific function.

cellular phone An 800- to 900-MHz radio communications system used to gain access to dial-up telephone circuits and vice versa. The system is divided into usually small coverage areas called "cells," which are interconnected via microwave or dedicated telephone circuits.

cellulitis Inflammation of the skin, characterized most commonly by local heat, redness, pain, swelling, and occasionally fever, malaise, chills, and headache.

cementum The bonelike connective tissue that covers the roots of the teeth and helps to support them.

centigram A metric unit of mass equal to one hundredth of a gram.

centimeter (cm) A metric unit of length equal to one hundredth of a meter, or 0.3937 inches.

central cord syndrome A spinal cord injury commonly seen with hyperextension or flexion cervical injuries; characterized by greater motor impairment of the upper than lower extremities.

central nervous system (CNS) The brain and spinal cord, which are encased in and protected by bone.

central nervous system ischemic response An increase in blood pressure caused by vasoconstriction where oxygen levels are too low, carbon dioxide levels are too high, or pH is too low in the medulla.

central thermoreceptors Nerve endings that are sensitive to heat; located in or near the anterior hypothalamus.

centrifugation Separating components of different densities contained in a liquid by spinning them at high speeds.

centriole Usually paired organelles lying in the centrosome.

centrosome A specialized zone of cytoplasm close to the nucleus that contains two centrioles.

cephalic presentation A classification of fetal position in which the head of the fetus is at the uterine cervix. Also known as *vertex presentation.*

cephalopelvic disproportion An obstetric condition in which a newborn's head is too large or a mother's birth canal too small to permit normal labor or birth.

cephalothorax The united head and thorax of a spider.

cerebella cortex The outer portion of the cerebellum.

cerebellum The second largest part of the brain, which plays an essential role in producing normal movements.

cerebral Pertaining to the brain.

cerebral aqueduct The narrow conduit between the third and fourth ventricles in the midbrain that conveys cerebral spinal fluid.

cerebral cortex A thin layer of gray matter made up of

neuron dendrites and cell bodies that compose the surface of the cerebrum.

cerebrospinal fluid (CSF) Fluid that fills the subarachnoid space in the brain and spinal cord and in the cerebral ventricles.

cerebrum The largest and uppermost part of the brain, which controls consciousness, memory, sensations, emotions, and voluntary movements.

certification or **registration** The process by which an agency or association grants recognition to an individual for meeting specific requirements to participate in an activity.

cerumen A yellowish or brownish waxy secretion produced in the external ear canal. Also known as "earwax."

ceruminous gland The gland that produces a waxy substance, *cerumen* (earwax).

cervical Pertaining to the neck.

cervical node One of the lymph glands in the neck.

cervical plexus The network of nerves formed by the ventral primary divisions of the first four cervical nerves.

cervical spondylosis A form of degenerative joint and disk disease affecting the cervical vertebrae and resulting in compression of the associated nerve roots.

cervical vertebrae The first seven segments of the vertebral column, designated C1 to C7.

cervicitis Acute or chronic inflammation of the uterine cervix.

cervix The lower part of the uterus.

Chadwick's sign The bluish coloration of the vulva and vagina that develops after the sixth week of pregnancy as a normal result of local venous congestion; an early sign of pregnancy.

chancre A skin lesion, usually of primary syphilis, that begins at the site of infection as a papule and develops into a red, bloodless, painless ulcer with a crater-like appearance.

channel An assigned frequency or pair of frequencies used to carry voice or data communications or both. In EMS, an ALS "MED" channel is a pair of radio frequencies, one used for transmitting, the other for receiving.

chemical name The exact designation of a chemical structure determined by the rules of chemical nomenclature.

chemoreceptor A sensory cell stimulated by a change in the concentration of chemicals to produce action potentials.

chemotaxis The response of leukocytes to products formed in immunologic reactions; a part of the inflammatory response.

CHEMTREC (Chemical Transportation Emergency Center) A public service of the Chemical Manufacturers Association; provides immediate advice to on-scene personnel regarding hazardous materials management.

Cheyne-Stokes respiration A regular, periodic pattern of breathing with equal intervals of apnea followed by a crescendo-decrescendo sequence of respirations.

chickenpox See **varicella.**

child abuse The physical, sexual, or emotional maltreatment of a child.

cholecystokinin A hormone that stimulates the contraction of the gallbladder and the secretion of pancreatic juice.

cholinergic Of or pertaining to nerve fibers that elaborate acetylcholine at the myoneural junctions.

chondrocytes Cartilage cells.

chorioamnionitis An inflammatory reaction in the amniotic membranes caused by organisms in the amniotic fluid.

chorionic gonadotropin A chemical component of urine of pregnant women.

choroid The portion of the vascular tunic associated with the sclera of the eye.

choroid plexus A network of brain capillaries that are involved in producing cerebral spinal fluid.

chromatin granules The material within the cell nucleus from which chromosomes are formed.

chronic obstructive pulmonary disease (COPD) A progressive and irreversible condition characterized by diminished inspiratory and expiratory capacity of the lungs.

chronic pain Pain that continues or recurs over a prolonged period, caused by various disease or abnormal conditions.

chronic pulmonary hypertension A condition of abnormally high pressure within the pulmonary circulation.

chronotropic Pertaining to agents that affect the heart rate; a drug that increases heart rate is said to have a positive chronotropic effect.

chyme The semifluid mass of partly digested food passed from the stomach into the duodenum.

ciliary body A structure continuous with the choroid layer that contains smooth muscle cells and functions in accommodation.

ciliated tissue Any tissue that projects cilia from its surface, such as portions of the epithelium in the respiratory tract.

circle of Willis The circle of interconnected blood vessels at the base of the brain.

circumduction Movement in a circular motion.

circumflex artery The subdivision of the left coronary artery that feeds the lateral and posterior portions of the left ventricle as well as part of the right ventricle.

citrate Any salt or ester of citric acid.

classic heat stroke A severe, sometimes fatal condition resulting from the failure of the temperature regulating capacity of the body; caused by prolonged exposure to the sun or to high temperatures.

clavicle A long, curved horizontal bone just above the first rib, forming the ventral portion of the shoulder girdle.

clinical perineum The portion of the perineum between the vaginal and anal openings.

clitoris Erectile tissue located in the vestibule of the vagina.

coarse ventricular fibrillation Fibrillatory waves greater than 3 mm in amplitude.

coccygeal bone The four segments of the vertebral column that fuse to form the adult coccyx; designated as C_1 to C_4.

coccygeal plexus A network of coccygeal nerves.

cochlea Part of the bony labyrinth of the inner ear.

coitus See *copulation.*

collagen The ropelike protein of the extracellular matrix.

collecting duct A straight tubule that extends from the cortex of the kidney to the tip of the renal pyramid.

Colles' fracture A fracture of the radius at the epiphysis within 1 inch of the joint of the wrist, easily recognized by the dorsal and lateral position of the hand that it causes.

colloid A state of matter in which large molecules or aggregates of molecules that do not precipitate are dispersed in another medium.

command (ICS term) The individual in charge of the incident scene. Also known as *incident commander.*

command post (ICS term) The area from which directs operations for an incident.

communicability period A stage of infection that begins when the latent period ends and continues as long as the agent is present and can potentially spread to other hosts.

communication The transmission and reception of information, resulting in common understanding.

communications center A facility used to dispatch emergency equipment and coordinate communications between field units and personnel.

compact bone Hard, dense bone that is usually found at the surface of skeletal structures, as distinguished from cancellous bone.

compartment syndrome The result of a crush injury usually caused by compressive forces or blunt trauma to muscle groups confined in tight fibrous sheaths with minimal ability to stretch, for example, below the knee or above the elbow.

competitive antagonist An agent with an affinity for the same receptor site as an agonist. The competition with the agonist for the site inhibits the action of the agonist; increasing the concentration of the agonist tends to overcome the inhibition.

complement One of 11 complex, enzymatic serum proteins; causes lysis in an antigen-antibody reaction.

complete abortion An abortion in which the patient has passed all of the products of conception.

complete breech A delivery presentation that occurs when the fetus has both knees and hips flexed; the buttocks are the presenting part.

compliance A measure of the distensibility of lung volume produced by a unit pressure change.

concentration gradient The concentration difference between two points in a solution divided by the distance between the points.

concha The three bony ridges on the lateral wall of the nasal cavity.

condyle A rounded projection on a bone, usually for articulation with another bone.

cone A photoreceptor in the retina of the eye; responsible for color vision.

confabulation The invention of stories to makeup for gaps in memory.

congenital rubella syndrome A serious disease that affects approximately 25% of infants born to women infected with rubella during the first trimester of pregnancy; associated with multiple congenital anomalies, mental retardation, and an increased risk of death from congenital heart disease and sepsis during the first 6 months of life.

conjugate gaze Deviation of both eyes to either side at rest; implies a structural lesion.

conjunctiva A mucous membrane covering the anterior surface of the eyeball and lining of the eyelids.

conjunctivitis Inflammation of the conjunctiva, caused by bacterial or viral infection, allergy, or environmental factors.

connective tissue Tissues that support and bind other body tissues and parts.

conservation of energy law The principle that energy can neither be created nor destroyed; it can only change from one form (mechanical, thermal, electrical, or chemical) to another.

constipation Difficulty in passing stools or incomplete or infrequent passage of hard stools.

contracture deformity An abnormal, usually permanent condition of a joint, characterized by flexion and fixation and caused either by atrophy and shortening of muscle fibers or by loss of elasticity of the skin.

contraindication A medical or physiologic factor that makes it harmful to administer a medication that would otherwise have therapeutic value.

contrastimulant A factor that works against stimulation.

contrecoup An injury occurring at a site opposite the side of impact.

control console Typically, a desk-mounted, enclosed piece of equipment that contains the mechanical and electronic controls used to operate a radio base station.

copulation The sexual union of two people of the opposite sex in which the penis is introduced into the vagina. Also known as **coitus.**

cord presentation A presentation that occurs when the cord slips down into the vagina or presents externally after the amniotic membranes have ruptured.

cornea The convex, transparent, anterior part of the eye.

corniculate cartilage A conical nodule of elastic cartilage surrounding the apex of each arytenoid cartilage.

coronary artery One of two arteries that arise from the base of the aorta and carry blood to the muscle of the heart.

coronary sinus A short trunk that receives most of the veins of the heart and empties into the right atrium.

cor pulmonale An abnormal cardiac condition characterized by hypertrophy of the right ventricle of the heart as a result of hypertension of the pulmonary circulation.

corpus callosum An arched mass of white matter in the depths of the longitudinal fissure; made up of the transverse fibers connecting the cerebral hemispheres.

corpus luteum A yellow endocrine body formed in the ovary at the site of a ruptured vesicular follicle immediately after ovulation.

corpus luteum cyst A type of cyst prone to rupture that forms as a result of hemorrhage in a mature corpus luteum.

costal margin The margin of lower limit of the ribs.

costochondral Pertaining to the junction of the ribs and cartilage.

countershock A high-intensity, short-duration electric shock applied to the area of the heart, resulting in total cardiac depolarization.

coup Local damage that occurs at the site of impact.

couplet Two PVCs in a row. Also known as a **salvo.**

coverage The area covered by radio communication. The generally accepted national emergency system standard is the "90/90" standard. This means that 90% of the coverage area will have communication 90% of the time. Coverage is usually expressed as dead (no coverage), marginal (spotty), good (few problems), or excellent (no problems).

Cowper's gland See *bulbourethral gland.*

coxae The hip joints; the head of the femur and the acetabulum of the innominate bone.

crackle A fine, bubbling sound heard on auscultation of the lung; produced by air entering distal airways and alveoli that contain serous secretions.

cranial nerve One of 12 pairs of nerves that originate from a nucleus within the brain.

cranial vault The eight skull bones that surround and protect the brain; brain case.

craniectomy Surgical removal of bone fragments from the cranium.

cremaster muscle A thin muscle layer spreading out over the spermatic cord in a series of loops; functions to draw the testis up toward the superficial inguinal ring in response to cold or stimulation of the nerve.

crenate The shrinking of red blood cells caused by exposure to a hypertonic solution.

cricoid cartilage The most inferior laryngeal cartilage.

cricothyroid membrane The membrane joining the thyroid and cricoid cartilages.

cricothyrotomy An emergency incision into the larynx.

croup An acute viral infection of the upper and lower respiratory tract that occurs primarily in infants and young children 3 months to 3 years of age; characterized by hoarseness; fever; harsh, brassy cough; inspiratory stridor; and varying degrees of respiratory distress. Also known as *laryngotracheobronchitis.*

crown The portion of human tooth covered by enamel.

crowning The phase at the end of labor in which the fetal head is seen at the opening of the vagina.

crush injury Injury from exposure of tissue to a compressive force sufficient to interfere with the normal structure and metabolic function of the involved cells and tissues.

crush syndrome A life-threatening and sometimes preventable complication of prolonged immobilization or compression; a pathologic process that causes destruction, alteration, or both, or muscle tissue.

crystalloid A substance in a solution that can be diffused through a semipermeable membrane.

crystalluria The presence of crystals in the urine.

CSF rhinorrhea CSF leakage caused by ethmoid cribriform plate fracture.

cubic centimeter (cc) A metric unit of length equal to one hundredth of a meter.

cumulative action The effect that occurs when several doses of a drug are administered or when absorption occurs more quickly than removal by excretion, metabolism, or both.

cuneiform cartilage A small rod of elastic cartilage above the corniculate cartilages in the larynx.

CUPS system A method of patient status coding that assigns patients to one of four categories: CPR, unstable, potentially unstable, and stable.

Cushing reflex An attempt by the body to compensate for a decline in cerebral perfusion pressure by a rise in mean arterial pressure.

Cushing's syndrome A metabolic disorder resulting from the chronic and excessive production of cortisol by the adrenal cortex or by the administration of glucocorticoids in large doses for several weeks or longer.

Cushing's triad Increased systolic pressure, widened pulse pressure, and a decrease in the pulse and respiratory rate that result from increased intracranial pressure.

cuticle The skin fold covering the root of the nail.

cyanotic Having bluish discoloration.

cystic medial necrosis Degenerative changes in the connective tissue of the aortic media.

cystitis Inflammation of the urinary bladder and ureters.

cytochrome oxidase A respiratory enzyme that functions in the transfer of electrons from cytochromes to oxygen, thus activating oxygen, which unites with hydrogen to form water.

cytology The study of cells.

cytomegalovirus (CMV) A member of a group of large species-specific herpes-type viruses with a wide variety of disease effects.

cytoplasm All of the substance of a cell other than the nucleus.

cytoplasmic membrane The plasma membrane.

cytotoxic Pertaining to a pharmacologic compound or other agent that destroys or damages tissue cells.

dartos muscle A layer of smooth muscle in the skin of the scrotum; raises and lowers testes in the scrotum in response to changes in ambient temperature.

deciduous tooth Any of the 20 teeth that appear normally during infancy.

decompression sickness A painful, sometimes fatal syndrome caused by the formation of nitrogen bubbles in the tissues of divers, caisson workers, or aviators who move too rapidly from environments of higher to those of lower atmospheric pressures.

dedicated line A special telephone circuit designated for specific point-to-point communication purposes such as alerting EMS quarters.

deep frostbite A cold injury that results in significant tissue loss even with appropriate therapy; associated with subdermal layers and deep tissues.

defense mechanism An unconscious, intrapsychic reaction to protect to the self from a stressful situation.

defibrillator A device used to depolarize fibrillating myocardial cells, thus allowing them to repolarize uniformly.

degradation The physical destruction or decomposition of a clothing material caused by use, ambient conditions, or exposure to chemicals.

delta cell A constituent of the islet of Langerhans; secretes somatostatin.

delta wave Widened, abnormal slurring or notching of the onset of the QRS complex; indicates anomalous spread of the impulse and is a diagnostic finding for Wolff-Parkinson-White syndrome.

deltoid muscle A large, thick triangular muscle that covers the shoulder joint.

dendrite The branching processes of a neuron that receives stimuli and conducts potentials toward the cell body.

dentin The chief material of teeth, surrounding the pulp and situated inside the enamel and cementum.

deoxyribonucleic acid (DNA) A type of nucleic acid that comprises the genetic material of cells.

depersonalization Forced emotional estrangement.

depolarization A change in electrical charge difference across the cell membrane that causes the difference to be smaller or closer to 0 mV; a phase of the action potential in which the membrane potential moves toward 0 or becomes positive.

depressant A substance that decreases or lessens a body function or activity.

depressed fracture Any fracture of the skull in which fragments are depressed below the normal surface of the skull.

depression A mood disturbance characterized by feelings of sadness, despair, and discouragement resulting from and normally proportionate to some personal loss or tragedy.

dermatitis Inflammation of the skin.

dermatome The skin surface area supplied by a single spinal nerve.

dermis Dense, irregular connective tissue that forms the deep layer of the skin.

descending colon The segment of the colon that extends from the end of the transverse colon at the splenic flexure on the left side of the abdomen down to the beginning of the sigmoid colon in the pelvis.

desensitization Emotional insensitivity.

diabetes insipidus A metabolic disorder characterized by extreme polyuria and polydypsia, caused by deficient production or secretion of antidiuretic hormone (ADH) or inability of the kidney tubules to respond to ADH.

diabetes mellitus A complex disorder of carbohydrate, fat, and protein metabolism that is primarily a result of partial or complete lack of insulin secretion by the beta cells of the pancreas or of defects of the insulin receptors.

diad The combination of sarcoplasmic reticulum and T tubules.

diagnosis Knowing completely.

dialysate A solution used in dialysis.

dialysis fistula An artificial passage, as in an arteriovenous fistula, used to gain access to the patient's blood stream for hemodialysis.

diaphragm The dome-shaped musculofibrous partition that separates the thoracic and abdominal cavities.

diaphragmatic hernia The protrusion of part of the stomach through an opening in the diaphragm.

diaphysis The shaft of a long bone, consisting of a tube of compact bone enclosing the medullary cavity.

diarrhea The frequent passage of loose, watery stools; generally the result of increased motility in the colon.

diencephalon The parts of the brain between the cerebral hemispheres and the mesencephalon.

diffusion The process in which solid, particulate matter in a fluid moves from an area of higher concentration to an area of lower concentration, resulting in an even distribution of the particles in the fluid.

diplopia Double vision.

direct laryngoscopy Visual examination of the larynx with a laryngoscope.

disease period A stage of infection that follows the incubation period and is of variable, disease-specific duration.

disequilibrium Unstable equilibrium; motion sickness.

disequilibrium syndrome A group of neurologic findings that sometimes occurs during or immediately after dialysis; thought to result from a disproportionate decrease in osmolality of the extracellular fluid compared to that of the intracellular compartment in the brain or cerebral spinal fluid.

disoriented Unaware of surroundings.

dissecting aortic aneurysm Localized dilation of the aorta characterized by a longitudinal dissection between the outer and middle layers of the vascular wall.

dissection Separation of an arterial wall, producing a tear in the intima and establishing communication with the lumen; usually affects the thoracic aorta.

disseminated intravascular coagulation (DIC) A grave coagulopathy resulting from the overstimulation of the body's clotting and anticlotting processes in response to disease or injury, such as septicemia, acute hypotension, poisonous snake bites, obstetric emergencies, severe trauma, or hemorrhage.

distribution The transport of a drug through the blood stream to various tissues of the body and ultimately to its site of action.

disulfiram-ethanol reaction A potentially life-threatening physiologic response caused by disulfiram and ethanol that produces ill effects on the gastrointestinal, cardiovascular, and autonomic nervous systems; disulfiram is prescribed to some alcoholic patients to assist them maintain abstinence.

diverticulum A pouchlike herniation through the muscular wall of a tubular organ; may be present in the stomach, small intestine, or, most commonly, the colon.

Do not resuscitate (DNR) A physician order instructing emergency care providers not to attempt resuscitation of a patient in the event of cardiac or respiratory failure. Also known as a **no-code order.**

dorsal root A that conveys afferent nerve processes to the spinal cord.

dorsal root ganglia See **spinal ganglia.**

dorsogluteal site An area made up of several gluteal muscles; used as an injection site.

dram A unit of mass equal to an apothecaries' measure of 60 grains or one-eighth, or in the avoirdupois system, one-sixteenth ounce or 27.34 grains.

dromotropic Pertaining to agents that affect conduction velocity through the conducting tissues of the heart; a drug that speeds conduction is said to have a positive dromotropic effect.

drowning Death by asphyxia after submersion.

drug Any substance injected into a muscle, blood vessel, or cavity of the body, taken by mouth or applied topically to treat or prevent a disease or condition.

drug absorption A process in which drug molecules move from the site of entry into the body to the general circulation.

drug abuse Self-medication or self-administration of a drug in chronically excessive amounts, resulting in psychological or physical dependence or both; functional impairment, and deviation from approved social norms.

drug allergy A systemic reaction to a drug, resulting from previous sensitizing exposure and the development of an immunologic mechanism.

drug dependence A state in which intense physical or emotional disturbance is produced if a drug is withdrawn; previously termed *habituation.*

drug interaction The modified effects of one drug by the prior or concurrent administration of another drug, thereby increasing or decreasing either the pharmacologic or physiologic action of one or both drugs; may be beneficial or detrimental.

drug protein complex A complex formed by the attachment of a drug to proteins, mainly albumin.

drug receptor Any part of a cell, usually an enzyme or large protein molecule, with which a drug molecule interacts to trigger its desired response or effect.

ductus arteriosus A vascular channel in the fetus that joins the pulmonary artery directly to the descending aorta.

ductus deferens A thick, smooth muscular tube that allows sperm to exit from the epididymis through the ejaculatory duct. Also known as *vas deferens.*

ductus venosus The continuation of the umbilical vein through the liver to the inferior vena cava.

duodenum The first subdivision of the small intestine.

duplex A system with the ability to transmit and receive traffic simultaneously through two different frequencies, one to transmit and one to receive. Similar in function to telephone communications in that two parties at either end of the communications link can talk simultaneously without blocking either message.

duplex/multiplex system A communications system with the ability to transmit and receive simultaneously with concurrent transmission of voice and telemetry.

dura mater The outermost layer of the meninges.

duration of action The period from the onset of drug action to the time when a drug effect is no longer seen.

dysconjugate gaze Deviation of the eyes to opposite sides at rest; implies a structural brain stem dysfunction in the pathways that traverse the brain stem from the upper midbrain to at least the level of the lower pons.

dyshemoglobinemia Hemoglobin saturated with compounds other than oxygen, for example, carbon monoxide and methemoglobinemia.

dysmenorrhea Pain associated with menstruation.

dyspareunia Pain with intercourse.

dyspnea Difficulty breathing.

dysrhythmia Variation from a normal rhythm.

EACOM/HEAR Emergency Administrative Communications (EACOM; General Electric), or Hospital Emergency Administrative Radio (HEAR; Motorola). These radio systems use 1500-Hz rotary-pulse dialing, which transmits specific groups of rotary tone pulses for the purpose of selectively addressing hospital-based receivers in particular regions throughout the United States. Most ambulance services have access to this system.

eardrum The cellular membrane that separates the external from the middle ear. Also known as *tympanic membranae.*

ectoparasite An organism that lives on the outside of the body of the host, such as a louse.

ectopic Out of place.

ectopic foci Cardiac dysrhythmias caused by irritation of an excitation impulse at a site other than the sinus node.

ectopic pregnancy An abnormal pregnancy in which the conceptus implants outside the uterine cavity.

eczema Superficial dermatitis of unknown cause.

effacement The shortening of the vaginal portion of the cervix and thinning of its walls as it is stretched and dilated by the fetus during labor.

efferent division The nerve fibers that send impulses from the central nervous system to the periphery.

efficacy An intrinsic activity that refers to a drug's ability to initiate biologic activity as a result of such binding.

Einthoven's triangle An equilateral triangle formed by the patient's right arm, left arm, and left leg; used in electrode sensor placement for ECG monitoring.

ejaculatory duct A duct formed by the joining of the

ductus deferens and the duct from the seminal vesicle that allows sperm to enter the urethra.

ejection The forceful expulsion of blood from the ventricle of the heart.

elastin Major connective tissue protein of elastic tissue that has a structure like a coiled spring.

elder abuse The infliction of physical pain, injury, debilitating mental anguish, unreasonable confinement, or willful deprivation by a caretaker of services necessary to maintain the mental and physical health of an elderly patient.

electroconvulsive therapy The induction of a brief convulsion by passing an electric current through the brain to treat of affective disorders.

electrolyte A cation or anion in solution that conducts an electrical current.

elevation Movement of a structure in a superior direction.

ellipsoid joint A modified ball-and-socket joint in which the articular surfaces are ellipsoid rather than spherical in shape.

embolectomy A surgical incision into an artery for the removal of an embolus or clot.

embryo In humans, the stage of prenatal development between the time of implantation of the fertilized ovum until the end of the seventh or eighth week.

emergency medical services (EMS) A national network of services coordinated to provide aid and medical assistance from primary response to definitive care; involves personnel trained in rescue, stabilization, transportation, and advanced treatment of traumatic or medical emergencies.

emissary veins The small vessels in the skull that connect the sinuses of the dura with the veins on the exterior of the skull through a series of anastomoses.

emphysema An abnormal condition of the pulmonary system characterized by overinflation and destructive changes of alveolar walls, resulting in a loss of lung elasticity and decreased gases.

enamel A hard white substance that covers the dentin of the crown of the tooth.

encephalitis An inflammatory condition of the brain, usually caused by an infection transmitted by the bite of an infected mosquito, may also result from lead or other poisoning or from hemorrhage.

endolymph Fluid found within the membranous labyrinth.

endometriosis An abnormal gynecologic condition characterized by ectopic growth and function of endometrial tissue; thought to result from fragments of endometrium from the lining of the uterus that are regurgitated during menstruation backward through the fallopian tubes into the peritoneal cavity, where they attach and grow as small cystic structures.

endometritis An inflammatory condition of the endometrium, usually caused by bacterial infection.

endometrium The mucous membrane lining of the uterus; changes in thickness and structure with the menstrual cycle.

endoplasmic reticulum (ER) A network of connecting sacs or canals that wind through a cell's cytoplasm, serving as a miniature circulatory system for the cell.

endotoxin A toxin contained in the cell walls of some microorganisms, especially gram-negative bacteria.

endotracheal intubation An airway management procedure in which an endotracheal tube is inserted through the mouth or nose into the trachea. Used to maintain a patent airway; to prevent aspiration of material from the digestive tract; to permit suctioning of tracheobronchial secretions; to administer positive-pressure ventilation; and to administer certain medications when other means of vascular access are unavailable.

enhanced automaticity Cause of dysrhythmias in Purkinje fibers and other myocardial cells with a high resting membrane potential; results from an acceleration of phase 4 depolarization commonly produced by an abnormally high leakage of sodium ions into the cells, causing the cells to reach threshold prematurely.

enophthalmos Recessed globe.

enteral route A route of drug administration along any portion of the gastrointestinal tract.

enzyme A protein produced by living cells that catalyzes chemical reactions in organic matter.

eosinophil A white blood cell that inhibits inflammation; readily stains with acidic dyes.

epicardium See *visceral pericardium.*

epicondyle A projection on the surface of a bone above its condyle.

epidermis The outer portion of skin; formed of epithelial tissue that rests on or covers the dermis.

epididymis A tightly coiled tube that lies along the top and behind the testes where sperm mature.

epidural hematoma Accumulation of blood between the dura mater and the cranium.

epidural space The space above or on the dura.

epiglottis A lidlike cartilage overhanging the entrance to the larynx.

epiglottitis Inflammation of the epiglottis; a severe form of the condition affecting primarily children is characterized by fever, sore throat, stridor, croupy cough, and an erthymatous epiglottis.

epilepsy A group of neurologic disorders characterized by recurrent episodes of convulsive seizures, sensory disturbances, abnormal behavior, loss of consciousness, or some combination of these.

epinephrine Adrenalin; the secretion of the adrenal medulla.

epiphyseal line A dense plate in a bone that is no longer growing, indicating the former site of the epiphyseal plate.

epiphyseal plate The site of bone elongation. Also known as the *growth pate.*

epiphysis The head of a long bone that is separated from the shaft of the bone by the epiphyseal plate until the bone stops growing, the plate is obliterated, and the shaft and the head are united.

epistaxis Bleeding from the nose.

epithelial tissue The cellular covering of internal and

external surfaces of the body, including the lining of vessels and other small cavities.

Epstein-Barr virus (EBV) The herpesvirus that causes infectious mononucleosis.

erection The condition of hardness, swelling, and elevation observed in the penis and to a lesser degree in the clitoris, usually caused by sexual arousal.

erythrocyte A red blood cell.

escape beat An automatic beat of the heart that occurs after an interval longer than the duration of the dominant heartbeat cycle.

eschar A scab or dry crust resulting from a thermal or chemical burn.

escharotomy Surgical incision into necrotic tissue resulting from a severe burn; sometimes necessary to prevent edema from building up sufficient interstitial pressure to impair capillary filling and cause ischemia.

esophageal gastric tube airway (EGTA) or **esophageal obturator airway (EOA)** An airway adjunct that occludes the esophagus and prevents air from entering the stomach and vomitus from entering the trachea.

esophageal reflux A chronic disease manifested by various sequelae associated with reflux of the stomach and duodenal contents into the esophagus.

esophageal stricture An abnormal temporary or permanent narrowing of the esophagus secondary to inflammation, external pressure, or scarring.

esophageal varices A complex of longitudinal, tortuous veins at the lower end of the esophagus that become large and swollen as a result of portal hypertension; these veins are especially susceptible to ulceration and hemorrhage.

esophagus The muscular canal extending from the pharynx to the stomach.

estimated date of confinement Delivery date for the fetus.

estrogen One of a group of hormonal steroid compounds that promote the development of female secondary sex characteristics.

ethmoid bone The very light and spongy bone at the base of the cranium, forming most of the walls of the superior part of the nasal cavity.

ethmoid sinus One of the numerous small, thin-walled cavities in the ethmoid bone of the skull, rimmed by the frontal maxilla and lacrimal, sphenoidal, and palatine bones.

ethylene glycol A chemical used in automobile antifreeze preparations.

eustachian tube See *auditory tube.*

eversion Turning outward.

evisceration The protrusion of an internal organ through a wound or surgical incision, especially in the abdominal wall.

excitability The property of a cell that enables it to react to irritation or stimulation.

excretion The elimination of toxic or inactive metabolites, primarily by the kidney; the intestine, lungs, and mammary glands, sweat glands, and salivary glands may also be involved.

excursion Movement from side to side.

exertional heat stroke An abnormal condition characterized by weakness, vertigo, nausea, muscle cramps, and loss of consciousness; caused by depletion of body fluid and electrolytes resulting from exposure to intense heat or the inability to acclimatize to heat.

exocrine Secreting into a duct; opposite of "endocrine."

exophthalmos An abnormal condition characterized by marked protrusion of the eyeballs.

exothermic Marked or accompanied by the evolution of heat.

exotoxin A toxin secreted or excreted by a living organism.

expiratory center The region of the medulla that is electrically active during nonquiet expiration.

expiratory reserve volume The maximum volume of air that can be exhaled after a normal expiration.

extension Sstretching out.

external anal sphincter A sphincter muscle located at the tip of the coccyx and surrounding fascia; prevents the movement of feces out of the rectum until it is relaxed.

external auditory canal The passage for sound impulses passing through the ear.

external auditory meatus The canal of the external ear. Also known as *external auditory canal.*

external ear The portion of the ear that includes the auricle and external auditory meatus; terminates at the eardrum.

external jugular vein One of a pair of large vessels in the neck that receive most of the blood from the exterior of the cranium and deep tissues of the face.

external urinary sphincter The smooth muscle that surrounds the urethra as the urethra extends through the pelvic floor; controls the flow of urine through the urethra.

extracellular Occurring outside of a cell or cell tissues or in cavities or spaces between cell layers or groups of cells.

extracellular matrix Nonliving chemical substances located between connective tissue cells.

extrapyramidal reaction A response to a treatment or drug characterized by involuntary movement, changes in muscle tone, and abnormal posture.

extravasated The passage or escape of blood, serum, or lymph into the tissues.

extubation Removal of an endotracheal tube.

exudate Fluid, cells, or other substances that have been slowly discharged from cells or blood vessels through small pores or breaks in cell membranes.

face presentation An abnormal presentation in which the brow or forehead of the fetus is the first part of the body to enter the birth canal. Also known as *brow presentation.*

facial bones The 14 bones that form the structure of the face in the anterior skull, they do not contribute to the cranial vault.

facial nerve palsy Partial or total loss of the functions of the facial muscles or the loss of sensation of the face.

facies A facial expression or appearance.

facilitated diffusion A carrier-mediated process that moves substances into or out of cells from a high to a low concentration.

fallopian tube See *uterine tube.*

false rib See **rib.**

false imprisonment Intentional and unjustifiable detention of a person.

false vocal cord See *vestibular fold.*

fascia The loose areolar connective tissue found beneath the skin or dense connective tissue that encloses and separates muscle.

fascicle A small bundle or cluster of nerve or muscle fibers that provides pathways for impulse conduction.

fasciotomy Incision of a fascia to relieve elevated intracompartmental pressure.

febrile seizure A seizure that results from fever.

fecalith A hard, impacted mass of feces in the colon.

feces Waste material discharged from the intestines.

femoral vein A large vein in the thigh originating in the popliteal vein and accompanying the femoral artery in the proximal two thirds of the thigh.

femur The thigh bone, which extends from the pelvis to the knee; the largest and strongest bone in the body.

fetus Unborn young, from the third month of the intrauterine period until birth.

fibrinogen A soluble blood protein converted into insoluble fibrin during clotting.

fibrocartilage Cartilage that consists of a dense matrix of white collagenous fibers.

fibrosis An abnormal condition in which fibrous connective tissue spreads over or replaces normal smooth muscle or other normal organ tissue.

fibrous connective tissue A connective tissue that consists mainly of bundles of strong, white collagenous fibers arranged in parallel rows.

fibrous joint See *joint.*

fibrous pericardium Fibrous outer layer of the

fibrous tunic The sclera and cornea.

fibula The bone of the leg, lateral to and smaller than the tibia.

Fick principle The principle, used to determine cardiac output, according to which the amount of oxygen uptake of each unit of blood as it passes through the lungs equals the oxygen concentration difference between arterial and mixed venous blood.

filtration Movement caused by a pressure gradient of a liquid through a filter that prevents some or all of the substances in the liquid from passing through.

fimbria A fringelike structure located at the border of the uterine tube.

fine ventricular fibrillation Fibrillatory waves less than 3 mm in amplitude.

first stage of labor The stage of labor that begins with the onset of regular contractions and ends with complete dilation of the cervix.

flat bones Bones that have a thin, flattened shape. Examples are certain skull bones, ribs, sternum, and scapulae.

flatulence The presence of an excessive amount of air or gas in the stomach or intestinal tract, causing distention of the organs and in some cases mild to moderate pain.

flexion Bending.

floating rib See *rib.*

flora Microorganisms that live on or in the body to compete with disease-producing microorganisms and provide a natural immunity against certain infections.

flutter waves Abnormal P waves in a "sawtooth" or "picket fence" pattern; represent atrial depolarization in an abnormal direction followed by atrial repolarization.

focal seizure See *Jacksonian seizure.*

fontanelle A space covered by a tough membrane between the bones of an infant's cranium.

foramen ovale An opening in the septum between the right and left atria in the fetal heart; provides a bypass for blood that would otherwise flow to the fetal lungs.

foramina A passage in the occipital bone through which the spinal cord enters the spinal column.

formed elements Cells and cell fragments of blood.

formic acid A colorless, pungent liquid found in nature in ants and other insects.

fourth ventricle The ventricle located in the superior region of the medulla; continuous with the central canal of the spinal cord.

frank breech See *front breech.*

fraternal twins Two offspring born of the same pregnancy from two ova released simultaneously from the ovary and fertilized at the same time.

French scale system A scale used to denote size of catheters and other tubular instruments, each unit is roughly equivalent to 0.33 mm in diameter.

frequency The number of repetitive cycles per second completed by a radio wave.

frequency modulation (FM) A deviation of carrier frequency in accordance with the strength of applied audio. FM is less susceptible to some types of interference than AM and is typically used in EMS communications.

frontal bone The single cranial bone that forms the front of the skull.

frontal lobe The largest of the five lobes that comprise each of the two cerebral hemispheres; significantly influences personality and is associated with higher mental activities such as planning, judgment, and conceptualization.

frontal plane An imaginary plane that divides the body into front and back or anterior and posterior positions. Also known as *coronal plane.*

frontal sinus One of a pair of small cavities in the frontal bone of the skull that communicates with the nasal cavity.

front breech A presentation that occurs when the fetal hips are flexed and the legs extend in front of the fetus; the buttocks are the presenting part. Also known as *frank breech.*

frostnip The mildest form of cold injury; may be treated without loss of tissue.

functional residual capacity The expiratory reserve volume plus the residual volume; reflects the amount of gas remaining in the lungs at the end of a normal expiration.

fundus The bottom or rounded end of a hollow organ, such as the fundus of the uterus.

fusion beat A PVC that occurs at approximately the same time that an electrical impulse of the underlying rhythm is activating the ventricles, thereby causing ventricular depolarization to occur simultaneously in two directions; results in a QRS complex that has the characteristics of both the PVC and the QRS complex of the underlying rhythm.

gallbladder A pear-shaped excretory sac on the visceral surface of the right lobe of the liver; serves as a reservoir for bile.

gallows humor Morbid or cynical humor.

ganglia A group of nerve cell bodies in the peripheral nervous system.

gap junction A small channel between cells that allows the passage of ions and small molecules between cells.

gastric gland A gland located in the mucus of the fundus and body of the stomach.

gastrin A polypeptide hormone that stimulates the flow of gastric juice and contributes to the stimulus causing bile and pancreatic enzyme secretion.

gastroenteritis The inflammation of the stomach and intestines that accompanies numerous gastrointestinal disorders.

gastrostomy An artificial opening into the stomach.

gating protein A protein that controls the rate at which ions move through an ion channel.

general gas law The characteristic of gas that it flows from an area of higher pressure or concentration to an area of lower pressure or concentration. Also known as *Boyle's law.*

generic name The official, established name assigned to a drug. Also known as a *nonproprietary name.*

genitalia Reproductive organs.

German measles See *rubella.*

gerontology The study of the problems of all aspects of aging.

gestation The period from the fertilization of the ovum until birth.

gestational diabetes mellitus (GDM) A disorder characterized by an impaired ability to metabolize carbohydrate, usually caused by a deficiency of insulin. It occurs in pregnancy and disappears after delivery, but in some cases returns years later.

gingiva The portion of the oral mucosa surrounding the tooth.

gingival hypertrophy Swelling of the gums; often associated with chronic *phenytoin* therapy.

gingivostomatitis Multiple, painful ulcers on the gums and mucous membranes of the mouth; the result of a herpesvirus infection.

Glasgow coma scale A standardized system for assessing the degree of conscious impairment in the critically ill and for predicting the duration and ultimate outcome of coma.

glia limitans A supporting structure of nervous tissue consisting of large, star-shaped cells.

gliding joint See *plane joint.*

globule A small spheric mass.

globulin One of a broad category of simple proteins classified by solubility, mobility, and size.

glomerular filtration rate (GFR) The amount of plasma that filters into Bowman's capsules per minute.

glomerulus The mass of capillary loops at the beginning of each nephron.

glossopharyngeal nerve Either of a pair of cranial nerves essential to the sense of taste, to sensation in some viscera, and to secretion from certain glands.

glottic opening The vocal cords and the space between them.

glottis The space between the vocal cords.

glucocorticoid An adrenocortical steroid hormone that increases glyconeogenesis, exerts an antiinflammatory effect, and influences many body functions.

glucosuria The abnormal presence of glucose in the urine resulting from large amounts of carbohydrate, kidney disease, or a metabolic disease such as diabetes mellitus.

gluteus medius muscle The muscle that originates between the anterior and posterior gluteal lines of the ilium and inserts in the greater trochanter of the femur.

glycolysis An anaerobic process during which glucose is converted to pyruvic acid.

glycoprotein Any of a large group of conjugated proteins in which the nonprotein substance is a carbohydrate.

goblet cell One of the many specialized cells that secrete mucus and form glands of the epithelium of the stomach, intestine, and parts of the respiratory tract.

goiter A hypertrophic thyroid gland, usually evident as a pronounced swelling in the neck.

golden hour The critical period during which surgical intervention for the trauma patient can enhance survival and reduce complications.

Golgi apparatus Specialized endoplasmic reticulum that concentrates and packages materials for secretion from the cell.

gomphosis An articulation by the insertion of a conic process into a socket, such as the insertion of the root of a tooth into an alveolus of the mandible or maxilla.

gonad A gamete-producing gland, such as an ovary or testis.

gout A disease associated with an inborn error of uric acid metabolism that increases production of or interferes with excretion of uric acid. Also known as *hyperuricemia.*

graafian follicle See *vesicular follicle.*

grain The smallest unit of mass in apothecaries' weights, being the same in all and equal to 4.79891 mg.

gram (g) A metric unit of mass equal to one thousandth of a kilogram.

gram-negative sepsis Sepsis caused by gram negative bacteria when the bacterium dies and is broken down in the body.

grand mal seizure An epileptic seizure characterized by a generalized involuntary muscular contraction and cessation of respiration followed by tonic and clonic spasms of the muscles.

grand multipara A woman who has had seven deliveries or more.

granulosa cell A cell in the layer surrounding the primary follicle.

gravida The number of all current and past pregnancies.

great vessels The large arteries and veins entering and leaving the heart. They include the aorta, the pulmonary arteries and veins, and the superior and inferior venae cavae.

Guillain-Barré syndrome A relatively rare disease affecting the peripheral nervous system, especially the spinal nerves, but also the cranial nerves; associated with a viral infection or immunization.

habituation See *drug dependence.*

hair follicle An invagination of the epidermis into the dermis that contains the root of the hair and receives the ducts of sebaceous and apocrine glands.

hair papilla A small, cup-shaped cluster of cells located at the base of the follicle where hair growth begins.

hair root The part of the hair that lies hidden in the follicle.

hair shaft The visible part of the hair.

half duplex The use of two different frequencies: one to transmit and one to receive, that cannot be used simultaneously.

half-life (t½) The amount of time required to reduce a drug level to one half its initial value.

hard palate The floor of the nasal cavity that separates the nasal cavity from the oral cavity.

head of bone An eminence on a bone by which it articulates with another bone.

hemasite A small, button-shaped indwelling vascular device usually placed in the upper arm or proximal, anterior thigh; similar to an AV graft, but has an external rubber septum sutured to the skin through which a dialysis catheter is inserted for treatment.

hemiblock Failure in conduction of cardiac impulse in either of two main divisions of the left branch of the bundle of His; interruption may occur in either the anterior (superior) or posterior (inferior) division.

hemiparesis One-sided weakness.

hemoagglutinin An agglutinin that clumps red blood corpuscles.

hemodialysis A procedure in which impurities or wastes are removed from the blood, used in treating renal insufficiency and various toxic conditions.

hemoglobin A complex protein-iron compound in the blood that carries oxygen to the cells from the lungs and carbon dioxide away from the cells to the lungs.

hemolytic anemia A condition in which there is reduced delivery of oxygen to tissues caused by increased hemolysis of erythrocytes.

hemophilia A group of heredity bleeding disorders in which one of the factors necessary for blood coagulation is deficient.

hemophilia A Caused by a deficiency of coagulation factor VIII; considered the classic type of hemophilia.

hemophilia B Caused by a deficiency of coagulation factor IX.

hemopneumothorax See *pneumohemothorax.*

hemopoietic tissue Tissue related to the process of formation and development of various types of blood cells.

hemoptysis Coughing up blood from the respiratory tract.

hemorrhage Flowing of blood.

hemorrhoid A varicosity in the lower rectum or anus caused by congestion in the veins of the hemorrhoidal plexus.

hemostasis The termination of bleeding by mechanical or chemical means or by substances that arrest the blood flow.

hemostatic An agent that reduces bleeding by speeding clot formation.

hemothorax A collection of blood in the pleural space, which causes the lung to collapse.

hemotympanum Blood behind the tympanic membrane from fractures of the temporal bone.

heparin A substance that inhibits blood clotting; obtained from the liver.

heparin lock A peripheral vascular access device that has no attached IV tubing; used to ensure ready access to peripheral veins for the brief administration of medications or when frequent IV therapy is indicated on an outpatient basis, for example, chemotherapy.

hepatic artery The branch of the aorta that delivers blood to the liver.

hepatic encephalopathy A type of brain damage caused by liver disease and consequent ammonia intoxication.

hepatic portal system The system that transports blood from the digestive tract to the liver.

hepatitis An inflammatory condition of the liver, characterized by jaundice, hepatomegaly, anorexia, abdominal and gastric discomfort, abnormal liver function, clay-colored stools, and dark urine. Viruses responsible for hepatitis are hepatitis A virus (HAV), hepatitis B virus (HBV), hepatitis C virus (HCV), hepatitis D virus (HDV), and hepatitis E virus (HEV).

hepatomegaly Enlargement of the liver.

Hering-Breuer reflex A reflex in which afferent impulses from stretch receptors in the lungs arrest inspiration; expiration then occurs.

hernia Protrusion of any organ through an abdominal

opening in the muscle wall of the cavity that surrounds it.

herniation A protrusion of a body organ or portion of an organ through an abnormal opening in a membrane, muscle, or other tissue.

herpes simplex virus type 1 (HSV-1) An infection caused by the herpes simplex virus; tends to occur in the facial area, particularly around the mouth and nose.

herpes simplex virus type 2 (HSV-2) An infection caused by the herpes simplex virus; usually limited to the genital region.

hertz (Hz) A unit of frequency equal to 1 cycle per second.

hexaxial reference system The system of intersecting lines of the standard limb leads and three other intersecting lines of reference: aVR, aVL, and aVF leads.

hiatal hernia Protrusion of a portion of the stomach upward through the diaphragm.

Hickman catheter A long, indwelling catheter sometimes used by patients with cancer, gastrointestinal dysfunction, debilitating diseases, and those who need intermittent intravenous administration of antibiotics, nutritional supplements, or other intravenous medications.

high-altitude cerebral edema (HACE) The most severe form of acute high-altitude illness; characterized by a progression of global cerebral signs in the presence of acute mountain sickness that are probably related to increased intracranial pressure.

high-altitude pulmonary edema (HAPE) An illness thought to be related, at least in part, to increased pulmonary artery pressure that develops in response to hypoxia; results in the release of leukotrienes, which increase pulmonary arteriolar permeability, and in leakage of fluid into extravascular locations.

high-grade AV block Occurs when at least two consecutive AV impulses (atrial P waves) fail to be conducted to the ventricles.

hilum A depression or pit at the part of an organ where the vessels and nerves enter.

hinge joint A joint that consists of a convex cylinder in one bone applied to a corresponding concavity in another bone. These joints permit movement in one plane only.

histamine An amine released by mast cells and basophils that promotes inflammation.

homeostasis A state of equilibrium in the body with respect to functions and composition of fluids and tissues.

human immunodeficiency virus (HIV) The viral agent responsible for acquired immunodeficiency syndrome (AIDS).

humerus The largest bone of the upper arm, comprising a body, head, and condyle

hyaline cartilage Gelatinous, glossy cartilage tissue; thinly covers the articulating ends of bones, connects the ribs to the sternum, and supports the nose, trachea, and part of the larynx.

hydrocephalus A pathologic condition characterized by an abnormal accumulation of cerebral spinal fluid, usually under increased pressure, within the cranial vault, with subsequent dilation of the ventricles.

hydrochloric acid (HCl) The acid in gastric juice.

hydrogen ion The acidic element in a solution.

hymen A mucous membrane that may partially or entirely occlude the vaginal outlet.

hymenoptera A large, highly specialized order of insects that includes wasps, bees, and ants.

hyoid bone The U-shaped bone between the mandible and larynx.

hypercalcemia A greater-than-normal concentration of calcium in the blood.

hypercholesterolemia Increased serum cholesterol.

hypercoagulability A tendency of the blood to coagulate more rapidly than normal.

hyperkalemia A greater-than-normal concentration of potassium in the blood.

hyperkaluria A high potassium concentration in the urine.

hypermagnesemia A condition that results from an abnormally high concentration of magnesium in the blood plasma.

hypernatremic A greater-than-normal concentration of sodium in the blood.

hyperosmolar hyperglycemic nonketotic coma (HHNK) A diabetic coma in which the level of ketone bodies is normal; caused by hyperosmolarity of extracellular fluid, resulting in dehydration of intracellular fluid.

hyperparathyroidism A condition of increased parathyroid function.

hyperphosphatemia High levels of alkaline phosphate in the blood.

hyperpolarization An increase in the charge difference across the cell membrane; causes the charge difference to move away from 0 mV.

hypertensive crisis A sudden, severe increase in blood pressure to a level exceeding 200/120 mm Hg.

hypertensive encephalopathy A set of symptoms, including headache, convulsions, and coma, associated with glomerulonephritis.

hyperthermia Abnormal excess body temperature.

hyperthyroidism A condition characterized by increased activity of the thyroid gland.

hypertonic A solution that causes cells to shrink.

hyperuricemia See *gout.*

hyperventilation A persistent, rapid, and deep respiration that often results in hyperpnea.

hypocalcemia A lower-than-normal concentration of calcium in the blood.

hypochlorhydria A deficiency of hydrochloric acid in the stomach's gastric juice.

hypoglycemia A lower-than-normal amount of glucose in the blood.

hypokalemia A lower-than-normal concentration of potassium in the blood.

hypomagnesemia A condition that results from an abnormally low concentration of magnesium in the blood plasma.

hyponatremia A lower-than-normal concentration of sodium in the blood.

hypoparathyroidism A condition of diminished parathyroid function.

hypopituitarism An abnormal condition caused by diminished activity of the pituitary gland; marked by excessive deposits of fat or acquisition of adolescent characteristics.

hypothalamus A portion of the diencephalon of the brain that activates, controls, and integrates the peripheral autonomic nervous system, endocrine processes, and many somatic functions such as body temperature, sleep, and appetite.

hypothermia An abnormal body temperature below 95° F (35° C).

hypothyroidism A condition characterized by decreased activity of the thyroid gland.

hypotonic A solution that causes cells to swell.

hypotonicity of the muscles Decreased muscle tone or tension.

hypovolemic shock A form of shock most frequently caused by hemorrhage, but also by dehydration.

hypoxia Inadequate, reduced tension of cellular oxygen, characterized by cyanosis, tachycardia, hypotension, peripheral vasoconstriction, and mental confusion.

hypoxic drive The low arterial oxygen pressure stimulus to respiration that is mediated through the carotid bodies.

I band See **isotropic band.**

iatrogenic Caused by treatment or diagnostic procedures.

identical twins Two offspring born of the same pregnancy and developed from a single fertilized ovum that splits into equal halves during the early phase of embryonic development, giving rise to separate fetuses.

idiopathic epilepsy See **primary epilepsy.**

idiosyncrasy An abnormal or peculiar response to a drug; thought to result from genetic enzymatic deficiencies or other unique physiologic variables that lead to abnormal mechanisms of drug metabolism or altered physiologic effects of the drug.

idioventricular rhythm A ventricular escape rhythm that results when impulses from higher pacemakers fail to reach the ventricles or when the rate of discharge of higher pacemakers become less than that of the ventricles.

ileocecal sphincter The valve between the ilium of the small intestine and the cecum of the large intestine.

ileum The distal portion of the small intestine.

ileus An obstruction of the intestines.

iliac crest The upper free margin of the ilium.

ilium One of the three bones that make up the innominate bone.

immersion hypothermia Hypothermia from immersion in cold water.

immunity Insusceptibility to a particular disease or condition.

immunization The process of rendering a person immune or of becoming immune.

immunoglobulin Any of five structurally and antigenically distinct antibodies present in the serum and external secretions of the body, including IgA, IgD, IgE, IgG, and IgM.

implied consent The presumption that an unconscious or incompetent person would consent to lifesaving care.

incident command system (ICS) A management program designed to control, direct, and coordinate emergency response operations and resources.

incomplete abortion An abortion in which the patient has passed some but not all of the products of conception.

incomplete breech The presentation that occurs when the fetus has one or both hips incompletely flexed, resulting in the presentation of one or both lower extremities, often a foot.

incubation period A stage of infection, during which the organism reproduces, that begins with invasion of the agent and ends when the disease process begins.

incus The middle of the three ossicles in the middle ear.

induced abortion The intentional termination of a pregnancy.

inferior nasal concha bone One of three bony ridges on the lateral wall of the nasal cavity.

inferior venae cavae The vein that returns blood from the lower limbs and the greater part of the pelvic and abdominal organs to the right atrium.

infertility The inability to produce offspring.

infiltration The process whereby a fluid passes into tissues.

influenza A highly contagious infection of the respiratory tract transmitted by airborne droplet infection. Three main types of the virus have been identified by researchers: types A, B, and C.

informed consent Consent obtained from a patient after explaining all facts necessary for the patient to make a reasonable decision.

inguinal canal The passage through the lower abdominal wall that transmits the spermatic cord in the male and the round ligament in the female.

inguinal node One of approximately 18 nodes in the group of lymph glands in the upper femoral triangle of the thigh.

inner ear The part of the ear that contains the sensory organs for hearing and balance.

insertion The more movable attachment point of a muscle.

inspiratory capacity The sum of the tidal volume and the inspiratory reserve volume.

inspiratory center The region of the medulla that stimulates inspiration.

inspiratory reserve volume The maximum volume of air that can be inspired after a normal inspiration.

insulin A hormone secreted by the pancreatic islets.

integumentary system The largest organ system of the

body. It consists of the skin and accessory structures such as hair, nails, and a variety of glands.

interatrial septum Separates the right and left atria of the heart.

intercalated disk Cell-to-cell attachment with gap junctions between cardiac muscle cells.

intercellular Occurring between or among cells.

interference Any undesired radio signal on a radio frequency. It may arise from other radio transmitters or other sources of electromagnetic radiation. "Nuisance interference" is interference that can be heard but does not override system signals. "Destructive interference" overrides system signals.

internal anal sphincter A sphincter muscle located at the caudal end of the rectum.

internal carotid artery Each of two arteries that enter the cranial vault through the carotid canals.

internal jugular vein One of a pair of veins in the neck; each collects blood from one side of the brain, the face, and the neck, and both unite with the subclavian vein to form the brachiocephalic vein.

internal mammary artery One of the pair of arteries that arise from the first portions of the subclavian arteries; supplies the pectoral muscles, breasts, pericardium, and abdominal muscles. Also known as *internal thoracic artery*.

internal thoracic artery See *internal mammary artery*.

internal urinary sphincter The smooth muscle of the bladder located at the junction of the urethra with the urinary bladder; controls the flow of urine through the urethra.

interneuron See *motor neuron*.

internodal tract Pathways between the segments of a nerve fiber.

interpolated PVC A PVC that falls between two sinus beats without interrupting the rhythm.

interstitial fluid Fluid that occupies the space outside the blood vessels.

interventricular foramina One of two passageways between the two lateral ventricles and the third ventricle.

interventricular septum The tissue that separates the right and left ventricles of the heart.

intervertebral disk One of the fibrous disks between all adjacent spinal vertebrae except the atlas and axis; serves as a "shock absorber" for the vertebral column; provide additional support for the body; and prevents the vertebral bodies from rubbing against each other.

intracellular Occurring within cell membranes.

intraocular pressure Pressure within the eye that keeps the eye inflated.

intraosseous infusion (IO infusion) Placement of a rigid needle into a bone and the infusion of fluid and medication directly into the bone marrow.

intrapleural Within the pleura.

intrapleural pressure See *intrathoracic pressure*.

intrapulmonic pressure The pressure of the gas within the alveoli; varies slightly above and below 760 mm Hg.

intrathoracic pressure The pressure in the pleural space; usually 751 to 754 mm Hg. Also known as *intrapleural pressure*.

intrinsic factor The factor secreted by the parietal cells of the gastric glands and required for adequate absorption of vitamin B_{12}.

invagination Infolding or in-pocketing.

invasion of privacy Making public without legal justification details about a person's private life that might reasonably expose that person to ridicule, notoriety, or embarrassment.

inversion Turning inward.

involuntary muscle A muscle that is not normally consciously controlled. See *smooth muscle*.

ion An atom or group of atoms carrying a charge of electricity by virtue of having gained or lost one or more electrons.

ipsilateral Pertaining to the same side of the body.

iris The colored portion of the eye that can be seen through the cornea.

irregular bones Bones that are not representative of the other three categories (long, short, or flat bones). Examples include vertebrae and facial bones.

ischium One of the three parts of the hip bone, which joins the ilium and the pubis to form the acetabulum.

islets of Langerhans Clusters of cells within the pancreas that produce insulin, glucagon, and pancreatic polypeptide.

isolette A self-contained incubator unit that provides controlled heat, humidity, and oxygen for the isolation and care of premature and low-birth-weight neonates.

isometric contraction A muscle contraction in which the length of the muscle does not change, but the tension produced increases.

isotonic solution A solution that causes cells to neither shrink nor swell.

isotonic contraction A muscle contraction in which the tension produced by the muscle stays the same, but the muscle length becomes shorter.

Jacksonian seizure A transitory disturbance in motor, sensory, or autonomic function resulting from abnormal neuronal discharges in a localized part of the brain. Also known as a *focal seizure*.

jaundice A yellow discoloration of the skin, mucous membranes, and sclerae of the eyes, caused by a greater-than-normal amount of bilirubin in the blood.

jejunum One of the three portions of the small intestine.

joint Any one of the connections between bones; Classified according to structure and movability as fibrous, cartilaginous, or synovial. Fibrous joints are immovable; cartilaginous joints are slightly movable; synovial joints are freely movable.

joint capsule A well-defined structure that encloses a joint.

Joule's law The principle that the amount of heat produced is directly proportional to the square of the current strength, times the resistance of the tissue, times the duration of the current flow.

J point The point at which the T wave takes off from the QRS complex.

jugular notch The superior margin of the manubrium; easily palpated at the anterior base of the neck. Also known as the **suprasternal notch.**

Kaposi's sarcoma A malignant, multifocal neoplasm of reticuloendothelial cells that begins as soft, brownish or purple papules on the feet and slowly spreads in the skin, metastasizing to the lymph nodes and viscera; associated with diabetes, malignant lymphoma, AIDS, and other disorders.

Kehr's sign A common complaint associated with splenic injury in which pain is noted in the left shoulder; thought to be caused by referred pain secondary to irritation of the adjacent diaphragm from splenic hematoma or hemoperitoneum.

Kent fibers See *bundle of Kent.*

ketoacidosis Acidosis accompanied by the accumulation of ketones in the body, resulting from faulty carbohydrate metabolism.

ketoacids Compounds containing the carbonyl and carboxyl groups.

ketonuria Presence in the urine of excessive amounts of ketone bodies.

kidney The organ that cleanses the body of the waste products continually produced by metabolism.

kilogram (kg) A metric unit of mass equal to 1000 grams or 2.2046 pounds.

kilohertz (KHz) A unit of frequency equal to 1000 cycles per second.

kinematics The process of predicting injury patterns that may result from the forces and motions of energy.

kinin Serum protein that causes vasodilation and increases vascular permeability.

Koplik's spots Small red spots with bluish-white centers on the lingual and buccal mucosa, characteristic of measles.

Korsakoff's psychosis A form of amnesia often seen in alcoholics, characterized by a loss of short-term memory and an inability to learn new skills.

Krebs' cycle A sequence of enzymatic reactions involving the metabolism of carbon chains of sugar, fatty acids, and amino acids to yield carbon dioxide, water, and high-energy phosphate bonds.

Kussmaul's respiration An abnormally deep, very rapid sighing respiratory pattern characteristic of diabetic ketoacidosis or other metabolic acidosis.

kyphosis An abnormal condition of the vertebral column characterized by increased convexity in the curvature of the thoracic spine as viewed from the side.

labial frenulum A medial fold of mucous membrane connecting the inside of each lip to the corresponding gum.

labia majora Two rounded folds of skin surrounding the labia minora and the vestibule.

labia minora Two longitudinal folds of mucous membrane enclosed by the labia majora and bounding the vestibule.

lacrimal bone One of the smallest and most fragile bones of the face, located in the anterior part of the medial wall of the orbit.

lacrimal canal The canal that carries excess tears away from the eye.

lacrimal gland The tear gland located in the superolateral corner of the orbit.

lacrimal sac An enlargement of the lacrimal canal that leads into the nasolacrimal duct.

lacrimation Excessive tear production.

lactation The secretion of milk from the breasts to nourish an infant or child.

lactic acid A three-carbon molecule derived from pyruvic acid as a product of anaerobic respiration.

lactiferous duct The duct that drains the grapelike cluster of milk-secreting glands in the breast.

lanugo hair Soft, downy hair covering a normal fetus.

laparoscopy Examination of the abdominal cavity with a laparoscope.

large intestine The portion of the digestive tract comprising the cecum; appendix; ascending, transverse, and descending colons, and rectum.

laryngectomy Surgical removal of the larynx, performed to treat cancer of the larynx.

laryngopharynx The lowest part of the pharynx.

laryngoscope An endoscope for visualization of the larynx.

laryngoscopy Examination of the larynx via a laryngoscope.

laryngotracheobronchitis See *croup.*

larynx The voice box, located just below the pharynx.

latent period A stage of infection that begins with pathogenic invasion of the body and ends when the agent can be shed or communicated.

latent period of drug action See *onset of action.*

lateral recumbent position The position in which the patient is lying on his or her right or left side.

lateral ventricle A large fluid-filled space in each cerebral hemisphere.

laxative A substance that causes evacuation of the bowel by increasing the bulk of the feces, by softening the stool, or by lubricating the intestinal wall.

lead An electrode sensor attached to the body to record electrical activity, especially of the heart and brain.

LeFort fracture Three patterns of injury that can be produced in the midface region.

left anterior descending artery The subdivision of the left coronary artery that supplies the left auricle and its appendix and supplies branches to both ventricles and numerous small branches to the pulmonary artery and commencement of the aorta.

legend A prescription drug.

legionellosis An acute bacterial pneumonia caused by infection with *Legionella pneumophila;* characterized by influenza-like illness followed within a week by high fever, chills, muscle aches, and headache.

Lenegre's disease See *Lev's disease.*

lens The crystalline lens of the eye.

leukemia A malignant neoplasm of blood-forming organs.

leukocyte White blood cell.

Lev's disease Third-degree block in the elderly from chronic degenerative changes in the conduction system; not usually associated with increased parasympathetic tone or drug toxicity. Also known as *Lenegre's disease.*

libel Publishing in writing false statements about someone, knowing them to be false, with malicious intent or with reckless disregard for their falsity.

licensure The process by which a government agency grants permission to an individual to engage in an occupation or profession.

ligament A band of white, fibrous tissue connecting bones.

ligamentum arteriosum A fibrous cord from the pulmonary artery to the branch of the aorta; the remains of the ductus arteriosus of the fetus.

limbic system The parts of the brain involved with emotions and olfaction.

linear fracture A fracture that extends parallel to the long axis of a bone but does not displace the bone tissue.

lingual tonsil A collection of lymphoid tissue on the posterior portion of the dorsum of the tongue.

lipid bilayer The central layer of the cytoplasmic membrane; composed of a double layer of lipid molecules.

lipodystrophy Any abnormality in the metabolism or distribution of fats.

lipoprotein A conjugated protein in which lipids form an integral part of the molecule; synthesized primarily in the liver.

liquefaction Conversion of solid tissues to a fluid or semifluid state.

liter (l) A metric unit of capacity equal to 1 cubic decimeter, 61.025 cubic inches, or 1.0567 liquid quarts.

Littre's gland The inner surface of the membrane lining the urethra; presents the orifices of numerous mucous glands and follicles situated in the submucous tissue.

loading dose A large quantity of drug that temporarily exceeds the body's capacity to excrete the drug.

lobule A small lobe or subdivision of a lobe.

long bones Bones that are longer than they are wide. Examples of long bones are the humerus, ulna, radius, femur, tibia, fibula, and phalanges.

long saphenous vein One of a pair of the longest veins in the body; begins in the medial marginal vein in the dorsum of the foot and ends in the femoral vein.

loop diuretic A group of powerful, short-acting agents that inhibit sodium and chloride reabsorption in the loop of Henle, resulting in an excessive loss of potassium and water and an increase in the excretion of sodium.

loop of Henle The U-shaped portion of the renal tubule.

lower esophageal sphincter The ring of muscle located at the inferior end of the esophagus that regulates the passage of materials out of the esophagus.

lucid interval A period of relative mental clarity between periods of decreased consciousness or irrationality.

lumbarsacral plexus The combination of all the ventral primary divisions of the lumbar, sacral, and coccygeal nerves.

lumbar vertebrae The five largest segments of the movable part of the vertebral column; designated L1 to L5.

lumen A cavity or channel within any organ or structure of the body.

lung One of a pair of light, spongy organs in the thorax, the main component of the respiratory system.

lunula The crescent-shaped white area of the nail; most visible on the thumbnail.

lymph capillary Tiny, blind-ended tubes distributed in the tissue spaces.

lymph node An encapsulated mass of lymph tissue found among lymph vessels.

lymphangitis An inflammation of one or more lymphatic vessels.

lymphocyte A type of white blood cell formed in lymphoid tissue.

lymphoma A neoplasm of lymphoid tissue; usually malignant.

lyse To produce decomposition.

lysis The process by which a cell swells and ruptures.

lysosome A membranous-walled organelle that contains enzymes, enabling it to function as an intracellular digestive system.

macrodrip tubing An apparatus used to deliver measured amounts of intravenous solutions at specific flow rates based on the size of drops of the solution. The drops delivered by a macrodrip are larger than those delivered by a microdrip.

macromolecule A molecule of colloidal size, such as a protein, nucleic acid, or polysaccharide.

macrophage A phagocytic cell in the immune system.

maintenance dose The amount of a drug required to keep a desired steady state of drug concentration in the tissues.

major incident An emergency event in which available resources are insufficient to manage the number of casualties or the nature of the emergency.

malar eminence The zygomatic or cheek bone.

malleolus A rounded, bony process, such as the protuberance on each side of the ankle.

malleus The largest of the three ossicles in the middle ear.

Mallory-Weiss syndrome A condition characterized by massive bleeding after a tear in the mucous membrane at the junction of the esophagus and the stomach.

mamma The breast; the organ of milk secretion.

mammalian diving reflex A reflex triggered by immersing the face in cold water; diverts blood from the arms and legs to the central circulation and lowers heart rate as a result of vagal stimulation.

mammary gland An external accessory sex organ in females; breasts.

mandible A large bone constituting the lower jaw.

mania A phase of bipolar disorder characterized by elation, agitation, hyperexcitability, hyperactivity, and increased speed of thought or speech.

manic Pertaining to a specific psychosis.

manic-depressive disorder A disorder marked by alternating periods of mania and depression. Also known as *bipolar disorder*.

manubriosternal junction The point at which the manubrium joins the body of the sternum; location of second rib. Also known as *sternal angle*.

manubrium One of the three bones of the sternum, presenting a broad quadrangular shape that narrows caudally at its articulation with the superior end of the body of the sternum.

Marfan's syndrome An abnormal condition characterized by elongation of the bones, often with associated abnormalities of the eyes and cardiovascular system.

mastectomy Surgical removal of one or both breasts, performed to remove a malignant tumor.

mastication Chewing, tearing, or grinding food with the teeth while it is mixed with saliva.

mastoid air cell One of several spaces within the mastoid process of the temporal bone; connects to the middle ear by ducts.

maxilla One of a pair of large bones that form the upper jaw.

maxillary sinus One of the pair of large air cells forming a pyramidal cavity in the body of the maxilla.

McBurney's point A site of extreme sensitivity in acute appendicitis situated in the normal area of the appendix, approximately 2 inches from the right anterior-superior spine of the ilium, on a line between that spine and the umbilicus.

mean arterial pressure The arithmetic mean of the blood pressure in the arterial portion of the circulation minus intracranial pressure.

meconium aspiration syndrome The inhalation of meconium by the fetus or newborn which can block the air passages and result in failure of the lungs to expand, or cause other pulmonary dysfunction.

meconium staining The presence of fetal stool in amniotic fluid.

mediastinitis Inflammation of the mediastinum.

mediastinum A portion of the thoracic cavity in the middle of the thorax, between the pleural sacs containing the two lungs. It extends from the sternum to the vertebral column and contains all the thoracic viscera except the lungs.

mediated transport mechanism A mechanism that uses carrier molecules to move large water-soluble molecules or electrically charged molecules across cell membranes.

medical control The authority responsible for ensuring that actions taken on behalf of ill or injured people are medically appropriate; including prospective, concurrent, and retrospective aspects of EMS, quality improvement, hiring, and education.

medulla The lowest part of the brain stem, which controls vital functions; an enlarged extension of the spinal cord. Also known as the *medulla oblongata*.

medulla oblongata See *medulla*.

medullary cavity A large, marrow-filled cavity in the diaphysis of a long bone.

megahertz (MHz) A unit of frequency equal to 1 million cycles per second. EMS radios transmit and receive on frequencies measured in megahertz.

melanocyte A body cell capable of producing melanin.

melena Abnormal black, tarry stools containing digested blood.

membranous labyrinth A membranous structure within the inner ear; forms the cochlea, vestibule, and semicircular canals.

menarche The first menstruation and the commencement of the cyclic menstrual function.

meninges Fluid-containing membranes surrounding the brain and spinal cord.

merocrine gland A gland that secretes products with no loss of cellular material; an example is a water-producing sweat gland.

mesencephalon See *midbrain*.

mesentery The double layer of peritoneum extending from the abdominal wall to the abdominal viscera, conveying vessels and nerves.

mesovarium A short peritoneal fold connecting the ovary with the broad ligament of the uterus.

metacarpal One of five bones extending from the carpus to the phalanges.

metarteriole One of the small peripheral blood vessels that contain scattered groups of smooth muscle fibers in their walls; located between the arterioles and the true capillaries.

metatarsal Any one of the five bones comprising the metatarsus.

meter (m) A metric unit of length equal to 39.37 inches.

methanol A chemical widely used as a solvent and in the production of formaldehyde.

methemoglobin A form of hemoglobin in which the iron component has been oxidized from the ferrous to the ferric state.

methemoglobinemia The presence of methemoglobin in the blood, causing cyanosis as a result of the red cell's inability to release oxygen.

microdrip tubing An apparatus for delivering relatively small amounts of intravenous solutions at specific flow rates. The drops delivered by a microdrip are smaller than those delivered by a macrodrip.

microgram (mcg, μg) A metric unit of mass equal to equal to one millionth of a gram.

microinfarct A very small infarct caused by obstruction of circulation in capillaries, arterioles, or small arteries.

microorganism Any tiny, usually microscopic entity capable of carry on living processes. Examples include bacteria, fungi, protozoa, and viruses.

microthrombus A minute thrombus.

microtubule A hollow tube that helps to support the cytoplasm of the cell; a component of certain cell organelles such as centrioles, spindle fibers, cilia, and flagella.

microwave Radio waves with frequencies of 890 MHz and upward. The signals are generated by special equipment that depends on line-of-sight placement to operate properly. Microwave channels may have a wide band to carry a large number of simultaneous transmissions.

midbrain One of the three parts of the brain stem. Also known as the *mesencephalon*.

middle cerebral artery The artery that supplies a large portion of the lateral cerebral cortex.

middle ear An air-filled space within the temporal bone that contains the auditory ossicles.

milliequivalent (mEq) One thousandth of a gram equivalent.

milligram (mg) A metric unit of mass equal to one thousandth of a gram.

millimeter (mm) A metric unit of length equal to one thousandth of a meter.

mineralocorticoid A hormone secreted by the adrenal cortex that maintains normal blood volume, promotes sodium and water retention, and increases urine secretion of potassium and hydrogen ions.

minim A measure of volume in the apothecaries' system, originally 1 drop of water. Sixty minims equal 1 fluid dram. One minim equals 0.06 ml.

minimal effective concentration The lowest plasma concentration that produces the desired drug effect.

minute alveolar ventilation The amount of inspired gas available for gas exchange during 1 minute.

minute volume The tidal volume times the respiratory rate, or the amount of gas inhaled or exhaled in 1 minute.

missed abortion The retention of the fetus in utero for 4 or more weeks after fetal death.

mitochondria Small spherical, rod-shaped, or thin filamentous structures in the cytoplasm of cells; a site of ATP production.

mitosis Cell division resulting in two daughter cells with exactly the same number and type of chromosomes as the mother cell.

mitral valve See *bicuspid valve*.

mittelschmerz Abdominal pain in the region of the ovary during ovulation; usually occurs midway through the menstrual cycle.

MMR vaccine The abbreviation for measles, mumps, and rubella virus vaccine live.

mobile data terminal (MDT) A computer, connected through a modem ("black box") with a radio, that sends and receives pretyped messages to printers, computer screens, or both. Some MDTs have graphics (floor plans) and data-base (hazardous materials) capabilities. MDTs rely on a host computer interfaced to a base station.

mobile or **vehicular repeater** A mobile radio unit capable of automatically retransmitting any radio traffic originated by a handheld portable, by other mobiles, or by base stations. This repeater may be one-way or two-way and may be known as a *PAC-RAT* (Motorola) or an *extender*.

mobile relay station A fixed-base station that automatically retransmits mobile or portable radio communications back to the receiving frequency of other portables, mobiles, and base stations operating in the same system. Also known as a "repeater."

mole A standard unit used to measure the amount of a substance.

monocyte A type of white blood cell found in lymph nodes, spleen, bone marrow, and loose connective tissue.

mons pubis The prominence caused by a pad of fatty tissue over the symphysis pubis in the female.

morphology The study of the physical shape and size of a specimen, plant, or animal.

motor neuron A neuron that innervates skeletal, smooth, or cardiac muscle fibers. Also known as an *interneuron*.

mucin The chief ingredient in mucus.

mucus The viscus, slippery secretion of mucous membranes and glands.

multifocal PVC A premature ventricular contraction that originates from multiple sites in the ventricles.

multigravida A woman who has had two or more pregnancies.

multipara A woman who has had two or more deliveries.

multiplex A system with the ability to simultaneously transmit two or more different types of information in either or both directions over the same frequency, for example, telemetry and voice.

muscarinic receptor A class of cholinergic receptor molecule specifically activated by muscarine in addition to acetylcholine.

muscular tissue A primary tissue type characterized by its contractile abilities.

mutagenic Any chemical or physical environmental agent that induces a genetic mutation or increases the mutation rate.

mutual aid An agreement with neighboring emergency agencies indicating that a mutual exchange of equipment and manpower will be available when called upon.

myalgia Diffuse muscle pain, usually accompanied by malaise, occurring in many infectious diseases.

myasthenia Muscle weakness.

myasthenia gravis An abnormal condition characterized by chronic fatigue and weakness of muscles, especially in the face and throat; results from a defect in the nerve impulses at the myoneural junction.

myelinated axon A nerve fiber having a myelin sheath.

myeloblast Bone marrow cell.

myoclonus A spasm of a muscle or group of muscles.

myoepithelium Tissue made up of contractile epithelial cells.

myofibril A slender, striated strand of smooth muscle.

myofilament An extremely fine molecular threadlike structure that helps to form the myofibril of muscle, thick myofibrils are formed of myosin, and thin myofilaments are formed of actin.

myometrium The muscular layer wall of the uterus.

myosin A cardiac and skeletal muscle protein; comprises approximately half of the proteins that occur in muscle tissue.

nail bed The end of a finger or toe covered by the nail; abundant in blood vessels.

nail body The visible part of the nail.

nares Nostrils.

nasal bone The bony partition that separates the nasal cavity into left and right parts. Also known as *nasal septum.*

nasal septum A partition that separates the right and left nasal cavities.

nasogastric tube Any tube passed into the stomach through the nose.

nasolacrimal duct A duct that leads from the lacrimal sac to the nasal cavity.

nasopharynx The uppermost portion of the tube just behind the nasal cavities.

nasotracheal Accessing the trachea through the nasal cavity.

near-drowning Submersion with at least temporary survival.

nebulizer A device for producing a fine spray of medication for inhalation therapy.

negligence Failure to use such care as a reasonably prudent EMS provider would use in similar circumstances. A deviation from a standard of care.

nematocyst A venomous stinging cell.

neoplasm Abnormal growth; a malignant or benign tumor.

nephron The functional unit of the kidney.

nerve A bundle of nerve fibers and accompanying connective tissue located outside the central nervous system.

nerve tract Bundles of parallel axons with associated sheaths in the central nervous system.

nervous tissue A major tissue type characterized by it conductile abilities.

nervous tunic The retina.

neuralgia Pain along a nerve.

neurogenic shock Shock resulting from vasomotor paralysis below the level of injury. Also known as *spinal cord shock.*

neuroglia Cells in the nervous system other than neurons.

neurohormone A hormone secreted by a neuron.

neuromuscular junction A specialized synapse between a motor neuron and a muscle fiber.

neuron The functional unit or the nervous system, consisting of the nerve cell body, the dendrites, and the axon.

neuropathy A disease of the peripheral nerves.

neurosis Any faulty or inefficient way of coping with anxiety or inner conflict; may ultimately lead to a neurotic disorder.

neutrophil A small, phagocytic white blood cell with a lobed nucleus and small granules in the cytoplasm; stains readily with neutral dyes.

Newton's first law of motion The principle that an object, whether at rest or in linear motion, remains in that state unless force is applied.

Newton's second law of motion The principle that force is equal to mass times acceleration or deceleration.

nicad batteries Nickel cadmium rechargeable batteries used in portable radios.

nicotinic receptor A class of cholinergic receptor molecules that are specifically activated by nicotine and acetylcholine.

nit The egg of a parasitic insect, particularly a louse.

nitrogen narcosis A condition of depressed central nervous system functions brought about by high partial pressure of nitrogen.

nocturia Particularly excessive urination at night.

node of Ranvier The short interval in the myelin sheath of a nerve fiber between adjacent Schwann cells.

noncardiogenic pulmonary edema See *adult respiratory distress syndrome.*

noncompensatory pause The pause that occurs when the next expected P wave of the underlying cardiac rhythm appears earlier than it would have if the SA node had not been disturbed by a conduction abnormality.

noncompetitive antagonist An agent that combines with different parts of the receptor mechanism and inactivates the receptor so that the agonist cannot be effective regardless of its concentration.

nonconducted PAC A premature atrial contraction blocked at the AV node.

nonelectrolyte A substance with no electrical charge.

nonproprietary name See *generic name.*

nonstriated muscle See *smooth muscle.*

noradrenalin An adrenergic hormone produced by the adrenal medulla, similar in chemical and pharmacologic properties to epinephrine. Acts to increase blood pressure by vasoconstriction, but does not affect cardiac output. Also known as *norepinephrine.*

nuclear membrane A double membrane structure surrounding and enclosing the nucleus. Also known as *nuclear envelope.*

nucleolus Any one of the somewhat rounded, dense well-defined nuclear bodies with no surrounding membrane; contains ribosomal RNA and protein.

nucleoplasm The protoplasm of the nucleus, as contrasted with that of the cell.

nucleus The central controlling body within a living cell.

nullipara A woman who has never borne a child.

obesity An abnormal increase in the proportion of fat cells, mainly in the viscera and subcutaneous tissues of the body.

obligate Necessary; compulsory.

obturator foramen A large opening on each side of the lower portion of the hip bone, formed posteriorly by the ischium, superiorly by the ilium, and anteriorly by the pubis.

occipital bone The cuplike bone at the back of the skull, marked by a large opening, the foramen magnum, that communicates with the vertebral canal.

occipital lobe One of the five lobes of each cerebral hemisphere.

occiput posterior presentation An abnormal presentation in which the infant's head is delivered face up instead of face down.

oculomotor nerve The third cranial nerve, which contains both sensory and motor fibers; provides for movement in most of the muscles of the eye, for constriction of the pupil, and for accommodation of the eye to light.

odontoid process The toothlike projection that rises perpendicularly from the upper surface of the body of the second cervical vertebra or axis, which serves as a pivot point for the rotation of the atlas.

official name Usually the same as the generic name. The official name of a drug is followed by the initials "USP" or "NF," denoting its listing in one of the official publications.

off-line medical control The establishment and monitoring of all medical components of an EMS system, including protocols, standing orders, educational programs, and the quality and delivery of on-line medical control.

olecranon fossa The depression in the posterior surface of the humerus that receives the olecranon of the ulna when the forearm is extended.

olecranon process The large bony process of the ulna. Also known as the **olecranon.**

olfactory Of or pertaining to the sense of smell.

olfactory bulb The tissue that receives the olfactory nerves from the nasal cavity.

olfactory membranes Membranes that contain the receptors for the sense of smell; located in the roof of the nasal cavity.

olfactory recess The extreme superior region of the nasal cavity.

olfactory tract The nerve tract that projects from the olfactory bulb to the olfactory cortex.

oliguria A diminished capacity to form or pass urine.

omphalocele Congenital herniation of intraabdominal viscera through a defect in the abdominal wall around the umbilicus.

oncotic pressure See *blood colloid osmotic pressure.*

on-line medical control The medical control physician who directly supervises prehospital care activities via radio or telephone. On-line medical control is also responsible for the activities of the emergency department staff and other designated physicians at the medical control hospital.

onset of action The interval between the time a drug is administered and the first sign of its effects. Also known as the *latent period of drug action.*

oocyte An incompletely developed ovum.

open vault fracture A fracture that results in direct communication between a scalp laceration and cerebral substance.

opiate A narcotic drug that contains opium, derivatives of opium, or any of several semisynthetic or synthetic drugs with opiumlike activity.

opioid Any synthetic narcotic that has opiatelike activities but is not derived from opium.

opposition Movement of the thumb and little finger toward each other.

optic nerve The nerve that carries visual signals from the eye to the crossing of the optic tracts.

orchitis Painful inflammation of the testicle.

organ A structure made up of two or more kinds of tissues, organized to perform a more complex function than can any one tissue alone.

organelle Any one of various particles of living substance bound within most cells, such as the mitochondria, the Golgi apparatus, the endoplasmic reticulum, the lysosomes, and the centrioles.

organ of Corti The organ of hearing; located in the cochlea and filled with endolymph.

oriented Aware of one's surroundings.

origin The less movable attachment point of a muscle.

oropharyngeolaryngeal axis The three axes of the mouth, pharynx, and trachea; a patient position used for direct visualization of the larynx.

oropharynx The portion of the pharynx located behind the mouth.

orotracheal Gaining access to the trachea through the oral cavity.

osmolality The osmotic concentration of a solution.

osmosis Diffusion of solvent (water) through a membrane from a less-concentrated solution to a more-concentrated solution.

osmotic pressure The force required to prevent the movement of water across a selectively permeable membrane.

otorrhea Any discharge from the external ear.

ovarian follicle The spherical cell aggregation in the ovary containing an oocyte.

ovarian ligament The bundle of fibers passing to the uterus from the ovary.

ovary One of the pair of female gonads found on each side of the lower abdomen beside the uterus.

ovulation Release of an ovum or secondary oocyte from the vesicular follicle.

oxyhemoglobin Oxygenated hemoglobin.

pacemaker cell Certain myocardial cells capable of initiating an electrical impulse.

packaging The completion of emergency care procedures needed to transfer a patient from the scene to the ambulance.

Paget's disease A common, nonmetabolic disease of bone of unknown cause, characterized by excessive bone destruction and unorganized bone repair.

paging equipment Equipment typically using tone activation with one-way transmission to receive-only units.

palatine bone One of a pair of bones of the skull forming the posterior part of the hard palate, part of the nasal cavity, and the floor of the orbit of the eye.

palatine tonsil One of two large oval masses of lymphoid tissue embedded in the lateral wall of the oropharynx.

pancreatic juice The fluid secretion of the pancreas produced by the stimulation of food in the duodenum.

para The number of past pregnancies that have remained viable to delivery.

parainfluenza virus One of a group of viruses isolated from patients with upper respiratory tract disease of varying severity in infants and young children; may cause croup, tracheobronchitis, bronchiolitis, bronchopneumonia, pharyngitis, and the common cold.

paralytic ileus The decrease in or absence of intestinal peristalsis that may occur after abdominal surgery, illness, or injury; the most common cause of intestinal obstruction.

parametritis An inflammatory condition of tissue of the structures around the uterus.

parasagittal plane An imaginary vertical plane passing through the body parallel to the medial plane; divide the body into left and right portions.

parasympathetic nervous system The subdivision of the autonomic nervous system usually involved in activating vegetative functions such as digestion, defecation, and urination.

parasympatholytic Anticholinergic: producing effects resembling those of interruption or blockade of the parasympathetic nerve supply to effector organs or tissues.

parasympathomimetic agent An agent whose effects mimic those resulting from stimulation of parasympathetic nerves, especially the effects produced by acetylcholine.

parasystole An independent ectopic rhythm whose pacemaker cannot be discharged by impulses of the dominant rhythm because of an area of depressed conduction surrounding the parasystolic focus.

parenteral Not in or through the digestive system.

parietal Of or pertaining to the outer wall of a cavity or organ.

parietal bone One of a pair of bones that form the side of the cranium.

parietal lobe The portion of each cerebral hemisphere that occupies the parts of the lateral and medial surfaces covered by the parietal bone.

parietal pericardium The portion of serous pericardium lining the fibrous pericardium.

parietal peritoneum The layer of peritoneum lining the abdominal walls.

parkinsonism A neurologic disorder characterized by tremor, muscle rigidity, hypokinesia, a slow shuffling gait, and difficulty in chewing, swallowing, and speaking; frequently occurs in patients treated with antipsychotic drugs.

parotitis Inflammation or infection of one or both parotid salivary glands.

paroxysm Frequent episodes of atrial tachycardia.

paroxysmal nocturnal dyspnea A sudden episode of dyspnea that occurs after lying down.

paroxysmal supraventricular tachycardia (PSVT) An ectopic rhythm in excess of 100 beats per minute and usually faster than 170 beats per minute that begins abruptly with a premature atrial or junctional beat and is supported by an AV nodal reentry mechanism or by an AV reentry mechanism involving an accessory pathway.

partial antagonist An agent that has affinity and some efficacy but that may antagonize the action of other drugs that have greater efficacy.

partial pressure The pressure exerted by a single gas; denoted by a P preceding the gas (for example, P_{O_2}).

partial reabsorption The amount of drug reabsorbed from the renal tubule by passive diffusion.

parturition The process of giving birth.

passive glomerular filtration The renal process whereby fluid in the blood is filtered across the capillaries of the glomerulus and into the urinary space of Bowman's capsule.

patella A flat, triangular bone at the front of the knee joint; kneecap.

peak plasma level The highest plasma concentration attained from a dose.

pectoral girdle See *shoulder girdle.*

pectus deformity Malformation of the chest wall.

pediatric trauma score An injury severity index that grades six components commonly seen in pediatric trauma patients: size (weight), airway, central nervous system, systolic blood pressure, open wound, and skeletal injury.

pelvic girdle The encircling bony structure supporting the lower limbs.

penetration The flow of a hazardous liquid chemical through zippers, stitched seams, pinholes, or other imperfections in a material.

penis The external reproductive organ of the male.

pepsin The principal digestive enzyme of gastric juice.

pepsinogen A proenzyme formed and secreted by certain cells of the gastric mucosa.

peptide bond A chemical bond between amino acids.

periappendiceal abscess A cavity containing pus and inflamed tissue around the vermiform appendix.

pericardial fluid A viscous fluid contained within the pericardial cavity between the visceral and parietal pericardium; serves as a lubricant.

pericardial friction rub A dry, grating sound heard with a stethoscope during auscultation; suggestive of pericarditis.

pericardial sac The sac that surrounds the heart.

pericardial tamponade Compression of the heart produced by the accumulation in the pericardial sac of fluid or blood.

pericardiocentesis A procedure for withdrawing fluid from the pericardial sac.

pericarditis Inflammation of the pericardium.

pericardium The membrane that surrounds the heart.

perilymph The fluid contained within the bony labyrinth.

perinatal Occurring at or near the time of birth.

periodontal membrane The membrane that surrounds the root of the tooth.

periosteum Tough connective tissue covering the bone.

periostitis Inflammation of the periosteum; characterized by tenderness and swelling of the affected bone, pain, fever, and chills.

peripheral nervous system (PNS) A major subdivision of the nervous system consisting of nerves and ganglia.

peripheral thermoreceptors Nerve endings sensitive to heat, located in the skin and some mucous membranes; usually categorized as cold or warm receptors.

peripheral vascular resistance The total resistance against which blood must be pumped. Also known as "afterload."

peristalsis The coordinated, rhythmic and serial contraction of smooth muscle that forces food through the digestive tract, bile through the bile duct, and urine through the ureters.

peritoneal cavity The potential space between the parietal and visceral layers of the peritoneum. Normally, the two layers are in contact.

peritonitis Inflammation of the peritoneum.

peritubular capillary The capillary network located in the cortex of the kidney.

permeable A condition of being pervious so that fluids and other substances can pass through, as occurs in a semipermeable membrane.

permeation The process by which a hazardous liquid chemical moves through a material on a molecular level.

persistent generalized lymphadenopathy (PGL) Enlarged lymph nodes involving two noncontiguous sites other than inguinal nodes; a common feature in early HIV infection.

petit mal seizure An epileptic seizure characterized by a sudden, momentary loss of consciousness occasionally accompanied by minor muscle spasms of the neck or upper extremities.

pH An inverse logarithm of the hydrogen ion concentration.

phagocytosis The process of ingestion by cells of solid substances such as other cells, bacteria, bits of necrosed tissue, and foreign particles.

phalanges Any bone of a finger or toe.

pharmacodynamics The study of how a drug acts on a living organism.

pharmacokinetics The study of the action and effects of drugs within the body, including the routes and mechanisms of absorption and excretion, the rate at which a drug's action begins and duration of the effect, and biotransformation.

pharyngeal tonsil One of two collections of aggregated lymphoid nodules on the posterior wall of the nasopharynx.

Phase 0 The rapid depolarization phase; represents the very rapid upstroke of the action potential that occurs when the cell membrane reaches the threshold potential (approximately −70 mV).

Phase 1 The early rapid repolarization phase; the phase in which the fast sodium channels close, the flow of sodium ions into the cell terminates, and the loss of potassium from the cell continues.

Phase 2 The plateau phase; the prolonged phase of slow repolarization of the action potential.

Phase 3 The terminal phase of rapid repolarization; results in the inside of the cell becoming markedly negative and the membrane potential returning to approximately −90 mV, or its resting level.

Phase 4 The period between action potentials when the membrane has returned to its RMP.

phencyclidine psychosis A true psychiatric emergency with clinical syndromes ranging from a catatonic and unresponsive state to bizarre and violent behavior; may occur after a single low-dose exposure to phencyclidine and may last from several days to weeks.

phlebitis Inflammation of a vein, often accompanied by formation of a clot. Also known as *thrombophlebitis.*

phonation The production of speech sounds.

phospholipid One of a class of compounds, widely distributed in living cells, containing phosphoric acid, fatty acids, and a nitrogenous base.

photophobia Abnormal sensitivity to light.

physical dependence An adaptive physiologic state occurring after prolonged use of many drugs; discontinuation causes withdrawal syndromes that are relieved by readministering the same drug or a pharmacologically related drug.

physiologic dead space The sum of the anatomic dead space plus the volume of any nonfunctional alveoli.

pia mater The innermost layer of the meninges that directly covers the brain.

Pickwickian syndrome An abnormal condition characterized by obesity, decreased pulmonary function, somnolence, and polycythemia.

pigmented retina The pigmented portion of the retina.

piloerection Erection of the hairs of the skin in response to cold environment, emotional stimulus, or irritation of the skin.

pinna See *auricle.*

pituitary gland The small gland attached to the hypothalamus, that supplies numerous hormones that govern many vital processes.

pivot joint A joint that consists of a relatively cylindrical bony process that rotates within a ring composed partly of bone and partly of ligament.

placard A four-sided, diamond-shaped sign displayed on hazardous material containers; usually yellow, red, orange, white, or green; contains a four-digit United Nations identification number (UN number) and a legend to indicate container contents.

placebo An inactive substance or a less-than-effective dose of a harmless substance; used in experimental drug studies to compare the effects of the inactive substance with those of the experimental drug.

placenta A highly vascular fetal organ through which the fetus absorbs oxygen, nutrients, and other substances and excretes carbon dioxide and other wastes.

placental barrier A protective biologic membrane that separates the blood vessels of the mother and fetus; provides some protection to the fetus by preventing the passage of certain drugs.

placenta previa A condition of pregnancy in which the placenta is implanted abnormally in the uterus so that it impinges on or covers the internal os of the uterine cervix.

plane joint A joint that consists of two opposed flat surfaces that are approximately equal in size. Also known as a *gliding joint.*

plasma The fluid portion of blood.

plasma protein binding A type of drug reservoir in which drugs attach to proteins, mainly albumin, and form a drug protein complex. The albumin molecule is too large to diffuse through the membrane of the blood vessel, trapping the bound drug in the blood stream and thereby forming a circulating drug reservoir.

plateau phase Prolongation of the depolarization phase of cardiac muscle cell membrane; results in a prolonged refractory period.

platelet A fragment of a cell; contains granules in the central part and clear protoplasm peripherally, but has no definite nucleus.

pleural fluid Serous fluid found in the pleural cavity; helps to reduce friction when the pleural membranes rub together.

pleural space The potential space between the visceral and parietal layers of the pleurae.

plexus A network of intersecting nerves and blood vessels or lymphatic vessels.

pneumatic antishock garment (PASG) A garment used to manage hypovolemia and decreased tissue perfusion.

pneumococcus A gram-positive diplococcal bacterium of the species *Diplococcus pneumoniae;* the most common cause of bacterial pneumonia.

pneumocystis carinii pneumonia (PCP) A bacterial pneumonia caused by infection with the parasite *Pneumocystis carinii,* usually seen in infants or debilitated or immunosuppressed people; characterized by fever, cough, tachypnea, and frequently, cyanosis.

pneumohemothorax A collection of air and blood in the pleural space. Also known as a **hemopneumothorax.**

pneumotaxic center A group of neurons in the pons that have an inhibitory effect on the inspiratory center.

pneumothorax A collection of air or gas in the pleural space that causes the lung to collapse.

poikilothermy Body temperature varying according to ambient temperature.

poison Any substance that produces harmful physiologic or psychologic effects.

poliomyelitis An infectious disease caused by one of three polio viruses. Asymptomatic, mild, and paralytic forms of the disease occur.

poliovirus hominis The causative organism of poliomyelitis.

polyarthritis Inflammation of several joints.

polycythemia An abnormal increase in the number of erythrocytes in the blood.

polyphagia Excessive eating.

polyuria Excessive secretion of urine.

pons The part of the brain stem between the medulla and the midbrain.

portal vein A vein that ramifies like an artery in the liver and ends in capillary-like sinusoids that convey the blood to the inferior vena cava through the hepatic veins.

positive-end expiratory pressure (PEEP) Ventilation controlled by a flow of air delivered in cycles of constant pressure through the respiratory cycle.

posterior cerebral artery The artery that supplies the posterior portion of the cerebrum.

posterior chamber of the eye The chamber of the eye between the iris and the lens.

posterior communicating artery The artery that branches off each internal carotid artery and connects with the ipsilateral posterior cerebral artery.

posterior superior iliac spine One of two bony segments that form the iliac crest.

postpartum The maternal period after delivery.

postpartum hemorrhage More than 500 ml of blood loss after delivery of the newborn.

postsynaptic neuron The membrane of a nerve that is in close association with a presynaptic terminal.

potassium ion The predominate intracellular cation; helps to regulate neuromuscular excitability and muscle contraction.

potassium-sparing agent A group of medications that promote sodium and water loss without an accompanying loss of potassium.

potential difference The difference in electrical potential, measured as the charge difference across the cell membrane.

potentiation The enhancement of effect caused by the concurrent administration of two drugs in which one drug increases the effect of the other drug.

precapillary sphincter The smooth muscle sphincter that regulates blood flow through a capillary.

precipitous delivery A rapid spontaneous delivery of less than 3 hours from onset of labor to birth; results from overactive uterine contractions and little maternal soft tissue or bony resistance.

precordial thump A CPR technique used to restore circulation in monitored ventricular fibrillation or stable ventricular tachycardia.

pregravid Before pregnancy.

prehospital care report A document used in the prehospital setting to record all patient care activities and circumstances related to an emergency response.

preload The amount of blood returning to the ventricle.

premature atrial contraction (PAC) A cardiac dysrhythmia characterized by an atrial beat occurring before the expected excitation; indicated on the electrocardiogram as an early P wave.

premature junctional contraction (PJC) A single contraction that occurs during sinus rhythm earlier than the next expected sinus beat; caused by premature discharge of an ectopic focus in the AV junctional tissue.

premature rupture of membranes (PROM) Rupture of the amniotic sac before the onset of labor, regardless of gestational age.

premature ventricular contraction (PVC) A cardiac dysrhythmia characterized by a ventricular beat preceding the expected electrical impulse; indicated on the electrocardiogram as an early, wide QRS complex without a preceding related P wave.

prenatal Existing or occurring before birth.

prepuce In males, the free fold of skin that covers the glans penis; the foreskin. In females, the external fold of the labia minora that covers the clitoris.

presenting part The part of the fetus that lies closest to the internal os of the cervix.

presynaptic neuron The nerve terminal that contains neurotransmitter vesicles.

presynaptic terminal The enlarged axon terminal.

priapism Painful, persistent erection of the penis.

primary bronchus One of the two tubes arising at the inferior end of the trachea; each primary bronchus extends into one of the lungs.

primary epilepsy Epilepsy for which the cause is unknown. Also known as *idiopathic epilepsy.*

primary follicle The ovarian follicle that contains the primary oocyte.

primary oocyte The oocyte before the first meiotic division.

prime mover A muscle that plays a major role in accomplishing movement.

primigravida A woman who is pregnant for the first time.

primipara A woman who has given birth only one time.

PR interval The time elapsing between the beginning of the P wave and the beginning of the QRS complex in the electrocardiogram.

Prinzmetal's angina An atypical form of angina that occurs at rest rather than with effort; associated with gross ST elevation in the electrocardiogram that disappears when the pain subsides.

prodromal stage The early period of labor before uterine contractions become forceful and frequent enough to result in progressive dilation of the uterine cervix.

progesterone A steroid sex hormone prescribed to treat various menstrual disorders, functional uterine bleeding, and repeated spontaneous abortions.

progestin Any group of hormones secreted by the corpus luteum, placenta, or adrenal cortex that have a progesterone-like effect on the uterus.

prolapsed umbilical cord An umbilical cord that protrudes beside or ahead of the presenting part of the fetus.

proliferative phase The time between the end of menses and ovulation characterized by rapid division of endometrial cells and the development of follicles in the ovary.

pronation Rotation of the forearm so that the anterior surface is down.

prone position The position in which the patient is lying on his or her stomach (facedown).

proprietary name See *trade name.*

proprioception Information about the position of the body and its various parts.

prostaglandin A class of naturally occurring fatty acids that affect body functions such as vasodilation, stimulation and contraction of uterine smooth muscle, and promotion of inflammation and pain.

prostate gland The gland that lies just below the male bladder; its secretion is one of the components of semen.

prosthesis An artificial replacement for a missing part of the body, such as an artificial limb.

prothrombin A chemical that is part of the clotting cascade, the precursor of thrombin.

protoplasm The living substance of a cell.

protraction Movement in the anterior direction

pseudoaneurysm A condition resembling an aneurysm, caused by enlargement and tortuosity of a vessel.

pseudomembranous colitis A life-threatening form of diarrhea caused by *Clostridium difficile.*

psoas muscle A long muscle originating from the transverse processes of the lumbar vertebrae and the fibrocartilage and sides of the vertebral bodies of the lower thoracic vertebrae and the lumbar vertebrae.

psoriasis A common, chronic, inheritable skin disorder characterized by circumscribed red patches covered by thick, dry, adherent scales that result from excessive development of epithelial cells.

psychologic dependence Emotional reliance on a drug; manifestations range from a mild desire for a drug, to craving and drug-seeking behavior, to repeated compulsive use of a drug for its subjectively satisfying or pleasurable effects.

psychology The science or study of behavior.

psychomotor seizure An epileptic seizure manifested by impaired consciousness of variable degree, the patient carries out a series of coordinated acts that are inappropriate, bizarre, and serve no useful purpose, about which the patient is amnesic.

psychosis Any major mental disorder of organic or emotional origin characterized by extreme derangement or disorganization of the personality, often accompanied by severe depression, agitation, regressive behavior, illusions, delusions, and hallucinations; the individual loses touch with reality and is incapable of functioning normally in society.

puberty The period of life when the ability to reproduce begins.

pubis One of a pair of pubic bones that with the ischium and the ilium form the hip bone and join the pubic bone from the opposite side at the pubic symphysis.

pulmonary artery The artery that carries deoxygenated blood from the right ventricle into the lung.

pulmonary capacity The sum of two or more pulmonary volumes.

pulmonary edema The accumulation of extravascular fluid in lung tissues and alveoli.

pulmonary embolism The blockage of a pulmonary artery by foreign matter such as fat, air, tumor tissue, or a thrombus that usually arises from a peripheral vein.

pulmonary hypertension A condition of abnormally high pressure within the pulmonary circulation.

pulmonary overpressurization syndrome (POPS) A condition that results from expansion of trapped air in the lungs; may lead to alveolar rupture and extravasation of air into extraalveolar locations.

pulmonary semilunar valve A valve that guards the orifice between the right ventricle and the pulmonary artery.

pulmonary surfactant Certain lipoproteins that reduce the surface tension of pulmonary fluids, allowing the exchange of gases in the alveoli of the lungs and contributing to the elasticity of pulmonary tissue.

pulmonary trunk The large elastic artery that carries blood from the right ventricle of the heart to the right and left pulmonary arteries.

pulmonary vein Any vein that carries oxygenated blood from the lung to the left atrium.

pulmonary ventilation The movement of air in and out of the lungs, bringing oxygen to the lungs and removing carbon dioxide.

pulmonic pressure Right-sided pressure.

pulp The soft, spongy chamber of the tooth.

pulse pressure The difference between systemic and pulmonic pressure.

pulsus paradoxus An abnormal decrease in systolic blood pressure that drops more than 10 to 15 mm Hg during inspiration compared to expiration; the first phase of Beck's triad.

punctate Spotted; marked with points of puncture.

punctum The opening of each lacrimal canal.

pupil The opening in the center of the iris that regulates the amount of light entering the eye.

purified protein derivative (PPD) A dried form of tuberculin used in testing for past or present infection with tubercle bacilli.

Purkinje fibers Myocardial fibers that are a continuation of the bundle of His and extend into the muscle walls of the ventricles.

pustule A small, circumscribed elevation of skin containing fluid, which is usually purulent.

P wave The first complex of the electrocardiogram, representing depolarization of the atria.

pyelolithotomy Removal of stone from a kidney by surgical incision.

pyloric sphincter A thickened, muscular ring in the stomach, separating the pylorus from the duodenum.

pyorrhea Discharge of pus.

pyrogen Any substance or agent that tends to cause a rise in body temperature.

pyruvate The end product of glycolysis; may be metabolized to lactate or acetyl CoA.

QRS complex The principle deflection in the electrocardiogram, representing ventricular depolarization.

QT interval The time elapsing from the beginning of the QRS complex to the end of the T wave, representing the total duration of electrical activity of the ventricles.

rabies An acute, usually fatal, viral disease of the central nervous system of animals; transmitted from animals to people by infected blood, tissue, or most commonly, saliva.

raccoon's eyes Ecchymosis of one or both orbits caused by fracture of the base of the sphenoid sinus.

radial tuberosity A large, oblong elevation at the distal end of the radius.

radioulnar syndesmosis The articulation of the radius and ulna, consisting of a proximal articulation, a distal articulation, and three sets of ligaments.

range The general perimeter of coverage, beyond which coverage is nonexistent or severely degraded to an unusable level. Measured in miles.

reabsorption The process of absorbing again that occurs in the kidneys.

reactive hyperemia Increased blood flow associated with increased metabolic activity.

receptor A reactive site on the cell surface or within the cell that combines with a drug molecule to produce a biologic effect.

reciprocity The practice of granting an individual licensure or certification/registration based on licensure or certification/registration by another state, agency, or association.

rectum The segment of the large intestine, continuous with the descending sigmoid colon, just proximal to the anal canal.

rectus femoris muscle A muscle of the anterior thigh; one of the four parts of the quadriceps femoris.

red marrow Specialized soft tissue found in many bones of infants and children, in the spongy bone of the proximal epiphyses of the humerus and femur and in the sternum, ribs, and vertebral bodies of adults. It is essential in the manufacture of red blood cells.

red measles See **rubeola.**

reentry The reactivation of tissue by a returning impulse; the sustaining mechanism in some cases of ventricular bigeminy or trigeminy, ventricular tachycardia, and paroxysmal supraventricular tachycardia.

referred pain Visceral pain felt at a site distant from its origin, for example, pain from a myocardial infarction felt in the patient's arm.

reflex An automatic response to a stimulus that occurs without conscious thought; produced by a reflex arc.

reflex arc The smallest portion of the nervous system that is capable of receiving a stimulus and producing a response.

refractory period The period after effective stimulation during which excitable tissue fails to respond to a stimulus of threshold intensity.

refractory shock Shock that is resistent to treatment, but is still reversible.

relative hypovolemia Inadequate preload as a result of vasodilation.

relative refractory period The portion of the action potential after the absolute refractory period during which another action potential can be produced with a greater-than-threshold stimulus strength.

renal calculus Kidney stone.

renal calyx The first unit in the system of the ducts of the kidney carrying urine from the renal pyramid of the cortex to the renal pelvis for excretion through the ureters.

renal capsule The cortical substance separating the renal pyramids.

renal corpuscle The glomerulus and Bowman's capsule that encloses it.

renal cortex The outer layer of the kidney, containing approximately 1.25 million renal tubules, which remove body waste in the form of urine.

renal medulla The inner layer of the kidney.

renal papilla The apex of the renal pyramid.

renal pelvis The funnel-shaped expansion of the upper end of the ureter that receives the calyces.

renal pyramid One of a number of pyramidal masses seen on longitudinal section of the kidney; contains part of the loop of Henle and the collecting tubules.

renal tubule One of the collecting tubules in the kidney.

renin-angiotensin-aldosterone mechanism Renin, released from the kidneys in response to low blood pressure, converts angiotensinogen to angiotensin I. Angiotensin I is converted by angiotensin-converting enzyme to angiotensin II, which causes vasoconstriction, resulting in increased blood pressure. Angiotensin II also increases aldosterone secretion which increases blood pressure by increasing blood volume.

repolarization The phase of the action potential in which the membrane potential moves from its maximum degree of depolarization toward the value of the resting membrane potential.

reposition To move a structure to its original position.

rescue To free from confinement or danger.

residual volume The volume of air remaining in the lungs after a maximum expiratory effort.

resin The enzyme that converts angiotensinogen to angiotensin I.

respiration The process of the molecular exchange of oxygen and carbon dioxide within the body's tissues.

respiratory bronchiole The smallest bronchiole that connects the terminal bronchiole to the alveolar duct.

respiratory membrane The membrane in the lungs across which gas exchange occurs with the blood.

respiratory syncytial virus (RSV) A single-strand virus that is a common cause of epidemics of acute bronchiolitis, bronchopneumonia, and the common cold in young children and sporadic acute bronchitis and mild upper respiratory tract infections in adults.

resting membrane potential (RMP) The electrical charge difference inside a cell membrane measured relative to just outside the cell membrane.

reticular Relating to a fine network of cells or collagen fibers.

reticular activating system A functional system in the brain essential for wakefulness, attention, concentration, and introspection.

reticular formation An area in the medulla where bits of gray and white matter mix intricately.

retina The nervous tunic of the eye; continuous with the optic nerve.

retraction Movement in the posterior direction

retrograde amnesia The loss of memory for events that occurred before the event that precipitated the amnesia.

retroperitoneum Behind the peritoneum.

retrovirus Any of a family of viruses that converts genetic RNA to DNA after entering the host cell.

revised trauma score An injury severity index that uses the Glasgow coma scale and measurements for systolic blood pressure and respiratory rate.

rheumatoid lungs Rheumatoid arthritis with emphasis on nonarticular changes, for example, pulmonary interstitial fibrosis, pleural effusion, and lung nodules.

Rh factor An antigenic substance present in the erythrocytes of most people; a person lacking the Rh factor is Rh negative.

rhonchi Abnormal sounds heard on auscultation of a respiratory airway obstructed by thick secretions, muscular spasm, neoplasm, or external pressure.

rib One of the 12 pairs of elastic arches of bone forming a large part of the thoracic skeleton. The first seven ribs on each side are called **true ribs** because they articulate directly with the sternum. The remaining five ribs are called **false ribs;** the first three attach ventrally to the ribs and the last two ribs are free at their ventral extremities and are called **floating ribs.**

ribonucleic acid (RNA) A nucleic acid, found in both the nucleus and cytoplasm of cells, that transmits genetic instructions from the nucleus to the cytoplasm. In the cytoplasm, RNA functions in the assembly of proteins.

ribosome The "factory" of a cell where protein is synthesized.

right lymphatic duct A vessel that conveys lymph from the right upper quadrant of the body into the blood stream in the neck at the junction of the right internal jugular and the right subclavian veins.

rod A photoreceptor in the retina of the eye; responsible for noncolor vision in low-intensity light.

R-on-T phenomenon The occurrence of a ventricular depolarization during a vulnerable period of relative refractoriness.

root The lowest part of the tooth; covered by cementum.

rotation Movement of a structure about its axis

rouleaux formation An aggregation of red cells in what looks like a stack of coins or checkers.

round ligament The remains of the umbilical vein.

R prime (R′) A subsequent positive deflection in the QRS complex that extends above the baseline and that is taller than the first R wave.

rubella A contagious viral disease characterized by fever, symptoms of mild upper respiratory tract infection, lymph node enlargement, and a diffuse, fine, red maculopapular rash; spread by droplet infection. Also known as *German measles.*

rubeola An acute, highly contagious viral disease involving the respiratory tract; characterized by a spreading maculopapular cutaneous rash; occurs primarily in young children who have not been immunized. Also known as *red measles.*

ruptured ovarian cyst A ruptured globular sac filled with fluid or semisolid material that develops in or on the ovary.

rupture of membranes Rupture of the amniotic sac; usually occurs toward the end of the first stage of labor.

salpingitis An inflammation or infection of the fallopian tube.

sacral bone Composed of the five segments of the vertebral column that are fused in the adult to form the sacrum; designated as S1 to S5.

sacral promontory The projecting portion of the pelvis at the base of the sacrum.

sacral sparing The preservation of sensory or voluntary motor function of the perineum, buttocks, scrotum, or anus.

saddle joint A joint that consists of two saddle-shaped articulating surfaces oriented at right angles to one another.

sagittal plane An imaginary plane that runs vertically through the middle of the body, producing right and left sections.

salicylate Any one of widely prescribed drugs derived from salicylic acid (for example, aspirin).

salivary amylase A digestive enzyme found in saliva which begins the chemical digestion of carbohydrates.

salivary gland One of the three pairs of glands that pour their secretions into the mouth, thus aiding the digestive process.

salpingitis An inflammation or infection of the fallopian tube.

saltatory conduction Conduction in which action potentials jump from one node of Ranvier to the next node of Ranvier.

salvos See *couplets.*

sarcoidosis A chronic disorder of unknown origin characterized by the formation of lesions in the lung, spleen, liver, skin, mucous membranes, and the lacrimal and salivary glands.

sarcolemma Part of a myofibril between adjacent Z lines.

sarcomere The contractile unit of skeletal muscle, containing thick and thin myofilaments.

sarcoplasmic reticulum Endoplasmic reticulum of the muscle.

scapula One of the pair of large, flat triangular bones that form the dorsal part of the shoulder girdle.

schizophrenia Any one of a large group of psychotic disorders characterized by gross distortions of reality, disturbances of language and communication, withdrawal from social interaction, and the disorganization and fragmentation of thought, perception, and emotional reaction.

Schwann cell A cell that forms a myelin sheath around each nerve fiber of the peripheral nervous system.

sciatic nerve A long nerve originating in the sacral plexus and extending through the muscles of the thigh, leg, and foot, with numerous branches.

scoliosis A lateral curvature of the spine.

scrotum The pouchlike sac that contains the testes.

sebaceous gland A gland of the skin, usually associated with a hair follicle that produces sebum.

sebum The secretion of sebaceous glands; prevents drying and protects against some bacteria.

secondary bronchus A branch from a primary bronchus that conducts air to each lobe of the lungs.

secondary epilepsy Epilepsy that can be traced to trauma, infection, a cerebrovascular disorder, or another illness that contributes to or causes the seizure disorder.

secondary follicle The follicle in which the secondary oocyte is surrounded by granulosa cells.

second stage of labor The stage of labor measured from full dilation of the cervix to delivery of the infant.

secretin The hormone that stimulates secretion of pancreatic juice.

secretion A general term for a substance produced inside a cell and released from the cell.

secretory phase The portion of the menstrual cycle extending from the time of formation of the corpus luteum after ovulation to the time when menstrual flow begins.

sector A subdivision of the incident command system encompassing a specific area of responsibility as deemed necessary by the incident commander.

sedative-hypnotic A drug that reversibly depresses the activity of the central nervous system, used chiefly to induce sleep and relieve anxiety.

self-contained breathing apparatus (SCBA) A respiratory protection device that provides an enclosed system of air.

Sellick's maneuver Cricoid cartilage pressure directed posteriorly to compress the trachea against the cervical vertebra, thereby occluding the esophagus; useful to limit risk of aspiration during an intubation procedure.

semen Male reproductive fluid.

semicircular canal A structure located in the inner ear that generates a nerve impulse when the head moves.

seminal vesicle One of two glandular structures that empty into the ejaculatory ducts; its secretion is one of the components of semen.

semipermeable membrane A membrane that is pervious such that fluids and other substances can pass through it.

sensory layer The portion of the retina containing rods and cones. Also known as the *sensory retina.*

sensory retina See *sensory layer.*

septic shock A form of shock that most often results from a serious systemic bacterial infection.

septum A thin wall dividing two cavities or masses of soft tissue.

serotonin A hormone and neurotransmitter released from platelets when blood vessel walls are damaged.

serous membrane One of the many thin sheets of tissue that line closed cavities of the body, such as the pleura lining the thoracic cavity, the peritoneum lining the abdominal cavity, and the pericardium lining the sac that encloses the heart.

serous pericardium The thin, inner layer of the pericardium that surrounds the heart.

serum Blood plasma, minus its clotting factors.

sexual assault A forcible act of sexual contact with the body of another person, male or female, without his or her consent.

shipping paper A description of a hazardous material that includes the substance name, classification, and

UN identification number; generally required to be carried in the transporting vehicle (motor vehicle, train, vessel, or aircraft).

short bones Bones that are approximately as broad as they are long. Examples are the carpal bones of the wrist and the tarsal bones of the ankle.

shoulder dystocia An obstacle to delivery that occurs when the fetal shoulders press against the maternal symphysis pubis, blocking shoulder delivery.

shoulder girdle The encircling bony structure supporting the upper limbs. Also known as the *pectoral girdle.*

shoulder presentation The presentation that results when the long axis of the fetus lies perpendicular to that of the mother. Also known as *transverse presentation.*

shunting The redirection of a flow of body fluid from one cavity or vessel to another.

sickle cell anemia Anemia characterized by the presence of crescent-shaped erythrocytes and excessive hemolysis; an inheritable condition.

side effect An often unavoidable and undesirable effect of using therapeutic doses of a drug; actions or effects other than those for which the drug was originally given.

sighing An occasional deep, audible inspiration; usually insignificant.

sigmoid colon The segment of the colon that extends from the end of the descending colon in the pelvis to the juncture with the rectum.

silicosis A lung disorder caused by continued long-term inhalation of the dust of an inorganic compound, silicon dioxide; characterized by dyspnea and the development of nodular fibrosis in the lungs.

simplex A system with the ability to transmit or receive in one direction at a time; one party transmits, the other receives. Simultaneous transmission cannot occur without blocking a message.

sinoatrial node (SA node) An area of specialized heart tissue that generates the cardiac electrical impulse.

sinus One of several cavities in the bones of the skull that connect to the nasal cavities by small channels.

sinusoid A form of terminating blood channel, somewhat larger than a capillary, lined with reticuloendothelial cells.

sizeup To quickly assess an emergency scene and determine what resources are needed.

skeletal muscle Muscle tissue that appears microscopically to consist of striped myofibrils. Also known as *striated muscle* and *voluntary muscle.*

Skene's glands The largest of the glands that open into the urethra of women.

slander Verbally stating to others false statements about another, knowing them to be false and with malicious intent, or with reckless disregard for their falsity.

sleep apnea A sleep disorder characterized by periods in which attempts to breathe are absent.

slough To shed or cast off; tissue that has been shed.

slow reactive substance of anaphylaxis A bronchoconstrictor mediator released from mast cells; increases the production of prostaglandins.

small intestine The longest portion of the digestive tract; divided into the duodenum, jejunum, and ileum.

smooth muscle One of two kinds of muscle, composed of elongated, spindle-shaped cells in muscles not under voluntary control, such as smooth muscle of the intestines, stomach, and other visceral organs. Also known as *visceral muscle* and *nonstriated muscle.*

sniffing position The patient position used during orotracheal intubation whereby the patient's neck is flexed at C5 and C6, and the head is extended at C1 and C2.

sodium bicarbonate An antiacid, electrolyte, and urinary alkalinizing agent.

sodium ions Ions involved in acid-base balance, water balance, nerve impulse transmission, and muscle contraction.

sodium-potassium exchange pump The biochemical mechanism that uses energy derived from ATP to achieve the active transport of potassium ions opposite to that of sodium ions.

soft palate The posterior muscular portion of the palate, forming an incomplete septum between the mouth and the oropharynx and between the oropharynx and the nasopharynx.

somatic nervous system The part of the nervous system composed of nerve fibers that send impulses from the central nervous system to skeletal muscle.

somatic pain Pain that arises from skeletal muscles, ligaments, vessels, or joints.

somatomotor nerves Motor nerves to the skeletal muscles.

spasm An involuntary muscle contraction of sudden onset.

special emergency radio service (SERS) A specific group of radio frequencies designated by the FCC for use by emergency agencies.

sperm See *spermatozoon.*

spermatic cord A structure extending from the deep inguinal ring in the abdomen to the testes. Each cord comprises arteries, veins, lymphatics, nerves, and the excretory duct of the testis.

spermatogenesis The process of development of spermatozoa.

spermatozoon The male sex cell, composed of a head and tail; contains genetic information transmitted by the male.

sphenoid bone The bone at the base of the skull, anterior to the temporal bones and the basilar part of the occipital bone.

sphenoid sinus One of a pair of cavities in the sphenoid bone, lined with mucous membrane continuous with that of the nasal cavity.

sphincter Ring-shaped muscle.

sphygmomanometer The device used to measure blood pressure.

spinal cord shock See *neurogenic shock.*

spinal ganglia The structures that contain the cell bodies of sensory neurons. Also known as *dorsal root ganglia.*

spinal nerve One of 31 pairs of nerves formed by the joining of the dorsal and ventral routes that arise from the spinal cord.

spinous process A part of the vertebrae projecting backward from the vertebral arch, giving attachment to muscles of the back.

spleen A large, highly vascular lymphatic organ situated in the upper part of the abdominal cavity between the stomach and the diaphragm. It responds to foreign substances in the blood, destroys worn-out erythrocytes, and is a storage site for red blood cells.

spondylosis A condition of the spine characterized by fixation or stiffness of the vertebral joint.

spontaneous abortion An abortion that usually occurs before the twelfth week of gestation; lay term: miscarriage.

S prime (S′) A subsequent negative deflection in the QRS complex that extends below the baseline.

squelch A radio receiver circuit used to suppress the audio portion of unwanted radio signals or radio noises below a predetermined carrier strength level.

staging area A designated area where incident-assigned vehicles are directed and held until needed.

standing orders Specific treatment protocols that may be used by prehospital emergency care providers in the absence of on-line medical control when delay in treatment would harm the patient.

stapes The smallest of the three ossicles in the middle ear.

staphylococcal infection An infection caused by any one of several pathogenic species of *Staphylococcus*, commonly characterized by the formation of abscesses of the skin or other organs.

Starling's law of the heart A rule that the force of the heartbeat is determined by the length of the fibers comprising the myocardial walls.

stasis A disorder in which the normal flow of fluid through a vessel of the body is slowed or halted.

status epilepticus A medical emergency characterized by continual convulsive seizures occurring without intervals of consciousness.

stellate wound A star-shaped wound.

sternal angle The point at which the manubrium joins the body of the sternum. Also known as the *angle of Louis*.

sternoclavicular joint The double gliding joint between the sternum and the clavicle.

sternum The elongated, flattened bone forming the middle portion of the thorax.

steroid A member of a large family of lipids, including some reproductive hormones, vitamins, and cholesterol.

stimulant A drug that enhances or increases body function or activity.

Stokes-Adams syndrome A condition characterized by sudden episodes of loss of consciousness caused by incomplete heart block; seizures may accompany the episodes.

stoma A surgically created artificial opening of an internal organ on the surface of the body.

stomach The major organ of digestion, located in the right upper quadrant of the abdomen.

stratum basale The innermost layer of the epidermis.

stratum corneum The most superficial layer of the epidermis.

stratum granulosum The layer of the epidermis that lies just beneath the stratum corneum, except in the palms of the hands and soles of the feet, where it lies just beneath the stratum lucidum.

stratum lucidum The layer of the epidermis that lies just beneath the stratum corneum; present only in the thick skin of the palms of the hands and soles of the feet.

stratum spinosum The layer of the epidermis that lies on top of the stratum basale and beneath the stratum granulosum.

streptococcal infection An infection caused by pathogenic bacteria of one of several species of the genus *Streptococcus* or their toxins.

stress A nonspecific mental or physical strain caused by any emotional, physical, social, economic, or other factor that initiates a physiologic response.

stressor Any factor that causes wear and tear on the body's physical or mental resources.

stretch mark See *stria*.

stria A streak or a linear scar that often results from rapidly developing tension in the skin. Also known as a *stretch mark*.

striated muscle See *skeletal muscle*.

stroke volume The volume of blood pumped out of one ventricle in a single heartbeat.

ST segment The early part of repolarization in the electrocardiogram of the right and left ventricles.

stylet A thin metal probe for inserting into or passing through a needle, tube, or catheter; sometimes used to change the configuration of an endotracheal tube.

styloid process A bony projection.

subarachnoid space The area below the arachnoid membrane but above the pia matter that contains cerebral spinal fluid.

subclavian vein The continuation of the axillary vein in the upper body; extends from the lateral border of the first rib to the sternal end of the clavicle, where it joins the internal jugular to form the brachiocephalic vein.

subcutaneous tissue The adherent layer of adipose tissue, just below the dermal layer. Also known as the *hypodermis*.

subdural space The space between the dura matter and arachnoid.

subendocardial infarction See *transmural infarction*.

subgaleal hematoma A collection of blood beneath the strong sheet of fibrous connective tissue that joins the frontal and occipitofrontal muscles.

sublingual route The route of medication administration in which the is placed under the tongue so that the tablet dissolves in salivary secretions.

subluxation A partial dislocation.

sudden death A death that occurs within the first 24 hours after the onset of illness or injury.

sudden infant death syndrome (SIDS) The unexpected and sudden death of an apparently normal and healthy infant that occurs during sleep and with no physical or autopsic evidence of disease.

sudoriferous gland See *sweat gland.*

summation The combined effect of two drugs that equals the sum of the individual effects of each agent.

superficial frostbite A cold injury with at least some minimal tissue loss; usually involves the dermis and shallow subcutaneous layers.

superficial pain Pain that arises from the skin or mucous membrane.

superior venae cavae The vein that returns blood from the head and neck, upper limbs, and thorax to the right atrium.

supination Rotation of the forearm so that the anterior surface is up.

supine hypotension syndrome Hypotension that occurs in pregnant women who are in a supine position; results when the uterus compresses the inferior vena cava, producing decreased cardiac filling and decreased cardiac output.

supine position The position in which the patient is lying on his or her back (faceup).

suprasternal notch The superior margin of the manubrium which can be easily felt at the anterior base of the neck. Also known as the *jugular notch.*

surface tension The tendency of the surface of a liquid to minimize the area of its surface by contracting.

suspensory ligament The band of peritoneum that extends from the ovary to the body wall; contains the ovarian vessels and nerves.

suture A border or joint between two bones of the cranium.

sweat gland A structure that produces sweat or viscus organic secretions. Also known as a *sudoriferous gland.*

sympathetic nervous system A subdivision of the autonomic nervous system, usually involved in preparing the body for physical activity.

sympatholytic Antiadrenergic: blocking transmission of impulses from the adrenergic postganglionic fibers to effector organs or tissues.

sympathomimetic A pharmacologic agent that mimics the effects of sympathetic-nervous-system stimulation of organs and structures by acting as an agonist or by increasing the release of the neurotransmitter norepinephrine at postganglionic nerve endings.

symphysis A cartilaginous joint.

symphysis pubis The slightly moveable interpubic joint of the pelvis, consisting of two bones separated by a disk of fibrocartilage and connected by two ligaments. Also known as the **pubic symphysis.**

synapse Functional membrane-to-membrane contact of a nerve cell with another nerve cell, muscle cell, gland cell, or sensory receptor; functions in transmitting action potentials from one cell to another.

synaptic cleft The space between the presynaptic and postsynaptic membranes.

synaptic vesicle A secretory vesicle in the presynaptic terminal containing neurotransmitter substances.

synchondrosis A cartilaginous joint between two immovable bones, such as the symphysis pubis, the sternum, and the manubrium.

syncytium Cardiac muscle cells that are so tightly bound together and their membranes so permeable to electrical impulse that they act as a mass of merged cells or a single cell.

syndesmosis A fibrous articulation in which two bones are connected by interosseous ligaments.

synergism The combined action of two drugs that is greater than the sum of each individual agent acting independently.

synergist A muscle that works with other muscles to cause movement.

synovial fluid A thin, lubricating film that allows considerable movement between articulating bones.

synovial joint See *joint.*

synovial membrane The inner layer of an articular capsule surrounding a freely movable joint.

syphilis A sexually transmitted disease characterized by distinct stages of effects over a period of years; any organ system may be involved.

systemic circulation Blood flow from the left ventricle to all parts of the body and back to the right atrium.

systemic pressure Left-sided pressure.

tabes dorsalis An abnormal condition characterized by the slow degeneration of all or part of the body and the progressive loss of peripheral reflexes.

tachycardia A heart rate greater than 100 beats per minute.

tachyphylaxis A phenomenon in which the repeated administration of some drugs results in a marked decrease in their effectiveness.

tachypnea A persistent respiratory rate that exceeds 20 breaths per minute.

talus The second-largest tarsal bone; ankle bone.

tardive dyskinesia An abnormal condition characterized by involuntary, repetitious movements of the muscles of the face, limbs, and trunk.

tarsal Pertaining to the area of articulation between the foot and the leg.

taste bud Any one of many peripheral taste organs distributed over the tongue and roof of the mouth.

telemetry The transmission and reception of physiologic data by radio or telephone, for example, electrocardiograms (ECGs).

temporal bone One of a pair of large bones forming part of the lower cranium and containing various cavities and recesses associated with the ear.

temporal lobe The lateral region of the cerebrum; contains the center for smell and some association areas for memory and learning.

ten code A code sometimes used in radio communications that uses the number 10 plus another number to relay a particular message.

tendon A band or cord of dense connective tissue that connects muscle to bone or other structures; characterized by strength and nonstretchability.

tenosynovitis Inflammation of a tendon sheath.

tension pneumothorax Accumulation of air or gas

within the pleural cavity, which if not relieved can lead to lung collapse.

teratogenic Any substance, agent, or process that interferes with normal prenatal development.

term A pregnancy that has reached 40 weeks gestation.

terminal bronchiole The end of the conducting airway.

termination of action The point at which a drug effect is no longer seen.

tertiary segmental bronchus The bronchus that extends from the secondary bronchus and conducts air to each lobule of the lung.

testes The male gonads that produce the male sex cells or sperm.

testicular torsion The axial rotation of the spermatic cord that occludes blood supply to the testicle, epididymis, and other structures.

testosterone The male sex hormone.

tetralogy of Fallot A congenital cardiac anomaly that consists of four defects: pulmonic stenosis, ventricular septal defect, malposition of the aorta so that it rises from the septal defect or the right ventricle, and right ventricular hypertrophy.

thalamus Tissue located just above the hypothalamus that helps to produce sensations, associates sensations with emotions, and plays a part in arousal.

therapeutic abortion The legal termination of a pregnancy for reasons of maternal well-being.

therapeutic action The desired, intended action of a drug.

therapeutic index A measurement of the relative safety of a drug.

therapeutic range The range of plasma concentrations that are most likely to produce the desired drug effect with the least likelihood of toxicity; the range between minimal effective concentration and toxic level.

thermogenesis Production of heat, especially by the cells of the body.

thermolysis Dissipation of body heat by radiation, evaporation, conduction, or convection.

thiazide A group of diuretics that are moderately effective in lowering blood pressure.

third stage of labor The stage of labor that begins with delivery of the infant and ends when the placenta has been expelled and the uterus has contracted.

third ventricle The ventricle located in the center of the diencephalon, between the two halves of the thalamus.

thoracentesis Puncturing of pleural space.

thoracic duct The common trunk of all the lymphatic vessels of the body, except those on the right side of the head and neck, the thorax, right upper limb, right lung, right side of the heart, and the diaphragmatic surface of the liver.

thoracic vertebrae The 12 bony segments of the spinal column of the upper back, designated T1 to T12.

thoroughfare channel The channel for blood through a capillary bed from an arteriole to a venule.

threatened abortion An abortion diagnosed when a patient has some uterine bleeding with an intrauterine pregnancy in which the internal cervical os is closed; may stabilize and end in normal delivery or progress to an incomplete or complete abortion.

threshold potential The value of the membrane potential at which an action potential is produced as a result of depolarization in response to a stimulus.

thrombectomy The removal of a thrombus from a blood vessel.

thrombin An enzyme formed in plasma as part of the clotting process; causes fibrinogen to change to fibrin, which is essential in the formation of a clot.

thrombocytes Cell fragments.

thrombocytopenia An abnormal hematologic condition in which the number of platelets is reduced; the most common cause is a bleeding disorder.

thromboembolism A condition in which a blood vessel is blocked by an embolus carried in the blood stream from the site of formation of the clot.

thrombogenesis Clot formation.

thrombolytic agent A drug that dissolves clots after their formation by promoting the digestion of fibrin.

thrombophlebitis See *phlebitis*.

thrombus An aggregation of platelets, fibrin, clotting factors, and the cellular elements of the blood attached to the interior wall of a vein or artery, sometimes occluding the lumen of the vessel.

thymectomy Excision of the thymus.

thymus A single, unpaired gland, located in the mediastinum; the primary central gland of the lymphatic system.

thyroid cartilage The largest laryngeal cartilage; forms the laryngeal prominence, or Adam's apple.

thyroid membrane The fibrous membrane that joins the hyoid and the thyroid cartilages.

tibia The second longest bone of the skeleton, located at the medial side of the leg.

tibial tuberosity A large, oblong elevation at the proximal end of the tibia that attaches to the ligament of the patella.

tidal volume The volume of air inspired or expired in a single, resting breath.

tissue binding A type of drug reservoir in which drug pooling occurs in fat tissue and bone.

T lymphocyte A thymus-derived lymphocyte of immunologic importance; responsible for cell-mediated immunity.

tolerance A physiological response requiring that a drug dosage be increased to produce the same effect formerly produced by a smaller dose; exists when there is a decreased physiologic response to the repeated administration of a drug or chemically related substance.

tone The audio signal or carrier wave of controlled amplitude and frequency used for equipment control purposes or to selectively signal a receiver, such as activating a pager. Tones are measured in Hertz.

tonsil A large collection of lymphatic tissue beneath the mucous membrane of the oral cavity and pharynx.

tonsillectomy Surgical removal of the tonsils.

tonsillitis Inflammation of the tonsils.

torr A measurement in millimeters of mercury.

torsades de pointes An unusual bidirectional ventricular tachycardia.

total lung capacity The sum of the inspiratory and expiratory reserve volumes plus the tidal volume and residual volume.

total pressure The combination of pressures exerted by all the gases in any mixture of gas.

toxic level The plasma concentration at which a drug is likely to produce serious adverse effects.

toxic shock A severe acute disease caused by infection with strains of *Staphylococcus aureus*.

trachea A cylindric tube in the neck composed of cartilage and membrane; conveys air to the lungs.

tracheal stenosis Constriction of the trachea.

tracheostomy An opening through the neck into the trachea through which an indwelling tube may be inserted.

trade name The copyrighted name of a drug, designated by the drug company that sells the medication. Also known as *brand name* or *proprietary name*.

tragus A projection of the cartilage of the auricle at the opening of the external auditory meatus.

transceiver A combination transmitter and receiver with a switching circuit or duplexer to use a single antenna.

transcutaneous cardiac pacing (TCP) The use of an artificial pacemaker to substitute for a natural pacemaker of the heart that is blocked or dysfunctional. In the prehospital setting, a transcutaneous pacemaker is used to treat symptomatic bradycardia, heart block associated with reduced cardiac output that is unresponsive to atropine, pacemaker failure, and asystole.

transient dysphagia A temporary impairment of speech.

transmural infarction A myocardial infarction that extends through the full thickness of the myocardium, including the endocardium and epicardium. Also known as *subendocardial infarction*.

transudate A fluid passed through a membrane as a result of a difference in hydrostatic pressure.

transverse colon The segment of the colon that extends from the end of the ascending colon at the hepatic flexure on the right side across the midabdomen to the beginning of the descending colon at the splenic flexure on the left side.

transverse plane An imaginary plane that divides the body into top and bottom or superior and inferior sections. Also known as the *horizontal plane*.

transverse presentation See *shoulder presentation*.

transverse process The bony segment that extends laterally from each side of the vertebral arch.

trauma An injury caused by a transfer of energy from some external source to the human body.

trauma score An injury severity index used to predict outcome for patients with blunt or penetrating injuries.

traumatic iridoplegia Traumatic dilation, or less commonly, constriction, of the pupil.

treatment protocols Guidelines that define the scope of prehospital intervention practiced by emergency care providers.

triaxial reference system Three intersecting lines of reference used in standard limb leads.

trichomoniasis A vaginal infection caused by the protozoan *Trichomonas vaginalis*, characterized by itching, burning, and frothy, pale yellow to green vaginal discharge.

tricuspid valve The valve located between the right atrium and ventricle.

trigeminal nerve Either of the largest pair of cranial nerves, essential for chewing and the general sensibility of the face.

trigone The triangular smooth area at the base of the bladder between the openings of two ureters and that of the urethra.

trimester One of three periods of approximately 3 months into which pregnancy is divided.

triplets Three PVCs in a row.

trochanter One of the two bony projections at the proximal end of the femur that serve as the attachment point for various muscles.

trochlea The medial aspect of the humerus; articulates with the ulna.

trophoblast A cell layer forming the outer layer of the blastocyst, which erodes the uterine mucosa during implantation; contributes to the formation of the placenta.

true rib See *rib*.

true vocal cord See *vocal cord*.

truncal obesity Obesity that preferentially affects or is isolated in the trunk of the body, as opposed to the extremities.

trunking system A radio system consisting of base stations on different channels connected to each other with small computers that work with special mobile and portable signaling to allow multiple simultaneous conversations. Systems are available for VHF, UHF, and 800 MHz.

T tubule Tubelike invagination of the sarcolemma that conducts action potentials toward the center of the cylindrical muscle fibers.

tubal ligation One of several sterilization procedures in which both fallopian tubes are blocked to prevent conception from occurring.

tubercle A nodule or small eminence, such as that on a bone or that produced by infection from tubercle bacilli.

tunic One of the enveloping layers of a part; one of the coats of a blood vessel; one of the coats of the eye; one of the coats of the digestive tract.

tunica adventitia The outermost fibrous coat of a vessel or an organ that is derived from the surrounding connective tissue.

tunica intima The innermost coat of a blood vessel.

tunica media The middle coat, usually muscular, of an artery or other tubular structure.

turbinate The concha nasalis.

T wave Deflection in the electrocardiogram after the QRS complex, representing ventricular repolarization.

tympanic membrane See *eardrum.*

type and crossmatch A test used to determine the patient's ABO group and Rh type.

ulceration The formation of a craterlike lesion on the skin or mucous membranes.

ultra high frequency (UHF) Radio frequency between 300 and 3000 MHz. The 460-MHz range is most commonly used for EMS communications.

umbilicus The point on the abdomen at which the umbilical cord joined the fetal abdomen.

unifocal PVC A premature ventricular contraction that originates from a single ectopic pacemaker site.

unipolar lead A lead composed of a single positive electrode and a reference point.

universal donor A person with blood of type O, Rh factor negative.

universal recipient A person with blood type AB who can receive any of the four types of blood.

unmyelinated axon A nerve fiber lacking a myelin sheath.

untoward effect A side effect that proves harmful to the patient.

upper esophageal sphincter The ring of muscle located at the superior opening of the esophagus that regulates the passage of materials into the esophagus.

urea A nitrogen-containing waste product.

uremia The presence of excessive amounts of urea and other nitrogenous waste products in the blood, such as occurs in renal failure.

uremic frost A pale, frostlike deposit of white crystals on the skin caused by kidney failure and uremia.

ureter One of a pair of tubes that carry the urine from the kidney into the bladder.

urethra A small tubular structure that drains urine from the bladder. In men, it also serves as a passageway for semen during ejaculation.

uric acid A product of the metabolism of protein present in the blood and excreted in the urine.

urinary bladder The muscular, membranous sac in the pelvis that stores urine for discharge through the urethra.

urogenital triangle The anterior portion of the perianal region; contains the openings of the urethra and vagina in the female and the root structures of the penis in the male.

uterine inversion A rare event in which the uterus turns inside out after birth.

uterine rupture A rare event in which the wall of the uterus ruptures when it is unable to withstand the strain placed on it.

uterine tube One of a pair of ducts opening at one end into the uterus and the other end into the peritoneal cavity, over the ovary. Also known as a *fallopian tube.*

uterosacral ligament A primary ligament that holds the uterus in place.

uterus The hollow, pear-shaped internal female organ of reproduction.

uvula The cone-shaped process hanging down from the soft palate that helps prevent food and liquid from entering the nasal cavities.

U wave Gradual deviation from the T wave in the electrocardiogram, thought to represent the final stage of repolarization of the ventricles.

vaginitis An inflammation of the vaginal tissues.

vagus nerve Either of the longest pair of cranial nerves essential for speech, swallowing, and the sensibilities and functions of many parts of the body.

vallecula A furrow between the glossoepiglottic folds on each side of the posterior oropharynx.

varicella An acute, highly contagious viral disease caused by a herpesvirus, varicella-zoster virus; occurs primarily in young children and is characterized by crops of pruritic vesicular eruptions on the skin. Also known as *chickenpox.*

varicella-zoster virus (VZV) A member of the herpesvirus family that causes the disease varicella (chickenpox) and herpes zoster (shingles).

varicocele A collection of varicose veins in the scrotum.

vascular tunic The choroid, ciliary body, and iris.

vas deferens See *ductus deferens.*

vasomotor Of or pertaining to the nerves and muscles that control the diameter of the lumen of blood vessels.

vasopressin mechanism The mechanism by which ADH secretion increases when blood pressure drops or plasma osmolarity increases; reduces urine production and stimulates vasoconstriction.

vastus lateralis muscle The largest of the four muscles of the quadriceps femoris, situated on the lateral side of the thigh.

vein A vessel carrying blood toward the heart.

venostasis Retardation of venous flow in a part.

venous capillary The ends of capillaries closest to venules.

venous sinus One of many sinuses that collect blood from the dura mater and drain it into the internal jugular vein.

ventral root The nerve that conveys efferent nerve processes away from the spinal cord.

ventricle A small cavity.

ventricular bigeminy A cardiac dysrhythmia characterized by two ventricular beats in rapid succession followed by a longer interval.

ventricular quadrigeminy A dysrhythmia that occurs when every fourth complex is a PVC.

ventricular tachycardia (VT) Tachycardia that usually originates in the Purkinje fibers.

ventricular trigeminy A cardiac dysrhythmia characterized by three ventricular beats in rapid succession followed by a longer interval.

ventrogluteal muscle The muscle that overlies the iliac crest and the anterior superior iliac spine.

venule Small blood vessels that collect blood from the capillaries and join to form veins.

vermiform appendix See *appendix.*

vertebral arch The dorsal, bony arch of a vertebra, composed of the laminae and pedicles; protects the spinal cord.

vertebral artery Each of the two arteries branching from the subclavian arteries.

vertebral body A bony disk that serves as the weight-bearing portion of the vertebrae.

vertex presentation See *cephalic presentation.*

vertigo A sensation of faintness or an inability to maintain normal balance in a standing or seated position.

very high frequency (VHF) Radio frequencies between 30 and 300 MHz (usually 150-MHz range). The VHF spectrum is further divided into "high" and "low" bands.

vesicular follicle The secondary follicle in which the oocyte attains its full size. Also known as the *graafian follicle.*

vesiculation The formation of vesicles.

vestibular fold One of two folds of mucous membrane stretching across the laryngeal cavity; helps close the glottis. Also known as the *false vocal cord.*

vestibule The portion of the inner ear adjacent to the oval window between the semicircular canals and the cochlea.

vestibule of the ear The middle region of the middle ear.

vestibule of the vagina The space behind the labia minora, containing the opening of the vagina, the urethra, and the vestibular glands.

vestibulocochlear nerve The eighth cranial nerve, formed by the cochlear and vestibular nerves; extends to the brain.

visceral Pertaining to internal organs enclosed within a body cavity, primarily the abdominal organs.

visceral pain Deep pain that arises from smooth vasculature or organ systems.

visceral pericardium The portion of the serous pericardium covering the heart surface. Also known as the *epicardium.*

visceral peritoneum The layer of peritoneum covering the abdominal organs.

vital capacity The volume of gas moved on deepest inspiration and expiration, or the sum of the inspiratory reserve volume, the tidal volume, and the expiratory reserve volume.

vitamin D A fat-soluble vitamin essential for the normal formation of bones and teeth, and for the absorption of calcium and phosphorus from the gastrointestinal tract.

vitamin K A fat-soluble compound essential for the synthesis of several related proteins involved in the clotting of blood.

vitreous humor The transparent jellylike material that fills the space between the lens and the retina.

vocal cord One of two folds of elastic ligaments covered by mucous membrane stretching from the thy-

roid cartilage to the arytenoid cartilage; vibration of the vocal cords is responsible for voice production. Also known as a *true vocal cord.*

voluntary muscle A muscle that is consciously controlled. See *skeletal muscle.*

vomer bone The bone forming the posterior and inferior part of the nasal septum.

vulva The external genitals of the female.

wandering atrial pacemaker The passive transfer of pacemaker sites from the sinus node to other latent pacemaker sites in the atria and AV junction.

water vapor pressure The partial pressure exerted by water molecules after they have been converted into a gas.

watt The unit of measurement of a transmitter's power output.

Wenckebach Mobitz type-I second-degree AV block; a progressive beat-to-beat prolongation of the PR interval, finally resulting in a nonconducted P wave. At this point, the sequence recurs.

wheeze A form of rhonchus characterized by a high-pitched musical quality; caused by high-velocity airflow through narrowed airways.

windchill chart An index developed to calculate the cooling effects of the ambient temperature based on thermometer readings and the wind speed.

withdrawal syndrome A predictable set of signs and symptoms that occurs after a decrease in the usual dose of a drug or its sudden cessation

xiphoid process The smallest of three parts of the sternum, articulating caudally with the body of the sternum and laterally with the seventh rib.

yellow marrow Specialized soft tissue (mainly adipose) found in the compact bone of most adult epiphyses.

Z line The delicate membrane-like structure found at either end of a sarcomere.

zone of coagulation In a burn wound, the central area that has sustained the most intense contact with the thermal source. In this area, coagulation necrosis of the cells has occurred and the tissue is nonviable.

zone of hyperemia An area in which blood flow is increased as a result of the normal inflammatory response to injury; lies at the periphery of the zone of stasis.

zone of stasis The area of burn tissue that surrounds the critically injured area; consists of tissue that is potentially viable despite the serious thermal injury.

zygomatic process See *zygomatic bone.*

zygomatic bone One of a pair of bones that forms the prominence of the cheek, the lower part of the orbit of the eye, and parts of the temporal bone. Also known as *zygomatic process.*

zygote The developing ovum from the time it is fertilized until it is implanted in the uterus as a blastocyst.

CREDITS AND ACKNOWLEDGMENTS

Division openers: Don McKenna/White Cat Studio.

Chapter 1 openers: Ronald Olschwanger; Mark Fisher, Port Orange, Fla; and Acadian Ambulance Service, Inc.

Sidebar 1-2: Reprinted with permission of the National Association of Emergency Medical Technicians.

Chapter 2 openers: Ronald Olschwanger, James Silvernail, and O'Fallon Fire Protection District.

Fig 2-2: American Medical Association: Guidelines for cardiopulmonary resuscitation and emergency cardiac care, 1992, American Medical Association.

Fig 2-3: Courtesy Wheeled Coach, Orlando, Fla.

Figs 2-4, 2-5: Courtesy Air Rescue Consortium of Hospitals, St. Louis, Mo.

Chapter 3 openers: Ronald Olschwanger and James Silvernail.

Chapter 4 openers: Kim McKenna, James Silvernail, and Larry Ashby.

Table 4-1: Department of Transportation: Emergency medical technician - paramedic: national standard curriculum, Washington, D.C., 1985, U.S. D.O.T. NHTSA.

Fig 4-8: Courtesy Medical Priority Consultants Inc., Salt Lake City, Utah.

Chapter 5 openers: Colin Williams, Ronald Olschwanger, and O'Fallon Fire Protection District.

Figs 5-1, 5-2, 5-3: Courtesy O'Fallon, (Mo.) Fire Protection District, St. Charles (Mo.) County Hazmat Team and St. Peters (Mo.) Fire Protection District. Photographer Martin Henderson.

Chapter 6 openers: Maryland Institute for Emergency Medical Services Systems, James Silvernail, and Ken Hines.

Fig 6-2: Courtesy Mettag Products, Starke, Fla.

Fig 6-3: Courtesy Hoag Memorial Hospital, Newport Beach, Calif.

Figs 6-4, 6-5: Lee: Flight nursing: principles and practice, St. Louis, 1991, Mosby.

Chapter 7 openers: Maryland Institute for Emergency Medical Services Systems, O'Fallon Fire Protection District, and Ken Hines.

Fig 7-1: Bronstein: Mosby's emergency care for hazardous material exposure, St. Louis, 1988, Mosby.

Figs 7-2, 7-3, 7-4: Courtesy O'Fallon, (Mo.) Fire Protection District, St. Charles (Mo.) County Hazmat Team and St. Peters (Mo.) Fire Protection District. Photographer Martin Henderson.

Table 7-1: Department of Transportation: Emergency medical technician - paramedic: national standard curriculum, Washington, D.C., 1985, U.S. D.O.T. NHTSA.

Chapter 8 openers: Thomas Cooper, William Greenblatt Photography, and Ronald Olschwanger.

Chapter 9 openers: Maryland Institute for Emergency Medical Services Systems and Acadian Ambulance Service, Inc.

Chapter 10 openers: Maryland Institute for Emergency Medical Services Systems; Frances Councill, Crawfordville, Fla; and Acadian Ambulance Service, Inc.

Fig 10-Un1 (in Table 10-1): Seely: Anatomy and physiology, ed 2, St. Louis, 1992, Mosby.

Fig 10-Un2 (in Table 10-9): Thibodeau: Structure and function of the body, ed 9, St. Louis, 1992, Mosby.

Fig 10-1: Sims/Illustrator Terry Cockerham

Fig 10-2: Sims/ Illustrators Terry Cockerham and Michael Schenk

Figs 10-3, 10-4: Illustrator Nadine Sokol

Fig 10-5: Illustrator Christine Oleksyk

Figs 10-6, 10-7: Thibodeau: Structure and function of the body, ed 9, St. Louis, 1992, Mosby.

Fig 10-9: Sims/Illustrator David J. Mascaro and Associates

Fig 10-10: Thibodeau: Structure and function of the body, ed 9, St. Louis, 1992, Mosby.

Figs 10-11, 10-12, 10-14, 10-16: Illustrator David J. Mascaro and Associates

Fig 10-17: Sims/Illustrator David J. Mascaro and Associates

Fig 10-18: Illustrator David J. Mascaro and Associates

Fig 10-19: Sims/Illustrator Rusty Jones

Figs 10-20, 10-21, 10-22, 10-23, 10-24: Sims/Illustrator Terry Cockerham

Fig 10-26: Illustrator John V. Hagen

Fig 10-27: Thibodeau: Structure and function of the body, ed 9, St. Louis, 1992, Mosby.

Fig 10-28: Illustrator David J. Mascaro and Associates

Figs 10-29, 10-30, 10-31: Thibodeau: Structure and function of the body, ed 9, St. Louis, 1992, Mosby.

Fig 10-32: Stevens: Histology, London, England, 1992, Gower Medical Publishing.

Fig 10-33: Thibodeau: Structure and function of the body, ed 9, St. Louis, 1992, Mosby.

Fig 10-34: Sims/Illustrator G. David Brown

Fig 10-35: Sims/Illustrator Michael Schenk

Fig 10-36: Thibodeau: Structure and function of the body, ed 9, St. Louis, 1992, Mosby.

Fig 10-37: Sims/Illustrators Cynthia Turner Alexander and Terry Cockerham

Fig 10-38: Sims/Illustrator Rusty Jones

Fig 10-39: Thibodeau: Structure and function of the body, ed 9, St. Louis, 1992, Mosby.

Fig 10-40: Illustrator David J. Mascaro and Associates

Fig 10-41: Thibodeau: Structure and function of the body, ed 9, St. Louis, 1992, Mosby.

Fig 10-42: Illustrator Christine Oleksyk

Fig 10-43: Seely; Anatomy and physiology, ed 2, St. Louis, 1992, Mosby.

Figs 10-44, 10-45: Thibodeau: Structure and function of the body, ed 9, St. Louis, 1992, Mosby.

Fig 10-46: Thibodeau: Anatomy and physiology, ed 2, St. Louis, 1993, Mosby.

Fig 10-47: Sims/Illustrator Karen Waldo

Fig 10-48: Thibodeau: Structure and function of the body, ed 9, St. Louis, 1992, Mosby.

Figs 10-49, 10-50: Sims/Illustrator Jody L. Fulks

Figs 10-51, 10-52, 10-53, 10-54: Thibodeau: Structure and function of the body, ed 9, St. Louis, 1992, Mosby.

Figs 10-55, 10-56: Illustrator Ronald J. Ervin

Figs 10-57, 10-58: Thibodeau: Structure and function of the body, ed 9, St. Louis, 1992, Mosby.

Fig 10-59: Sims/Illustrator Kevin A. Sommerville

Figs 10-60, 10-61, 10-62: Thibodeau: Structure and function of the body, ed 9, St. Louis, 1992, Mosby.

Figs 10-63, 10-64: Sims/Illustrator Marsha J. Dohrmann

Table 10-2: Thibodeau: Structure and function of the body, ed 9, St. Louis, 1992, Mosby.

Tables 10-3, 10-5: Seely: Anatomy and physiology, ed 2, St. Louis, 1992, Mosby.

Table 10-6: Adapted from Seely: Anatomy and physiology, ed 2, St. Louis, 1992, Mosby.

Tables 10-7, 10-8, 10-9: Thibodeau: Structure and function of the body, ed 9, St. Louis, 1992, Mosby.

Chapter 11 openers: Ronald Olschwanger and Maryland Institute for Emergency Medical Services Systems.

Figs 11-5, 11-6, 11-7, 11-9, 11-10, 11-11, 11-12, 11-15: Seidel: Mosby's guide to physical examination, ed 2, St. Louis, 1991, Mosby.

Table 11-2: Sheehy: Emergency Nursing, ed 3, St. Louis, 1992, Mosby.

Table 11-4: Simon: Prehospital pediatric life support, St. Louis, 1989, Mosby.

Chapter 12 openers: Mark Fisher, Port Orange, Fla; Larry Ashby; and City EMS.

Fig 12-1: Sims/Illustrator Jody L. Fulks

Fig 12-2: Thibodeau: Structure and function of the body, ed 9, St. Louis, 1992, Mosby.

Fig 12-3: Seidel: Mosby's guide to physical examination, ed 2, St. Louis, 1991, Mosby.

Fig 12-4: Seely: Anatomy and physiology, ed 2, St. Louis, 1992, Mosby.

Fig 12-5: Wilson: Respiratory disorders, St. Louis, 1990, Mosby.

Fig 12-8: Thibodeau: Structure and function of the body, ed 9, St. Louis, 1992, Mosby.

Figs 12-9, 12-10: Seely: Anatomy and physiology, ed 2, St. Louis, 1992, Mosby.

Fig 12-11: Thibodeau: Structure and function of the body, ed 9, St. Louis, 1992, Mosby.

Fig 12-12: Illustrator Trent Stephens

Fig 12-25: Courtesy Brunswick Biomedical Technologies, Inc., Wareham, Mass.

Fig 12-27: Courtesy Respironics Inc., Monroeville, Pennsylvania.

Figs 12-36, 12-37: Gorback: Emergency airway management, Philadelphia, 1990, B.C. Decker.

Figs 12-38, 12-39: Courtesy Michael Gorback, M.D.

Figs 12-40, 12-41: Courtesy Armstrong Medical Industries, Inc., Lincolnshire, Ill.

Fig 12-42: Gorback: Emergency airway management, Philadelphia, 1990, B.C. Decker.Fig 12-45: Courtesy Fenem Inc., New York, N.Y.

Figs 12-47, 12-48: Gorback: Emergency airway management, Philadelphia, 1990, B.C. Decker.

Figs 12-50, 12-52, 12-53, 12-54, 12-55, 12-59: Courtesy Life Support Products Inc., Irvine, Calif.

Fig 12-61: doCarmo: Basic EMT skills and equipment, St. Louis, 1988, Mosby.

Fig 12-68: Courtesy Ohmeda, Louisville, Co.

Chapter 13 openers: Thomas Cooper, Larry Ashby, and Ronald Olschwanger.

Fig 13-2: Thibodeau: Structure and function of the body, ed 9, St. Louis, 1992, Mosby.

Figs 13-3, 13-4: Illustrator Barbara Cousins

Fig 13-5: Illustrator Nadine Sokol

Fig 13-6: Illustrator Christine Oleksyk

Fig 13-12: Berne: Physiology, ed 3, St. Louis, 1993, Mosby.

Fig 13-13: Seely: Anatomy and physiology, ed 2, St. Louis, 1992, Mosby.

Figs 13-14, 13-15: Illustrator Christine Oleksyk

Fig 13-16: Hardaway: Shock, Littleton, Mass., 1988, PSG Publishing Co., Inc.

Fig 13-20: Courtesy Jobst Institute, Inc., Toledo, Ohio.

Fig 13-24: Illustrators Molly Babich and John Daugherty

Chapter 14 openers: Ronald Olschwanger; Mary J. Myers, Houston; and Julie Long.

Figs 14-1, 14-2, 14-3: McKenry: Mosby's pharmacology in nursing, ed 18, St. Louis, 1992, Mosby.

Fig 14-4: Clark: Pharmacological basis of nursing, ed 4, St. Louis, 1993, Mosby.

Figs 14-5, 14-7: McKenry: Mosby's pharmacology in nursing, ed 18, St. Louis, 1992, Mosby.

Figs 14-10, 14-11, 14-12, 14-13, 14-14, 14-15: Clark: Pharmacological basis of nursing, ed 4, St. Louis, 1993, Mosby.

Fig 14-17: Courtesy Medical Technology Products Inc., Huntington Station, N.Y.

Fig 14-23: Illustrator Barbara CousinsFig 14-24: Seely: Anatomy and physiology, ed 2, St. Louis, 1992, Mosby.

Box 14-3: McKenry: Mosby's pharmacology in nursing, ed 18, St. Louis, 1992, Mosby.

Table 14-1: Courtesy Sterling Winthrop, Inc., New York, N.Y.

Table 14-2: Seely: Anatomy and physiology, ed 2, St. Louis, 1992, Mosby.

Tables 14-3, 14-4: McKenry: Mosby's pharmacology in nursing, ed 18, St. Louis, 1992, Mosby.

Chapter 15 openers: Terry O'Gara, Port Orange, Fla; Mary J. Myers, Houston; and Maryland Institute for Emergency Medical Services Systems.

Fig 15-1: National Safety Council (1992). Accident Facts 1992 edition, Itasco, Ill.

Figs 15-5, 15-7: Moylan: Principles of trauma surgery, ed 2, New York, N.Y., 1992, Gower Medical Publishing.

Fig 15-8: London: A colour atlas of diagnosis after recent injury, Ipswich, England, 1990, Wolfe Medical Publications Ltd.

Fig 15-9: Moylan: Principles of trauma surgery, ed 2, New York, N.Y., 1992, Gower Medical Publishing.

Figs 15-10, 15-11, 15-12: London: A colour atlas of diagnosis after recent injury, Ipswich, England, 1990, Wolfe Medical Publications Ltd.

Fig 15-13: Sheehy: Emergency nursing, ed 3, St. Louis, 1992, Mosby.

Fig 15-14: London: A colour atlas of diagnosis after recent injury, Ipswich, England, 1990, Wolfe Medical Publications Ltd.

Fig 15-15: Ragge: Immediate eye care, Torrington Place, London, England, 1990, Wolfe Medical Publications Ltd.

Fig 15-16: London: A colour atlas of diagnosis after recent injury, Ipswich, England, 1990, Wolfe Medical Publications Ltd.

Figs 15-17, 15-18: Ragge: Immediate eye care, Torrington Place, London, England, 1990, Wolfe Medical Publications Ltd.

Fig 15-19: Thibodeau: Structure and function of the body, ed 9, St. Louis, 1992, Mosby.

Figs 15-20, 15-22, 15-23: London: A colour atlas of diagnosis after recent injury, Ipswich, England, 1990, Wolfe Medical Publications Ltd.

Fig 15-25: Sheehy: Emergency nursing, ed 3, St. Louis, 1992, Mosby.

Fig 15-26: Snell: Clinical anatomy for emergency medicine, St. Louis, 1993, Mosby.

Fig 15-27: London: A colour atlas of diagnosis after recent injury, Ipswich, England, 1990, Wolfe Medical Publications Ltd.

Figs 15-28, 15-29: Moore: Early care of the injured patient, ed 4, Philadelphia, 1990, B.C. Decker.

Fig 15-30: Courtesy Gary Quick, M.D.

Fig 15-37: Courtesy California Medical Products Inc., Long Beach, Calif.

Fig 15-38B: Courtesy Ferno Washington, Wilmington, Ohio.

Fig 15-44: Courtesy Life Support Products Inc., Irvine, Calif.

Figs 15-47, 15-48, 15-50, 15-56: London: A colour atlas of diagnosis after recent injury, Ipswich, England, 1990, Wolfe Medical Publications Ltd.

Fig 15-58: Moylan: Principles of trauma surgery, ed 2, New York, N.Y., 1992, Gower Medical Publishing.

Fig 15-59: Illustrator David J. Mascaro and Associates

Figs 15-63, 15-69: London: A colour atlas of diagnosis after recent injury, Ipswich, England, 1990, Wolfe Medical Publications Ltd.

Tables 15-2, 15-3, 15-4: Moore: Early care of the injured patient, ed 4, Philadelphia, 1990, B.C. Decker.

Chapter 16 openers: Ken Hines and William Greenblatt Photography.

Fig 16-2: Thibodeau: Structure and function of the body, ed 9, St. Louis, 1992, Mosby.

Fig 16-5: doCarmo: Basic EMT skills and equipment, St. Louis, 1988, Mosby.

Figs 16-10 through 16-21: London: A colour atlas of diagnosis after recent injury, Ipswich, England, 1990, Wolfe Medical Publications Ltd.

Figs 16-24, 16-25, 16-26: Courtesy St. Johns Mercy Medical Center, St. Louis, Mo.

Fig 16-27: Trott: Wounds and lacerations, St. Louis, 1991, Mosby.

Fig 16-28: Lee: Flight nursing: principles and practice, St. Louis, 1991, Mosby.Fig 16-30: JEMS, March 1992, p. 52, Jems Communications Inc., Carlsbad, Calif.

Fig 16-31: Courtesy Michael Graham, M.D.

Table 16-1: Courtesy American Burn Association, Valhalla, N.Y.

Chapter 17 openers: City EMS, Acadian Ambulance Service, Inc., and Thomas Cooper.

Fig 17-1: Courtesy Boehringer Laboratories Inc., Norristown, PA.

Figs 17-2 through 17-10: Wilson: Respiratory disorders, St. Louis, 1990, Mosby.

Chapter 18 openers: Ronald Olschwanger, Thomas Cooper, and William Greenblatt Photography.

Fig 18-1: Sims/Illustrator Rusty Jones

Fig 18-2: Thibodeau: Structure and function of the body, ed 9, St. Louis, 1992, Mosby.

Fig 18-3: Sims/Illustrator Joan Beck

Fig 18-4: Seely: Anatomy and physiology, ed 2, St. Louis, 1992, Mosby.

Figs 18-5, 18-6: Illustrator Christine Oleksyk

Fig 18-7: Huszar: Basic dysrhythmias, ed 2, St. Louis, 1994, Mosby.

Fig 18-8: Illustrator Barbara Cousins

Fig 18-9: Illustrator Ronald J. Ervin

Figs 18-10, 18-11: Marriott: Advanced concepts in arrhythmias, ed 2, St. Louis, 1989, Mosby.

Fig 18-12: Rowlands, Clinical electrocardiography, New York, 1991, Gower Medical Publishing.

Figs 18-13, 18-14, 18-15: Grauer: Practical guide to ECG interpretation, St. Louis, 1992, Mosby.

Fig 18-16: Goldberger: Treatment of cardiac emergencies, ed 5, St. Louis, 1990, Mosby.

Fig 18-17: Huszar: Basic dysrhythmias, ed 2, St. Louis, 1994, Mosby.

Figs 18-18, 18-19, 18-20, 18-21: Grauer: Practical guide to ECG interpretation, St. Louis, 1992, Mosby.

Figs 18-22 through 18-33, 18-41: Huszar: Basic dysrhythmias, ed 2, St. Louis, 1994, Mosby.

Figs 18-36, 18-38, 18-51: JAMA 1992; 268: 2199-2275. Copyright 1992, American Medical Association.

Fig 18-53: Huszar: Basic dysrhythmias, ed 2, St. Louis, 1994, Mosby.

Fig 18-54: Atwood: Introduction to basic cardiac dysrhythmias, St. Louis, 1990, Mosby.

Figs 18-55, 18-56, 18-57: Huszar: Basic dysrhythmias, ed 2, St. Louis, 1994, Mosby.

Figs 18-59, 18-60: JAMA 1992; 268: 2199-2275. Copyright 1992, American Medical Association.

Fig 18-62: Huszar: Basic dysrhythmias, ed 1, St. Louis, 1988, Mosby.

Fig 18-64: JAMA 1992; 268: 2199-2275. Copyright 1992, American Medical Association.

Figs 18-69, 18-70: Huszar: Basic dysrhythmias, ed 1, St. Louis, 1988, Mosby.

Fig 18-72: Huszar: Basic dysrhythmias, ed 2, St. Louis, 1994, Mosby.

Fig 18-74: Grauer: Practical guide to ECG interpretation, St. Louis, 1992, Mosby.

Figs 18-75, 18-76, 18-77, 18-78: JEMS, May 1990, p. 42, 43, Jems Communications Inc., Carlsbad, Calif.

Figs 18-82, 18-84: Grauer: Practical guide to ECG interpretation, St. Louis, 1992, Mosby.

Figs 18-85, 18-86: JAMA 1992; 268: 2199-2275. Copyright 1992, American Medical Association.

Fig 18-87: Illustrator David J. Mascaro and Associates

Fig 18-88: Goldberger: Treatment of cardiac emergencies, ed 5, St. Louis, 1990, Mosby.

Fig 18-89: Sheehy: Emergency nursing, ed 3, St. Louis, 1992, Mosby.

Fig 18-93: Courtesy Michigan Instruments, Grand Rapids, Mich.

Fig 18-94: Courtesy Darox Corporation, San Diego, Calif.

Fig 18-96: Courtesy Cardiac Pacemakers Inc., St. Paul, Minn.

Fig 18-97: Courtesy Matrx Medical Inc., Orchard Park, N.Y.

Chapter 19 openers: Acadian Ambulance Service, Inc., James Silvernail, and William Greenblatt Photography.

Fig 19-1: Thibodeau: Structure and function of the body, ed 9, St. Louis, 1992, Mosby.

Figs 19-2, 19-3: Seely: Anatomy and physiology, ed 2, St. Louis, 1992, Mosby.

Table 19-1: Seely: Anatomy and physiology, ed 2, St. Louis, 1992, Mosby.

Table 19-2: Clark: Pharmacological basis of nursing, ed 4, St. Louis, 1993, Mosby.

Chapter 20 openers: City EMS, Colin Williams, and Ronald Olschwanger.

Figs 20-1, 20-2, 20-3, 20-4: Thibodeau: Structure and function of the body, ed 9, St. Louis, 1992, Mosby.

Figs 20-5, 20-6: Sims/Illustrator Karen Waldo

Fig 20-7: Sims/Illustrator Scott Bodell

Fig 20-8A: London: A colour atlas of diagnosis after recent injury, Ipswich, England, 1990, Wolfe Medical Publications Ltd.

Fig 20-8B: Courtesy Gary Quick, M.D.

Chapter 21 openers: Ronald Olschwanger, Acadian Ambulance Service, Inc., and William Greenblatt Photography.

Fig 21-1: Thibodeau: Structure and function of the body, ed 9, St. Louis, 1992, Mosby.

Fig 21-7: Courtesy Quinton Instrument Co., Seattle, Wash.

Fig 21-8: Courtesy Pharmacia Deltec, Inc., St. Paul, Minn.

Chapter 22 openers: Acadian Ambulance Service, Inc.; Katherine P. Williams, Williamstown, NJ; and City EMS.

Fig 22-1: Grimes: Infectious diseases, St. Louis, 1991, Mosby.

Fig 22-3: Courtesy Gary Quick, M.D.

Chapter 23 openers: Thomas Cooper, Ronald Olschwanger, and City EMS.

Fig 23-1: Courtesy Saint Louis Zoo, St. Louis, Mo.

Figs 23-2, 23-3, 23-4: Auerbach, Management of wilderness and environmental emergencies, ed 2, St. Louis, 1989, Mosby.

Figs 23-5, 23-6: Courtesy Saint Louis Zoo, St. Louis, Mo.

Figs 23-7, 23-8, 23-9: Auerbach: A medical guide to hazardous marine life, ed 2, St. Louis, 1991, Mosby.

Table 23-1: Ho: Current emergency diagnosis and treatment, ed 3, Norwalk, CT, 1990, Appleton and Lange.

Table 23-2: Dillmann: Designer drugs: an update of street drug names, JEMS, July 1988, p. 46, Jems Communications Inc., Carlsbad, Calif.

Table 23-3: Clark: Pharmacological basis of nursing, ed 4, St. Louis, 1993, Mosby.

Chapter 24 openers: Larry Ashby; Terry O'Gara, Port Orange, Fla; and O'Fallon Fire Protection District.

Figs 24-2, 24-3, 24-4: Grimes: Infectious diseases, St. Louis, 1991, Mosby.

Figs 24-5, 24-6, 24-7, 24-9: Courtesy The Centers for Disease Control, 1990. In Grimes: Infectious diseases, St. Louis, 1991, Mosby.

Fig 24-8: Morse: Atlas of sexually transmitted disease, London, England, 1990, Gower Medical Publishing.

Fig 24-10: Auerbach, Management of wilderness and environmental emergencies, ed 2, St. Louis, 1989, Mosby.

Figs 24-11, 24-12, 24-13: Courtesy The Centers for Disease Control, 1990. In Grimes: Infectious diseases, St. Louis, 1991, Mosby.

Fig 24-14: Courtesy Gary Quick, M.D.

Sidebar 24-1: Guidelines for Prevention of Transmission of HIV and Hepatitis B Virus to Health Care and Public-Safety Workers. U.S. Department of Health and Human Services, Centers for Disease Control, National Institute of Occupational Safety and Health: Guidelines for prevention of transmission of human immunodeficiency virus and hepatitis B virus to health-care and public-safety workers, Washington, DC, 1989, DHHS, CDC, NHOSH.

Table 24-1: Adapted from "Examples of Recommended personal protective equipment for worker protection against HIV and HBV transmission in prehospital setting, Centers for Disease Control, February 1989.

Table 24-2: Centers for Disease Control, Morbidity and Mortality Weekly Report, June 23, 1989.

Chapter 25 openers: Ronald Olschwanger and Acadian Ambulance Service, Inc.

Fig 25-1: JAMA 1992; 268: 2199-2275. Copyright 1992, American Medical Association.

Figs 25-2, 25-3, 25-4, 25-5: Auerbach, Management of wilderness and environmental emergencies, ed 2, St. Louis, 1989, Mosby.

Table 25-1: Sheehy: Emergency nursing, ed 3, St. Louis, 1992, Mosby.

Chapter 26 openers: William Greenblatt Photography, Maryland Institute for Emergency Medical Services Systems, and City EMS.

Chapter 27 openers: William Greenblatt Photography, City EMS, and James Silvernail.

Sidebar 27-1: Adapted from Lewandowski: "Psychosocial Aspects of Pediatric Critical Care" in Hazinski: Nursing care of the critically ill child, ed 2, St. Louis, 1992, Mosby.

Fig 27-1: Courtesy Gary Quick, M.D.

Figs 27-2, 27-3: JAMA 1992; 268: 2199-2275. Copyright 1992, American Medical Association.

Figs 27-4, 27-5, 27-6: Barkin: Pediatric emergency medicine: concepts and clinical practice, St. Louis, 1992, Mosby.

Table 27-1: Adapted from Kennedy: "Renal Disorders" in Hazinski: Nursing care of the critically ill child, ed 2, St. Louis, 1992, Mosby.

Table 27-5: Barkin: Pediatric emergency medicine: concepts and clinical practice, St. Louis, 1992, Mosby.

Tables 27-6, 27-7: JAMA 1992; 268: 2199-2275. Copyright 1992, American Medical Association.

Chapter 28 openers: William Greenblatt Photography, City EMS, and James Silvernail.

Figs 28-1, 28-2, 28-3, 28-4, 28-5: Thibodeau: Structure and function of the body, ed 9, St. Louis, 1992, Mosby.

Figs 28-6, 28-7: Seidel: Mosby's guide to physical examination, ed 2, St. Louis, 1991, Mosby.

Fig 28-9: Thibodeau: Structure and function of the body, ed 9, St. Louis, 1992, Mosby.

Figs 28-11, 28-12, 28-13: Al-Azzawi: Color atlas of childbirth and obstetric techniques, London, England, 1990, Wolfe Publishing Ltd.

Figs 28-14, 28-15: Reproduced with permission. Textbook of Neonatal Resuscitation, 1990, copyright American Heart Association.

Fig 28-17: Courtesy St. Louis Children's Hospital, St. Louis, Mo.

Table 28-2: Seidel: Mosby's guide to physical examination, ed 2, St. Louis, 1991, Mosby.

Chapter 29 openers: St. Louis Children's Hospital.

Figs 29-1, 29-2, 29-3: Seidel: Mosby's guide to physical examination, ed 2, St. Louis, 1991, Mosby.

Chapter 30 openers: William Greenblatt Photography, Ronald Olschwanger, and Ken Hines.

Cover: Acadian Ambulance Service, Inc.; William Greenblatt Photography; Thomas Cooper; Byron Rhodes, Orlando, Fla; Mary J. Myers, Houston; Ken Hines; and Bishop at Phototake (New York).

INDEX

Betaxin; *see* Thiamine
Beverages, alcoholic, 771
Bicarbonate
  in blood, 295
  excess in metabolic alkalosis, 298-299, *299*
Biceps brachialis muscle, 136
Biceps brachii muscle, 136
Bicuspid valve, 153
Bike chemist, defined, 763t
Bile, secretion of, 165
Bioethics
  defined, 3
  purpose of, 7
Biological half-life, 354-356, *355*
Biotelemetry, characteristics of, 35
Biotransformation, drug, 349
  in children, 371
  defined, 335
  in older adult, 372
Biot's respiration, characteristics of, 195
BIPA; *see* Berman intubating-pharyngeal
    airway
Birth control pills, deep vein thrombosis
    associated with, 389
Bites
  Arachnida, 750-753
  arthropod; *see* Arthropods, bites from
  complications of, 498
  insect, anaphylaxis caused by, 725
  management of, 498
  reptile, 755-757
  snake, 655-756
    management of, 756-757
  tick, 754-755
Bitolterol, bronchodilator effects of, 391
Black widow spider, *752*
  bites of, 751-752
    management of, 752
    signs and symptoms of, 752
Bladder
  adrenergic stimulation of, 383t
  male, *168*
  during pregnancy, 872
  structure and function of, 167-168
  sympathetic and parasympathetic
    stimulation of, 377t
  trauma to, 472
Blast injury, 410-411
  from changes in environmental pressure,
    410
  from flying debris, 411
  from victim propulsion, 411
Bleeding; *see also* Hemorrhage
  arterial, characteristics of, 489
  from gastrointestinal disorders, 706-707
  internal, immediate transfer of patient
    with, 186
  during pregnancy, third-trimester, 881-883
  vaginal, during pregnancy, 880
  variceal, 706-707
Blindness from diabetes mellitus, 674
Blisters in frostbite, *815*
Blood
  carbon dioxide content of, 231, 233
  characteristics of, 117
  components of, 149-151, 286-287
  drugs affecting, 388-389
  formed elements of, 149-150
  gloves for handling items soiled by, 182
  in homeostasis, 149
  normal arterial, 299
  oxygen content of, 231
  oxygen transport by, conditions affecting,
    234
  oxygenation of
    abnormal conditions affecting, 234
    factors affecting, 233
  pH of, 295
  sympathetic and parasympathetic
    stimulation of, 377t
  venous, oxygen tension of, 231
Blood alcohol content, 771
Blood brain barrier, characteristics of, 348-349
Blood cells, classification of, 150t

Blood colloid osmotic pressure, 301
Blood flow; *see also* Circulation
  capillary, 303
  cerebral, 434-435
    factors affecting, 435
  regulation of
    nervous control of, 305
    peripheral vascular resistance and,
      284-285
    by tissues, 303, 305
    viscosity in, 285
Blood gases, analysis of, 299-300
Blood grouping, 322, *322*
Blood plasma; *see* Plasma
Blood pressure
  assessment of, 187
    with auscultation, 187
    with palpation, 188
  average, by age, 188t
  diastolic, 187
    assessment of, 187-188
  regulation of
    atrial natriuretic factor in, 308
    baroreceptors in, 305
    hormonal mechanisms of, 306
    renin-angiotensin-aldosterone mechanism
      in, *307*
  systolic, 187
    minimal, 185
    in shock, 317
Blood tests, alcohol content in, 771
Blood vessels
  adrenergic stimulation of, 383t
  atherosclerosis of, 636-637
  coronary, anatomy of, 151
  of neck, injuries to, 441
  sympathetic and parasympathetic
    stimulation of, 377t
  sympathetic innervation of, 301
Blowout fractures, 422-423, *423*
BLS; *see* Basic life support
Blue bloaters, 522, *523*; *see also* Bronchitis,
    chronic
Blue blood, defined, 763t
Blue velvet, defined, 763t
Blunt trauma, 401-402
  from automobile accidents, 402-404
  from blast injuries, 410-411
  change-of-speed injuries in, 401
  defined, 399
  to eye, assessment of, 427-428
  force in, 401
  to neck, 439
  pericardial tamponade from, 468-469
  from sports injuries, 410
  from vertical falls, 411
Body(ies)
  directional terms for, 111
  overview of, 109-113
  regions of, 110
  systems overview of, 108-179
  terminology related to, 109-110
Body cavities, 110-113, *112*
Body fluid(s)
  extracellular, 287
  gloves for handling of, 182
  imbalance of, 292
  intracellular, 287
  loss of, in burn shock, 506
  movement of, 288-292
    by diffusion, 291
    by osmosis, 288-291
  reabsorption of, 308-309
Body mass, drug action and, 352
Body movement
  biomechanics of, 128-129, *130-131,* 131
  types of, 129
Body packing, defined, 763t
Body planes, *110*
Body temperature
  assessment of, 188-189
    types of, 189
  maintenance of, 186

Body temperature—cont'd
  regulation of, 805, 806-807, 809
    arteriovenous anastomoses in, 300-301
  respiratory effects of, 237
Boehringer valve in adult respiratory distress
    syndrome management, 522
Bone(s)
  carpal, *125,* 126
  characteristics and classification of, 116-117
  of foot, *127,* 127-128
  gunshot injuries to, 417
  injuries of, from child abuse, 851
  of lower extremity, *126,* 127
  of pelvic girdle, *126,* 127
  of skull, *122*
  of upper extremity, *125*
  of vertebral column, *123*
  of wrist, *127*
Bone marrow, fluid and drug administration
    in, in children, 857-858
Bony labyrinth, 178
Botulism, signs and symptoms of, 742
Bowel; *see also* Intestine(s)
  penetrating trauma to, 472
Bowel habits, determining, 210
Bowel sounds, assessment of, 203-204
Bowman's capsule, 166
Boyle's law, 424, 818, 820
Bradycardia
  defined, 184
  in shock, 317
  sinus; *see* Sinus bradycardia
Bradycardia decision tree, *854*
Bradydysrhythmias from poisoning, 733
Bradypnea, characteristics of, 195
Brain
  anatomy of, 433
  arterial blood supply to, 685-686, *686*
  contusions of, from compression injuries,
    406
  divisions of, 138t, 687
  edema of, signs and symptoms of, 434
  glucose uptake by, 670
  hemorrhage of, 434-437
    types of, 435-437, *436*
  injury to
    assessment of patient with, 216
    from child abuse, 850-851
  ischemia of, 434
  meningeal coverings of, *141*
  penetrating injury to, 437
    assessment and neurological evaluation
      of, 437-439
    circulation after, 438
    drug therapy after, 439
    fluid therapy after, 438-439
  structures of, *138*
  trauma to, 433-439; *see also* Head injury
    from head-on collisions, 403
  vascular tone in, regulation of, 435
  venous sinuses associated with, *686,* 687
  ventricles of, 687, *687*
Brainstem
  components of, 138-139
  function of, 138t
Breach of duty, 23
Breast(s)
  female, anatomy of, 174, *174*
  during pregnancy, 872-873
Breath odor, significance of, 191
Breath sounds
  abnormal, 199-201
  absent, 199
  adventitious, 200, *200*
  assessment of, 196
  bronchial, 199
  bronchovesicular, 199
  in cardiovascular assessment, 635
  continuous, 200-201
  diminished, 199
  discontinuous, 200
  in ill versus well patients, *199*
  normal, 196, *198,* 199
  vesicular, 196, 199

OTHER MOSBY PRODUCTS OF INTEREST

BOOK CODE	AUTHOR/TITLE	PUB DATE
21764	ACLS: Video Series	7/93
00200	Allison: Advanced Life Support Skills	7/93
07067	American Red Cross CPR for the Professional Rescuer Text	3/93
21231	American Red Cross Emergency Response Text	3/93
21241	American Red Cross First Aid: Instructor's Resource Kit—IBM	3/91
21135	American Red Cross First Aid: Responding to Emergencies Text	3/91
23788	American Safety Video Publishers: ACLS Update	11/93
23789	American Safety Video Publishers: EZ ECGs	2/94
23793	American Safety Video Publishers: HazMat for EMS	3/94
07405	American Safety Video Publishers: Learning ECGs Video Series	12/93
07172	American Safety Video Publishers: PALS Plus: Pediatric Advanced Life Support	12/92
07296	American Safety Video Publishers: PALS Plus: Pediatric Emergencies	12/92
07257	American Safety Video Publishers: PASS ACLS	12/92
23795	American Safety Video Publishers: PASS CPR!	12/93
23797	American Safety Video Publishers: PASS EMT!	12/93
23791	American Safety Video Publishers: PASS Paramedic!	12/93

08093	American Safety Video Publishers: Rescue Company—First Due Video Series	12/93
08077	American Safety Video Publishers: Engine Company—First Due Video Series	12/93
24448	American Safety Video Publishers: Truck Company—First Due Video Series	7/94
00258	Atwood: Introduction to Cardiac Dysrhythmias	3/90
00383	Auerbach-Geehr: Management of Wilderness and Environmental Emergencies, 2/e	12/88
00385	Auf der Heide: Disaster Response	6/89
01185	Bosker: The 60-Second EMT	11/87
01808	Bosker: Geriatric Emergency Medicine	7/90
07813	Bronstein: Emergency Care for Hazardous Materials Exposure, 2/e	6/94
01458	doCarmo: Basic EMT Skills and Equipment	8/88
01473	Emergidose Slideguides: Pocket Adult/Pediatric Emergency Drugs Guide, 5/e	7/91
01478	Emergidose Slideguides: Binder Adult/Pediatric Emergency Drugs Guide, 5/e	7/91
01472	Emergidose Slideguides: Pocket Pediatric/Neonatal Emergency Drugs Guide, 2/e	8/91
01471	Emergidose Slideguides: Binder Pediatric/Neonatal Emergency Drugs, 2/e	7/91
01969	Gonsoulin: Prehospital Drug Therapy	9/93
01932	Gosselin-Smith: Mosby's First Responder Workbook, 2/e	10/88
00174	Grauer: ACLS Teaching Kit: An Instructor's Resource	12/89
01979	Grauer: ACLS Volume 1, Volume 2, and Pocket Reference	3/93
07069	Grauer: ACLS Volume 1: Certification Preparation, 3/e	3/93

07070	Grauer: ACLS Volume 2: A Comprehensive Review, 3/e	3/93
01980	Grauer: ACLS: Mega Code Review Study Cards, 2/e	3/93
07685	Grauer: ACLS: Pocket Reference	3/93
02002	Grauer: ECG Interpretation Pocket Reference	9/91
02159	Grauer: Practical Guide to ECG Interpretation	9/91
07203	Huszar: Basic Dysrhythmia Interpretation and Management, 2/e	5/94
02927	Huszar: Early Defibrillation	6/91
03353	Judd: First Responder: Textbook/Workbook Package, 2/e	10/88
08077	Kidd: Engine Company: 1st Due Video Series	11/93
08093	Kidd: Rescue Company: 1st Due Video Series	11/93
06195	Krebs: When Violence Erupts	4/90
06138	Lee: Flight Nursing: Principles and Practice	9/90
05853	Mack: EMT Certification Preparation	2/90
03375	Madigan: Prehospital Emergency Drugs Pocket Reference	3/90
05791	Miller: Manual of Prehospital Emergency Medicine	3/92
03351	Moore: Vehicle Rescue and Extrication	9/90
05854	NAEMSP/Kuehl: Prehospital Systems and Medical Oversight, 2/e	7/94
06579	NAEMSP/Swor: Quality Management in Prehospital Care	1/93
23884	NAEMT: Pre-hospital Trauma Life Support, 3/e	6/94
04284	Rothenberg: Advanced Medical Life Support	11/87
04315	Sanders: Mosby's Paramedic Textbook	5/94
04314	Sanders/McKenna: Workbook to Accompany Mosby's Paramedic Textbook	5/94

00443	Seidel: Mosby's Guide to Physical Examination, 3/e	12/90
04894	Simon: Pediatric Life Support	11/88
06343	Smith: Water Rescue: Basic Skills for Emergency Responders	1/94
05321	Ward: Prehospital Treatment Protocols	3/89
03525	Yvorra: Mosby's Emergency Dictionary	10/88